THE WASHINGTON MANUAL® OF MEDICAL THERAPEUTICS

33rd Edition

Department of Medicine
Washington University School of Medicine
St. Louis, Missouri

Editors

Corey Foster, MD

Neville F. Mistry, MD

Parvin F. Peddi, MD

Shivak Sharma, MD

. Wolters Kluwer | Lippincott Williams & Wilkins
Health

Philadelphia · Baltimore · New York · London
Buenos Aires · Hong Kong · Sydney · Tokyo

Acquisitions Editor: Avé McCracken
Managing Editor: Michelle M. LaPlante
Vendor Manager: Alicia Jackson
Manufacturing Manager: Benjamin Rivera
Marketing Manager: Kimberly Schonberger
Design Coordinator: Teresa Mallon
Cover Designer: Becky Baxendell
Production Services: Aptara, Inc.
Printer: RR Donnelley

33rd Edition

Adhesive binding:
ISBN: 9781608310036
ISBN: 1608310035

Spiral binding:
ISBN: 9781605470146
ISBN: 1605470147

The Washington Manual® is an intent-to-use mark belonging to Washington University in St. Louis to which international legal protection applies. The mark is used in this publication by LWW under license from Washington University.

To purchase additional copies of this book, call our customer service department at (800) 638-3030 or fax orders to (301) 223-2320. International customers should call (301) 223-2300.

Visit Lippincott Williams & Wilkins on the Internet: at LWW.com. Lippincott Williams & Wilkins customer service representatives are available from 8:30 am to 6 pm, EST.

We dedicate this Manual to the outstanding medicine housestaff at Washington University/Barnes-Jewish Hospital—their wisdom, dedication, and compassion continue to inspire us each and every day.

Contents

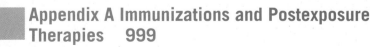
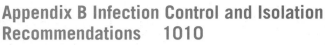

Contributors

Jennifer Alexander-Brett, MD, PhD
Clinical Fellow
Division of Pulmonary & Critical Care

Beau Ances, MD, PhD, MS
Assistant Professor of Neurology

Hilary M. Babcock, MD, MPH
Assistant Professor of Medicine
Division of Infectious Diseases

Benico Barzilai, MD
Professor of Medicine
Division of Cardiovascular Medicine

Morey Blinder, MD
Associate Professor of Medicine
Division of Hematology

Stephan Brenner, MD
Resident
Department of Emergency Medicine

Angela L. Brown, MD
Assistant Professor of Medicine
Department of Internal Medicine

Bernard C. Camins, MD
Assistant Professor of Medicine
Division of Infectious Diseases

Luke Carlstrom, MD
Clinical Fellow
Division of Pulmonary & Critical Care

Mario Castro, MD
Professor of Medicine
Division of Pulmonary & Critical Care

Murali Chakinala, MD
Associate Professor of Medicine
Division of Pulmonary & Critical Care

Alexander Chen, MD
Instructor of Medicine
Division of Pulmonary & Critical Care

Steven Cheng, MD
Assistant Professor of Medicine
Division of Nephrology

Ara Chrissian, MD
Clinical Fellow
Division of Pulmonary & Critical Care

William E. Clutter, MD
Associate Professor of Medicine
Division of Endocrinology

Daniel H. Cooper, MD
Clinical Fellow
Division of Cardiovascular Medicine

Daniel Coyne, MD
Professor of Medicine
Division of Nephrology

Lee Demertzis, MD
Clinical Fellow
Division of Pulmonary & Critical Care

Vladimir Despotovic, MD
Clinical Fellow
Division of Pulmonary & Critical Care

Charles Eby, MD
Associate Professor
Department of Pathology & Immunology

Gregory A. Ewald, MD
Associate Professor of Medicine
Division of Cardiovascular Medicine

Mitchell N. Faddis, MD, PhD
Associate Professor of Medicine
Division of Cardiovascular Medicine

Corey Foster, MD
Chief Resident, Ambulatory Services
Division of Medical Education

Victoria J. Fraser, MD
Professor of Medicine
Division of Infectious Diseases

Brian F. Gage, MD
Associate Professor of Medicine
Division of General Medical Sciences

Anne C. Goldberg, MD
Associate Professor of Medicine
Division of Endocrinology

Seth Goldberg, MD
Clinical Fellow
Division of Nephrology

Boone Goodgame, MD
Assistant Professor of Medicine
Division of Oncology

Ramaswamy Govindan, MD
Associate Professor of Medicine
Division of Oncology

Ritu Gupta, MD
Clinical Fellow
Division of Allergy & Immunology

Christopher J. Gutjahr, MD
Instructor of Medicine
Division of Hospital Medicine

C. Prakash Gyawali, MD
Associate Professor of Medicine
Division of Gastroenterology

José E. Hagan, MD
Clinical Fellow
Division of Infectious Diseases

S. Eliza Halcomb, MD
Assistant Professor
Department of Emergency Medicine

Katherine E. Henderson, MD
Assistant Professor of Clinical Medicine
Department of Medicine

Raksha Jain, MD
Clinical Fellow
Division of Pulmonary & Critical Care

Shirley Joo, MD
Assistant Professor of Medicine
Division of Allergy and Immunology

Susan M. Joseph, MD
Instructor of Medicine
Division of Cardiovascular Medicine

Andrew Kates, MD
Associate Professor of Medicine
Division of Cardiovascular Medicine

Andrew Kau, MD
Clinical Fellow
Division of Allergy & Immunology

Nigar Kirmani, MD
Professor of Medicine
Division of Infectious Diseases

Marine H. Kollef, MD
Professor of Medicine
Division of Pulmonary & Critical Care

Kory Lavine, MD
Resident
Department of Medicine

Brian R. Lindman, MD
Clinical Fellow
Division of Cardiovascular Medicine

Mauricio Lisker-Melman, MD
Professor of Medicine
Division of Gastroenterology

Ahmad Manasra, MD
Senior Assistant Resident
Department of Internal Medicine

Stacy A. Mandras, MD
Clinical Fellow
Division of Cardiovascular Medicine

Janet McGill, MD
Associate Professor of Medicine
Division of Endocrinology

Scott T. Micek, PharmD, BCPS
Department of Pharmacy
Barnes-Jewish Hospital

Brent W. Miller, MD
Associate Professor of Medicine
Division of Nephrology

Neville F. Mistry, MD
Chief Resident, Kipnis-Daughaday Firm C
Division of Medical Education

Hector Molina, MD
Associate Professor
Division of Rheumatology

Daniel Morgensztern, MD
Assistant Professor of Medicine
Division of Oncology

Michael E. Mullins, MD
Assistant Professor of Emergency Medicine
Department of Medicine

Meena Murugappan, MD
Clinical Fellow
Division of Pulmonary & Critical Care

Diana Nurutdinova, MD
Instructor in Medicine
Division of Infectious Diseases

E. Turner Overton, MD
Assistant Professor of Medicine – Infectious Diseases

Parvin F. Peddi, MD
Chief Resident, Karl-Flance Firm B
Division of Medicine Education

Christopher Phillips, MD
Clinical Fellow
Division of Rheumatology

Reshma Rangwala, MD
Instructor in Medicine
Division of Hospital Medicine

Dominic Reeds, MD
Assistant Professor in Medicine
Director, Clinical Nutrition Support Service

David J. Ritchie, PharmD
Clinical Pharmacist
Division of Infectious Diseases

Daniel B. Rosenbluth, MD
Professor of Medicine and Pediatrics
Division of Pulmonary & Critical Care

Tonya Russell, MD
Assistant Professor of Medicine
Division of Pulmonary & Critical Care

Bala Sankarpandian, MD
Clinical Fellow
Division of Nephrology

Carlos A.Q. Santos, MD
Instructor of Medicine
Division of Infectious Diseases

Anil B. Seetharam, MD
Clinical Fellow
Division of Gastroenterology

Robert M. Senior, MD
Professor of Medicine and Cell Biology and Physiology
Division of Pulmonary & Critical Care

Shivak Sharma, MD
Chief Resident, Shatz-Strauss Firm A
Division of Medical Education

Victoria Sharma, MD
Senior Resident
Department of Neurology

Devin Sherman, MD
Clinical Fellow
Division of Pulmonary & Critical Care

Mark Thoelke, MD
Associate Professor
Division of Hospital Medicine

Roger Yusen, MD, MPH
Associate Professor of Medicine
Division of Pulmonary & Critical Care

Chairman's Note

The rate of increase of medical knowledge places an enormous burden on physicians to keep up with recent advances, particularly in novel therapies that will improve patient outcomes. The *Washington Manual® of Medical Therapeutics* provides an easily accessible source of current information that covers a practical clinical approach to the diagnosis, investigation, and treatment of common medical conditions that internists encounter on a regular basis. The pocket-book size of the *Manual* ensures that it will continue to be of enormous assistance to interns, residents, medical students, and other practitioners in need of readily accessible practical clinical information. It meets an important unmet need in an era of information overload.

I acknowledge the authors, which include house officers, fellows, and attendings at Washington University/Barnes-Jewish Hospital. Their efforts and outstanding skill are evident in the quality of the final product. In particular, I am proud of our editors: Corey Foster, Neville F. Mistry, Parvin Peddi, and Shivak Sharma; and the series editors: Katherine Henderson and Tom De Fer, who have worked tirelessly to produce another outstanding edition of the *Manual*. I also recognize Melvin Blanchard, MD, Chief of the Division of Medical Education in the Department of Medicine at Washington University, for his guidance and advice. I am confident that this *Manual* will meet its desired goal of providing practical knowledge that can be directly applied to improving patient care.

Kenneth S. Polonsky, MD
Adolphus Busch Professor
Chairman, Department of Medicine
Washington University School of Medicine
St. Louis, Missouri

Preface

It is our pleasure to introduce the 33rd edition of *The Washington Manual of Medical Therapeutics*. "The Manual," as it is fondly labeled here at Washington University, developed from a simple handbook for senior medical students and housestaff. Since its inception, the *Manual* has been edited by Chief Residents. Wayland MacFarlane, MD, was the initial editor, producing the text in 1943. In 1962, Dr. Robert Packman oversaw the first major revision of the *Manual*, transforming it from a short textbook to a portable reference.

Over the past 65 years, the *Manual* has met with tremendous success, becoming the best-selling medical text in the world. It has been translated into more than a dozen languages and can be found in all corners of the globe. As a testament to the rapid advancement of medicine, the *Manual* has also grown significantly in size and content. As the practice of medicine and the use of portable technologies coevolve, the *Manual* must adapt to meet the needs of physicians. To that end, we have revised the outline format used in the last edition, hoping to organize information in a logical and readily accessible format. In our quest to polish the 33rd edition of the *Manual*, we have sought to retain the virtues that have made the work a success: a concise discussion of pathophysiology, an accurate discussion of current therapies, and ease of reading. Alongside the format modifications, we have carefully updated the content of the *Manual* to reflect advancing technologies and therapeutics.

The Washington Manual of Medical Therapeutics has established a tradition of excellence that we aspire to preserve. No discussion of the *Manual* would be complete without mention of the Washington University medicine housestaff, fellows, medical students, and attendings. We are inspired daily by their brilliance, compassion, and dedication. It is truly an honor that they turn to the *Manual* for guidance. We are deeply indebted for the substantial support and direction that Katherine Henderson and Tom De Fer, the series editors, provided in the creation of this edition of the *Manual*. We also thank Avé McCracken and the editorial staff at Lippincott Williams & Wilkins for their assistance and patience with our busy schedules.

We have had the honor and pleasure of serving as Chief Residents of the Shatz-Strauss, Karl-Flance, and Kipnis-Daughaday firms and the Wohl Clinic of the Department of Medicine at Washington University. Our Firm Chiefs, Megan Wren, William Clutter, and Geoffrey Cislo, have been instrumental over the course of the year, serving as mentors and role models. Our program director, Melvin Blanchard, has been a great help in the production of the *Manual*. Our Chairman of Medicine, Kenneth Polonsky, provided guidance and support in the creation of this text. We thank our families for their support and inspiration. To Raquel, Gabriel, and Isabel; Srinivas; Victoria—our gratitude is beyond measure. To my late father, Dr. Farookh Mistry, I will never forget your kindness, wisdom, and encouragement.

Corey Foster, MD
Neville F. Mistry, MD
Parvin F. Peddi, MD
Shivak Sharma, MD

1

Patient Care in Internal Medicine

Mark Thoelke and Christopher J. Gutjahr

General Care of the Hospitalized Patient

GENERAL PRINCIPLES

- Although a general approach to common problems can be outlined, **therapy must be individualized.** All diagnostic and therapeutic procedures should be explained carefully to the patient, including the potential risks, benefits, and alternatives. This explanation minimizes anxiety and provides the patient and the physician with appropriate expectations.
- The period of hospitalization represents a complex interplay of multiple caregivers that subjects the patient to potential harm by **medical errors and iatrogenic complications.** Every effort must be made to minimize these risks. Basic measures include:
  - Use of standardized abbreviations and dose designations
  - Excellent communication between physicians and other caregivers
  - Institution of appropriate prophylactic precautions
  - Prevention of nosocomial infections, including attention to hygiene and discontinuation of unnecessary catheters
  - Medicine reconciliation at all transfers of care
- **Hospital orders**
  - **Admission orders** should be written promptly after evaluation of a patient. Each set of orders should bear the **date and time** of writing and the legible signature of the physician. Consideration should be given to including a **printed signature** and a **contact number.** All orders should be clear, concise, organized, and legible. Computer order entry will facilitate aspects of this process.
  - To ensure that no important therapeutic measures are overlooked, the **content and organization** of admission orders may follow the outline below (the **mnemonic ADC VANDALISM**):
    - **A**dmitting service, location, and physician responsible for the patient
    - **D**iagnoses
    - **C**ondition of the patient
    - **V**ital signs with frequency
    - **A**ctivity limitations
    - **N**ursing instructions (e.g., Foley catheter to gravity drainage, wound care, daily weights)
    - **D**iet. Remember that "npo" may preclude oral medications unless specified
    - **A**llergies, sensitivities, and previous drug reactions
    - **L**aboratory tests and radiographic studies
    - **I**V fluids, including composition and rate
    - **S**edatives, analgesics, and other PRN medications
    - **M**edications, including dose, frequency, route, and indication. State "First dose now" when appropriate
  - **Orders should be reevaluated frequently** and altered as patient status dictates.

- **Discharge**
  - **Discharge planning** begins at the time of admission. Assessment of the patient's social situation and potential discharge needs should be made.
  - **Early coordination** with nursing, social work, and case coordinators/managers facilitates efficient discharge and a complete postdischarge plan.
  - **Patient education** should occur regarding changes in medications and other new therapies. Compliance with treatment is influenced by patient's understanding of that treatment.
  - **Prescriptions** should be written for all new medication, and the patient should be provided with a complete medication list including instructions and indications.
  - **Communication** with physicians who will be resuming care of the patient after discharge is important for optimal follow-up care.

PROPHYLACTIC MEASURES

Venous Thromboembolism Prophylaxis

GENERAL PRINCIPLES

Epidemiology

Venous thromboembolism (VTE) is the most common preventable cause of death in hospitalized patients. Roughly 75% of fatal pulmonary emboli occur in nonsurgical patients. **Risk factors** for VTE include advanced age, previous VTE, trauma, conditions associated with prolonged immobility (major surgery, stroke, paralysis), obesity, heart failure, malignancy, pregnancy, inflammatory bowel disease, and coagulation factor deficiency.

Prevention

- All able patients should be encouraged to ambulate several times a day.
- Acutely ill patients with severe respiratory disease, with congestive heart failure (CHF), or who are bedridden and have additional risk factors described above should be considered for **prophylactic dosing** of low-dose unfractionated heparin (UFH; 5,000 units SC q8h or q12) or low-molecular-weight heparin (LMWH; enoxaparin, 40 mg SC or 4,000 units SC daily, or dalteparin, 5,000 units SC daily), or fondaparinux 2.5 mg SC daily.
- Aspirin alone is not adequate deep vein thrombosis (DVT) prophylaxis.
- At-risk patients with contraindications to anticoagulation prophylaxis should receive mechanical prophylaxis with intermittent pneumatic compression or graded compression stockings (*Chest 2008 Jun;133(6 Suppl):381S–453S*).
- Treatment of VTE is reviewed in Chapter 17, Disorders of Hemostasis and Thrombosis.

Pressure Ulcers

GENERAL PRINCIPLES

Epidemiology

Pressure ulcers typically occur within the first 2 weeks of hospitalization and can develop within 2 to 6 hours. There has been a 63% increase in incidence of pressure ulcers over the last decade. Once they develop, pressure ulcers are difficult to heal and have been associated with increased mortality (*J Gerontol A Biol Sci Med Sci 1997; 52:M106*).

Prevention

Prevention is the key to management of pressure ulcers. The majority of pressure ulcers are preventable. Evidence for best practices is lacking, making pressure ulcers a "never event" a questionable goal. Measures include:

- **Risk factor assessment,** including immobility, limited activity, incontinence, impaired nutritional status, impaired circulation, and altered level of consciousness.
- **Skin care,** including daily inspection with particular attention to bony prominences and minimizing exposure to moisture from incontinence, perspiration, or wound drainage. Moisturizers should be applied to dry sacral skin.
- Nutritional supplements in patients at risk.
- Interventions aimed at **relieving or redistributing pressure,** including frequent repositioning (minimum of every 2 hours, or every 1 hour for wheelchair-bound patients), pillows or foam wedges between bony prominences, maintenance of the head of the bed at the lowest degree of elevation, and use of lifting devices when moving patients. **Pressure-reducing devices** (foam, dynamic air mattresses) and pressure-relieving devices (low-air-loss, air-fluidized beds) can also be used (*JAMA 2006; 296:974*).

DIAGNOSIS

Clinical Presentation

Physical Examination
National Pressure Ulcer Advisory Panel Staging:

- **Suspected deep tissue injury:** Purple or maroon localized area of discolored intact skin or blood-filled blister due to damage of underlying soft tissue from pressure and/or shear. The area may be preceded by tissue that is painful, firm, mushy, boggy, warmer, or cooler as compared to adjacent tissue.
- **Stage I:** Intact skin with nonblanchable redness of a localized area usually over a bony prominence. Darkly pigmented skin may not have visible blanching; its color may differ from the surrounding area.
- **Stage II:** Partial thickness loss of dermis presenting as a shallow open ulcer with a red pink wound bed, without slough. May also present as an intact or open/ruptured serum-filled blister.
- **Stage III:** Full thickness tissue loss. Subcutaneous fat may be visible but bone, tendon, or muscle are not exposed. Slough may be present but does not obscure the depth of tissue loss. May include undermining and tunneling.
- **Stage IV:** Full thickness tissue loss with exposed bone, tendon, or muscle. Slough or eschar may be present on some parts of the wound bed. Often include undermining and tunneling.
- **Unstageable:** Full thickness tissue loss in which the base of the ulcer is covered by slough (yellow, tan, gray, green, or brown) and/or eschar (tan, brown, or black) in the wound bed.

TREATMENT

- **Initial interventions** include use of pressure-relieving devices, occlusive dressings, pain control, normal saline for cleansing, use of topical agents that promote wound healing (DuoDERM, silver sulfadiazine [Silvadene], bacitracin zinc, Neosporin, Polysporin), avoidance of agents that delay healing (antiseptic agents, such as Dakin solution, hydrogen peroxide; wet-to-dry gauze), and removal of necrotic debris.
- **Adequate nutrition** with particular attention to protein intake (1.25 to 1.50 g protein/kg/d), vitamin C (500 mg PO daily), and zinc sulfate (220 mg PO daily) supplementation in the presence of deficiencies may also facilitate healing.
- For clean pressure ulcers that continue to produce exudate or are not healing after 2 to 4 weeks of therapy, consider a 2-week trial of **topical antibiotic** (e.g., silver sulfadiazine, double antibiotic).
- **Other adjunctive therapies** for nonhealing ulcers include electrical stimulation, radiant heat, negative pressure therapy, and surgical intervention (*JAMA 2008;300: 2647*).

Other Precautions

GENERAL PRINCIPLES

Prevention

- **Fall precautions** should be written for patients who have a history of falls or are at high risk of a fall (i.e., those with dementia, syncope, orthostatic hypotension). Falls are the most common accident in hospitalized patients, frequently leading to injury. Fall risk should not be equated with confinement to bed, which may lead to debilitation and higher risk of future falls.
- **Seizure precautions** should be considered for patients with a history of seizures or those at risk of seizing. Precautions include padded bed rails and an oral airway at the bedside.
- **Restraint orders** are written for patients who are at risk of injuring themselves or interfering with their treatment due to disruptive or dangerous behaviors. Restraint orders must be reviewed and renewed every 24 hours. Physical restraints may exacerbate agitation. Bed alarms or sitters are alternatives in appropriate settings.

ACUTE INPATIENT CARE

- New or recurrent symptoms that require evaluation and management frequently develop in hospitalized patients.
- Evaluation should generally include a directed history, including a complete description of the symptom (i.e., alleviating and precipitating factors, quality of the symptom, associated symptoms, and the course of the symptom, including acuity of onset, severity, duration, and previous episodes); physical examination; review of the medical problem list; review of medications with attention to recent medication discontinuation, addition, or dosage adjustment; and consideration of recent procedures.

- Further evaluation should be directed by the initial assessment, the acuity and severity of the complaint, and the diagnostic possibilities.
- An approach to selected common complaints is presented in this section.

Chest Pain

GENERAL PRINCIPLES

Chest pain is a common complaint in the hospitalized patient, and the severity of chest discomfort does not always correlate with the gravity of its cause. Chest pain should be evaluated to distinguish potentially life-threatening conditions such as pulmonary embolus, myocardial infarction, and aortic dissection from less serious cases.

DIAGNOSIS

Clinical Presentation

History

History should be taken in the context of the patient's other medical conditions, particularly previous cardiac or vascular history, cardiac risk factors, and factors that would predispose to a pulmonary embolus.

Physical Examination

Physical examination is ideally conducted during an episode of pain and includes vital signs (with bilateral BP measurements if considering aortic dissection), a careful cardiopulmonary and abdominal examination, and inspection and palpation of the chest for possible trauma, rash, and reproducibility of the pain.

Diagnostic Testing

Assessment of **oxygenation status, chest radiography, and electrocardiogram (ECG)** is appropriate in most patients. Serial cardiac enzymes should be obtained if there is suspicion of ischemia. Spiral computed tomography (CT) and VQ scans are employed to diagnose pulmonary embolus.

TREATMENT

- If **cardiac ischemia** is a concern, initial therapy should include supplemental oxygen, aspirin, and administration of nitroglycerin, 0.4 mg SL, or morphine sulfate, 1 to 2 mg IV, or both. Treatment of ischemic heart disease is discussed in Chapter 3, Preventative Cardiology and Ischemic Heart Disease.
- If a **gastrointestinal (GI) source** of chest pain is suspected, a combination of Maalox and diphenhydramine (30 mL of each in a 1:1 mix) can be administered.
- **Costochondritis** or other **musculoskeletal pain** typically responds to nonsteroidal anti-inflammatory drug (NSAID) therapy.
- **Prompt empiric anticoagulation** while awaiting testing should be considered if there is high suspicion for myocardial infarction or pulmonary embolism (barring contraindication).

Dyspnea

GENERAL PRINCIPLES

Dyspnea is most commonly caused by a cardiopulmonary abnormality, such as CHF, cardiac ischemia, bronchospasm, pulmonary embolus, infection, mucus plugging, and aspiration. Dyspnea must be promptly and carefully evaluated.

DIAGNOSIS

Clinical Presentation

History
Initial evaluation should include a review of the medical history for underlying pulmonary or cardiovascular disease, and a directed history.

Physical Examination
A detailed cardiopulmonary examination should take place, including vital signs with comparison of current findings to those documented earlier.

Diagnostic Testing

- Oxygen assessment should take place promptly. Arterial blood gas measurement provides more information than pulse oximetry. Chest radiography is useful in most patients.
- Other diagnostic and therapeutic measures should be directed by the findings in the initial evaluation and the severity of the suspected diagnosis.

TREATMENT

Therapeutic measures should be directed by the findings in the initial evaluation and the severity of the suspected diagnoses.

Acute Hypertensive Episodes

GENERAL PRINCIPLES

Etiology

- Acute hypertensive episodes in the hospital are most often caused by inadequately treated essential hypertension.
- Volume overload and pain may exacerbate hypertension and should be recognized appropriately and treated.
- Hypertension associated with withdrawal syndromes (e.g., alcohol, cocaine, etc.) and rebound hypertension associated with sudden withdrawal of antihypertensive medications (i.e., clonidine, α-adrenergic antagonists) should be considered. These entities should be treated as discussed in Chapter 3, Preventative Cardiology and Ischemic Heart Disease.

TREATMENT

Treatment decisions should consider baseline BP, presence of symptoms (e.g., chest pain or shortness of breath), and current and baseline antihypertensive medications.

Fever

GENERAL PRINCIPLES

Etiology

Fever accompanies many illnesses and is a valuable marker of disease activity.

DIAGNOSIS

Clinical Presentation

History

History should include chronology of the fever and associated symptoms, medications, potential exposures, and a complete social and travel history.

Physical Examination

- **Physical examination** should include **oral or rectal temperature** monitoring from a consistent site. In the hospitalized patient, special attention should be paid to any rash, new murmur, abnormal fluid accumulation, intravascular lines, and indwelling devices such as gastric tubes or Foley catheters.
- In the **neutropenic patient,** the skin, oral cavity, and perineal area should be examined carefully for breaches of mucosal integrity. For management of neutropenic fever, see Chapter 19, Medical Management of Malignant Disease.

Differential Diagnosis

- Infection is a primary concern; drug reaction, malignancy, VTE, vasculitis, and tissue infarction are other possibilities but are diagnoses of exclusion.
- The differential diagnosis for fever is very broad, and the pace and complexity of the workup depend on the diagnostic considerations taken in the context of the clinical stability and immune status of the host.

Diagnostic Testing

- Testing includes culture of blood and urine, complete blood count (CBC) with differential, serum chemistries with liver function tests, and urinalysis.
- Diagnostic evaluation generally includes chest radiography.
- Cultures of abnormal fluid collections, sputum, cerebrospinal fluid, and stool should be sent if clinically indicated. Cultures are ideally obtained prior to initiation of antibiotics; however, antibiotics should not be delayed if serious infection is suspected.

TREATMENT

- **Antipyretic drugs** may be given to decrease associated discomfort. Not all fevers require treatment. Aspirin (325 mg) and acetaminophen are the drugs of choice (325 to 650 mg PO or per rectum q4h). **Aspirin should be avoided in adolescents** with possible viral infections because this combination has been associated with Reye's syndrome.
- **Tepid water baths** are effective in treating hyperpyrexia. Use of hypothermic (cooling) blankets and ice packs are uncomfortable and should generally be discouraged.
- **Empiric antibiotics** should be considered in hemodynamically unstable patients in whom infection is a primary concern and in neutropenic and asplenic patients.

- **Heat stroke and malignant hyperthermia** are medical emergencies that require prompt recognition and treatment (see Chapter 24, Medical Emergencies).

Pain

GENERAL PRINCIPLES

Definition

Pain is subjective, and therapy must be individualized. Chronic pain may not be associated with any objective physical findings. **Pain scales** should be employed for quantitation.

Classification

- Acute pain usually requires only temporary therapy.
- For chronic pain, nonnarcotic preparations should be used when possible.
- Anticonvulsants and antidepressants are more useful than narcotics for neuropathic pain. If pain is refractory to conventional therapy, then nonpharmacologic modalities, such as nerve blocks, sympathectomy, and relaxation therapy, may be appropriate.

TREATMENT

Medications

- **Acetaminophen**
  - **Effects:** Antipyretic and analgesic actions but no anti-inflammatory or antiplatelet properties.
  - **Preparations and dosage:** Acetaminophen, 325 to 1,000 mg q4–6h (maximum dose, 4 g/d), is available in tablet, caplet, liquid, and rectal suppository form. It should be used at low doses in patients with liver disease.
  - **Adverse effects**
    - The principal advantage of acetaminophen is its lack of gastric toxicity.
    - **Hepatic toxicity** may be serious, however, and acute overdose with 10 to 15 g can cause fatal hepatic necrosis (see Chapter 16, Liver Diseases, and Chapter 24, Medical Emergencies).
- **Aspirin**
  - **Effects: Aspirin** has analgesic, antipyretic, anti-inflammatory, and antiplatelet effects.
  - **Preparations and dosages:**
    - Aspirin is given in a dosage of 325 to 650 mg PO q4h PRN (maximum dose, 4 g/d) for relief of pain.
    - Rectal suppositories (300 to 600 mg q3–4h) may be irritating to the mucosa and have variable absorption.
    - Enteric-coated tablets and nonacetylated salicylates may cause less injury to the gastric mucosa than buffered or plain aspirin.
  - **Adverse effects**
    - Dose-related **side effects** include tinnitus, dizziness, and hearing loss.
    - Dyspepsia and GI bleeding can develop and may be severe.
    - Hypersensitivity reactions, including bronchospasm, laryngeal edema, and urticaria, are uncommon, but patients with asthma and nasal polyps are more susceptible.
    - **Patients with allergic or bronchospastic reactions to aspirin should not be given NSAIDs.**

- ○ Chronic excessive use can result in interstitial nephritis and papillary necrosis.
- ○ Aspirin should be used with caution in patients with hepatic or renal disease, bleeding disorders, and pregnancy, and those who are receiving anticoagulation therapy.
- ○ **Antiplatelet effects** may last for up to 1 week after a single dose.
- **NSAIDs**
  - **Effects: NSAIDs** have analgesic, antipyretic, and anti-inflammatory properties mediated by inhibition of cyclooxygenase. All NSAIDs have similar efficacy and toxicities, with a side-effect profile similar to that of the salicylates.
  - **Adverse effects**
    - ○ NSAIDs may blunt the cardioprotective effects of aspirin.
    - ○ **NSAIDs should be used with caution in patients with impaired renal or hepatic function** (see Chapter 22, Arthritis and Rheumatologic Diseases). **Ketorolac** is an analgesic that can be given IM or IV (15 to 30 mg q8h) and is often used postoperatively; however, parenteral therapy should not exceed 5 days. Nephrotoxicity is more pronounced with IM than with PO administration.
- **Cyclooxygenase-2 (COX-2) inhibitors**
  - **Effects: COX-2 inhibitors** act primarily on COX-2, an inducible form of cyclooxygenase and an important mediator of pain and inflammation. COX-2 inhibitors have little significant effect on the gastric mucosa. COX-2 inhibitors offer no analgesic advantage over other NSAIDs.
  - **Preparations and dosages:** The currently available selective COX-2 inhibitor is **celecoxib. Meloxicam** is also available but is less selective for COX-2.
  - **Adverse effects**
    - ○ Chronic, high-dose COX-2 inhibitor use has been shown to increase death from MI (*NEJM 2006;355:873*).
    - ○ COX-2 inhibitors should not be used in patients who have allergic or bronchospastic reactions to aspirin or other NSAIDs.
    - ○ Celecoxib is contraindicated in patients with allergic-type **reactions to sulfonamides.**
- **Opioid analgesics**
  - **Effects:** Opioid analgesics are pharmacologically similar to opium or morphine and are the drugs of choice when analgesia without antipyretic action is desired.
  - **Preparations and dosages:** Table 1 lists equianalgesic dosages.

Table 1	Equipotent Doses of Opioid Analgesics			
Drug	Onset (min)	Duration (hr)	IM/IV/SC (mg)	PO (mg)
Fentanyl	7–8	1–2	0.1	NA
Levorphanol	30–90	4–6	2	4
Hydromorphone	15–30	2–4	1.5–2.0	7.5
Methadone	30–60	4–12	10	20
Morphine	15–30	2–4	10	30[a]
Oxycodone	15–30	3–4	NA	20
Meperidine	10–45	2–4	75	300
Codeine	15–30	4–6	120	200

Note: Equivalences are based on single-dose studies.
NA, not applicable.
[a]An IM:PO ratio of 1:2 to 1:3 used for repetitive dosing.

- **Constant pain**
  - **Constant pain** requires continuous (around-the-clock) analgesia with supplementary (PRN) doses for breakthrough pain at doses of roughly one-third of the basal dose. Medication dosages should be maintained at the lowest level that provides adequate analgesia. If frequent PRN doses are required, the maintenance dose should be increased, or the dosing interval should be decreased.
  - **If adequate analgesia** cannot be achieved at the maximum recommended dose of one narcotic or if the side effects are intolerable, the patient should be changed to another preparation beginning at one-half of the equianalgesic dose to account for incomplete cross-tolerance.
  - **Oral medications** should be used when possible.
  - **Parenteral and transdermal administration** are useful in the setting of dysphagia, emesis, or decreased GI absorption.
  - **Continuous IV administration** provides steady blood levels and allows for rapid dose adjustment.
  - Agents with short half-lives, such as morphine, should be used. Narcotic-naïve patients should be started on the lowest possible doses, whereas patients with demonstrated tolerance will require higher doses.
  - **Patient-controlled analgesia** is often used to control pain in a postoperative or terminally ill patient.
  - Advantages of patient-controlled analgesia include enhancement in pain relief, decrease in anxiety, and decrease in the total narcotic dose. Opioid-naïve patients should not have basal rates prescribed due to risk of overdose.
- **Selected drugs**
  - **Codeine** is usually given in combination with aspirin or acetaminophen. It is also an effective cough suppressant at a dosage of 10 to 15 mg PO q4–6h.
  - **Oxycodone and propoxyphene** are also usually prescribed orally in combination with aspirin or acetaminophen. Available tablets include oxycodone with acetaminophen (5 mg/325 mg PO q6h), oxycodone with aspirin (5 mg/325 mg PO q6h), and propoxyphene with acetaminophen (50 mg/325 mg or 100 mg/ 650 mg q6h).
  - **Immediate-release and sustained-release morphine sulfate** preparations (immediate-release, 5 to 30 mg PO q2–8h; sustained-release, 15 to 120 mg PO q12h; or a rectal suppository) can be used. The liquid form can be useful in patients who have difficulty in swallowing pills. Larger doses of morphine may be necessary to control pain as tolerance develops. Morphine should be used with caution in renal insufficiency.
  - **Meperidine** (50 to 150 mg PO, SC, or IM q2–3h) causes less biliary spasm, urinary retention, and constipation than morphine but results in more respiratory depression and is a myocardial depressant. It is **contraindicated in patients who are taking monoamine oxidase inhibitors and is cautioned in individuals with renal failure** (accumulation of active metabolites causes CNS excitement and seizures). Repetitive dosing is more likely to cause seizures; therefore, chronic administration is not recommended. Coadministration of **hydroxyzine** (25 to 100 mg IM q4–6h) may decrease nausea and potentiate the analgesic effect of meperidine.
  - **Methadone** is very effective when administered orally and suppresses the symptoms of withdrawal from other opioids because of its extended half-life. Despite its long elimination half-life, its analgesic duration of action is much shorter.

- ○ **Hydromorphone** (2 to 4 mg PO q4–6h; 1 to 2 mg IM, IV, or SC q4–6h) is a potent morphine derivative. It is also available as a 3-mg rectal suppository.
- ○ **Fentanyl** is available in a transdermal patch with sustained release over 72 hours. Initial onset of action is delayed. Respiratory depression may occur more frequently with fentanyl.
- ○ **Mixed agonist–antagonist agents** (butorphanol, nalbuphine, oxymorphone, pentazocine) offer few advantages and produce more adverse effects than do the other agents.
- **Precautions**
  - ○ **Opioids are relatively contraindicated** in acute disease states in which the pattern and degree of pain are important diagnostic signs (e.g., head injuries, abdominal pain). They may also increase intracranial pressure.
  - ○ **Opioids should be used with caution** in patients with hypothyroidism, Addison disease, hypopituitarism, anemia, respiratory disease (e.g., chronic obstructive pulmonary disease [COPD], asthma, kyphoscoliosis, severe obesity), severe malnutrition, debilitation, or chronic cor pulmonale.
  - ○ Opioid dosage should be adjusted for patients with impaired hepatic function.
  - ○ Drugs that potentiate the adverse effects of opioids include phenothiazines, antidepressants, benzodiazepines, and alcohol.
  - ○ **Tolerance** develops with chronic use and coincides with the development of physical dependence.
  - ○ **Physical dependence** is characterized by a withdrawal syndrome (anxiety, irritability, diaphoresis, tachycardia, GI distress, and temperature instability) when the drug is stopped abruptly. It may occur after only 2 weeks of therapy.
  - ○ Administration of an opioid antagonist may precipitate withdrawal after only 3 days of therapy. Withdrawal can be minimized by tapering the medication slowly over several days.
- **Adverse and toxic effects**
  - ○ Although individuals may tolerate some preparations better than others, at equianalgesic doses, few differences in side effects exist.
  - ○ **CNS effects** include sedation, euphoria, and pupillary constriction.
  - ○ **Respiratory depression** is dose related and is especially pronounced after IV administration.
  - ○ **Cardiovascular effects** include peripheral vasodilation and hypotension, especially after IV administration.
  - ○ **GI effects** include constipation, nausea, and vomiting. Patients who are receiving opioid medications should be provided with stool softeners and laxatives. Nausea and vomiting can be limited by keeping the patient in a recumbent position. Benzodiazepines, dopamine antagonists (e.g., prochlorperazine, metoclopramide, etc.), and ondansetron can be used as antiemetics. Opioids may precipitate toxic megacolon in patients with inflammatory bowel disease.
  - ○ **Urinary retention** may be caused by increased bladder, ureter, and urethral sphincter tone.
  - ○ **Pruritus** occurs most commonly with spinal administration.
- **Opioid overdose**
  - ○ **Naloxone,** an opioid antagonist, should be readily available for administration in the case of accidental or intentional overdose. For details of administration, see Chapter 24, Medical Emergencies.

  ○ Side effects include hyper- or hypotension, irritability, anxiety, restlessness, tremulousness, nausea, and vomiting.
  ○ Naloxone can also precipitate seizure activity and cardiac arrhythmias.
* **Alternative medications**
  * **Tramadol:** Tramadol is similar to opioids but has less potential for addiction and abuse.
    ○ **Preparations and dosages:** Between 50 and 100 mg PO q4–6h can be used for acute pain. For elderly patients and those with renal or liver dysfunction, dosage reduction is recommended.
    ○ **Adverse effects:** Because CNS effects include sedation, concomitant use of alcohol, sedatives, or narcotics should be avoided. Nausea, dizziness, constipation, and headache may also occur. Respiratory depression has not been described at prescribed dosages but may occur with overdose. **Tramadol should not be used in patients who are taking a monoamine oxidase inhibitor.**
  * **Anticonvulsants** (e.g., gabapentin, valproate) **and tricyclic antidepressants** (e.g., amitriptyline) are PO agents that can be used to treat neuropathic pain.
  * **Topical anesthetics** (e.g., lidocaine) may provide analgesia to a localized region (e.g., postherpetic neuralgia).

Altered Mental Status

GENERAL PRINCIPLES

Etiology
Mental status changes have a broad differential diagnosis that includes neurologic (e.g., stroke, delirium), metabolic (e.g., hypoxemia, hypoglycemia), toxic (e.g., drug effects, alcohol withdrawal), and other etiologies. Infection (e.g., urinary tract infections, pneumonia, etc.) is a common cause in the elderly and patients with underlying neurologic disease.

DIAGNOSIS

Clinical Presentation
History
* **Focus** particularly on medications, underlying dementia, neurologic or psychiatric disorders, and a history of alcohol and drug use.
* Directed history should be obtained from the patient; family and nursing personnel may be able to provide additional details.

Physical Examination
Physical examination generally includes vital signs, a search for sites of infection, a complete cardiopulmonary examination, and a detailed neurologic examination including mental status evaluation.

Diagnostic Testing
* Testing includes blood glucose, serum electrolytes, creatinine, CBC, urinalysis, oxygen assessment, and chest radiograph.

- Other evaluation, including culture, lumbar puncture, toxicology screen, thyroid function tests, B_{12} levels, and syphilis serologies, should be directed by initial findings and diagnostic possibilities.
- If indicated by initial findings and diagnostic possibilities, the following should be obtained:
  - CT of the head (initially, a noncontrast study is appropriate)
  - Electroencephalogram (EEG)
  - ECG

TREATMENT

Management of specific disorders is discussed in Chapter 23, Neurologic Disorders.

Medications

Agitation and psychosis may be features of a change in mental status. The antipsychotic, haloperidol and the benzodiazepine, lorazepam are commonly used in the **acute management** of these symptoms. The newer-generation antipsychotics **(risperidone, olanzapine, quetiapine, clozapine, ziprasidone)** are alternative agents that may lead to decreased incidence of extrapyramidal symptoms. All of these agents may pose risks to the elderly if given for long term.

- **Haloperidol** is the initial drug of choice for acute management of agitation and psychosis. The initial dose of 0.5 to 5 mg (0.25 mg in **elderly patients**) PO and 2 to 10 mg IM or IV can be repeated every 30 to 60 minutes until the desired effect is achieved. Sedation is usually achieved with 10 to 20 mg PO or IM. **IV infusions** (1 to 40 mg/hr) can also be used as an alternative to bolus injections. Compared with other antipsychotics with similar efficacy, haloperidol has fewer active metabolites and fewer anticholinergic, sedative, and hypotensive effects, although it may have more extrapyramidal side effects. In low dosages, haloperidol rarely causes hypotension, cardiovascular compromise, or excessive sedation.
  - **Prolongation of the QT interval** with development of torsades de pointes may be seen with high-dose IV therapy. In patients who are receiving IV therapy, QT_c and electrolytes (primarily potassium and magnesium) should be monitored. Use should be discontinued with prolongation of $QT_c > 450$ milliseconds or 25% above baseline.
  - **Postural hypotension** may occasionally be acute and severe after IM administration. If significant hypotension occurs, administration of IV fluids with the patient in the Trendelenburg position is usually sufficient. If **vasopressors** are required, norepinephrine or phenylephrine should be used, as dopamine may exacerbate the psychotic state.
  - **Neuroleptic malignant syndrome** is an infrequent, potentially lethal complication of antipsychotic drug therapy. Clinical manifestations include rigidity, akinesia, altered sensorium, fever, tachycardia, and alteration in BP. Severe muscle rigidity can cause rhabdomyolysis and acute renal failure. **Laboratory abnormalities** include elevations in creatine kinase, liver function tests, and white blood cell count (see Chapter 23, Neurologic Disorders).
- **Lorazepam** is a benzodiazepine that is useful for agitation and psychosis in the setting of hepatic dysfunction and sedative or alcohol withdrawal, and in patients who are refractory to monotherapy with neuroleptics. The **initial dose** is 0.5 to 2.0 mg IV. The **key features** of lorazepam are its short duration of action and few

active metabolites. The use of lorazepam, as with all benzodiazepines, is limited by excess sedation, respiratory depression, and the potential to precipitate agitation in the elderly and in patients with liver disease and low albumin.

SPECIAL CONSIDERATIONS

Sundown syndrome

* **Sundown syndrome** refers to the appearance of worsening confusion in the evening and is associated with dementia, delirium, and unfamiliar environments.
* Behavioral interventions, such as increased lighting, maintenance of a familiar environment, and reorientation, should be attempted first.
* If behavioral interventions are ineffective, short-term antipsychotic therapy may be warranted.

Insomnia and Anxiety

GENERAL PRINCIPLES

Etiology

* **Insomnia and anxiety** may be attributed to a variety of underlying medical or psychiatric disorders, and symptoms may be exacerbated by hospitalization.
* Possible causes of **insomnia** to consider include mood and anxiety disorders, substance abuse disorders, common medications (i.e., β-blockers, steroids, bronchodilators, etc.), sleep apnea, hyperthyroidism, and nocturnal myoclonus.
* **Anxiety** may be seen in anxiety disorder, depression, substance abuse disorders, hyperthyroidism, and complex partial seizures.

TREATMENT

Medications

Selected medications for insomnia or anxiety, or both:

* **Benzodiazepines** are frequently used in management of anxiety and insomnia. Table 2 provides a list of selected benzodiazepines and their dosages.
  * **Pharmacology:** Most benzodiazepines undergo oxidation to active metabolites in the liver. **Lorazepam, oxazepam, and temazepam** undergo glucuronidation to inactive metabolites; therefore, these agents may be particularly useful in the elderly and in those with liver disease. **Benzodiazepine toxicity** is heightened by malnutrition, advanced age, hepatic disease, and concomitant use of alcohol, other CNS depressants, isoniazid, and cimetidine. Benzodiazepines with long half-lives may accumulate substantially, even with single daily dosing. This effect is a particular concern in the elderly, in whom the half-life may be increased two- to fourfold.
  * **Dosages**
    * **Relief of anxiety and insomnia** is achieved at the doses outlined in Table 2. Therapy should be started at the lowest recommended dosage with intermittent dosing schedules.

Table 2		Characteristics of Selected Benzodiazepines	
Drug	**Route**	**Usual Dosage**	**Half-life (hr)**
Alprazolam	PO	0.75–4.0 mg/24 hr (in three doses)	12–15
Chlordiazepoxide	PO	15–100 mg/24 hr (in divided doses)	5–30
Clorazepate	PO	7.5–60.0 mg/24 hr (in one to four doses)	30–100
Diazepam	PO	6–40 mg/24 hr (in one to four doses)	20–50
	IV	2.5–20.0 mg (slow IV push)	20–50
Flurazepam	PO	15–30 mg at bedtime	50–100
Lorazepam[a]	PO	1–10 mg/24 hr (in two to three doses)	10–20
	IV or IM	0.05 mg/kg (4 mg max)	10–20
Midazolam	IV	0.01–0.05 mg/kg	1–12
	IM	0.08 mg/kg	1–12
Oxazepam[a]	PO	10–30 mg/24 hr (in three to four doses)	5–10
Prazepam	PO	20–60 mg/24 hr (in three to four divided doses)	36–200
Temazepam[a]	PO	15–30 mg at bedtime	8–12
Triazolam[a]	PO	0.125–0.250 mg at bedtime	2–5

[a]Metabolites are inactive.

- **Side effects** include drowsiness, dizziness, fatigue, psychomotor impairment, and anterograde amnesia.
- The elderly are more sensitive to these agents and may experience falls, paradoxical agitation, and delirium.
- **IV administration of diazepam and midazolam** can be associated with hypotension and respiratory or cardiac arrest.
- **Respiratory depression** can occur even with oral administration in patients with respiratory compromise.
- **Tolerance** to benzodiazepines can develop.
- **Dependence** may develop after only 2 to 4 weeks of therapy.
- A **withdrawal syndrome** consisting of agitation, irritability, insomnia, tremor, palpitations, headache, GI distress, and perceptual disturbance begins 1 to 10 days after a rapid decrease in dosage or abrupt cessation of therapy and may last for several weeks.
- **Seizures and delirium** may also occur with sudden discontinuation of benzodiazepines. Although the severity and incidence of withdrawal symptoms appear to be related to dose and duration of treatment, withdrawal symptoms have been reported even after brief therapy at doses in the recommended range. Short-acting and intermediate-acting drugs should be decreased by 10% to 20% every 5 days, with a slower taper in the final few weeks; long-acting preparations can be tapered more quickly.

- **Overdose**
  - ○ **Flumazenil,** a benzodiazepine antagonist, should be readily available in case of accidental or intentional overdose. For details of administration, see Chapter 24, Medical Emergencies. Common side effects include dizziness, nausea, and vomiting.
  - ○ **Flumazenil should be used with caution in patients with a history of seizure disorder or if overdose with tricyclic antidepressants is suspected.**
- **Trazodone**
  - • **Trazodone** is an antidepressant that may be useful for the treatment of severe anxiety or insomnia.
  - • **Side effects**
    - ○ Highly sedating, causes postural hypotension, and is associated with ventricular ectopy and priapism. No deaths or cardiovascular complications have been reported in patients taking trazodone alone.
    - ○ A number of potential drug interactions can occur with trazodone.
- **Nonbenzodiazepine hypnotics** appear to act on the benzodiazepine receptor. These agents have been shown to be safe and effective for initiating sleep. All should be used with caution in patients with impaired respiratory function.
  - • **Zolpidem** is an imidazopyridine hypnotic agent that is useful for the treatment of insomnia. It has no withdrawal syndrome, rebound insomnia, or tolerance. Side effects include headache, daytime somnolence, and GI upset. The starting **dose** is 5 mg PO every night at bedtime for the elderly and 10 mg for other patients, titrating up to 20 mg as needed. Doses should be reduced in cirrhosis.
  - • **Zaleplon** has a half-life of approximately 1 hour and has no active metabolites. **Side effects** include drowsiness, dizziness, and impaired coordination. Zaleplon should be used with caution in those with compromised respiratory function. The starting dose is 5 mg PO at bedtime for the elderly or patients with hepatic dysfunction and 10 to 20 mg PO at bedtime for other patients.
  - • **Eszopiclone** offers a longer half-life compared to the above agents. Side effects include headache, somnolence, and dizziness. Starting dose is 2 mg, with reduced dosing in the elderly, debilitated, and patients with liver disease.
- **Antihistamines: Over-the-counter antihistamines** can be used for insomnia and anxiety, particularly in patients with a history of drug dependence. Anticholinergic side effects limit the utility, especially in the elderly.

PERIOPERATIVE MEDICINE

Preoperative Cardiac Evaluation

GENERAL PRINCIPLES

- The role of the medical consultant is to estimate the level of cardiac risk associated with a given procedure. "Clearance" cannot be readily granted, as **there is always some level of risk.**
- Based on the estimated risk, the consultant should then determine the need for further evaluation and prescribe possible interventions to mitigate risk.
- Though preoperative consultations often focus on cardiac risk, it is essential to remember that poor outcomes can result from significant disease in other organ

systems. **Evaluation of the entire patient is necessary to provide optimal perioperative care.**

Definition

Perioperative cardiac complications are generally defined as cardiac death, myocardial infarctions (both ST- and non-ST elevation), CHF, and clinically significant rhythm disturbances.

Epidemiology

- The incidence of perioperative cardiac complications varies markedly depending on the definitions employed and the population studied. Overall, an estimated 50,000 perioperative infarctions and 1 million other cardiovascular complications occur annually (*N Engl J Med 2001;345:1677*).
- Of those who have a perioperative MI, the risk of in-hospital mortality is estimated at 10% to 15% (*Chest 2006;130:584*).

Pathophysiology

- Autopsy data suggest fatal perioperative MIs occur via the same mechanism as non-perioperative MIs (*Int J Cardiol 1996;57:37*).
- Angiographic data suggest that existing stenoses may play a role with some perioperative events; however (*Am J Cardiol 1996;77:1126*), a significant number, maybe most, perioperative MIs are "stress" related and not due to plaque rupture (*J Cardiothorac Vasc Anesth 2003;17:90*).

DIAGNOSIS

Clinical Presentation

History

- The focus of the history is to identify factors/comorbid conditions that will affect perioperative risk.
- Current guidelines focus on identification of active cardiac disease and known risk **factors for perioperative events.**
  - Evidence of *active* cardiac conditions
    - Unstable/acute coronary syndrome?
    - Recent MI (defined as within 30 days)?
    - Symptoms of decompensated CHF?
    - Significant arrhythmias?
    - Severe valvular disease?
  - Clinical risk factors
    - Preexisting, stable CAD
    - Compensated CHF
    - Diabetes mellitus
    - Prior CVA or TIA
    - Renal insufficiency
  - Other
    - Age >70 years has been identified in several studies as a significant risk factor (*JAMA 2001;285:1865*; *Eur Heart J 2008;29:394*). Not uniformly accepted as an independent risk factor.
    - Abnormal ECG

- ○ Nonsinus rhythm (rate controlled and stable)
- ○ Hypertension, poorly controlled

Physical Examination
- A complete physical exam is essential.
- Specific attention should be paid to:
  - **Vital signs**—particularly blood pressure and evidence of **hypertension.**
    - ○ Systolic blood pressure < 180 and diastolic blood pressure < 110 are generally considered acceptable.
    - ○ The management of stage III hypertension (SBP >180 or DBP < 110) is controversial. Postponing elective surgery to allow adequate BP control in this setting is acceptable, but this is poorly studied and how long to wait after treatment is instituted is unclear.
  - Evidence of **CHF** (elevated JVP, crackles, S3, etc.).
  - **Murmurs** suggestive of **significant valvular lesions,** particularly aortic stenosis (AS):
    - ○ Symptomatic stenotic lesions such as mitral stenosis and AS are thought to be associated with the greatest risk.
    - ○ **Aortic stenosis**
      - Severe AS (valve area <0.7 cm^2 or mean gradient $\geq$ 50 mm Hg) is associated with an approximate 30% incidence of cardiac morbidity with a mortality of approximately 10% (*Am J Med 2004;116:8*; *Am J Cardiol 1998;81:448*).
      - The risk of asymptomatic, moderate AS appears to be less, and surgery can be considered in this group with careful evaluation (*Chest 2005;128:2944*).
    - ○ **Mitral stenosis**
      - Not well studied in the perioperative setting.
      - Percutaneous valvotomy should be considered with severe stenosis.
    - ○ Symptomatic **regurgitant lesions** are generally tolerated perioperatively and can be managed medically *as long as the patient is well compensated* preoperatively.

Diagnostic Criteria (Fig. 1)
- **Step 1: Establish the urgency of surgery**
  - Emergency surgery proceeds to OR.
  - Evaluate preoperatively and suggest management strategies as time will allow.
  - Important to note that many surgeries, though not absolutely emergent, are urgent and are unlikely to allow for a time-consuming evaluation.
- **Step 2: Assess for active cardiac conditions**
  - As defined above (see History)
  - Acute coronary syndrome (ST-elevation MI, NSTEMI, unstable angina)
  - Decompensated heart failure
  - Unstable arrhythmias
  - Severe valvular disease
  - If present, postponing surgery to allow for further management is recommended.
- **Step 3: Determine the surgery-specific risk**
  - If the surgery is inherently *low risk*, patients can generally undergo the procedure without further evaluation.
  - Though professional judgement is required, surgical risk can generally be divided as follows:
    - ○ **Low-risk surgeries** (<1% expected risk of adverse cardiac events) include superficial procedures, cataract surgery, breast surgery, endoscopic procedures, and most procedures that can be performed in an ambulatory setting.

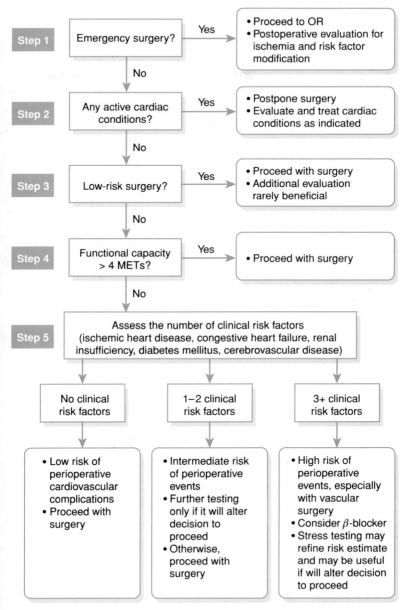

Figure 1. Cardiac evaluation algorithm for noncardiac surgery. (Adapted from the 2007 ACC/AHA guidelines on perioperative evaluation for noncardiac surgery. *Circulation* 2007;116:e418.)

- ○ **Intermediate risk surgeries** (1% to 5% risk of adverse cardiac events) include carotid endarterectomy, intraperitoneal surgeries, intrathoracic surgeries, orthopedic surgeries, head and neck surgeries, and prostate surgery.
- ○ **Vascular surgery** involving extremity revascularization and aortic surgeries is generally found to carry the highest risk (>5% risk of adverse cardiac events).
- **Step 4: Assess the patient's functional capacity**
  - Poor functional capacity (<4 METs) is associated with an increased risk of perioperative cardiac events (*Arch Intern Med 1999;159:2185*; *Chest 1999;116: 355*).
  - Likewise, patients with good functional capacity are unlikely to suffer serious cardiovascular complications.
  - Though exercise testing is the gold standard, functional capacity can be reliably estimated by patient self-report (*Am J Cardiol 1989;64:651*).
  - Examples of activities that suggest at least a moderate functional capacity (>4 METs) include:
    - ○ Climbing one to two flights of stairs
    - ○ Able to walk up a hill
    - ○ Walk a block at a brisk pace
  - **Patients with a functional capacity of >4 METs *without symptoms* can proceed to surgery with relatively low risk.**
- **Step 5: Assess the patient's clinical risk factors**
  - The number of risk factors combined with the surgery-specific risk (intermediate vs. vascular) determines further management.
  - The clinical risk factors are adapted from the *Revised Cardiac Risk Index (RCRI)* (*Circulation 1999;100:1043*):
    - ○ Ischemic heart disease
    - ○ History of TIA or CVA
    - ○ History of CHF
    - ○ Renal insufficiency (Cr ≥ 2.0)
    - ○ Diabetes mellitus
- Patients with **no clinical risk factors** are inherently *low risk* (<1% risk of cardiac events) and are unlikely to benefit from further intervention. They may proceed to surgery.
  - Patients with **one or two clinical risk factors** are generally at *intermediate risk* and may proceed to surgery.
    - ○ Perioperative heart rate control with β-blockers can be considered for this group, though this is controversial.
    - ○ Stress testing may provide a better estimate of cardiovascular risk, and so may be considered if knowledge of this increased risk would change management (*J Am Coll Cardiol 2006;48:964*).
    - ○ It is important to note that revascularization is unlikely to improve upon this risk and is not recommended solely to reduce perioperative risk (see Revascularization below) (*N Engl J Med 2004;351:2795*).
  - Patients with **three or more clinical risk factors** are at *high risk* of adverse cardiac events, particularly when undergoing vascular surgery.
    - ○ Perioperative heart rate control with β-blockers is recommended, but this is controversial.
    - ○ Stress testing can provide a better estimate of the degree of risk and can be considered if a more precise estimate of risk will alter the decision to proceed with the planned surgery.

• Despite the increased risk, there is evidence that preoperative revascularization fails to improve perioperative cardiovascular outcomes in this population (see Revascularization below) (*N Engl J Med 2004;351:2795*; *J Am Coll Cardiol 2007;49: 1763*).

Diagnostic Testing

• **12-Lead electrocardiogram**
  • The value of a routine ECG is controversial, and it is often unnecessary.
  • The current ACC/AHA guidelines recommend an ECG in:
    ○ Class I: Patients with 1+ risk factors undergoing vascular surgery and patients with PVD, CAD, or CVD undergoing intermediate risk surgery.
    ○ Class II: Patients without risk factors undergoing vascular surgery and patients with other clinical risk factors undergoing intermediate risk surgery (*Circulation 2007;116:e418*).
  • If there is concern for underlying CAD or if surveillance for ischemia postoperatively is planned, a preoperative ECG should be obtained.
• **Resting echocardiogram**
  • In general, the indications for echocardiographic evaluation in the preoperative setting are no different than in the nonoperative setting. **An echo is not routinely necessary.**
  • Murmurs found on physical exam suggestive of significant underlying valvular disease should be evaluated by echo.
  • An assessment of left ventricular function should be considered when there is clinical concern for underlying CHF not previously diagnosed or if there is concern for deterioration since the last exam.
• **Stress evaluation**
  • The decision to pursue a stress evaluation should be guided by an assessment of preoperative.
  • Risk as detailed below (see Risk Stratification). **Routine stress evaluation of all patients undergoing surgery is not warranted.**
  • Even if revascularization is not warranted (see Revascularization below), a stress evaluation does add to the evaluation of the potentially high-risk patient. **A positive test indicates a substantially increased risk of a perioperative cardiac event, while a negative study suggests a lower risk than that predicted by clinical factors alone** (*JAMA 2001;285:1865*).
• **Exercise stress testing**
  ○ If the patient is able to exercise adequately, exercise testing is the first choice.
  ○ Patients must be able to exercise to 85% of their predicted maximal heart rate.
  ○ The **presence of a left bundle branch block decreases the accuracy of exercise testing.** Vasodilator nuclear imaging is preferred in this instance.
  ○ **Exercise ECG stress**
    - Though not as frequently pursued, this test can still be useful.
    - Patients **must have no baseline ECG abnormalities that preclude interpretation of the test.**
  ○ **Exercise-echo** and **exercise-nuclear perfusion** stress testing
    - Neither is clearly superior to the other.
    - Patient comorbidities (e.g., obesity impeding echo windows) and additional questions to be answered (e.g., valvular disease making an echo more useful) should be considered in selecting the modality.

- **Pharmacologic stress testing**
  - ○ **Vasodilator nuclear perfusion imaging** and **dobutamine echocardiography** are the generally available options.
  - ○ As with exercise testing, neither is clearly superior to the other for risk stratification.
- Consideration must be given to patient comorbidities that make utilization of a modality's pharmacologic agent undesirable (e.g., supraventricular arrhythmias with dobutamine and bronchospasm with adenosine).

TREATMENT

Medications

- **β-Blockers**
  - **Evidence**
    - ○ Multiple relatively small studies have provided support for the benefit of perioperative β-blockade. Some benefit has been shown in patients with or at risk for CAD undergoing noncardiac surgeries (*N Engl J Med 1996;335:1713*). The most pronounced benefit has been in high-risk patients undergoing vascular surgery (*N Engl J Med 1999;341:1789*), particularly where β-blocker dose was titrated to heart rate control (*J Am Coll Cardiol 2006;48:964*; *Circulation 2006;114(Suppl):I344*).
    - ○ However, the large POISE trial, while confirming the decrease in cardiac events with aggressive perioperative β-blockade, showed an alarming increase in overall mortality and stroke risk (*Lancet 2008;371:1839*). Though the mechanism is not certain, it is likely related to perioperative hemodynamic instability associated with new exposure to β-blockers.
    - ○ The major difference between the studies showing benefit and the POISE trial was the β-blocker regimen utilized. The POISE trial employed a relatively high dose of extended-release metoprolol beginning on the day of surgery. The others started a long-acting β-blocker days to weeks prior to the surgery and titrated the dose preoperatively.
  - **Recommendations**
    - ○ The ACC/AHA recommendations for perioperative β-blockade were released before the POISE trial was published and cannot be considered current. An update is expected.
    - ○ For now, treatment of patients at high risk for perioperative myocardial injury (three or more risk factors and/or a positive stress evaluation) seems reasonable, particularly those undergoing vascular surgery.
    - ○ The benefit of perioperative beta-blockade appears to be correlated to reductions in heart rate (*Anesth Analg 2008;106:1039*). Thus, doses large enough to lower the resting heart rate to the range of 50 to 60 bpm are probably the most beneficial. However, starting the medication as early as possible prior to surgery with careful titration of dose preoperatively is strongly preferred. This should be done with careful attention to blood pressure, as the risk of hypotension obviously increases with escalating doses of the medication.
    - ○ Patients already taking β-blockers should be continued on their medication. Withholding β-blockers in those already taking them is not recommended.
    - ○ Attention should be paid to the presence of contraindications to β-blocker use.

- **Statins**
  - **Evidence**
    - It had been previously recommended to hold statins (HMG-CoA reductase inhibitors) perioperatively because of concerns of increased risk of rhabdomyolysis. It appears now that this is unfounded (*Am J Cardiol 2005;95:658*).
    - Two trials have shown a decrease in perioperative cardiac events with statins in patients undergoing vascular surgery.
    - The only published prospective study of perioperative statin use involved the administration of atorvastatin to patients scheduled to undergo vascular surgery. The atorvastatin group demonstrated an 18% absolute reduction versus placebo in the occurrence at 6 months of the composite end point of cardiac death, nonfatal MI, stroke, and unstable angina (*J Vasc Surg 2004;39: 967*).
    - Prepublication results from the larger DECREASE III trial showed a decrease in perioperative myocardial ischemia in patients undergoing high-risk vascular surgery when treated with extended-release fluvastatin (*J Am Coll Cardiol 2008;52:2032*).
  - **Recommendations**
    - Patients undergoing vascular surgery may benefit from initiation of statin therapy perioperatively (ACC/AHA class IIa recommendation).
    - Other potential population targets for statin therapy would appear to be chiefly patients who would otherwise benefit from aggressive lipid lowering such as diabetics or those with known cardiac disease.
    - A class IIb indication is given to patients with one or more clinical risk factors undergoing intermediate risk surgeries.
- **α_2-Agonists**
  - **Evidence**
    - Multiple studies of the perioperative cardiovascular benefit of α_2-agonists have been performed. These included a variety of agents. As clonidine is the α_2-agonist of choice in the United States, it will be the focus here.
    - A meta-analysis of the perioperative use of clonidine concluded that clonidine was able to decrease the incidence of perioperative ischemia in both cardiac and noncardiac surgeries (*Anesthesiology 2002;96:323*). The study was not able to address the effect on perioperative infarctions or mortality.
    - A subsequent trial of perioperative clonidine use was also able to show a decrement in the incidence of perioperative ischemia and also showed improvements in both 30-day and 2-year mortality (*Anesthesiology 2004;101:284*). However, the results lose significance when all perioperative β-blocker use is excluded.
  - **Recommendations**
    - It appears clonidine does have cardioprotective benefits, but the evidence is not conclusive.
    - The use of α_2-agonists as a risk-reduction strategy in patients at risk for adverse cardiac outcomes when β-blockers are contraindicated appears a reasonable consideration.
    - If given, no particular administration protocol is clearly superior. The protocol used in the study cited above consisted of clonidine 0.2 mg orally on the evening prior with the concurrent placement of a 0.2-mg/d clonidine patch (one time only). An additional 0.2-mg dose of clonidine was given on the morning of surgery due to the expected lag in onset of action of the transdermal preparation. Hemodynamics need to be monitored closely.

- **Aspirin**
  - For discussion, see Perioperative Anticoagulation and Antithrombotic Management.
  - Also see Revascularization below.
- **Revascularization:** The best available data on preoperative revascularization come from the CARP trial—a prospective study of patients scheduled to undergo vascular surgery (*N Engl J Med 2004;351:2795*):
  - The patients studied all had angiographically proven significant coronary artery disease.
  - Patients were randomized to revascularization (coronary artery bypass grafting [CABG] in 41% and percutaneous intervention in 59%) versus no revascularization.
  - Notable exclusions from the study population were patients found to have significant left main disease, severe LV dysfunction, severe AS, and the presence of severe coexisting illnesses.
  - There was no difference between the groups in the occurrence of myocardial infarction or death at 30 days or in mortality with long-term follow-up.
  - Patients with three or more clinical risk factors and extensive ischemia on stress testing were evaluated in a separate small study (*J Am Coll Cardiol 2007;49:1763*). High event rates were seen in both the revascularization and no revascularization arms, and there was no benefit seen with revascularization.
  - Taken together, these studies suggest the risk of adverse cardiac events is not altered by attempts at preoperative revascularization—even in high-risk populations.
  - A notable possible exception are patients with left main disease, who appeared to have benefited from preoperative revascularization in a subset analysis of the CARP trial data (*Am J Cardiol 2008;102:809*).
  - Based on these results, **a strategy of routinely pursuing coronary revascularization as a method of decreasing perioperative cardiac risk cannot be recommended.**
  - However, careful screening of patients is still essential to **identify those high-risk subsets** who may obtain a survival benefit from revascularization **independent of their need for noncardiac surgery,** such as those with underlying left main coronary artery disease.
  - Additional considerations in patients **who have undergone PCI (percutaneous coronary intervention) preoperatively** apply:
    - If a **bare metal stent** is utilized, the risk of adverse cardiac outcomes perioperatively is greatly increased in the weeks following the PCI (*J Am Coll Cardiol 2000;35:1288; J Am Coll Cardiol 2003;42:234*). This is thought largely to be due to the occurrence of in-stent thrombosis, possibly associated with cessation of antiplatelet therapy for the surgery.
      - Any subsequent surgery needs to be delayed for a *minimum* of 2 weeks, though 6 weeks is preferred.
      - There is limited evidence that patients with older stents still have increased risk of adverse cardiac events if aspirin is discontinued at a later date (*J Am Coll Cardiol 2005;45:456*). Thus, *minimization of the time off of aspirin or, preferably, perioperative continuation is recommended.*
    - The risk of in-stent thrombosis with **drug-eluting stents** is even longer lasting. Moreover, the point at which this risk may decrease has not been able to be clearly defined (*Anesthesiology 2008;109:596*).

- The greatest predictor of thrombosis of a DES appears to be premature discontinuation of dual antiplatelet therapy with aspirin and a thienopyridine (*JAMA 2005;293:2126*).
- Thus, the currently recommended delay of elective surgical procedures after placement of a DES is 12 months of dual antiplatelet therapy (*Circulation 2007;115:813*).
- For procedures that must be performed and mandate cessation of thienopyridine therapy, continuation of aspirin therapy perioperatively if at all possible is recommended. A recent review concluded that if aspirin is continued, short-term discontinuation of thienopyridine therapy may be relatively safe (*Circulation 2009;119:1634*).
  - For angioplasty alone, studies have conflicted, with a 2-week waiting period appearing to be safe (*Am J Cardiol 2005;96:512*) and a longer period appearing to be more appropriate in another (*Am J Cardiol 2006;97:1188*). The ACC/AHA guidelines suggest a 2 to 4 week delay.

MONITORING FOLLOW-UP

Postoperative infarction and surveillance

- Most events will occur within 48 to 72 hours of surgery, with the majority in the first 24 hours (*Anesthesiology 1998;88:572*; *Arch Surg 2003;138:596*; *CMAJ 2005;173: 779*).
- Most are *not* heralded by chest pain and may be clinically asymptomatic (*Anesthesiology 1990;72:153*).
- The current ACC/AHA guidelines recommend:
  - Obtaining ECGs postoperatively and on postoperative days 1 and 2 for patients with known or suspected CAD undergoing intermediate or high-risk surgeries.
  - **Troponin measurements** are only recommended in the setting of ECG changes or clinical symptoms.
  - There is no need to perform surveillance in low-risk surgeries.
- The utility of postoperative troponin assessment is controversial.
  - Several studies suggest an increased risk of cardiac events and death in patients with abnormal troponins postoperatively (*Eur Heart J 2005;26:2448*; *Anaesthesia 2004;59:318*).
  - The risk appears to be greatest in the 30-day perioperative period, but has been shown to last 12+ months.
  - Aggressive medical management triggered by a finding of elevated troponins in the otherwise asymptomatic patient may, therefore, be warranted.
- Symptomatic infarctions should be addressed according to standard therapy of acute coronary syndromes. The major caveat is that bleeding risk with anticoagulants must be carefully considered.

Perioperative Anticoagulation and Antithrombotic Management

GENERAL PRINCIPLES

- Patients receiving anticoagulants are frequently encountered perioperatively and are challenging to manage.

- The risk of thromboembolic events must be weighed against the risk of surgical bleeding. Patient preferences regarding the associated complications (e.g., increased risk of stroke vs. increased risk of reoperation to control hemorrhage) must be considered.
- The *perioperative risk of thromboembolism is greater than that expected* from extrapolation of annual rates in otherwise stable patients, likely due to a rebound hypercoagulable state from cessation of anticoagulants and hypercoagulability due to surgical trauma.
  - The risk of venous thromboembolic events may be increased up to 100-fold (*N Engl J Med 1997;336:1506*).
  - The risk of arterial thromboembolism also appears to be elevated based on event rates seen in bridging anticoagulation trials, though not likely to the extent seen for VTE (*Arch Intern Med 2004;164:1319; Circulation 2004;110:1658*).

DIAGNOSIS

- For patients found to be taking anticoagulating medications, *it is essential to determine the indication for the medication.* Management cannot be determined without knowledge of the reason the patient is being treated.
- Any history of hypercoagulability and/or prior thromboembolism should be sought.
- The details of the planned surgery will need to be reviewed and the surgical team involved.
  - The surgeon's perspective on bleeding risk and the consequences of increased surgical bleeding will need to be determined.
  - *The use of regional anesthesia (e.g., epidural) can be greatly impacted by the use of anticoagulant medications.* The anesthesiologist will need to be involved early in the care of patients who may need perioperative treatment with anticoagulants.

TREATMENT

- Recommended management varies according to the indication for anticoagulation, medication used, and surgical bleeding risk.
- For **patients being treated with oral anticoagulants/vitamin K antagonists (VKA):**
  - Patients undergoing certain minor procedures can ***continue oral anticoagulation through the perioperative period:***
    - This is the recommended approach for patients with an indication for VKA therapy who are undergoing procedures at low risk for bleeding complications.
    - These include *minor dental procedures, cataract surgery, endoscopy without biopsy, arthrocentesis,* and *minor dermatologic procedures* (*Arch Int Med 2003;163:901; Chest 2008;133:299S*).
  - For surgical procedures associated with a more significant bleeding risk, **the VKA will need to be discontinued.**
    - Though the international normalized ratio (INR) at which surgery can be safely performed is subjective, *an INR of <1.5 is typically a reasonable goal.* This will need to be confirmed with the surgical team.
    - If the patient's INR goal is stable in the 2 to 3 target range, the VKA will typically need to be stopped 5 days preoperatively (*Ann Intern Med 1995;122:40*). If the patient's INR target is higher, an additional dose may need to be held.

○ The INR should be checked preoperatively. If a level <1.5 is not obtained on the day prior to surgery, a single 1-mg oral dose of vitamin K appears to be a safe and effective method of achieving an INR <1.5 on the anticipated day of surgery. There is no clear evidence this induces resistance to postoperative anticoagulation (*J Thromb Thrombolysis 2007;24:93*).

○ The VKA can generally be resumed 12 to 24 hours postoperatively if postoperative bleeding has been controlled (*Chest 2008;133:299S*).

○ **Bridging anticoagulation,** though frequently recommended, likely increases the risk of perioperative bleeding (*Arch Intern Med 2008;168:63*).

○ Bridging therapy refers to the administration of an alternative anticoagulation during the time the INR is anticipated to be below the therapeutic range:
  - Typically, this period is 2 days after the last dose of warfarin preoperatively until four doses of warfarin have been administered postoperatively.
  - Patient responses to VKA therapy are widely variable, so these are only approximations.
  - Measurement of the INR is recommended to guide therapy—particularly regarding decisions on cessation of bridging anticoagulation.
  - *Resumption of bridging therapy within 24 hours is probably safe for minor procedures.*
  - *For patients undergoing major surgery,* restarting bridging therapy within 24 hours of surgery is associated with unacceptably high bleeding rates (*J Thromb Haemost 2007;5:2211*). One option is to delay restarting bridging until 48 to 72 hours postoperatively. A second option is to resume the VKA postoperatively within 12 to 24 hours as above and forego bridging postoperatively (*Chest 2008;133:299S*).

• Choices for bridging therapy are generally the LMWHs and UFH. There is less experience in this setting with other agents (e.g., fondaparinux), and their use cannot be considered routine.

○ **LMWHs** have the advantages of relatively predictable pharmacokinetics in patients with normal renal function and ability to be administered subcutaneously.
  - Monitoring of anticoagulant effect is typically not required.
  - Subcutaneous administration allows for outpatient therapy in appropriate patients. This decreases the amount of time the patient must be hospitalized, and also has economic advantages (*Chest 2004;125:1642*).
  - The effect of LMWH can linger if a therapeutic anticoagulation dose is given <1 day prior to surgery (*Ann Intern Med 2007;146:184*). Thus, the last dose should be given 24 hours prior to surgery. Also, if the medication is being given on a once-daily regimen, the dose should be 50% of the usual dose (*Chest 2008;133:299S*).
  - **UFH** can be used in patients with renal disease, but typically it must be administered IV and requires frequent monitoring of the aPTT, necessitating hospitalization.
  - UFH should be stopped 4 hours prior to the planned surgical procedure to allow the anticoagulant effect to wane.

• Selection of patients to treat with bridging therapy and selecting the appropriate agent is controversial. The following are adapted from the American College of Chest Physicians guidelines for the management of perioperative anticoagulation, except where noted (*Chest 2008;133:299S*).

- ○ **Patients at *high risk of thromboembolic events should typically be treated with bridging therapy.*** Full-dose LMWH is recommended over UFH, though either is acceptable. Though the ACCP recommendation is evidence based, it should be noted that the older ACC/AHA guidelines on management of valvular disease continue to recommend IV UFH for bridging in patients with prosthetic valves (*Circulation 2006;114:e84*). This includes patients with:
  - Mechanical mitral valve
  - Older-generation mechanical valve (e.g., Starr–Edwards ball-in-cage valve) in aortic or mitral position
  - Any mechanical valve with a history of cardioembolism within the preceding 6 months
  - Nonvalvular atrial fibrillation with either a history of embolism in the last 3 months *or* CHADS$_2$ score ≥5 (*JAMA 2001;285:2921*); see Chapter 5, Cardiac Arrhythmias
  - Valvular atrial fibrillation
  - Recent VTE (<3 months)
  - Known thrombophilic state (e.g., protein C deficiency)
- ○ For patients at *moderate risk of thromboembolic events*, treatment with bridging is recommended, but options other than full anticoagulation are optional. Therapeutic anticoagulation with LMWH or UFH (as for high-risk patients) is preferred, but treatment with DVT prophylaxis dosing of LMWH is considered an acceptable alternative. This includes patients with:
  - Mechanical aortic valve (bileaflet) *with one or more* associated risk factors for thromboembolism: AF, CHF, hypertension, age ≥75, diabetes mellitus, and prior history of CVA or TIA
  - Atrial fibrillation with a CHADS$_2$ score of 3 or 4 (calculation as above) *or history of prior embolism with lower score*
  - History of VTE within preceding 3 to 12 months
  - Non–high-risk thrombophilia (e.g., heterozygous factor V Leiden mutation)
  - History of recurrent VTE
  - Active malignancy
- ○ **Patients at *low risk for thromboembolism* are not felt to require bridging therapy.** Treatment with DVT prophylaxis doses of LMWH is an alternative. This group includes patients with:
  - Mechanical aortic valve (bileaflet) *without associated risk factors* (as outlined above)
  - Nonvalvular atrial fibrillation with a CHADS$_2$ score ≤2 *and no history of embolism*
  - Prior VTE >12 months prior (without history of recurrent VTE or known hypercoagulable state)
- • **Patients being treated with aspirin**
  - • Controversy exists over the use of aspirin in the perioperative period.
  - • There is, however, surprisingly little evidence on the effect of aspirin on perioperative outcomes in noncardiac surgery. Studies of bleeding risk have conflicted.
    - ○ One study in orthopedic surgery patients (*Lancet 2000;355:1295*) and another in a variety of surgeries (*Am J Surg 1982;143:215*) found increased bleeding risk.
    - ○ A study of patients undergoing unplanned surgeries found no clear increase in bleeding (*Surg Gynecol Obstet 1983;156:439*).
    - ○ However, some evidence suggests that withdrawal of aspirin in patients with CAD may be associated with an increased risk of cardiac events (*Int J*

Cardiol 2000;76:257), particularly in those who have undergone prior cardiac stent placement (*J Am Coll Cardiol 2005;45:456*).

- ○ There is more evidence as applies to aspirin use in coronary artery bypass surgery, where early use of aspirin appears to improve outcomes (*N Engl J Med 2002; 347:1309*).

- **Recommendations**
  - ○ An assessment of the patient's cardiac risk and the bleeding risk of the surgical procedure must be undertaken.
  - ○ For planned surgeries where increased bleeding could result in significant morbidity (e.g., neurosurgery) or when the risk of stopping the medication is minimal (e.g., primary prevention), aspirin will need to be held 7 or more days prior to surgery to allow the anticoagulant effect of aspirin to resolve through new platelet generation.
  - ○ For patients with substantial cardiac risk, continuation of aspirin through the perioperative period is recommended if feasible. Special conditions apply if an intracoronary stent is in place (see Revascularization above).
  - ○ Regardless, the period during which patients with substantial cardiac risk will be off of aspirin should be minimized. Typically, aspirin can be restarted on the first postoperative day so long as adequate hemostasis has been obtained.
- **Patients being treated with thienopyridine**
  - • *Clopidogrel* is the most commonly encountered thienopyridine. *Ticlopidine* is used far less frequently because of an increased incidence of adverse effects.
  - • The increased bleeding risk of thienopyridines with surgery is best described with coronary artery bypass surgery. In the CURE trial, a 50% increase in major bleeding was described in the group that received clopidogrel within 5 days of surgery (*N Engl J Med 2001;345:494*).
  - • In other settings data are limited and conflicting reports have been presented (*J Thromb Thrombolysis 2004;17:21*). Increased bleeding was described in patients undergoing transbronchial biopsy while being treated with clopidogrel (*Chest 2006; 129:734*).
  - • **Recommendations**
    - ○ In general, because of the perception of increased bleeding risk with thienopyridines, most advise stopping them perioperatively unless the patient has undergone prior coronary stent placement (*Arch Surg 2009;144:69*). Based on the CURE trial data, clopidogrel should be stopped at least 5 days prior to the planned surgery.
    - ○ For a discussion of the management of thienopyridine therapy in patients who have undergone coronary artery stent placement, please see Preoperative Cardiac Evaluation, section on Revascularization.
- **Nonsteroidal anti-inflammatory medications**
  - • Most NSAID therapy is noncritical and can be temporarily interrupted to mitigate the effect on perioperative bleeding risk.
  - • The duration of time required for the reversible effect on platelet inhibition to resolve varies with the half-life of the medication.
  - • **Recommendations**
    - ○ NSAIDs should be discontinued preoperatively in time to allow five half-lives of the medication to expire before surgery.
    - ○ For medications with short half-lives such as ibuprofen, this could be as little as 1 day (*Ann Intern Med 2005;142:506*).

PERIOPERATIVE MANAGEMENT OF SPECIFIC CONDITIONS

Hypertension

GENERAL PRINCIPLES

- Severe hypertension (BP > 180/110) preoperatively often results in wider fluctuations in intraoperative BP and has been associated with an increased rate of perioperative cardiac events (see Preoperative Cardiac Evaluation).
- Antihypertensive agents that the patients are taking prior to admission for surgery may have an impact on the perioperative period:
  - When the patient is receiving β-blockers or clonidine chronically, withdrawal of these medications may result in tachycardia and rebound hypertension, respectively.
  - Evidence suggests that holding angiotensin-converting enzyme inhibitors and angiotensin II receptor blockers on the day of surgery may reduce perioperative hypotension. This is believed to be due to the effect of this class of medication in blunting the compensatory activation of the renin–angiotensin system perioperatively.

TREATMENT

- Hypertension in the postoperative period is a common problem with multiple possible causes.
  - All *remediable causes of hypertension*, such as pain, agitation, hypercarbia, hypoxia, hypervolemia, and bladder distention, should be excluded or treated.
  - Poor control of essential hypertension secondary to discontinuation of medications the patient was previously taking, in the immediate postoperative period, is not uncommon. Reviewing the patient's home medication list is recommended.
  - A rare cause of perioperative hypertension is *pheochromocytoma*, particularly if its presence was unrecognized. Patients can develop an acute hypertensive crisis perioperatively. Treatment with **phentolamine** or **nitroprusside** is recommended in this situation. Preoperative treatment when the diagnosis is suspected to minimize this risk is recommended. This is classically accomplished by titration of **phenoxybenzamine** preoperatively.
- Many parenteral antihypertensive medications are available for patients who are unable to take medications orally. Transdermal clonidine is also an option, but the onset of action is delayed.

Pacemakers and Implantable Cardioverter Defibrillators (ICDs)

GENERAL PRINCIPLES

- The use of electrocautery intraoperatively can have adverse effects on the function of implanted cardiac devices.
- A variety of errors can occur from resetting of the device to inadvertent discharge of an ICD.

- Complications are rare, but are more likely with abdominal and thoracic surgeries.

DIAGNOSIS

- The type of device (i.e., pacemaker or ICD) and manufacturer should be determined.
- The initial indication for placement and the patient's underlying rhythm should be determined. Ideally, this can be determined from the history and an electrocardiogram.
- When the device was last formally interrogated should be ascertained.
- The device should be interrogated within 3 to 6 months of a significant surgical procedure.

TREATMENT

If the patient is pacemaker dependent, the device should be reprogrammed to an asynchronous mode (e.g., VOO, DOO) for the surgery.

- The application of a magnet will cause most pacemakers to revert to an asynchronous pacing mode, but if this is the planned management, it should be tested preoperatively, especially in the pacemaker-dependent patient.
- It should be noted that the effect of a magnet on ICDs is typically different than the effect on pacemakers, in that it affects the antitachycardia function but does not alter the pacing function of most models. If the pacing function of an ICD needs to be altered perioperatively, the device will need to be reprogrammed.
- The antitachycardia function of an ICD will typically need to be programmed off for surgical procedures where electrocautery may cause interference with device function, leading to the potential of unintentional discharge.
  - The effect of a magnet on this function is variable, so programming is the preferred management.
  - Continuous monitoring for arrhythmia during the period when this function is suspended is essential.
- Continuous ECG and pulse monitoring is recommended during surgery. Pulse monitoring should not be affected by electrocautery interference.
- Postoperative interrogation may be necessary, particularly if the device settings were changed perioperatively or if the patient is pacemaker dependent.
- *Consultation with an electrophysiologist is strongly recommended if there is any uncertainty regarding the perioperative management of a device.*

Pulmonary Disease and Preoperative Pulmonary Evaluation

GENERAL PRINCIPLES

Epidemiology

- Clinically significant postoperative *pulmonary complications are probably more common* than cardiac complications (*Am J Respir Crit Care Med 2005;171:514*), and the occurrence of one may increase the chance of the other occurring (*Am J Med 2003; 115:515*).

- Though definitions vary, clinically significant pulmonary complications generally include *pneumonia, respiratory failure, bronchospasm, atelectasis, and exacerbation* of underlying chronic lung disease.
- Postoperative respiratory failure can be a life-threatening complication, with a 30-day mortality rate as high as 26.5% (*J Am Coll Surg 2007;204:1188*).

Etiology

Both patient-dependent risk factors and surgery-specific risk factors combine to produce the level of risk. These are reviewed in detail in a 2006 guideline from the American College of Physicians (*Ann Intern Med 2006;144:575*).

Risk Factors

- **Procedure-related risk factors**
  - The **surgical site** is generally considered the greatest determinant of risk, with *upper abdominal* and *thoracic* surgeries imparting the greatest risk (*N Engl J Med 1999;340:937*). Surgical procedures not involving the torso can also impart increased risk of pulmonary complications. Examples include neurosurgery (*Ann Surg 2000;232:242*) and surgeries involving the mouth and palate (*J Am Coll Surg 2007;204:1188*).
  - The **surgery duration** also imparts risk, with prolonged procedures increasing the risk of pulmonary complications (*Arch Int Med 1992;152:967*).
  - The **type of anesthesia** utilized appears to affect pulmonary risk as well. Though somewhat controversial, it appears neuraxial anesthesia carries less risk of pneumonia (*BMJ 2000;321:1*) and respiratory failure (*Lancet 2002;359:1276*).
- **Patient-dependent risk factors**
  - **Chronic lung disease,** particularly COPD, has reliably been found to be a risk factor for postoperative pulmonary complications. Unsurprisingly, patients with progressively more severe disease appear to be at increased risk for more serious complications (*Chest 1993;104:1445*). However, even patients with advanced lung disease can safely undergo surgery if it is deemed necessary (*Br Med J 1975;3:670*). Thus, **there is no identified degree of COPD that precludes surgery.**
  - Data on non-COPD chronic lung disease are not well studied.
    - **Asthma** that is compensated does *not* appear to be a significant risk factor.
    - **Interstitial lung disease** likely places patients at higher risk, but it is not well studied in patients undergoing general surgery (*Chest 2007;132:1637*). Restriction associated with **obesity** does not appear to be a significant risk factor (*Ann Intern Med 2006;144:575*).
    - **Pulmonary hypertension** is associated with significant morbidity in patients undergoing surgery (*J Am Coll Cardiol 2005;45:1691*; *Br J Anaesth 2007;99:184*).
  - **Poor general health status** is associated with increased perioperative pulmonary risk. Multiple measures of general health status have been correlated with poor pulmonary outcomes.
  - **Advanced age** has also been identified as a predictor of postoperative pulmonary complications. The degree to which medical comorbidities confound this information is unclear, but multiple studies have found a significant association and it is included as a factor in risk prediction models, particularly age >60 years (*Ann Surg 2000;232:242*; *Ann Intern Med 2001;135:847*).

- **Smoking** is a risk factor for pulmonary complications. The degree of tobacco abuse correlates with the degree of risk (*Am J Respir Crit Care Med 2003;167:741*).
- **Obstructive sleep apnea** is increasingly being recognized as a risk factor for perioperative complications, both pulmonary and cardiac (*Chest 2008;133:1128*). The most frequent pulmonary complication appears to be hypoxemia (*Anesthesiology 2008;108:822*). Unrecognized sleep apnea may pose an even greater risk (*Mayo Clin Proc 2001;76:897*).

DIAGNOSIS

Clinical Presentation

History

- The preoperative pulmonary evaluation should focus on evaluating the presence of and severity of patient-dependent risk factors.
  - Any history of chronic lung disease should be detailed. An effort should be made to determine the patient's baseline and whether there has been any recent deterioration, such as increased cough or sputum production.
  - Any symptoms of a current upper respiratory infection should be ascertained. Though not an absolute contraindication to surgery, it seems prudent to postpone purely elective procedures until such infections have resolved.
  - A full smoking history should be obtained.
- As noted, comorbid conditions impact the likelihood of pulmonary complications. Therefore, a complete medical history is necessary.

Physical Examination

- A complete physical examination should be part of any preoperative evaluation.
- Attention should be paid to evidence of chronic lung disease such as increased anteroposterior (AP) dimensions of the chest and the presence of adventitious lung sounds, particularly wheezing.
- The maximum laryngeal height should be determined. A value of <4 cm has been associated with pulmonary complications. Persistent coughing after a voluntary cough is also an indicator of increased risk (*Am J Respir Crit Care Med 2003;167: 741*).

Diagnostic Criteria

- Unlike the situation for preoperative cardiac risk stratification, relatively few tools for quantifying preoperative pulmonary risk are available.
- In general, patients are deemed to be at an elevated risk of complications if they are undergoing high-risk procedures as noted above and have one or more of the identified patient-dependent risk factors. To what degree their risk is elevated remains, by and large, a subjective assessment. It does appear that the risk of increasing numbers of risk factors is additive, such that patients with multiple risk factors are at increasingly high levels of risk.
- Risk indices for predicting postoperative respiratory failure (*Ann Surg 2000;232:242*) and postoperative pneumonia (*Ann Intern Med 2001;135:847*) have been developed. Though somewhat cumbersome, these represent the best available objective risk prediction tools. The former was refined in a more recent study, but it remains somewhat unwieldy for routine clinical use (*J Am Coll Surg 2007;204: 1188*).

Diagnostic Testing

Laboratories

- **Pulmonary function tests (PFTs)**
  - The value of preoperative PFTs is unclear and controversial outside of lung resection surgery, where its role is better defined.
  - Though PFTs can clearly be used to define lung disease, in the setting of nonpulmonary surgery there is concern that they add little beyond what can be gathered clinically (*Chest 1997;111:1536*).
  - Firm recommendations for or against PFTs cannot be made.
  - However, in patients with unexplained pulmonary symptoms and patients with lung disease and an unclear baseline, PFTs should be considered.
- **Arterial blood gas (ABG) analysis**
  - It is unclear that ABG results add to the estimate of preoperative pulmonary risk beyond other clinically derived variables.
  - In general, an ABG is not an integral part of the preoperative pulmonary evaluation.
  - An ABG should be obtained *when otherwise clinically necessary*, such as to determine if a patient's lung disease is compensated.
- **Chest radiography**
  - The value of a routine chest radiograph is variable.
  - Many findings deemed abnormal are chronic and do not affect management (*Can J Anesth 2005;52:568*).
  - In general, a chest radiograph is recommended only if otherwise clinically indicated.
- **Serum albumin**
  - A decreased serum albumin level has been shown to be a strong predictor of increased pulmonary risk (*Ann Intern Med 2006;144:581*), though a more recent large study found a lesser risk than suggested previously (*J Am Coll Surg 2007;204: 1188*).
  - Though studies vary in definition, a level <3.5 mg/dL appears to be indicative of increased risk.
  - Despite the evidence identifying a decreased albumin level as a strong predictor of perioperative risk, there is at present no conclusive evidence that enteral or parenteral **nutritional supplementation** decreases risk (*Ann Intern Med 2006;144: 596*).

TREATMENT

- **Modifiable patient-related risk factors**
  - The effect of preoperative **smoking cessation** on pulmonary complications has been largely described in cardiothoracic surgeries, where a benefit to smoking cessation at least 2 months prior to surgery has been shown (*Mayo Clin Proc 1989;64:609*). The effect on a general surgical population is less clear, as most of the benefit of smoking cessation has been related to improvements in nonpulmonary outcomes such as fewer wound complications (*Ann Surg 2008;248:739*). Nevertheless, given the long-term benefits of smoking cessation, all patients should be counseled to stop smoking even if <8 weeks from surgery. Previous concerns about a paradoxical increase in complications appear unwarranted (*Chest 2005;127:1977*).
  - **COPD therapy** should be optimized. Symptoms should be aggressively treated preoperatively. Although not all patients with COPD respond to corticosteroid therapy, a preoperative course of **steroids** is reasonable for symptomatic patients

already receiving **maximal bronchodilator therapy** who are not at their best personal baseline level. Patients *with recent sputum changes* may benefit from a preoperative course of **antibiotics.**

- **Modifiable procedure-related risk factors**
  - Consideration of alternative procedures with the lowest possible pulmonary risk should be undertaken for high-risk patients.
  - **Laparoscopic procedures** may yield fewer pulmonary complications (*Br J Anaesth 1996;77:448*). Typically, though, the pulmonary benefits demonstrated with laparoscopic procedures have been in laboratory variables such as spirometry, and it is unclear if this will lead consistently to fewer clinical pulmonary complications.
  - Where possible, use of **neuraxial/regional** anesthetic methods may be preferable in higher-risk patients.
- **Postoperative interventions**
  - **Lung expansion maneuvers,** such as incentive spirometry or deep breathing exercises, should be employed. Intensive preoperative training has been shown to reduce pulmonary complications in patients undergoing coronary artery bypass (*JAMA 2006;296:1851*). Whether the same would be true in a general surgical population or with less intensive training is not clear. However, the intervention is benign and is probably helpful.
  - **Noninvasive positive pressure ventilation (NPPV)** is an option for both the prevention and treatment of postoperative respiratory failure. CPAP was shown in a recent review to decrease postoperative pulmonary complications in patients undergoing abdominal surgery (*Ann Surg 2008;247:617*) and in those undergoing thoracoabdominal aortic surgery (*Chest 2005;128:821*). For patients who do develop postoperative respiratory failure, there is evidence to suggest NPPV will improve pulmonary outcomes (*JAMA 2005;293:589*). The best studied of the NPPV modalities is CPAP, but other modalities have also been used (*Chest 2005;128:2688*). The optimal modality and delivery system is undefined. Because of the potential complications of its use, patients being treated with NPPV require intensive monitoring.
  - **Appropriate analgesia** is essential to prevent splinting, but oversedation needs to be carefully avoided. There is some evidence to suggest that epidural analgesia can reduce postoperative pulmonary complications relative to other regimens (*Arch Surg 2008;143:990*).
  - A strategy of **selective nasogastric tube placement** rather than routine use has also been shown to decrease the risk of pulmonary complications (*Cochrane Database Syst Rev 2007(3)*). Communication with the surgical team is important to determine if this is an appropriate consideration.
  - Appropriate **DVT prophylaxis** is strongly encouraged.

Anemia and Transfusion Issues in Surgery

GENERAL PRINCIPLES

- Blood products represent a finite and costly resource.
- Transfusion of blood products is associated with substantial risks including transmission of bloodborne infections, transfusion-related acute lung injury (TRALI), transfusion reactions, and immunosuppressive effects.

Epidemiology

Preoperatively, anemia is present in 5% to 76% of patients, with the wide variance related to the definition of anemia and type of surgery studied (*Am J Med 2004; 116(S):58S*). Regardless, it is a common clinical occurrence.

DIAGNOSIS

- Patients should be asked about a history of anemia or hematologic disease. Any history of a bleeding diathesis should be noted.
- Any clinical signs of anemia (e.g., pallor) or coagulopathy (e.g., petechiae) should be duly noted.
- Prior medical records and testing should be reviewed.
- In patients without findings from the initial evaluation to suggest a hematologic abnormality, the degree of testing is controversial.
  - For low-risk procedures, it is not clear that otherwise asymptomatic individuals require any preoperative testing, and there is no evidence that routine testing before low-risk procedures increases safety (*N Engl J Med 2000;342:168*).
  - For higher-risk procedures, particularly those with a more substantial bleeding risk, a baseline CBC and coagulation profile is typically obtained. If recent results are available, repeating the tests is likely unnecessary.
  - Further testing of patients found to have significant anemia or coagulopathy should be performed as clinically indicated.

TREATMENT

It is essential to remember that volume resuscitation and control of active bleeding is the initial therapy of anemia, particularly in the perioperative period when acute blood loss is a common occurrence.

- Anemia to a hemoglobin concentration of 5 gm/dL, which is reasonably well tolerated in euvolemic, otherwise healthy individuals under stable, experimental conditions (*Anesthesiology 2000;93:1004*).
- Data from patients who refused transfusion are consistent with this finding, as nearly all deaths attributed to anemia occurred at a hemoglobin concentration <5 gm/dL (*Transfusion 1994;34:396*).
- How this applies to patients undergoing surgery is less clear.
  - Preoperative hemoglobin levels <10 gm/dL are associated with an increase in morbidity/mortality risk. The risk increases steadily with decreasing hemoglobin levels, with a pronounced surge in risk at levels <6 gm/dL (*Lancet 1996;348:1055*).
  - Postoperatively, in a cohort of patients who refused transfusion, no mortality was observed until the hemoglobin decreased below 7 gm/dL. A marked increase in risk was seen as hemoglobin levels dropped below the 5 gm/dL threshold (*Transfusion 2002;42:812*).
  - As these were observational studies, the degree to which the anemia was a causative factor—rather than a marker of illness—cannot be determined.
  - Increased surgical blood loss, as evidenced by the degree of decrease in hemoglobin from the preoperative to the postoperative values, was noted to be associated with increased morbidity and mortality.

- The benefit of transfusion at physiologically tolerable levels of anemia is unclear.
  - A study of intensive care unit patients suggested that the classic transfusion threshold of a hemoglobin of 10 g/dL was too liberal, as patients treated with a more "restrictive" strategy (with a trigger of 7 g/dL) had outcomes that were at least equivalent and in some cases better (*N Engl J Med 1999;336:933*). The applicability of this study to the perioperative setting is uncertain, particularly as postcardiac surgery patients were excluded from the trial.
  - Other observational studies have suggested that transfusion may actually increase the risk of adverse outcomes (*Crit Care Med 2006;34:1608; J Surg Res 2002;102:237*).
- It is generally agreed that transfusion is not required when the hemoglobin exceeds 10 gm/dL. Likewise, it is generally agreed that a hemoglobin <6 gm/dL necessitates transfusion (*Anesthesiology 2006;105:198*).
- The best strategy for patients with hemoglobin between 6 and 10 gm/dL is unclear.
  - Markers of intolerance of anemia (e.g., tachycardia) should be considered.
  - Evidence of end-organ dysfunction (e.g., myocardial ischemia) should prompt transfusion.
  - Preoperatively, consideration of the expected blood loss with the planned surgery may alter the threshold for transfusion.
  - The presence of cardiovascular disease may influence the decision to transfuse:
    - Concomitant cardiovascular disease appears to increase the risk of perioperative mortality for any given level of anemia (*Lancet 1996;348:1055*).
    - Two studies have demonstrated an increase in myocardial ischemia with a hematocrit <28% (*Transfusion 1998;38:924; Crit Care Med 1993;21:860*), though analysis of critically ill patients with cardiovascular disease showed no significant increase in adverse outcomes with a transfusion threshold of a hemoglobin of 7 gm/dL (*Crit Care Med 2001;29:227*). It is difficult to establish the effect of volume status on these results, particularly in the patients with anemia postoperatively.
    - Thus, no firm recommendations can be made. It appears reasonable to **consider transfusion at a hemoglobin <9 gm/dL in this population,** though other groups have recommended tolerance of a lower hemoglobin, suggesting a threshold for transfusion of 8 gm/dL (*Br J Haematol 2001;113:24*).

Other Nonoperative Therapies

Measures to *reduce the need for allergenic blood* should be utilized where feasible.

- Preoperative **autologous blood donation** should be considered for elective procedures where the anticipated need for transfusion is high.
- **Preoperative erythropoietin** can be considered in patients with decreased hemoglobin concentration (*N Engl J Med 1997;336:933*). Patients need to have adequate iron stores when this is utilized; supplemental iron therapy may be required. There are also concerns about increased risk for deep venous thrombosis in patients treated with erythropoietin preoperatively that have been included in an FDA-mandated "black box" warning that limit its use in this setting (*Med Lett Drugs Ther 2007;49:37*).
- **Intraoperative measures** include *normovolemic hemodilution* for surgeries with high expected blood loss. This approach has the advantage of requiring minimal preoperative preparation (*Arch Pathol Lab Med 2007;1331:695*). *Intraoperative blood salvage and autotransfusion* and *positional blood pooling* are the other options.

- Avoidance of perioperative hypothermia may also limit blood loss and, thereby, decrease transfusion requirements (*Anesthesiology 2008;108:71*).

SPECIAL CONSIDERATIONS

Patients with **sickle cell anemia** should generally be transfused to a hemoglobin of 10 gm/dL preoperatively to decrease the incidence of complications.

Liver Disease

GENERAL PRINCIPLES

- Patients with hepatic dysfunction suffer from an increased risk of morbid outcomes when undergoing surgery.
- Patients with underlying liver disease are at substantial risk for acute hepatic decompensation postoperatively.
- The myriad systemic effects of liver dysfunction result in an increased frequency of other complications as well, such as bleeding and infection.

Classification

- The best validated measure of perioperative risk in patients *with cirrhosis* is the **Child–Pugh score,** reflecting increased risk with greater degrees of hepatic dysfunction.
  - A large review of patients undergoing a variety of surgical procedures clearly identified a demarcation between Child's class A (score <7) and those with more severe class B and C disease (*Anesthesiology 1999;90:42*).
    - 30-day mortality was 9.4% in the Child's class A group versus 16.7% in classes B and C (combined). Other complications were also significantly more common.
    - Interestingly, the type of cirrhosis appears to have an impact as well, as **patients with primary biliary cirrhosis and primary sclerosing cholangitis appear to tolerate surgery better.**
  - Other studies have shown further that patients with Child's class C disease have extremely high operative risk, with perioperative mortality exceeding 80% with abdominal surgery in this group (*Surgery 1997;122:730*).
- The MELD score may also be an indicator of postoperative mortality in cirrhotics. One study in cholecystectomy found a MELD score ≥8 to be a marker of increased risk relative to the Child–Pugh score (*Clin Gastroenterol Hepatol 2004;2:1123*). Other studies have found the Child–Pugh score to be superior, however (*Clin Gastroenterol Hepatol 2004;2:719*).

DIAGNOSIS

Clinical Presentation
History
- As part of the preoperative history and physical, evidence of liver disease should be sought.
- Historical details suggesting a risk for hepatic disease such as alcohol or drug abuse and prior blood transfusion should be sought.
- Other indicators of a risk for liver disease may be noted in the preoperative evaluation (e.g., family history of hemochromatosis).

Physical Examination

Physical examination evidence of liver dysfunction should be noted. Some should be obvious, such as icterus and abdominal distension with ascites, but other abnormalities such as spider nevi, palmar erythema, and testicular atrophy may be more subtle.

Diagnostic Testing

Laboratories

- Because of the low prevalence and because significant disease is usually clinically suspected, routine laboratory screening for hepatic dysfunction in patients presenting for surgery who are without clinically suspected or known liver disease is not recommended (*Med Clin N Am 2003;87:211*).
- Patients with known or suspected liver disease should undergo a thorough evaluation of liver function including **hepatic enzyme levels, albumin** and **bilirubin** measurements, and **evaluation for coagulopathy.**
- **Renal function,** including electrolytes, blood urea nitrogen (BUN), and creatinine measurements, should also be evaluated.

TREATMENT

- Patients with **acute viral or alcoholic hepatitis** tolerate surgery poorly, and *delaying surgery until recovery is recommended* if possible.
- Patients with **chronic hepatitis** without evidence of hepatic decompensation generally tolerate surgery well.
- Based on the high perioperative mortality rates in patients with **advanced cirrhosis,** nonoperative alternatives should be strongly considered.
- For patients who do require surgery, steps should be taken to optimize the preoperative status.
  - **Coagulopathy** should be corrected.
    - Vitamin K should be administered if the INR is elevated. As the coagulopathy may well be refractory to this measure in the setting of liver disease, fresh frozen plasma and cryoprecipitate may be required.
    - **Thrombocytopenia** is a common occurrence and should generally be corrected if severe. The general recommendation for most surgical procedures is a minimum platelet count of 50,000. However, in the setting of liver disease, the coexistence of platelet dysfunction should be considered, particularly if there is clinical bleeding with an otherwise adequate platelet count.
  - Renal and electrolyte abnormalities should be addressed.
    - Careful attention should be paid to **volume status.**
    - Nephrotoxic substances, such as NSAIDs and aminoglycosides, should be avoided.
    - Patients with cirrhosis often have **hypokalemia** and **alkalosis.** These conditions should be corrected preoperatively to minimize the risks of cardiac arrhythmias and to limit encephalopathy.
    - If **hyponatremia** occurs, free water restriction may be required.
  - **Ascites** should be treated.
    - Ascites has been found to be an independent risk factor for postoperative pulmonary complications (*J Am Coll Surg 2007;204:1188*).
    - If time permits, **diuretic therapy** should be instituted.
    - **Paracentesis** should be considered preoperatively if diuretics are ineffective or if time constraints prevent their use.

- **Encephalopathy** should be treated.
  - **Lactulose** titrated to two to three soft bowel movements per day should be started in patients with encephalopathy.
  - Protein restriction has been recommended for individuals who respond poorly to lactulose but should be done cautiously, because excessive restriction may actually contribute to malnutrition.
  - **Sedatives and other narcotics** can precipitate or worsen encephalopathy. They should be used only cautiously and dose reductions should be considered.
  - **Hypokalemia** should be avoided.
- Adequate **nutrition** should be provided.

Diabetes Mellitus

GENERAL PRINCIPLES

- Medical and surgical patients with hyperglycemia are at increased risk for poor outcomes (*J Clin Endocrinol Metab 2002;87:978*).
- Poor preoperative glucose control, as indicated by elevated hemoglobin A1c levels, is associated with an increased risk of surgical infections (*Arch Surg 2006;141:375*). Hyperglycemia postoperatively also appears to be associated with an increased risk of postoperative infection (*JPEN J Parenter Enteral Nutr 1998;22:77*).
- There is some suggestion, particularly in patients undergoing cardiothoracic surgery, that more aggressive medical management of hyperglycemia mitigates the risk of infection (*Ann Thor Surg 1997;63:356*) and possibly mortality (*J Thorac Cardiovasc Surg 2003;125:1007*).
- That hyperglycemia is a marker for poor outcomes appears to be relatively clear. However, whether aggressive management truly improves outcomes is uncertain. Trial results have been mixed.
  - In a population of mostly surgical patients requiring critical care, impressive reductions in mortality were demonstrated in a single institution study (*N Engl J Med 2001;345:1359*). The results of this trial prompted widespread adoption of aggressive insulin protocols in surgical ICUs.
  - However, a recent larger multicenter trial (NICE-SUGAR) of both surgical and medical critical care patients was unable to show improvements in outcome and actually found a slight increase in risk with aggressive treatment of hyperglycemia (*N Engl J Med 2009;360:1283*).
- Diabetics are at increased risk for cardiovascular disease. Appropriate risk stratification for cardiac complications of surgery is vital to the perioperative evaluation of these patients.

Classification

- Establishing the etiology of hyperglycemia has important implications for subsequent patient care.
  - **Stress hyperglycemia** can occur in the perioperative setting because of the body's response to surgery with the release of counterregulatory hormones and cytokines that impede glucose metabolism. These patients need adequate glucose control during the perioperative period, but are unlikely to require such treatment later.
  - Type 2 diabetes is notoriously underdiagnosed, however, and the notation of perioperative hyperglycemia may be the first indication of its presence.
- It is also essential to distinguish between type 1 and type 2 diabetes mellitus.

- **Type 1 diabetics** will require a continuous supply of insulin regardless of glucose level and oral intake.
- The insulin requirement, if any, of **type 2 diabetics** during the perioperative period will vary.

DIAGNOSIS

Diagnostic Testing
Laboratories
- Most patients should have a **hemoglobin A1c** obtained.
  - This can assist in differentiating perioperative stress hyperglycemia from undiagnosed diabetes.
  - Knowledge of recent glycemic control in known diabetics is also helpful in determining what therapy is required.
- Evaluating **renal function** is also recommended given the increased prevalence of renal disease in diabetics.
- Cardiovascular risk stratification may require other evaluations (see Preoperative Cardiovascular Evaluation).

TREATMENT

- Elective surgery in patients with uncontrolled diabetes mellitus should preferably be scheduled after acceptable glycemic control has been achieved.
- If possible, the operation should be scheduled for early morning to minimize prolonged fasting.
- Frequent monitoring of blood glucose levels is required in all situations.
- **Type 1 diabetes**
  - Some form of basal insulin is required at all times.
  - On the evening prior to surgery, the regularly scheduled basal insulin should be continued. If taken in the morning, it is still recommended to give the regularly scheduled basal insulin without dose adjustment (*Diabetes Care 2004;27:553*). However, patients who are very tightly controlled may be at increased risk for hypoglycemia and will need to be monitored closely. A decrease in the last preoperative basal insulin dose may be considered in this circumstance.
  - Glucose infusions (e.g., D5-containing fluids) can be administered to avoid hypoglycemia while the patient is NPO and until tolerance of oral intake postoperatively is established.
  - For complex procedures and procedures requiring a prolonged NPO status, a continuous insulin infusion will likely be necessary.
  - *Caution should be exercised with the use of subcutaneous insulin* in the intraoperative and critical care settings, as alterations in tissue perfusion may result in variable absorption.
- **Type 2 diabetes**
  - Treatment of type 2 diabetics varies according to their preoperative requirements and the complexity of the planned procedure (*Med Clin N Am 2003;87:175*).
  - Consideration should be given to the efficacy of the patients' current regimen. If they are not well controlled at baseline, then an escalation in therapy may be required.
    - **Diet-controlled type 2 diabetes**
      - This can generally be managed without insulin therapy.

- Glucose values should be checked regularly and elevated levels (>180 mg/dL) can be treated with intermittent doses of short-acting insulin.
○ **Type 2 diabetes managed with oral therapy**
  - **Short-acting sulfonylureas** and **other oral agents** should be withheld on the operative day.
  - **Metformin** and **long-acting sulfonylureas** (e.g., chlorpropamide) should be withheld 1 day before planned surgical procedures. Metformin is generally held for 48 hours postoperatively. Renal function should be normal prior to resuming treatment. Other oral agents can be resumed when patients are tolerating their preprocedure diet.
  - Most patients can be managed without an insulin infusion.
  - Glucose values should be checked regularly and elevated levels (>180 mg/dL) can be treated with intermittent doses of short-acting insulin.
○ **Type 2 diabetes managed with insulin**
  - If it is anticipated the patient will be able to eat postoperatively, basal insulin is still given on the morning of surgery.
  - If given as long-acting insulin (e.g., glargine insulin) and the patient usually takes the dose in the morning, 50% to 100% of the usual dose can be given.
  - If the patient utilizes intermediate-acting insulin (e.g., NPH), one-half to two-thirds of the usual morning dose is given to avoid periprocedural hyperglycemia.
  - Dextrose-containing IV fluids may be required to avoid hypoglycemia.
  - Patients undergoing major procedures will typically require an insulin drip perioperatively.
  - The usual insulin treatment can be reintroduced once oral intake is established postoperatively.
- **Target glucose levels**
  - There are no generally agreed-upon target glucose levels applicable to the entire postsurgical population.
    ○ Previous recommendations for aggressive glucose control in the critical care setting (*Diabetes Care 2008;31S:S12*) were published prior to the aforementioned NICE-SUGAR trial.
    ○ In a general medical–surgical population, recurring glucose values >200 mg/dL were associated with a poor outcome (*J Clin Endocrinol Metab 2002;87:978*).
  - Pending further research, a goal of maintaining glucose levels <180 mg/d in the postoperative setting seems reasonable. It should be noted that this may still require intensive treatments such as insulin infusion.
  - In patients treated with sliding scale insulin, it is essential to monitor the response to therapy. Patients who are hyperglycemic consistently are unlikely to have adequate glucose control with intermittent treatment alone, and a basal/bolus regimen should be introduced if hyperglycemia is persistent (*Diabetes Care 2007;30: 2181*).

Adrenal Insufficiency and Corticosteroid Management

GENERAL PRINCIPLES

- Surgery is a potent activator of the hypothalamic–pituitary axis, and patients with adrenal insufficiency may lack the ability to respond appropriately to surgical stress.

- Patients receiving corticosteroids as medical therapy for indications other than adrenal dysfunction may develop adrenal insufficiency. Case reports of presumed adrenal insufficiency from the 1950s led to the widespread use of perioperative "stress-dose" steroids in this population (*J Am Med Assoc 1952;149:1542*; *Ann Intern Med 1953;39:116*).

Pathophysiology

- The subtype of adrenal insufficiency has implications on management.
  - **Tertiary adrenal insufficiency** due to exogenous corticosteroid administration is the most common adrenal problem encountered. These patients should have intact mineralocorticoid function and therefore, if treated, should require only glucocorticoid supplementation (*N Engl J Med 2003;348:727*).
  - Likewise, **secondary adrenal insufficiency** should not result in mineralocorticoid deficiency. The possibility of deficits in other hormones due to pituitary disease should be considered.
  - **Primary adrenal insufficiency** requires replacement of both mineralocorticoids and glucocorticoids.
- The dose and duration of exogenous corticosteroids required to produce clinically significant tertiary adrenal insufficiency is highly variable, but general principles can be outlined (*Med Clin N Am 2003;87:175*).
  - Daily therapy with **5 mg or less of prednisone** (or its equivalent), **alternate-day corticosteroid therapy,** and **any dose given for** <3 weeks *should not result in clinically significant adrenal suppression.*
  - Patients receiving >**20 mg/d of prednisone (or equivalent) for** >**3 weeks** and patients who are clinically "**cushingoid" in appearance** can be expected to have *significant suppression of adrenal responsiveness.*
  - The function of the hypothalamic–pituitary axis *cannot be readily predicted* in **patients receiving doses of prednisone 5 to 20 mg for** >**3 weeks.**

DIAGNOSIS

Clinical Presentation

History
- The dose and duration of prior corticosteroid therapy should be clarified.
- The coexistence of diseases that suggest the possibility of primary adrenal insufficiency should be sought (e.g., autoimmune thyroid disease, malignant tumors that metastasize to the adrenal such as lung cancer, etc.).

Physical Examination
Physical exam findings suggestive of adrenal hypofunction such as hyperpigmentation should be noted. As above, inspection for features of a "cushingoid" appearance should be performed.

Diagnostic Testing

Laboratories
- For patients in whom clinical prediction of adrenal function is difficult, a **cosyn-tropin stimulation test** can be performed to determine adrenal responsiveness.

- **Electrolyte abnormalities** should be sought in patients with *primary adrenal insufficiency*. Patients with *other forms of adrenal insufficiency are unlikely to manifest the classic hyperkalemia and hyponatremia* due to intact mineralocorticoid function.

TREATMENT

- **Patients expected to have an intact adrenal function** (as outlined above) should take their regularly scheduled dose of corticosteroid. No further treatment is required.
- Whether patients should otherwise be treated depends on the type of adrenal insufficiency encountered and the anticipated surgical stress.
  - For **patients with primary disease of the hypothalamic–pituitary–adrenal (HPA) axis,** adrenal supplementation is generally recommended. These recommendations are based on extrapolation from small studies in the literature, expert opinion, and clinical experience (*JAMA 2002;287:236*).
    - **Minor surgical stress** (e.g., colonoscopy, cataract surgery): Administer 25 mg hydrocortisone or 5 mg methylprednisolone IV on the day of the procedure only.
    - **Moderate surgical stress** (e.g., cholecystectomy, hemicolectomy): Administer 50 to 75 mg hydrocortisone or 10 to 15 mg methylprednisolone IV on the day of the procedure and taper quickly over 1 to 2 days to the usual dose.
    - **Major surgical stress** (e.g., major cardiothoracic surgery, Whipple procedure): Administer 100 to 150 mg hydrocortisone or 20 to 30 mg methylprednisolone IV on the day of the procedure and taper to the usual dose over the next 1 to 2 days.
    - **Critically ill patients undergoing emergent surgery** (e.g., sepsis, hypotension): Administer 50 to 100 mg hydrocortisone IV every 6 to 8 hours or 0.18 mg/kg/hr as a continuous infusion plus 50 mg/d of fludrocortisone until the shock has resolved. Then gradually taper the dose, monitoring vital signs and serum sodium closely.
    - Additional **mineralocorticoid supplementation** for patients with primary adrenal insufficiency may or may not be necessary, depending on the dose and mineralocorticoid potency of the corticosteroid given.
  - For patients with adrenal insufficiency due to exogenous steroid administration, the necessity of further treatment is controversial.
    - Two trials of glucocorticoid supplementation in patients receiving exogenous steroids undergoing surgery found no evidence of adrenal crisis when the patients' baseline steroid dose was continued (*Surgery 1997;121:123*; *J Clin Periodontol 1999;26:577*).
    - Several other observational studies examined perioperative cessation of all steroids in this population and found clinical adrenal insufficiency to be a very rare occurrence even then (*Arch Surg 2008;143:1222*). Patients who did develop clinical symptoms of adrenal insufficiency all responded to treatment with supplemental steroids.
    - Based on this evidence, *continuation of the patients' baseline steroid dose without additional steroid treatment* is a reasonable treatment strategy. Patients should be monitored closely for signs/symptoms of adrenal insufficiency.
    - Some still recommend supplemental steroid therapy in this population. If this management strategy is pursued, treatment as outlined above for patients with primary disease of the HPA axis is reasonable.

Chronic Renal Insufficiency and End-Stage Renal Disease

GENERAL PRINCIPLES

- **Chronic renal insufficiency (CRI)** is an independent risk factor for **perioperative cardiac complications,** so all patients with renal disease need appropriate cardiac risk stratification (*JAMA 2001;285:1865*).
- **Patients with end-stage renal disease (ESRD)** have a substantial mortality risk when undergoing surgery (*Arch Intern Med 1994;154:1674*).
- Most general anesthetic agents have no appreciable nephrotoxicity or effect on renal function other than that mediated through hemodynamic changes (*Anesthesiol Clin 2006;24:523*).

TREATMENT

- **Volume status**
  - Every effort should be made to **achieve euvolemia** preoperatively to reduce the incidence of volume-related complications intra- and postoperatively (*Med Clin N Am 2003;87:193*).
  - Though this typically entails removing volume, some patients may be hypovolemic and require hydration.
  - Patients with CRI not receiving hemodialysis may require treatment with loop diuretics.
  - Patients being treated with **hemodialysis** should undergo dialysis preoperatively.
    - This is commonly performed on the day prior to surgery.
    - Hemodialysis can be performed on the day of surgery as well, but the possibility that transient electrolyte abnormalities and hemodynamic changes postdialysis can occur should be considered.
- **Electrolyte abnormalities**
  - **Hyperkalemia** in the preoperative setting should be treated, particularly as tissue breakdown associated with surgery may elevate the potassium level further postoperatively.
    - For patients on dialysis, preoperative dialysis should be utilized.
    - For patients with CRI not undergoing dialysis, alternative methods of potassium excretion will be necessary.
      - **Loop diuretics** can be utilized, particularly if the patient is also hypervolemic.
      - **Sodium polystyrene sulfonate (SPS) resins** can also be utilized. The possibility that *intestinal necrosis* with SPS resins occurs more frequently in the perioperative setting has been suggested (*Am J Kidney Dis 1992;20:159*).
  - Although chronic **metabolic acidosis** has not been associated with elevated perioperative risk, some local anesthetics have reduced efficacy in acidotic patients. Preoperative metabolic acidosis should be corrected with sodium bicarbonate infusions or dialysis.
- **Bleeding diathesis**
  - **Platelet dysfunction** has long been associated with uremia.
    - The value of a preoperative bleeding time in predicting postoperative bleeding has been questioned (*Blood 1991;77:2547*). A preoperative bleeding time is, therefore, not recommended.

○ Patients who evidence perioperative bleeding should, however, be treated.
  - **Dialysis** for patients with ESRD will improve platelet function.
  - **Desmopressin** (0.3 μg/kg IV or intranasally) can be utilized.
  - **Cryoprecipitate,** 10 U over 30 minutes IV, is an additional option.
  - In patients with coexisting anemia, **red blood cell transfusions** can improve uremic bleeding.
  - For patients **with a history of prior uremic bleeding,** preoperative desmopressin or **conjugated estrogens** (0.5 mg/kg/d IV for 5 days) should be considered.
- **Heparin** given with dialysis can increase bleeding risk. *Heparin-free dialysis* should be discussed with the patient's nephrologist when surgery is planned.

Acute Renal Failure

GENERAL PRINCIPLES

Surgery has been associated with an increased risk of **acute renal failure (ARF)** (*Med Clin N Am 2003;87:193*).

- Patients with **CRI** are at increased risk of ARF.
- ARF among patients with normal preoperative renal function is a relatively rare event, but is associated with increased mortality when it occurs (*Anesthesiology 2007;107:892*).

DIAGNOSIS

- The approach to ARF in the perioperative setting is not substantially different from that in the nonoperative setting.
- However, certain additional factors have to be considered when evaluating the cause in the perioperative setting:
  - **Intraoperative hemodynamic changes,** particularly hypotension, should be considered.
    ○ Intraoperative factors associated with ARF postoperatively include vasopressor use and diuretic use (*Anesthesiology 2007;107:892*).
    ○ A careful review of the operative record is advised.
  - Certain procedures can have an adverse effect on the renal function (e.g., aortic clamping procedures). Therefore, careful attention to the details of the procedure is necessary.
  - The possibility that bleeding is responsible for a prerenal state deserves special attention.

TREATMENT

For a detailed discussion regarding the management of acute renal failure, please refer to Chapter 10, Renal Diseases.

2

Nutrition Support
Dominic Reeds

Nutrient Requirements

GENERAL PRINCIPLES

- **Energy**
  - **Total daily energy expenditure** (TEE) is composed of resting energy expenditure (normally ~70% of TEE), the thermic effect of food (normally ~10% of TEE), and energy expenditure of physical activity (normally ~20% of TEE).
  - **Malnutrition** and **hypocaloric feeding** decrease resting energy expenditure to values 15% to 20% below those expected for actual body size, whereas metabolic stressors, such as inflammatory diseases or trauma, often increase energy requirements (usually by <50% of pre-illness values).
  - It is impossible to determine **daily energy requirements** precisely with predictive equations because of the complexity of factors that affect metabolic rate. Judicious use of predictive equations can provide a reasonable estimate that should be modified as needed based on the patient's clinical course.
  - The **Harris–Benedict equation** provides a reasonable estimate of resting energy expenditure (in kcal/d) in healthy adults. The equation takes into account the effect of body size and lean tissue mass (which is influenced by gender and age) on energy requirements and can be used to estimate total daily energy needs in hospitalized patients:

$$\text{Men} = 66 + (13.7 \times W) + (5 \times H) - (6.8 \times A)$$
$$\text{Women} = 665 + (9.6 \times W) + (1.8 \times H) - (4.7 \times A)$$

  where W is the weight in kg, H the height in cm, and A is the age in years.
  - Energy requirements per kilogram of body weight are inversely related to body mass index (BMI) (Table 1). The lower range within each category should be considered in insulin-resistant, critically ill patients unless they are depleted in body fat.
  - **Ideal body weight** can be estimated based on height. For men, 106 lb is allotted for the first 5 ft, then 6 lb is added for each inch above 5 ft; for women, 100 lb is given for the first 5 ft, with 5 lb added for each additional inch.
- **Protein**
  - Protein intake of 0.8 g/kg/d meets the requirements of 97% of the adult population.
  - Protein requirements are affected by several factors, such as the amount of nonprotein calories provided, overall energy requirements, protein quality, and the patient's nutritional status. Protein requirements increase as nonprotein caloric intake declines and patients who are being permissively underfed should receive up to 2 g per kilogram of ideal body weight per day to minimize loss of lean body mass.
  - Inadequate amounts of any of the essential amino acids result in inefficient utilization.

Table 1	Estimated Energy Requirements for Hospitalized Patients Based on Body Mass Index
BMI (kg/m²)	Energy Requirements (kcal/kg/d)
15	35–40
15–19	30–35
20–24	20–25
25–29	15–20
≥30	<15

Note: These values are recommended for critically ill patients and all obese patients; add 20% of total calories in estimating energy requirements in non–critically ill patients.

- Illness increases the efflux of amino acids from skeletal muscle; however, increasing protein intake to >1.2 g/kg/d of prehospitalization body weight in critically ill patients may not reduce the impact of illness on loss of lean body mass (*Crit Care Med 1998;26(9):1529*).
- Table 2 gives approximate protein requirements during different clinical conditions.
- **Essential fatty acids**
  - The liver can synthesize most fatty acids, but humans lack the desaturase enzyme needed to produce the n-3 and n-6 fatty acid series. Therefore, linoleic acid should constitute at least 2% and linolenic acid at least 0.5% of the daily caloric intake to prevent the occurrence of essential fatty acid deficiency.
  - The plasma pattern of increased triene-to-tetraene ratio (>0.4) can be used to detect essential fatty acid deficiency.
  - Patients who are unable to receive intravenous (IV) or oral lipid solutions may receive a daily topical application of 1 tbsp of safflower oil to provide essential fatty acids.
- **Carbohydrates**
  - Certain tissues, such as bone marrow, erythrocytes, leukocytes, renal medulla, eye tissues, and peripheral nerves, cannot metabolize fatty acids and require glucose (~40 g/d) as a fuel. Other tissues such as the brain prefer glucose (~120 g/d).

Table 2	Recommended Daily Protein Intake
Clinical Condition	Protein Requirements (g/kg IBW/d)[a]
Normal	0.8
Metabolic "stress" (illness/injury)	1.0–1.5
Acute renal failure (undialyzed)	0.8–1.0
Hemodialysis	1.2–1.4
Peritoneal dialysis	1.3–1.5

IBW, ideal body weight.
[a] Additional protein intake may be needed to compensate for excess protein loss in specific patient populations such as those with burn injury, open wounds, and protein-losing enteropathy or nephropathy. Lower protein intake may be necessary in patients with chronic renal insufficiency who are not treated by dialysis and certain patients with hepatic encephalopathy.

- **Major minerals**
  Major minerals are important for ionic equilibrium, water balance, and normal cell function. The following are the daily recommended intakes (enteral and parenteral values, respectively):
  - Sodium, 0.5 to 5.0 g and 60 to 150 mEq
  - Potassium, 2 to 5 g and 60 to 100 mEq
  - Magnesium, 300 to 400 mg and 8 to 24 mEq
  - Calcium, 800 to 1,200 mg and 5 to 15 mEq
  - Phosphorus, 800 to 1,200 mg and 12 to 24 mEq
- **Micronutrients (trace elements and vitamins)**
  Trace elements and vitamins are essential constituents of enzyme complexes. The recommended dietary intake for trace elements, fat-soluble vitamins, and water-soluble vitamins (Table 3) is set at two standard deviations above the estimated mean so that it will cover the needs of 97% of the healthy population. See Table 3 for specific micronutrient deficiency symptoms.

SPECIAL CONSIDERATIONS

- Both the amount and location of prior gut resection influences nutrient needs. Patients with an inadequate length of functional small bowel ($<\sim$150 cm) either from resection or medical disease require additional vitamins and minerals if they are not receiving parenteral nutrition. Table 4 provides guidelines for supplementation in these patients.
- Distal ileum resection can cause rapid development of B_{12} deficiency.
- Proximal gut resection (stomach or duodenum) can result in iron, calcium, and copper deficiency.
- Patients with excessive gastrointestinal (GI) tract losses require additional fluids and electrolytes. An assessment of fluid losses due to diarrhea, ostomy output, and fistula volume should be made to help determine fluid requirements. Knowledge of fluid losses is also useful in calculating intestinal mineral losses by multiplying the volume of fluid loss by an estimate of intestinal fluid electrolyte concentration (Table 5).

Assessment of Nutritional Status

GENERAL PRINCIPLES

- Patients should be assessed for protein-energy malnutrition as well as specific nutrient deficiencies.
- A thorough history and physical exam combined with appropriate laboratory studies is the best approach to evaluate nutritional status.

DIAGNOSIS

Clinical Presentation

History

- Assess for changes in diet pattern (size, number, and content of meals). If present, the reason for altered food intake should be investigated.

Table 3	Trace Mineral, Fat-Soluble Vitamin, and Water-Soluble Vitamin Requirements and Assessment of Deficiency			
Nutrient	Recommended Daily Enteral Intake in Normal Adults	Recommended Daily Parenteral Intake in Normal Adults	Symptoms or Signs of Deficiency	Laboratory Evaluation
Chromium	30–200 mcg	10–20 mcg	Glucose intolerance, peripheral neuropathy, encephalopathy	Serum chromium
Copper	2 mg	0.3 mg	Anemia, neutropenia, osteoporosis, diarrhea	Serum copper, plasma ceruloplasmin
Iodine	150 mcg	70–140 mcg	Hypothyroidism, goiter	Urine iodine, thyroid-stimulating hormone
Iron	10–15 mg	1.0–1.5 mg	Microcytic hypochromic anemia	Serum iron and total iron-binding capacity, serum ferritin
Manganese	1.5 mg	0.2–0.8 mg	Hypercholesterolemia, dementia, dermatitis	Serum manganese
Selenium	50–200 mcg	20–40 mcg	Cardiomyopathy, muscle weakness	Serum selenium, blood glutathione peroxidase activity
Zinc	15 mg	2.5–4.0 mg	Growth retardation, delayed sexual maturation, hypogonadism, alopecia, acro-orificial skin lesion, diarrhea, mental status changes	Plasma zinc
Vitamin K (phylloquinone)	50–100 mcg	100 mcg	Easy bruising/bleeding	Prothrombin time

Vitamin			Deficiency symptoms	Laboratory test
Vitamin A (retinol)	5,000 International Units	3,300 International Units	Night blindness, Bitot's spots, keratomalacia, follicular hyperkeratosis, xerosis	Serum retinol
Vitamin D (ergocalciferol)	400 International Units	200 International Units	Rickets, osteomalacia, osteoporosis, bone pain, muscle weakness, tetany	Serum 25-hydoxy-vitamin D
Vitamin E (α-tocopherol)	10–15 International Units	10 International Units	Hemolysis, retinopathy, neuropathy, abnormal clotting	Serum tocopherol: total lipid (triglyceride and cholesterol) ratio
Vitamin B_1 (thiamine)	1.0–1.5 mg	3 mg	Beriberi; cardiac failure, Wernicke's encephalopathy, peripheral neuropathy, fatigue, ophthalmoplegia	RBC transketolase activity
Vitamin B_2 (riboflavin)	1.1–1.8 mg	3.6 mg	Cheilosis, sore tongue and mouth, eye irritation, seborrheic dermatitis	RBC glutathione reductase activity
Vitamin B_3 (niacin)	12–20 mg	40 mg	Pellagra (dermatitis, diarrhea, dementia), sore mouth and tongue	Urinary N-methyl-nicotinamide
Vitamin B_5 (pantothenic acid)	5–10 mg	10 mg	Fatigue, weakness, paresthesias, tenderness of heels and feet	Urinary pantothenic acid
Vitamin B_6 (pyridoxine)	12 mg	4 mg	Seborrheic dermatitis, cheilosis, glossitis, peripheral neuritis, convulsions, hypochromic anemia	Plasma pyridoxal phosphate

(continued)

Table 3 Trace Mineral, Fat-Soluble Vitamin, and Water-Soluble Vitamin Requirements and Assessment of Deficiency (*Continued*)

Nutrient	Recommended Daily Enteral Intake in Normal Adults	Recommended Daily Parenteral Intake in Normal Adults	Symptoms or Signs of Deficiency	Laboratory Evaluation
Vitamin B$_7$ (biotin)	100–200 mcg	60 mcg	Seborrheic dermatitis, alopecia, mental status change, seizures, myalgia, hyperesthesia	Plasma biotin
Vitamin B$_9$ (folic acid)	400 mcg	400 mcg	Megaloblastic anemia, glossitis, diarrhea	Serum folic acid, RBC folic acid
Vitamin B$_{12}$ (cobalamin)	5 mcg	5 mcg	Megaloblastic anemia, paresthesias, decreased vibratory or position sense, ataxia, mental status changes, diarrhea	Serum cobalamin, serum methylmalonic acid
Vitamin C (ascorbic acid)	100 mg	100 mg	Scurvy, petechia, purpura, gingival inflammation, and bleeding, weakness, depression	Plasma ascorbic acid, leukocyte ascorbic acid

Table 4	Guidelines for Vitamin and Mineral Supplementation in Patients with Severe Malabsorption	
Supplement	Dose	Route
Prenatal multivitamin with minerals[a]	1 tablet daily	PO
Vitamin D[a]	50,000 units two to three times per week	PO
Calcium[a]	500 mg elemental calcium tid–qid	PO
Vitamin B_{12}[b]	1 mg daily	PO
	100–500 mcg q1–2 mo	SC
Vitamin A[b]	10,000–50,000 units daily	PO
Vitamin K[b]	5 mg/d	PO
	5–10 mg/wk	SC
Vitamin E[b]	30 units/d	PO
Magnesium gluconate[b]	108–169 mg elemental magnesium qid	PO
Magnesium sulfate[b]	290 mg elemental magnesium one to three times per week	IM/IV
Zinc gluconate or zinc sulfate[b]	25 mg elemental zinc daily plus 100 mg elemental zinc per liter intestinal output	PO
Ferrous sulfate[b]	60 mg elemental iron tid	PO
Iron dextran[b]	Daily dose based on formula or table	IV

[a]Recommended routinely for all patients.
[b]Recommended for patients with documented nutrient deficiency or malabsorption.

- Unintentional weight loss of >10% body weight in the last 6 months is associated with a poor clinical outcome (*Am J Med 1980;69:491*).
- Look for evidence of **malabsorption** (diarrhea, weight loss).
- For symptoms of specific **nutrient deficiencies,** see Table 3.
- Consider factors that may increase metabolic stress (infection, inflammatory disease, malignancy, etc.).
- Assess patient's functional status (e.g., bedridden, suboptimally active, very active).

Table 5	Electrolyte Concentrations in Gastrointestinal Fluids			
Location	Na (mEq/L)	K (mEq/L)	Cl (mEq/L)	HCO_3 (mEq/L)
Stomach	65	10	100	—
Bile	150	4	100	35
Pancreas	150	7	80	75
Duodenum	90	15	90	15
Mid–small bowel	140	6	100	20
Terminal ileum	140	8	60	70
Rectum	40	90	15	30

Physical Examination
- Patients can be classified by BMI as underweight (<18.5 kg/m^2), normal weight (18.5 to 24.9 kg/m^2), overweight (25.0 to 29.9 kg/m^2), class I obesity (30.0 to 34.9 kg/m^2), class II obesity (35.0 to 39.9 kg/m^2), or class III obesity ($\geq$40.0 kg/m^2) (*Obes Res 1998;6(Suppl 2):S53*).
- Patients who are **extremely underweight** (BMI < 14 kg/m^2) or those **with rapid, severe weight loss** (even with supranormal BMI) have a high risk of death and should be considered for admission to the hospital for nutritional support.
- Look for **tissue depletion** (loss of body fat and skeletal muscle wasting).
- Assess **muscle function** (strength testing of individual muscle groups).
- **Fluid status:** Evaluate patients for dehydration (hypotension, tachycardia, mucosal xerosis, etc.) or excess body fluid (edema or ascites).
- Evaluate patient for sources of protein or nutrient losses: large wounds, burns, nephrotic syndrome, surgical drains, etc. Quantify the volume of drainage and the concentration of fat and protein content.

Diagnostic Testing
Laboratories
- Perform laboratory studies to determine specific nutrient deficiencies only when clinically indicated, as the plasma concentration of many nutrients may not reflect true body stores (Table 3).
- Plasma albumin and prealbumin concentration should not be used to assess patients for protein-calorie malnutrition or to monitor the adequacy of nutrition support. While levels of these plasma proteins correlate with clinical outcome, inflammation and injury can alter their synthesis and degradation, consequently limiting their utility in nutritional assessment (*Crit Care Med 1982;10:305*; *Gastroenterology 1990; 99:1845*).
- Most hospitalized patients are vitamin D deficient and caregivers should have a low threshold for checking plasma 25-OH vitamin D levels (*N Engl J Med 1998: 338:777*).

Enteral Nutrition

GENERAL PRINCIPLES

Whenever possible, **oral/enteral** feeding is preferred to parenteral **feeding** because it limits mucosal atrophy, maintains immunoglobulin A (IgA) secretion, and prevents cholelithiasis. Additionally, oral/enteral feeds are less expensive than parenteral nutrition.

- **Types of feedings**
  - **Hospital diets** include a regular diet and those modified in either nutrient content (amount of fiber, fat, protein, or sodium) or consistency (liquid, puréed, soft). There are ways that food intake can often be increased:
    - Encourage patients to eat.
    - Provide assistance at mealtime.
    - Allow some food to be supplied by relatives and friends.
    - Limit missed meals for medical tests and procedures.

- ○ Avoid unpalatable diets. Milk-based formulas (e.g., Carnation Instant Breakfast) contain milk as a source of protein and fat and tend to be more palatable than other defined formula diets.
  - ○ Use of calorically dense supplements, for example, Ensure or Boost.
- **Defined liquid formulas**
  - **Polymeric formulas** are appropriate for most patients. They contain nitrogen in the form of whole proteins and include blenderized food, milk-based, and lactose-free formulas. Lactose-free formulas (e.g., Osmolite, Ensure) are the most commonly used polymeric formulas in hospitalized patients. These formulas are available as standard iso-osmolar solutions, containing approximately 1 kcal/mL, 16% calories as protein, 55% calories as carbohydrate, and 30% calories as fat. Other formulas are available with modified nutritional content including high-nitrogen, high-calorie, fiber-enriched, and low-potassium/phosphorus/magnesium formulas.
  - **Semielemental (oligomeric) formulas** (e.g., Propeptide, Peptamen) contain hydrolyzed protein in the form of small peptides and free amino acids. While these formulas may have benefit in the patients who have exocrine pancreatic insufficiency or short gut, pancreatic enzyme replacement is a less-expensive, equally effective intervention in most of these patients.
  - **Elemental monomeric formulas** (e.g., Vivonex, Glutasorb) contain nitrogen in the form of free amino acids and small amounts of fat (<5% of total calories) and are hyperosmolar (550 to 650 mOsm/kg). These formulas are not palatable and require either tube feeding or mixing with other foods or flavorings for oral ingestion. Free amino acids are poorly absorbed, and as a result, absorption of monomeric formulas is not clinically superior to that of oligomeric or polymeric formulas in patients with adequate pancreatic digestive function. These formulas may exacerbate osmotic diarrhea in patients with short gut.
  - **Oral rehydration solutions** stimulate sodium and water absorption by taking advantage of the sodium–glucose cotransporter present in the brush border of intestinal epithelium. Oral rehydration therapy can be useful in patients with severe GI fluid and mineral losses, such as those with short bowel syndrome (*Clin Ther 1990;12(Suppl A):129*). In these patients, it is particularly important that the sodium concentration of the solution be between 90 and 120 mEq/L to avoid intestinal sodium secretion and negative sodium and water balance. The characteristics of several oral rehydration solutions are listed in Table 6.
- **Tube feeding**
  - Tube feeding is useful in patients who have a **functional GI tract** but who cannot or will not ingest adequate nutrients.
  - The type of tube feeding approach selected (nasogastric, nasoduodenal, nasojejunal, gastrostomy, jejunostomy, pharyngostomy, and esophagostomy tubes) depends on physician experience, clinical prognosis, gut patency and motility, risk of aspirating gastric contents, patient preference, and anticipated duration of feeding.
  - Short-term (<6 weeks) tube feeding can be achieved by placement of a soft, small-bore nasogastric or nasoenteric feeding tube. Tube feeding can be used to supplement oral intake. Although nasogastric feeding is usually the most appropriate route, orogastric feeding in patients with nasal injury or gross nasal deformity and nasoduodenal or nasojejunal feeding in those with gastroparesis can also be used. Nasoduodenal and nasojejunal feeding tubes can be placed at the bedside with a success rate approaching 90% when inserted by experienced personnel (*Nutr Clin Pract 2001;16:258*).

Table 6	Characteristics of Selected Oral Rehydration Solutions						
Product	Na (mEq/L)	K (mEq/L)	Cl (mEq/L)	Citrate (mEq/L)	kcal/L	CHO (g/L)	mOsm
Equalyte	78	22	68	30	100	25	305
CeraLyte 70	70	20	98	30	165	40	235
CeraLyte 90	90	20	98	30	165	40	260
Pedialyte	45	20	35	30	100	20	300
Rehydralyte	74	19	64	30	100	25	305
Gatorade	20	3	NA	NA	210	45	330
WHO[a]	90	20	80	30	80	20	200
WashingtonUniversity[b]	105	0	100	10	85	20	250

Note: Mix formulas with sugar-free flavorings as needed for palatability.
NA, not applicable; WHO, World Health Organization.
[a]WHO formula: Mix $^3/_4$ tsp sodium chloride, $^1/_2$ tsp sodium citrate, $^1/_4$ tsp potassium chloride, and 4 tsp glucose (dextrose) in 1 L ($4^1/_4$ cups) distilled water.
[b]Washington University formula: Mix $^3/_4$ tsp sodium chloride, $^1/_2$ tsp sodium citrate, and 3 tbsp + 1 tsp Polycose powder in 1 L ($4^1/_4$ cups) distilled water.

- Long-term (>6 weeks) tube feeding usually requires a gastrostomy or jejunostomy tube that can be placed endoscopically, radiologically, or surgically, depending on the clinical situation and local expertise.
  - **Percutaneous gastrostomy and jejunostomy** can be performed using endoscopic or fluoroscopic techniques.
  - **Surgical gastrostomy and jejunostomy** can be performed by open and laparoscopic techniques and are particularly useful when endoscopic and radiologic approaches are technically not possible.
- **Feeding schedules:** Patients who have feeding tubes in the stomach can often tolerate intermittent bolus or gravity feedings, in which the total amount of daily formula is divided into four to six equal portions.
- **Bolus feedings** are given by syringe as rapidly as tolerated.
- **Gravity feedings** are infused over 30 to 60 minutes.
- The patient's upper body should be elevated by 30 to 45 degrees during feeding and for at least 2 hours afterwards. Tubes should be flushed with water after each feeding. Intermittent feedings are useful for patients who cannot be positioned with continuous head-of-the-bed elevation or who require greater freedom from feeding. Patients who experience nausea and early satiety with bolus gravity feedings may require continuous infusion at a slower rate.
- **Continuous feeding** can often be started at 20 to 30 mL/hr and advanced by 10 mL/hr every 6 hours until the feeding goal is reached. Patients who have gastroparesis often tolerate gastric tube feedings when they are started at a slow rate (e.g., 10 mL/hr) and advanced by small increments (e.g., 10 mL/hr every 8 to 12 hours). Patients with severe gastroparesis may require passage of the feeding tube tip past the ligament of Treitz. **Continuous feeding should always be used when feeding directly into the duodenum or jejunum to avoid distention, abdominal pain, and dumping syndrome.**
- **Jejunal feeding** may be possible in closely monitored patients with mild to moderate **acute pancreatitis** (*J Am Coll Nutrition 1995;14(6):662*).

- **Contraindications:** The intestinal tract cannot be used effectively in some patients due to:
  - Persistent nausea or vomiting
  - Intolerable postprandial abdominal pain or diarrhea
  - Mechanical obstruction or severe hypomotility
  - Severe malabsorption
  - Presence of high-output fistulas

COMPLICATIONS

- **Mechanical complications**
  - **Nasogastric feeding tube misplacement** occurs more commonly in unconscious patients. Intubation of the tracheobronchial tree has been reported in up to 15% of patients. Intracranial placement can occur in patients with skull fractures.
  - **Erosive tissue damage** can lead to nasopharyngeal erosions, pharyngitis, sinusitis, otitis media, pneumothorax, and GI tract perforation.
  - **Tube occlusion** is often caused by inspissated feedings or pulverized medications given through small-diameter (<No. 10 French) tubes. Frequent flushing of the tube with 30 to 60 mL of water and avoiding administration of pill fragments or "thick" medications help to prevent occlusion. Techniques used to unclog tubes include the use of a small-volume syringe (10 mL) to flush warm water or pancreatic enzymes (Viokase dissolved in water) through the tube.
- **Hyperglycemia**
  - Achieving tight control of blood glucose (<110 mg/dL) in critically ill patients may improve outcomes; however, it increases the risk of hypoglycemia (*N Engl J Med 2001;345:1359*).
  - Subcutaneously administered insulin can usually maintain good glycemic control. IV insulin drip protocols may be used to control blood glucose in critically ill patients with anasarca or hemodynamic instability to ensure adequate insulin absorption.
  - Intermediate-duration insulin (e.g., NPH) can often be used safely once tube feedings reach 1,000 kcal/d. Long-duration insulin (e.g., detemir, glargine) should be used with caution in critically ill patients because changes in clinical status may affect pharmacokinetics and increase the risk of sustained hypoglycemia.
  - Patients who are receiving bolus feeds should receive short-acting insulin at the time of the feed.
  - Patients who are being given continuous (24 hours a day) feeding should receive intermediate- or long-duration insulin every 12 to 24 hours when clinically stable.
- **Pulmonary aspiration**
  - The etiology of **pulmonary aspiration** can be difficult to determine in tube-fed patients because aspiration can occur from refluxed tube feedings or oropharyngeal secretions that are unrelated to feedings.
  - Addition of food coloring to tube feeds **should not be used** for the diagnosis of aspiration. This method is insensitive for diagnosis, and several case reports suggest that food coloring can be absorbed by the GI tract in critically ill patients, which can lead to serious complications and death (*N Engl J Med 2000;343:1047*).
  - Gastric residuals are poorly predictive of aspiration risk.
  - Prevention of reflux: Decrease gastric acid secretion with pharmacologic therapy (H2 blocker, PPI), elevate head of bed during feeds, and avoid gastric feeding in

high-risk patients (e.g., those with gastroparesis, frequent vomiting, gastric outlet obstruction).

- **GI complications**
  - Nausea, vomiting, and abdominal pain are common.
  - **Diarrhea** is often associated with antibiotic therapy (*JPEN 1991;15:27*) and the use of liquid medications that contain nonabsorbable carbohydrates, such as sorbitol (*Am J Med 1990;88:91*). If diarrhea from tube feeding persists after proper evaluation of possible causes, a trial of antidiarrheal agents or fiber is justified. Diarrhea is common in patients who receive tube feeding and occurs in up to 50% of critically ill patients.
  - Diarrhea in patients with short gut, who do not have other causes such as *Clostridium difficile* infection, may be minimized by use of small, frequent meals that do not contain concentrated sweets (e.g., soda). Intestinal transit time should be maximized to allow nutrient absorption using tincture of opium, loperamide, or diphenoxylate. Low-dose clonidine (0.025 to 0.05 mg orally twice a day) may be used to reduce diarrhea in hemodynamically stable patients with short bowel syndrome (*JPEN 2004;28(4):265*).
  - **Intestinal ischemia/necrosis** has been reported in patients receiving tube feeding. These cases have occurred predominantly in critically ill patients receiving vasopressors for blood pressure support in conjunction with enteral feeding. There are no reliable clinical signs for diagnosis, and the mortality rate is high. **Caution should be used when enterally feeding critically ill patients requiring pressors.**

Parenteral Nutrition

GENERAL PRINCIPLES

- Patients who are unable to consume "adequate" nutrients for a "prolonged" period of time by oral or enteral routes require parenteral nutritional therapy to prevent the adverse effects of malnutrition.
- The decision to use parenteral nutrition can be difficult because the precise definition of "adequate" and "prolonged" is not clear and depends on the patient's body fat, lean tissue mass, preexisting medical illnesses, and level of metabolic stress.
- In general, parenteral nutrition should be considered if energy intake has been or is anticipated to be inadequate (<50% of daily requirements) for more than 7 to 10 days and enteral feeding is not feasible. The efficacy of this approach has not been tested in clinical trials.
- Routine use of immediate postoperative total parenteral nutrition (TPN) does not appear to improve outcomes in unselected patients (*Ann Surg 1993;217(2):185*).
- **Recommendations**
  - **Central parenteral nutrition (CPN)**
    - The infusion of hyperosmolar (usually >1,500 mOsm/L) nutrient solutions requires a large-bore, high-flow vessel to minimize vessel irritation and damage.
    - Percutaneous subclavian vein **catheterization** with advancement of the catheter tip to the junction of the superior vena cava and right atrium is the most commonly used technique for CPN access. The internal jugular, saphenous, and femoral veins are also used, although less desirable due to decreased patient

comfort and difficulty in maintaining sterility. Catheters that are tunneled under the skin prior to entering the vascular tree are preferred in patients who are likely to receive >8 weeks of TPN to reduce the risk of mechanical failure.

o Peripherally inserted central venous catheters (which reduce the risk of pneumothorax) are increasingly used to provide CPN in patients with adequate antecubital vein access. These catheters are not suitable for patients in whom CPN is anticipated to be necessary for an extended duration (>6 months).

- **CPN macronutrient solutions**
  o Crystalline **amino acid solutions** containing 40% to 50% essential and 50% to 60% nonessential amino acids (usually with little or no glutamine, glutamate, aspartate, asparagine, tyrosine, and cysteine) are used to provide protein needs (Table 2). Infused amino acids are oxidized and should be included in the estimate of energy provided as part of the parenteral formulation.
  o Some amino acid solutions have been modified for specific disease states such as those enriched in branched-chain amino acids for use in patients who have hepatic encephalopathy and solutions that contain mostly essential amino acids for use in patients with renal insufficiency.
  o **Glucose** (dextrose) in IV solutions is hydrated; each gram of dextrose monohydrate provides 3.4 kcal. While there is no absolute requirement for glucose in most patients, providing >150 g glucose per day maximizes protein balance.
  o **Lipid emulsions** are available as a 10% (1.1 kcal/mL) or 20% (2.0 kcal/mL) solution and provide energy as well as a source of essential fatty acids. Emulsion particles are similar in size and structure to chylomicrons and are metabolized like nascent chylomicrons after acquiring apoproteins from contact with circulating endogenous high-density lipoprotein particles. Lipid emulsions are as effective as glucose in conserving body nitrogen economy once absolute tissue requirements for glucose are met. The optimal percentage of calories that should be infused as fat is not known, but 20% to 30% of total calories is reasonable for most patients. The rate of infusion should not exceed 1.0 kcal/kg/hr (0.11 g/kg/hr) because most complications associated with lipid infusions have been reported when providing more than this amount (*Curr Opin Gastroenterol 1991;7:306*). A rate of 0.03 to 0.05 g/kg/hr is adequate for most patients who are receiving continuous CPN. Lipid emulsions should not be given to patients who have triglyceride concentrations of >400 mg/dL. Moreover, patients at risk for hypertriglyceridemia should have serum triglyceride concentrations checked at least once during lipid emulsion infusion to ensure adequate clearance. Underfeeding obese patients by the amount of lipid calories that would normally be given (e.g., 20% to 30% of calories) facilitates mobilization of endogenous fat stores for fuel and may improve insulin sensitivity. IV lipids should still be administered twice per week to these patients to provide essential fatty acids.

COMPLICATIONS

- **Mechanical complications**
  - Complications at time of line placement include pneumothorax, air embolism, arterial puncture, hemothorax, and brachial plexus injury.
  - Thrombosis and pulmonary embolus: Radiologically evident subclavian vein thrombosis occurs commonly; however, clinical manifestations (upper extremity

edema, superior vena cava syndrome) are rare. Fatal microvascular pulmonary emboli can be caused by nonvisible precipitate in parenteral nutrition solutions. Inline filters should be used with all solutions to minimize the risk of these emboli.

- **Metabolic complications:** Usually caused by overzealous or inadequate nutrient administration:
  - Fluid overload
  - Hypertriglyceridemia
  - Hypercalcemia
  - Specific nutrient deficiencies. Consider providing supplemental **thiamine** (100 mg for 3 to 5 days) during initiation of CPN in patients with risk for thiamine deficiency (e.g., alcoholism).
  - Hypoglycemia
  - **Hyperglycemia** should be avoided because it is associated with an increased risk of infection. Blood glucose goals for closely monitored intensive care unit (ICU) patients are ideally 80 to 120 mg/dL. Management of patients with hyperglycemia or type 2 diabetes (*Mayo Clin Proc 1996;71:587*) can be performed in the following way:
    ○ If blood glucose is >200 mg/dL, consider obtaining better control of blood glucose before starting CPN.
    ○ If CPN is started, (a) limit dextrose to <200 g/d, (b) add 0.1 units of regular insulin for each gram of dextrose in CPN solution (e.g., 15 units for 150 g), (c) discontinue other sources of IV dextrose, and (d) order routine, regular insulin with blood glucose monitoring by fingerstick every 4 to 6 hours or IV regular insulin infusion with blood glucose monitoring by fingerstick every 1 to 2 hours.
    ○ In outpatients who use insulin, an estimate of the reduction in blood sugar that will be caused by the administration of 1 unit of insulin may be calculated by dividing 1,500 by the total daily insulin dose (e.g., for a patient receiving 50 units of insulin as an outpatient, 1 unit of insulin may be predicted to reduce plasma glucose concentration by 1,500/50 = 30 mg/dL).
    ○ If blood glucose remains >200 mg/dL and the patient has been requiring SC insulin, add 50% of the supplemental short-acting insulin given in the last 24 hours to the next day's CPN solution and double the amount of SC insulin sliding-scale dose for blood glucose values >200 mg/dL.
    ○ The insulin-to-dextrose ratio in the CPN formulation should be maintained while the CPN dextrose content is changed.
- **Infectious complications**
  - Catheter-related sepsis is the most common life-threatening complication in patients who receive CPN and is most commonly caused by skin flora: *Staphylococcus epidermidis* and *Staphylococcus aureus*.
  - In **immunocompromised patients** and those with long-term (>2 weeks) CPN, *Enterococcus*, *Candida* species, *Escherichia coli*, *Pseudomonas*, *Klebsiella*, *Enterobacter*, *Acinetobacter*, *Proteus*, and *Xanthomonas* should be considered.
  - The principles of **evaluation and management** of suspected catheter-related infection are outlined in the Infectious Disease section.
  - Although antibiotics are often infused through the central line, the **antibiotic lock technique** has been used successfully to treat and prevent central catheter-related infections (*Nutrition 1998;14:466*; *Antimicrob Agents Chemother*

1999;43:2200). This technique involves local delivery of antibiotics in the catheter without systemic administration.

- **Hepatobiliary complications.** Although these abnormalities are usually benign and transient, more serious and progressive disease may develop in a small subset of patients, usually after 16 weeks of CPN therapy or in those with short bowel (*Diseases of the Liver. 7th ed. Philadelphia: JB Lippincott, 1993:1505*).
  - Biochemical: Elevated aminotransferases and alkaline phosphatase are commonly seen.
  - Histologic alterations: Steatosis, steatohepatitis, lipidosis, phospholipidosis, cholestasis, fibrosis, and cirrhosis have all been seen.
  - Biliary complications usually occur in patients who receive CPN for >3 weeks.
    - Acalculous cholecystitis
    - Gallbladder sludge
    - Cholelithiasis
    - Routine efforts to prevent hepatobiliary complications in all patients receiving long-term CPN include providing a portion (20% to 40%) of calories as fat, cycling CPN so that the glucose infusion is stopped for at least 8 to 10 hours per day, encouraging enteral intake to stimulate gallbladder contraction and maintain mucosal integrity, avoiding excessive calories, and preventing hyperglycemia.
    - If abnormal liver biochemistries or other evidence of liver damage occurs, evaluation for other possible causes of liver disease should be performed.
    - If mild hepatobiliary complications are noted parenteral nutrition does not need to be discontinued, but the same principles used in preventing hepatic complications can be applied therapeutically.
    - When cholestasis is present, copper and manganese should be deleted from the CPN formula to prevent accumulation in the liver and basal ganglia. A 4-week trial of metronidazole or ursodeoxycholic acid has been reported to be helpful in some patients.

- **Metabolic bone disease**
  - Metabolic bone disease has been observed in patients receiving long-term (>3 months) CPN.
  - Patients may be asymptomatic. Clinical manifestations include bone fractures and pain (*Annu Rev Nutr 1991;11:93*). Demineralization may be seen in radiologic studies. Osteopenia, osteomalacia, or both may be present.
  - The precise causes of metabolic bone disease are not known, but several mechanisms have been proposed, including aluminum toxicity, vitamin D toxicity, and negative calcium balance.
  - Several therapeutic options should be considered in patients who have evidence of bone abnormalities.
  - Remove vitamin D from the CPN formulation if the parathyroid hormone and 1,25-hydroxy vitamin D levels are low.
  - Reduce protein to <1.5 g/kg/d because amino acids cause hypercalciuria.
  - Maintain normal magnesium status because magnesium is necessary for normal parathormone action and renal conservation of calcium.
  - Provide oral calcium supplements of 1 to 2 g/d.
  - Consider bisphosphonate therapy to decrease bone resorption.

- **Peripheral parenteral nutrition**
  - Peripheral parenteral nutrition is often considered to have limited usefulness because of the high risk of thrombophlebitis.

- Appropriate adjustments in the management of peripheral parenteral nutrition can increase the life of a single infusion site to >10 days. The following guidelines are recommended:
  - Provide at least 50% of total energy as a lipid emulsion piggybacked with the dextrose–amino acid solution.
  - Add 500 to 1,000 U heparin and 5 mg hydrocortisone per liter (to decrease phlebitis).
  - Place a fine-bore 22- or 23-gauge polyvinylpyrrolidone-coated polyurethane catheter in as large a vein as possible in the proximal forearm using sterile technique.
  - Place a 5-mg glycerol trinitrate ointment patch (or 1/4 in. of 2% nitroglycerin ointment) over the infusion site.
  - Infuse the solution with a volumetric pump.
  - Keep the total infused volume <3,500 mL/d.
  - Filter the solution with an inline 1.2-m filter (*Nutrition 1994;10:49*).
- **Long-term home parenteral nutrition**
  - Long-term home parenteral nutrition is usually given through a **tunneled catheter** or an implantable subcutaneous port inserted in the subclavian vein.
  - **Nutrient formulations** can be infused overnight to permit daytime activities in patients who are able to tolerate the fluid load. IV lipids may not be necessary in patients who are able to ingest and absorb adequate amounts of fat.
- **Monitoring nutrition support**
  - Adjustment of the nutrient formulation is often needed as medical therapy or clinical status changes.
  - When nutrition support is initiated, other sources of **glucose** (e.g., peripheral IV dextrose infusions) should be stopped and the volume of other IV fluids adjusted to account for CPN.
  - Vital signs should be checked every 8 hours.
  - In certain patients, body weight, fluid intake, and fluid output should be followed daily.
  - Serum electrolytes (including phosphorus) should be measured every 1 or 2 days after CPN is started until values are stable and then rechecked weekly.
  - Serum glucose should be checked up to every 4 to 6 hours by fingerstick until blood glucose concentrations are stable and then rechecked weekly.
  - If lipid emulsions are being given, **serum triglycerides** should be measured during lipid infusion in patients at risk for hypertriglyceridemia to demonstrate adequate clearance (triglyceride concentrations should be <400 mg/dL).
  - Careful attention to the catheter and catheter site can help to prevent **catheter-related infections.**
    - Gauze dressings should be changed every 48 to 72 hours or when contaminated or wet, but transparent dressings can be changed weekly.
    - Tubing that connects the parenteral solutions with the catheter should be changed every 24 hours.
    - A 0.22-μm filter should be inserted between the IV tubing and the catheter when **lipid-free CPN** is infused and should be changed with the tubing.
    - A 1.2-μm filter should be used when a total nutrient admixture containing a **lipid emulsion** is infused.
    - When a **single-lumen** catheter is used to deliver CPN, the catheter should not be used to infuse other solutions or medications (with the exception of compatible antibiotics) and it should not be used to monitor central venous pressure.

○ When a **triple-lumen** catheter is used, the distal port should be reserved solely for the administration of CPN.

Refeeding the Severely Malnourished Patient

COMPLICATIONS

Initiating nutritional therapy in patients who are severely malnourished and have had minimal nutrient intake can have adverse clinical consequences and precipitate the refeeding syndrome.

- **Hypophosphatemia, hypokalemia, and hypomagnesemia:** Rapid and marked decreases in these electrolytes occur during initial refeeding because of insulin-stimulated increases in cellular mineral uptake from extracellular fluid. For example, plasma phosphorus concentration can fall below 1 mg/dL and cause death within hours of initiating nutritional therapy if adequate phosphate is not given (*Am J Clin Nutr 1981;34:393*).
- **Fluid overload** and **congestive heart failure** are associated with decreased cardiac function and insulin-induced increased sodium and water reabsorption in conjunction with nutritional therapy containing water, glucose, and sodium. Renal mass may be reduced, limiting the ability to excrete salt or water loads.
- **Cardiac arrhythmias:** Patients who are severely malnourished often have bradycardia. Sudden death from ventricular tachyarrhythmias can occur during the first week of refeeding in severely malnourished patients and may be associated with a prolonged QT interval (*Ann Intern Med 1985;102:49*) or plasma electrolyte abnormalities. Patients with EKG changes should be monitored on telemetry, possibly in an ICU.
- **Glucose intolerance:** Starvation causes insulin resistance such that refeeding with high-carbohydrate meals or large amounts of parenteral glucose can cause marked elevations in blood glucose concentration, glucosuria, dehydration, and hyperosmolar coma. In addition, carbohydrate refeeding in patients who are depleted in thiamine can precipitate Wernicke's encephalopathy.
- **Recommendations**
- Careful **evaluation** of cardiovascular function and plasma electrolytes (history, physical examination, electrocardiogram, and blood tests) and correction of abnormal plasma electrolytes are **important before initiation of feeding.**
- Refeeding by the oral or enteral route involves the frequent or continuous administration of small amounts of food or an isotonic liquid formula.
- Parenteral supplementation or complete parenteral nutrition may be necessary if the intestine cannot tolerate feeding.
- During initial refeeding, fluid intake should be limited to approximately 800 mL/d plus insensible losses. Adjustments in fluid and sodium intake are needed in patients who have evidence of fluid overload or dehydration.
- Changes in body weight provide a useful guide for evaluating the efficacy of fluid administration. Weight gain greater than 0.25 kg/d or 1.5 kg/wk probably represents fluid accumulation in excess of tissue repletion. Initially approximately 15 kcal/kg, containing approximately 100 g carbohydrate and 1.5 g protein per kilogram of actual body weight, should be given daily.
- The rate at which the caloric intake can be increased depends on the severity of the malnutrition and the tolerance to feeding. In general, increases of 2 to 4 kcal/kg every 24 to 48 hours are appropriate.

- Sodium should be restricted to approximately 60 mEq or 1.5 g/d, but liberal amounts of phosphorus, potassium, and magnesium should be given to patients who have normal renal function.
- All other nutrients should be given in amounts needed to meet the recommended dietary intake (Table 3).
- Body weight, fluid intake, urine output, plasma glucose, and electrolyte values should be **monitored daily** during early refeeding (first 3 to 7 days) so that nutritional therapy can be appropriately modified when necessary.

Preventative Cardiology and Ischemic Heart Disease

Angela L. Brown, Anne C. Goldberg, Katherine E. Henderson, Kory Lavine, Andrew Kates, and Neville F. Mistry

Hypertension

GENERAL PRINCIPLES

Definition

Hypertension is defined as the presence of a blood pressure (BP) elevation to a level that places patients at increased risk for target organ damage in several vascular beds including the retina, brain, heart, kidneys, and large conduit arteries (Table 1).

Classification

- **Normal BP** is defined as systolic blood pressure (SBP) < 120 mm Hg and diastolic blood pressure (DBP) < 80 mm Hg; pharmacologic intervention is not indicated.
- **Prehypertension** is defined as SBP 120 to 139 mm Hg or DBP 80 to 89 mm Hg. These patients should engage in comprehensive lifestyle modifications to delay progression or prevent the development of hypertension. Pharmacologic therapy should be initiated in prehypertensive patients with evidence of target organ damage or diabetes.
- **In stage 1** (SBP 140 to 159 mm Hg or DBP 90 to 99 mm Hg) **and stage 2** (SBP > 160 mm Hg or DBP > 100 mm Hg) **hypertension,** pharmacologic therapy should be initiated in addition to lifestyle modification to lower BP below 140/90 mm Hg in patients without diabetes or chronic kidney disease. In patients with diabetes or chronic kidney disease, BP should be lowered below 130/80 mm Hg. Patients with BP levels more than 20/10 mm Hg above their treatment target will often require more than one medication to achieve adequate control. Patients with an average BP of 200/120 mm Hg or greater require immediate therapy and, if symptomatic end-organ damage is present, hospitalization.
- **Hypertensive crisis** includes hypertensive emergencies and urgencies. It usually develops in patients with a previous history of elevated BP but may arise in those who were previously normotensive. The severity of a hypertensive crisis correlates not only with the absolute level of BP elevation, but also with the rapidity of development, because autoregulatory mechanisms have not had sufficient time to adapt.
- **Hypertensive urgencies** are defined as a substantial increase in BP, usually with a DBP >120 mm Hg, and occur in approximately 1% of hypertensive patients. Hypertensive urgencies (i.e., upper levels of stage 2 hypertension, hypertension with optic disk edema, progressive end-organ complications rather than damage, and severe perioperative hypertension) warrant BP reduction within several hours (*JAMA 2003;289:2560–2572*).

Table 1	Manifestations of Target Organ Disease
Organ System	**Manifestations**
Large vessels	Aneurysmal dilation
	Accelerated atherosclerosis
	Aortic dissection
Cardiac	
Acute	Pulmonary edema, myocardial infarction
Chronic	Clinical or ECG evidence of CAD; LVH by ECG or echocardiogram
Cerebrovascular	
Acute	Intracerebral bleeding, coma, seizures, mental status changes, TIA, stroke
Chronic	TIA, stroke
Renal	
Acute	Hematuria, azotemia
Chronic	Serum creatinine > 1.5 mg/dL, proteinuria > 1+ on dipstick
Retinopathy	
Acute	Papilledema, hemorrhages
Chronic	Hemorrhages, exudates, arterial nicking

CAD, coronary artery disease; ECG, electrocardiogram; LVH, left ventricular hypertrophy; TIA, transient ischemic attack.

- **Hypertensive emergencies** include **accelerated hypertension,** typically defined as an SBP > 210 mm Hg and DBP > 130 mm Hg presenting with headaches, blurred vision, or focal neurologic symptoms, and **malignant hypertension** (which requires the presence of papilledema). Hypertensive emergencies require immediate BP reduction by 20% to 25% to prevent or minimize end-organ damage (i.e., hypertensive encephalopathy, intracranial hemorrhage, unstable angina [UA] pectoris, acute myocardial infarction [MI], acute left ventricular failure with pulmonary edema, dissecting aortic aneurysm, progressive renal failure, or eclampsia).
- **Isolated systolic hypertension,** defined as an SBP > 140 mm Hg and normal DBP, occurs frequently in the elderly (beginning after the fifth decade and increasing with age). Nonpharmacologic therapy should be initiated with medications added as needed to lower SBP to <140 mm Hg. Patient tolerance of antihypertensive therapy should be assessed frequently.

Epidemiology

- The public health burden of hypertension is enormous, affecting an estimated 60.5 million Americans adults (*Wong ND. Arch Intern Med 2007;167:2431–2436*). Indeed, for nonhypertensive individuals aged 55 to 65 years of age, the lifetime risk of developing hypertension is 90% (*Vasan RS, et al. JAMA 2002;287:1003–1010*).
- Data derived from the Framingham study have shown that hypertensive patients have a fourfold increase in cerebrovascular accidents, as well as a sixfold increase in congestive heart failure (CHF) when compared to normotensive control subjects.
- Disease-associated morbidity and mortality, including atherosclerotic cardiovascular disease, stroke, heart failure (HF), and renal insufficiency, increase with higher levels of SBP and DBP.

- Over the past three decades, aggressive treatment of hypertension has resulted in a substantial decrease in death rates from stroke and coronary heart disease. Unfortunately, rates of end-stage renal disease and hospitalization for CHF have continued to increase. BP control rates remain poor with only 34% of treated hypertensive patients below their goal BP level (*Ong KL, et al. HTN 2007;49:69–75*).

Etiology

Of all hypertensive patients, more than 90% have primary or essential hypertension; the remainder have secondary hypertension due to causes such as renal parenchymal disease, renovascular disease, pheochromocytoma, Cushing's syndrome, primary hyperaldosteronism, coarctation of the aorta, obstructive sleep apnea, and uncommon autosomal dominant or autosomal recessive diseases of the adrenal–renal axis that result in salt retention.

Risk Factors

BP rises with age. Other contributing factors include overweight/obesity, increased dietary sodium intake, decreased physical activity, increased alcohol consumption, and lower dietary intake of fruits, vegetables, and potassium.

Prevention

Prevention should be focused on risk factor modification. Strategies must address cultural and social barriers related to health care delivery and behavioral modification.

DIAGNOSIS

Clinical Presentation

- BP elevation is usually discovered in asymptomatic individuals during routine health visits.
- Optimal detection and evaluation of hypertension requires accurate noninvasive BP measurement, which should be obtained in a seated patient with the arm resting level with the heart. A calibrated, appropriately fitting BP cuff (inflatable bladder encircling at least 80% of the arm) should be used because falsely high readings can be obtained if the cuff is too small.
- Two readings should be taken, separated by 2 minutes. SBP should be noted with the appearance of Korotkoff sounds (phase I) and DBP with the disappearance of sounds (phase V).
- In certain patients, the Korotkoff sounds do not disappear but are present to 0 mm Hg. In this case, the initial muffling of Korotkoff sounds (phase IV) should be taken as the DBP. One should be careful to avoid reporting spuriously low BP readings due to an auscultatory gap, which is caused by the disappearance and reappearance of Korotkoff sounds in hypertensive patients and may account for up to a 25-mm Hg gap between true and measured SBP. Hypertension should be confirmed in both arms, and the higher reading should be used.

History

- The history should seek to discover secondary causes of hypertension and note the presence of medications that can affect BP (e.g., decongestants, oral contraceptives, appetite suppressants, nonsteroidal anti-inflammatory agents, exogenous

thyroid hormone, recent alcohol consumption, caffeine anabolic steroids, and illicit stimulants such as cocaine).
- A diagnosis of secondary hypertension should be considered in the following situations:
  - Age at onset younger than 30 or older than 60 years
  - Hypertension that is difficult to control after therapy has been initiated
  - Stable hypertension that becomes difficult to control
  - Clinical occurrence of a hypertensive crisis
  - The presence of signs or symptoms of a secondary cause such as hypokalemia or metabolic alkalosis that is not explained by diuretic therapy
- In patients who present with significant hypertension at a young age, a careful family history may give clues to forms of hypertension that follow simple Mendelian inheritance.

Physical Examination
The physical examination should include investigation for target organ damage or a secondary cause of hypertension by noting the presence of carotid bruits, an S_3 or S_4, cardiac murmurs, neurologic deficits, elevated jugular venous pressure, rales, retinopathy, unequal pulses, enlarged or small kidneys, cushingoid features, and abdominal bruits. Overweight/obesity should be assessed by measurement of height and weight, and/or abdominal waist circumference.

Differential Diagnosis
- Hypertension may be part of several important syndromes of withdrawal from drugs, including alcohol, cocaine, and opioid analgesics. Rebound increases in BP also may be seen in patients who abruptly discontinue antihypertensive therapy, particularly β-adrenergic antagonists and central α_2-agonists (see Complications).
- Cocaine and other sympathomimetic drugs (e.g., amphetamines, phencyclidine hydrochloride) can produce hypertension in the setting of acute intoxication and when the agents are discontinued abruptly after chronic use. Hypertension is often complicated by other end-organ insults, such as ischemic heart disease, stroke, and seizures. Phentolamine is effective in acute management, and sodium nitroprusside or nitroglycerin can be used as an alternative (Table 2). β-Adrenergic antagonists should be avoided due to the risk of unopposed α-adrenergic activity, which can exacerbate hypertension.

Diagnostic Testing
Laboratories
Tests are needed to help identify patients with possible target organ damage, to help assess cardiovascular risk, and to provide a baseline for monitoring the adverse effects of therapy:

- Urinalysis
- Hematocrit
- Plasma glucose
- Serum potassium
- Serum creatinine
- Calcium
- Uric acid
- Fasting lipid levels

Table 2	Commonly Used Antihypertensive Agents by Functional Class		
Drugs by Class	**Properties**	**Initial Dose**	**Usual Dosage Range (mg)**
β-Adrenergic antagonists			
Atenolol[a,b]	Selective	50 mg PO daily	25–100
Betaxolol	Selective	10 mg PO daily	5–40
Bisoprolol[a]	Selective	5 mg PO daily	2.5–20
Metoprolol	Selective	50 mg PO bid	50–450
Metoprolol XL	Selective	50–100 mg PO daily	50–400
Nebivolol	Selective with vasodilatory properties	5 mg PO daily	5–40
Nadolol[a]	Nonselective	40 mg PO daily	20–240
Propranolol[b]	Nonselective	40 mg PO bid	40–240
Propranolol LA	Nonselective	80 mg PO daily	60–240
Timolol[b]	Nonselective	10 mg PO bid	20–40
Carteolol[a]	ISA	2.5 mg PO daily	2.5–10
Penbutolol	ISA	20 mg PO daily	20–80
Pindolol	ISA	5 mg PO daily	10–60
Labetalol	α- and β-antagonist properties	100 mg PO bid	200–1,200
Carvedilol	α- and β-antagonist properties	6.25 mg PO bid	12.5–50
Acebutolol[a]	ISA, selective	200 mg PO bid, 400 mg PO daily	200–1,200
Calcium channel antagonists			
Amlodipine	DHP	5 mg PO daily	2.5–10
Diltiazem		30 mg PO qid	90–360
Diltiazem SR		60–120 mg PO bid	120–360
Diltiazem CD		180 mg PO bid	180–360
Diltiazem XR		80 mg daily	180–480
Isradipine	DHP	2.5 mg PO bid	2.5–10
Nicardipine[b]	DHP	20 mg PO tid	60–120
Nicardipine SR	DHP	30 mg PO bid	60–120
Nifedipine	DHP	10 mg PO tid	30–120
Nifedipine XL (or CC)	DHP	30 mg PO daily	30–90
Nisoldipine	DHP	20 mg PO daily	20–40
Verapamil[b]		80 mg PO tid	80–480
Verapamil COER		80 mg PO daily	180–480
Verapamil SR		120–140 mg PO daily	120–480
Angiotensin-converting enzyme inhibitors			
Benazepril[a]		10 mg PO bid	10–40
Captopril[a]		25 mg PO bid–tid	50–450

(continued)

Table 2	Commonly Used Antihypertensive Agents by Functional Class (*Continued*)		

Drugs by Class	Properties	Initial Dose	Usual Dosage Range (mg)
Enalapril[a]		5 mg PO daily	2.5–40
Fosinopril		10 mg PO daily	10–40
Lisinopril[a]		10 mg PO daily	5–40
Moexipril		7.5 mg PO daily	7.5–30
Quinapril[a]		10 mg PO daily	5–80
Ramipril[a]		2.5 mg PO daily	1.25–20
Trandolapril		1–2 mg PO daily	1–4
Angiotensin II receptor blocker			
Candesartan		8 mg PO daily	8–32
Eprosartan		600 mg PO daily	600–800
Irbesartan		150 mg PO daily	150–300
Olmesartan		20 mg PO daily	20–40
Losartan		50 mg PO daily	25–100
Telmisartan		40 mg PO daily	20–80
Valsartan		80 mg PO daily	80–320
Diuretics			
Bendroflumethiazide	Thiazide diuretic	5 mg PO daily	2.5–15
Benzthiazide	Thiazide diuretic	25 mg PO bid	50–100
Chlorothiazide	Thiazide diuretic	500 mg PO daily (or IV)	125–1,000
Chlorthalidone	Thiazide diuretic	25 mg PO daily	12.5–50
Hydrochlorothiazide	Thiazide diuretic	12.5 mg PO daily	12.5–50
Hydroflumethiazide	Thiazide diuretic	50 mg PO daily	50–100
Indapamide	Thiazide diuretic	1.25 mg PO daily	2.5–5.0
Methyclothiazide	Thiazide diuretic	2.5 mg PO daily	2.5–5.0
Metolazone	Thiazide diuretic	2.5 mg PO daily	1.25–5
Polythiazide	Thiazide diuretic	2.0 mg PO daily	1–4
Quinethazone	Thiazide diuretic	50 mg PO daily	25–100
Trichlormethiazide	Thiazide diuretic	2.0 mg PO daily	1–4
Bumetanide	Loop diuretic	0.5 mg PO daily (or IV)	0.5–5
Ethacrynic acid	Loop diuretic	50 mg PO daily (or IV)	25–100
Furosemide	Loop diuretic	20 mg PO daily (or IV)	20–320
Torsemide	Loop diuretic	5 mg PO daily (or IV)	5–10
Amiloride	Potassium-sparing diuretic	5 mg PO daily	5–10
Triamterene	Potassium-sparing diuretic	50 mg PO bid	50–200
Eplerenone	Aldosterone antagonist	25 mg PO daily	25–100
Spironolactone	Aldosterone antagonist	25 mg PO daily	25–100

(continued)

Table 2	Commonly Used Antihypertensive Agents by Functional Class (*Continued*)		
Drugs by Class	**Properties**	**Initial Dose**	**Usual Dosage Range (mg)**
α-Adrenergic antagonists			
Doxazosin		1 mg PO daily	1–16
Prazosin		1 mg PO bid–tid	1–20
Terazosin		1 mg PO at bedtime	1–20
Centrally acting adrenergic agents			
Clonidine[b]		0.1 mg PO bid	0.1–1.2
Clonidine patch		TTS 1/wk (equivalent to 0.1 mg/d release)	0.1–0.3
Guanfacine		1 mg PO daily	1–3
Guanabenz		4 mg PO bid	4–64
Methyldopa[b]		250 mg PO bid–tid	250–2,000
Direct-acting vasodilators			
Hydralazine		10 mg PO qid	50–300
Minoxidil		5 mg PO daily	2.5–100
Miscellaneous			
Reserpine[b]		0.5 mg PO daily	0.01–0.25

DHP, dihydropyridine; ISA, intrinsic sympathomimetic activity; TTS, transdermal therapeutic system.
[a] Adjusted in renal failure.
[b] Available in generic form.

- Electrocardiogram (ECG)
- Chest radiography
- Echocardiography may be of value for certain patients to assess cardiac function or detection of left ventricular hypertrophy (LVH)

TREATMENT

Behavioral

- **Nonpharmacologic therapy.** Lifestyle modifications should be encouraged in all hypertensive patients regardless of whether they require medication. These changes may have beneficial effects on other cardiovascular risk factors. Some of these lifestyle modifications include cessation of smoking, reduction in body weight if the patient is overweight, judicious consumption of alcohol, adequate nutritional intake of minerals and vitamins, reduction in sodium intake, and increased physical activity.

Medications

- **Initial drug therapy.** Data from the ALLHAT trial have shown decreased cardiovascular and cerebrovascular morbidity and mortality with the use of thiazide diuretics (*JAMA 2002;288:2981–2997*); thus, this class of drug is favored as first-line therapy unless there is a contraindication to their use or the characteristics of a patient's profile (concomitant disease, age, race) mandate the institution of a different agent.

Calcium channel antagonists and angiotensin-converting enzyme (ACE) inhibitors have a low side-effect profile and have been shown to decrease BP to degrees similar to those observed with diuretics and β-adrenergic antagonists. In ALLHAT, reductions in morbidity and mortality were similar to diuretics making them reasonable initial agents. In patients with stage 2 hypertension, therapy may be initiated with a two-drug combination, typically a thiazide diuretic plus a calcium antagonist, ACE inhibitor, or β-adrenergic antagonists. Initial drug choice may be affected by coexistent factors, such as age, race, angina, HF, renal insufficiency, LVH, obesity, hyperlipidemia, gout, and bronchospasm. Cost and drug interactions should also be considered. The BP response is usually consistent within a given class of agents; therefore, if a drug fails to control BP, another agent from the same class is unlikely to be effective. At times, however, a change within drug class may be useful in reducing adverse effects. The lowest possible effective dosage should be used to control BP, adjusted every 1 to 3 months as needed.

- **Additional therapy.** When a second drug is needed, it should generally be chosen from among the other first-line agents. A diuretic should be added first, as doing so may enhance effectiveness of the first drug, yielding more than a simple additive effect.

- **Adjustments of a therapeutic regimen.** In considering a modification of therapy because of inadequate response to the current regimen, the physician should investigate other possible contributing factors. Poor patient compliance, use of antagonistic drugs (i.e., sympathomimetics, antidepressants, steroids, nonsteroidal anti-inflammatory drugs [NSAIDs], cyclosporine, caffeine, thyroid hormones, cocaine, erythropoietin), inappropriately high sodium intake, or increased alcohol consumption should be considered before antihypertensive drug therapy is modified. Secondary causes of hypertension must be considered when a previously effective regimen becomes inadequate and other confounding factors are absent.

- **Diuretics** (Table 2) are effective agents in the therapy of hypertension, and data have accumulated to demonstrate their safety and benefit in reducing the incidence of stroke and cardiovascular events.

  - **Several classes of diuretics** are available, generally categorized by their site of action in the kidney. Thiazide and thiazide-like diuretics (e.g., hydrochlorothiazide, chlorthalidone) block sodium reabsorption predominantly in the distal convoluted tubule by inhibition of the thiazide-sensitive Na/Cl cotransporter. Loop diuretics (e.g., furosemide, bumetanide, ethacrynic acid, and torsemide) block sodium reabsorption in the thick ascending loop of Henle through inhibition of the Na/K/2Cl cotransporter and are the most effective agents in patients with renal insufficiency (estimated glomerular filtration rate [eGFR] < 35 mL/min/1.73 m^2). Spironolactone and eplerenone, potassium-sparing agents, act by competitively inhibiting the actions of aldosterone on the kidney. Triamterene and amiloride are potassium-sparing drugs that inhibit the epithelial Na$^+$ channel in the distal nephron to inhibit reabsorption of Na$^+$ and secretion of potassium ions. Potassium-sparing diuretics are weak agents when used alone; thus, they are often combined with a thiazide for added potency. Aldosterone antagonists may have an additional benefit in improving myocardial function in HF; this effect may be independent of its effect on renal transport mechanisms.

  - **Side effects** of diuretics vary by class. Thiazide diuretics can produce weakness, muscle cramps, and impotence. Metabolic side effects include hypokalemia, hypomagnesemia, hyperlipidemia (with increases in low-density lipoproteins [LDLs] and triglyceride levels), hypercalcemia, hyperglycemia, hyperuricemia, hyponatremia, and, rarely, azotemia. Thiazide-induced pancreatitis has also been reported. Metabolic side effects may be limited when thiazides are used in low doses (e.g., hydrochlorothiazide, 12.5 to 25.0 mg/d). Loop diuretics can cause electrolyte abnormalities such as hypomagnesemia, hypocalcemia, and hypokalemia, and can also produce irreversible ototoxicity (usually dose related and more common with parenteral therapy). Spironolactone and eplerenone can produce hyperkalemia; however, the gynecomastia that may occur in men and breast tenderness in women are not seen with eplerenone. Triamterene (usually in combination with hydrochlorothiazide) can cause renal tubular damage and renal calculi. Unlike thiazides, potassium-sparing and loop diuretics do not cause adverse lipid effects.

- β-**Adrenergic antagonists** (Table 2) are effective antihypertensive agents and are part of medical regimens that have been proven to decrease the incidence of stroke, MI, and HF.
  - The **mechanism of action** of β-adrenergic antagonists is competitive inhibition of the effects of catecholamines at β-adrenergic receptors, which decreases heart rate and cardiac output. These agents also decrease plasma renin and cause a resetting of baroreceptors to accept a lower level of BP. β-Adrenergic antagonists cause release of vasodilatory prostaglandins, decrease plasma volume, and may also have a central nervous system (CNS)-mediated antihypertensive effect.
  - **Classes of β-adrenergic antagonists** can be subdivided into those that are cardioselective, with primarily β_1-blocking effects, and those that are nonselective, with β_1- and β_2-blocking effects. At low doses, the cardioselective agents can be given with caution to patients with mild chronic obstructive pulmonary disease, diabetes mellitus (DM), or peripheral vascular disease. At higher doses, these agents lose their β_1 selectivity and may cause unwanted effects in these patients. β-Adrenergic antagonists can also be categorized according to the presence or absence of partial agonist or intrinsic sympathomimetic activity (ISA). β-Adrenergic antagonists with ISA cause less bradycardia than do those without it. In addition, there are agents with mixed properties having both α- and β-adrenergic antagonist actions (labetalol and carvedilol). Nebivolol is highly selective β-adrenergic antagonist that is vasodilatory through an unclear mechanism.
  - **Side effects** include high-degree atrioventricular (AV) block, HF, Raynaud's phenomenon, and impotence. Lipophilic β-adrenergic antagonists, such as propranolol, have a higher incidence of CNS side effects including insomnia and depression. Propranolol can also cause nasal congestion. β-Adrenergic antagonists can cause adverse effects on the lipid profile; increased triglyceride and decreased high-density lipoprotein (HDL) levels occur mainly with nonselective β-adrenergic antagonists but generally do not occur when β-adrenergic antagonists with ISA are used. Pindolol, a selective β-adrenergic antagonist with ISA, may actually increase HDL and nominally increase triglycerides. Side effects of labetalol include hepatocellular damage, postural hypotension, a positive antinuclear antibody (ANA) test, a lupus-like syndrome, tremors, and potential hypotension in the setting of halothane anesthesia. Carvedilol appears to have a similar side-effect profile to other β-adrenergic antagonists. Both labetalol and carvedilol have negligible effects on lipids. Rarely, reflex tachycardia may occur because of the initial vasodilatory effect of labetalol and carvedilol. Because β-receptor density is increased with chronic antagonism, abrupt withdrawal of these agents can precipitate angina pectoris, increases in BP, and other effects attributable to an increase in adrenergic tone.
- **Selective α-adrenergic antagonists** such as prazosin, terazosin, and doxazosin have replaced nonselective α-adrenergic antagonists such as phenoxybenzamine

(Table 2) in the treatment of essential hypertension. Based on the ALLHAT trial, these drugs appear to be less efficacious than diuretics, calcium channel blockers, and ACE inhibitors in reducing primary end points of cardiovascular disease when used as monotherapy (*JAMA 2002;283:1967–1975*; *JAMA 2002;288:2981–2997*).

- **Side effects** of these agents include a "first-dose effect," which results from a greater decrease in BP with the first dose than with subsequent doses. Selective α_1-adrenergic antagonists can cause syncope, orthostatic hypotension, dizziness, headache, and drowsiness. In most cases, side effects are self-limited and do not recur with continued therapy. Selective α_1-adrenergic antagonists may improve lipid profiles by decreasing total cholesterol and triglyceride levels and increasing HDL levels. Additionally, these agents can improve the negative effects on lipids induced by thiazide diuretics and β-adrenergic antagonists. Doxazosin specifically may be less effective in lowering SBP than thiazide diuretics and may additionally be associated with a higher risk of cardiovascular disease, particularly HF and stroke in patients with hypertension and at least one additional risk factor for coronary artery disease (CAD) (*JAMA 2002;283:1967–1975*).

- **Centrally acting adrenergic agents** (Table 2) are potent antihypertensive agents. In addition to its oral dosage forms, clonidine is available as a transdermal patch that is applied weekly.
  - **Side effects** may include bradycardia, drowsiness, dry mouth, orthostatic hypotension, galactorrhea, and sexual dysfunction. Transdermal clonidine causes a rash in up to 20% of patients. These agents can precipitate HF in patients with decreased left ventricular function, and abrupt cessation can precipitate an acute withdrawal syndrome (AWS) of elevated BP, tachycardia, and diaphoresis (see Complications). Methyldopa produces a positive direct antibody (Coombs) test in up to 25% of patients, but significant hemolytic anemia is much less common. If hemolytic anemia develops secondary to methyldopa, the drug should be withdrawn. Severe cases of hemolytic anemia may require treatment with glucocorticoids. Methyldopa also causes positive ANA test results in approximately 10% of patients and can cause an inflammatory reaction in the liver that is indistinguishable from viral hepatitis; fatal hepatitis has been reported. Guanabenz and guanfacine decrease total cholesterol levels, and guanfacine can also decrease serum triglyceride levels.

- **Reserpine, guanethidine, and guanadrel** (Table 2) were among the first effective antihypertensive agents available. Currently, these drugs are not regarded as first- or second-line therapy because of their significant side effects.
  - **Side effects** of reserpine include severe depression in approximately 2% of patients. Sedation and nasal stuffiness also are potential side effects. Guanethidine can cause severe postural hypotension through a decrease in cardiac output, a decrease in peripheral resistance, and venous pooling in the extremities. Patients who are receiving guanethidine with orthostatic hypotension should be cautioned to arise slowly and to wear support hose. Guanethidine can also cause ejaculatory failure and diarrhea.

- **Calcium channel antagonists** (Table 2) are effective agents in the treatment of hypertension. Generally, they have no significant CNS side effects and can be used to treat diseases, such as angina pectoris, that can coexist with hypertension. **Due to the concern that the use of short-acting dihydropyridine calcium channel antagonists may increase the number of ischemic cardiac events, they are not indicated for hypertension management** (*JAMA 1995;274:620–625*); long-acting agents are considered safe in the management of hypertension (*Am J Cardiol 1996;77:81–82*).

- **Classes of calcium channel antagonists** include diphenylalkylamines (e.g., verapamil), benzothiazepines (e.g., diltiazem), and dihydropyridines (e.g., nifedipine). The dihydropyridines include many newer second-generation drugs (e.g., amlodipine, felodipine, isradipine, and nicardipine), which are more vasoselective and have longer plasma half-lives than nifedipine. Verapamil and diltiazem have negative cardiac inotropic and chronotropic effects. Nifedipine also has a negative inotropic effect but in clinical use this effect is much less pronounced than that of verapamil or diltiazem because of peripheral vasodilation and reflex tachycardia. Less negative inotropic effects have been observed with the second-generation dihydropyridines. All calcium channel antagonists are metabolized in the liver; thus in patients with cirrhosis, the dosing interval should be adjusted accordingly. Some of these drugs also inhibit the metabolism of other hepatically cleared medications (e.g., cyclosporine). Verapamil and diltiazem should be used with caution in patients with cardiac conduction abnormalities as they can worsen HF in patients with decreased left ventricular function.
- **Side effects** of verapamil include constipation, nausea, headache, and orthostatic hypotension. Diltiazem can cause nausea, headache, and rash. Dihydropyridines can cause lower extremity edema, flushing, headache, and rash. Calcium channel antagonists have no significant effects on glucose tolerance, electrolytes, or lipid profiles. In general, calcium channel antagonists should not be initiated in patients immediately after MI because of increased mortality in all but the most stable patients without evidence of HF.
- **Inhibitors of the renin–angiotensin system** (Table 2) are effective antihypertensive agents in a broad array of patients.
  - **ACE inhibitors** may have beneficial effects in patients with concomitant HF or kidney disease. One study has also suggested that ACE inhibitors (ramipril) may significantly reduce the rate of death, MI, and stroke in patients without HF or low ejection fraction (*N Engl J Med 2000;342:145–153*). Additionally, they can reduce hypokalemia, hypercholesterolemia, hyperglycemia, and hyperuricemia caused by diuretic therapy and are particularly effective in states of hypertension associated with a high renin state (e.g., scleroderma renal crisis).
  - **Side effects** associated with the use of ACE inhibitors are infrequent. They can cause a dry cough (up to 20% of patients), angioneurotic edema, and hypotension, but they do not cause levels of lipids, glucose, or uric acid to increase. ACE inhibitors that contain a sulfhydryl group (e.g., captopril) may cause taste disturbance, leukopenia, and a glomerulopathy with proteinuria. Because ACE inhibitors cause preferential vasodilation of the efferent arteriole in the kidney, worsening of renal function may occur in patients who have decreased renal perfusion or who have preexisting severe renal insufficiency. ACE inhibitors can cause hyperkalemia and should be used with caution in patients with a decreased GFR who are taking potassium supplements or who are receiving potassium-sparing diuretics.
  - **Angiotensin receptor blockers (ARBs)** are a class of antihypertensive drugs that are effective in diverse patient populations (*N Engl J Med 1996;334:1649–1654*). Several of these agents are now approved for the management of mild to moderate hypertension (Table 2). Additionally, ARBs may be useful alternatives in patients with HF who are unable to tolerate ACE inhibitors (*N Engl J Med 2001;345:1667–1675*).
    - **Side effects** of ARBs occur rarely but include angioedema, allergic reaction, and rash.

- **Direct-acting vasodilators** are potent antihypertensive agents (Table 2) now reserved for refractory hypertension or specific circumstances, such as the use of hydralazine in pregnancy. Hydralazine in combination with nitrates is useful in treating patients with hypertension and HF (see Chapter 4, Heart Failure, Cardiomyopathy, and Valvular Heart Disease).
  - **Side effects** of hydralazine therapy may include headache, nausea, emesis, tachycardia, and postural hypotension. Asymptomatic patients may have a positive ANA test result and a hydralazine-induced systemic lupus-like syndrome may develop in approximately 10% of patients. Patients who may be at increased risk for this latter complication include (i) those treated with excessive doses (e.g., >400 mg/d), (ii) those with impaired renal or cardiac function, and (iii) those with the slow acetylation phenotype. Hydralazine should be discontinued if clinical evidence of a lupus-like syndrome develops and a positive ANA test result is present. The syndrome usually resolves with discontinuation of the drug, leaving no adverse long-term effects. Side effects of minoxidil include weight gain, hypertrichosis, hirsutism, ECG abnormalities, and pericardial effusions.
- **Parenteral antihypertensive agents** are indicated for the immediate reduction of BP in patients with hypertensive emergencies. Judicious administration of these agents (Table 3) may also be appropriate in patients with hypertension complicated by HF or MI. These drugs are also indicated for individuals who have perioperative hypertensive urgency or are in need of emergency surgery. If possible, an accurate baseline BP should be determined before the initiation of therapy. In the setting of hypertensive emergency, the patient should be admitted to an intensive care unit (ICU) for close monitoring, and an intra-arterial monitor should be used when available. Although parenteral agents are indicated as a first line in hypertensive emergencies, oral agents may also be effective in this group; the choice of drug and route of administration must be individualized. If parenteral agents are used initially, oral medications should be administered shortly thereafter to facilitate rapid weaning from parenteral therapy.
  - **Sodium nitroprusside,** a direct-acting arterial and venous vasodilator, is the drug of choice for most hypertensive emergencies (Table 3). It reduces BP rapidly and is easily titratable, and its action is short lived when discontinued. Patients should be monitored very closely to avoid an exaggerated hypotensive response. Therapy for more than 48 to 72 hours with a high cumulative dose or renal insufficiency may cause accumulation of thiocyanate, a toxic metabolite. Thiocyanate toxicity may cause paresthesias, tinnitus, blurred vision, delirium, or seizures. Serum thiocyanate levels should be kept at <10 mg/dL. Patients on high doses (>2 to 3 mg/kg/min) or those with renal dysfunction should have serum levels of thiocyanate drawn after 48 to 72 hours of therapy. In patients with normal renal function or those receiving lower doses, levels can be drawn after 5 to 7 days. Hepatic dysfunction may result in accumulation of cyanide, which can cause metabolic acidosis, dyspnea, vomiting, dizziness, ataxia, and syncope. Hemodialysis should be considered for thiocyanate poisoning. Nitrites and thiosulfate can be administered intravenously for cyanide poisoning.
  - **Nitroglycerin** given as a continuous IV infusion (Table 3) may be appropriate in situations in which sodium nitroprusside is relatively contraindicated, such as in patients with severe coronary insufficiency or advanced renal or hepatic disease. It is the preferred agent for patients with moderate hypertension in the setting of acute coronary ischemia or after coronary artery bypass surgery because of its more favorable effects on pulmonary gas exchange and collateral coronary blood

Table 3 Parental Antihypertensive Drug Preparations

Drug	Administration	Onset	Duration of Action	Dosage	Adverse Effects and Comments
Fenoldopam	IV infusion	<5 min	30 min	0.1–0.3 mcg/kg/min	Tachycardia, nausea, vomiting
Sodium nitroprusside	IV infusion	Immediate	2–3 min	0.5–10 mcg/kg/min (initial dose, 0.25 mcg/kg/min for eclampsia and renal insufficiency)	Hypotension, nausea, vomiting, apprehension. Risk of thiocyanate and cyanide toxicity increased in renal and hepatic insufficiency, respectively; levels should be monitored. Must shield from light.
Diazoxide	IV bolus	15 min	6–12 hr	50–100 mg q5–10 min, up to 600 mg	Hypotension, tachycardia, nausea, vomiting, fluid retention, hyperglycemia. May exacerbate myocardial ischemia, heart failure, or aortic dissection.
Labetalol	IV bolus	5–10 min	3–6 hr	20–80 mg q5–10 min, up to 300 mg	Hypotension, heart block, heart failure, bronchospasm, nausea, vomiting, scalp tingling, paradoxical pressor response. May not be effective in patients receiving α- or β-antagonists.
Nitroglycerin	IV infusion	1–2 min	3–5 min	0.5–2 mg/min	Headache, nausea, vomiting. Tolerance may develop with prolonged use.
	IV infusion			5–250 mcg/min	

(continued)

Table 3   Parental Antihypertensive Drug Preparations (*Continued*)

Drug	Administration	Onset	Duration of Action	Dosage	Adverse Effects and Comments
Esmolol	IV bolus IV infusion	1–5 min	10 min	500 mcg/kg/min for first 1 min 50–300 mcg/kg/min	Hypotension, heart block, heart failure, bronchospasm.
Phentolamine	IV bolus	1–2 min	3–10 min	5–10 mg q5–15 min	Hypotension, tachycardia, headache, angina, paradoxical pressor response.
Hydralazine (for treatment of eclampsia)	IV bolus	10–20 min	3–6 hr	10–20 mg q20 min (if no effect after 20 mg, try another agent)	Hypotension, fetal distress, tachycardia, headache, nausea, vomiting, local thrombophlebitis. Infusion site should be changed after 12 hr.
Methyldopate (for treatment of eclampsia)	IV bolus	30–60 min	10–16 hr	250–500 mg	Hypotension
Nicardipine	IV infusion	1–5 min	3–6 hr	5 mg/hr, increased by 1.0–2.5 mg/hr q15 min, up to 15 mg/hr	Hypotension, headache, tachycardia, nausea, vomiting.
Enalaprilat	IV bolus	5–15 min	1–6 hr	0.6255 mg q6h	Hypotension

flow. In patients with severely elevated BP, sodium nitroprusside remains the agent of choice. Nitroglycerin reduces preload more than afterload and should be used with caution or avoided in patients who have inferior MI with right ventricular infarction and are dependent on preload to maintain cardiac output.

- **Labetalol** can be administered parenterally (Table 3) in hypertensive crisis, even in patients in the early phase of an acute MI, and is the drug of choice in hypertensive emergencies that occur during pregnancy. When given intravenously, the β-adrenergic antagonist effect is greater than the α-adrenergic antagonist effect. Nevertheless, symptomatic postural hypotension may occur with IV use, thus patients should be treated in a supine position. Labetalol may be particularly beneficial during adrenergic excess (e.g., clonidine withdrawal, pheochromocytoma, postcoronary bypass grafting). As the half-life of labetalol is 5 to 8 hours, intermittent IV bolus dosing may be preferable to IV infusion. IV infusion can be discontinued before oral labetalol is begun. When the supine DBP begins to rise, oral dosing can be initiated at 200 mg PO, followed in 6 to 12 hours by 200 to 400 mg PO, depending on the BP response.

- **Esmolol** is a parenteral, short-acting, cardioselective β-adrenergic antagonist (Table 3) that can be used in the treatment of hypertensive emergencies in patients in whom β-blocker intolerance is a concern. Esmolol is also useful for the treatment of aortic dissection. β-Adrenergic antagonists may be ineffective when used as monotherapy in the treatment of severe hypertension and are frequently combined with other agents (e.g., with sodium nitroprusside in the treatment of aortic dissection).

- **Nicardipine** is an effective IV calcium antagonist preparation (Table 3) approved for use in postoperative hypertension. Side effects include headache, flushing, reflex tachycardia, and venous irritation. Nicardipine should be administered via a central venous line. If it is given peripherally, the IV site should be changed q12h. Fifty percent of the peak effect is seen within the first 30 minutes, but the full peak effect is not achieved until after 48 hours of administration.

- **Enalaprilat** is the active deesterified form of enalapril (Table 3) that results from hepatic conversion after an oral dose. Enalaprilat (as well as other ACE inhibitors) has been used effectively in cases of severe and malignant hypertension. However, variable and unpredictable results have also been reported. ACE inhibition can cause rapid BP reduction in hypertensive patients with high renin states such as renovascular hypertension, concomitant use of vasodilators, and scleroderma renal crisis; thus, Enalaprilat should be used cautiously to avoid precipitating hypotension. Therapy can be changed to an oral preparation when IV therapy is no longer necessary.

- **Diazoxide and hydralazine** are only rarely used in hypertensive crises and offer little or no advantage to the agents discussed previously. It should be noted, however, that hydralazine is a useful agent in pregnancy-related hypertensive emergencies because of its established safety profile.

- **Fenoldopam** is a selective agonist to peripheral dopamine-1 receptors, and it produces vasodilation, increases renal perfusion, and enhances natriuresis. Fenoldopam has a short duration of action; the elimination half-life is <10 minutes. The drug has important application as parental therapy for high-risk hypertensive surgical patients and the perioperative management of patients undergoing organ transplantation.

- **Oral loading of antihypertensive agents** has been used successfully in patients with hypertensive crisis when urgent but not immediate reduction of BP is indicated.

- **Oral clonidine loading** is achieved by using an initial dose of 0.2 mg PO followed by 0.1 mg PO q1h to a total dose of 0.7 mg or a reduction in diastolic pressure of 20 mm Hg or more. BP should be checked at 15-minute intervals over the first hour, 30-minute intervals over the second hour, and then hourly. After 6 hours, a diuretic can be added, and an 8-hour clonidine dosing interval can be begun. Sedative side effects are significant.
- Sublingual nifedipine has an onset of action within 30 minutes but can produce wide fluctuations and excessive reductions in BP. Because of the potential for adverse cardiovascular events (stroke/MI), sublingual nifedipine should be avoided in the acute management of elevated BP. Side effects include facial flushing and postural hypotension.

Lifestyle/Risk Modification

General considerations and goals. The goal of treatment for hypertension is to prevent long-term sequelae (i.e., target organ damage). Barring an overt need for immediate pharmacologic therapy, most patients should be given the opportunity to achieve a reduction in BP over an interval of 3 to 6 months by applying nonpharmacologic modifications and pharmacologic therapies if needed. The primary goal is to reduce BP to <140/90 mm Hg while concurrently controlling other modifiable cardiovascular risk factors. As isolated systolic hypertension is also associated with increased cerebrovascular and cardiac events, the therapeutic goal in this subset of patients should be to lower BP to <140 mm Hg systolic. Treatment should be more aggressive in patients with chronic kidney disease or diabetes, with a goal BP of <130/80. Discretion is warranted in prescribing medication to lower BP that may affect cardiovascular risk adversely in other ways (e.g., glucose control, lipid metabolism, uric acid levels). In the absence of hypertensive crisis, BP should be reduced gradually to avoid end-organ (e.g., cerebral) ischemia.

SPECIAL CONSIDERATIONS

- **Protocol**
  - **Hypertensive crisis.** In hypertensive emergency, control of acute or ongoing end-organ damage is more important than the absolute level of BP. BP control with a rapidly acting parenteral agent should be accomplished as soon as possible (within 1 hour) to reduce the chance of permanent organ dysfunction and death. A reasonable goal is a 20% to 25% reduction of mean arterial pressure or a reduction of the diastolic pressure to 100 to 110 mm Hg over a period of minutes to hours. A precipitous fall in BP may occur in patients who are elderly, volume depleted, or receiving other antihypertensive agents, and caution should be used to avoid cerebral hypoperfusion. BP control in hypertensive urgencies can be accomplished more slowly. The initial goal of therapy in urgency should be to achieve a DBP of 100 to 110 mm Hg. Excessive or rapid decreases in BP should be avoided to minimize the risk of cerebral hypoperfusion or coronary insufficiency. Normal BP can be attained gradually over several days as tolerated by the individual patient.
- **Aortic dissection**
  - Acute, proximal aortic dissection (type A) is a surgical emergency, whereas uncomplicated, distal dissection (type B) can be treated successfully with medical therapy alone. All patients, including those treated surgically, require acute and chronic antihypertensive therapy to provide initial stabilization and to prevent complications (e.g., aortic rupture, continued dissection). Medical therapy of chronic stable

aortic dissection should seek to maintain SBP at or below 130 to 140 mm Hg if tolerated. Antihypertensive agents with negative inotropic properties, including calcium channel antagonists, β-adrenergic antagonists, methyldopa, clonidine, and reserpine, are preferred for management in the postacute phase.

- ○ **Sodium nitroprusside** is considered the initial drug of choice because of the predictability of response and absence of tachyphylaxis. The dose should be titrated to achieve an SBP of 100 to 120 mm Hg or the lowest possible BP that permits adequate organ perfusion. Nitroprusside alone causes an increase in left ventricular contractility and subsequent arterial shearing forces, which contribute to ongoing intimal dissection. Thus, when using sodium nitroprusside, adequate simultaneous β-**adrenergic antagonist therapy** is essential, regardless of whether systolic hypertension is present. Traditionally, propranolol has been recommended. **Esmolol,** a cardioselective IV β-adrenergic antagonist with a very short duration of action, may be preferable, especially in patients with relative contraindications to β-antagonists. If esmolol is tolerated, a longer-acting β-adrenergic antagonist should be used.
- ○ **IV labetalol** has been used successfully as a single agent in the treatment of acute aortic dissection. Labetalol produces a dose-related decrease in BP and lowers contractility. It has the advantage of allowing for oral administration after the acute stage of dissection has been managed successfully.
- ○ **Trimethaphan camsylate,** a ganglionic blocking agent, can be used as a single IV agent if sodium nitroprusside or β-adrenergic antagonists cannot be tolerated. Unlike sodium nitroprusside, trimethaphan reduces left ventricular contractility. Because trimethaphan is associated with rapid tachyphylaxis and sympathalgia (e.g., orthostatic hypotension, blurred vision, and urinary retention), other drugs are preferable.
- **Individual patient considerations.** Cultural and other individual differences among patients must be considered in planning a therapeutic regimen. Although classification of adult BP is somewhat arbitrary, it may nevertheless be useful in making clinical decisions (Table 4).
  - **The elderly hypertensive patient** (older than 60 years) is generally characterized by increased vascular resistance, decreased plasma renin activity, and greater LVH than in younger patients. Often elderly hypertensive patients have coexisting medical problems that must be considered in initiating antihypertensive therapy. Drug doses should be increased slowly to avoid adverse effects and hypotension. Diuretics as initial therapy have been shown to decrease the incidence of stroke, fatal MI, and overall mortality in this age group (*JAMA 1991;265:3255–3264*). Calcium channel antagonists decrease vascular resistance, have no adverse effects on lipid levels, and are also good choices for elderly patients. ACE inhibitors and ARBs may be effective agents in this population.
  - **Black hypertensive patients** generally have a lower plasma renin level, higher plasma volume, and higher vascular resistance than do white patients. Thus, black patients respond well to diuretics, alone or in combination with calcium channel antagonists. ACE inhibitors, ARBs, and β-adrenergic antagonists are also effective agents in this population particularly when combined with a diuretic.
  - **The obese hypertensive patient** is characterized by more modest elevations in vascular resistance, higher cardiac output, expanded intravascular volume, and lower plasma renin activity at any given level of arterial pressure. Weight reduction is the primary goal of therapy and is effective in reducing BP and causing regression of LVH.

Table 4	Classification of Blood Pressure for Adults Aged 18 Years and Older[a]	
Category	Systolic Pressure (mm Hg)	Diastolic Pressure (mm Hg)
Normal[b]	<120 and	<80
Prehypertension	120–139 or	80–89
Hypertension[c]		
Stage 1	140–159 or	90–99
Stage 2	>160 or	>100

Isolated systolic hypertension is defined as a systolic BP of 140 mm Hg or more and a diastolic BP of <90 mm Hg and staged appropriately (e.g., 170/85 mm Hg is defined as stage 2 isolated systolic hypertension). In addition to classifying stages of hypertension on the basis of average BP levels, the clinician should specify the presence or absence of target organ disease and additional risk factors. This specificity is important for risk classification and management.
[a]Not taking antihypertensive drugs and not acutely ill. When systolic and diastolic pressures fall into different categories, the higher category should be selected to classify the individual's blood pressure (BP) status.
[b]Optimal BP with respect to cardiovascular risk is <120 mm Hg systolic and <80 mm Hg diastolic. However, unusually low readings should be evaluated for clinical significance.
[c]Based on the average of two or more readings taken at each of two or more visits after an initial screening.
From The Seventh Report of the Joint National Committee on Prevention, Detection, Evaluation, and Treatment of High Blood Pressure: the JNC 7 report. Chobanian AV, Bakris GL, Black HR, et al.; National Heart, Lung, and Blood Institute Joint National Committee on Prevention, Detection, Evaluation, and Treatment of High Blood Pressure; National High Blood Pressure Education Program Coordinating Committee. *JAMA* 2003 May 21;289(19):2560–2572. Epub 2003 May 14. Erratum in: *JAMA* 2003 Jul 9;290(2):197, with permission.

- **The diabetic patient** with nephropathy may have significant proteinuria and renal insufficiency, which can complicate management (see Chapter 10, Renal Diseases). Control of BP is the most important intervention shown to slow loss of renal function. ACE inhibitors should be used as first-line therapy, as they have been shown to decrease proteinuria and to slow progressive loss of renal function independent of their antihypertensive effects. ACE inhibitors may also be beneficial in reducing the rates of death, MI, and stroke in diabetics who have cardiovascular risk factors but lack left ventricular dysfunction. Hyperkalemia is a common side effect in diabetic patients treated with ACE inhibitors, especially in those with moderate to severe impairment of their GFR. ARBs are also effective antihypertensive agents and have been shown to slow the rate of progression to end-stage renal disease, thus supporting a renal protective effect (*N Engl J Med 2001 Sep 20;345(12):861–869*).
- **The hypertensive patient with chronic renal insufficiency** has hypertension that usually is partially volume dependent. Retention of sodium and water exacerbates the existing hypertensive state, and diuretics are important in the management of this problem. With a serum creatinine > 2.5 mg/dL, loop diuretics are the most effective class.
- **The hypertensive patient with LVH** is at increased risk for sudden death, MI, and all-cause mortality. Although there is no direct evidence, regression of LVH could be expected to reduce the risk for subsequent complications. ACE inhibitors appear to have the greatest effect on regression.
- **The hypertensive patient with CAD** is at increased risk for UA and MI. β-Adrenergic antagonists can be used as first-line agents in these patients as they can

decrease cardiac mortality and subsequent reinfarction in the setting of acute MI and can decrease progression to MI in those who present with UA. β-Adrenergic antagonists also have a role in secondary prevention of cardiac events and in increasing long-term survival after MI. Care should be exercised in those with cardiac conduction system disease. Calcium channel antagonists should be used with caution in the setting of acute MI, as studies have shown conflicting results from their use. ACE inhibitors are also useful in patients with CAD and decrease mortality in individuals who present with acute MI, especially those with left ventricular dysfunction, and more recently have been shown to decrease mortality in patients without left ventricular dysfunction.

- **The hypertensive patient with HF** is at risk for progressive left ventricular dilatation and sudden death. In this population, ACE inhibitors decrease mortality (*N Engl J Med 1992;327:685–691*), and in the setting of acute MI, they decrease the risk of recurrent MI, hospitalization for HF, and mortality (*N Engl J Med 1992;327:669–677*). ARBs have similar beneficial effects, and they appear to be an effective alternative in patients who are unable to tolerate an ACE inhibitor (*N Engl J Med 2001;345:1667–1675*). Nitrates and hydralazine also decrease mortality in patients with HF irrespective of hypertension, but hydralazine can cause reflex tachycardia and worsening ischemia in patients with unstable coronary syndromes and should be used with caution. Calcium channel antagonists should generally be avoided in patients in whom negative inotropic effects would affect their status adversely.

- **Pregnancy and hypertension**
  - Hypertension in the setting of pregnancy is a special situation because of the potential for maternal and fetal morbidity and mortality associated with elevated BP and the clinical syndromes of preeclampsia and eclampsia. The possibility of teratogenic or other adverse effects of antihypertensive medications on fetal development also should be considered.
  - **Classification of hypertension** during pregnancy has been proposed by the American College of Obstetrics and Gynecology (*N Engl J Med 1996;335:257–265*).
    - **Preeclampsia or eclampsia.** Preeclampsia is a condition defined by pregnancy, hypertension, proteinuria, generalized edema, and, occasionally coagulation and liver function abnormalities after 20 weeks gestation. Eclampsia encompasses these parameters in addition to generalized seizures.
    - **Chronic hypertension.** This disorder is defined by a BP > 140/90 mm Hg before the 20th week of pregnancy.
    - **Transient hypertension.** This condition results in increases in BP without associated proteinuria or CNS manifestations. BP returns to normal within 10 days of delivery.
  - **Therapy.** Treatment of hypertension in pregnancy should begin if the DBP is >100 mm Hg.
    - Nonpharmacologic therapy, such as weight reduction and vigorous exercise, is not recommended during pregnancy.
    - Alcohol and tobacco use should be strongly discouraged.
    - Pharmacologic intervention with methyldopa is recommended as first-line therapy because of its proven safety. Hydralazine and labetalol are also safe and can be used as alternative agents; both can be used parenterally.
    - Other antihypertensives have theoretical disadvantages, but none except the ACE inhibitors have been proven to increase fetal morbidity or mortality.

○ If a patient is suspected of having preeclampsia or eclampsia, urgent referral to an obstetrician who specializes in high-risk pregnancy is recommended.

○ Monoamine oxidase inhibitors (MAOIs). MAOIs used in association with certain drugs or foods can produce a catecholamine excess state and accelerated hypertension. Interactions are common with tricyclic antidepressants, meperidine, methyldopa, levodopa, sympathomimetic agents, and antihistamines. Tyramine-containing foods that can lead to this syndrome include certain cheeses, red wine, beer, chocolate, chicken liver, processed meat, herring, broad beans, canned figs, and yeast. Nitroprusside, labetalol, and phentolamine have been used effectively in the treatment of accelerated hypertension associated with monoamine oxidase inhibitor use (Table 3).

COMPLICATIONS

Withdrawal syndrome associated with discontinuation of antihypertensive therapy. In substituting therapy in patients with moderate to severe hypertension, it is reasonable to increase doses of the new medication in small increments while tapering the previous medication to avoid excessive BP fluctuations. On occasion, an AWS develops, usually within the first 24 to 72 hours. Occasionally BP rises to levels that are much higher than those of baseline values. The most severe complications of AWS include encephalopathy, stroke, MI, and sudden death. The AWS is associated most commonly with centrally acting adrenergic agents (particularly clonidine) and β-adrenergic antagonists but has been reported with other agents as well including diuretics. Rarely should BP medications be withdrawn; rather, in discontinuing therapy these drugs should be tapered over several days to weeks unless other medications are used to substitute in the interim. Discontinuation of antihypertensive medications should be done with caution in patients with preexisting cerebrovascular or cardiac disease. Management of AWS by reinstitution of the previously administered drug is generally effective. Sodium nitroprusside (Table 2) is the treatment of choice when parenteral administration of an antihypertensive agent is required or when the identity of the previously administered agent is unknown. In the AWS caused by clonidine, β-adrenergic antagonists should not be used because unopposed α-adrenergic activity will be augmented and may exacerbate hypertension. However, labetalol (Table 2) may be useful in this situation.

PATIENT EDUCATION

Patient education is an essential component of the treatment plan and promotes patient compliance. Physicians should emphasize that:

• Lifelong treatment is usually required.
• Symptoms are an unreliable gauge of severity of hypertension.
• Prognosis improves with proper management.
• Lifestyle modifications are essential.

MONITORING/FOLLOW-UP

• BP measurements should be performed on multiple occasions under nonstressful circumstances (e.g., rest, sitting, empty bladder, comfortable temperature) to obtain an accurate assessment of BP in a given patient.

- Hypertension should not be diagnosed on the basis of one measurement alone, unless it is >210/120 mm Hg or accompanied by target organ damage. Two or more abnormal readings should be obtained, preferably over a period of several weeks, before therapy is considered.
- Care should also be used to exclude pseudohypertension, which usually occurs in elderly individuals with stiff, noncompressible vessels. A palpable artery that persists after cuff inflation (Osler sign) should alert the physician to this possibility.
- Home and ambulatory BP monitoring can be used to assess a patient's true average BP, which correlates better with target organ damage. Circumstances in which ambulatory BP monitoring might be of value include:
  - Suspected "white-coat hypertension" (increases in BP associated with the stress of physician office visits) should be evaluated carefully.
  - Evaluation of possible "drug resistance" where suspected.

Dyslipidemia

GENERAL PRINCIPLES

- Lipids are sparingly soluble molecules that include cholesterol, fatty acids, and their derivatives.
- Plasma lipids are transported by lipoprotein particles composed of proteins called **apolipoproteins,** and **phospholipids, cholesterol esters,** and **triglycerides.**
- Human plasma lipoproteins are separated into **five major classes** based on density:
  - Chylomicrons (least dense)
  - Very-low-density lipoproteins (VLDLs)
  - Intermediate-density lipoproteins (IDLs)
  - Low-density lipoproteins (LDLs)
  - High-density lipoproteins (HDLs)
  - A sixth class, lipoprotein(a) [Lp(a)], resembles LDL in lipid composition and has a density that overlaps LDL and HDL
- Physical properties of plasma lipoproteins are summarized in Table 5.

Table 5	Physical Properties of Plasma Lipoproteins		
Lipoprotein	**Lipid Composition**	**Origin**	**Apolipoproteins**
Chylomicrons	TG, 90%; chol, 3%	Intestine	B-48; C-I, C-II, C-III; E
VLDL	TG, 55%; chol, 20%	Liver	B-100; C-I, C-II, C-III; E
IDL	TG, 30%; chol, 35%	Metabolic product of VLDL	B-100; C-I, C-II, C-III; E
LDL	TG, 10%; chol, 50%	Metabolic product of IDL	B-100
HDL	TG, 5%; chol, 20%	Liver, intestine	A-I, A-II, A-IV; C-I, C-II, C-III; E
Lp(a)	TG, 10%; chol, 50%	Liver	B-100; Apo(a)

Chol, cholesterol; HDL, high-density lipoprotein; IDL, intermediate-density lipoprotein; LDL, low-density lipoprotein; Lp(a), lipoprotein(a); TG, triglyceride; VLDL, very-low-density lipoprotein.
[a]Balance of particle composition: protein and phospholipid.

- **Atherosclerosis and lipoproteins.** Nearly 90% of patients with coronary heart disease (CHD) have some form of dyslipidemia. Increased levels of LDL, remnant lipoproteins, and Lp(a) as well as decreased levels of HDL have all been associated with an increased risk of premature vascular disease (*J Am Coll Cardiol 1992;19:792–802*; *Circulation 1998;97:2519–2526*).
- **Clinical dyslipoproteinemias**
  - Most dyslipidemias are multifactorial in etiology and reflect the effects of uncharacterized genetic influences coupled with diet, activity, smoking, alcohol use, and comorbid conditions such as obesity and DM.
  - Differential diagnosis of the major lipid abnormalities is summarized in Table 6.
  - The major genetic dyslipoproteinemias are reviewed in Table 7 (*Circulation 1974; 49:476–488*; *J Lipid Res 1990;31:1337–1349*; *Clin Invest 1993;71:362–366*).
- **Standards of care for hyperlipidemia**
  - LDL cholesterol–lowering therapy, particularly with hydroxymethylglutaryl-coenzyme A (HMG-CoA) reductase inhibitors, lowers the risk of CHD-related death, morbidity, and revascularization procedures in hypercholesterolemic patients with (secondary prevention) (*Lancet 1994;344:1383–1389*; *N Engl J Med 1996;335:1001–1009*; *N Engl J Med 1998;339:1349–1357*; *Lancet 2002;360:7–22*) or without (primary prevention) known CHD (*Lancet 2002;360:7–22*; *N Engl J Med 1995;333:1301–1307*; *JAMA 1998;279:1615–1622*; *Lancet 2003;361: 1149–1158*; *Lancet 2004;364:685–696*).
  - Identification and management of high LDL cholesterol is the primary goal of the National Cholesterol Education Program's (NCEP's) third expert report

Table 6	Differential Diagnosis of Major Lipid Abnormalities	
Lipid Abnormality	**Primary Disorders**	**Secondary Disorders**
Hypercholesterolemia	Polygenic, familial hypercholesterolemia, familial defective apo B-100	Hypothyroidism, nephrotic syndrome
Hypertriglyceridemia	Lipoprotein lipase deficiency, apo C-II deficiency, familial hypertriglyceridemia	Diabetes mellitus, obesity, metabolic syndrome, alcohol use, oral estrogen
Combined hyperlipidemia	Familial combined hyperlipidemia, type III hyperlipoproteinemia	Diabetes mellitus, obesity, metabolic syndrome, hypothyroidism, nephrotic syndrome
Low HDL	Familial alpha lipoproteinemia, Tangier disease, familial HDL deficiency, lecithin:cholesterol acyltransferase deficiency	Diabetes mellitus, metabolic syndrome, hyper-triglyceridemia, smoking

HDL, high-density lipoprotein.

Table 7	Review of Major Genetic Dyslipoproteinemias			
Type of Genetic Dyslipidemia	Typical Lipid Profile	Type of Inheritance	Phenotypic Features	Other Information
Familial hyper-cholesterolemia (FH)	• Increased total (>300 mg/dL) and LDL (>250 mg/dL) cholesterol • Homozygous form (rare) can have total cholesterol >600 mg/dL and LDL >550 mg/dL	Autosomal dominant	• Premature CAD • Tendon xanthomas • Xanthelasmas • Premature arcus corneae	Due to mutations of the LDL receptor that lead to defective uptake and degradation of LDL
Familial combined hyperlipidemia (FCH)	• High levels of VLDL, LDL, or both • LDL apo B-100 level >130 mg/dL	Autosomal dominant	• Premature CAD • Patients do *not* develop tendon xanthomas	Genetic and metabolic defects are not established
Familial defective apolipoprotein B-100	• Similar to familial hypercholesterolemia		• Similar to familial hypercholesterolemia	Most all cases are due to a glutamine for arginine mutation at amino acid 3500 of apo B-100
Type III hyperlipoproteinemia (familial dysbetalipoproteinemia)	• Symmetric elevations of cholesterol and triglycerides (300–500 mg/dL) • Elevated VLDL to triglyceride ratio (>0.3)	Autosomal recessive	• Premature CAD • Tuberous or tuberoeruptive xanthomas • Planar xanthomas of the palmar creases are essentially pathognomonic	Many homozygotes are normolipidemic and emergence of hyperlipidemia often requires a secondary metabolic factor such as diabetes mellitus, hypothyroidism, or obesity

(continued)

Table 7   Review of Major Genetic Dyslipoproteinemias (*Continued*)

Type of Genetic Dyslipidemia	Typical Lipid Profile	Type of Inheritance	Phenotypic Features	Other Information
Chylomicronemia syndrome	• Most patients have triglycerides in the range of 150–500 mg/dL • Clinical manifestations occur when triglycerides exceed 1,500 mg/dL	• Onset before puberty indicates deficiency of lipoprotein lipase or apo C-II, both autosomal recessive • Familial hypertriglyceridemia is an autosomal dominant disorder caused by overproduction of VLDL triglycerides and manifests in adults	• Eruptive xanthomas • Lipemia retinalis • Pancreatitis • Hepatosplenomegaly	Familial hypertriglyceridemia and FCH patients may develop chylomicronemia syndrome in the presence of secondary factors such as obesity, alcohol use, or diabetes

CAD, coronary artery disease; LDL, low-density lipoprotein; VLDL, very-low-density lipoprotein.

on cholesterol management in adults, or Adult Treatment Program III (ATP III) (*JAMA 2001;285:2486–2497*).
- The ATP III executive summary and full report can be viewed online at www. nhlbi.nih.gov/guidelines/cholesterol/.

DIAGNOSIS

Screening

- Screening for hypercholesterolemia should begin **in all adults aged 20 years or older.**
- Screening is best performed with a lipid profile (total cholesterol, LDL cholesterol, HDL cholesterol, and triglycerides) obtained after a 12-hour fast.
- If a fasting lipid panel cannot be obtained, total and HDL cholesterol should be measured.
- Measurement of fasting lipids is indicated if the total cholesterol is ≥200 mg/dL or HDL cholesterol is ≤40 mg/dL.
- If lipids are unremarkable and the patient has no major risk factors for CHD (Table 8), then screening can be performed every 5 years (*JAMA 2001;285:2486–2497*).
- Patients hospitalized for an acute coronary syndrome (ACS) or coronary revascularization should have a lipid panel obtained within 24 hours of admission if lipid levels are unknown.
- Individuals with hyperlipidemia should be evaluated for potential **secondary causes,** including hypothyroidism, DM, obstructive liver disease, chronic renal disease, or nephrotic syndrome, or medications such as estrogens, progestins, anabolic steroids, and corticosteroids.

TREATMENT

- **Therapeutic lifestyle change**
  - ATP III thresholds for initiating cholesterol-lowering therapy with **therapeutic lifestyle change** (TLC, diet and exercise) and **hypolipidemic drugs** are summarized in Table 9 (*Circulation 2004;110:227–239*).

Table 8	Major Risk Factors That Modify LDL Goals

Cigarette smoking
Hypertension (blood pressure ≥ 140/90 mm Hg or on antihypertensive medication)
Low HDL cholesterol (<40 mg/dL)[a]
Family history of premature CHD (CHD in male first-degree relative <age 55 yr; CHD in female first-degree relative <age 65 yr)
Age (men ≥ 45 yr; women ≥ 55 yr)

CHD, coronary heart disease; HDL, high-density lipoprotein; LDL, low-density lipoprotein.
[a]HDL cholesterol ≥60 mg/dL counts as a "negative" risk factor; its presence removes one risk factor from the total count.
Modified from Expert Panel on Detection, Evaluation, and Treatment of High Blood Cholesterol in Adults. Executive Summary of the Third Report of the National Cholesterol Education Program (NCEP) Expert Panel on Detection, Evaluation, and Treatment of High Blood Cholesterol in Adults (Adult Treatment Panel III). *JAMA* 2001;285:2486–2497.

Table 9	ATP III Low-Density LDL-C Goals and Thresholds for Therapeutic Lifestyle Changes and Drug Therapy		
Category	**LDL-C Goal**	**Start TLC**	**Start Drug Therapy**
Very high risk	<70 mg/dL	Any LDL-C	LDL-C ≥70 mg/dL
High risk	<100 mg/dL	≥100 mg/dL	≥100 mg/dL (consider if baseline LDL-C < 100 mg/dL)
Moderately high risk	<130 mg/dL (<100 mg/dL optional)	≥130 mg/dL	≥130 mg/dL (optional if baseline LDL-C 100–129 mg/dL)
Moderate risk	<130 mg/dL	≥130 mg/dL	≥160 mg/dL
Lower risk	<160 mg/dL	≥160 mg/dL	≥190 mg/dL (optional if baseline LDL-C 160–189 mg/dL)

ATP III, Adult Treatment Panel III; LDL-C, low-density lipoprotein cholesterol; TLC, therapeutic lifestyle changes.
Modified from Grundy SM, Cleeman C, Merz NB, et al. Implications of recent clinical trials for the National Cholesterol Education Program Adult Treatment Panel III Guidelines. *Circulation* 2004;110:227–239.

- ○ All patients requiring cholesterol treatment should implement a diet restricted in total and saturated fat intake in accordance with ATP III recommendations (Table 10) (*JAMA 2001;285:2486–2497*).
- ○ Moderate exercise and weight reduction is also recommended.
- ○ A registered dietitian may be helpful to plan and start a saturated fat–restricted and weight loss–promoting diet.
- • **Treatment targets**
  - • **High risk and very high risk**
    - ○ The ATP III LDL cholesterol treatment target for all high-risk patients is <100 mg/dL (*JAMA 2001;285:2486–2497*).
    - ○ For CHD patients in the **very-high-risk** category, an LDL cholesterol <70 mg/dL is a therapeutic option (*Circulation 2004;110:227–239*).
    - ○ An LDL cholesterol of ≥100 mg/dL is now identified as the threshold for simultaneous treatment with TLC and lipid-lowering agents (*Circulation 2004;110:227–239*).
    - ○ Based on outcomes in the Heart Protection Study (HPS), lipid-lowering drug therapy is also an option for patients with CHD and baseline LDL cholesterol < 100 mg/dL (*Lancet 2002;360:7–22*).
    - ○ If a high-risk patient has hypertriglyceridemia or low HDL cholesterol, a fibrate or nicotinic acid (niacin) may be added to cholesterol-lowering therapy (*Circulation 2004;110:227–239*).
  - • **Moderately high risk**
    - ○ Patients with two or more non-LDL cholesterol risk factors and a Framingham point score predicting a 10-year CHD risk of 10% to 20% are considered at **moderately high risk** of CHD.

Table 10	Nutrient Composition of the Therapeutic Lifestyle Change Diet
Nutrient	**Recommended Intake**
Saturated fat[a]	<7% of total calories
Polyunsaturated fat	Up to 10% of total calories
Monounsaturated fat	Up to 20% of total calories
Total fat	25–35% of total calories
Carbohydrate[b]	50–60% of total calories
Fiber	20–30 g/d
Protein	Approximately 15% of total calories
Cholesterol	<200 mg/d
Total calories (energy)[c]	Balance energy intake and expenditure to maintain desirable body weight/prevent weight gain

[a]Trans fatty acids are another low-density lipoprotein (LDL)–raising fat that should be kept at a low intake.
[b]Carbohydrate should be derived predominantly from foods rich in complex carbohydrates, including grains (especially whole grains), fruits, and vegetables.
[c]Daily energy expenditure should include at least moderate physical activity (contributing approximately 200 kcal/d).
From Executive Summary of the Third Report of the National Cholesterol Education Program (NCEP) Expert Panel on Detection, Evaluation, and Treatment of High Blood Cholesterol in Adults (Adult Treatment Panel III). *JAMA* 2001;285:2486–2497, with permission.

- ○ Pharmacotherapy should be initiated if LDL cholesterol is ≥130 mg/dL.
  - ○ ATP III identifies an LDL cholesterol target < 100 mg/dL as optional for this group, with drug therapy to be considered for patients with baseline LDL cholesterol 100 to 129 mg/dL.
  - ○ Patients with two or more risk factors and a 10-year risk <10% are candidates for drug therapy when LDL cholesterol remains ≥160 mg/dL despite TLC (*Circulation 2004;110:227–239*).
- **Low risk**
  - ○ For **low-risk patients** (0 to 1 risk factors), cholesterol-lowering therapy should be considered if the LDL cholesterol is ≥190 mg/dL, especially for patients who have undergone a 3-month trial of TLC.
  - ○ Patients with very high LDL concentrations (≥190 mg/dL) often have a hereditary dyslipidemia and require treatment with multiple lipid-lowering agents. These patients should be referred to a lipid specialist, and family members should be screened with a fasting lipid battery.
  - ○ When LDL cholesterol is 160 to 189 mg/dL, drug therapy should be considered if the patient has a significant risk factor for cardiovascular disease, such as heavy tobacco use, poorly controlled hypertension, strong family history of early CHD, or low HDL cholesterol (*Circulation 2004;110:227–239*).
- **Assessing response to therapy**
  - **Response to therapy should be assessed after 6 weeks** and the dose of medication titrated if the LDL cholesterol treatment target is not achieved.
  - The initial dose of a cholesterol-lowering drug should be sufficient to achieve a 30% to 40% reduction in LDL cholesterol.

Table 11	ATP III Diagnostic Criteria for the Metabolic Syndrome
Risk Factor	**ATP III[a] Definition**
Carbohydrate metabolism	Fasting glucose $\geq$ 110 mg/dL (alternatively >100 mg/dL)
Abdominal obesity[b]	Men, waist > 40 in.
	Women, waist > 35 in.
Dyslipidemia	Triglycerides $\geq$ 150 mg/dL
	Men, HDL cholesterol < 40 mg/dL
	Women, HDL cholesterol < 50 mg/dL
Hypertension	BP $\geq$ 130/85 mm Hg

ATP III, Adult Treatment Panel III; BP, blood pressure; HDL, high-density lipoprotein.
[a]To qualify for the diagnosis of metabolic syndrome by ATP III criteria, a patient must meet at least three of the five criteria (hyperglycemia, abdominal obesity, high triglycerides, low HDL cholesterol, high blood pressure).
[b]Waist circumferences in Asian and South Asian patients may require different cutpoints.
Modified from Executive Summary of the Third Report of the National Cholesterol Education Program (NCEP) Expert Panel on Detection, Evaluation, and Treatment of High Blood Cholesterol in Adults (Adult Treatment Panel III). *JAMA* 2001;285:2486–2497.

- If target LDL cholesterol has not been reached after 12 weeks, current therapy should be intensified by further dose titration, adding another lipid-lowering agent, or referral to a lipid specialist.
- Patients at goal should be monitored every 4 to 6 months.
- **Metabolic syndrome**
  - The constellation of abdominal obesity, hypertension, glucose intolerance, and an atherogenic lipid profile (hypertriglyceridemia; low HDL cholesterol; and small, dense LDL cholesterol) characterizes a condition called the **metabolic syndrome.** ATP III diagnostic criteria for the metabolic syndrome are summarized in Table 11 (*JAMA 2001;285:2486–2497*; http://www.idf.org/home/index.cfm?node=1429).
  - Approximately 22% of Americans qualify for a diagnosis of the metabolic syndrome by ATP III criteria. Prevalence is increased in older individuals, women, Hispanic Americans, and African Americans (*JAMA 2002;287:356–359*).
  - Multiple studies have demonstrated an association between cardiovascular events and death and all-cause mortality with the metabolic syndrome (*Am J Med 2006; 119:812–819*).
  - ATP III recognizes the metabolic syndrome as a **secondary treatment** target after LDL cholesterol is controlled (*JAMA 2001;285:2486–2497*).
  - The report recommends treating the underlying causes of metabolic syndrome (overweight/obesity, physical inactivity) by implementing weight loss and aerobic exercise and managing cardiovascular risks, such as hypertension, that may persist despite lifestyle changes (*JAMA 2001;285:2486–2497*).
- **Hypertriglyceridemia**
  - Recent analyses suggest that hypertriglyceridemia is an **independent cardiovascular risk factor** (*Circulation 2007;115:450–458*; *Ann Intern Med 2007;147:377–385*).
  - Hypertriglyceridemia is often observed in the metabolic syndrome, and there are many potential etiologies for hypertriglyceridemia, including obesity, DM, renal

insufficiency, genetic dyslipidemias, and therapy with oral estrogen, glucocorticoids, or β-blockers.

- The ATP III classification of serum triglyceride levels is as follows (*JAMA 2001; 285:2486–2497*):
  - ○ Normal: <150 mg/dL
  - ○ Borderline-high: 150 to 199 mg/dL
  - ○ High: 200 to 499 mg/dL
  - ○ Very high: ≥500 mg/dL
- Treatment of hypertriglyceridemia depends on the degree of severity.
  - ○ For patients with very high triglycerides, triglyceride reduction through a very low fat diet (≤15% of calories), exercise, weight loss, and drugs (fibrates, niacin) is the primary goal of therapy to prevent acute pancreatitis.
  - ○ When patients have a lesser degree of hypertriglyceridemia, control of LDL cholesterol is the primary aim of initial therapy. TLC is emphasized as the initial intervention to lower triglycerides (*JAMA 2001;285:2486–2497*).
- **Non-HDL cholesterol**
  - Non-HDL cholesterol is a secondary treatment target.
  - A patient's non-HDL cholesterol is calculated by subtracting HDL cholesterol from total cholesterol.
  - Target non-HDL cholesterol is 30 mg/dL higher than the LDL cholesterol target.
  - LDL and non-HDL cholesterol treatment targets for various degrees of cardiovascular risk are summarized in Table 12 (*JAMA 2001;285:2486–2497*; *Circulation 2004;110:227–239*).
- **Low HDL cholesterol**
  - One of the modifications from ATP II includes redefining low HDL cholesterol as <40 mg/dL.
  - Low HDL cholesterol is an **independent CHD risk factor** that is identified as a non-LDL cholesterol risk and included as a component of the Framingham scoring algorithm (*JAMA 1986;256:2835–2838*).
  - Etiologies for low HDL cholesterol include physical inactivity, obesity, insulin resistance, DM, hypertriglyceridemia, cigarette smoking, high-carbohydrate diets (>60% calories), and certain medications (β-blockers, anabolic steroids, progestins).

Table 12	Comparison of LDL-C and Non-HDL-C Goals by CHD Risk Category	
Category	**LDL-C Target (mg/dL)**	**Non-HDL-C Target (mg/dL)**
Very high risk	<70	<100
High risk	<100	<130
Moderately high risk	<130	<160
Moderate risk	<130	<160
Low risk	<160	<190

CHD, coronary heart disease; HDL-C, high-density lipoprotein cholesterol; LDL-C, low-density lipoprotein cholesterol.
Modified from Grundy SM, Cleeman C, Merz NB, et al. Implications of recent clinical trials for the National Cholesterol Education Program Adult Treatment Panel III Guidelines. *Circulation* 2004;110:227–239.

- Because therapeutic interventions for low HDL cholesterol are of limited efficacy, ATP III identifies **LDL cholesterol as the primary target of therapy for patients with low HDL cholesterol.**
- Low HDL cholesterol often occurs in the setting of hypertriglyceridemia and metabolic syndrome. Management of these conditions may result in improvement of HDL cholesterol.
- Aerobic exercise, weight loss, smoking cessation, menopausal estrogen replacement, and treatment with niacin or fibrates may elevate low HDL cholesterol (*JAMA 2001;285:2486–2497*).
- **Lipid-lowering therapy and age**
  - The risk of a fatal or nonfatal cardiovascular event increases with age, and most cardiovascular events occur in patients aged 65 years and older.
  - Secondary prevention trials with the HMG-CoA reductase inhibitors have demonstrated significant clinical benefit for patients aged 65 to 75 years.
  - The HPS failed to show an age threshold for primary or secondary prevention with statin therapy. Patients aged 75 to 80 years at study entry experienced a nearly 30% reduction in major vascular events (*Lancet 2002;360:7–22*).
  - The Prospective Study of Pravastatin in the Elderly (PROSPER) trial found a significant reduction in major coronary events among patients aged 70 to 82 years with vascular disease or CHD risks treated with pravastatin (*Lancet 2002;360:1623–1630*).
  - **ATP III does not place age restrictions** on treatment of hypercholesterolemia in elderly adults.
  - ATP III recommends TLC for young adults (men aged 20 to 35 years; women aged 20 to 45 years) with an LDL level ≥ 130 mg/dL. Drug therapy should be considered in the following high-risk groups:
    - Men who both smoke and have elevated LDL levels (160 to 189 mg/dL).
    - All young adults with an LDL ≥ 190 mg/dL.
    - Those with an inherited dyslipidemia (*JAMA 2001;285:2486–2497*).
- **Treatment of elevated LDL cholesterol**
  - **HMG-CoA reductase inhibitors (statins)**
    - Statins (Table 13) are the treatment of choice for elevated LDL cholesterol (*JAMA 2001;285:2486–2497*; *N Engl J Med 1999;341:498–511*; *Ann Pharmacother 2002;36:1907–1917*; *Circulation 2002;106:1024–1028*; *JAMA 1984;251:351–364*).

Table 13	Currently Available Statins					
Name	**Atorvastatin**	**Fluvastatin**	**Lovastatin**	**Pravastatin**	**Rosuvastatin**	**Simvastatin**
Dose range (mg PO/d)	10–80	20–80	10–80	10–80	5–40	10–80
Triglyceride effect (%)	↓ 13–32	↓ 5–35	↓ 2–13	↓ 3–15	↓ 10–35	↓ 12–36
LDL effect (%)	↓ 38–54	↓ 17–36	↓ 29–8	↓ 19–34	↓ 41—65	↓ 28–46
HDL effect (%)	↑ 4.8–5.5	↑ 0.9–12	↑ 4.6–8	↑ 3–9.9	↑ 10–14	↑ 5.2–10

HDL, high-density lipoprotein; LDL, low-density lipoprotein; ↑, increased; ↓, decreased.

- The lipid-lowering effect of statins appears within the first week of use and becomes stable after approximately 4 weeks of use.
- Common side effects (5% to 10% of patients) include GI upset (e.g., abdominal pain, diarrhea, bloating, constipation), and muscle pain or weakness, which can occur without creatinine kinase elevations. Other potential side effects include malaise, fatigue, headache, and rash (*N Engl J Med 1999;341:498–511*; *JAMA 1984;251:351–364*).
- Elevations of liver transaminases two to three times the upper limit of normal are dose dependent and reversible with discontinuation of the drug.
  - Liver enzymes should be measured before initiating therapy, at 8 to 12 weeks after dose initiation or titration, then every 6 months.
  - The medication should be discontinued if liver transaminases elevate to more than three times the upper limit of normal (*Circulation 2002;106:1024–1028*).
- Because some of the statins undergo metabolism by the cytochrome P450 enzyme system, taking them in combination with other drugs metabolized by this enzyme system increases the risk of **rhabdomyolysis** (*N Engl J Med 1999;341:498–511*; *Circulation 2002;106:1024–1028*).
  - Among these drugs are fibrates (greater risk with gemfibrozil), itraconazole, ketoconazole, erythromycin, clarithromycin, cyclosporin, nefazodone, and protease inhibitors (*Circulation 2002;106:1024–1028*).
  - Statins may also interact with large quantities of grapefruit juice to increase the risk of myopathy, although the precise mechanism of this interaction is unclear.
  - Simvastatin can increase levels of warfarin and digoxin. Rosuvastatin may also increase warfarin levels.
- **Bile acid sequestrant resins**
  - Currently available bile acid sequestrant resins include the following:
    - **Cholestyramine**: 4 to 24 g PO/d in divided doses before meals.
    - **Colestipol**: tablets, 2 to 16 g PO/d; granules, 5 to 30 g PO/d in divided doses before meals.
    - **Colesevelam**: 625-mg tablets; 3 tablets PO bid or 6 tablets PO daily with food (maximum, 7 tablets PO/d).
  - Bile acid sequestrants typically lower LDL levels by 15% to 30% and thereby lower the incidence of CHD (*N Engl J Med 1999;341:498–511*; *JAMA 1984;251:351–364*). These agents should not be used as monotherapy in patients with triglyceride levels > 250 mg/dL because they can raise triglyceride levels. They may be combined with nicotinic acid or statins.
  - Common side effects of resins include constipation, abdominal pain, bloating, nausea, and flatulence.
  - Bile acid sequestrants may decrease oral absorption of many other drugs, including warfarin, digoxin, thyroid hormone, thiazide diuretics, amiodarone, glipizide, and statins.
    - Colesevelam interacts with fewer drugs than the older resins.
    - Other medications should be given 1 hour before or 4 hours after resins.
- **Nicotinic acid (Niacin)**
  - Niacin can lower LDL cholesterol levels by ≥15%, lower triglyceride levels 20% to 50%, and raise HDL cholesterol levels by up to 35% (*Circulation 2007;115:450–458*; *Arch Intern Med 1994;154:1586–1595*).
  - Crystalline niacin is given 1 to 3 g PO/d in two to three divided doses with meals. Extended-release niacin is dosed at night. The starting dose is 500 mg PO, and

the dose may be titrated monthly in 500-mg increments to a maximum of 2,000 mg PO (administer dose with milk or crackers).

○ Common side effects of niacin include flushing, pruritus, headache, nausea, and bloating. Other potential side effects include elevation of liver transaminases, hyperuricemia, and hyperglycemia.
- Flushing may be decreased with use of aspirin 30 minutes before the first few doses.
- Hepatotoxicity associated with niacin is partially dose dependent and appears to be more prevalent with over-the-counter time-release preparations.

○ Avoid use of niacin in patients with gout, liver disease, active peptic ulcer disease, and uncontrolled DM.
- Niacin can be used with care in patients with well-controlled DM (HgA$_{1c}$ ≤ 7%).
- Serum transaminases, glucose, and uric acid levels should be monitored every 6 to 8 weeks during dose titration, then every 4 months.

- **Ezetimibe**
  ○ Ezetimibe is currently the only available cholesterol absorption inhibitor.
  ○ It appears to act at the brush border of the small intestine and inhibits cholesterol absorption.
  ○ The recommended dosing is 10 mg PO once daily. No dosage adjustment is required for renal insufficiency, mild hepatic impairment, or in elderly patients.
  ○ Ezetimibe may provide an additional 25% mean reduction in LDL when combined with a statin and provides an approximately 18% decrease in LDL when used as monotherapy (*Am J Cardiol 2002;90:1092–1097*; *Eur Heart J 2003;24:729–741*; *Am J Cardiol 2002;90:1084–1091*; *Mayo Clin Proc 2004;79: 620–629*).
  ○ It is not recommended for use in patients with moderate to severe hepatic impairment.
  ○ There appear to be few side effects associated with ezetimibe.
    - In clinical trials, there was no excess of rhabdomyolysis or myopathy when compared with statin or placebo alone.
    - There is a low incidence of diarrhea and abdominal pain compared to placebo. Liver function monitoring is not required with monotherapy because there appears to be no significant impact on liver enzymes when this drug is used alone.
    - Liver enzymes should be monitored when used in conjunction with a statin, as there appears to be a slight increased incidence of enzyme elevations with combination therapy.
  ○ Long-term clinical outcome trials of ezetimibe are ongoing. There has been one short-term surrogate outcome trial suggesting a lack of additive effectiveness with regard to carotid intima-media thickness (*N Engl J Med 2008;358:1431–1443*). The clinical utility of these results has been questioned and the matter is currently unresolved.

- **Treatment of hypertriglyceridemia**
  - **Nonpharmacologic treatment**
    ○ Nonpharmacologic treatments are important in the therapy of hypertriglyceridemia.
    ○ Nonpharmacologic approaches include the following:
      - Changing oral estrogen replacement to transdermal estrogen

- Decreasing alcohol intake
- Encouraging weight loss and exercise
- Controlling hyperglycemia in patients with DM
- Avoiding simple sugars and very high carbohydrate diets

- **Pharmacologic treatment**
  - Pharmacologic treatment of isolated hypertriglyceridemia consists of a fibric acid derivative or niacin.
  - Statins may be effective for patients with mild to moderate hypertriglyceridemia and concomitant LDL cholesterol elevation (*N Engl J Med 2007;357:1009–1017*).
  - **Fibric acid derivatives**
    - Currently available fibric acid derivatives include **Gemfibrozil**: 600 mg PO bid before meals; **Fenofibrate:** typically 48 to 145 mg PO/d.
    - Fibrates generally lower triglyceride levels 30% to 50% and increase HDL levels 10% to 35%. They can lower LDL levels by 5% to 25% in patients with normal triglyceride levels, but may actually increase LDL levels in patients with elevated triglyceride levels.
    - Common side effects include dyspepsia, abdominal pain, cholelithiasis, rash, and pruritus. Fibrates may potentiate the effects of warfarin (*N Engl J Med 1999;341:498–511*).
    - Gemfibrozil given in conjunction with statins may increase the risk of rhabdomyolysis (*Circulation 2002;106:1024–1028*; *Am J Med 2004;116:408–416*; *Am J Cardiol 2004;94:935–938*; *Am J Cardiol 2005;95:120–122*; *Lancet 2005;366:1849–1861*).
  - **Omega-3 fatty acids**
    - Omega-3 fatty acids from fish oil can lower triglycerides in high doses (*J Clin Invest 1984;74:82–89*; *J Lipid Res 1990;31:1549–1558*).
    - The active ingredients are eicosapentaenoic acid (EPA) and docosahexaenoic acid (DHA).
    - To lower triglyceride levels, 1 to 6 g of EPA plus DHA is needed daily.
    - Main side effects are burping, bloating, and diarrhea.
    - A prescription form of omega-3 acid fatty acids is available and is indicated for triglycerides over 500 mg/dL; four tablets contain about 3.6 g of omega-3 acid ethyl esters and can lower triglycerides by 30%.
    - In practice, omega-3 fatty acids are being used as an adjunct to statin or other drugs in patients with moderately elevated triglyceride levels.
    - The combination of omega-3 fatty acids plus statin has the advantage of avoiding the risk of myopathy seen in the statin–fibrate combination (*Am J Cardiol 2008;102:429–433*; *Am J Cardiol 2008;102:1040–1045*).
- **Treatment of low HDL cholesterol**
  - Low HDL cholesterol often occurs in the setting of hypertriglyceridemia and metabolic syndrome. Management of accompanying high LDL cholesterol, hypertriglyceridemia, and the metabolic syndrome may result in improvement of HDL cholesterol (*Circulation 2001;104:3046–3051.*)
  - Treatment specifically targeted at raising low HDL cholesterol levels may reduce the risk of cardiovascular events (*JAMA 2007;298:786–798*).
  - Nonpharmacologic therapies are the mainstay of treatment including:
    - Smoking cessation
    - Exercise
    - Weight loss

Table 14	ATP III Categories of CHD Risk
Category	**Definition**
Very high risk	CHD and: • Multiple risk factors (especially diabetes) • Severe and poorly controlled risk factors (especially continued cigarette smoking) • Multiple risk factors of the metabolic syndrome • Acute coronary syndromes
High risk	CHD or CHD risk equivalent
Moderately high risk	2+ risk factors and 10-yr CHD risk 10–20%
Moderate risk	2+ risk factors and 10-yr CHD risk <10%
Lower risk	0–1 risk factors

ATP III, Adult Treatment Panel III; CHD, coronary heart disease.
Modified from Grundy SM, Cleeman C, Merz NB, et al. Implications of recent clinical trials for the National Cholesterol Education Program Adult Treatment Panel III Guidelines. *Circulation* 2004;110:227.

- In addition, medications known to lower HDL levels should be avoided such as β-blockers, progestins, and androgenic compounds.
- **Niacin is the most effective pharmacologic agent for increasing HDL levels** (*J Lipid Res 1990;31:1549–1558*).

Lifestyle/Risk Modification

Risk assessment

- A major innovation of ATP III is a formal method of CHD risk assessment. ATP III now recognizes **five categories of CHD risk**: very high, high, moderately high, moderate, and lower risk. These CHD risk categories are defined in Table 14.
- DM, noncoronary atherosclerosis (symptomatic cerebrovascular disease, peripheral artery disease, abdominal aortic aneurysm), or multiple risk factors conferring a 10-year CHD risk of more than 20% are considered **CHD risk equivalents in ATP III** (*Circulation 2004;110:227–239*).
- Risk assessment for patients without known CHD or CHD risk equivalents begins with consideration of five risk factors summarized in Table 8 (*JAMA 2001;285:2486–2497*).
- A Framingham point score should be determined for any individual with two or more non-LDL cholesterol risk factors. **Framingham point score** algorithms for men and women are summarized in Table 15 (*JAMA 2001;285:2486–2497*; *Circulation 2004;110:227–239*; *Circulation 1998;97:1837–1847*).
- Patients with multiple non-LDL cholesterol CHD risk factors are then divided into those with a **10-year CHD risk >20%, 10% to 20%, or <10%.**
- Presently, emerging risk factors (e.g., obesity, sedentary lifestyle, prothrombotic and proinflammatory factors, and impaired fasting glucose) do not impact risk assessment, although they may influence clinical judgment when determining therapeutic options.

Table 15	Estimate of 10-Year risk (Framingham Point Scores) for Men and Women

Estimate of 10-yr Risk for Men

Age (yr)	Points
20–34	−9
35–39	−4
40–44	0
45–49	3
50–54	6
55–59	8
60–64	10
65–69	11
70–74	12
75–79	13

			Points		
Total Cholesterol	**Age 20–39**	**Age 40–49**	**Age 50–59**	**Age 60–69**	**Age 70–79**
<160	0	0	0	0	0
160–199	4	3	2	1	0
200–239	7	5	3	1	0
240–279	9	6	4	2	1
≥280	11	8	5	3	1

			Points		
	Age 20–39	**Age 40–49**	**Age 50–59**	**Age 60–69**	**Age 70–79**
Nonsmoker	0	0	0	0	0
Smoker	8	5	3	1	1

HDL (mg/dL)	Points	Systolic BP (mm Hg)	Points if Untreated	Points if Treated
≥60	−1	<120	0	0
50–59	0	120–129	0	1
40–49	1	130–139	1	2
<40	2	140–159	1	2
		≥160	2	3

Point Total	10-yr Risk (%)	Point total	10-yr Risk (%)
<0	<1	9	5
0	1	10	6
1	1	11	8
2	1	12	10
3	1	13	12
4	1	14	16
5	2	15	20
6	2	16	25
7	3	≥17	≥30
8	4		

(continued)

Table 15	Estimate of 10-Year risk (Framingham Point Scores) for Men and Women (*Continued*)

Estimate of 10-yr Risk in Women

Age (yr)	Points
20–34	–7
35–39	–3
40–44	0
45–49	3
50–54	6
55–59	8
60–64	10
65–69	12
70–74	14
75–79	16

			Points		
Total Cholesterol	Age 20–39	Age 40–49	Age 50–59	Age 60–69	Age 70–79
<160	0	0	0	0	0
160–199	4	3	2	1	1
200–239	8	6	4	2	1
240–279	11	8	5	3	2
≥280	13	10	7	4	2

			Points		
	Age 20–39	Age 40–49	Age 50–59	Age 60–69	Age 70–79
Nonsmoker	0	0	0	0	0
Smoker	9	7	4	2	1

HDL (mg/dL)	Points	Systolic BP (mm Hg)	Points if Untreated	Points if Treated
≥60	–1	<120	0	0
50–59	0	120–129	1	3
40–49	1	130–139	2	4
<40	2	140–159	3	5
		≥160	4	6

Point Total	10-yr Risk (%)	Point Total	10-yr Risk (%)
<9	<1	17	5
9	1	18	6
10	1	19	8
11	1	20	11
12	1	21	14
13	2	22	17
14	2	23	22
15	3	24	27
16	4	≥25	≥30

BP, blood pressure; HDL, high-density lipoprotein.
From Executive Summary of the Third Report of the National Cholesterol Education Program (NCEP) Expert Panel on Detection, Evaluation, and Treatment of High Blood Cholesterol in Adults (Adult Treatment Panel III). *JAMA* 2001;285:2486–2497, with permission.

CORONARY ARTERY DISEASE

General Coronary Artery Disease and Stable Exertional Angina

GENERAL PRINCIPLES

Definition

- Coronary artery disease (CAD) is most commonly defined as a >50% luminal stenosis of any epicardial coronary artery.
- Chronic stable angina is the typical manifestation of ischemic heart disease in nearly half of patients with CAD.

Epidemiology

- CAD is the leading cause of morbidity and mortality in Western Society.
- Prevalence of CAD in the United States was 7.6% as of 2006 (*American Heart Association, Heart Disease and Stroke Statistics 2009 Update*).
- Of the 16.8 million individuals in the United States carrying a diagnosis of CAD, 7.9 million presented as MI and 9.8 million as angina pectoris.
- CAD was responsible for 35.3% of all U.S. deaths in 2005.
- An estimated 785,000 Americans will have a first MI and 470,000 will have a recurrent MI in 2009. Another 195,000 will have a silent MI.

Etiology

- CAD most commonly results from luminal obstruction by atheromatous plaque.
- Other causes include congenital coronary abnormalities, myocardial bridging, vasculitis, prior radiation therapy, cocaine use, aortic stenosis, hypertrophic cardiomyopathy, coronary vasospasm, spontaneous coronary dissection, and syndrome X.

Pathophysiology

- CAD manifestations include stable angina, ACS, CHF, sudden cardiac death, and silent ischemia.
- ACS represents a continuum of clinical presentations ranging from UA to ST-segment elevation MI (STEMI). ACS most often results from acute thrombosis of a coronary artery at the site of atheromatous plaque rupture or ulceration.
- Stable angina most often results from fixed coronary lesions that produce a mismatch between myocardial oxygen supply and demand. This mismatch is accentuated by increasing cardiac workload.
- Anginal symptoms usually develop when a fixed stenosis reaches 70% or greater. In the setting of increased myocardial demand or diminished oxygen supply, the fixed stenosis does not permit adequate distal perfusion and ischemia results, manifesting itself as angina.

Risk Factors

- Hypertension
- Diabetes mellitus: The incidence of CAD in patients with diabetes is two to four times that of the general population. Insulin resistance, such as that seen with the metabolic syndrome, is associated with increased risk of CAD.

- Obesity increases the risk of CAD and is associated with additional cardiac risk factors, including hypertension, diabetes, and lipid abnormalities. A body mass index of >25 kg/m^2 is considered overweight and >30 kg/m^2 is obese.
- Dyslipidemia: Elevated LDL, low HDL, and elevated triglycerides are independent risk factors for CAD.
- Family history of premature CAD: Defined as first-degree male relative with CAD before age 55 or female relative before age 65.
- Tobacco use is associated with a marked increase in risk of CAD. The risk is reversible and smoking cessation restores the risk of CAD to that of a nonsmoker within approximately 15 years (*Arch Intern Med 1994 Jan 24;154(2):169–175*).

Prevention

- Aspirin (75 to 162 mg/d) should be considered in patients at higher risk of cardiovascular events ($>10\%$ risk of stroke or MI over 10 years). The U.S. Preventative Services Task Force recommends aspirin be used for men aged 45 to 79 and women aged 55 to 79 (http://www.ahrq.gov/clinic/USpstf/uspsasmi.htm#related).
- Regular cardiovascular risk assessment commencing at age 20 and recurring every 5 years. The **Framingham Risk Score** is a commonly used algorithm for estimating risk of CAD (http://hp2010.nhlbihin.net/ATPiii/calculator.asp?usertype=prof).
- Risk factor modification including tobacco cessation, treatment of hypertension, diabetes, obesity, and lipid control.
- Initiation of statin therapy may limit the risk of developing CAD in addition to subsequent MI and cardiac mortality in select patients who have an elevated CRP (*NEJM 2008;359:2195*).
- Current exercise guidelines recommend a minimum of 30 minutes of moderate-intensity aerobic physical activity 5 days per week in addition to activities of daily living (*Circulation 2007;116:1081–1093*).
- Hormone replacement therapy is not indicated for either primary or secondary CAD prevention in postmenopausal women.

Associated Conditions

- Stable angina
- Unstable angina
- Non–ST-segment elevation MI (NSTEMI)
- ST-segment elevation MI
- Congestive heart failure

DIAGNOSIS

Clinical Presentation

History

- Angina: Typical angina has three features: (i) substernal chest discomfort or heaviness with a characteristic quality and duration that is (ii) precipitated by stress and (iii) relieved by rest or nitroglycerin (NTG).
  - Atypical angina has two of these three features.
  - Noncardiac chest pain meets one or none of these characteristics.
- The severity of angina may be quantified using the Canadian Cardiovascular Society (CCS) classification system (Table 16).

Table 16	Canadian Cardiovascular Society Classification System
Class	**Definition**
CCS 1	Angina with strenuous activity
CCS 2	Angina with moderate activity (walking greater than two blocks or one flight of stairs)
CCS 3	Angina with mild activity (walking less than two blocks or one flight of stairs)
CCS 4	Angina that occurs with any activity or at rest

Anginal symptoms may include typical chest discomfort or anginal equivalents.
CCS, Canadian Cardiovascular Society.
From *Coronary Artery Dis* 2004;15:111, with permission.

- Associated symptoms may include dyspnea, diaphoresis, nausea, vomiting, and dizziness.
- Female patients and those with diabetes or chronic kidney disease may have minimal or atypical symptoms that serve as anginal equivalents. Such symptoms include dyspnea, epigastric pain, and nausea.
- A careful history usually provides sufficient information to establish an appropriate pretest probability of CAD. For instance, in men and older women, the presence of typical angina in association with other cardiac risk factors is strongly predictive of CAD (Table 17).

Physical Examination
- Clinical exam should include measurement of BP, heart rate, and arterial pulses.
- Cardiac exam findings including murmurs and gallops are of high importance.
- Clinical stigmata of hyperlipidemia such as corneal arcus and xanthelasmas should be noted.
- Signs of heart failure including an S_3 gallop, rales on lung exam, elevated jugular venous pulsation, and peripheral edema may also be present.

Table 17	Pretest Probability of Coronary Disease (%)					
	Nonanginal Chest Pain		**Atypical Angina**		**Typical Angina**	
Age (yr)	**Men**	**Women**	**Men**	**Women**	**Men**	**Women**
30–39	4	2	34	12	76	26
40–49	13	3	51	22	87	55
50–59	20	7	65	31	93	73
60–69	27	14	72	51	94	86

Pretest probability of CAD in Symptomatic Patients According to Age and Sex (Combined Diamond/Forrester and CASS Data). ACC/AHA 2002 Guideline Update for the Management of Patients with Chronic Stable Angina.

Diagnostic Criteria

Angina is primarily a clinical diagnosis that is made based on history, clinical presentation and known risk of coronary artery disease. This diagnosis is often supported by diagnostic testing as outlined below.

- First level list item 1
  - Second level list item 1

Differential Diagnosis

- A wide range of disorders may manifest with chest discomfort and may include both cardiovascular and noncardiovascular etiologies (Table 18).
- A careful history focused on cardiac risk factors, physical exam, and initial laboratory evaluation usually narrows the differential diagnosis.
- Despite these efforts, further diagnostic testing is often required to determine the likelihood of CAD (see stress testing).

Table 18	Differential Diagnosis of Chest Pain
Diagnosis	**Comments**
Cardiovascular	
Aortic stenosis	Anginal episodes can occur with severe aortic stenosis.
HCM	Subendocardial ischemia may occur with exercise and/or exertion.
Prinzmetal's angina	Coronary vasospasm that may be elicited by exertion or emotional stress.
Syndrome X	Ischemic chest pain in the presence of normal coronary arteries that is thought to be related to microvascular disease.
Pericarditis	Pleuritic chest pain associated with pericardial inflammation from infectious or autoimmune disease.
Aortic dissection	May mimic anginal pain and/or involve the coronary arteries.
Cocaine use	Results in coronary vasospasm and/or thrombus formation.
Other	
Anemia	Marked anemia can result in a myocardial O_2 supply–demand mismatch.
Thyrotoxicosis	Increase in myocardial demand may result in an O_2 supply–demand mismatch.
Esophageal disease	GERD and esophageal spasm can mimic angina (responsive to NTG).
Biliary colic	Gallstones can usually be visualized on abdominal sonography.
Pneumonia	Usually visualized on chest x-ray. The pain may be pleuritic.
Musculoskeletal	Costochondritis (Tsetse's syndrome).

HCM, hypertrophic cardiomyopathy; GERD, gastroesophageal reflux disease; NTG, nitroglycerin.

Diagnostic Testing

- **Stress testing and indications**
  - Patients without known CAD:
    - Not indicated in asymptomatic patients as a screening test.
    - Patients with anginal symptoms.
    - Asymptomatic intermediate-risk patients who plan on beginning a vigorous exercise program or those with high-risk occupations (e.g., airline pilot).
    - Asymptomatic high-risk patients with risk factors such as diabetes or peripheral vascular disease.
  - Patients with known CAD:
    - Post-MI risk stratification (see section on STEMI).
    - Preoperative risk assessment.
    - Recurrent anginal symptoms despite medical therapy or revascularization.
    - Routine screening in asymptomatic patients after revascularization is controversial.
- **Exercise stress testing (ETT)**
  - The test of choice for evaluating most patients of intermediate risk for CAD (Table 17).
  - Bruce Protocol: Consists of 3-minute stages of increasing treadmill speed and incline. BP, heart rate, and ECG are monitored throughout the study and the recovery period.
  - Specificity and sensitivity of 70% to 80% if the patient has a normal resting ECG and reaches the target heart rate (85% of maximal predicted heart rate for age).
  - The study is considered positive if:
    - New ST-segment depressions of >1 mm in multiple leads
    - Hypotensive response to exercise
    - Sustained ventricular arrhythmias are precipitated by exercise
  - The Duke Treadmill Score provides prognostic information for patients presenting with chronic angina (Table 19).
- **Stress testing with imaging**
  - Recommended for patients with the following baseline ECG abnormalities:
    - Preexcitation (Wolf–Parkinson–White syndrome)
    - Left ventricular hypertrophy (LVH)
    - Left bundle branch block (LBBB) or paced rhythm
    - Intraventricular conduction delay (IVCD)

Table 19	Exercise Stress Testing: Duke Treadmill Score	
Score	**Minutes exercised − [5 × maximum ST-segment deviation] − [4 × anginal score]** **Angina score: 0 = none, 1 = not test limiting, 2 = test limiting**	
>5	Annual mortality 0.25%	Medical therapy
−10 to 4	Annual mortality 1.25%	Further testing based on risk factors and imaging
<−10	Annual mortality >5%	Coronary angiography

In general β-blockers, other nodal blocking agents, and nitrates should be discontinued prior to stress testing.
From *NEJM* 1991;325:849, with permission.

- ◦ Digoxin effects
- ◦ Resting ST-segment or T-wave changes
- **Myocardial perfusion imaging.** Commonly utilizes tracers Thalium-201 or technetium-99m in conjunction with exercise or pharmacologic stress. Perfusion imaging allows the diagnosis and localization of areas of ischemia and allows determination of ejection fraction. Myocardial viability can also be assessed via this technique. Nuclear perfusion stress imaging has a sensitivity of 85% to 90% and specificity of 70%.
- **Echocardiographic imaging.** Exercise or dobutamine stress testing can be performed with echocardiography to aid in the diagnosis of CAD. As with nuclear imaging, echocardiography adds to the sensitivity and specificity of the test by revealing areas with wall motion abnormalities. The technical quality of this study can be limited by imaging quality (i.e., obesity). Stress echocardiography has a sensitivity of 75% and specificity of 85% to 90%.
- **Magnetic resonance perfusion imaging** with adenosine utilizing contrast enhancement is another tool to evaluate myocardial ischemia and viability.
- **Pharmacologic stress testing**
  - In patients who are unable to exercise, pharmacologic stress testing may be preferable.
  - Dipyridamole, adenosine, and regadenoson are vasodilators that are commonly used in conjunction with myocardial perfusion scintigraphy. These agents are the agents of choice in patients with LBBB or paced rhythm on ECG due to the increased incidence of false-positive stress tests with either exercise or dobutamine infusion.
  - Dobutamine is a positive inotrope commonly used with echocardiographic stress tests.
- **Contraindications to stress testing**
  - Acute MI within 2 days
  - UA not previously stabilized by medical therapy
  - Cardiac arrhythmias causing symptoms or hemodynamic compromise
  - Symptomatic severe aortic stenosis
  - Symptomatic heart failure
  - Acute pulmonary embolus, myocarditis, pericarditis, or aortic dissection

Diagnostic Procedures
Coronary Angiography

- The gold standard for evaluating coronary anatomy that quantifies the presence and severity of atherosclerotic lesions.
- Should be performed in patients with known or suspected angina with a markedly positive stress test or who have survived sudden cardiac death.
- Can be used to evaluate patients who are suspected of having a nonatherosclerotic cause of ischemia (e.g., coronary anomaly, coronary dissection, radiation vasculopathy).
- Consider cardiac catheterization in patients who have recurrent chest pain despite aggressive medical therapy for angina.
- Can assist in the diagnosis of vasospasm.
- Intravascular ultrasound (IVUS): Can assess plaque burden, providing definitive assessment of the coronary vasculature at time of catheterization.
- Coronary flow reserve as measured by Doppler or pressure techniques aids in the assessment of the functional significance of a stenotic lesion.

- Left ventricular catheterization: Allows measurement of LV filling pressure, aortic valve gradient, and an assessment of regional wall motion via contrast ventriculography.
- Noninvasive alternatives to coronary angiography include coronary CT angiography and magnetic resonance angiography. These modalities are currently under intensive study. Compared to invasive coronary angiography, CT angiography has a sensitivity of 80% to 90% and specificity of 85% (*Circulation 2006;114:2334*). This modality is limited by radiation exposure, requirement for HR less than 70 bpm, and presence of coronary calcification or stents.

TREATMENT

- The major goal of treatment in patients with stable angina is to prevent MI, cardiac death, and to reduce symptoms.
- A combination of lifestyle modification, medical therapy, and coronary revascularization should be employed. A recommended strategy for the evaluation and management of the patient with stable angina can be found in Figure 1.
- **Medical treatment** is aimed at improving myocardial oxygen supply, reducing myocardial oxygen demand, controlling exacerbating factors (anemia, valvular disease), and limiting the development of further atherosclerotic disease.
  - Aspirin (75 to 162 mg/d) reduces cardiovascular events including repeat revascularization, MI, and cardiac death by approximately 33% (*BMJ 1994;308:81; Lancet 1992;114:1421*).
    - Aspirin desensitization may be performed in selected patients with aspirin allergy.
    - Clopidogrel (75 mg/d) can be used in patients who are allergic or intolerant of aspirin.
    - Dual therapy with aspirin and clopidogrel may reduce the incidence of adverse cardiac outcomes in high-risk patients such as those with a prior MI (*NEJM 2006;354:1706; JACC 2007;49:1982*).
  - β-Adrenergic antagonists (Table 20) control anginal symptoms by decreasing heart rate and myocardial work leading to reduced myocardial oxygen demand.
    - The dosage can be adjusted to result in a resting heart rate of 50 to 60 bpm.
    - Use of β-blockers is contraindicated in patients with severe active bronchospasm, significant AV block, marked resting bradycardia, or poorly compensated HF.
    - β-Blockers may worsen coronary vasospasm and should be avoided in such patients.
  - Calcium channel blockers can be used either in conjunction with or in lieu of β-blockers in the presence of contraindications or adverse effects (Table 21).
    - Calcium antagonists are often used in conjunction with β-blockers if the latter are not fully effective at relieving anginal symptoms. Both long-acting dihydropyridines and nondihydropyridine agents can be used.
    - Calcium channel blockers are effective agents for the treatment of coronary vasospasm.
    - The use of short-acting dihydropyridines (nifedipine) should be avoided due to the potential to increase the risk of adverse cardiac events (*Circulation 1995;92:1326*).
  - Nitrates, either long-acting formulations for chronic use or sublingual preparations for acute anginal symptoms, can be used as adjunctive antianginal agents (Table 22).
    - Sublingual preparations should be used at the first indication of angina or prophylactically before engaging in activities that are known to precipitate angina.

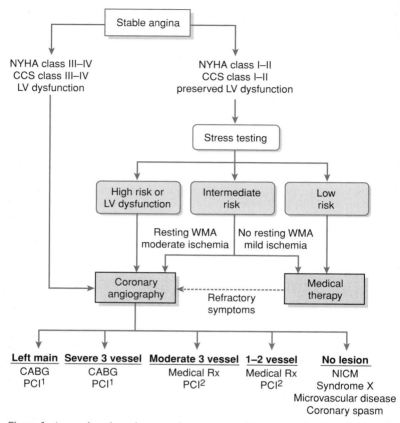

Figure 1. Approach to the evaluation and management of the patient of stable angina. Patients with clinical heart failure, severe limiting angina, and those with LV dysfunction should undergo coronary angiography to define underlying coronary artery disease. Patients without the above features may undergo further risk stratification with stress testing. Following stress testing, patients may undergo either coronary angiography or empiric medical therapy depending on their risk profile. Patients initially treated with medical therapy who have refractory systems should undergo angiography. [1]PCI results in equivalent cardiovascular outcomes to CABG with the exception of increased target vessel revascularization. [2]PCI should be reserved for patients who have high-grade lesions, severe ischemia, and those refractory to medical therapy. NYHA, New York Heart Association; CCS, Canadian Cardiovascular Society Classification (angina); LV, left ventricle; WMA, wall motion abnormality; CABG, coronary artery bypass grafting; PCI, percutaneous coronary intervention; NICM, nonischemic cardiomyopathy.

Patients should seek prompt medical attention if angina occurs at rest or fails to respond to the third sublingual dose.

○ Nitrate tolerance resulting in reduced therapeutic response may occur with all nitrate preparations. The institution of a nitrate-free period of 10 to 12 hours (usually at night) can enhance treatment efficacy.

Table 20	β-Blockers Commonly Used for Ischemic Heart Disease	
Drug	**β-Receptor Selectivity**	**Dose**
Propranolol	β_1 and β_2	20–80 mg bid
Metoprolol	β_1	50–200 mg bid
Atenolol	β_1	50–200 mg daily
Nebivolol	β_1	5–40 mg daily
Nadolol	β_1 and β_2	40–80 mg daily
Timolol	β_1 and β_2	10–30 mg tid
Acebutolol	β_1	200–600 mg bid
Bisoprolol	β_1	10–20 mg daily
Esmolol (IV)	β_1	50–300 mcg/kg/min
Labetalol	Combined α, β_1, β_2	200–600 mg bid
Pindolol	β_1 and β_2	2.5–7.5 mg tid
Carvedilol	Combined α, β_1, β_2	3.125–25 mg bid

- ACE inhibitors may have additive benefit in the treatment of stable angina.
  - A reduction of exercise-induced myocardial ischemia has been reported with the addition of an ACE inhibitor in patients with stable angina and normal LV function receiving optimal β-blocker therapy (*NEJM 2004;351:2048*; *Lancet 2003;362:782*).
  - ACEI therapy in high-risk patients with vascular disease or diabetes and at least one other cardiovascular risk factor reduced the rate of death, MI, or stroke (*NEJM 2000;342:145*).
- Ranolazine is a novel antianginal agent that does not depend upon reductions in heart rate or BP. Its exact mechanism of action is unknown; however, it appears to have effect on cardiomyocyte metabolism and sodium ion channel function.

Table 21	Calcium Channel Blockers Commonly Used for Ischemic Heart Disease	
Drug	**Duration of Action**	**Usual Dosage**
Dihydropyridines		
Nifedipine		
Slow release	Long	30–180 mg/d
Amlodipine	Long	5–10 mg/d
Felodipine (SR)	Long	5–10 mg/d
Isradipine (SR)	Medium	2.5–10 mg/d
Nicardipine	Short	20–40 mg tid
Nondihydropyridines		
Diltiazem		
Immediate release	Short	30–80 mg qid
Slow release	Long	120–360 mg/d
Verapamil		
Immediate release	Short	80–160 mg tid
Slow release	Long	120–480 mg/d

Table 22	Nitrate Preparations Commonly Used for Ischemic Heart Disease		
Preparation	**Dosage**	**Onset (min)**	**Duration**
Sublingual nitroglycerin	0.3–0.6 mg prn	2–5	10–30 min
Aerosol nitroglycerin	0.4 mg prn	2–5	10–30 min
Oral isosorbide dinitrate	5–40 mg tid	30–60	4–6 hr
Oral isosorbide mononitrate	10–20 mg bid	30–60	6–8 hr
Oral isosorbide mononitrate SR	30–120 mg daily	30–60	12–18 hr
2% Nitroglycerin ointment	0.5–2.0 in. tid	20–60	3–8 hr
Transdermal nitroglycerin patches	5–15 mg daily	>60	12 hr
Intravenous nitroglycerin	10–200 mcg/min	<2	During infusion

It has shown benefit in the symptomatic relief of refractory angina (*Clin Ther 2006;28:1996*).

- Cholesterol-lowering agents including statins, fibrates, bile acid sequestrants, and niacin reduce recurrent events and improve overall outcome in patients with established CAD.
    - HMG-CoA reductase inhibitors (statins) are the best studied agents and have been shown to limit atherosclerotic burden and reduce cardiac outcomes in patients with CAD (*Lancet 2002;360:7*; 4S: *Lancet 1994;344:1383*; *NEJM 1996; 355:1001*).
    - Recent studies have demonstrated that more intensive statin therapy is superior in preventing cardiovascular outcomes (*NEJM 2005;352:1425*; *NEJM 2004; 350:1495*).
- **Coronary revascularization**
    - In general, medical therapy with at least two, and preferably three, classes of antianginal agents should be attempted before this approach is considered a failure and coronary revascularization pursued.
    - In patients with stable angina and preserved LV function, medical therapy results in similar cardiovascular outcomes when compared to percutaneous coronary intervention (PCI). Of the patients who receive medical therapy only, there is a higher need for revascularization to control anginal symptoms (*NEJM 2007;256:1503*; RITA-2: *Lancet 1997;350:461*).
    - PCI and/or coronary artery bypass graft (CABG) surgery is indicated in patients who present with the following:
        - Angina refractory to medical therapy
        - Angina and reduced LV function
        - Severe activity limiting angina (CCS class III–IV)
        - Angina in the presence of left main or severe three-vessel CAD
    - The choice between PCI and CABG is dependent on the coronary anatomy, medical comorbidities, and patient preference. CABG is preferred in diabetics with multivessel disease and LV dysfunction (BARI: *NEJM 1996;335:217*).
        - The Syntax trial compared PCI versus CABG in patients with previously untreated three-vessel CAD or left main CAD. The study demonstrated an

increased risk of major adverse cardiac and vascular events in the PCI group attributable to repeat intervention (Syntax: *N Engl J Med 2009 March 5;360: 961*).

○ CABG carries a 1% to 3% mortality rate, 5% to 10% incidence of perioperative MI, and a small risk of perioperative stroke. The use of internal mammary artery grafts is associated with 90% graft patency at 10 years, compared with 40% to 50% for saphenous vein grafts. The long-term patency of a radial artery graft is 80% at 5 years. After 10 years of follow-up, 50% of patients develop recurrent angina or other adverse cardiac events related to late vein graft failure or progression of native CAD (*NEJM 1996;334:216*).

○ The risks of elective PCI include <1% mortality, a 2% to 5% rate of nonfatal MI, and <1% need for emergent CABG for an unsuccessful procedure. Patients undergoing PCI have shorter hospital stays and similar outcomes with respect to subsequent cardiac events and mortality compared to those undergoing CABG. PCI does have a higher rate of target lesion stenosis that can be minimized using drug-eluting stents (DES) (*NEJM 2005;352:2174*).

- **Alternative therapies** are available for patients with chronic stable angina who are refractory to medical management and who are not candidates for further percutaneous or surgical revascularization.

  - Transmyocardial laser revascularization has been delivered by percutaneous and epicardial surgical techniques. Surgical transmyocardial laser revascularization has been shown to improve symptoms in patients with stable angina, although the mechanism that is responsible is controversial. No benefit has been demonstrated in terms of increasing myocardial perfusion or mortality.

  - Therapeutic angiogenesis is a novel approach that aims to facilitate the growth of collateral blood vessels by delivering proangiogenic growth factors (VEGF and FGF) to the myocardium. Small studies have suggested some benefit in exercise capacity and myocardial perfusion.

PATIENT EDUCATION

- Compliance with medications, diet, and exercise should be stressed to patients. All patients should be encouraged to participate in cardiac rehab as well as meet with a registered dietician.
- Patients with known CAD should present for evaluation if any change in chest pain pattern, frequency, or intensity develops.
- Patients should also be evaluated if they report the presence of any HF symptoms including dyspnea, orthopnea, or paroxysmal nocturnal dyspnea.

MONITORING/FOLLOW-UP

- Close patient follow-up is a critical component of the treatment of CAD as lifestyle modification and secondary risk factor reduction require serial reassessment and interventions.
- Relatively minor changes in anginal symptoms can be safely treated with titration and/or addition of antianginal medications.
- Significant changes in anginal complaints (frequency, severity, or time to onset with activity) should be evaluated by either stress testing (usually in conjunction with an imaging modality) or cardiac catheterization as warranted.

• Patients with angina refractory to medical therapy should be considered for coronary revascularization if the anatomy is amenable to revascularization.

Acute Coronary Syndrome—Unstable Angina and Non–ST-segment Elevation MI

GENERAL PRINCIPLES

Definition

• Acute coronary syndrome (ACS) refers to any constellation of clinical symptoms that are compatible with acute myocardial ischemia. For simplicity, ACS can be divided into STEMI, NSTEMI, and UA.
• STEMI results from complete and prolonged occlusion of an epicardial coronary blood vessel and is defined based on ECG criteria (ST-segment elevation greater than 0.1 mV in at least two contiguous leads or a new LBBB).
• NSTEMI and UA are considered to be closely related conditions whose pathogenesis and clinical presentations are similar but differ in severity. NSTEMI usually results from severe coronary artery narrowing, transient occlusion, or microembolization of thrombus and/or atheromatous material. If the stenosis is not severe enough or the occlusion does not persist long enough to cause myocardial necrosis (as indicated by positive biomarkers), the syndrome is labeled UA.
  • Approximately three-fourths of patients presenting with UA/NSTEMI will have an abnormal ECG, more often seen as labile ST-segment depression or T-wave inversions, or less frequently transient ST-segment elevations.
  • The diagnosis of UA confers a 10% to 20% risk of progression to acute MI in the untreated patient. Medical treatment reduces this risk to 5% to 7%.
• NSTEMI is defined by an elevation of cardiac enzymes (creatine kinase MB [CK-MB] or troponin) and the absence of persistent ST-segment elevation. In the absence of elevated cardiac enzymes, the syndrome is termed UA.
• The management of ACS should focus on rapid diagnosis, risk stratification, and institution of therapies that restore coronary blood flow and reduce myocardial ischemia.

Epidemiology

• ACS accounts for almost 1.6 million hospitalizations each year (*Circulation 2006;113:e85; JACC 2007;50:e1*).
• Among patients with ACS, approximately 60% have UA and 40% have MI, either NSTEMI or STEMI.
• Of the patients with MI, two-thirds present with an NSTEMI and the remaining one-third present with an acute STEMI.
• At 1 year, patients with UA/NSTEMI are at considerable risk for death (~6%), recurrent MI (~11%), and need for revascularization (~50% to 60%). It is important to note that although the short-term mortality of STEMI is greater than that of NSTEMI, the long-term mortality is the same (*JACC 2007;50:e1; JAMA 1996;275: 1104*).

Pathophysiology

• Myocardial ischemia results from decreased myocardial oxygen supply and/or increased demand. In the majority of cases, NSTEMI is due to a sudden decrease in blood supply via partial occlusion of the affected vessel. In some cases, marked increased myocardial oxygen demand may lead to NSTEMI, as seen in severe anemia or hypertensive crisis.

- UA/NSTEMI most often represents acute atherosclerotic plaque rupture and superimposed thrombus formation. Alternatively, it may also be due to progressive mechanical obstruction from advancing atherosclerotic disease, in-stent restenosis (ISR), or bypass graft disease.
- Atherosclerotic plaques that are prone to rupture are termed vulnerable plaques. Vulnerable plaques often do not cause critical stenosis and thus may be difficult to identify by angiography alone. Experimental imaging modalities that may identify vulnerable plaques prior to rupture are currently being evaluated.
- Plaque rupture may be triggered by local and/or systemic inflammation as well as shear stress. Rupture leads to exposure of lipid-rich subendothelial components to circulating platelets and inflammatory cells serving as a potent substrate for thrombus formation.
- Less common causes include dynamic obstruction of the coronary artery due to vasospasm (Prinzmetal angina), syndrome X, coronary vasculitis, dissection, embolus, and myocardial bridge.

Risk Factors

- The approach to clinical testing, pharmacologic treatment, and timing of possible invasive therapy is guided by the probability of progression to MI and/or reinfarction and risk of subsequent mortality.
- Patients at highest risk for progression to MI include those with:
  - Rest angina
  - Associated dynamic ischemic ECG changes (ST-segment deviations or T-wave inversions)
  - Continued symptoms despite initiation of medical therapy
- Several clinical tools have been developed to estimate a patient's risk of MI and cardiac mortality, including the TIMI (Thrombolysis in Myocardial Infarction) and GRACE (Global Registry of Acute Coronary Events) risk score.
- The TIMI risk score can be used to determine the patient's short-term risk of death or nonfatal MI (*JAMA 2000;284:835*). Patients can be classified as low, intermediate, or high risk on the basis of their clinical profile (Fig. 2).
  - Low-risk patients (TIMI 0 or 1) may be observed with cardiac monitoring in a chest pain or observation unit.
    - If the patient remains chest pain free, has normal cardiac enzymes, and has no clinical signs of HF, a noninvasive stress test should be obtained for further risk stratification.
    - Patients should have negative cardiac enzymes for 24 hours prior to stress testing. If a patient presents with positive cardiac enzymes and noninvasive testing is selected, a submaximal or pharmacologic stress test 72 hours after the peak value may be performed.
    - Low-risk patients with a positive stress test should be managed with medication and invasive testing individualized based on clinical status and the severity of the ischemic burden.
  - Intermediate- and high-risk patients should be admitted to the hospital for observation and management.
    - Patients with ongoing symptoms should be admitted to the ICU for more aggressive monitoring with consideration for urgent cardiac catheterization.

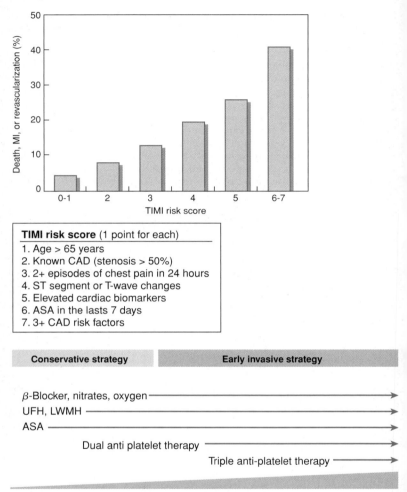

Figure 2. Top. 14-day rates of death, MI, or urgent revascularization from the TIMI 11B and ESSENCE trials based on increasing TIMI risk score. Coronary artery disease (CAD) risk factors include family history of CAD, diabetes, hypertension, hyperlipidemia, and tobacco use. TIMI, Thrombolysis in Myocardial Infarction; MI, myocardial infarction. (Adapted from *JAMA 2000;284:835–842.*) **Bottom.** Differing management strategies in patients with ACS based on TIMI risk score. UFH, unfractionated heparin; LWMH, low-molecular-weight heparin; ASA, aspirin; dual antiplatelet therapy includes either ASA and clopidogrel or ASA and a glycoprotein IIb/IIIa inhibitor; triple antiplatelet therapy denotes ASA, clopidogrel, and a glycoprotein IIb/IIIa inhibitor.

  ○ Intermediate- and high-risk patients should undergo noninvasive stress testing or coronary angiography based on their clinical course and risk profile (see below).

DIAGNOSIS

Initial assessment of the patient with UA/NSTEMI includes the clinical presentation (history and physical examination), 12-lead ECG, and measurement of cardiac-specific biomarkers (troponin or CK-MB).

Clinical Presentation
History
- The three principal presentations for UA are **rest angina** (angina occurring at rest and prolonged, usually >20 minutes), **new-onset angina,** and **progressive angina** (previously diagnosed angina that has become more frequent, lasts longer, or occurs with less exertion). New-onset and progressive angina should occur with at least mild to moderate activity (CCS class III severity).

Physical Examination
- Evaluation and management should be individualized based on the patient's clinical presentation, risk factors, and ECG. A physical exam should be performed focusing on objective evidence of HF, including peripheral hypoperfusion, heart murmur, elevated jugular venous pulsation, pulmonary edema, and peripheral edema.
- The presence of severe underlying coronary disease is suggested in patients with refractory chest discomfort, clinical evidence of LV dysfunction such as CHF, hypotension, and new ECG changes that are consistent with myocardial ischemia.

Laboratories
Biochemical makers
- A CBC, fasting glucose, and lipid profile should be obtained in all patients with suspected CAD.
- High-sensitivity CRP, lipoprotein A, and homocysteine are all associated with increased risk of CAD; however, these markers have not yet been embraced in standard of care guidelines.

Diagnostic Testing
Electrocardiography
- A baseline ECG should be recorded in all patients with suspected CAD. A normal tracing does not exclude the presence of disease.
- Possible indicators of CAD include significant Q waves, ST-segment changes, and T-wave inversions.
- If the patient is experiencing anginal symptoms, serial ECGs should be obtained to assess for dynamic ischemic changes.

Imaging
- Chest x-ray can be helpful by providing information on heart size and lung parenchyma.
- Should be obtained in patients with evidence of CHF, valvular heart disease, or aortic disease.

- Echocardiogram permits measurement of global LV systolic, wall motion abnormalities, diastolic function, and valvular disease. LV function may guide appropriate medical or surgical therapy, rehabilitation, and work status.
- May be helpful in establishing pathophysiologic mechanisms and guiding therapy in patients with heart failure in addition to angina.
- Additional imaging modalities including coronary calcium screening (CAC) and carotid intima-media thickness may play an important role in the at-risk patient, but have limited role in the symptomatic patient.

Laboratories
Measurement of cardiac-specific markers

- Cardiac biomarkers are essential in the diagnosis of UA/NSTEMI and should be obtained in all patients who present with chest discomfort suggestive of ACS. In patients with negative cardiac markers within 6 hours of the onset of pain, a second sample should be drawn within 6 to 12 hours. The most commonly measured markers are troponins, CK-MB, and myoglobin (Table 23).
- Cardiac-specific troponin is the preferred marker and should be measured in all patients.
  - Troponin T and I assays are highly specific and sensitive markers of myocardial necrosis. Serum troponin levels are usually undetectable in normal individuals, and any elevation is considered abnormal.
  - MI size and risk of subsequent cardiac death is directly proportional to the absolute increase in cardiac-specific troponin (*NEJM 1996;335:1333*; *Circulation 1998;98:1853*).

Table 23	Cardiac Biomarkers		
	Detectable	**Peak**	**Return to Baseline**
Troponin I, T	3–6 hr	24–36 hr	5–14 d
CK-MB	2–6 hr	12–18 hr	24–48 hr
Myoglobin	1–2 hr	6–8 hr	12–24 hr

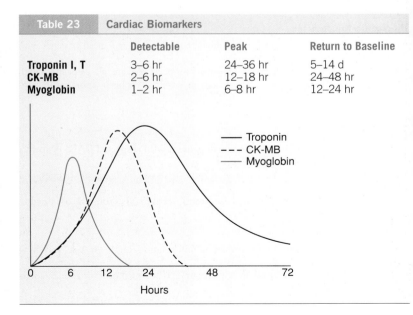

- CK-MB is also an acceptable marker of myocardial necrosis, but lacks specificity, as it is present in both skeletal and cardiac muscle cells.
  - Specificity can be improved by using the CK-MB/total CK fraction. A CK-MB fraction greater than 2.5% is suggestive of myocardial injury.
  - CK-MB is a useful assay for detecting postinfarct ischemia, as a fall and subsequent rise in enzyme levels suggests reinfarction.
  - Similarly, CK-MB levels are often followed after percutaneous revascularization. Small rises in CK-MB often represent distal microembolization, while large rises suggest more significant complications, such as acute stent thrombosis.
- Myoglobin is released more rapidly following myocardial damage than either CK-MB, troponin T, or troponin I, but lacks specificity.
- Lactate dehydrogenase (LDH), alanine transaminase (ALT), and aspartame transaminase (AST) are nonspecific markers of myocardial necrosis and should not be used.
- C-reactive protein levels may aid in initial risk assessment in ACS patients and predict mortality independent of troponin elevations (*JACC 1998;31:1460*).

Electrocardiography

- A 12-lead ECG should be obtained immediately in patients with ongoing chest discomfort and as rapidly as possible in patients whose chest discomfort subsided prior to evaluation.
- Approximately 50% of patients with UA/NSTEMI have significant ECG abnormalities, including transient ST-segment elevations, ST depressions, and T-wave inversions (*JACC 2007;50:e1*).
  - ST-segment depression >0.05 mV (0.5 mm) in two contiguous leads is a sensitive indicator of myocardial ischemia, especially if dynamic and associated with symptoms.
  - Symmetrical T-wave inversions of >0.2 mV (2 mm) across the precordium (Wellens' waves) are strongly suggestive for myocardial ischemia and particularly worrisome for a critical lesion in the left anterior descending (LAD) artery distribution.
  - Nonspecific ST-segment changes or T-wave inversions (those that do not meet voltage criteria) are less helpful.

TREATMENT

- **Goals of therapy.** In addition to prompt risk stratification, patients presenting with UA/NSTEMI should receive medications that reduce myocardial ischemia through reduction in myocardial oxygen demand, improvement in coronary perfusion, and prevention of further thrombus formation.
- **Early conservative versus invasive strategies.** Two different strategies have evolved for patients with UA/NSTEMI (Fig. 3).
  - **Early conservative strategy.** The patient is treated with medical therapy at maximally tolerated doses and coronary angiography is reserved for patients with evidence of recurrent ischemia despite medical therapy or a positive stress test. Although the choice should always be individualized to a particular patient, in general, an early conservative approach can be used in low-risk patients and selected intermediate-risk patients without adverse effects on clinical outcomes.
  - **Early invasive strategy.** Patients are routinely referred for coronary angiography and subsequent revascularization, as warranted. High-risk patients, including those

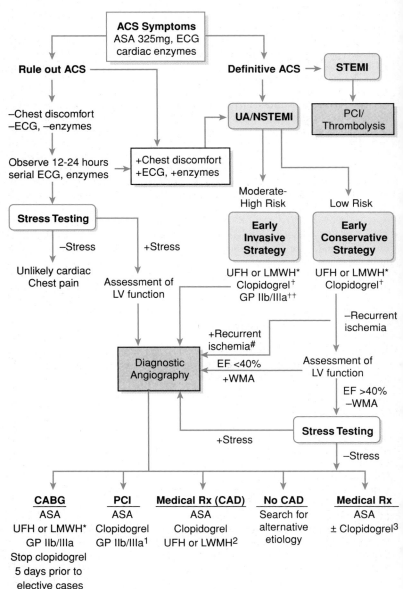

with recurrent ischemia on medical therapy, evidence of myocardial injury, CHF, LV dysfunction, sustained ventricular tachycardia (VT), or prior coronary revascularization (PCI within 6 months or CABG), are best assessed with an early invasive approach. Angiography in these individuals defines coronary anatomy and directs the choice of revascularization options, if appropriate.

- An early invasive strategy is also warranted in low- or intermediate-risk patients with repeated ACS presentations despite appropriate therapy. Cardiac catheterization provides the means to distinguish between those with no significant coronary disease and those with anatomy that is amenable to revascularization.

- Multiple clinical trials and meta-analysis have demonstrated the benefit of an early invasive strategy in high-risk (and possibly intermediate risk) patients, especially those with refractory angina, new or dynamic ST-segment changes, elevated cardiac enzymes, diabetes, and high TIMI risk scores (*Lancet 1999;354:708*; *NEJM 2001;344:1879*; *JAMA 2003;290:1593*; *Lancet 2002;360:743*; *NEJM 2009;360:2165*; *JAMA 2005;293:2908*).

- Patients with mild to moderate renal insufficiency (creatinine clearance greater than 30) also benefit from an early invasive strategy. No benefit was seen in patients with a creatinine clearance less than 30 or those receiving dialysis (*Circulation 2009;120:851*).

Medications

The goal of pharmacologic treatment is to provide relief from chest pain and limit thrombus formation through inhibition of platelet activation and aggregation.

- This approach should include antiplatelet, anticoagulant, and antianginal medications (Table 24).
- All patients presenting with UA/NSTEMI should be restricted to bedrest and provided supplemental oxygen as needed.
- **Antiplatelet therapy** (Table 25)

Figure 3. Diagnostic and therapeutic approach to patients presenting with ACS focusing on antiplatelet and antithrombotic therapy. *Bivalirudin and fondaparinux are appropriate alternatives to UFH and LMWH. †Clopidogrel should be given when there is a reasonable certainty that the patient will not require CABG. GP IIb/IIIa inhibitors can be used as an alternative to clopidogrel when dual antiplatelet therapy is indicated and need for CABG is possible. In this setting, clopidogrel can be given after diagnostic angiography. ††GP IIb/IIIa inhibitors can be administered, in addition to ASA and clopidogrel, in high-risk patients. #Indicators of recurrent ischemia include worsening chest pain, increasing cardiac enzymes, and dynamic ECG changes. ¹GP IIb/IIIa inhibitors should be continued per cath lab protocols. ²UFH, LWMH, or alternative agents should be continued for 48 to 72 hours. ³Clopidogrel should be given to patients with likely CAD who elected for a conservative approach and to patients who presented with myocardial injury. ACS, acute coronary syndrome; STEMI, ST-segment elevation myocardial infarction; NSTEMI: non–ST-segment elevation myocardial infarction; Rx, treatment; UFH, unfractionated heparin; LMWH, low-molecular-weight heparin; GP IIb/IIIa, glycoprotein IIb/IIIa inhibitor; EF, ejection fraction; CAD, coronary artery disease; CABG, coronary artery bypass grafting; PCI, percutaneous coronary intervention; WMA, wall motion abnormality. (Adapted from the ACC/AHA 2007 Guidelines for the Management of Patients With Unstable Angina/Non-ST-Elevation Myocardial Infarction.)

Table 24	Initial Medical Regimen for Unstable Angina/NSTEMI	
Medications	**Route**	**Dosage**
Nitroglycerin	Sublingual	0.3–0.6 mg prn
	Aerosol	0.4 mg prn
	Intravenous	10–200 mcg/min
Oxygen	Nasal canula	2–4 L as needed
Morphine	Intravenous	2–4 mg prn
β-Blocker (metoprolol)	Intravenous	5 mg (3 doses)
	Oral	25 mg qid
Aspirin	Oral	325 mg
Heparin	Intravenous	4,000 unit bolus, 12–14 units/kg/hr

- All patients should receive **aspirin (ASA)** unless a contraindication exists.
  - ASA effectively blocks platelet aggregation within minutes and should be administered **immediately** by EMS or on arrival to the ER.
  - The only contraindications to ASA therapy are a history of documented drug allergy and active bleeding. Patients with an ASA allergy should immediately receive clopidogrel (see below), and an allergy consultation should be obtained for possible desensitization.
- **Clopidogrel** (Plavix), **Ticlopidine** (Ticlid), and **Prasugrel** (Effient) are ADP receptor antagonists that inhibit platelet activation and aggregation. Clopidogrel is preferred over ticlopidine because of a lower risk of gastrointestinal bleeding, neutropenia, and thrombotic thrombocytopenic purpura (TTP). Prasugrel was recently approved by the FDA for treatment of patients following ACS.
  - Clopidogrel can be used in patients who are intolerant or allergic to aspirin.
  - A minimum of 1 month of therapy should be given if medical or percutaneous treatment is planned and ideally continued for at least 1 year. The length of treatment will depend upon the type of stent placed (see section on STEMI).
  - The issue of CABG surgery is of particular concern with regards to clopidogrel administration and timing. It is currently recommended that clopidogrel be withheld from patients for at least 5 days prior to CABG, given the risk of bleeding and its long drug half-life.
    - A recent multicentered study demonstrated that the increased risk of bleeding from clopidogrel therapy may be restricted to the first 2 to 3 days following drug cessation (*JACC 2008;52(21):1693*).
    - Intermediate- to high-risk patients should receive dual antiplatelet therapy upon presentation regardless of their likelihood of requiring CABG. Glycoprotein IIb/IIIa antagonists (see below) are potent IV agents with a short plasma half-life and are thus attractive alternatives to clopidogrel in this setting.
  - Clopidogrel resistance is a newly recognized entity that confers increased risk of adverse outcomes in patients presenting with ACS. A polymorphism in the CYP2C19 gene has been associated with decreased platelet inhibition and increased risk of major adverse cardiovascular outcomes in patients receiving clopidogrel (*NEJM 2009;360:354; NEJM 2009;360:363*).
    - Reduced CYP2C19 activity leads to impaired cytochrome P450–mediated conversion of clopidogrel to its active metabolite.

Table 25	Antiplatelet Agents in Unstable Angina/NSTEMI	
Medication	**Dosage**	**Comments**
Aspirin (ASA)	162–325 mg daily	Aspirin reduces subsequent MI and cardiac death in patients with unstable angina.
Clopidogrel (Plavix)	300–600 mg loading dose, 75 mg daily	In combination with ASA, clopidogrel (300 mg loading dose, then 75 mg/d) decreased the composite end point of cardiovascular death, MI, or stroke by 18% to 30% in patients with UA/NSTEMI (*NEJM 2001;345:494; Lancet 2001;358:527; JAMA 2002;288:2411*). There may be further beneft in using a clopidogrel loading dose of 600 mg without an increased risk of bleeding in patients undergoing PCI (*Circulation 2005;111:2099*).
Ticlopidine (Ticlid)	250 mg bid	
Prasugrel	60 mg loading dose, 10 mg daily	Prasugrel has increased anti-platelet potency compared to clopidogrel. Prasugrel reduced the incidence of cardiovascular death, myocardial infarction, and stroke (9.9% vs. 12.1%) at the expense of increased major (2.4% vs. 1.1%) and fatal bleeding (0.4% vs. 0.1%), compared to clopidogrel (*NEJM 2007; 357:2001*).
Eptifibatide (Integrilin)[a]	180 mcg/kg IV bolus, 2 mcg/kg/min[a,b]	Eptifibatide reduces the risk of death or MI in patients with ACS undergoing either invasive or noninvasive therapy in combination with ASA and heparin (*NEJM 1998;339:436; Circulation 2000;101:751*). Compared to abciximab and tirofiban, eptifibatide has the most consistent effects on platelet inhibition with shortest on-time and drug half-life (*Circulation 2002;106:1470–1476*).

(*continued*)

Table 25	Antiplatelet Agents in Unstable Angina/NSTEMI (*Continued*)	
Medication	**Dosage**	**Comments**
Tirofiban (Aggrastat)	0.4 mcg/kg IV bolus, 0.1 mcg/kg/min[a,b]	Tirofiban reduces the risk of death or MI in patients with ACS undergoing either invasive or noninvasive therapy in combination with ASA and heparin (*Circulation 1997; 96:1445; NEJM 1998;338: 1498; NEJM 1998;338:1488*).
Abciximab (ReoPro)	0.25 mg/kg IV bolus, 10 mcg/min[a,c]	Abciximab reduces the risk of death or MI in patients with ACS undergoing coronary intervention (*NEJM 1994;330:956; Lancet 1997;349:1429; NEJM 1997; 336:1689*). It should not be used in patients in whom percutaneous intervention is not planned (*Lancet 2001;357:1915*). Platelet inhibition may be reversed by platelet transfusion.

[a]The recommended duration of treatment is 72 to 96 hours following presentation or at least 12 hours after any percutaneous intervention.
[b]Infusion doses should be decreased by 50% in patients with a GFR less than 30 mL/min and avoided in patients on HD.
[c]Abciximab may be used in patients with ESRD, as it is not cleared by the kidney.

- - Clopidogrel resistance can be screened for using point-of-care platelet inhibition assays or genotyping.
  - Proposed strategies to combat clopidogrel resistance include elevated clopidogrel dosing and first-line use of prasugrel, which does not require cytochrome P450–mediated conversion to an active metabolite.
- Prasugrel has increased potency and results in greater and more uniform platelet inhibition compared to clopidogrel. While it decreased adverse outcomes in patients following ACS, prasugrel treatment increased bleeding rates and should be avoided in patients older than 75 years, less than 60 kg, and those with prior stroke or TIA.
  - ○ **Glycoprotein IIb/IIIa (GP IIb/IIIa) antagonists** block the interaction between platelets (GP IIb/IIIa receptor) and fibrinogen, thus targeting the final common pathway for platelet aggregation. GP IIb/IIIa inhibitors (abciximab, eptifibatide, or tirofiban) should be considered in the treatment of all high-risk patients with refractory UA/NSTEMI, especially those with significant ST-T changes or elevated cardiac enzymes.
    - GP IIb/IIIa antagonists should be used in conjunction with therapeutically dosed unfractionated heparin (UFH) or enoxaparin.
    - The utility of GP IIb/IIIa antagonists in conjunction with ASA, clopidogrel, and heparin therapy appears to be restricted to patients with elevated

cardiac biomarkers and those with diabetes (*JAMA 2006;295:1531*; *Circulation 2001;104:2767*; *NEJM 2009;360:2176*).

- GP IIb/IIIa antagonists may be used as an alternative to clopidogrel in intermediate- to high-risk patients presenting with UA/NSTEMI that may require surgical revascularization.

- GP IIb/IIIa antagonists increase the risk of major bleeding, especially when used in combination with clopidogrel.

- Thrombocytopenia, which can be severe, is an uncommon complication of all these agents and should prompt discontinuation of the drug.

- **Anticoagulant therapy** (Table 26)
  - Anticoagulation is a key component in the management of patients with ACS and should be routinely used in conjunction with ASA. Available therapeutic agents include **intravenous UFH, enoxaparin** (low-molecular-weight heparin [LMWH], **fondaparinux,** and **bivalirudin** (Angiomax).
  - **UFH and LMWH** minimize thrombus formation by inhibiting factors IIa and Xa, respectively. The use of both agents is limited by heparin-induced thrombocytopenia (HIT).
  - **Fondaparinux** is a synthetic polysaccharide that contains the same pentasaccharide sequence found in UFH and LMWH. It selectively inhibits factor Xa and does not bind PF4, making HIT unlikely with its use.
  - **Bivalirudin (Angiomax)** is a direct thrombin inhibitor. Bivalirudin can be given in conjunction with ASA and clopidogrel in patients presenting with UA/NSTEMI who will undergo an early invasive strategy.
    - Bivalirudin is particularly useful in the management of both cardiac and cardiac surgery patients with HIT.
  - **Thrombolytic therapy** is not indicated in UA/NSTEMI and has been shown to increase mortality.

- **Anti-ischemic therapy** (Table 27)
  - **Nitroglycerin** reduces myocardial oxygen demand and enhances myocardial oxygen delivery. The choice of preparation depends on the severity of symptoms.
    - Treatment can be initiated at the time of presentation with sublingual nitroglycerin.
    - Less stable patients or those who require additional agents to control significant hypertension should be treated with intravenous nitroglycerin until pain relief, hypertension control, or both are achieved.
  - **β-Adrenergic blockers** limit cardiac ischemia by reducing myocardial oxygen demand and should be started early in the absence of contraindications. In high-risk patients, intravenous, followed by oral, preparations can be used. Treatment with an oral preparation alone is acceptable, especially if the patient is intermediate to low risk or is unable to tolerate intravenous agents.
    - The goals of therapy are to reduce the heart rate to 60 bpm and maintain an SBP greater than 90 to 100 mm Hg.
    - Contraindications to β-blocker therapy include advanced AV block, active bronchospasm, decompensated CHF, cardiogenic shock, hypotension, and bradycardia.
  - **Calcium channel blockers** can be used as third-line agent in patients continuing to have chest pain in the setting of adequate β-blocker and nitrate therapy.
    - Nifedipine, amlodipine, diltiazem, and verapamil appear to have similar coronary dilatory properties. Neither of these agents has demonstrated an effect on mortality or recurrent MI.

Table 26	Anticoagulant Medications	
Medication	**Dosage**	**Comments**
Heparin (UFH)	60 units/kg IV bolus (maximum dose: 4,000 units), 12–14 units/kg/hr	Heparin therapy, when used in conjunction with ASA, has been shown to reduce the early rate of death or MI by up to 60% (*JAMA 1996;276:811*). The activated partial thromboplastin time (aPTT) should be adjusted to maintain a value of 1.5–2.0 times control.
Enoxaparin (LMWH)	1 mg/kg SC bid[a]	LMWH is at least as efficacious as UFH and may further reduce the rate of death, MI, or recurrent angina (*NEJM 1997;337:447*). LMWH may increase the rate of bleeding (*JAMA 2004;292:45*) and cannot be reversed in the setting of refractory bleeding. LMWH does not require monitoring for clinical effect. If cardiac catheterization is planned, then the dose should be withheld on the morning of procedure.
Fondaparinux	2.5 mg SC daily	Fondaparinux has efficacy similar to that of LMWH with possibly reduced bleeding rates (*NEJM 2006;354:1464*).
Bivalirudin (Angiomax)[b]	0.75 mg/kg IV bolus, 1.75 mg/kg/hr	When used in conjunction with ASA and clopidogrel, bivalirudin is at least as effective as the combination of ASA, UFH, clopidogrel, and GP IIb/IIIa antagonists with decreased bleeding rates (*NEJM 2006;355:2203*). Monitoring is required with a goal aPTT of 1.5–2.5 times control.

[a]LMWH should be given at reduced dose (50%) in patients with a serum creatinine greater than 2 mg/dL or GFR less than 30 mL/min.
[b] Bivalirudin requires dosage adjustment in patients with a GFR less than 30 mL/min or those on hemodialysis.

Table 27	Antianginal Medications	
Medication	**Dosage**	**Comments**
Nitroglycerin (NTG)	SL: 0.4 mg every 5 min Topical: 0.5–2 in. IV: 10–200 mcg/min	Significant antianginal effects are not seen above 200 mcg/min, but doses of up to 400 mcg/min can be used for BP control. Nitroglycerin is contraindicated in patients who have used PDE5 inhibitors (e.g., within 24 hr of sildenafil or 48 hr of tadalafil) given the risk of severe hypotension. Appropriate timing for vardenafil dosing with nitrates is unknown and should be avoided. Nitrates are relatively contraindicated in patients who are preload dependent, including those with severe aortic stenosis and hypertrophic obstructive cardiomyopathy.
Morphine	2–4 mg IV	IV narcotics are effective agents for relief of anginal symptoms and should be used if NTG does not provide complete relief or cannot be titrated further due to hypotension or headache.
β-Blockers	Metoprolol: 5 mg IV (3 doses) 25 mg PO qid Bisoprolol: 10–20 mg PO daily Carvedilol: 3.125–25 mg PO bid Atenolol: 50–200 mg PO daily Propranolol: 20–80 mg PO bid Esmolol: 50–300 mcg/kg/min Nebivolol: 5–40 mg PO daily	β-Adrenergic blockade reduces the risk of recurrent ischemia, myocardial infarction, and mortality in patients with UA/NSTEMI (*J Interv Cardiol 2003;16:299*). The efficacy of β-blockade is limited by the development of cardiogenic shock. Those at risk include patients greater than 70 yr of age, SBP less than 120 mm Hg, and heart rate greater than 110 bpm or less than 60 bpm. In such cases, oral agents at reduced doses may be cautiously used (*Lancet 2005;366:1622*).

(continued)

Table 27	Antianginal Medications (*Continued*)	
Medication	**Dosage**	**Comments**
Calcium channel blockers	Nifedipine 30–180 mg daily Amlodipine 5–10 mg daily Diltiazem 30–80 mg qid Verapamil 80–160 mg tid	Short-acting nifedipine preparations should be avoided in the absence of adequate concurrent β-blocker therapy because of increased risk of myocardial infarction and death. Verapamil and diltiazem should be avoided in patients with evidence of severe LV dysfunction, pulmonary congestion, or AV block.

- Calcium channel blockers are useful in vasospastic angina, cocaine-induced vasospasm, and among patients in whom β-blockade is contraindicated.
- **Ranolazine** is a novel antianginal agent that is useful in the treatment of chronic stable angina. Addition of ranolazine to standard medical therapy does not reduce recurrent ischemia, MI, or death in patients presenting with UA/NSTEMI (*JAMA 2007;297:1775*).
- **Blood transfusion** improves oxygen-carrying capacity and myocardial oxygen supply. The potential benefit of routine blood transfusions in patients presenting with an NSTEMI is based on limited clinic data (*NEJM 2001;345:1230*).
  - The recommended target hemoglobin and hematocrit is 10 mg/dL and 30%, respectively.
  - Patients presenting with UA/NSTEMI who are actively bleeding and/or significantly anemic should be transfused routinely.
- **Other medical therapies**
  - **ACE inhibitors** are effective antihypertensive agents and have been shown to reduce mortality in patients with CAD and LV systolic dysfunction.
    - ACE inhibitors should be used in patients with LV dysfunction (EF <40%), hypertension, or diabetes presenting with ACS. ARBs are appropriate in patients who cannot tolerate ACE inhibitors (*NEJM 2003;349:1893*).
  - **HMG-CoA reductase inhibitors (statins)** are potent lipid-lowering agents that reduce the incidence of ischemia, MI, and death in patients with CAD. Statins should be routinely administered within 24 hours of presentation in patients presenting with ACS.
    - Statin therapy reduces adverse outcomes through lipid lowering, anti-inflammatory, and atherosclerotic plaque–stabilizing effects.
    - Aggressive statin therapy reduces the risk of recurrent ischemia, MI, and death in patients presenting with ACS (*JAMA 2001;285:1711*).
    - The reduction in adverse outcomes following early initiation of aggressive lipid lowering to target LDL less than 70 therapy can be seen within 30 days following initial presentation (*NEJM 2004;350:1495*). Aggressive LDL lowering also reduces the incidence of peri-procedural MI following PCI (*JACC 2007;49: 1272*).

- **NSAIDS** are associated with an increased risk of death, MI, myocardial rupture, hypertension, and HF in large meta-analyses (*Circulation 2006;113:2906*). Adverse outcomes have been observed for both nonselective and COX-2 selective agents.
  - ○ NSAIDS should be discontinued in patients presenting with UA/NSTEMI.
  - ○ Acetaminophen is an acceptable alternative for the treatment of osteoarthritis and other musculoskeletal pain.

Other Nonoperative Therapies

- **Revascularization**
- The indications for PCI and CABG in patients with UA/NSTEMI are similar to those for individuals with stable angina.
  - ○ Patients who are optimally managed with CABG include those with:
    - Significant left main CAD
    - Three-vessel disease and abnormal LV function (EF <50%)
    - Two-vessel disease with a significant proximal LAD artery stenosis and abnormal LV function
    - Diabetes and multivessel disease
  - ○ Patients with multivessel coronary disease requiring revascularization can be treated with CABG or PCI. Patients who are treated with CABG tend to have a lower incidence of angina, less need for subsequent revascularization, but increased risk of stroke. There is no difference in the rates of cardiac death or MI between the two treatment strategies with either the use of bare metal stents (BMS) or DES. While the preferred treatment of unprotected left main disease remains CABG, however, recent data do suggest an important role for PCI (*Circulation 2008;118:1146*; *NEJM 2009;360:961*).
  - ○ The decision between PCI and CABG should be based on the extent and complexity of coronary disease, medical comorbidities, and patient preference.
- If there is uncertainty regarding the hemodynamic significance of a coronary lesion, fractional flow reserve (FFR) can be performed to quantify the functional severity of blood flow limitation. This modality has been shown to reduce death, recurrent MI, or revascularization compared to conventional PCI at 1 year in patients with multivessel CAD (*NEJM 2009;360:213*).
- DES significantly reduce the rate of ISR and adverse cardiac outcomes compared to BMS (*NEJM 2003;349:1315*; *Circulation 2003;108:788*). However DES imparts an additional risk of late stent thrombosis, most notably following the discontinuation of clopidogrel therapy within 1 year following stent placement (*JAMA 2007;297:159*).
- The management of patients following PCI is discussed in detail in the section on hypertension, dyslipidemia and stable angina.

Lifestyle/Risk Modification

Risk factor modification is addressed in detail in the section on STEMI and should include attention to smoking cessation, weight loss, exercise, control of hypertension, diabetes, and hyperlipidemia.

COMPLICATIONS

The highest rate of progression to MI or development of recurrent MI is in the first 2 months after presentation with the index episode. Beyond that time point, most patients have a clinical course similar to those with chronic stable angina.

MONITORING/FOLLOW-UP

- It is incumbent on the entire hospital staff (physicians, nurses, dietitians, pharmacists, and rehabilitation specialists) to prepare the patient for hospital discharge. The patient should be discharged on a medical regimen that takes advantage of proven methods of secondary prevention. The patient should also be provided a sublingual or spray formulation of nitroglycerin and instructed on its appropriate use.
- Arrangements for follow-up care should also be established before hospital discharge.

ST-Segment Elevation Myocardial Infarction

GENERAL PRINCIPLES

- STEMI is a medical emergency caused by acute occlusion of an epicardial coronary artery. Vessel occlusion is most often due to atherosclerotic plaque rupture and subsequent thrombus formation.
- Compared to UA/NSTEMI, STEMI is associated with a higher in-hospital and long-term morbidity and mortality. Left untreated, the mortality rate of uncomplicated STEMI can exceed 30% and the presence of mechanical complications (papillary muscle rupture, ventricular septal defect [VSD], and free wall rupture) increases the mortality rate to 90%. Over the past few decades, there has been a dramatic improvement in short-term mortality to the current rate of 6% to 10%.
- Ventricular fibrillation accounts for approximately 50% of mortality and occurs within the first hour from symptom onset.
- Keys to treatment of STEMI include rapid recognition and diagnosis, coordinated mobilization of health care resources, and prompt reperfusion therapy.
- Mortality is directly related to total ischemia time and restoration of coronary blood flow.

Prevention

Secondary prevention. The strategies outlined for primary prevention and the management of stable angina have also been shown to decrease the rates of repeat infarction, progression to CHF, and incidence of cardiovascular deaths in patients with known CAD (see stable angina).

DIAGNOSIS

Clinical Presentation

Clinical stratification on initial presentation

- Multiple risk assessment tools have been developed to stratify patients presenting with acute STEMI into low-, intermediate-, and high-risk groups based on history, physical exam, and hemodynamic monitoring (Fig. 4).
- The Killip classification system utilizes history and physical exam findings (S_3 gallop, pulmonary congestion, and cardiogenic shock) to predict 30-day mortality in the absence of reperfusion therapy (*Am J Cardiol 1967;20:457*). In contrast, the TIMI risk score for STEMI incorporates a combination of history and physical to predict 30-day mortality in patients who receive thrombolytic therapy (*Circulation 2000;102:2031*). The Forrester classification system uses invasive

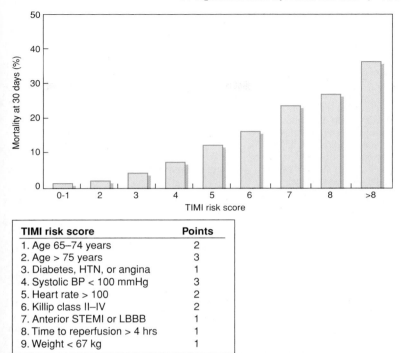

Figure 4. Risk indices for ST-segment elevation MI. Killip classification in acute MI. **Top.** TIMI risk score for STEMI (*Circulation 2000;102:2031*). **Bottom.** Killip classification system (*Am J Cardiol 1967;20:457*). The TIMI risk score incorporates prognosis following coronary reperfusion with thrombolytic therapy. The Killip classification system was devised before reperfusion therapy was routinely used. HTN, hypertension; BP, blood pressure.

hemodynamic data including cardiac index and pulmonary capillary wedge pressure (*NEJM 1976;295:1356*).

History

- Chest pain from STEMI resembles angina, but lasts longer, is more intense, and is not relieved by rest or sublingual nitroglycerin. Chest discomfort may be accompanied by dyspnea, diaphoresis, palpitations, nausea, vomiting, fatigue, and/or syncope.

Table 28	Key Information in the Patient Presenting with STEMI	
History and Physical Exam	Laboratory Values	Records
Inquire about the exact time of chest pain onset	Complete blood cell count	Prior ECGs
Consider other etiologies of chest pain with ST-segment elevation (i.e., aortic dissection, cocaine use)	Basic chemistry panel	Last cardiac catheterization
Identify absolute and relative contraindications to PCI and thrombolysis	PTT, PT and INR	CABG operative report
Evaluate for signs of heart failure, mechanical complications of MI, aortic dissection, and neurologic disease	Cardiac enzymes	Prior echocardiogram

- It is imperative to determine the time of symptom onset, as this is critical in determining the appropriate means of reperfusion (Table 28).
- STEMI may have atypical presentations particularly in women, elderly and postoperative patients as well as those with diabetes and chronic or end-stage kidney disease. Such patients may experience atypical or no chest pain and may instead present with confusion, dyspnea, unexplained hypotension, or CHF.
- If the patient has a history of previous cardiac catheterization or revascularization, it is important to obtain these records, as these can provide valuable information with respect to PCI planning, particularly in the setting of previous coronary artery bypass grafting. However, this should not delay definitive therapy.
- Review absolute and relative contraindications to thrombolytic therapy (see below) and potential issues complicating primary PCI (IV contrast allergy, PVD/peripheral revascularization, renal dysfunction, CNS disease, pregnancy, and bleeding diathesis).
- Inquire about recent cocaine use. In this setting, aggressive medical therapy with nitroglycerin, coronary vasodilators, and benzodiazepines should be administered before reperfusion therapy is considered.

Physical Examination

Physical examination should be directed at identifying hemodynamic instability, pulmonary congestion, mechanical complications of MI, and other causes of acute chest discomfort.

- The identification of a new systolic murmur may suggest the presence of ischemic mitral regurgitation (MR) or a VSD.
- A limited neurologic exam to detect baseline cognitive and motor deficits and a vascular examination (lower extremity pulses and bruits) will aid in determining candidacy for reperfusion treatment.
- Cardiogenic shock due to right ventricular myocardial infarction (RVMI) may be clinically suspected by the presence of hypotension, elevated jugular venous pressure,

and absence of pulmonary congestion. While RVMI may be seen in isolation, it more commonly complicates inferior/posterior MI.
- Bilateral arm BPs should be obtained to assess for the presence of aortic dissection.

Diagnostic Criteria

STEMI requires the presence of at least two of the following criteria:

- History of prolonged chest discomfort or anginal equivalent (30 minutes)
- Presence of ≥1 mm ST-segment elevation in two consecutive ECG leads or new LBBB
- Presence of elevated cardiac biomarkers

Diagnostic Testing

Laboratories

Blood samples should be sent for cardiac enzymes (Troponin, CK-MB), complete blood cell count, coagulation studies (PTT, prothrombin time [PT], international normalized ratio [INR]), creatinine, electrolytes including magnesium, and type and screen. A fasting lipid profile should be obtained in all patients with STEMI for secondary prevention.

- Initial cardiac enzymes (including high-sensitivity troponin assays) may be normal, depending upon the time in relation to symptom onset. In general, cardiac enzymes should have little role in the initial decision making process and awaiting these studies may lead to unnecessary delays in delivering therapy.
- CK-MB can be used to confirm that myocardial injury occurred within the previous 48 hours, as troponin levels may remain elevated for several days after MI. CK-MB is also useful to detect periprocedural infarctions.
- The risk of subsequent cardiac death is directly proportional to the increase in cardiac-specific troponins, even when CK-MB levels are not elevated. Cardiac enzymes should be measured daily until the peak level has been reached to determine the extent of myocardial damage.
- Routine use of cardiac noninvasive imaging is not recommended for the initial diagnosis of STEMI. When the diagnosis is in question, a transthoracic echocardiogram (TTE) can be performed to document regional wall motion abnormalities. If not adequately evaluated by TTE, a transesophageal echocardiogram (TEE) can be obtained to assess for acute complications of MI and presence of aortic dissection.
- A portable chest radiograph is useful to assess for pulmonary edema and evaluate for other causes of chest pain including aortic dissection. Importantly, a normal mediastinal width does not exclude aortic dissection, especially if clinically suspected.

Electrocardiography

The ECG is paramount to the diagnosis of STEMI and should be obtained within 5 minutes of presentation. If the diagnosis of STEMI is in doubt, serial ECGs may help elucidate the diagnosis. Classic findings include (Table 29):

- **T waves.** Peaked upright T waves may be the first ECG manifestation of myocardial injury.
- **ST-segment changes**
  - Convex ST-segment elevation ≥ 1 mm in two consecutive leads with peaked or inverted T waves is usually indicative of myocardial injury and correlates with the territory of injured myocardium (Fig. 8).

Table 29	ECG-Based Anatomic Distribution	
ST Elevation	**Myocardial Territory**	**Coronary Artery**
V_1–V_6 or LBBB	Anterior and septal walls	Proximal LAD or left main
V_1–V_2	Septum	Proximal LAD or septal branch
V_2–V_4	Anterior wall	LAD
V_5–V_6	Lateral wall	LCX
II, III, aVF	Inferior wall	RCA or LCX
I, aVL	High lateral wall	Diagonal or proximal LCX

LBBB, left bundle branch block; LAD, left anterior descending artery; LCX, left circumflex artery; RCA, right coronary artery.

- Posterior wall MI is recognized by ST-segment depression in leads V_1 to V_3, ST-segment elevation in V_7 to V_9 and is treated as a STEMI.
- RVMI is diagnosed with ST-segment elevation in lead V_4R.
- ECG criteria for ischemic changes in patients with preexisting LBBB or RV-pacing can be found in Table 30.
- **Q waves.** Development of new pathologic Q waves (>40 milliseconds) is considered diagnostic for MI, but may occur in patients with prolonged ischemia.
- A new LBBB suggests anterior wall injury.
- Infarction of the left circumflex territory may be electrocardiographically silent.
- The presence of reciprocal ST-segment depression opposite of the infarct territory increases the specificity for acute MI.
- **ECG changes that mimic MI.** ST-segment elevation and Q waves may result from numerous etiologies other than acute MI including prior MI with aneurysm formation, aortic dissection, LV hypertrophy, pericarditis, myocarditis, and pulmonary embolism (Table 31). It is critical to obtain prior ECGs to clarify the diagnosis.

TREATMENT

- **Acute management.** Prompt treatment should be initiated as soon as the diagnosis is suspected, as mortality and subsequent HF are directly related to ischemia time (Fig. 5). All medical centers should utilize an AHA/ACC guideline–based STEMI protocol. Centers that are not primary PCI capable should have protocols in place to

Table 30	Criteria for ST-segment Elevation for Prior LBBB or RV-paced Rhythm

ECG change

ST-segment elevation greater than 1 mm in the presence of a positive QRS complex (concordant with the QRS)

ST-segment elevation greater than 5 mm in the presence of a negative QRS complex (disconcordant with the QRS)

ST-segment depression greater than 1 mm in V_1–V_3.

Sgarbossa's (GUSTO) criteria: *Am J Cardiol 1996;77:423; NEJM 1996;334:481; PACE 2001; 24:1289.*

Table 31	Differential Diagnosis of ST-Segment Elevation

Cardiac Etiologies	Other Etiologies
Prior MI with aneurysm formation	Pulmonary embolism
Aortic dissection with coronary involvement	Hyperkalemia
Pericarditis	
Myocarditis	
LV hypertrophy or aortic stenosis (with strain[a])	
Hypertrophic cardiomyopathy	
Coronary vasospasm (cocaine, Prinzmetal angina)	
Early repolarization (normal variant)	
Brugada syndrome	

[a]Strain may occur in numerous settings including systemic hypertension, hypotension, tachycardia, exercise, and sepsis.

meet accepted time to therapy guidelines for either administration of thrombolytic therapy with subsequent transfer or rapid transfer to a primary PCI-capable facility.

- **Before presentation to the hospital.** The general public should be informed of the signs and symptoms consistent with an acute MI that should lead them to seek urgent medical care. Availability of "911" access and emergency medical services facilitates delivery of patients to emergency medical care.
- **In the emergency department,** an acute MI protocol should be activated that includes a targeted clinical examination and a 12-lead ECG completed within 10 minutes of arrival.
- **Immediate management.** The goal of immediate management in patients with STEMI is to identify candidates for reperfusion therapy. The goal is a door-to-needle time of <30 minutes or door-to-balloon time of <90 minutes. Other key priorities include relief of ischemic pain as well as recognition and treatment of hypotension, pulmonary edema, and arrhythmia.
- **General measures** include continuous BP, pulse oximetry, and telemetry monitoring.
  - Supplemental oxygen should be administered if saturations are <90%. If necessary, institution of mechanical ventilation decreases the work of breathing and reduces myocardial oxygen demand.
  - Two peripheral IV catheters should be inserted upon arrival.
  - Serial ECGs should be obtained for patients who do not have ST-segment elevation on the initial ECG, but experience ongoing chest discomfort as they may demonstrate evolving ST-segment elevation.

Medications

Upstream medical therapy should include administration of antiplatelet and anticoagulant medications as well as agents that reduce myocardial ischemia (Table 32).

- **Aspirin (ASA)** should be given immediately to all patients with suspected acute MI. ASA treatment resulted in relative reduction in cardiovascular mortality by 23% and the incidence of nonfatal MI by 49% (*Lancet 1988;2:349*).
- **Clopidogrel** reduces mortality, reinfarction, and acute stent thrombosis without an increase in serious bleeding or intracranial hemorrhage when given in conjunction

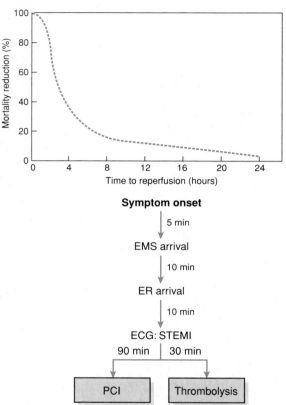

Figure 5. The benefit of coronary reperfusion is inversely related to ischemia time. **Top.** Graphic representation of mortality benefit of coronary reperfusion as a function of ischemia time. (Adapted from *JAMA 2005;293:979.*) **Bottom.** Recommended timeline of events following chest pain onset as a according to ACC/AHA guidelines (*Circulation 2008;117:296*).

with thrombolytic therapy or PCI (*Lancet 2005;366:1607*; *NEJM 2005;352:1179*; *JAMA 2005;294:1224*). Clopidogrel can be given as an alternative to aspirin in the setting of true aspirin allergy (anaphylaxis). Subsequent allergy consultation for aspirin desensitization should be obtained as ASA and clopidogrel treatment is superior to either agent alone.

- **Prasugrel** may be used as an alternative to clopidogrel. In patients who presented with STEMI, prasugrel decreased adverse cardiac outcomes without an increase in major bleeding events compared to clopidogrel (300 mg loading dose, 75 mg maintenance dose) (*NEJM 2007;357:2002*; *Lancet 2009;373:723*).
- **Glycoprotein (GP) IIb/IIIa inhibitors** have shown limited efficacy and increased bleeding rates when used in conjunction with ASA and clopidogrel prior to primary

Table 32	Upstream Medical Therapy	
Medication	Dosage	Comments
Aspirin (ASA)	162–325 mg	Nonenteric coated formulations (chewed or crushed) given orally or rectally facilitate rapid drug absorption and platelet inhibition.
Clopidogrel	300–600 mg loading dose, 75–150 mg daily	600 mg loading dose followed by 7 d of 150 mg maintenance dose may reduce the incidence of stent thrombosis and MI compared to the standard 300 mg loading dose and 75 mg maintenance dose.
		Caution should be used in the elderly as clinical trials validating clopidogrel use in STEMI either did not include elderly patients or did not use a loading dose.
Prasugrel	60 mg loading dose 10 mg daily	Compared to clopidogrel, prasugrel is a quicker acting and more potent antiplatelet agent with improved efficacy, but did significantly increase CABG bleeding rates.
		Prasugrel should not be used in patients greater than 75 yr old, less than 60 kg, or with a history of stroke/TIA.
Unfractionated heparin (UFH)	60 units/kg IV bolus, 12 units/kg/hr	UFH should be given to all patients undergoing PCI and those receiving thrombolytics with the exception of streptokinase.
		The maximum IV bolus is 4,000 units.
Enoxaparin (LMWH)	30 mg IV bolus, 1 mg/kg SC bid	Patients greater than 75 yr of age should not be given a loading dose and receive 0.75 mg SC bid.
		An additional loading dose of 0.3 mg/kg should be given if the last dose of LMWH was more than 8 hr prior to PCI. The use of LMWH is only validated in thrombolysis and rescue PCI.

(continued)

Table 32	Upstream Medical Therapy (*Continued*)	
Medication	**Dosage**	**Comments**
Bivalirudin	0.75 mg/kg IV bolus, 1.75 mg/kg/hr	Bivalirudin has been validated in patients undergoing PCI and has not been studies in conjunction with thrombolysis. Patients who received a heparin bolus prior to bivalirudin had a lower incidence of stent thrombosis than those who only received bivalirudin.
Fondaparinux	2.5 mg IV bolus, 2.5 mg SC daily	Shown to be superior to UFH when used during thrombolysis with decreased bleeding rates. Fondaparinux increases the risk of catheter thrombosis when used during PCI (*JAMA 2006;295:1519*).
Nitroglycerin	0.4 mg SL or aerosol infusion: 10–200 mcg/min	Sublingual or aerosol nitroglycerin can be given every 5 min for a total of three doses in the absence of hypotension. IV nitroglycerin can be used for uncontrolled chest discomfort.
Metoprolol	5 mg IV (3 doses), 25 mg PO qid	β-Blockers should also be avoided in patients with evidence of heart failure, hemodynamic instability, marked first-degree AV block, advanced heart block, and bronchospasm.

PCI (see facilitated PCI). However, it may be reasonable to use GP IIb/IIIa inhibitors as an alternative to clopidogrel, particularly in patients who present with acute complications of MI requiring surgery (ischemic MR, ruptured papillary muscle, or VSD).

- **Anticoagulant therapy (UFH, LMWH, or bivalirudin)** should be initiated in all patients with acute MI regardless of the choice of PCI, thrombolytic, or medical therapy.
  - LMWH (enoxaparin) is an alternative to UFH with more predictable kinetics and easier route of administration that has shown efficacy in conjunction with thrombolysis and PCI (*Lancet 2001;358:605; NEJM 2006;354:1477; JACC 2007;49:2238*). UFH is preferred during PCI as real-time therapeutic monitoring of LWMH in the catheterization laboratory is often not possible.

- **Bivalirudin** should be given to patients with HIT and has equivalent efficacy to UFH with respect to overall mortality when given in combination with ASA and clopidogrel in patients undergoing primary PCI. Bivalirudin reduced bleeding rates at the expense of an increased frequency of acute stent thrombosis (*NEJM 2008;358:2218*; *Lancet 2009;374:1149*).
- UFH or LMWH should be administered to patients receiving selective fibrinolytic agents (alteplase, reteplase, or tenecteplase). UFH has been shown to increase bleeding without improving mortality in patients who receive streptokinase.
- **Nitroglycerin** should be administered to patients with ischemic chest pain. Nitroglycerin should either be avoided or used with caution in patients with:
  - Hypotension (SBP < 90 mm Hg)
  - RVMI
  - HR greater than 100 or less than 50 bpm
  - Documented use of phosphodiesterase inhibitors
- **Morphine** (2 to 4 mg IV) can be used for refractory chest pain that is not responsive to nitroglycerin. Adequate analgesia decreases levels of circulating catecholamines and reduces myocardial oxygen consumption.
- **β-Adrenergic blockade** improves myocardial ischemia, limits infarct size, and reduces major adverse cardiac events including mortality, recurrent ischemia, and malignant arrhythmias. IV β-blockers can increase mortality in patients with HF, cardiogenic shock (Killip II or greater), age older than 70 years, SBP less than 120 mm Hg, HR greater than 110 or less than 60 bpm (*Lancet 2005;366:1622*). Oral β-blockers may be used with caution in select patients.
- **Acute coronary reperfusion**
  - The majority of patients who suffer an acute STEMI have thrombotic occlusion of the infarct-related coronary artery. Early restoration of coronary perfusion limits infarct size, preserves LV function, and reduces mortality.
    - All patients who present with a STEMI within 12 to 24 hours of symptom onset should be considered for immediate reperfusion therapy.
    - Unless spontaneous resolution of ischemia occurs (as determined by resolution of chest discomfort and normalization of ST elevation), the choice of reperfusion strategy includes thrombolysis, primary PCI, or emergent CABG (Fig. 6).
    - The choice of reperfusion therapy should almost be considered of secondary importance to the overall goal of achieving reperfusion in a timely fashion as the morbidity and mortality associated with an acute MI are linearly related to the time to treatment.
    - In general, primary PCI is the preferred reperfusion strategy when available within 90 minutes of medical contact (including transfer to a PCI-capable facility). If cardiac catheterization is not readily available, thrombolytic therapy should be administered within 30 minutes of medical contact.
    - **PCI** is preferred over thrombolysis in patients who:
      - Are <75 years of age and present with cardiogenic shock within 36 hours of MI and PCI can be performed within 18 hours of shock
      - Have a contraindication to fibrinolytic therapy
      - Are at high risk of death or development of CHF
      - Underwent recent PCI or prior CABG
    - **Thrombolysis** may be preferred if patients are presenting to the hospital within the first 2 hours of symptom onset.
  - **Primary PCI** is the preferred reperfusion strategy when performed in a timely fashion at an appropriate facility. Compared to thrombolytic therapy, PCI offers

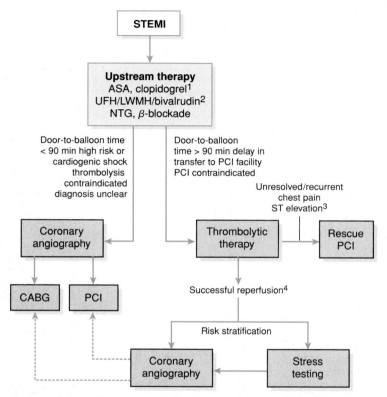

Figure 6. Strategies for coronary reperfusion and risk assessment. [1]Prasugrel may be used in place of clopidogrel in patients undergoing PCI. [2]UFH may be used with either PCI or thrombolytic therapy, while bivalirudin has only been studied with PCI and LMWH has only been validated for thrombolytic therapy and rescue PCI. [3]Patients who do not experience chest pain relief or ST-segment normalization 60 to 90 minutes following thrombolysis should undergo rescue PCI. [4]Signs of successful reperfusion include chest pain relief, 50% reduction in ST-segment elevation and idioventricular rhythm. ASA, aspirin; UFH, unfractionated heparin; LMWH, low-molecular-weight heparin; NTG, nitroglycerin; PCI, percutaneous coronary intervention; CABG, coronary artery bypass graft.

superior vessel patency and improved survival regardless of lesion location or patient age (*NEJM 1997;336:1621*; *Lancet 2003;361:13*).

○ Primary PCI should be considered if an available catheterization facility can provide a door-to-balloon time of less than 90 minutes. Optimally, operators should perform greater than 75 PCIs per year at experienced centers with a volume that exceeds 200 PCIs per year.

○ Patients who present to a facility where cardiac catheterization is not available should be immediately transferred to a PCI-capable center with an estimated total door-to-balloon time of less than 90 minutes. In this setting, primary

PCI significantly lowered the incidence of death, MI, or stroke compared to on-site thrombolysis (*NEJM 2003;249:733*; *JACC 2002;39:1713*; *Eur Heart J 2000;21:823*). If the estimated transfer time will exceed a total door-to-balloon time of 90 minutes, on-site thrombolysis should be performed (see below).

○ PCI is also indicated in patients who present with cardiogenic shock, refractory arrhythmias, have contraindications to thrombolytic therapy, or if the diagnosis is uncertain.

○ Treatment is optimal when the angioplasty is performed within 12 hours of symptom onset and may be effective beyond that point if symptoms persist.

○ Additional advantages of primary PCI include immediate assessment of coronary anatomy, atherosclerotic disease burden, and LV function.

○ If the patient has multivessel coronary disease, the appropriateness and timing of complete revascularization should be determined after the infarct-related artery is opened and the patient stabilized.
  - If the functional significance of coronary lesions is not readily apparent, an invasive (FFR) or noninvasive (stress testing) assessment should be undertaken.
  - Complete revascularization is best performed in a staged manner to minimize contrast-mediated renal toxicity.

○ Coronary stenting is superior to balloon angioplasty alone and reduces the rates of target vessel revascularization (*NEJM 1999;341:1949*; *NEJM 2002;346:957*). DES further reduce the need for target vessel revascularization without increasing the incidence of stent thrombosis (*Circulation 2009;120:964*; *JACC 2008;51:618*; *JAMA 2008;299:1788*).

○ Abciximab infusion at the time of PCI should be routinely used as it reduces the rate of death, MI, and urgent revascularization by approximately 50% (*Circulation 1998;98:734*; *NEJM 2001;344:1895*; *JACC 2003;42:1879*). Recommended anticoagulation strategies for PCI are shown in Figure 7.
  - Eptifibatide and tirofiban may have similar efficacy to abciximab (*Am J Cardiol 2004;94:35*; *JAMA 2008;299:1788*; *JACC 2008;51:529*).
  - Bivalirudin is an acceptable alternative to the use of combined heparin and GP IIb/IIIa inhibitor during PCI with lower bleeding rates (*NEJM 2008;358:2218* *JAMA 2003;19:853*).

○ Facilitated PCI, a strategy of reduced dose of GP IIb/IIIa inhibitors and/or thrombolytic agent prior to PCI, should not be routinely employed as it does not improve efficacy and significantly increases bleeding rates (*Lancet 2006;367:569*; *NEJM 2008;358:2205*; *Lancet 2006;367:579*).

• **Thrombolytic therapy** offers the advantages of availability and rapid administration. The primary disadvantage of thrombolytic therapy is the risk of intracranial hemorrhage, uncertainty of whether normal coronary flow has been restored, and reocclusion of the infarct-related artery.

○ Thrombolytic therapy is most effective if given within 12 hours of the symptom onset with a pooled relative mortality reduction of 18% (*Lancet 1994;343:311*; *Lancet 1987;2:871*). Beyond 12 hours, thrombolysis yields little benefit.

○ Thrombolytic therapy is not indicated for patients with resolved chest pain or those with ST-segment depression.

○ Absolute and relative contraindications to thrombolytic therapy are listed in Table 33.

○ Multiple thrombolytic agents are available and are classified into two groups based on their selectivity for fibrin substrates. Fibrin-selective agents include **recombinant tissue plasminogen activator** (rt-PA), **reteplase** (r-PA), and

Upstream therapy ASA, clopidogrel[1] UFH (bolus)	Upstream therapy ASA, clopidogrel[1] UFH (bolus)	Upstream therapy ASA, clopidogrel[1] LMWH (bolus)
ⅴ	ⅴ	ⅴ
PCI UFH	PCI bivalrudin	PCI LMWH ± UFH
ⅴ	ⅴ	ⅴ
Abciximab	Bivalrudin	Abciximab

Advantages	proven efficacy	lower bleeding rates mortality benefit[2]	ease of administration
Disadvantages	higher bleeding rates	increased stent thrombosis without UFH bolus	only validated in rescue PCI[3] inconsistent anticoagulation

Figure 7. Recommended strategies for upstream therapy prior to PCI. [1] Prasugrel may be used in place of clopidogrel in patients undergoing PCI. GP IIb/IIIa inhibitors may be used instead of clopidogrel in patients who present with mechanical complications of MI and require urgent cardiac surgery. [2] In comparison to UFH + GP IIb/IIIa inhibitor, bivalirudin improves mortality and decreases bleeding in patients presenting with STEMI. A heparin bolus should be given prior to bivalirudin to decrease the rate of stent thrombosis (*NEJM 2008;358:2218*). [3] LMWH has only been studied in rescue PCI and has not been validated for primary PCI (*NEJM 2006;354:1477*). ASA, aspirin; UFH, unfractionated heparin; LMWH, low-molecular-weight heparin; NTG, nitroglycerin; PCI, percutaneous coronary intervention.

Table 33	Contraindications to Thrombolytic Therapy

Absolute Contraindications	Relative Contraindications
History of intracranial hemorrhage or hemorrhagic stroke	Prior ischemic stroke more than 3 mo ago
Ischemic stroke within 3 mo	Allergy or previous use of streptokinase (greater than 5 d ago)[a]
Known structural cerebrovascular lesion (AVMs, aneurysms, tumor)	Recent internal bleeding (2–4 wk)
Closed head injury within 3 mo	Prolonged/traumatic CPR more than 10 min
Aortic dissection	Major surgery within 3 wk
Severe uncontrolled hypertension (SBP > 180 mm Hg, DBP > 110 mm Hg)	Active peptic ulcer disease
Active bleeding or bleeding diathesis	Noncompressible vascular punctures
Acute pericarditis	Severe menstrual bleeding
	History of intraocular bleeding
	Pregnancy

AVM, arteriovenous malformation; CPR, cardiopulmonary resuscitation; DBP, diastolic blood pressure; SBP, systolic blood pressure.
[a] Thrombolytics other than streptokinase may be used.

tenecteplase (TNK-tPA). **Streptokinase** is the only nonselective agent in use. Further details and dosing information can be found in Table 34.

- The **choice of thrombolytic agent** is guided by considerations of efficacy, bleeding risk, availability, ease of administration, and cost. Compared with streptokinase, rt-PA is associated with a slightly greater risk of intracranial hemorrhage but offers the net clinical benefit of additional 10 lives saved per 1,000 patients treated (*NEJM 1993;329:673*).

- Fibrin-selective agents should be used in combination with anticoagulant therapy (UFH, LMWH, fondaparinux, or bivalirudin). Recent studies have demonstrated that LMWH and fondaparinux may be superior to UFH (*Lancet 2001;358:605*; *Circulation 2002;105:1642*; *NEJM 2006;354:1477*; *JAMA 2006;295:1519*). Addition of UFH to streptokinase does not improve outcomes (*NEJM 1993;329:673*).

○ The therapeutic efficacy of thrombolytic treatment can be monitored by clinical response (resolution of chest pain), improvement in ST-segment elevation, or by the presence of accelerated idioventricular rhythm.

- Thrombolytic therapy does not achieve coronary artery patency in 30% of patients. In contrast, primary PCI results in restoration of normal coronary flow (TIMI 3) in greater than 95% of cases.

○ Individuals with persistent angina or persistent ischemic changes on the ECG (<50% reduction in ST-segment elevation) 60 to 90 minutes after the initiation of thrombolytic therapy should be considered for urgent coronary angiography and PCI (rescue PCI).

- Rescue PCI reduces the incidence of death, reinfarction, and HF by nearly 50% (*Circulation 1994;90:2280*; *NEJM 2005;353:2758*).

- Routine coronary angiography within 24 hours of thrombolysis has reduced adverse cardiac events compared to rescue PCI (*Lancet 2004;264:1045*). Routine PCI has also proved beneficial for patients who receive thrombolysis as an initial therapy and are subsequently transferred to a PCI-capable facility (*Lancet 2008;371:559*). This strategy should be differentiated from facilitated PCI where thrombolytic agents are administered immediately before primary PCI.

○ The most common complication of thrombolytic therapy is bleeding. Intracranial hemorrhage occurs in 0.7% to 0.9% of cases and may result in death or permanent neurologic defects.

- The risk of intracranial hemorrhage is increased twofold in patients older than 75 years, less than 70 kg, on anticoagulation therapy (Coumadin), or with severe hypertension (BP > 170/90).

- Any patient who experiences a sudden change in neurologic status should undergo urgent head CT and all anticoagulant and thrombolytic therapies discontinued. Fresh frozen plasma should be given to patients with intracerebral hemorrhage. Cryoprecipitate may also be used to replenish fibrinogen and factor VIII levels. Platelet transfusions can be useful in patients with markedly prolonged bleeding times. Neurologic and neurosurgical consultation should be obtained immediately.

- Major bleeding complications that require blood transfusion occur in approximately 10% of patients.

- Venipuncture should be limited and arterial puncture avoided in patients treated with thrombolytic therapy for 24 hours after the initiation of treatment.

Table 34   Thrombolytic Agents

Medication	Dosage	Comments
Streptokinase (SK)	1.5 million units IV over 60 min	Produces a generalized fibrinolytic state (not clot specific).
		SK reduces mortality following STEMI: 18% relative risk reduction and 2% absolute risk reduction (*Lancet 1987;2:871*).
		Allergic reactions including skin rashes, fever, and anaphylaxis may be seen in 1–2% of patients. Isolated hypotension occurs in 10% of patients and usually responds to volume expansion.
		Because of the development of antibodies, patients who were previously treated with streptokinase should be given an alternate thrombolytic agent.
Recombinant tissue plasminogen activator (rt-PA)	15 mg IV bolus 0.75 mg/kg over 30 min (maximum 50 mg) 0.50 mg/kg over 60 min (maximum 35 mg)	Fibrin selective agent with improved clot specificity compared to SK.
		Does not cause allergic reactions or hypotension.
		Mortality benefit compared to SK at the expense of an increased risk of intracranial hemorrhage (*NEJM 1993;329:673*)
Reteplase (r-PA)	Two 10-unit IV boluses administered 30 min apart	Fibrin selective agent with a longer half-life but reduced clot specificity compared to rt-PA.
		Mortality benefit equivalent to that of rt-PA (*NEJM 1997;337:1118*).
Tenecteplase (TNK-tPA)	0.50 mg/kg IV bolus (total dose 30–50 mg)	Genetically engineered variant of rt-PA with slower plasma clearance, improved fibrin specificity, and higher resistance to plasminogen activator inhibitor-1 (PAI-1).
		Mortality benefit equivalent to that of rt-PA with reduced bleeding rates (*Lancet 1999;354:716*).
		Monitoring is required with a goal aPTT of 1.5–2.5 times control.

- **Emergency CABG** is a high-risk procedure that should be considered only if the patient has severe left main disease or refractory ischemia in the setting of failed PCI or coronary anatomy that is not amenable to PCI. Emergency surgery should also be considered for patients with acute mechanical complications of MI including papillary muscle rupture, severe ischemic MR, VSD, ventricular aneurysm formation in the setting of intractable ventricular arrhythmias, or ventricular free wall rupture.

Peri-infarct Management

- **The coronary care unit (CCU)** was the first major advance in the modern era of treatment of acute MI. The majority of patients benefit from the specialized training of the nursing and support staff in the CCU. Most patients with acute MI should be observed for 24 to 48 hours in the CCU.
- Bedrest is appropriate intermediate care for the first 24 hours after presentation with an acute MI. After 24 hours, clinically stable patients can progressively advance their activity as tolerated.
- Patients should have continuous telemetry monitoring to detect for recurrent ischemia and arrhythmias. Daily evaluation should include assessment for recurrent chest discomfort and HF symptoms, physical exam focusing on new murmurs and evidence of HF, and routine ECGs.
- A baseline echocardiogram should be obtained to document ejection fraction, wall motion abnormalities, valvular lesions, and presence of ventricular thrombus.
- **Hemodynamic monitoring** may be useful to optimize medical therapy in unstable patients (see below).
- **Cardiac pacing** may be required in the setting of an acute MI. Rhythm disturbance may be transient in nature, in which case temporary pacing is sufficient until a stable rhythm returns (see below).

Post-MI Medical Therapy

- **Aspirin** is the preferred antiplatelet agent after MI and should be used indefinitely. Doses of 75 to 325 mg/d have been shown to reduce the risk of recurrent MI, stroke, and cardiac death.
- **Clopidogrel** (75 mg/d) or **Prasugrel** (10 mg/d) should be given for a minimum of 1 month in patients who receive a BMS and for at least 1 year in patients who receive a DES.
- **β-Blockers** confer a mortality benefit following acute MI. Treatment should begin as soon as possible (preferably within the first 24 hours) and continued indefinitely.
- **ACE inhibitors** provide a reduction in short-term mortality and incidence of CHF and recurrent MI when initiated within the first 24 hours of an acute MI (*Lancet 1994;343:1115*; *Lancet 1995;345.669*).
  - Patients with ejection fraction less than 40%, large anterior MI, and prior MI derive the most benefit from ACE-inhibitor therapy.
  - Therapy may be initiated with captopril and titrated as BP permits. Conversion to a more long-acting agent is appropriate prior to discharge.
  - Contraindications include hypotension, acute renal failure, bilateral renal artery stenosis, and hyperkalemia. Care must be taken to avoid hypotension.
  - Angiotensin II receptor blockers can be used in patients who are intolerant of ACE inhibitors with equivalent efficacy.
- **HMG-CoA reductase inhibitors** should be started in all patients in the absence of contraindications. Several trials have shown the benefit of early and aggressive use of

statins following AMI. The goal is at least 50% reduction in LDL or LDL less than 70 mg/dL.

- **Aldosterone receptor antagonists (Aldactone and eplerenone)** have shown benefit in post-MI patients with LV ejection fraction of less than 40% (*NEJM 1999;341:709; NEJM 2003;348:1309*). Caution should be used in patients with hyperkalemia and renal insufficiency.

SPECIAL CONSIDERATIONS

Risk assessment

- Patients who present greater than 24 hours after symptom onset and those who receive thrombolysis or medical therapy alone should undergo further risk assessment. Patients may be evaluated using either a noninvasive (stress testing) or invasive (coronary angiography) strategy.
- **Stress testing** can be used to determine prognosis, residual ischemia, and functional capacity.
  - A submaximal exercise stress test can be performed as early as 4 to 6 days following MI. Pharmacologic stress testing (preferably nuclear perfusion imaging) may also be used and is optimal for evaluating ischemic burden.
  - Alternatively, stress testing can be performed after hospital discharge (2 to 6 weeks) for low-risk patients.
  - Coronary angiography should be performed in patients with limiting angina, significant ischemic burden, and those with poor functional capacity.
- **Cardiac catheterization without prior noninvasive assessment** is an alternative approach for high-risk individuals who presented greater than 24 hours after symptom onset or those managed medically. At the time of catheterization, decisions on revascularization should be made based on the patient's anatomy, ventricular function, and clinical status.
  - Recent studies have failed to show any benefit of opening totally occluded arteries greater than 3 days following acute MI in clinically stable patients (*NEJM 2006;355:2395–2407*). In this population, assessment of myocardial viability should be performed prior to PCI.
  - Angioplasty of a totally occluded infarct-related artery may be considered in clinically unstable patients, those with rest angina, NYHA class III–IV HF, or those with multivessel disease.
- Patients treated medically who experience complications of MI, including recurrent angina/ischemia, HF, significant ventricular arrhythmia, or a mechanical complication of the MI, should proceed directly to coronary angiography to define their anatomy and offer an appropriate revascularization strategy.
- **Special clinical situations**
  - **RVMI** is seen in approximately 50% of patients with an acute inferior MI. Roughly half of these patients have hemodynamic compromise as a result of right ventricular involvement.
    - Clinical signs may include hypotension, cardiogenic shock, elevated jugular venous pulsation, Kussmaul sign (an increase in jugular venous pressures with inspiration), and right-sided third or fourth heart sounds. The lung fields are often clear in the absence of a large inferior infarct or MR.
    - Right precordial ECG leads should be obtained and analyzed for ST elevation (V_4R is the most sensitive and specific lead and is transient).

Table 35	Risk Factors for ISR and Stent Thrombosis
ISR	**Stent Thrombosis**
Diabetes	Clopidogrel discontinuation
Chronic kidney disease	Clopidogrel resistance
Prior restenosis	Diabetes
Prior stent placed in the setting of ACS	Chronic kidney disease
Small luminal diameter (<2.5 mm)	Malignancy
Long lesion length	Prior brachytherapy
Proximal LAD lesion	Small luminal diameter (<3 mm)
Saphenous vein graft lesion	Long lesion length
Residual stenosis following prior	Bifurcation lesion
intervention	Margin dissection
	Incomplete wall apposition
	Overlapping stents

ISR, in-stent restenosis; ACS, acute coronary syndrome; LAD, left anterior descending artery.

- ○ LV filling pressures are typically normal or decreased, the right atrial pressures are elevated (>10 mm Hg), and the cardiac index is depressed. In some patients, elevated right atrial pressures may not be evident until IV fluids are administered.
- ○ Initial therapy is intravenous fluids. If hypotension persists, inotropic support with dobutamine and/or an intra-aortic balloon pump (IABP) may be necessary. Invasive hemodynamic monitoring is critical in the hypotensive patient as it guides volume status and the need for inotropic and mechanical support.
- ○ In patients with heart block and AV dyssynchrony, sequential AV pacing may have a marked beneficial effect.
- • **ISR and stent thrombosis** are disease entities unique to patients who have previously undergone coronary angioplasty. Risk factors for ISR and stent thrombosis can be found in Table 35.
  - ○ ISR is a result of intimal hyperplasia and occurs within 6 to 9 months following balloon angioplasty and stent deployment. Progressive exertional angina is the typical presenting symptom. Prior to BMS, the incidence of target lesion restenosis 1 year following balloon angioplasty was 35% to 40%. BMS placement reduced the rate of angiographic restenosis to 20% to 30% and DES have further reduced the 1-year restenosis rate to 3% to 5%.
    - - DES placement is the treatment of choice for ISR. Several DES systems are available including paclitaxel (TAXUS), sirolimus (CYPHER), and everolimus (Xience) eluting stents. The TAXUS and CYPHER stents are the best studied and significantly reduce ISR rates (*NEJM 2002;346:1773*; *NEJM 2003;349:1315*; *JAMA 2005;294:1215*), with the CYPHER stent producing the lowest rates of lumen loss (*JAMA 2006;295:895*; *Circulation 2006;114:2148*). Early studies with the Xience stent have demonstrated improved results compared to the TAXUS stent (*JAMA 2008;299:1903*; *Circulation 2009;119:680*).
    - - Other proposed treatments for ISR including rotational atherectomy and brachytherapy produce inferior results compared to DES placement, and in the case of brachytherapy increase the risk of stent thrombosis (*JAMA 2006;295:1264*; *JAMA 2006;295:1253*).

○ Stent thrombosis occurs with BMS or DES, and is due to poor endothelial repair. Stent thrombosis commonly presents either as an ACS or as sudden cardiac death. The etiology of stent thrombosis is based on the time from prior coronary intervention (*JAMA 2005;293:2126*; *JACC 2009;53:1399*).

- Acute stent thrombosis occurs within 24 hours and is due to mechanical procedural complications as well as inadequate anticoagulation and antiplatelet therapies.

- Subacute stent thrombosis (24 hours to 30 days) is a consequence of inadequate platelet inhibition and mechanical stent complications. Cessation of clopidogrel therapy during this time yields a 30- to 100-fold risk of stent thrombosis.

- Late (30 days to 1 year) and very late (greater than 1 year) stent thrombosis occur principally with DES and are associated with clopidogrel cessation (four- to sixfold increased risk) and resistance.

- Given the high mortality rate, the best treatment for stent thrombosis is prevention. In general, PCI with thrombus aspiration and repeat stent deployment is recommended. Screening for clopidogrel resistance and initiation of more potent antiplatelet regimens such as prasugrel or clopidogrel 150 mg in combination with cilostazol is warranted (*JACC 2005;46:1833*; *Circulation* 2009;119:3207).

• **Ischemic MR** is a poor prognostic indicator following MI that most often presents with HF. It is associated with posterior infarcts and resultant posterior papillary muscle involvement. The presence of MR following MI significantly increases mortality (*Ann Intern Med 1992;117:10*; *Am J Med 2006;119:103*).

○ The mechanism of acute MR includes papillary muscle dysfunction or leaflet tethering due to posterior wall akinesis.

○ Progressive MR following MI may develop as a result of LV chamber dilation, apical remodeling, or posterior wall dyskinesis. These changes lead to leaflet tethering or mitral annular dilation.

○ Echocardiography is the diagnostic modality of choice. Ischemic MR is not always readily identified on physical exam and may have unusual characteristics due to the posteriorly directed regurgitant jet. TEE may be required to access the severity and mechanism of MR.

○ Initial treatment involves aggressive afterload reduction and revascularization. Stable patients should receive a trial of medical therapy and undergo surgery only if they fail to improve. Early surgical intervention is warranted for patients with severe ischemic MR and HF as well as those who are unlikely to benefit from revascularization.

• **STEMI** in the setting of recent **cocaine use** presents a unique and challenging management situation (*Circulation 2008;117:1897–1907*). ST elevation can result from myocardial ischemia due to coronary vasospasm, in situ thrombus formation, and/or increased myocardial oxygen demand. The common pathophysiology is excessive stimulation of α- and β-adrenergic receptors. Chest pain due to cocaine use usually occurs within 3 hours, but may be seen several days following use.

○ Oxygen, aspirin, and heparin (UFH or LMWH) should be administered to all patients with cocaine-associated STEMI.

○ Nitrates should be used preferentially to treat vasospasm. Additionally, benzodiazepines may confer additional relief by decreasing sympathetic tone.

○ **Selective β_1-adrenergic blockers** are contraindicated due to the potential for unopposed α-adrenergic activity.

- Phentolamine (α-adrenergic antagonist) and calcium channel blockers may reverse coronary vasospasm and are recommended as second-line agents.
- The use of reperfusion therapy is controversial and should be reserved for those patients whose symptoms persist despite initial medical therapy.
  - Primary PCI is the preferred approach for the patient with persistent symptoms and ECG changes despite aggressive medical therapy. It is important to note that coronary angiography and intervention carry a significant risk of worsening vasospasm.
  - Fibrinolytic therapy should be reserved for patients who are clearly having a STEMI who cannot undergo PCI.

COMPLICATIONS

Complications following acute MI

Myocardial damage predisposes the patient to several potential adverse consequences and complications that should be considered if the patient experiences new clinical signs and/or symptoms. These include recurrent chest pain, cardiac arrhythmias, cardiogenic shock, and mechanical complications of MI.

- **Recurrent chest pain** may be due to ischemia in the territory of the original infarction, pericarditis, myocardial rupture, or pulmonary embolism.
  - Recurrent angina is experienced by 20% to 30% of patients after MI who receive fibrinolytic therapy and up to 10% of patients in the early time period following percutaneous revascularization. These symptoms may represent recurrence of ischemia or infarct extension.
    - Assessment of the patient may include evaluation for new murmurs or friction rubs, ECG to assess for new ischemic changes, cardiac enzymes (troponin and CK-MB), echocardiography, and repeat coronary angiography if indicated.
    - Patients with recurrent chest pain should continue to receive ASA, clopidogrel, heparin, nitroglycerin, and β-adrenergic antagonist therapy.
    - If recurrent angina is refractory to medical treatment, repeat coronary angiography and intervention should be considered along with possible placement of an IABP.
  - **Acute pericarditis** occurs 24 to 96 hours after MI in approximately 10% to 15% of patients. The associated chest pain is often pleuritic and may be relieved in the upright position. A friction rub may be noted on clinical examination and the ECG may show diffuse ST-segment elevation. Treatment is directed at pain management.
    - Aspirin is generally considered a first-line agent. NSAIDs such as indomethacin (25 to 50 mg qid) may be used if aspirin is not effective.
    - Glucocorticoids (prednisone, 1 mg/kg daily) may be useful if symptoms are severe and refractory to initial therapy. Steroid use should be deferred until at least 4 weeks after acute MI due to their adverse impact on infarct healing and risk of ventricular rupture (*Am Heart J 1981;101:750*). Colchicine may be beneficial for recurrent symptoms.
    - Heparin should be avoided in the setting of pericarditis with or without effusion as it may lead to pericardial hemorrhage.
  - **Dressler syndrome** is thought to be an autoimmune process characterized by malaise, fever, pericardial pain, leukocytosis, elevated sedimentation rate, and often

a pericardial effusion. In contrast to acute pericarditis, Dressler syndrome occurs 1 to 8 weeks after MI. Treatment is identical to acute pericarditis.

- **Arrhythmias.** Cardiac rhythm abnormalities are common following MI and may include conduction block, atrial arrhythmias, and ventricular arrhythmias. Arrhythmias that result in hemodynamic compromise require prompt, aggressive intervention. If the arrhythmia precipitates refractory angina or HF, urgent therapy is warranted. For all rhythm disturbances exacerbating conditions should be addressed, including electrolyte imbalances, hypoxia, acidosis, and adverse drug effects. (Details on specific arrhythmias can be found in Table 36.)
  - **Transcutaneous and transvenous pacing.** Conduction system disease that progresses to complete heart block or results in symptomatic bradycardia can be effectively treated with cardiac pacing. A transcutaneous pacing device can be used under emergent circumstances, and a temporary transvenous system can be used for longer-duration therapy.
    - Absolute indications for temporary transvenous pacing include asystole, symptomatic bradycardia, recurrent sinus pauses, complete heart block, and incessant VT.
    - Temporary transvenous pacing may also be warranted for new trifascicular block, new Mobitz II block, and for patients with LBBB who require a pulmonary artery catheter, given the risk of developing complete heart block.
  - **Implantable cardioverter-defibrillators (ICDs)** should not routinely be implanted in patients with reduced LV function following MI or those with ventricular tachycardia/fibrillation (VT/VF) in the setting of ischemia or immediately following reperfusion.
    - Routine insertion of ICDs into patients with reduced LV function immediately following MI does not improve outcomes (*NEJM 2004;351:2481*).
    - In contrast, patients who continue to have depressed LV function (EF <35%) greater than 1 month following MI benefit from ICD therapy (*NEJM 2005;352: 225*).
    - ICD therapy is also indicated for patients with recurrent episodes of sustained VT or VF despite coronary reperfusion.
- **Cardiogenic shock** is an infrequent but serious complication of MI and is defined as hypotension in the setting of inadequate ventricular function to meet the metabolic needs of the peripheral tissue. Risk factors include prior MI, older age, diabetes, and anterior infarction. Organ hypoperfusion may manifest as progressive renal failure, dyspnea, diaphoresis, or mental status changes. Hemodynamic monitoring reveals elevated filling pressures (wedge pressure >20 mm Hg) and depressed cardiac index (<2.5 L/kg/min).
- Patients with cardiogenic shock in the setting of MI have a mortality in excess of 50%. Such patients may require invasive hemodynamic monitoring and advanced therapeutic modalities including inotropic and mechanical support (Fig. 8).
- **Dobutamine** is the inotrope of choice for patients with relatively preserved SBP (>90 mm Hg) as it both increases myocardial contractility and decreases ventricular afterload.
- **Dopamine** is the preferred therapeutic agent in patients with an SBP less than 80 mm Hg. Addition of norepinephrine or phenylephrine may be required in markedly hypotensive patients (SBP <70 mm Hg).
- **Milrinone** should be added in patients who are either not responding to dobutamine or who are experiencing excessive tachycardia in response to dobutamine. It should not be routinely used in patients with renal insufficiency.

Table 36	Arrhythmias Complicating MI	
Arrhythmia	**Treatment**	**Comments**
Intraventricular conduction delays	None	The left anterior fascicle is most commonly affected because of isolated coronary blood supply. Bifascicular and trifascicular block may progress to complete heart block and other rhythm disturbances.
Sinus bradycardia	None Atropine 0.5 mg Temporary pacing[a]	Sinus bradycardia is common in patients with RCA infarcts. In the absence of hypotension or significant ventricular ectopy, observation is indicated.
AV block	Temporary pacing[a]	First-degree AV block usually does not require specific treatment. Mobitz I second-degree block occurs more often with inferior MI. The block is usually within the His bundle and does not require treatment unless symptomatic bradycardia is present. Mobitz II second-degree AV block originates below the His bundle and is more commonly associated with anterior MI. Because of the significant risk of progression to complete heart block, patients should be observed in the CCU and treated with temporary pacing if symptomatic. Third-degree AV block complicates large anterior and RV infarcts. In patients with anterior MI, third-degree heart block often occurs 12–24 hr after initial presentation and may appear suddenly. Temporary pacing is recommended because of the risk of progression to ventricular asystole.

(*continued*)

Table 36	Arrhythmias Complicating MI (*Continued*)	
Arrhythmia	**Treatment**	**Comments**
Sinus tachycardia	None[b]	Sinus tachycardia is common in patients with acute MI and is often due to enhanced sympathetic activity resulting from pain, anxiety, hypovolemia, anxiety, heart failure, or fever. Persistent sinus tachycardia suggests poor underlying ventricular function and is associated with excess mortality.
Atrial fibrillation and flutter	β-Blockers Anticoagulation Cardioversion	Atrial fibrillation and flutter are observed in up to 20% of patients with acute MI. Because atrial fibrillation and atrial flutter are usually transient in the acute MI period, long-term anticoagulation is often not necessary after documentation of stable sinus rhythm.
Accelerated junctional rhythm	None	Accelerated junctional rhythm occurs in conjunction with inferior MI. The rhythm is usually benign and warrants treatment only if hypotension is present. Digitalis intoxication should be considered in patients with accelerated junctional rhythm.
Ventricular premature depolarizations (VPDs)	β-Blockers if symptomatic[c]	VPDs are common in the course of an acute MI. Prophylactic treatment with lidocaine or other antiarrhythmics has been associated with increased overall mortality and is not recommended (*NEJM 1989; 321:406*).
Accelerated idioventricular rhythm (AIVR)	None	Commonly seen within 48 hr of successful reperfusion and is not associated with an increased incidence of adverse outcomes. If hemodynamically unstable, sinus activity may be restored with atropine or temporary atrial pacing.

(*continued*)

Table 36	Arrhythmias Complicating MI (*Continued*)	
Arrhythmia	Treatment	Comments
Ventricular tachycardia (VT)	Cardioversion for sustained VT Lidocaine or amiodarone for 24–48 hr[d]	Nonsustained ventricular tachycardia (NSVT, <30 sec) is common in the first 24 hr after MI and is only associated with increased mortality when occurring late in the post-MI course. Sustained VT (>30 sec) during the first 48 hr after acute MI is associated with increased in-hospital mortality.
Ventricular fibrillation (VF)	Unsynchronized cardioversion Lidocaine or amiodarone for 24–48 hr[d]	VF occurs in up to 5% of patients in the early post-MI period and is life threatening.

[a]Atropine and temporary pacing should only be used for symptomatic or hemodynamically unstable patients.
[b]The use of β-blockers in the setting of sinus tachycardia and poor LV function may result in decompensated heart failure.
[c]β-Blockers should be used with caution in the setting of bradycardia and frequent VPDs as they may increase the risk of polymorphic VT.
[d]Lidocaine should be used as a 1 mg/kg bolus followed by a 1 to 2 mg/kg/hr infusion. Amiodarone should be given as a 150 to 300 mg bolus followed by an infusion of 1 mg/kg/hr for 6 hours and then 0.5 mg/kg/hr for 18 hours.

- Patients in whom contraindications do not exist should be considered for insertion of an IABP, as inotropes increase myocardial oxygen consumption and may worsen ischemia (Table 37).
- All patients with cardiogenic shock should undergo echocardiography to evaluate for mechanical complications of MI (see below).
- For patients who present with cardiogenic shock, an early revascularization strategy is superior to initial medical stabilization. This benefit did not extend to patients older than 75 years (*NEJM 1999;341:625*).
- Select patients with refractory HF who fail to respond to inotropes and require prolonged mechanical support may be considered for either cardiac transplant or placement of a LV assist device (LVAD).
- Patients with large anterior infarcts, documented LV thrombus, or chronic atrial fibrillation should receive continued anticoagulant therapy. Heparin (UFH or LMWH) can be used until a therapeutic INR of 2 to 3 is achieved.
- Patients with anterior apical akinesis or documented LV thrombus as assessed by echocardiography at the time of discharge should receive Coumadin for 3 to 6 months unless other indications warrant its continued use. The dose of aspirin should be reduced to 81 mg to decrease bleeding risk.
- If **HIT** develops, heparin should be discontinued immediately and anticoagulation performed with a direct thrombin inhibitor (bivalirudin or argatroban).

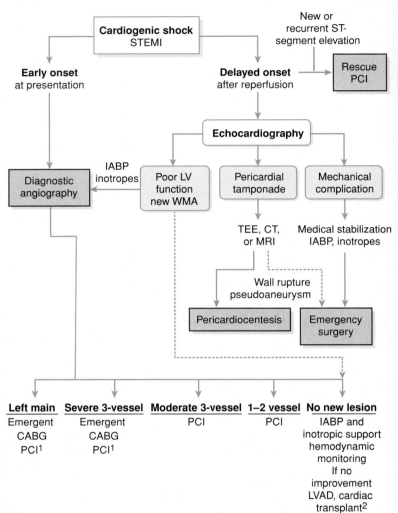

Figure 8. Recommended diagnostic and therapeutic strategy for patients presenting with STEMI and cardiogenic shock. [1] PCI may be preferable if CABG cannot be readily performed or if surgery imposes unacceptable risk. [2] Advanced heart therapy modalities including percutaneous LV assist devices (TandemHeart, Impella), external ventricular assist devices, and extracorporeal membrane oxygenation (ECMO) may be required prior to placement of a permanent LVAD or cardiac transplant. PCI, percutaneous coronary intervention; WMA, wall motion abnormality; TEE, transesophageal echocardiography; IABP, intra-aortic balloon counterpulsation; LVAD, left ventricular assist device; CABG, coronary artery bypass graft.

Table 37	Intra-Aortic Balloon Counterpulsation	
Indications	**Contraindications**	**Monitoring**
Cardiogenic shock, pump failure	Aortic insufficiency	Daily chest x-ray, platelet count, and creatinine
Papillary muscle rupture	Severe peripheral vascular disease	Regular evaluation of lower extremity pulses
Severe ischemic mitral regurgitation	Systemic infection, sepsis	Heparin infusion (PTT)
VSD		
Facilitation of unprotected left main and LAD angioplasty or CABG		
Complex PCI with severe underlying CAD		

VSD, ventricular septal defect; LAD, left anterior descending artery; CABG, coronary artery bypass graft; PCI, percutaneous coronary intervention.

- **Mechanical complications**
  - **Aneurysm.** After MI, the affected area of the myocardium may undergo infarct expansion and thinning, forming an aneurysm. The wall motion may become dyskinetic, and the endocardial surface is at risk for mural thrombus formation.
    - LV aneurysm is suggested by persistent ST elevation on the ECG and may be diagnosed by imaging studies including ventriculography, echocardiography, and MRI.
    - Anticoagulation is warranted to lower the risk of embolic events, especially if a mural thrombus is present (see above).
    - Surgical intervention may be appropriate if the aneurysm results in HF or ventricular arrhythmias that are not satisfactorily managed with medical therapy.
  - **Ventricular pseudoaneurysm.** Incomplete rupture of the myocardial free wall can result in formation of a ventricular pseudoaneurysm. In this case, blood escapes through the myocardial wall and is contained within the visceral pericardium. In the post-CABG patient, hemorrhage from frank ventricular rupture may be contained within the fibrotic pericardial space producing a pseudoaneurysm.
    - Echocardiography (TTE with contrast or TEE) is the preferred diagnostic test to assess for a pseudoaneurysm, often allowing differentiation from a true aneurysm.
    - Prompt surgical intervention for pseudoaneurysms is advised because of the high incidence of myocardial rupture.
  - **Free wall rupture** represents a catastrophic complication of acute MI accounting for 10% of early deaths. Rupture typically occurs within the first week after MI and presents with sudden hemodynamic collapse. This complication can occur after anterior or inferior MI but is more commonly seen in hypertensive women with a first-large transmural MI, treated late with fibrinolytic therapy, and given NSAIDs or glucocorticoids.
    - Echocardiography may identify patients with particularly thinned ventricular walls at risk for rupture.
    - Pericardiocentesis and intra-aortic balloon pump support may be necessary for patients awaiting emergent surgical correction.
    - Despite optimal intervention, mortality of free wall rupture remains greater than 90%.

- **Papillary muscle rupture** is a rare complication after MI and is associated with abrupt clinical deterioration. The posterior medial papillary muscle is most commonly affected due to its isolated vascular supply, but anterolateral and right ventricular papillary rupture have been reported. Of note, papillary muscle rupture may be seen in the setting of a relatively small MI.
  - The diagnostic test of choice is echocardiography with Doppler imaging as physical exam reveals a murmur in only ~50% of cases.
  - Initial medical therapy should include aggressive afterload reduction. Patients with refractory HF and those with hemodynamic instability may require inotropic support with dobutamine and/or intra-aortic balloon counterpulsation. Surgical repair is indicated in the majority of patients.
- **Ventricular septal rupture** (or defect) formation is most commonly associated with anterior MI. The perforation may follow a direct course between the ventricles or a serpiginous route through the septal wall.
  - Diagnosis can be made by echocardiography with Doppler imaging and often requires TEE.
  - Diagnosis should be suspected in the postinfarct patient who develops HF symptoms and a new holosystolic murmur.
  - Stabilization with afterload reduction, inotropic support, and/or intra-aortic balloon pump may be necessary for hemodynamically unstable patients until definitive therapy with surgical repair can be performed.
  - In hemodynamically stable patients, surgery is best deferred for at least a week to improve patient outcome. Left untreated, mortality approaches 90%.
  - Percutaneous device closure in the cardiac catheterization laboratory can be performed on a compassionate basis in select patients with an unacceptable surgical risk.

MONITORING/FOLLOW-UP

Routine office visits 1 month after discharge and every 3 to 12 months thereafter are suggested for the patient presenting with an acute MI.

- Patients should be instructed to seek more frequent or urgent follow-up evaluation if they experience any noticeable change in their clinical status.
- Specific plans for long-term follow-up care should be individualized based upon clinical status, anatomy, prior interventions, and change in symptoms.
- A stress imaging study is appropriate for patients who have a significant change in clinical status (either HF or angina). Routine testing is not warranted in patients without change in clinical status or in those with an estimated annual mortality (by prior risk assessment) of <1%.
- Coronary angiography should be considered for patients with significant ischemic burden on stress testing that is potentially amenable to revascularization or those with marked limitations of ordinary activity despite maximal medical therapy.

4 Heart Failure, Cardiomyopathy, and Valvular Heart Disease

Brian R. Lindman, Stacy A. Mandras, Benico Barzilai, Susan M. Joseph, and Gregory A. Ewald

Heart Failure

GENERAL PRINCIPLES

Definition

Heart failure (HF) is a clinical syndrome in which either structural or functional abnormalities in the heart impair its ability to meet the metabolic demands of the body. HF is a progressive disorder and is associated with extremely high morbidity and mortality.

Classification

- HF may be due to abnormalities in myocardial contraction (systolic dysfunction), relaxation and filling (diastolic dysfunction), or both.
- Almost half of patients admitted with HF have preserved systolic function.
- HF may be classified either by ACC/AHA HF stage or by New York Heart Association (NYHA) Functional Class (Tables 1 and 2).

Epidemiology

- In the United States there are approximately 5 million people living with HF.
- Over 550,000 new cases of HF are diagnosed each year.
- HF accounts for over 1 million hospitalizations per year.
- Estimated 1- and 5-year mortality is 30% and 50%, respectively.

Etiology

- Coronary artery disease (CAD) is the most frequent cause of HF in the United States, accounting for over 50% of cases (*Arch Intern Med 2001;161:996*). Diabetes and hypertension are other major contributors.
- Other causes include valvular heart disease, toxins induced (alcohol, cocaine, chemotherapy), myocarditis (infectious or autoimmune), familial cardiomyopathy, infiltrative disease (amyloidosis, sarcoidosis, hemochromatosis), peripartum cardiomyopathy, hypertrophic cardiomyopathy [HCM], constrictive pericardial disease, high-output states (i.e., arteriovenous malformation or fistula), generalized myopathy (Duchenne or Becker muscular dystrophy), tachycardia-induced cardiomyopathy, and idiopathic cardiomyopathy.
- HF is often precipitated by dietary and medication noncompliance; however, myocardial ischemia, HTN, arrhythmias (particularly atrial fibrillation), infection, volume overload, alcohol/toxins, thyroid disease, drugs (nonsteroidal

Table 1	American College of Cardiology/American Heart Association Guidelines of Evaluation and Management of Chronic Heart Failure in Adults	

Stage	Description	Treatment
A	No structural heart disease and no symptoms but risk factors: CAD, HTN, DM, cardio toxins, familial cardiomyopathy	Lifestyle modification—diet, exercise, smoking cessation; treat hyperlipidemia and use ACEI for HTN
B	Abnormal LV systolic function, MI, valvular heart disease but no HF symptoms	Lifestyle modifications, ACEI, β-adrenergic blockers
C	Structural heart disease and HF symptoms	Lifestyle modifications, ACEI, β-adrenergic blockers, diuretics, digoxin
D	Refractory HF symptoms to maximal medical management	Therapy listed under A, B, C and mechanical assist device, heart transplantation, continuous IV inotropic infusion, hospice care in selected patients

ACEI, angiotensin-converting enzyme inhibitor; CAD, coronary artery disease; DM, diabetes mellitus; HF, heart failure; HTN, hypertension; LV, left ventricular; MI, myocardial infarction. Adapted from Hunt SA, Baker DW, Chin MH, et al. ACC/AHA guidelines for the evaluation and management of chronic heart failure in the adult: executive summary. *J Am Coll Cardiol* 2005;46:1116–1143.

anti-inflammatory drugs [NSAIDs], calcium channel blockers [CCBs], doxorubicin), and pulmonary embolism are also potential triggers.

Pathophysiology

- HF begins with injury to or stress on the heart.
- Regardless of etiology, the myocardial injury is associated with adverse remodeling, manifested as an increase in left ventricular (LV) size (dilation) and/or mass

Table 2	New York Heart Association Functional Classification

NYHA class	Symptoms
I (mild)	No symptoms or limitation while performing ordinary physical activity (walking, climbing stairs, etc.)
II (mild)	Mild symptoms (mild shortness of breath, palpitations, fatigue, and/or angina) and slight limitation during ordinary physical activity
III (moderate)	Marked limitation in activity due to symptoms, even during less-than-ordinary activity (walking short distances [20–100 m]). Comfortable only at rest
IV (severe)	Severe limitations with symptoms even while at rest. Mostly bedbound patients

(hypertrophy), and a change in shape (the heart becomes more spherical). These changes in geometry result in hemodynamic stresses on the heart and further impair cardiac function.

- Compensatory adaptations occur, including activation of the renin-angiotensin-aldosterone system (RAAS) and vasopressin (antidiuretic hormone), which lead to increased sodium retention and peripheral vasoconstriction. The sympathetic nervous system is also activated, with increased levels of circulating catecholamines, resulting in increased myocardial contractility. Ultimately these neurohormonal pathways result in direct cellular toxicity, fibrosis, arrhythmias, and pump failure.
- The reduction in cardiac output results in organ hypoperfusion, and pulmonary and systemic venous congestion.

DIAGNOSIS

Clinical Presentation

- Affected patients most commonly present with symptoms of HF including:
  - Dyspnea (on exertion and/or at rest)
  - Fatigue
  - Exercise intolerance
  - Orthopnea, paroxysmal nocturnal dyspnea
  - Systemic or pulmonary venous congestion (lower extremity swelling or cough/wheezing)
  - Presyncope, palpitations, and angina may also be present
- Other presentations include incidental detection of asymptomatic cardiomegaly or symptoms related to coexisting arrhythmia, conduction disturbance, thromboembolic complications, or sudden death (*J Am Coll Cardiol 1989;13:1219*; *N Engl J Med 1994;331:1564*).
- Clinical manifestations of HF vary depending on the rapidity of cardiac decompensation, underlying etiology, age, and comorbidities of the patient.
- Extreme decompensation presents as hypoperfusion of vital organs with renal failure (decreased urine output), mental status changes (confusion and lethargy), and cardiogenic shock.

Physical Examination
- Systemic and pulmonary venous congestion result in lower extremity edema, pulmonary crackles, jugular venous distension, diminished carotid upstrokes, pleural and pericardial effusions, hepatic congestion, and ascites.
- Third or fourth heart sound may be present, as well as the holosystolic murmurs of tricuspid or mitral regurgitation (MR).

Diagnostic Testing

Laboratories
- Initial laboratory studies should include complete blood count, comprehensive metabolic panel (including electrolytes, BUN, creatinine, calcium, magnesium, fasting glucose, and liver function tests), fasting lipid profile, urinalysis, and thyroid function tests.
- B-type natriuretic peptide (BNP) is released by myocytes in response to stretch, volume overload, and increased filling pressures. Elevated BNP is present in patients with asymptomatic LV dysfunction as well as symptomatic HF.

- BNP levels have been shown to correlate with HF severity and predict survival (*N Engl J Med 2002;347:161*). A serum BNP > 400 is consistent with HF; however, specificity is reduced in patients with renal dysfunction. A serum BNP level < 100 has a good negative predictive value to exclude HF in patients presenting with dyspnea (*Curr Opin Cardiol 2006;21:208*).
- Additional laboratory testing in a patient with new-onset HF without CAD should include diagnostic tests for HIV, hepatitis, and hemochromatosis. When clinically suspected, serum tests for rheumatologic diseases (ANA, ANCA, etc.), amyloidosis (SPEP/UPEP), or pheochromocytoma should be considered (*Circulation 2009;119:1977*).

Electrocardiography

An electrocardiogram (ECG) should be performed to look for evidence of ischemia (ST-T wave abnormalities), previous myocardial infarction (MI) (Q waves), conduction delays, and arrhythmias (supraventricular and ventricular).

Imaging

- Chest radiography should also be performed to evaluate the presence of pulmonary edema or cardiomegaly, and rule out other etiologies of dyspnea (pneumonia, pneumothorax).
- An echocardiogram should be performed to assess LV function and structure, evaluate valvular heart disease, and exclude cardiac tamponade.
- LV function may also be evaluated using radionuclide ventriculography or cardiac catheterization with ventriculography.
- Cardiac magnetic resonance imaging (MRI) may also be useful in assessing ventricular function and evaluating the presence of valvular heart disease, infiltrative cardiomyopathies (amyloid and sarcoid), myocarditis, and previous MI.

Diagnostic Procedures

- Coronary angiography should be performed in patients with angina or evidence of ischemia by ECG or stress testing unless the patient is not a candidate for revascularization (*Circulation 2009;119:1977*).
- Right heart catheterization with placement of a pulmonary artery (PA) catheter may help guide therapy in patients with hypotension and evidence of shock.
- Cardiopulmonary exercise testing with measurement of peak oxygen consumption is useful in assessing functional capacity and in identifying candidates for heart transplantation (*Circulation 2009;83:778; J Heart Lung Transplant 2003;22:70*).
- Endomyocardial biopsy may be useful in making the diagnosis if infiltrative cardiomyopathy is suspected; however in most cases of nonischemic cardiomyopathy, only nonspecific findings of hypertrophy or fibrosis are seen and biopsy results rarely alter management (*Eur Heart J 2007;28:3076; Circulation 2009;119:1977*).

TREATMENT

Medications

- In general, pharmacologic therapy in chronic HF is aimed at blocking the neurohormonal pathways that contribute to the progression of HF, and reducing symptoms, hospitalizations, and mortality.
- The cornerstone of medical therapy for HF includes vasodilators, β-adrenergic blockade, and diuretic therapy for volume overload. Most patients require a multidrug regimen.

Table 3	Drugs Commonly Used for Treatment of Heart Failure	
Drug	**Initial dose**	**Target**
Angiotensin-converting enzyme inhibitors		
Captopril	6.25–12.5 mg q6–8h	50 mg tid
Enalapril	2.5 mg bid	10 mg bid
Fosinopril	5–10 mg daily; can use bid	20 mg daily
Lisinopril	2.5–5.0 mg daily; can use bid	10–20 mg bid
Quinapril	2.5–5.0 mg bid	10 mg bid
Ramipril	1.25–2.5 mg bid	5 mg bid
Trandolapril	0.5–1.0 mg daily	4 mg daily
Angiotensin receptor blockers		
Valsartan[a]	40 mg bid	160 mg bid
Losartan	25 mg daily; can use bid	25–100 mg daily
Irbesartan	75–150 mg daily	75–300 mg daily
Candesartan[a]	2–16 mg daily	2–32 mg daily
Olmesartan	20 mg daily	20–40 mg daily
Thiazide diuretics		
HCTZ	25–50 mg daily	25–50 mg daily
Metolazone	2.5–5.0 mg daily or bid	10–20 mg total daily
Loop diuretics		
Bumetanide	0.5–1.0 mg daily or bid	10 mg total daily (maximum)
Furosemide	20–40 mg daily or bid	400 mg total daily (maximum)
Torsemide	10–20 mg daily or bid	200 mg total daily (maximum)
Aldosterone antagonists		
Eplerenone	25 mg daily	50 mg daily
Spironolactone	12.5–25.0 mg daily	25 mg daily
β-Blockers		
Bisoprolol	1.25 mg daily	10 mg daily
Carvedilol	3.125 mg q12h	25–50 mg q12h
Metoprolol succinate	12.5–25.0 mg daily	200 mg daily
Digoxin	0.125–0.25 mg daily	0.125–0.25 mg daily

HCTZ, hydrochlorothiazide.
[a]Valsartan and Candesartan are the only U.S. Food and Drug Administration–approved angiotensin II-receptor blockers in the treatment of heart failure.

- **β-Adrenergic receptor antagonists (β-blockers)** (Table 3). β-Blockers are a critical component of HF therapy and work by blocking the toxic effects of chronic adrenergic stimulation on the heart.
  - Many large randomized trials have documented the beneficial effects of β-blockers on functional status, disease progression, and survival in patients with NYHA class II–IV symptoms.
  - Improvement in ejection fraction (EF), exercise tolerance, and functional class are common after the institution of a β-blocker.

- Typically, 2 to 3 months of therapy is required to observe significant effects on LV function, but reduction of cardiac arrhythmia and incidence of sudden cardiac death (SCD) may occur much earlier (*JAMA 2003;289:712*).
- β-Blockers should be instituted at a low dose and titrated with careful attention to blood pressure (BP) and heart rate. Some patients experience volume retention and worsening HF symptoms that typically respond to transient increases in diuretic therapy.
- Individual β-blockers have unique properties, and the beneficial effect of β-blockers may not be a class effect. Therefore, one of three β-blockers with proven benefit on mortality in large clinical trials should be used (*Circulation 2009;119: 1977; Circulation 2005;112:e154*):
  - **Carvedilol** (*N Engl J Med 2001;344:1651; Lancet 2003;362:7*)
  - **Metoprolol succinate** (*JAMA 2000;283:1295*)
  - **Bisoprolol** (*Lancet 1999;353:9*)
- **Vasodilators**
- **Vasodilator therapy** is a mainstay of treatment in patients with HF. The RAAS and sympathetic nervous system, as well as increased secretion of arginine vasopressin increase arterial vasoconstriction (afterload) and venous vasoconstriction (preload) in patients with HF. Agents with predominantly venodilatory properties decrease preload and ventricular filling pressures. In the absence of LV outflow tract obstruction, arterial vasodilators reduce afterload by decreasing systemic vascular resistance (SVR), resulting in increased cardiac output, decreased ventricular filling pressure, and decreased myocardial wall stress. The efficacy and toxicity of vasodilator therapy depend on intravascular volume status and preload. Vasodilators should be used with caution in patients with a fixed cardiac output [e.g., aortic stenosis (AS) or HCM] or with predominantly diastolic dysfunction.
  - **Oral vasodilators** should be the initial therapy in patients with symptomatic chronic HF and in patients in whom parenteral vasodilators are being discontinued. When treatment with oral vasodilators is being initiated in hypotensive patients, it is prudent to use agents with a shorter half-life.
- **ACE (angiotensin-converting enzyme) inhibitors** (Table 3) attenuate vasoconstriction, vital organ hypoperfusion, hyponatremia, hypokalemia, and fluid retention attributable to compensatory activation of the renin-angiotensin system. They are the first choice for antagonism of the RAAS.
  - Multiple large clinical trials have clearly demonstrated that ACE inhibitors improve symptoms and survival in patients with LV systolic dysfunction (*Circulation 2009;119:1977; Circulation 2005;112:e154*).
    - ACE inhibitors may also prevent the development of HF in patients with asymptomatic LV dysfunction and in those at high risk of developing structural heart disease or HF symptoms (i.e., patients with CAD, diabetes mellitus, HTN). Currently, no consensus has been reached regarding the optimal dosing of ACE inhibitors in HF, although higher doses have been shown to reduce morbidity without improving overall survival (*Circulation 1999;100:2312*).
    - Absence of an initial beneficial response to treatment with an ACE inhibitor does not preclude long-term benefit.
    - Most ACE inhibitors are excreted by the kidneys, necessitating careful dose titration in patients with renal insufficiency. Acute renal insufficiency may occur in patients with bilateral renal artery stenosis. Additional adverse effects include rash, angioedema, dysgeusia, increases in serum creatinine, proteinuria, hyperkalemia, leukopenia, and cough.

- ○ Oral potassium supplements, potassium salt substitutes, and potassium-sparing diuretics should be used with caution during treatment with an ACE inhibitor.
  - ○ Agranulocytosis and angioedema are more common with captopril than with other ACE inhibitors, particularly in patients with associated collagen vascular disease or serum creatinine >1.5 mg/dL.
  - ○ *ACE inhibitors are contraindicated in pregnancy.*
- **Angiotensin II receptor blockers (ARBs)** (Table 3) inhibit the renin-angiotensin system via specific blockade of the angiotensin II receptor.
  - ARBs reduce morbidity and mortality associated with HF in patients who are not receiving an ACE inhibitor (*N Engl J Med 2001;345:1667; Lancet 2000;355:1582; Lancet 2003;362:777*), and therefore should be instituted when ACE inhibitors are not tolerated (*Circulation 2009;119:1977; Circulation 2005;112:e154*).
  - In contrast to ACE inhibitors, they do not increase bradykinin levels, which may be responsible for the cough associated with ACE inhibitors.
  - Caution should be exercised when ARBs are used in patients with renal insufficiency and bilateral renal artery stenosis because hyperkalemia and acute renal failure can develop.
  - Renal function and potassium levels should be periodically monitored.
  - *ARBs are contraindicated in pregnancy.*
- **Hydralazine** acts directly on arterial smooth muscle to produce vasodilation and to reduce afterload. In combination with nitrates, hydralazine improves survival in patients with HF (*N Engl J Med 1986;314:1547*).
  - A **combination of hydralazine and isosorbide dinitrate** (starting dose: 37.5/20 mg three times daily) when added to standard therapy with β-blockers and ACE inhibitors has been shown to reduce mortality in black patients (*N Engl J Med 2004;351:2049*).
  - Reflex tachycardia and increased myocardial oxygen consumption may occur, requiring cautious use in patients with ischemic heart disease.
- **Nitrates** are predominantly venodilators and help relieve symptoms of venous and pulmonary congestion. They reduce myocardial ischemia by decreasing ventricular filling pressures and by directly dilating coronary arteries. Nitrate therapy may precipitate hypotension in patients with reduced preload.
- **Parenteral vasodilators** should be reserved for patients with severe HF or those who are unable to take oral medications. Intravenous vasodilator therapy may be guided by central hemodynamic monitoring (PA catheterization) to assess efficacy and avoid hemodynamic instability. Parenteral agents should be started at low doses, titrated to the desired hemodynamic effect, and discontinued slowly to avoid rebound vasoconstriction.
- **Nitroglycerin** is a potent vasodilator, with effects on venous and, to a lesser extent, arterial vascular beds. It relieves pulmonary and systemic venous congestion and is an effective coronary vasodilator. Nitroglycerin is the preferred vasodilator for treatment of HF in the setting of *acute MI* or *unstable angina.*
- **Sodium nitroprusside** is a direct arterial vasodilator with less potent venodilatory properties. Its predominant effect is to reduce afterload, and it is particularly effective in patients with HF who are hypertensive or who have severe aortic or mitral valvular regurgitation. Nitroprusside should be used cautiously in patients with myocardial ischemia because of a potential reduction in regional myocardial blood flow (*coronary steal*).
  - The initial dose of **0.25 mcg/kg/min** can be titrated (**maximum dose of 10 mcg/kg/min**) to the desired hemodynamic effect or until hypotension develops. The

half-life of nitroprusside is 1 to 3 minutes, and its metabolism results in the release of cyanide, which is metabolized by the liver to thiocyanate and is then excreted via the kidney.

- *Toxic levels* of thiocyanate (>10 mg/dL) may develop in patients with renal insufficiency. Thiocyanate toxicity is manifested as nausea, paresthesias, mental status changes, abdominal pain, and seizures.
- *Methemoglobinemia* is a rare complication of treatment with nitroprusside.
- **Recombinant BNP (nesiritide)** is an arterial and venous vasodilator.
  - Intravenous infusion of nesiritide reduces right atrial and LV end-diastolic pressures (LVEDP) and SVR and results in an increase in cardiac output.
  - It is administered as a 2-mcg/kg IV bolus, followed by a continuous IV infusion starting at 0.01 mcg/kg/min. Nesiritide is approved for use in acute HF exacerbations and relieves HF symptoms early after its administration (*JAMA 2002;287:1531*).
  - It should not be used to improve renal function or to enhance diuresis. *Nesiritide is not recommended for intermittent outpatient use.*
  - *Hypotension* is the most common side effect of nesiritide, and its use should be avoided in patients with systemic hypotension (systolic BP < 90 mm Hg) or evidence of cardiogenic shock. Episodes of hypotension should be managed with discontinuation of nesiritide and cautious volume expansion or pressor support if necessary.
- **Enalaprilat** is an active metabolite of the ACE inhibitor enalapril that is available for IV administration. Its onset of action is more rapid and its pharmacologic half-life shorter than that of enalapril. The initial dosage is 1.25 mg IV q6h, which can be titrated to a maximum dosage of 5 mg IV q6h. Patients who take diuretics or those with impaired renal function (serum creatinine > 3 mg/dL, creatinine clearance < 30 mL/min) should initially receive 0.625 mg IV q6h. When dosing is being converted from IV to PO administration, enalaprilat, 0.625 mg IV q6h, is approximately equivalent to enalapril, 2.5 mg PO daily.
- **α-Adrenergic receptor antagonists** have not been shown to improve survival in HF, and hypertensive patients treated with doxazosin as first-line therapy had an increased risk of developing HF (*JAMA 2000;283:1967*).
- **Digitalis glycosides** increase myocardial contractility and may attenuate the neurohormonal activation associated with HF. Digoxin decreases the number of HF hospitalizations without improving overall mortality (*N Engl J Med 1997;336:525*).
  - Discontinuation of digoxin in patients who are stable on a regimen of digoxin, diuretics, and an ACE inhibitor may result in clinical deterioration (*N Engl J Med 1993;329:1*).
  - The usual daily dose is 0.125 to 0.25 mg and should be decreased in patients with renal insufficiency. Clinical benefits may not be related to the serum levels, and, although serum digoxin levels of 0.8 to 2.0 ng/mL are considered "therapeutic," toxicity can occur in this range.
  - *The toxic–therapeutic ratio is narrow,* and serum levels should be followed closely, particularly in patients with unstable renal function.
  - Observations suggest that women and patients with higher serum digoxin levels (1.2 to 2.0 ng/mL) have an increased mortality risk (*JAMA 2003;289:871; N Engl J Med 2002;347:1403*).
  - *Drug interactions with digoxin* are common. Oral antibiotics such as erythromycin and tetracycline may increase digoxin levels by 10% to 40%. Quinidine, verapamil, flecainide, and amiodarone also increase digoxin levels significantly.

- *Digoxin toxicity* may be caused or exacerbated by drug interactions, electrolyte abnormalities (particularly hypokalemia), hypoxemia, hypothyroidism, renal insufficiency, and volume depletion.
- **Diuretic therapy** (Table 3), in conjunction with restriction of dietary sodium and fluids, often leads to clinical improvement in patients with symptomatic HF. Frequent assessment of the patient's weight along with careful observation of fluid intake and output is essential during initiation and maintenance of therapy. Frequent complications of therapy include hypokalemia, hyponatremia, hypomagnesemia, volume contraction alkalosis, intravascular volume depletion, and hypotension. Serum electrolytes, BUN, and creatinine levels should be followed after institution of diuretic therapy. Hypokalemia may be life threatening in patients who are receiving digoxin or in those who have severe LV dysfunction that predisposes them to ventricular arrhythmias. Potassium supplementation or a potassium-sparing diuretic should be considered in addition to careful monitoring of serum potassium levels.
- **Thiazide diuretics (hydrochlorothiazide, chlorthalidone)** can be used as initial agents in patients with normal renal function in whom only a mild diuresis is desired. **Metolazone**, unlike other thiazides, exerts its action at the proximal as well as the distal tubule and may be useful in combination with a loop diuretic in patients with a low glomerular filtration rate.
- **Loop diuretics (furosemide, torsemide, bumetanide, ethacrynic acid)** should be used in patients who require significant diuresis and in those with markedly decreased renal function.
  - Furosemide reduces preload acutely by causing direct venodilation when administered IV, making it useful for managing severe HF or acute pulmonary edema.
  - Use of loop diuretics may be complicated by hyperuricemia, hypocalcemia, ototoxicity, rash, and vasculitis. Furosemide and bumetanide are sulfa derivatives and may rarely cause drug reactions in sulfa-sensitive patients. Ethacrynic acid can generally be used safely in such patients.
- **Potassium-sparing diuretics** do not exert a potent diuretic effect when used alone.
- **Spironolactone** (12.5 to 25 mg daily) is an aldosterone receptor antagonist that has been shown to improve survival and decrease hospitalizations in NYHA class III–IV patients with low EF (*N Engl J Med 1999;341:709*) and is therefore indicated in such patients if the creatinine is <2.5 mg/dL and potassium is <5.0 mEq/L (*Circulation 2009;119:1977*).
  - The potential for development of life-threatening hyperkalemia exists with the use of these agents. Gynecomastia may develop in 10% to 20% of men treated with spironolactone. Serum potassium must be monitored closely after initiation; concomitant use of ACE inhibitors and NSAIDs and the presence of renal insufficiency increase the risk of hyperkalemia.
- **Eplerenone**, a selective aldosterone receptor antagonist without the hormonal side effects of spironolactone, is Food and Drug Administration (FDA)-approved drug for treatment of HTN and HF and reduces mortality in patients with HF associated with acute MI (*N Engl J Med 2003;348:1309*).
- **Inotropic agents**
  - **Sympathomimetic agents** are potent drugs that are primarily used to treat severe HF. Beneficial and adverse effects are mediated by stimulation of myocardial β-adrenergic receptors. The most important adverse effects are related to the arrhythmogenic nature of these agents and the potential for exacerbation of myocardial ischemia. Treatment should be guided by careful hemodynamic and ECG monitoring. Patients with refractory chronic HF may benefit symptomatically

Table 4	Inotropic Agents	
Dose	**Mechanism**	**Effects/Side Effects**
1–3 mcg/kg/min	Dopaminergic receptors	Splanchnic vasodilation
2–8 mcg/kg/min	β_1-Receptor agonist	+ Inotropic
7–10 mcg/kg/min	α-Receptor agonist	↑ SVR
2.5–15.0 mcg/kg/min	β_1-receptor agonist >β_2-receptor agonist >α-receptor agonist	+ Inotropic, ↓ SVR, tachycardia
50-mcg/kg bolus IV over 10 min, 0.375–0.75 mcg/kg/min	↑ cAMP	↓ SVR, + inotropic; atrial and ventricular tachyarrhythmias

cAMP, cyclic adenosine monophosphate; SVR, systemic vascular resistance; ↑, increased; ↓, decreased.
Needs dose adjustment for creatinine clearance.

from continuous ambulatory administration of IV inotropes as palliative therapy or as a bridge to mechanical ventricular support or cardiac transplantation. However, this strategy may increase the risk of life-threatening arrhythmias or indwelling catheter-related infections (*Circulation 2009;119:1977; Circulation 2005; 112:e154*).

○ **Dopamine** (Table 4) should be used primarily for stabilization of the hypotensive patient.

○ **Dobutamine** (Table 4) is a synthetic analog of dopamine. Dobutamine tolerance has been described, and several studies have demonstrated increased mortality in patients treated with continuous dobutamine. Dobutamine has no significant role in the treatment of HF resulting from diastolic dysfunction or a high-output state.

○ **Phosphodiesterase inhibitors** increase myocardial contractility and produce vasodilation by increasing intracellular cyclic adenosine monophosphate. **Milrinone** is currently available for clinical use and is indicated for treatment of refractory HF. Hypotension may develop in patients who receive vasodilator therapy or have intravascular volume contraction, or both. Milrinone may improve hemodynamics in patients who are treated concurrently with dobutamine or dopamine. Data suggest that in-hospital short-term milrinone administration in addition to standard medical therapy does not reduce the length of hospitalization or the 60-day death or rehospitalization rate when compared with placebo (*JAMA 2002;287:1541*).

Other Nonoperative Therapies

• **Coronary revascularization** reduces ischemia and may improve systolic function in some patients with CAD.

• **Cardiac resynchronization therapy** or **biventricular pacing** (see Chapter 5, Cardiac Arrhythmias) appears to be beneficial in patients with an EF of 35% or less, NYHA class III–IV HF, and conduction abnormalities (left bundle branch block and atrioventricular delay). It has been demonstrated to improve quality of life and reduce the risk of death in carefully selected patients (*N Engl J Med 2005;352: 1539*).

- **Implantable Cardiac Defibrillator (ICD)** placement is recommended for all HF patients with an EF ≤35% for primary prevention of SCD. Sudden death occurs six to nine times more often in patients with HF compared to the general population and is the leading cause of death in ambulatory HF patients.
  - Multiple large randomized trials have demonstrated a survival benefit of 1% to 1.5% per year in patients with both ischemic and nonischemic cardiomyopathy (*Circulation 2009;119:1977*; *N Engl J Med 2005;352:1539*).
  - Patients should receive at least 3 months of optimal medical therapy prior to reassessment of EF and implantation of an ICD.
  - Following an acute MI or revascularization, EF should be assessed following 40 days of optimal therapy prior to ICD implantation.
  - ICD therapy should be deferred in patients with advanced age, life-shortening comorbidities, and end-stage HF patients who are not candidates for transplantation.
- An **intraaortic balloon pump** (IABP) can be considered for patients in whom other therapies have failed, have transient myocardial dysfunction, or are awaiting a definitive procedure such as transplantation. Severe aortoiliac atherosclerosis and aortic valve insufficiency are contraindications to IABP placement.

Surgical Management

- **Ventricular assist devices (VADs)** require surgical implantation and are indicated for patients with severe HF after cardiac surgery, for individuals with intractable cardiogenic shock after acute MI, and as a "bridge to transplantation" for patients awaiting heart transplantation. Consideration of a LV assist device as permanent or "destination" therapy is reasonable in highly selected patients with refractory end-stage HF and an estimated 1-year mortality over 50% with medical therapy (*Circulation 2009;119:1977*).
  - Currently available devices vary with regard to degree of mechanical hemolysis, intensity of anticoagulation required, and difficulty of implantation. The decision to institute VAD circulatory support must be made in consultation with a cardiac surgeon who has experience with this procedure.
- **Cardiac transplantation** is an option for selected patients with severe end-stage HF that has become refractory to aggressive medical therapy and for whom no other conventional treatment options are available.
  - Approximately 2,200 heart transplants are performed each year in the United States.
  - Candidates considered for transplantation should generally be younger than 65 years (although selected older patients may also benefit), have advanced HF (NYHA class III–IV), have a strong psychological support system, have exhausted all other therapeutic options, and be free of irreversible extracardiac organ dysfunction that would limit functional recovery or predispose them to posttransplant complications (*J Am Coll Cardiol 1993;22:1*).
  - Survival rates post heart transplant are approximately 90%, 70%, and 50% at 1, 5, and 10 years since the induction of calcineurin-inhibitor based immunosuppression. Annual statistics can be found on the United Network for Organ Sharing Web site (www.unos.org).

- In general, functional capacity and quality of life improve significantly after transplantation.
- **Posttransplant complications** include acute and chronic rejection, typical and atypical infections, and adverse effects of immunosuppressive agents. Cardiac allograft vasculopathy (CAD/chronic rejection) and malignancy are the leading causes of death after the first posttransplant year.

Lifestyle/Risk Modification

- Dietary counseling for sodium and fluid restriction should be provided.
- Smoking cessation should be strongly encouraged.
- Exercise training is recommended in stable HF patients as an adjunct to pharmacologic treatment. Exercise training in patients with HF has been shown to improve exercise capacity (peak VO_2 max as well as 6-minute walk time), improve quality of life, and decrease neurohormonal activation. The HF-ACTION Trial randomized over 2,300 patients with HF to exercise training versus standard medical therapy, and demonstrated a decrease in the combined end point of all-cause death or hospitalization in the exercise group (*JAMA 2009;301:1451*; *JAMA 2009;301:1439*). Treatment programs should be individualized and include a warm-up period, 20 to 30 minutes of exercise at the desired intensity, and a cool-down period 3 to 5 days a week (*Circulation 2003;107:1210*).
- Weight loss should be recommended when appropriate.

SPECIAL CONSIDERATIONS

- **Fluid and free water restriction** (<1.5 L/d) is especially important in the setting of hyponatremia (serum sodium < 130 mEq/L) and volume overload.
- **Minimization of medications** with deleterious effects in HF should be attempted.
  - **Negative inotropes** (e.g., verapamil, diltiazem) should be avoided in patients with impaired ventricular contractility, as should over-the-counter β stimulants (e.g., compounds containing ephedra, pseudoephedrine hydrochloride).
  - **NSAIDs**, which antagonize the effect of ACE inhibitors and diuretic therapy, should be avoided if possible.
- **Administration of supplemental oxygen** may relieve dyspnea, improve oxygen delivery, reduce the work of breathing, and limit pulmonary vasoconstriction in patients with hypoxemia.
- **Sleep apnea** has prevalence as high as 37% in the HF population. Treatment with nocturnal positive airway pressure improves symptoms and EF (*N Engl J Med 2003;348:1233*; *Am J Respir Crit Care Med 2001;164:2147*).
- **Dialysis** or **ultrafiltration** may be beneficial in patients with severe HF and renal dysfunction who cannot respond adequately to fluid and sodium restriction and diuretics (*J Am Coll Cardiol 2007;49:675*). Other mechanical methods of fluid removal such as therapeutic thoracentesis and paracentesis may provide temporary symptomatic relief of dyspnea. Care must be taken to avoid rapid fluid removal and hypotension.
- **End-of-life considerations** may be necessary in the patient with advanced HF that is refractory to therapy. Discussions regarding the disease course, treatment options, survival, functional status, and advance directives should be addressed early in the treatment of the patient with HF. For those with end-stage disease (stage D, NYHA class IV) with multiple hospitalizations and severe decline in their functional status and quality of life, hospice and palliative care should be considered.

Acute Heart Failure and Cardiogenic Pulmonary Edema

GENERAL PRINCIPLES

Pathophysiology

Cardiogenic pulmonary edema (CPE) occurs when the pulmonary capillary pressure exceeds the forces that maintain fluid within the vascular space (serum oncotic pressure and interstitial hydrostatic pressure).

- Increased pulmonary capillary pressure may be caused by LV failure of any cause, obstruction to transmitral flow [e.g., mitral stenosis (MS), atrial myxoma], or, rarely, pulmonary veno-occlusive disease.
- Alveolar flooding and impairment of gas exchange follow accumulation of fluid in the pulmonary interstitium.

DIAGNOSIS

Clinical Presentation

- Clinical manifestations of CPE may occur rapidly and include dyspnea, anxiety, and restlessness.
- The patient may expectorate pink frothy fluid.
- Physical signs of decreased peripheral perfusion, pulmonary congestion, use of accessory respiratory muscles, and wheezing are often present.

Diagnostic Testing

Imaging
- Radiographic abnormalities include cardiomegaly, interstitial and perihilar vascular engorgement, Kerley B lines, and pleural effusions.
- The radiographic abnormalities may follow the development of symptoms by several hours, and their resolution may be out of phase with clinical improvement.

TREATMENT

- **Supplemental oxygen** should be administered initially to raise the arterial oxygen tension to **>60 mm Hg.**
  - **Mechanical ventilation** is indicated if oxygenation is inadequate by noninvasive means or if hypercapnia coexists.
  - Placing the patient in a sitting position improves pulmonary function.
  - Strict bed rest, pain control, and relief of anxiety can decrease cardiac workload.
- **Precipitating factors** should be identified and corrected, as resolution of pulmonary edema can often be accomplished with correction of the underlying process. The most common precipitants are:
  - Severe HTN
  - MI or myocardial ischemia (particularly if associated with MR)
  - Acute valvular regurgitation
  - New-onset tachyarrhythmias or bradyarrhythmias
  - Volume overload in the setting of severe LV dysfunction

Medications

- **Morphine sulfate** reduces anxiety and dilates pulmonary and systemic veins. Two to five milligrams can be given intravenously over several minutes and can be repeated every 10 to 25 minutes until an effect is seen.
- **Furosemide** is a venodilator that decreases pulmonary congestion within minutes of IV administration, well before its diuretic action begins. An initial dose of 20 to 80 mg IV should be given over several minutes and can be increased based on response, to a maximum of 200 mg in subsequent doses.
- **Nitroglycerin** is a venodilator that can potentiate the effect of furosemide. IV administration is preferable to oral and transdermal forms as it can be rapidly titrated.
- **Nitroprusside** is an effective adjunct in the treatment of acute CPE and is useful when CPE is brought on by acute valvular regurgitation or HTN (see Valvular Heart Disease). Pulmonary and systemic arterial catheterization should be considered to guide titration of nitroprusside therapy.
- **Inotropic agents**, such as dobutamine or phosphodiesterase inhibitors, may be helpful after initial treatment of CPE in patients with concomitant hypotension or shock.
- **Recombinant BNP (nesiritide)** is administered as an IV bolus followed by an IV infusion.
  - Nesiritide reduces intracardiac filling pressures by producing vasodilation and indirectly increases the cardiac output.
  - In conjunction with furosemide, nesiritide produces natriuresis and diuresis.

SPECIAL CONSIDERATIONS

- **Right heart catheterization** (e.g., Swan–Ganz catheter) may be helpful in cases in which a prompt response to therapy does not occur by allowing differentiation between cardiogenic and noncardiogenic causes of pulmonary edema via measurement of central hemodynamics and cardiac output. It may then be used to guide subsequent therapy.
- **Acute hemodialysis and ultrafiltration** may be effective, especially in the patient with significant renal dysfunction and diuretic resistance (*J Am Coll Cardiol 2007;49:675*; *Congest Heart Fail 2008;14:19*).

CARDIOMYOPATHY

Dilated Cardiomyopathy

GENERAL PRINCIPLES

Definition

Dilated cardiomyopathy (DCM) is a disease of heart muscle characterized by dilation of the cardiac chambers and reduction in ventricular contractile function.

Epidemiology

DCM is the most common form of cardiomyopathy and is responsible for approximately 10,000 deaths and 46,000 hospitalizations each year. The lifetime incidence of DCM is 36.5 cases per 100,000 persons.

Pathophysiology

- DCM may be secondary to progression of any process that affects the myocardium and dilation is directly related to neurohormonal activation. The majority of cases are idiopathic (*Am J Cardiol 1992;69:1458*).
- Dilation of the cardiac chambers and varying degrees of hypertrophy are anatomic hallmarks. Tricuspid and MR are common due to the effect of chamber dilation on the valvular apparatus.
- **Atrial and ventricular arrhythmias** are present in as many as one-half of these patients and are probably responsible for the high incidence of sudden death in this population.

DIAGNOSIS

Clinical Presentation

- Symptomatic HF (dyspnea, volume overload) is often present.
- A portion of patients with preclinical disease may be asymptomatic.
- The ECG is usually abnormal, but changes are typically nonspecific.

Diagnostic Testing

Imaging

- Diagnosis of DCM can be confirmed with echocardiography or radionuclide ventriculography.
- Two-dimensional and Doppler echocardiography is helpful in differentiating this condition from hypertrophic or restrictive cardiomyopathy (RCM), pericardial disease, and valvular disorders.

Diagnostic Procedures

Endomyocardial biopsy provides little information that affects treatment of patients with dilated cardiomyopathies and is not routinely recommended (*Circulation 2009;119:1977; Eur Heart J 2007;28:3076*).

TREATMENT

Medications

- The medical management of symptomatic patients is identical to that for HF from other causes.
- Therapeutic strategies include control of total body sodium and volume in addition to appropriate preload and afterload reduction using vasodilator therapy.
- β-Adrenergic antagonists should be used unless contraindicated.
- Immunizations against influenza and pneumococcal pneumonia are recommended.
- Chronic oral anticoagulation has not been shown to decrease the risk of thromboembolism in patients with LV dysfunction. Anticoagulation should be strongly considered in individuals with a history of thromboembolic events, atrial fibrillation, or evidence of an LV thrombus. The level of anticoagulation recommended varies but is generally an international normalized ratio of 2.0 to 3.0.
- Immunosuppressive therapy with agents such as prednisone, azathioprine, and cyclosporine for biopsy-proven myocarditis has been advocated by some, but efficacy has not been established (*Circulation 2009;119:1977; N Engl J Med 1995;333:269*).

Other Nonoperative Therapies

- DCM (of nonischemic origin) is associated with an increased incidence of **SCD** and **ventricular arrhythmia.** In comparison to NYHA class IV HF patients who are more likely to die of progressive pump failure, SCD is relatively more common in patients with mild to moderate symptoms.
- Suppression of asymptomatic ventricular premature beats or nonsustained ventricular tachycardia (NSVT) using antiarrhythmic drugs in patients with HF does not improve survival and may increase mortality as a result of the proarrhythmic effects of the drugs (*N Engl J Med 1989;321:406*; *N Engl J Med 2005;352:225*; *N Engl J Med 1995;333:77*).
- Primary prevention of SCD is recommended by implantation of an ICD in patients with DCM who continue to have an EF of 35% or less and NYHA class II–III symptoms despite maximal medical therapy for 3 months.
- Cardiac resynchronization therapy is beneficial in selected patients with symptomatic HF (*N Engl J Med 2005;352:1539*; *N Engl J Med 2004;350:2140*).

Surgical Management

- Cardiac transplantation should be considered for selected patients with HF due to DCM that is refractory to medical therapy.
- IABP or placement of a VAD may be necessary for stabilization of patients in whom cardiac transplantation is an option or before other definitive surgical therapies.
- Mitral valve annuloplasty or replacement can be used for symptomatic relief in patients with severe MR.

Diastolic Dysfunction

GENERAL PRINCIPLES

Definition

- **Diastolic dysfunction** refers to abnormality in the mechanical function of the heart during diastole or the relaxation phase of the cardiac cycle. Usually, this involves elevated filling pressures and impairment of ventricular filling.
- **Diastolic heart failure** (DHF) refers to the syndrome of HF in the presence of preserved systolic function.

Epidemiology

- Almost half of patients admitted to the hospital with HF have a normal or near-normal EF.
- DHF is most prevalent in elderly women, most of whom have HTN and/or DM. Many of these women also have CAD and/or atrial fibrillation.

Etiology

- The vast majority of patients with DHF have hypertension and LV hypertrophy.
- Myocardial disorders associated with DHF include RCM, obstructive and non-obstructive HCM, infiltrative cardiomyopathies, and constrictive pericarditis.

Pathophysiology

- Reduced ventricular compliance plays a major role in the pathophysiology of DHF.
- Abnormal sodium handling by the kidneys and arterial stiffness also contribute.

DIAGNOSIS

Diagnostic Testing

Imaging
- Differentiating between diastolic and systolic HF cannot be reliably accomplished without two-dimensional echocardiography.
- Diagnosis is based on echocardiographic criteria and Doppler findings of normal LV systolic function with impaired diastolic relaxation and elevated filling pressures.

TREATMENT

Treatment is directed toward improving the symptoms with diuretic therapy and correcting the precipitating factors (e.g., hypertension, CAD, tachycardia).

Hypertrophic Cardiomyopathy

GENERAL PRINCIPLES

Definition

Hypertrophic cardiomyopathy (HCM) is a myocardial disorder characterized by ventricular hypertrophy, diminished LV cavity dimensions, normal or enhanced contractile function, and impaired ventricular relaxation in the absence of an identifiable cause.

Epidemiology

- HCM is the most common inherited heart defect, occurring in 1 of 500 individuals.
- Approximately 500,000 people have HCM in the United States, yet most are unaware. An estimated 36% of young athletes who die suddenly have probable or definite HCM, making it the leading cause of SCD in young people in the United States, including trained athletes (*Circulation 2009;119:1977*).
- The idiopathic form of HCM has an early onset (as early as the first decade of life) without associated HTN.
- An acquired form also occurs in elderly patients with chronic HTN.

Pathophysiology

- The pathophysiologic change in HCM is myocardial hypertrophy that is typically predominant in the ventricular septum (asymmetric hypertrophy) but may involve all ventricular segments.
- Many cases of HCM have a genetic component, with mutations in the myosin heavy-chain gene that follow an autosomal dominant transmission with variable phenotypic expression and penetrance.
- HCM can be classified according to the presence or absence of LV outflow tract obstruction.
- LV outflow obstruction may occur at rest, but is enhanced by factors that increase LV contractility or decrease ventricular volume.
- Delayed ventricular diastolic relaxation and decreased compliance are common and may lead to pulmonary congestion.
- Myocardial ischemia is frequently secondary to a myocardial oxygen supply–demand mismatch.

- Systolic anterior motion of the anterior leaflet of the mitral valve is often associated with MR and may contribute to LV outflow tract obstruction.

DIAGNOSIS

Clinical Presentation

- Presentation varies, but may include dyspnea, angina, arrhythmias, syncope, cardiac failure, or sudden death.
- Sudden death is most common in children and young adults between the ages of 10 and 35 years and often occurs during periods of strenuous exertion.

History

Family history of HCM or sudden death is suggestive of the familial subtype.

Physical Examination

- Physical findings include bisferious carotid pulse (in the presence of obstruction).
- Forceful double or triple apical impulse and a coarse **systolic outflow murmur** localized along the left sternal border that is **accentuated by maneuvers that decrease preload** (e.g., standing, Valsalva maneuver) may also be found.

Diagnostic Testing

Electrocardiography

The ECG of HCM is usually abnormal, and invariably so in symptomatic patients with LV outflow tract obstruction. The most common abnormalities are ST segment and T-wave abnormalities, followed by evidence of left ventricular hypertrophy (*Am J Cardiol 2002;90:1020*).

Imaging

- Two-dimensional echocardiography and Doppler flow studies can establish the presence of a significant LV outflow gradient at rest or with provocation.
- Additional risk stratification should be pursued with 24- to 48-hour Holter monitoring and exercise testing.

TREATMENT

- Management is directed toward relief of symptoms and prevention of endocarditis, arrhythmias, and sudden death.
- Treatment in asymptomatic individuals is controversial, and no conclusive evidence has been found that medical therapy is beneficial.
- All individuals with HCM should avoid strenuous physical activity, including most competitive sports.

Medications

- β-Blockers may reduce symptoms of HCM by reducing myocardial contractility and heart rate. However, symptoms may recur during long-term therapy.
- Calcium channel antagonists, particularly verapamil and diltiazem, may improve the symptoms of HCM, primarily by augmentation of diastolic ventricular filling. Therapy should be initiated at low doses, with careful titration in patients with outflow obstruction. The dose should be increased gradually over several days to

weeks if symptoms persist. Dihydropyridines should be avoided in patients with LV outflow tract obstruction as a result of their vasodilatory properties.

- Diuretics may improve pulmonary congestive symptoms in patients with elevated pulmonary venous pressures. These agents should be used cautiously in patients with severe LV outflow obstruction because excessive preload reduction worsens the obstruction.
- Nitrates and vasodilators should be avoided because of the risk of increasing the LV outflow gradient.
- **Treatment of arrhythmias.** Atrial and ventricular arrhythmias occur commonly in patients with HCM. Supraventricular tachyarrhythmias are tolerated poorly and should be treated aggressively; cardioversion is indicated if hemodynamic compromise develops.
  - **Digoxin is relatively contraindicated** because of its positive inotropic properties and potential for exacerbating ventricular outflow obstruction.
  - Atrial fibrillation should be converted to sinus rhythm when possible, and anticoagulation is recommended if paroxysmal or chronic atrial fibrillation develops.
  - **Diltiazem, verapamil, or β-blockers** can be used to control the ventricular response before cardioversion. Procainamide, disopyramide, or amiodarone (see Chapter 5, Cardiac Arrhythmias) may be effective in the chronic suppression of atrial fibrillation.
  - Patients with NSVT detected on ambulatory monitoring are at increased risk for sudden death. However, the benefit of suppressing these arrhythmias with medical therapy has not been established, and the risk of a proarrhythmic effect of antiarrhythmic drugs exists.
  - ICD placement should be considered in high-risk patients: those with genetic mutations associated with SCD; prior SCD or sustained ventricular tachyarrhythmia; a history of syncope or near-syncope, recurrent or exertional, in young patients; multiple nonsustained episodes of VT on Holter recordings; hypotensive response to exercise; LV hypertrophy with a wall thickness >30 mm in young patients; and a history of sudden, premature death in close relatives (*JAMA 2007;298:405*). There is very limited benefit for invasive electrophysiologic testing in the risk stratification of patients with HCM.
- Symptomatic ventricular arrhythmias should be treated as outlined in Chapter 5, Cardiac Arrhythmias.
- Dual-chamber pacing (see Chapter 5, Cardiac Arrhythmias) improves symptoms in some patients with HCM. Alteration of the ventricular activation sequence via right ventricular (RV) pacing may minimize LV outflow tract obstruction secondary to asymmetric septal hypertrophy.
- Only 10% of the patients with HCM meet the criteria for pacemaker implantation, and the effect on decreasing the left ventricular outflow tract (LVOT) gradient is only 25%. Dual-chamber pacing has not been demonstrated to decrease morbidity and mortality in patients with HCM.

Surgical Management

- Surgical therapy is useful in the treatment of symptoms but has not been shown to alter the natural history of HCM.
- The most frequently used operative procedure involves septal myotomy–myectomy with or without mitral valve replacement (MVR).
- Alcohol septal ablation, a catheter-based alternative to surgical myotomy–myectomy, seems to be equally effective at reducing obstruction and providing symptomatic

relief when compared to the gold standard surgical procedure (*J Am Coll Cardiol 2007;50:831*).
- Cardiac transplantation should be reserved for patients with end-stage HCM with symptomatic HF.

PATIENT EDUCATION

Genetic counseling and family screening are recommended for first-degree relatives of patients at high risk for SCD, because the disease is transmitted as an autosomal dominant trait.

Restrictive Cardiomyopathy

GENERAL PRINCIPLES

Definition
- Restrictive cardiomyopathy (RCM) is characterized by a rigid heart with poor ventricular filling.
- Both infiltrative (amyloidosis or sarcoidosis) and noninfiltrative (diabetic or idiopathic) forms exist.
- Pericardial disease (constrictive pericarditis) can present in a similar fashion but carries a different prognosis and treatment options and so must be excluded.

Pathophysiology
- In amyloidosis, amyloid deposits in the interstitium replace the normal myocardial contractile units and cause restriction.
- Approximately 5% of sarcoidosis cases have cardiac involvement in which scar formation leads to restriction.
- Other etiologies included hemochromatosis, Gaucher's and Hurler's cardiomyopathies (rare, inherited glycogen storage diseases), hypereosinophilic syndrome, and carcinoid heart disease.

DIAGNOSIS

Diagnostic Testing
Electrocardiography
The classic ECG finding in amyloidosis is low voltage with poor R-wave progression. In sarcoidosis, conduction disease is often present.

Imaging
- In RCM, echocardiography with Doppler analysis may demonstrate thickened myocardium with normal or abnormal systolic function, abnormal diastolic filling patterns, and elevated intracardiac pressure.
- Cardiac MRI, PET, and CT are emerging as useful diagnostic tools as granulomas, inflammation, and edema may be seen in patients with cardiac sarcoid which appear to improve with therapy (*Am Heart J 2009;157:746*).

Diagnostic Procedures
- On cardiac catheterization, elevated RV and LV filling pressures are seen with a classic dip-and-plateau pattern in the RV and LV pressure tracing.

- RV endomyocardial biopsy may be diagnostic and should be considered in patients in whom a diagnosis is not established.

TREATMENT

- Specific therapy aimed at amelioration of the underlying cause should be initiated.
- Cardiac hemochromatosis may respond to reduction of total body iron stores via phlebotomy or chelation therapy with deferoxamine.
- Cardiac sarcoidosis may respond to glucocorticoid therapy, but prolongation of survival with this approach has not been established.
- In those with syncope and/or ventricular arrhythmias, placement of an ICD is indicated. Those patients with high-grade conduction disease also warrant pacemaker placement.
- No therapy is known to be effective in reversing the progression of cardiac amyloidosis. Digoxin should be avoided in patients with cardiac amyloidosis because of enhanced susceptibility to digoxin toxicity.

Peripartum Cardiomyopathy

GENERAL PRINCIPLES

Definition

- Peripartum cardiomyopathy (PPCM) is defined as LV systolic dysfunction diagnosed in the last month of pregnancy up to 5 months postpartum.
- The incidence of PPCM is 1 in 3,000 to 4,000 pregnancies in the United States

Etiology

- The etiology of PPCM remains unclear. There is evidence to support **viral triggers,** including coxsackievirus, parvovirus B19, adenovirus, and herpesvirus, which may replicate unchecked in the reduced immunologic state brought on by pregnancy.
- **Fetal microchimerism** has also been a suggested cause, in which fetal cells escape into the maternal circulation and induce an autoimmune myocarditis (*Lancet 2006;368:687*).
- Recently, a cleavage product of **prolactin** has also been implicated in the development of PPCM (*Cell 2007;128:589*).

Risk Factors

Risk factors that predispose a woman to PPCM include advanced maternal age, multiparity, multiple pregnancy, preeclampsia, and gestational hypertension. There is a higher risk in African-American women, but this may be confounded by the higher prevalence of hypertension in this population.

DIAGNOSIS

Clinical Presentation

- Clinically, women with PPCM present with the signs and symptoms of HF.
- As dyspnea on exertion and lower extremity edema are common in late pregnancy, PPCM may be difficult to recognize. Cough, orthopnea, and paroxysmal nocturnal dyspnea are warning signs that PPCM may be present, as is the presence of a displaced apical impulse and a new MR murmur on exam.

- Most commonly, patients present with New York Heart Association (NYHA) class III and IV HF, although more mild cases and sudden cardiac arrest also occur.

Diagnostic Testing

Electrocardiography
On ECG, LVH is often present, as are ST-T wave abnormalities.

Imaging
Diagnosis requires an echocardiogram with a depressed EF and/or LV dilatation.

TREATMENT

Medications

- The mainstay of treatment is afterload and preload reduction.
- **ACE inhibitors** are used in the postpartum patient, while hydralazine is used in the patient who is still pregnant.
- **β-Blockers** are used to reduce tachycardia, arrhythmia, and risk of SCD, and are relatively safe, though β_1-selective blockers (metoprolol and atenolol) are preferred because they avoid peripheral vasodilation and uterine relaxation.
- **Digoxin** is also safe during pregnancy and should be used to augment contractility and rate control, although levels need to be closely monitored in the pregnant patient.
- **Diuretics** are used for preload reduction and symptom relief and are also safe. In those with thromboembolism, **heparin** is required, followed by **Coumadin** after delivery.

OUTCOME/PROGNOSIS

- The prognosis in PPCM is better than that seen in other forms of nonischemic cardiomyopathy.
- The extent of ventricular recovery at 6 months post delivery can predict overall recovery, although continued improvement has been seen 2 to 3 years after diagnosis.
- Subsequent pregnancies in patients with PPCM are associated with significant deterioration in LV function and can even result in death. Family planning counseling is essential after the diagnosis of PPCM is made, and women who do not recover their LV function should be encouraged to consider forgoing future pregnancy.

PERICARDIAL DISEASE

Constrictive Pericarditis

GENERAL PRINCIPLES

- Constrictive pericarditis, as a cause of right-sided HF, often goes undiagnosed.
- Constrictive pericarditis is often difficult to distinguish from RCM.
- Multiple imaging modalities and invasive hemodynamics are often needed to confirm the diagnosis.

Etiology

- Common
  - Idiopathic

- Viral pericarditis (chronic or recurrent)
- Postcardiotomy
- Chest irradiation
- Less common
  - Autoimmune connective tissue disorders
  - End-stage renal disease, uremia
  - Malignancy (e.g., breast, lung, lymphoma)
  - Tuberculosis (most common cause in developing countries)

Pathophysiology

The pericardium is a fibrous sac surrounding the heart consisting of two layers, a thin visceral layer attached to the pericardium and a thicker parietal layer. The pericardial space is normally filled with 15 to 50 mL of fluid. In the setting of chronic inflammation, the pericardial layers become thickened, scarred, and calcified; the pericardial space is obliterated and the pericardium becomes noncompliant. This external constraint impairs cardiac filling and leads to an equalization of pressures in all four chambers.

DIAGNOSIS

Clinical Presentation

History

The clinical presentation of constrictive pericarditis is insidious, with gradual development of fatigue, exercise intolerance, and venous congestion; if it goes undiagnosed for a long period, it is not unusual for patients to have undergone an extensive GI/liver evaluation, including a liver biopsy (showing cirrhosis—"nutmeg liver") before the diagnosis is made.

Physical Examination

- Features of right-sided HF:
  - Lower extremity edema, hepatomegaly, ascites, and elevated Jugular Venous Pressure (JVP)
- Features more specific for constriction:
  - Increased JVP with prominent y descent
  - Kussmaul's sign: lack of expected decrease or obvious increase of JVP upon inspiration
  - Pericardial knock: early, loud, high-pitched S_3

Differential Diagnosis

- **Pericardial constriction**
  - Ventricular interdependence *present*
  - Abnormal pericardial features (thickened, adherent, and/or calcified)
  - Preserved (or increased) tissue Doppler velocities on echo
  - Pulmonary HTN mild or absent
  - Septal bounce seen on noninvasive imaging
  - Equalization of pressures in all cardiac chambers (LVEDP – RVEDP < 5 mm Hg)
  - RVEDP/RVSP > 1/3
  - BNP low or mildly elevated (usually <200, unless postcardiotomy or radiation with concomitant LV dysfunction)

- **Restrictive cardiomyopathy**
  - Ventricular interdependence *absent*
  - Abnormal myocardial features (infiltration, thickened, fibrotic, conduction system disease)
  - Decreased tissue Doppler velocities on echo
  - Pulmonary HTN present
  - Normal septal motion
  - LVEDP – RVEDP > 5 mm Hg
  - RVEDP/RVSP < 1/3
  - BNP elevated (>200)

Diagnostic Testing

- **Echo**
- First-line diagnostic test
- Helpful for distinguishing constriction from restriction (see above)
- Ventricular systolic function is often normal and can lead to the false assessment that the heart function is "normal" as not a cause of the patient's symptoms
- May require a fluid bolus to elicit some of the hemodynamic findings of constriction
- Features suggestive of constriction include:
  - Thickened, echogenic pericardium
  - Tethering of the pericardium to the myocardium
  - Dilated, incompressible IVC
  - Septal bounce
  - Inspiratory variation in mitral flow velocity curves
  - Expiratory reversal of hepatic vein flow
  - Preserved (or increased) tissue Doppler velocities of the mitral annulus
- **Cath**
  - Often required to make the diagnosis of constriction
  - Method of choice for an accurate hemodynamic assessment
- **CT and MRI**
  - Provide excellent anatomy of the pericardium (thickness and calcification)
  - An MRI and gated CT can show evidence of ventricular interdependence (septal bounce); this may be particularly important if echo images are poor
  - Can provide other anatomical information that may be helpful in making the diagnosis of constriction (i.e., engorgement of IVC and hepatic veins) and its etiology (i.e., lymph nodes, tumors)

TREATMENT

- Limited role for medical therapy: diuretics and low-salt diet to alleviate edema
- Patients with constriction often have a resting sinus tachycardia to maintain cardiac output in the setting of a reduced stroke volume (from reduced diastolic filling); β-blockers and CCBs to slow the heart rate should be avoided

Surgical Management

- **Surgical pericardiectomy is the only definitive treatment** and should be pursued once the diagnosis is made
- Five to fifteen percent operative mortality; the highest mortality is in those with more advanced HF symptoms
- A significant majority experience a symptomatic benefit from surgery

Cardiac Tamponade

GENERAL PRINCIPLES

Cardiac tamponade is a *clinical diagnosis* and is considered a medical emergency

Etiology
- More likely to cause tamponade:
  - Idiopathic pericarditis
  - Infection (bacterial, including mycobacteria; fungal; and viral, including HIV)
  - Neoplasms (sometimes initially diagnosed during a workup for a pericardial effusion)
- Postcardiotomy
- Autoimmune connective tissue disorders
- Uremia
- Trauma
- Radiation
- Myocardial infarction (subacute)
- Drugs (hydralazine, procainamide, isoniazid, phenytoin)
- Hypothyroidism

Pathophysiology
Fluid accumulation in the pericardial space increases the pericardial pressure; the pressure depends on the amount of fluid, the rate of accumulation, and the compliance of the pericardium. If there is a rapid accumulation of fluid (e.g., trauma or perforation during PCI), a small volume of fluid can raise the pericardial pressure substantially; if the accumulation of fluid is more insidious, the pericardium can stretch and a large amount of fluid can accumulate at a lower pressure. Tamponade develops when the pressure in the pericardial space is sufficiently high to interfere with cardiac filling, resulting in a decrease in cardiac output.

DIAGNOSIS

Clinical Presentation
History
- The diagnosis of cardiac tamponade should be suspected in patients with elevated jugular venous pressure, hypotension, and distant heart sounds (**Beck's triad**)
- Symptoms can include dyspnea, fatigue, anxiety, presyncope, chest discomfort, abdominal fullness, slowed sensorium, and a vague sense of being "uncomfortable;" patients often feel more comfortable sitting forward

Physical Examination
- Pulsus paradoxus >10 mm Hg
- Jugular venous distention
- Diminished heart sounds
- Tachycardia, hypotension, and signs of shock

Diagnostic Testing
- **EKG**
  - Low voltage

- Tachycardia
- Electrical alternans (due to the swinging of the heart within the pericardium; specific but not sensitive)
- **TTE**
  - First-line diagnostic test to diagnose an effusion and evaluate its hemodynamic significance
  - The size of the effusion can be misleading; its hemodynamic impact depends on the rate of fluid accumulation
  - Important to assess the location of the effusion and determine the width of the fluid rim around the heart; this has implications for the approach taken to drain the fluid
  - Features suggestive of a hemodynamically significant effusion:
    - Dilated, incompressible IVC
    - Significant respiratory variation of tricuspid and mitral inflow velocities
    - Early diastolic collapse of the right ventricle and collapse of the right atrium (during ventricular diastole)
    - Usually the effusion is circumferential
- **TEE**
  - Helpful when TTE images are poor or when there is a suspicion for a loculated effusion (particularly those that might develop at the atrial level after cardiac surgery)
- **CT and MRI**
  - Can be helpful in assessing the anatomical location of the effusion (particularly if loculated)
  - May be helpful in determining the etiology of the effusion and the content of the pericardial fluid
  - These imaging studies should be avoided in an unstable patient
- **RHC**
  - Usually not necessary to establish the diagnosis
  - Hemodynamic assessment showing equalization of atrial and ventricular diastolic pressures

TREATMENT

- Limited role for medical therapy
- Maintain adequate filling pressures with IV fluids
- Avoid diuretics, nitrates, and any other preload-reducing medications
- Avoid efforts to slow sinus tachycardia; it compensates for a reduced stroke volume to try to maintain adequate cardiac output
- If intubation is to be performed for respiratory distress before the fluid is drained, make sure volume status is replete and a pericardiocentesis needle is immediately available before any sedatives are given (a patient in particularly "severe tamponade" can arrest with the preload reduction from sedation)

Other Nonoperative Therapies

Percutaneous pericardiocentesis with echocardiographic guidance can be a relatively safe and effective way to drain the pericardial fluid if there is an adequate amount of fluid; the approach should be guided by where the predominant collection of fluid is located and is usually easiest when the effusion is anterior

Surgical Management

- Open pericardiocentesis with the creation of a window is a minimally invasive procedure and is preferred for recurring effusions, loculated effusions, or those not safely accessible percutaneously
- Allows pericardial biopsies to be taken which may be helpful in making a diagnosis

VALVULAR HEART DISEASE

Mitral Stenosis

GENERAL PRINCIPLES

- Mitral stenosis (MS) is characterized by incomplete opening of the mitral valve during diastole, which limits antegrade flow and yields a sustained diastolic pressure gradient between the left atrium (LA) and the left ventricle (LV).
- Because of antibiotics, the incidence of rheumatic heart disease (and MS) has decreased in the developed world.

Etiology

- **Rheumatic**
  - Predominant cause of MS
  - Two-thirds are females
  - May be associated with MR
  - Stenotic orifice often shaped like a "fish mouth"
  - Rheumatic fever can cause fibrosis, thickening, and calcification leading to fusion of the commissures, leaflets, chordae, and/or papillary muscles
- **Other causes**
  - SLE
  - Rheumatoid arthritis
  - Congenital
  - Substantial mitral annular calcification
  - Mitral valve prosthesis dysfunction or "patient-prosthesis" mismatch
  - Oversewn or small mitral annuloplasty ring
  - "Functional MS" may occur with obstruction of left atrial outflow due to:
    ○ Tumor, particularly myxoma
    ○ LA thrombus
    ○ Endocarditis with a large vegetation
    ○ Congenital membrane of the LA (i.e., cor triatriatum)

Pathophysiology

Physiologic states that either increase the transvalvular flow (enhance cardiac output) or decrease diastolic filling time (via tachycardia) can increase symptoms at any given valve area. Pregnancy, exercise, hyperthyroidism, atrial fibrillation with rapid ventricular response, and fever are examples in which either or both of these conditions occur. Symptoms are often first noticed at these times (Fig. 1).

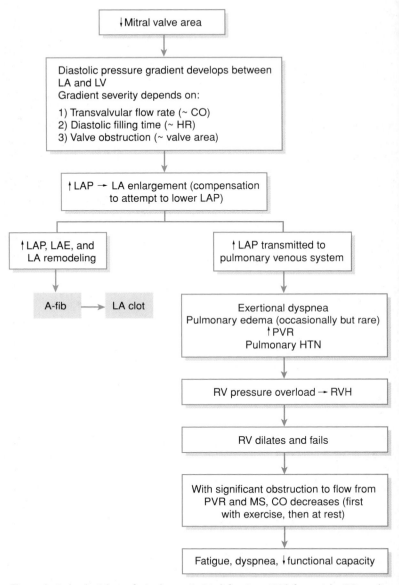

Figure 1. Pathophysiology of mitral stenosis. LA, left atrium; LV, left ventricle; CO, cardiac output; HR, heart rate; LAP, left atrial pressure; LAE, left atrial enlargement; PVR, pulmonary vascular resistance; RV, right ventricle; RVH, right ventricular hypertrophy; CO, cardiac output.

DIAGNOSIS

Clinical Presentation

History

After a prolonged asymptomatic period, depending on when they present, patients may report any of the following: dyspnea, decreased functional capacity, orthopnea and/or PND, fatigue, palpitations (often due to atrial fibrillation), systemic embolism, hemoptysis, chest pain, and/or signs and symptoms of infective endocarditis.

Physical Examination

Findings on physical exam will depend on the severity of valve obstruction and the associated adaptations that have had time to develop in response to it; they may include:

- Accentuation of S_1 may occur when the leaflets are flexible.
- Opening snap (OS)—caused by sudden tensing of the valve leaflets; the A_2-OS interval varies inversely with the severity of stenosis (shorter interval ~ more severe stenosis).
- Mid-diastolic rumble—low-pitched murmur heard best at the apex with the bell of the stethoscope; the severity of stenosis is related to the duration of the murmur, not intensity (more severe ~ longer duration).
- Loud P_2, TR murmur, PA tap, and/or RV heave can indicate pulmonary hypertension.
- ↑JVP, hepatic congestion, and peripheral edema can indicate varying degrees of right heart.

Diagnostic Testing

- **ECG**
  - P mitrale (P-wave duration in lead II ≥0.12 seconds indicating LAE)
  - Atrial fibrillation
  - RVH
- **CXR**
  - LAE
  - Enlarged RA/RV and/or enlarged pulmonary arteries
  - Calcification of the MV and/or annulus
- **TTE**
  - Assess etiology of MS
  - Assess leaflets and subvalvular apparatus to determine candidacy for percutaneous mitral balloon valvotomy (PMBV)
  - Determine mitral valve area and mean transmitral gradient
  - Estimate PA systolic pressure and evaluate RV size and function
- **Exercise testing with echo**
  - Helpful in clarifying functional capacity of those with an unclear history
  - Assess transmitral gradient and PA pressure with exercise when there is a discrepancy between resting Doppler findings, clinical findings, signs, and symptoms
- **TEE**
  - Assess presence or absence of clot and severity of MR in patients being considered for PMBV
  - Evaluate MV morphology and hemodynamics in patients with MS for whom TTE was suboptimal

- **Cath**
  - Indicated to determine severity of MS when clinical and echo assessment are discordant
  - Reasonable in patients with MS to assess the cause of severe pulmonary hypertension when out of proportion to the severity of MS as determined by noninvasive testing; can also assess the reversibility of pulmonary hypertension
- **Severe MS**
  - Mean gradient (mm Hg) > 10
  - PASP (mm Hg) > 50
  - Valve area (cm^2) < 1.0

TREATMENT

- **Medical**
  - Medical therapy is aimed at slowing progression of pulmonary HTN, preventing endocarditis, reducing the risk of thromboembolism, and reducing HF symptoms
  - For HF, intermittent diuretics and a low-salt diet are often adequate
  - For patients who develop symptoms only with exercise (likely associated with tachycardia), negative chronotropic agents such as β-blockers or non-dihydropyridine CCBs may be of benefit
  - Since most MS is rheumatic in origin, prophylaxis against rheumatic fever is appropriate
- **Atrial fibrillation**
  - Patients with MS are particularly prone to develop A-fib and/or flutter (30% to 40% of patients with MS)
  - Can exacerbate and worsen symptoms (particularly when there is a rapid ventricular response) due to a shortened diastolic filling period and loss of atrial kick
  - Therapy is mostly aimed at rate control and prevention of thromboembolism
  - Rate control: β-blockers or non-dihydropyridine CCBs tend to be more effective than digoxin for tachycardia associated with exertion
  - ACC/AHA Guidelines—Class I Indications for Anticoagulation for Prevention of Systemic Embolization in Patients with Mitral Stenosis:
    - MS and AF (paroxysmal, persistent, or permanent)
    - MS and a prior embolic event, even in sinus rhythm
    - MS with left atrial thrombus
  - Efforts to maintain sinus rhythm (through DCCV, ablation, or with drugs) are focused on those patients with symptoms from their AF, but can be particularly challenging in patients with MS.

Other Nonoperative Therapies

Percutaneous mitral balloon valvotomy (PMBV)

- ACC/AHA Guidelines—Class I Indications for PMBV
  - Symptomatic (NYHA class II, III, or IV) with moderate or severe MS and valve morphology favorable for PMBV in the absence of LA thrombus or moderate to severe MR
  - Asymptomatic with moderate or severe MS and valve morphology favorable for PMBV who have pHTN (PASP >50 mm Hg at rest or >60 mm Hg with exercise) in the absence of LA thrombus or moderate to severe MR
- Balloon inflation separates the commissures and fractures some of the nodular calcium in the leaflets, yielding an increased valve area

- Hemodynamic results often observed: transmitral gradient ↓50% to 60%, cardiac output ↑10% to 20%, and valve area increases from 1.0 to 2.0 cm²
- Contraindications: LA thrombus, moderate to severe MR, and an echo score of >8 (this score reflects the thickening, mobility, and calcification of the leaflets and subvalvular apparatus; this is a relative contraindication)
- Complications: death (~1%), stroke, cardiac perforation, severe MR requiring surgical correction, and residual ASD requiring closure
- When done in patients with favorable MV morphology, event-free survival (freedom from death, repeat valvotomy, or MV replacement) is 80% to 90% at 3 to 7 years (*Circulation 1992;85:448*)
- It compares favorably with surgical mitral commissurotomy (open or closed) and is the valvotomy procedure of choice in experienced centers in patients without contraindications

Surgical Management

- **ACC/AHA Guidelines—Class I Indications for Surgery for Mitral Stenosis**
  - MV surgery (repair if possible) is indicated in symptomatic patients (NYHA III or IV) with moderate or severe MS in a patient with acceptable operative risk when:
    ○ PMBV is unavailable
    ○ PMBV is contraindicated because of LA thrombus despite anticoagulation or because concomitant moderate to severe MR is present, or
    ○ Valve morphology is not favorable for PMBV
  - Symptomatic patients with moderate or severe MS who also have moderate to severe MR should receive valve replacement unless valve repair is possible at the time of surgery
- Surgical treatment is usually reserved for those who are not candidates for PMBV because of the presence of one or more contraindications to PMBV or because the percutaneous option is unavailable
- Surgical valvotomy can be done either closed (bypass unnecessary) or open (done under direct visualization on bypass)

OUTCOME/PROGNOSIS

MS usually progresses slowly with a long latent period (several decades) between rheumatic fever and the development of stenosis severe enough to cause symptoms. Ten-year survival of untreated patients with MS depends on the severity of symptoms at presentation: asymptomatic or minimally symptomatic patients have an 80% 10-year survival, whereas those with significant limiting symptoms have a 0% to 15% 10-year survival. Once severe pulmonary hypertension develops, mean survival is 3 years. The mortality of untreated patients is due mostly to progressive pulmonary and systemic congestion, systemic embolism, pulmonary embolism, and infection (in order of frequency).

Aortic Stenosis

GENERAL PRINCIPLES

- **Aortic stenosis** (AS) is the most common cause for obstruction of flow from the LV into the aorta—it is present in 2% of those >65 years of age and 4% of those >85 years of age.

- Other causes of obstruction occur above the valve (supravalvular) and below the valve (subvalvular), both fixed (i.e., subaortic membrane) and dynamic (i.e., HCM with obstruction).
- **Aortic sclerosis** is thickening of the aortic valve leaflets that cause turbulent flow through the valve and a murmur but no significant gradient; over time it can develop into AS.

Epidemiology

- **Calcific/degenerative**
  - Most common cause in United States
  - Trileaflet calcific AS usually presents in the 7th to 9th decades (mean age mid-70s)
  - Risk factors similar to CAD, exacerbated by abnormal Ca metabolism
  - Active biological process with bone formation in the valve
  - Calcification leading to stenosis affects both trileaflet and bicuspid valves
- **Bicuspid**
  - Occurs in 1% to 2% of population (congenital lesion)
  - Usually presents in the 6th to 8th decades (mean age mid-late 60s)
  - ~50% of patients needing AVR for AS have a bicuspid valve
  - More prone to endocarditis than trileaflet valves
  - Associated with aortopathies (i.e., dissection, aneurysm) in a significant proportion of patients
- **Rheumatic**
  - More common cause worldwide, much less common in the United States
  - Usually presents in the 3rd to 5th decades
  - Almost always accompanied by mitral valve disease

Pathophysiology

The pathophysiology for calcific AS involves both the valve and the ventricular adaptation to the stenosis. Within the valve, there is growing evidence for an active biological process that begins much like the formation of an atherosclerotic plaque and eventually leads to calcified bone formation (Fig. 2).

DIAGNOSIS

Clinical Presentation

History
- **The classic triad of symptoms includes angina, syncope, and HF.**
- Frequently patients will gradually limit themselves in ways that mask the presence of symptoms, but indicate a progressive and premature decline in functional capacity. In the setting of severe AS, these patients should be viewed as symptomatic.

Physical Examination
- Harsh systolic crescendo–decrescendo murmur heard best at the right upper sternal border and radiating to both carotids; time to peak intensity correlates with severity (later peak ~ more severe).
- Diminished or absent A_2 (soft S_2) suggests severe AS.
- An OS suggests bicuspid AS.
- S_4 reflects atrial contraction on a poorly compliant ventricle.
- Pulsus parvus et tardus: late-peaking and diminished carotid upstroke in severe AS.

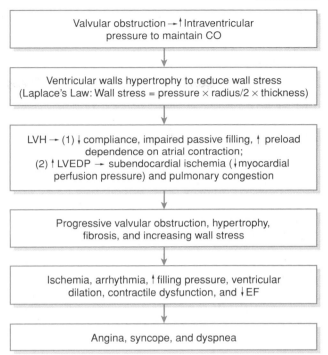

Figure 2. Pathophysiology of aortic stenosis. CO, cardiac output; LVH, left ventricular hypertrophy; LVEDP, left ventricular end-diastolic pressure; EF, ejection fraction.

- Gallavardin phenomenon is an AS murmur heard best at the apex (easily confused with MR).
- Between extremes, it is often difficult to assess AS severity on exam.

Diagnostic Testing

- **ECG:** LAE and LVH
- **CXR:** LVH, cardiomegaly, and calcification of the aorta, aortic valve, and/or coronaries
- **TTE**
  - Leaflet number, morphology, and calcification
  - Calculate valve area using continuity equation and measure transvalvular mean and peak gradients
- **Severe AS**
  - Peak jet velocity (m/s) >4.0
  - Mean gradient (mm Hg) >40
  - Valve area (cm^2) <1.0
- **Further evaluation in selected patients**
  - **TEE**
    - Clarify whether there is a bicuspid valve if unclear on TTE

- ○ Occasionally needed to evaluate for other or additional causes of LVOT obstruction
- **Exercise testing:** Performed in the patient presumed to be asymptomatic or in whom symptoms are unclear: evaluate for exercise capacity, abnormal blood pressure response (<20 mm Hg increase with exercise), or exercise induced symptoms
- **Dobutamine stress echo:** Useful to assess the patient with LV dysfunction with a small calculated valve area (suggesting severe AS) but a low (<30 to 40 mm Hg) mean transvalvular gradient (suggesting less severe AS)
  - ○ Can help distinguish truly severe AS from pseudo severe AS
  - ○ Assess for the presence of contractile reserve
- **Cath**
  - ○ In patients undergoing AVR who are at risk for CAD
  - ○ Evaluate for CAD in patients with moderate AS and symptoms of angina
  - ○ Hemodynamic assessment of severity of AS in patients in whom noninvasive tests are inconclusive or when there is discrepancy between noninvasive tests and clinical findings regarding AS severity (utilizes the Gorlin formula)
- **CTA:** CTA may be an alternative to cath to evaluate coronary anatomy prior to valve surgery (the role and accuracy of CTA is still being investigated)
- **BNP or NtBNP**
  - ○ Predicts symptom-free survival in asymptomatic patients and preoperative level predicts postoperative survival, functional class, and LV function (*Circulation 2004;109:2302*)
  - ○ BNP is higher in patients with truly severe AS versus pseudo severe AS and predicts survival among patients with low-flow, low-gradient AS (*Circulation 2007;115:2848*)

TREATMENT

- Severe symptomatic AS is a surgical disease; **currently, there are no medical treatments proven to decrease mortality or delay surgery**
- HTN: treat with appropriate antihypertensive agents cautiously to avoid hypotension
- ACEI: some data suggest that ACE inhibition may advantageously interfere with the valvular biology that leads to valve calcification
- Statins: some clinical evidence suggests statins may slow progression of AS (*J Am Coll Cardiol 2007;47:2141*), but the data are mixed and may depend on the severity of AS when the statin is initiated
- Avoid overdiuresis and loss of preload which may precipitate hypotension
- Use vasodilators, particularly nitroglycerin, very cautiously so as to avoid hypotension
- **Severe AS with decompensated HF**
  - Patients with severe AS and LV dysfunction may experience decompensated HF; depending on the clinical scenario, several options may help bridge the patient to definitive surgical management (AVR):
    - ○ IABP (contraindicated in patients with moderate to severe AR)
    - ○ Sodium nitroprusside
    - ○ Balloon aortic valvuloplasty
  - Each of the above measures provides some degree of afterload reduction, either at the level of the valve (valvuloplasty) or SVR (IABP, Nipride); this afterload reduction can facilitate forward flow; as the HF becomes more compensated and transient end-organ damage is reversed (i.e., renal failure, respiratory failure), operative mortality can decrease

- **Percutaneous**
  - Balloon aortic valvuloplasty has a limited role in the treatment of patients with severe AS; the improvement in valve area is modest and the clinical improvement that it provides usually lasts weeks to months
  - **Transcatheter aortic valve replacement (AVR)** has recently been introduced as an option for patients at high risk for AVR
    - Performed via a transfemoral or transapical approach
    - There are ongoing trials to assess the safety and efficacy of this approach in high-risk surgical candidates and those who are inoperable
    - These techniques and device characteristics are rapidly evolving

Surgical Management

- Symptomatic severe AS is a deadly disease; AVR is the only currently effective treatment
  - Certain associated high-risk features or the need for another cardiac surgical intervention may lead to the recommendation for an AVR even when the patient is asymptomatic or has less than severe AS
  - Operative mortality varies significantly depending on age, comorbidities, surgical experience, and concurrent surgical procedures to be performed
  - **ACC/AHA Guidelines—Class I Indications for AVR**
    - Symptomatic patients with severe AS
    - Patients with severe AS undergoing CABG
    - Patients with severe AS undergoing surgery on the aorta or other heart valves
    - Patients with severe AS and LV systolic dysfunction (EF <50%)

OUTCOME/PROGNOSIS

AS is a progressive disease typically characterized by an asymptomatic phase until the valve area reaches a minimum threshold, generally <1 cm^2. In the absence of symptoms, patients with AS have a good prognosis with a risk of sudden death estimated to be <1% per year. Predictors of decreased event-free survival (free of AVR or death) include higher peak aortic jet velocity, extent of valve calcification, and coexistent CAD. Once patients experience symptoms, their average survival is 2 to 3 years with a high risk of sudden death.

Mitral Regurgitation

GENERAL PRINCIPLES

- Prevention of mitral regurgitation (MR) is dependent on the integrated and proper function of the mitral valve (annulus and leaflets), subvalvular apparatus (chordae tendineae and papillary muscles), left atrium, and the ventricle; abnormal function or size of any one of these components can lead to MR.
- **Organic MR** refers to MR caused *primarily* by lesions to the valve leaflets and/or chordae tendineae (i.e., myxomatous degeneration, endocarditis, and rheumatic).
- **Functional MR** refers to MR caused *primarily* by ventricular dysfunction usually with accompanying annular dilatation (i.e., DCM and ischemic MR).
- It is critical to define the mechanism of MR and the time course (acute vs. chronic) as these significantly impact clinical management.

Etiology

- Degenerative (overlap with mitral valve prolapse syndrome)
  - Usually occurs as a primary condition (Barlow's disease or fibroelastic deficiency), but has also been associated with heritable diseases affecting the connective tissue including Marfan's syndrome, Ehlers–Danlos syndrome, osteogenesis imperfecta, etc.
  - May be familial or nonfamilial
  - Occurs in 1% to 2.5% of the population (based on stricter echo criteria)
  - Female to male 2:1
  - Either or both leaflets may prolapse
  - Most common reason for MV surgery
  - Myxomatous proliferation and cartilage formation can occur in the leaflets, chordae tendineae, and/or annulus
- Dilated Cardiomyopathy (DCM)
  - Mechanism of MR due to both:
    ○ Annular dilatation from ventricular enlargement
    ○ Papillary muscle displacement due to ventricular enlargement and remodeling prevents adequate leaflet coaptation
  - May occur in the setting of nonischemic DCM or ischemic DCM (there is often an overlap of mechanism for MR in the setting of previous infarction)
- Ischemic
  - **Ischemic MR is mostly a misnomer, as this is primarily postinfarction MR,** not MR caused by active ischemia (although MR can be do to ischemia alone or postinfarct MR can be exacerbated by ischemia)
  - Mechanism of MR usually involves one or both of the following:
    ○ Annular dilatation from ventricular enlargement
    ○ Local LV remodeling with papillary muscle displacement (both the dilatation of the ventricle and the akinesis/dyskinesis of the wall to which the papillary muscle is attached can prevent adequate leaflet coaptation)
  - Rarely, MR may develop acutely from papillary muscle rupture (more commonly of the posteromedial papillary muscle)
- Rheumatic
  - May be pure MR or combined MR/MS
  - Caused by thickening and/or calcification of the leaflets and chords
- Infective Endocarditis: Usually caused by destruction of the leaflet tissue (i.e., perforation)
- Other causes
  - Congenital (cleft, parachute, or fenestrated mitral valves)
  - Infiltrative diseases (i.e., amyloid)
  - Systemic Lupus Erythematosus (Libman–Sacks lesion)
  - HCM with obstruction
  - Mitral annular calcification
  - Paravalvular prosthetic leak
  - Drug toxicity (e.g., Phen-fen)
- Acute causes
  - Ruptured papillary muscle
  - Ruptured chordae tendineae
  - Infective endocarditis

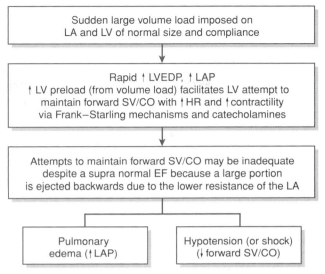

Figure 3. Acute mitral regurgitation. LA, left atrium; LV, left ventricle; LVEDP, left ventricular end-diastolic pressure; LAP, left atrial pressure; SV, stroke volume; CO, cardiac output; EF, ejection fraction.

Pathophysiology

- Acute MR (Fig. 3)
- Chronic MR (Fig. 4)

DIAGNOSIS

Clinical Presentation

History

- Acute MR
  - Most prominent symptom is relatively rapid onset of significant shortness of breath which may lead quickly to respiratory failure
  - Symptoms of reduced forward flow may also be present depending on the patient's ability to compensate for the regurgitant volume
- Chronic MR
  - The etiology of MR and the time at which the patient presents will influence the symptoms reported
  - In degenerative MR that has gradually progressed, the patient may be asymptomatic even when the MR is severe. As compensatory mechanisms fail, patients may note:
    ○ Dyspnea on exertion (may be due to pHTN and/or pulmonary edema)
    ○ Palpitations (from an atrial arrhythmia)
    ○ Fatigue
    ○ Volume overload

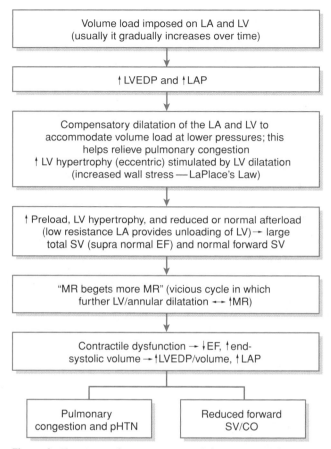

Figure 4. Chronic mitral regurgitation. LA, left atrium; LV, left ventricle; LVEDP, left ventricular end-diastolic pressure; LAP, left atrial pressure; SV, stroke volume; CO, cardiac output; EF, ejection fraction; pHTN, pulmonary hypertension.

- Patients with ischemic MR and MR due to a DCM may report similar symptoms; in general, these patients will tend to be more symptomatic because almost all of them have associated LV dysfunction

Physical Examination
- Acute MR
  - Tachypnea with respiratory distress
  - Tachycardia
  - Systolic murmur, usually at the apex—may not be holosystolic and may be absent
  - Relative hypotension (even shock)

- Chronic MR
  - Apical holosystolic murmur that radiates to the axilla
  - The murmur may radiate to the anterior chest wall if the posterior leaflet is prolapsed or toward the back if the anterior leaflet is prolapsed
  - In mitral valve prolapse, there is a midsystolic click heard before the murmur
  - S_2 may be widely split due to an early A_2
  - Other signs of CHF (LE edema, ⇑ central venous pressure, crackles, etc.)

Diagnostic Testing

- ECG
  - LAE, LVH/LVE
  - Atrial fibrillation
  - Pathologic Q waves from previous MI in ischemic MR
- CXR
  - Enlarged LA
  - Pulmonary edema
  - Enlarged pulmonary arteries
  - Cardiomegaly
- TTE
  - Assess etiology of MR
  - LA size and LV dimensions (should be dilated in chronic severe MR of any etiology)
  - Ejection fraction (LV dysfunction is present if EF $\leq 60\%$)
  - Qualitative and quantitative measures of MR severity
- TEE
  - Provides better visualization of the valve to help define anatomy, presence of endocarditis, and feasibility of repair
  - May help determine severity of MR when TTE is nondiagnostic, particularly in the setting of an eccentric jet
- 3D echo: May provide additional and more accurate anatomic insights that can guide repair
- Exercise Testing with Echo
  - Helpful in clarifying functional capacity of those with an unclear history
  - Assess severity of MR with exercise in patients with exertional symptoms that seem discordant with the assessment of MR severity at rest
  - Assess PA pressure with exercise
- MRI
  - Assess EF in patients with severe MR, but with an inadequate assessment of EF by echo
  - Assess quantitative measures of MR severity when echo is nondiagnostic
  - Viability assessment may play a role in considering therapeutic strategy in ischemic MR
- Nuclear
  - Assess EF in patients with severe MR, but with an inadequate assessment of EF by echo
  - Viability assessment may play a role in considering therapeutic strategy in ischemic MR
- Cath
  - Right heart cath to evaluate:
    - Pulmonary hypertension in patients with chronic severe MR

- ○ LA filling pressure in patients with unclear symptoms
- ○ Giant V waves on PCWP tracing may suggest severe MR
- Left heart cath:
  - ○ May influence therapeutic strategy in ischemic MR
  - ○ Evaluation of CAD in patients with risk factors undergoing MV surgery
  - Left ventriculogram can evaluate LV function and severity of MR
- CTA: CTA may be an alternative to LHC to evaluate coronary anatomy prior to valve surgery (the role and accuracy of CTA is still being investigated)

TREATMENT

- **Acute:**
  - While awaiting surgery, aggressive afterload reduction with IV nitroprusside or an IABP can diminish the amount of MR and stabilize the patient by promoting forward flow and reducing pulmonary edema
  - These patients are usually tachycardiac, but attempts to slow their heart rate should be avoided as they are often heart rate dependent for an adequate forward cardiac output
- **Chronic:** The role for medical therapy may differ depending on the etiology of the MR
  - **Degenerative MR:**
    - ○ In the asymptomatic patient with normal LV function and chronic severe MR due to leaflet prolapse, there is generally no accepted medical therapy
    - ○ In the absence of systemic HTN, there is no known indication for vasodilating drugs
    - ○ Whether ACEI or β-blockers delay ventricular remodeling and the need for surgery is being investigated in prospective studies
  - **Functional MR:**
    - ○ Treat as other patients with LV dysfunction
    - ○ ACEI and β-blockers are indicated and have been shown to reduce mortality and the severity of MR
    - ○ Some patients may also qualify for cardiac resynchronization therapy, which has also been shown to reduce the severity of MR
- **Percutaneous**
  - Various approaches target each of the interrelated components that can contribute to MR: annular dilatation, lack of leaflet coaptation, and ventricular remodeling causing papillary muscle displacement
  - Currently, the most developed device may be the placement of a mitral clip, which pinches the leaflets together in an attempt to enhance coaptation
  - This is a rapidly developing field with new devices and several trials in progress

Surgical Management

- ACC/AHA Guidelines—Class I Indications for Surgery in Mitral Regurgitation
- Symptomatic acute severe MR
- Chronic severe MR and NYHA functional class II, III, or IV symptoms in the absence of severe LV dysfunction (EF < 30%) and/or end-systolic dimension (ESD) > 55 mm
- Asymptomatic with chronic severe MR and mild-moderate LV dysfunction (EF 30% to 60%) and/or ESD ≥ 40 mm

- MV repair is recommended over MV replacement in the majority of patients with severe chronic MR who require surgery, and patients should be referred to surgical centers experienced in MV repair
- Surgery for MR is most commonly performed in patients with degenerative mitral valve disease
- Advances in surgical technique and lower operative mortality are causing some centers to operate earlier on patients with severe MR, even when they are asymptomatic
- Preoperative factors that increase operative and/or postoperative mortality include: worse NYHA functional class, LV dysfunction (EF < 60%), age, associated CAD, and atrial fibrillation
- Surgery for patients with ischemic MR and MR due to a DCM is more controversial and potentially more complex; the MR is largely due to a ventricular problem, so an isolated annuloplasty likely will not solve the problem; this is an active area of research and debate
- Certain patients with atrial fibrillation should be considered for a concomitant surgical MAZE procedure

Aortic Regurgitation

GENERAL PRINCIPLES

- Aortic regurgitation (AR) may result from pathology of the aortic valve, the aortic root, or both; it is important that both the valve and the root are evaluated to determine the appropriate management and treatment.
- AR usually develops insidiously with a long asymptomatic period; when it occurs acutely, it is often associated life threatening and must be managed aggressively.

Etiology
- More common
  - Bicuspid aortic valve
  - Rheumatic disease
  - Calcific degeneration
  - Infective endocarditis
  - Idiopathic dilatation of the aorta
  - Myxomatous degeneration
  - Systemic hypertension
  - Dissection of the ascending aorta
  - Marfan's syndrome
- Less common
  - Traumatic injury to the aortic valve
  - Collagen vascular diseases (ankylosing spondylitis, rheumatoid arthritis, Reiter's syndrome, giant cell aortitis, and Whipple's disease)
  - Syphilitic aortitis
  - Discrete subaortic stenosis
  - VSD with prolapse of an aortic cusp
- Acute
  - Infective endocarditis
  - Dissection of the ascending aorta
  - Trauma

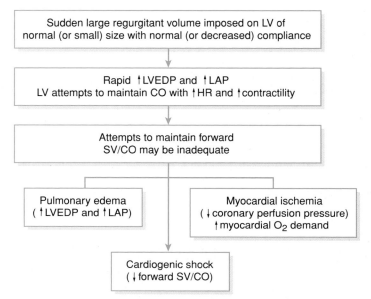

Figure 5. Acute aortic regurgitation. LV, left ventricle; LVEDP, left ventricular end-diastolic pressure; LAP, left atrial pressure; CO, cardiac output; HR, heart rate; SV, stroke volume.

Pathophysiology
- Acute AR (Fig. 5)
- Chronic AR (Fig. 6)

DIAGNOSIS

Clinical Presentation

History
- **Acute:** Patients with acute AR may present with **symptoms of cardiogenic shock and severe dyspnea.** Other presenting symptoms may be related to the cause of acute AR.
- **Chronic:** Symptoms depend on the presence of LV dysfunction and whether the patient is in the **compensated versus decompensated stage.** Compensated patients are typically asymptomatic, whereas those in the decompensated stage may note decreased exercise tolerance, dyspnea, fatigue, and/or angina.

Physical Examination
- Acute
  - **Tachycardia**
  - Wide pulse pressure may be present, but is often not present because forward stroke volume (and therefore systolic blood pressure) is reduced
  - Brief soft diastolic murmur heard best at 3rd left intercostal space (often not heard)

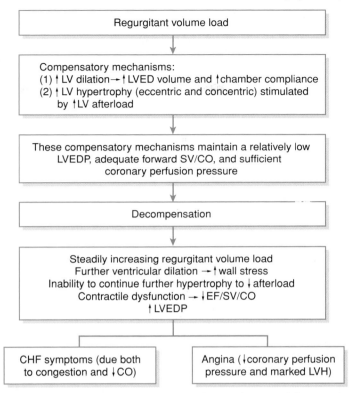

Figure 6. Chronic aortic regurgitation. LV, left ventricle; LVED, left ventricular end-diastolic; LVEDP, left ventricular end-diastolic pressure; EF, ejection fraction; SV, stroke volume; CO, cardiac output; CHF, congestive heart failure.

- Systolic flow murmur (due to volume overload and hyperdynamic LV)
- Look for evidence of aortic dissection, infective endocarditis, and Marfanoid characteristics
- Chronic
  - LV heave, and PMI is laterally displaced
  - Diastolic decrescendo murmur heard best at LSB leaning forward at end-expiration (severity of AR correlates with duration, not intensity, of the murmur)
  - Systolic flow murmur (due mostly to volume overload; concomitant AS may also be present)
  - Austin Flint murmur
  - Widened pulse pressure (often >100 mm Hg) with a low diastolic pressure; there are numerous eponyms for the characteristic signs related to a wide pulse pressure.

Diagnostic Testing

The diagnostic evaluation will likely depend somewhat on the acuity of the presentation, but will likely include:

- **ECG**
  - Tachycardia
  - LVH and LAE (more common in chronic AR)
  - New conduction block may suggest an aortic root abscess
- **CXR:** Look for pulmonary edema, widened mediastinum, and cardiomegaly
- **TTE**
  - LV systolic function
  - LV dimensions at end-systole and end-diastole
  - Leaflet number and morphology
  - Assessment of the severity of AR
  - Look for evidence of endocarditis or aortic dissection
  - Dimension of aortic root
- **TEE**
  - Clarify whether there is a bicuspid valve if unclear on TTE
  - Better sensitivity and specificity for aortic dissection than TTE
  - Clarify whether there is endocarditis ± root abscess if unclear on TTE
  - Better visualization of aortic valve in patients with a prosthetic aortic valve
- **Cath**
  - In patients undergoing AVR who are at risk for CAD
  - Assessment of LV pressure, LV function, and severity of AR (via aortic root angiography) is indicated in symptomatic patients in whom the severity of AR is unclear on noninvasive imaging or discordant with clinical findings

Imaging
MRI/CT
- Depending on the institution, either of these may be the imaging modality of choice for evaluating aortic dimensions and/or for evaluation of aortic dissection
- If echo assessment of the severity of AR is inadequate, MRI is useful for assessing the severity of AR
- CTA may be an alternative to cath to evaluate coronary anatomy prior to valve surgery (the role and accuracy of CTA are still being investigated)

TREATMENT

- **The role of medical therapy in patients with AR is limited;** there are currently no randomized, placebo-controlled data showing that vasodilator therapy delays the development of symptoms or
- LV dysfunction warranting surgery
- **Vasodilator therapy (i.e., nifedipine, ACEI, hydralazine) is indicated to reduce systolic blood pressure in hypertensive patients with AR**
- Other than for treating hypertension, vasodilator therapy has a potential role in three situations:
  - As chronic therapy in patients with severe AS who have symptoms or LV dysfunction but are not surgical candidates
  - As a short-term therapy to improve hemodynamics in patients with severe HF and severe LV dysfunction prior to surgery
  - May be considered for long-term therapy in asymptomatic patients with severe AS who have some LV dilatation but normal LV systolic function
- When endocarditis is suspected or confirmed, appropriate antibiotic coverage is critical

Surgical Management

- **ACC/AHA Guidelines—Class I Indications for Aortic Valve Replacement for AR**
  - **Symptomatic with severe AR irrespective of LV systolic function**
  - Asymptomatic with chronic severe AR and LV systolic dysfunction (EF ≤50%)
  - Chronic severe AR while undergoing CABG, surgery on the aorta, or other valve surgery
- Acute, severe AR is almost universally symptomatic and is treated surgically
- If the aortic root is dilated, it may be repaired or replaced at the time of AVR
  - For patients with a bicuspid valve, Marfan's syndrome (or related genetically triggered aortopathy), surgery on the aorta should occur at the time of AVR if the aortic root or ascending aorta is >4.5 cm
- Although worse NYHA functional class, LV dysfunction, and the chronicity of these abnormalities are predictors of higher operative and postoperative mortality, AVR is usually a better alternative than medical therapy in improving overall mortality and morbidity

OUTCOME/PROGNOSIS

- Asymptomatic patients with normal LV systolic function (*JACC 2006;48(3):e1–e148*)
  - Progression to symptoms and/or LV dysfunction <6% per year
  - Progression to asymptomatic LV dysfunction <3.5% per year
  - Sudden death <0.2% per year
- Asymptomatic patients with LV dysfunction
  - Progression to cardiac symptoms >25% per year
- Symptomatic patients
  - Mortality rate >10% per year

Prosthetic Heart Valves

GENERAL PRINCIPLES

The choice of valve prosthesis depends on many factors including the patient, surgeon, cardiologist and clinical scenario. With improvements in bioprosthetic valves, the recommendation for a mechanical valve in patients <65 years of age is no longer as firm and bioprosthetic valve use has increased in younger patients.

- **Mechanical**
  - Ball-and-cage (Starr–Edwards)—rarely, if ever, used today
  - Bileaflet (i.e., St. Jude, Carbomedics)—most commonly used
  - Single-tilting disk (i.e., Björk–Shiley, Medtronic Hall, Omnicarbon)
  - **Advantages:** structurally stable, long-lasting, relatively hemodynamically efficient (particularly bileaflet)
  - **Disadvantages:** need for anticoagulation, risk of bleeding, risk of thrombosis/embolism despite anticoagulation, severe hemodynamic compromise if disk thrombosis or immobility occurs (single-tilting disk), risk of endocarditis
- **Bioprosthetic**
  - Porcine aortic valve tissue (i.e., Hancock, Carpentier–Edwards)
  - Bovine pericardial tissue (i.e., Carpentier–Edwards Perimount)

Table 5

Valve and Duration	Aspirin (75–100 mg)	Warfarin (INR 2–3)	Warfarin (INR 2.5–3.5)	No Warfarin
Mechanical				
AVR—low risk				
<3 months	Class I	Class I	Class IIa	
>3 months	Class I	Class I		
AVR—high risk	Class I		Class I	
MVR	Class I		Class I	
Biological				
AVR—low risk				
<3 months	Class I	Class IIa		Class IIb
>3 months	Class I			Class IIa
AVR—high risk	Class I	Class I		
MVR—low risk				
<3 months	Class I	Class IIa		
>3 months	Class I			Class IIa
MVR—high risk	Class I	Class I		

- Stented or stentless
- **Advantages:** no need for anticoagulation, low thromboembolism risk, low risk of catastrophic valve failure
- **Disadvantages:** structural valve deterioration, imperfect hemodynamic efficiency, risk of endocarditis, still a small risk (0.7% per year) of thromboembolism without anticoagulation
- **Homograft (cadaveric)**
  - Rarely used for AV surgery; the only remaining use for aortic valve/root homograft may be in the setting AV endocarditis, particularly complex aortic root endocarditis
  - Most commonly used to replace the pulmonic valve

TREATMENT

Medications

Risk factors include atrial fibrillation, previous thromboembolism, LV dysfunction, and hypercoagulable condition. Low risk means no risk factors. INR should be maintained between 2.5 and 3.5 for aortic disk valves and Starr–Edwards valves regardless of risk factors (*JACC 2006;48(3):e1–e148*) (Table 5).

5 Cardiac Arrhythmias

Shivak Sharma, Daniel H. Cooper, and
Mitchell N. Faddis

TACHYARRHYTHMIAS

Approach to Tachyarrhythmias

GENERAL PRINCIPLES

- Tachyarrhythmias are commonly encountered in the inpatient setting.
- Approaching these rhythms in a prompt and stepwise manner will facilitate early recognition of the underlying arrhythmia and timely initiation of appropriate therapy.
- Clinical decision making is guided by patient symptoms and signs of hemodynamic stability.

Definition

Cardiac rhythms whose ventricular rate exceeds **100 beats per minute** (bpm).

Classification

Tachyarrhythmias are broadly classified based on the width of the QRS complex on the electrocardiogram (ECG):

- Narrow-Complex Tachyarrhythmia (QRS < 120 milliseconds): Arrhythmia (supraventricular tachycardia) originates within or above the atrioventricular (AV) node and rapidly activates ventricles via the normal His–Purkinje system.
- Wide-Complex Tachyarrhythmia (QRS ≥ 120 milliseconds): Arrhythmia originates outside the normal conduction system (ventricular tachycardia [VT]) or travels via an abnormal His–Purkinje system (supraventricular tachycardia with aberrancy) activating the ventricles in an abnormally slow manner.

Etiology

Mechanism divided into disorders of **impulse conduction** and **impulse formation**:

- **Disorders of Impulse Conduction: Reentry** accounts for the majority of tachyarrhythmias. It refers to conduction of the electrical activation wavefront retrograde into a myocardial region that was initially refractory to antegrade conduction of the wavefront. Differential refractory periods of myocardial tissue are a necessary component to allow reentry to occur. As a result of reentry, propagation of the activation wavefront around a myocardial circuit sustains the arrhythmia (e.g., VT).
- **Disorders of Impulse Formation: Enhanced automaticity** (e.g., accelerated junctional and accelerated idioventricular rhythm) **and triggered activity** (e.g., long QT syndrome and digitalis toxicity) are other less common mechanisms of tachyarrhythmias.

DIAGNOSIS

Clinical Presentation

- Tachyarrhythmias can be the cause of initial presentation at an outpatient or acute care setting.
- They can be associated with systemic illnesses in patients who are being evaluated in the emergency department or are being treated in an inpatient setting.

History

- Symptoms are an important facet of what guides clinical decision making.
- **Dyspnea, angina, lightheadedness or syncope and decreased level of consciousness** are alarming symptoms likely to guide the physician to a more immediate therapeutic option.
- Baseline symptoms that reflect **poor left ventricular (LV) function,** such as dyspnea on exertion (DOE), orthopnea, paroxysmal nocturnal dyspnea (PND), and lower extremity swelling, are critical to elucidate.
- **Palpitations:** Commonly associated with tachyarrhythmias, but important to inquire about the nature of their onset and termination.
  - Sudden onset and termination is highly suggestive of a tachyarrhythmia.
  - Symptom abatement with breath holding or Valsalva maneuver is suggestive of a supraventricular tachyarrhythmia. AV node is critical in the maintenance of this arrhythmia.
- History of **organic heart disease** (i.e., ischemic, nonischemic, valvular cardiomyopathy) or **endocrinopathy** (i.e., thyroid disease, pheochromocytoma) should be sought.
- History of **familial or congenital causes of arrhythmias** such as hypertrophic cardiomyopathy (HCM), congenital long QT syndrome, or other congenital heart disease should be addressed as well.
- **Medications:** Critical to obtain a complete list, including over-the-counter and herbal medications.

Physical Examination

- Signs of clinical stability or instability, including vital signs, mental status, peripheral perfusion, etc., are critical in guiding initial decision making.
- If clinically stable, then physical exam should be focused on determining underlying cardiovascular abnormalities that may make certain rhythms more or less likely.
- Findings of **congestive heart failure (CHF),** including elevated jugular venous pressure (JVP), pulmonary rales, peripheral edema, and S_3 gallop, make the diagnosis of malignant ventricular arrhythmias more likely.
- **Mitral valve prolapse** (MVP) is associated with supraventricular and ventricular arrhythmias and often produces a midsystolic click.
- **Hypertrophic obstructive cardiomyopathy** (HOCM) produces a harsh systolic crescendo–decrescendo ejection murmur heard best along the left sternal border (murmur increases with Valsalva and decreases with squatting), sustained PMI, S_4 gallop, and occasionally a paradoxically split S_2. HOCM is associated with atrial arrhythmias (atrial fibrillation [AF] in 20% to 25%), as well as malignant ventricular arrhythmias.
- If arrhythmia is sustained, here are some special considerations during physical exam:
  - **Palpate the pulse** and assess for rate and regularity.

- ○ If rate is about 150 bpm, suspect atrial flutter (AFl) with 2:1 block.
- ○ If rate is >150 bpm, suspect atrioventricular nodal reentrant tachycardia (AVNRT) or atrioventricular reentrant tachycardia (AVRT).
- ○ Ventricular arrhythmia rates are more variable.
- ○ If pulse is irregular with no pattern, suspect AF.
- ○ Irregular pulse with a discernible pattern (group beating) suggests the presence of second-degree heart block.
- **"Cannon" A waves:** Revealed on inspection of JVP and reflect atrial contraction against a closed tricuspid valve.
  - ○ If irregular, then suggestive of underlying AV dissociation and clue for VT.
  - ○ If regular in 1:1 ratio with peripheral pulse, then suggestive of AVNRT, AVRT, or a junctional tachycardia, all leading to retrograde atrial activation occurring simultaneously with ventricular contraction.

Diagnostic Testing

Laboratories

Serum electrolytes, complete blood count (CBC), thyroid function tests, serum concentration of digoxin (when applicable), and a **toxicology screen** should be considered for all patients.

Electrocardiography

- **A 12-lead ECG** is critical for the initial evaluation; may need to be repeated several times depending on changes in patient's clinical course.
- If the patient is clinically stable, obtain a 12-lead ECG and a **continuous rhythm strip** with leads that best demonstrate atrial activation (e.g., V_1, II, III, aVF).
- Examine the ECG for evidence of conduction abnormalities, such as preexcitation or bundle branch block, or signs of structural heart disease, such as prior myocardial infarction (MI).
- Comparison of the ECG obtained during arrhythmia with that at baseline can highlight subtle features of the QRS deflection that indicate the superposition of atrial and ventricular depolarization.
- Rhythm strip is very useful to document the response to interventions (e.g., vagal maneuvers, antiarrhythmic drug therapy, electrical cardioversion).

Imaging

Chest radiograph and **transthoracic echocardiogram** can help provide evidence of structural heart disease that may make ventricular arrhythmias more likely.

Diagnostic Procedures

- **Continuous ambulatory ECG monitoring**
  - 24 to 72 hours; useful for documenting symptomatic transient arrhythmias that occur with sufficient frequency.
  - Recording mode useful for assessment of patient's heart rate response to daily activities or antiarrhythmic drug treatment.
  - Correlation between patient-reported symptoms in a time-marked diary and heart rhythm recordings is the key to determine if symptoms are attributable to an arrhythmia.
- **In-hospital telemetry monitoring**
  - Mainstay of surveillance monitoring during the course of hospitalization for cardiac arrhythmia patients who are seriously ill or are having life-threatening arrhythmias.

- **Event recorders**
  - Weeks to months; useful for documenting symptomatic transient arrhythmias that occur infrequently.
  - A "loop" recorder is worn by the patient and continuously records the ECG. When activated by the patient or with an autodetection feature, the ECG recording is saved with the preceding 4 to 5 minutes of rhythm data.
  - An "event monitor" is connected only when the patient experiences symptoms.
  - An **implantable loop recorder or insertable loop recorder (ILR)** is a subcutaneous monitoring device, to provide automated or patient-activated recording of significant arrhythmic events that occur very infrequently over several months or for patients who are unable to activate external recorders.
- **Exercise ECG**
  - Useful for studying exercise-induced arrhythmias or to assess the sinus node response to exercise.
- **Electrophysiology study (EPS)**
  - Invasive, catheter-based procedure that is used to study a patient's susceptibility to arrhythmias or to investigate the mechanism of a known arrhythmia.
  - EPS is also combined with catheter ablation for curative treatment of many arrhythmia mechanisms.
  - The efficacy of EPS to induce and study arrhythmias is highest for reentrant mechanisms.

TREATMENT

Please refer to the treatment of individual tachyarrhythmias for hemodynamically stable patients and ACLS algorithm for tachycardias in Appendix C.

Supraventricular Tachyarrhythmias

GENERAL PRINCIPLES

- **Supraventricular tachyarrhythmias (SVT)** are often recurrent, occasionally persistent, and a frequent cause of visits to emergency departments and primary care physician offices.
- The evaluation of patients with SVT should always begin with prompt assessment of hemodynamic stability and clinical "substrate."
  - Young and healthy adults may tolerate tachyarrhythmias a lot better than a patient with LV systolic or diastolic dysfunction, valvular heart disease, or other cardiopulmonary comorbidity.
- The diagnostic and therapeutic discussion that follows is aimed at the hemodynamically stable patient. If patient is deemed clinically unstable based on clinical signs, symptoms, or hemodynamics, one should immediately proceed to cardioversion per advanced cardiac life support (ACLS) guidelines.

Definition

- Tachyarrhythmias that require atrial or AV nodal tissue, or both, for their initiation and maintenance are termed SVT.
- The QRS complex in most SVTs is narrow (QRS < 120 milliseconds). However, they can certainly present as wide-complex tachycardia (WCT) (QRS ≥ 120 milliseconds) in SVT with aberrancy or preexcited tachycardia.

Classification

- SVT can be classified in several ways—ECG appearance, underlying mechanism, AV node dependence, etc.
- A diagnostic approach to tachyarrhythmias as summarized in Figure 1 is a clinically useful classification to approach these patients.

Epidemiology

- Published incidence data can vary widely between studies and is difficult to quantify because of high rate of asymptomatic episodes in patients.
- The estimated prevalence and incidence of paroxysmal supraventricular tachycardia (PSVT) based on one population study are 2.25 per 1,000 and 35 per 100,000 person-years, respectively (*J Am Coll Cardiol 1998;31:150*).

DIAGNOSIS

What are the odds?—When approaching any diagnostic dilemma, it is always helpful to have a rough idea of how commonly or rarely a particular diagnosis presents in your patient population.

- **AF** is the most common narrow-complex tachycardia seen in the inpatient setting. **AFl** can often accompany AF and is diagnosed one-tenth as often as AF but is twice as prevalent as the paroxysmal SVTs. The other atrial tachyarrhythmias are far less common.
- In one case series, **AVNRT** was reported as the most common diagnosis of the paroxysmal SVTs (60%) followed by AVRT (30%) (*Crit Care Med 2000 Oct;28(10 Suppl):N129*).
- However, if your patient is younger than age 40, then AVRT, often in the context of Wolff–Parkinson–White (WPW) syndrome, is more likely.
- Please refer to Figure 1 for the diagnostic approach to tachyarrhythmias.

Clinical Presentation

The clinical presentation for SVT is similar to tachyarrhythmias in general and has been previously outlined in this section.

Differential Diagnosis

- **Atrial fibrillation**
  - The most common sustained tachyarrhythmia is discussed as a separate topic in this section.
- **Atrial flutter**
  - The second most common atrial arrhythmia, with estimated 200,000 new cases in the United States annually, is associated with increasing age, underlying heart disease, and male gender (*J Am Coll Cardiol 2000;36:2242*).
  - AFl usually presents as a **regular rhythm** but can be **irregularly irregular** when associated with variable AV block (2:1 to 4:1 to 3:1, etc.).
  - **Mechanism:** Reentrant circuit around functional or structural conduction barriers within the atria. Atrial rate is 250 to 350 bpm with conduction to ventricle that is usually not 1:1; most often 2:1. **(SVT with regular ventricular rate of 150 bpm should raise suspicion for AFl.)**
  - Like AF, AFl is commonly associated with the postcardiac surgery period, pulmonary disease, thyrotoxicosis, and atrial enlargement.

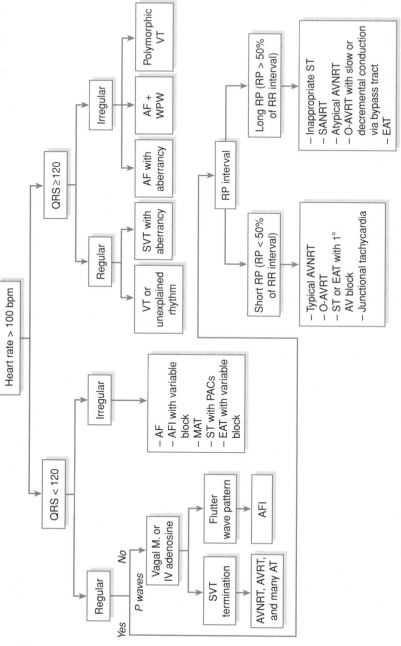

- **ECG:** In typical AFl, "sawtooth" pattern best visualized in leads II, III, and aVF with negative deflections in V_1.
- **Multifocal atrial tachycardia (MAT)**
  - **Irregularly irregular** SVT seen generally in elderly hospitalized patients with multiple comorbidities.
  - MAT is most often associated with chronic obstructive pulmonary disease (COPD) and heart failure, but also associated with glucose intolerance, hypokalemia, hypomagnesemia, drugs (e.g., theophylline), and chronic renal failure.
  - **ECG:** SVT with at least **three distinct P-wave morphologies,** generally best visualized in leads II, III, and V_1.
- **Sinus tachycardia (ST)**
  - ST with frequent premature atrial complexes (PACs) can lead to **irregularly irregular rhythm.**
  - It is also the most common mechanism of **long RP tachycardia.**
  - Most often, ST is a normal physiologic response to hyperadrenergic states (fever, pain, hypovolemia, anemia, hypoxia, etc.), but can also be induced by illicit drugs (cocaine, amphetamines, methamphetamine) and prescription drugs (theophylline, atropine, β-adrenergic agonists).
  - **Inappropriate ST** refers to persistently elevated sinus rate in the absence of an identifiable physical, pathologic, or pharmacologic influence.
- **Ectopic atrial tachycardia (EAT)**
  - EAT with variable block can present as an **irregularly irregular** rhythm and can be distinguished from AFl by an **atrial rate of 150 to 200 bpm.**
  - EAT with variable block is associated with **digoxin toxicity.**
  - EAT is characterized by a regular atrial activation pattern with a P-wave morphology originating outside of the sinus node complex resulting in a **long RP tachycardia.**
  - **Mechanism:** Enhanced automaticity, triggered activity, and, possibly microreentry.
- **AV nodal reentrant tachycardia (AVNRT)**
  - This reentrant rhythm occurs in patients who have functional dissociation of their AV node into "slow" and "fast" pathways. AVNRT can occur at any age, with a predilection for **middle age** and **female gender.** Structural heart disease is not a prerequisite.
- **"Typical" AVNRT**
  - More common; conduction proceeds antegrade down the slow pathway with retrograde conduction up the fast pathway, leading to **short RP tachycardia.**
  - **ECG:** P waves hidden in QRS complexes or buried at the end of QRS complexes creating a pseudo-r' (V_1) or pseudo-s' (II). Compare QRS and ST segment in tachycardia and sinus rhythm to find retrograde P waves.
- **"Atypical" AVNRT**
  - Less common; antegrade conduction proceeds over the fast AV nodal pathway with retrograde conduction over the slow AV nodal pathway, leading to a **long RP tachycardia.**
  - The retrograde P wave is inscribed well after the QRS complex in the second half of the RR interval.
- **AV reentrant tachycardia (AVRT)**
  - **Orthodromic AVRT (O-AVRT)** is the most common AVRT accounting for about 95% of all AVRT.
    - Accessory pathway-mediated reentrant rhythm occurs when antegrade conduction to the ventricle takes place through the AV node and retrograde conduction

to the atrium occurs through the accessory or "bypass" tract, leading to a **short RP tachycardia.**

- ○ **ECG:** Retrograde P waves are frequently seen after the QRS complex and are usually distinguishable from the QRS (i.e., separated by >70 milliseconds).
- ○ O-AVRT is the most common mechanism of SVT in patients with preexcitation syndromes, like WPW syndrome (defined by short PR and a delta wave on upstroke of QRS) present on sinus rhythm ECG.
- ○ O-AVRT can occur without preexcitation in which conduction through the bypass tract occurs only during tachycardia in a retrograde fashion ("concealed pathway").
- ○ Less commonly, retrograde conduction over the accessory pathway to the atrium proceeds slowly enough for atrial activation to occur in the second half of the RR interval, leading to a **long RP tachycardia.** The associated incessant tachycardia can cause tachycardia-induced cardiomyopathy.
- **Antidromic AVRT:** This reentrant form of SVT occurs when conduction to the ventricle is down an accessory bypass tract with retrograde conduction through the AV node or a second bypass tract.
  - ○ The QRS seems consistent with VT; however, the presence of preexcitation on the baseline QRS should be diagnostic for WPW syndrome. Antidromic AVRT is seen in <5% of patients with WPW syndrome.
- **Junctional tachycardia**
  - Arises from enhanced automaticity within the AV junction as the electrical impulses conduct to the ventricle and atrium simultaneously, similar to typical AVNRT, so that the retrograde P waves are frequently buried in the QRS complex.
  - Common in young children particularly after cardiac surgery.
- **Sinoatrial nodal reentrant tachycardia (SANRT)**
  - Reentrant circuit is localized at least partially within the sinoatrial (SA) node.
  - Abrupt onset and termination, triggered by a PAC.
  - **ECG:** P-wave morphology and axis are identical to the native sinus P wave during normal sinus rhythm.

TREATMENT

- Please refer to Table 1 for general therapeutic approach to common SVTs.
- Acute treatment of symptomatic SVT should follow the **ACLS protocol** as outlined in Appendix C.
- Chronic treatment should be aimed at either prevention of recurrence or prevention of the complications associated with the specific SVT.
- Many SVTs can be terminated by **AV nodal blocking agents or techniques** (Table 2), whereas AF, AFl, and some atrial tachycardias will persist with a slowing of the ventricular rate due to partial AV nodal blockade.
- **Correction of electrolyte abnormalities** like hypokalemia and hypomagnesemia may have therapeutic and preventive value in the treatment of some SVTs.
- **Radiofrequency ablation (RFA):** Definitive cure with high success rates from 85% to 95% for many SVTs, including AVNRT, accessory bypass tract-mediated tachycardias, focal atrial tachycardia, and AFl.
- Complication rates are dependent on the particular procedure and are usually <1% and include bleeding, groin hematomas, cardiac perforation or tamponade, stroke, pulmonary embolism, and complete heart block requiring permanent pacemaker (PPM).

Table 1	Treatment of Common SVTs

Treatment Strategies (*J Am Coll Cardiol 2003;42:1493*)

Atrial flutter (AFl)	Anticoagulation similar to AF; risk of thromboembolic complications is similar.
	Rate control with same agents as AF.
	If highly symptomatic or rate control difficult, electrical or chemical cardioversion is appropriate.
	If pacemaker present, overdrive atrial pacing can achieve cardioversion.
	Catheter ablation of typical right AFl with long-term success above 90% and rare complications.
Multifocal atrial tachycardia (MAT)	Therapy targeted at treatment of underlying pathophysiologic process.
	Maintain potassium and magnesium electrolyte balance.
	Antiarrhythmic, if symptomatic rapid ventricular response. Individualize β-adrenergic blockers vs. calcium channel blocker therapy.
	DC cardioversion is not effective.
Sinus tachycardia (ST)	Therapy targeted at treatment of underlying pathophysiologic process.
Ectopic atrial tachycardia (EAT)	**Acute therapy:** Identify and treat precipitating factors like digoxin toxicity; if hemodynamically stable, then β-blockers and calcium channel blockers. In rare cases amiodarone, flecainide, or sotalol.
	Chronic therapy: Rate control with β-adrenergic blockers and calcium channel blockers. If unsuccessful, options include catheter ablation (86% success rate), flecainide, propafenone, sotalol, or amiodarone.
AV nodal reentrant tachycardia (AVNRT)	Catheter ablation highly successful (96%) but has to be individualized to each patient.
	If medical therapy more desirable—β-adrenergic blockers, calcium channel blockers, and digoxin; then consider propafenone, flecainide, etc.
Orthodromic AV reentrant tachycardia (O-AVRT)	**Acute therapy:** Vagal maneuvers, adenosine, calcium channel blockers. If ineffective, then procainamide or β-blockers.
	Chronic suppressive therapy: Catheter ablation highly successful (95%) but has to be individualized to each patient. If medical therapy more desirable for prevention, flecainide and procainamide are indicated.
Antidromic AV reentrant tachycardia (A-AVRT)	**Acute therapy:** Avoid adenosine or other AV node–specific blocking agents. Consider ibutilide, procainamide, or flecainide.
	Chronic suppressive therapy: Accessory pathway catheter ablation is preferred and successful (95%). If medical therapy desired, consider flecainide and propafenone.

	Patient Preparation[a]	Mechanism	Dose/Duration/Details	Toxicity	Contraindication	Potentiators/Antagonists	Common Side Effects
Valsalva	Describe the procedure	Vagal stimulation during relaxation phase	Exhale forcefully against a closed airway for several seconds followed by relaxation	Well tolerated	Patient unable to follow commands	—	—
Carotid sinus massage	Check for carotid bruits and history of CVA; then place in recumbent position with neck extended	Vagal stimulation	First, apply enough pressure to simply feel carotid pulse with index and middle fingers. If no effect, then use rotating motion for 3–5 sec	Well tolerated. Risk of embolizing carotid plaque. **Never massage both carotids**	Recent TIA or stroke, or ipsilateral significant carotid artery stenosis or carotid artery bruit	—	—
Adenosine	Explain the potential side effects to the patient	AV nodal blocking agent. Short-acting (serum half-life 4–8 min)	Initial: 6 mg IV rapid bolus via antecubital vein, followed by 10–30 mL saline flush. If desired effect not achieved, can repeat 12 mg followed by 12 mg after 1–2 min intervals. Central venous line: 3 mg IV initial dose	Precipitate prolonged asystole in patients with sick sinus syndrome or second- or third-degree AV block	Significant bronchospasm	Potentiators: Dipyridamole and carbamazepine. **Effect pronounced in heart transplant recipients.** Antagonists: Caffeine and theophylline	Facial flushing, palpitations, chest pain, hypotension, exacerbation of bronchospasm.

Table 2   Common Vagal Maneuvers and Adenosine

[a]Patients should be under continuous ECG monitoring for each of these procedures. To enhance diagnostic value of rhythm strip, use leads V_1, II (atrial activity). AVNRT, AVRT, and many atrial tachycardias will terminate with vagal maneuvers or adenosine and in AFl, the appearance of flutter waveform will help diagnosis. Water immersion, eyeball pressure, coughing, gagging, deep breathing, etc. are other alternative vagal maneuvers.

- There is growing evidence but lack of large randomized trials with long-term follow-up, which suggests that catheter ablation as compared to antiarrhythmic therapy improves quality of life and is more cost-effective in the long term (*Am J Cardiol 1998;82:589*).

Atrial Fibrillation

GENERAL PRINCIPLES

- The medical management of **atrial fibrillation (AF)** requires careful consideration of three issues: **rate control, prevention of thromboembolic events, and rhythm control.** Recent studies have shown that there is no mortality advantage to a management strategy aimed at maintaining sinus rhythm (*N Engl J Med 2002;347:1825*). Therefore, the approach to AF in the minimally symptomatic patient is devoted to prevention of thromboembolus and pharmacologic control of the ventricular response to AF. Rhythm control is reserved for patients who remain symptomatic despite efforts to optimize the ventricular response to AF.
- **Rate control** of AF can be achieved with agents that limit conduction through the AV node. These include the nondihydropyridine calcium channel blockers (diltiazem, verapamil), β-adrenergic blockers, and digoxin. Refer to Table 3 for loading and dosing recommendations.
- **Prevention of thromboembolic events** is a central tenet of AF management and should begin with individual risk assessment of each patient. Chronic warfarin anticoagulation is currently the most effective therapy for attenuating the risk of stroke associated with AF; however, its initiation requires careful risk–benefit analysis to identify the patients who are at sufficient risk for embolic cerebrovascular accident (CVA) to outweigh the increased risk of hemorrhagic complications.
- **Rhythm control**
  ○ Pharmacologic control with antiarrhythmic drugs is most effective at preventing recurrence of AF and less effective at chemical cardioversion of AF.
  ○ Nonpharmacologic methods of rhythm control include catheter or surgical ablation techniques that block the initiation and maintenance of AF.

Definition

AF is an atrial tachyarrhythmia characterized by the predominantly uncoordinated activation of the atria with the consequent deterioration of atrial mechanical function. AF has a pattern on 12-lead ECG indicated by the absence of consistent P waves. Instead, there are rapid, low-amplitude oscillations or fibrillatory waves that vary in size, shape, and timing across the baseline of the ECG recording. The ventricular response to AF is characteristically irregular and often rapid in the presence of intact AV conduction. AF is the most common cardiac arrhythmia.

Classification

AF has been classified into four forms based upon the clinical presentation: first occurrence, paroxysmal, persistent, and permanent forms.

- **First occurrence** may be symptomatic or asymptomatic. The spontaneous conversion rate is high, measured >60% in hospitalized patients.
- **Paroxysmal** AF describes a recurrent form of AF in which individual episodes are <7 days and usually <48 hours in duration.

Table 3   Pharmacologic Agents Used for Heart Rate Control in Atrial Fibrillation

Drug	Loading Dose	Onset of Action	Maintenance Sose	Major Side Effects	Recommendation
Without evidence of accessory pathway					
Esmolol[a]	IV: 0.5 mg/kg over 1 min	5 min[b]	0.06–0.2 mg/kg/min	↓BP, ↓HR, HB, HF, bronchospasm	I
Metoprolol[a]	IV: 2.5–5.0 mg bolus over 2 min (up to three doses)	5 min	NA	↓BP, ↓HR, HB, HF, bronchospasm	I
	PO: Same as maintenance	4–6 h	25–100 mg bid		
Propranolol[a]	IV: 0.15 mg/kg	5 min	NA	↓BP, ↓HR, HB, HF, bronchospasm	I
	PO: Same as maintenance	60–90 min	80–240 mg/d in divided doses		
Diltiazem	IV: 0.25 mg/kg over 2 min	2–7 min	5–15 mg/hr	↓BP, HB, HF	I
	PO: Same as maintenance	2–4 hr	120–360 mg/d in divided doses; slow release available		
Verapamil	IV: 0.075–0.15 mg/kg over 2 min	3–5 min	NA	↓BP, HB, HF	I
	PO: Same as maintenance	1–2 hr	120–360 mg/d in divided doses; slow release available		

With evidence of accessory pathway[c]

Amiodarone	IV: 150 mg over 10 min	Days	1 mg/min × 6 h, then 0.5 mg/min	See below	IIa

In patients with heart failure and without accessory pathway

Digoxin	IV: 0.25 mg q2h, up to 1.5 mg PO: 0.5 mg/d	60 min or more 2 days	0.125–0.375 mg/d IV or orally	Digoxin toxicity, HB, ↓HR	I
Amiodarone[d]	IV: 150 mg over 10 min PO: 800 mg/d for 1 wk, 600 mg/d for 1 wk, 400 mg/d for 1 wk,	Days 1–3 wk	1 mg/min × 6 h, then 0.5 mg/min 100–400 mg PO daily	↓BP, HB, ↓HR, warfarin interaction; see text for description of dermatologic, thyroid, pulmonary, corneal, and liver side effects	Acute setting: IIa(IV) nonacute/chronic: IIb(PO)

NA, not applicable; ↓BP, hypotension; ↓HR, bradycardia; HB, heart block; HF, heart failure.

[a]Only representative members of the type of β-blockers are included in the table, but other similar agents could be used for this indication in appropriate doses.

[b]Onset is variable and some effects occur earlier.

[c]Conversion to sinus rhythm and catheter ablation of the accessory pathway are generally recommended; pharmacologic therapy for rate control may be appropriate therapy in certain patients. See text for discussion of AF in setting of preexcitation/WPW syndrome.

[d]Amiodarone can be useful to control the heart rate in patients with AF when other measures are unsuccessful or contraindicated.

Adapted from Fuster V, Ryden LE, Cannom DS, et al. ACC/AHA/ESC 2006 Guidelines for the Management of Patients With Atrial Fibrillation: A Report of the American College of Cardiology/American Heart Association Task Force on Practice Guidelines and the European Society of Cardiology Committee for Practice Guidelines (Writing Committee to Revise the 2001 Guidelines for the Management of Patients With Atrial Fibrillation). *Circulation* 2006;114:e257–e354.

- **Persistent** AF describes a recurrent form of AF in which individual episodes are >7 days in duration or require electrical cardioversion to terminate.
- **Permanent** AF describes the form of long-lasting AF, which has failed attempts at cardioversion, electrical or pharmacologic, or has been accepted due to contraindications for cardioversion or a lack of symptoms.

Epidemiology

- **AF** is the most common sustained tachyarrhythmia for which patients seek treatment and the most likely etiology for an irregularly irregular rhythm discovered on an inpatient ECG. AF is typically a disease of the elderly affecting >10% of those older than 75 years.
- Independent risk factors for AF in addition to advanced age include male sex, diabetes mellitus, cardiovascular disease such as CHF, valvular heart disease, hypertension, and previous MI (*JAMA 1994;271:840*). Below age 65, obesity and obstructive sleep apnea are important risk factors for new-onset AF (*J Am Coll Cardiol 2007; 49(5):565*). Although clinical hyperthyroidism is associated with new-onset AF, the prevalence is low in a population of patients with AF (*J Epidemiol 2008;18(5): 209*).
- Following cardiothoracic surgery, AF occurs in 20% to 50% of patients (*J Am Coll Cardiol 2006;48(4):8540*).

Pathophysiology

The precise mechanisms giving rise to AF are incompletely understood. The initiation of AF is commonly due to rapid, repetitive firing of an ectopic focus within the pulmonary veins with fibrillatory conduction to the bodies of the atria. The maintenance of persistent AF likely requires multiple reentrant circuits varying in location and timing to explain the self-perpetuating characteristic of AF. Structural and electrical remodeling of the left atrium associated with cardiovascular disease promotes ectopic activity and heterogeneous conduction patterns that provide the substrate for AF. AF, when present, also promotes structural and electrical remodeling in the atria that stabilizes the rhythm. Inflammation and fibrosis may play a major role in initiation and maintenance of AF. Inflammatory markers, such as interleukin-6 and C-reactive protein, are raised in AF and correlate with the duration of AF, success of cardioversion, and thrombogenesis.

Prevention

- Currently, there is a lack of prospective clinical trials that examine the value of primary prevention of nonpostoperative AF through treatment of associated conditions or risk factor modification. Retrospective analyses suggest lipid-lowering statin drugs may have a potent effect on reducing recurrent AF independent of lipid-lowering effect. A meta-analysis that included 3,557 patients enrolled in selected statin trials demonstrated a 61% reduction in the incidence of recurrent AF associated with **statin treatment** (*J Am Coll Cardiol 2008;51:828*). Angiotensin-converting enzyme inhibitor **(ACEI) and** angiotensin receptor blockers **(ARBs)** have been shown to prevent atrial remodeling in animals via suppression of the renin–angiotensin system. A meta-analysis of patients with CHF and hypertension treated with either ACEI or ARBs demonstrated a reduction in new-onset AF by 20% to 30% (*J Am Coll Cardiol 2005;45:1832*).
- A number of pharmacologic and nonpharmacologic strategies have been evaluated to prevent postoperative AF. Perioperative continuation of *β*-adrenergic antagonists

has been shown to reduce postoperative AF rates. **Amiodarone, sotalol, magnesium, or omega-3 fatty acids** used in the perioperative period have demonstrated a reduction in postoperative AF (*Ann Pharmacother 2007;41:587*).

DIAGNOSIS

AF is diagnosed by 12-lead ECG with a stereotypical pattern of an irregularly fluctuating baseline with an irregular, and often rapid, ventricular rate (>100 bpm). AF should be distinguished from other tachycardia mechanisms with an irregular ventricular response such as MAT and AFl with variable conduction.

Clinical Presentation

Symptoms associated with AF can range from severe (acute pulmonary edema, palpitations, angina, syncope) to nonspecific (fatigue) to none at all. Symptoms are usually secondary to the rapid ventricular response to AF rather than the loss of atrial systole. However, patients with significant ventricular systolic or diastolic dysfunction can have symptoms directly attributable to the loss of atrial systole. Prolonged episodes of tachycardia due to AF may lead to a **tachycardia-induced cardiomyopathy.**

TREATMENT

The medical management of AF is directed at three therapeutic goals: **rate control, prevention of thromboembolic events, and rhythm control** through maintenance of sinus rhythm. Recent studies have shown that there is no mortality advantage to a management strategy aimed at maintaining sinus rhythm (*N Engl J Med 2002;347:1825*). Therefore, the approach to the treatment of AF in the minimally symptomatic patient is devoted to prevention of thromboembolus and pharmacologic control of the ventricular response to AF. Pharmacologic maintenance of sinus rhythm is reserved for patients who remain symptomatic despite efforts to optimize the ventricular response to AF.

Medications

Medical management of AF should start with a consideration of appropriate antithrombotic therapy. Warfarin has been shown to be consistently superior to aspirin or aspirin in combination with clopidogrel for prevention of thromboembolus. Rate control of the ventricular response to AF is achieved with medications that limit conduction through the AV node such as **verapamil, diltiazem, β-adrenergic antagonists, and digoxin**. Rhythm control through maintenance of sinus rhythm can be attempted with selected antiarrhythmic drugs.

First Line
- **Prevention of thromboembolic complications** is a central tenet of AF management and should begin with individual risk assessment of each patient. Chronic warfarin anticoagulation is currently the most effective therapy for attenuating the risk of stroke associated with AF; however, its initiation requires careful risk–benefit analysis to identify the patients who are at sufficient risk for embolic CVA to outweigh the increased risk of hemorrhagic complications.
  - The **CHADS$_2$ score** is a validated, risk stratification tool that can categorize nonvalvular AF patients as low, intermediate, or high risk for stroke based on the presence

| Table 4 | Stroke Risk in Patients With Nonvalvular AF Not Treated With Anticoagulation According to the CHADS₂ Index |

CHADS₂ risk criteria	Score
Prior stroke or TIA	2
Age >75 yr	1
Hypertension	1
Diabetes mellitus	1
Heart failure	1

Patients (N = 1,733)	Adjusted stroke Rate (%/yr)[a] (95% CI)	CHADS₂ score	Risk category	Recommended Antithrombotic Therapy
120	1.9 (1.2–3.0)	0	Low	→ Aspirin 81–325 mg PO daily
463	2.8 (2.0–3.8)	1	Moderate	→ Aspirin or Warfarin
523	4.0 (3.1–5.1)	2	Moderate	→ Previous CVA/TIA/embolism?
337	5.9 (4.6–7.3)	3	High	- Yes = Warfarin
220	8.5 (6.3–11.1)	4	High	- No = Aspirin or Warfarin
65	12.5 (8.2–17.5)	5	High	→ Warfarin (INR 2.0–3.0)
5	18.2 (10.5–27.4)	6	High	

AF, atrial fibrillation; CHADS₂, cardiac failure, hypertension, age, diabetes, and stroke (doubled); CI, confidence interval; and TIA, transient ischemic attack; Aspirin, 81–325 mg PO daily; Warfarin, INR 2.0–3.0.
[a]The adjusted stroke rate was derived from multivariate analysis assuming no aspirin usage. Adapted from Fuster V, Ryden LE, Cannom DS, et al. ACC/AHA/ESC 2006 Guidelines for the Management of Patients With Atrial Fibrillation: A Report of the American College of Cardiology/American Heart Association Task Force on Practice Guidelines and the European Society of Cardiology Committee for Practice Guidelines (Writing Committee to Revise the 2001 Guidelines for the Management of Patients With Atrial Fibrillation). *Circulation* 2006;114: e257–e354. Data from Gage BF, Waterman AD, Shannon W, et al. Validation of clinical classification schemes for predicting stroke: results from the National Registry of Atrial Fibrillation. *JAMA* 2001;285:2864–2870.

of these risk factors: **C**HF, **H**ypertension (HTN), **A**ge >75, **D**iabetes mellitus, or prior **S**troke/TIAs (Table 4).
- In one study, high-risk patients have a 6% to 7% per year stroke risk that can be reduced to 3.6% per year if placed on aspirin 325 mg/d or reduced further to 2.3% per year if placed on therapeutic doses of warfarin (*Circulation 1991;84:527*). A general consensus exists that patients younger than 65 years without structural heart disease or hypertension (i.e., "lone AF") are at low risk (approximately 1% per year) and can be managed with daily aspirin (ASA) alone. The current American Heart Association (AHA)/American College of Cardiology (ACC)/European Society of Cardiology (ESC) recommendations for chronic antithrombotic therapy in AF are summarized in Table 5.
- The role of antithrombotic therapy leading up to and after restoration of sinus rhythm is discussed below in the context of cardioversion.
- **Rate control** of AF can be achieved with agents that prolong conduction through the AV node. These include the nondihydropyridine calcium channel blockers

		Class of Recommendation
Patient Features	**Antithrombotic Therapy**	
Age <60 yr, no heart disease (lone AF)	Aspirin (81–325 mg/d) or no therapy	I
Age <60 yr, heart disease but no RF[a]	Aspirin (81–325 mg/d)	I
Age 60–74 yr, no RF[a]	Aspirin (81–325 mg/d)	I
Age 65–74 yr with diabetes mellitus or CAD	Oral anticoagulation (INR 2.0–3.0)	I
Age 75 yr or older, women	Oral anticoagulation (INR 2.0–3.0)	I
Age 75 yr or older, men, no other RF	Oral anticoagulation (INR 2.0–3.0) or aspirin (81–325 mg/d)	I
Age 65 yr or older, heart failure	Oral anticoagulation (INR 2.0–3.0)	I
LV ejection fraction <35% or fractional shortening <25%, and hypertension	Oral anticoagulation (INR 2.0–3.0)	I
Rheumatic heart disease (mitral stenosis)	Oral anticoagulation (INR 2.0–3.0)	I
Prosthetic heart valves; prior thromboembolism	Oral anticoagulation (INR 2.0–3.0 or higher)	I
Persistent atrial thrombus on TEE	Oral anticoagulation (INR 2.0–3.0 or higher)	IIa

Table 5. Appropriate Anticoagulation in Various AF Populations

AF, atrial fibrillation; CAD, coronary artery disease; INR, international normalized ratio; TEE, transesophageal echocardiography.
[a]Risk factors for thromboembolism include heart failure (HF), left ventricular (LV) ejection fraction less than 35%, and history of hypertension.
Adapted from Fuster V, Ryden LE, Cannom DS, et al. ACC/AHA/ESC 2006 Guidelines for the Management of Patients With Atrial Fibrillation: A Report of the American College of Cardiology/American Heart Association Task Force on Practice Guidelines and the European Society of Cardiology Committee for Practice Guidelines (Writing Committee to Revise the 2001 Guidelines for the Management of Patients With Atrial Fibrillation). *Circulation* 2006;114:e257–e354.

(diltiazem, verapamil), β-adrenergic blockers, and digoxin. Refer to Table 3 for loading and dosing recommendations.

- **Digoxin** is useful in controlling the resting ventricular rate in AF in the setting of LV dysfunction and CHF and may be useful as adjunctive therapy in combination with calcium channel antagonists or β-adrenergic antagonists for optimum rate control of chronic AF. It is less useful for rate control during exertion.
- **Digitalis toxicity** is usually diagnosed clinically with presenting symptoms including **nausea, abdominal pain, vision changes, confusion, and delirium.** It is often seen in patients with renal dysfunction or in those patients on agents known to increase digoxin levels (verapamil, diltiazem, erythromycin, cyclosporine, etc.). **Paroxysmal atrial tachycardia with varying degrees of AV block and bidirectional VT** are the most commonly seen arrhythmias in association with digitalis toxicity. Treatment is supportive, by withholding the drug, insertion of temporary pacemakers for AV block, and **IV phenytoin for bidirectional VT.**

- **Nonpharmacologic rate control** of AF can be accomplished by AV nodal ablation in association with PPM implantation. This strategy should be reserved for patients who have failed pharmacologic rate control and rhythm control is either ineffective or contraindicated.

Second Line
- **Rhythm control of AF** is accomplished pharmacologically with antiarrhythmic drugs that modify impulse formation or propagation to prevent initiation of AF. Antiarrhythmic drugs are less effective at restoration of sinus rhythm through **pharmacologic cardioversion. The risk of thromboembolus associated with a pharmacologic cardioversion should be considered before beginning antiarrhythmic drug therapy.** Guidelines for anticoagulation are discussed below:
  - **Pharmacologic cardioversion** should be done in the hospital setting with continuous ECG monitoring because of a small risk of life-threatening tachyarrhythmias or bradyarrhythmias. Ibutilide is the only drug that is approved by the U.S. Food and Drug Administration for pharmacologic cardioversion. Clinical trials have shown a 45% conversion rate for AF and a 60% conversion rate for AFL. **Ibutilide** is associated with a 4% to 8% risk for Torsades de pointes (TdP), especially in the first 2 to 4 hours after administration of the drug. Because of this risk, patients must be monitored on telemetry with an external defibrillator immediately available during ibutilide infusion and for at least 4 hours after ibutilide infusion. The risk for TdP is higher in patients with cardiomyopathy and CHF. Ibutilide is given as an IV bolus, at a dosage of 1 mg (0.01 mg/kg if patient is <60 kg), **infused slowly over 10 minutes.** Faster administration can promote TdP. The efficacy of antiarrhythmics to achieve pharmacologic conversion drops sharply when AF is >7 days in duration. For shorter-duration AF episodes, dofetilide, sotalol, flecainide, and propafenone have some efficacy, while amiodarone has limited efficacy to achieve pharmacologic cardioversion.
  - **Maintenance of sinus rhythm** with antiarrhythmic agents is associated with a small risk for life-threatening proarrhythmia. As a result, antiarrhythmic therapy should be reserved for patients who have highly symptomatic AF in spite of adequate rate control. Antiarrhythmic agents are grouped by the predominate mechanism of action according to the Vaughan Williams classification. **Class I agents inhibit the fast sodium channel, class II agents are β-adrenergic antagonists, class III agents primarily block potassium channels, and class IV agents are calcium channel antagonists.** Commonly used antiarrhythmic agents, their major route of elimination, and dosing regimen are listed in Table 6. The most effective agents for maintenance of sinus rhythm are flecainide, propafenone, sotalol, dofetilide, and amiodarone.
    - **Flecainide** and **propafenone** are class Ic antiarrhythmic drugs that are useful for maintenance of sinus rhythm in patients with structurally normal hearts. In patients with structural heart disease, class Ic agents are associated with an increased mortality rate (*N Engl J Med 1989;321:406*), and both agents are potent negative inotropes that can provoke or exacerbate heart failure. Both agents prolong the QRS duration as an early manifestation of toxicity. The toxic drug levels correlate with heart rate due to preferential blockade of active sodium channels. This property is described as use dependence. Exercise ECG can be used to give additional information about dose safety at high heart rates. Flecainide should be used with caution without concomitant dosing with an AV nodal blocker because a paradoxical increase in the ventricular rate may occur

Table 6   Commonly Used Antiarrhythmic Drug

Class	Drug	Route of Administration (Elimination)[a]	Initial/Loading Dose	Maintenance Dose	Major Adverse Effects[a]/Comments
Ia	Procainamide	IV (R, H) PO (R, H)	15–18 mg/kg at 20 mg/min 50 mg/kg/24 h, Max: 5 g/24 h	1–4 mg/min IR: 250–500 mg q3–6h; SR: 500 mg q6; Procanbid: 1,000–2,500 mg q12h	GI, CNS, +ANA/SLE-like syndrome, fever, hematologic, anticholinergic. Follow QT$_c$, serum procainamide (4–8 mg/L) and NAPA levels (<20 mg/mL)
	Quinidine	PO (H)	Sulfate, 200–400 mg q6h; gluconate, 324–972 mg q8–12h	NA	↑QT, TdP, ↓BP, thrombocytopenia, cinchonism, GI upset
	Disopyramide	PO (H, R)	300–400 mg	IR: 100–200 mg q6h; SR: 200–400 mg q12h	Anticholinergic, HF
Ib	Lidocaine	IV (H)	1 mg/kg over 2 min (may repeat × 2 up to 3 mg/kg total)	1–4 mg/min	↓HR, CNS, GI. Adjust dose in pts w/ hepatic failure, AMI, HF, or shock
Ic	Mexilitine	PO (H)	400 mg one time dose	200–300 mg q8h	GI, CNS
	Flecainide	PO (H, R)	50 mg q12h	Increase by 50–100 mg/d every 4 days to max 400 mg/d	HF, GI, CNS, blurred vision
	Propafenone	PO (H)	IR:150 mg q8h ER: 225 mg q12h	IR: Increase at 3–4 day intervals up to 300 mg q8h; ER: may increase in 5 day intervals, up to 425 mg q12h	GI, dizziness

(continued)

Table 6	Commonly Used Antiarrhythmic Drug (*Continued*)			
Class	**Drug**	**Route of Administration (Elimination)**[a]	**Initial/Loading Dose**	**Maintenance Dose**	**Major Adverse Effects**[a]**/Comments**
III	Sotalol	PO (R)	80 mg q12h	May increase every 3 days up to 240–320 mg/d in two to three divided doses	↓HR, ↓BP, CHF, CNS. Limit QT$_c$ prolongation to <550 ms
	Dofetilide	PO (R, H)	CrCl (mL/min): Dose (mcg bid): >60: 500 40–60: 250 20–39: 125 <20: Contraindicated	Dose adjusted based on QT$_c$ 2–3 hr after inpatient doses 1 through 5. Chronic therapy requires calculation of QT$_c$ and CrCl every 3 months with adjustment as necessary	↑QT, VT/TdP, HA, dizziness. See text for further details on initiating and monitoring treatment.
	Ibutilide	IV (H)	1 mg (0.01 mg/kg if pt <60 kg) over 10 min; can repeat if no response 10 min after initial infusion	NA	↑QT, TdP, AV block, GI, HA
	Amiodarone	IV (H) PO (H)	IV: 150 mg over 10 min PO: 800 mg/d for 1 wk, then 600 mg/d for 1 wk, then 400 mg/d for 1 wk	1 mg/min × 6 h, then 0.5 mg/min 100–400 mg PO daily	↓BP, HB, ↓HR, warfarin interaction; see text for description of dermatologic, thyroid, pulmonary, corneal, and liver effects

NA, not applicable; R, renal; H, hepatic; ↓BP, hypotension; ↓HR, bradycardia; HB, heart block; HF, heart failure; VT, ventricular tachycardia; TdP, torsades de pointes, AMI, acute myocardial infarction, HA, headache; IR, immediate release; ER, extended release.
[a]Either common or life-threatening adverse effects of these medications are listed. This is not a comprehensive list of all possible adverse effects.

due to drug-induced conversion of AF to AFl. Propafenone is less prone to this phenomenon due to intrinsic β-adrenergic antagonism.

○ **Sotalol** is a class III antiarrhythmic agent that is useful for the maintenance of sinus rhythm. Sotalol is a mixture of stereoisomers (DL-); D-sotalol is a potassium channel blocker, while L-sotalol is a β-antagonist. Side effects reflect both mechanisms of action. In addition to QT interval prolongation leading to TdP, DL-sotalol may result in sinus bradycardia or AV conduction abnormalities. Sotalol should not be used in patients with decompensated CHF due to the negative inotropic effect or with a prolonged QT interval.

○ **Dofetilide** is a class III antiarrhythmic agent that is useful for the maintenance of sinus rhythm. Dofetilide blocks the rapid component of the delayed rectifier potassium current, I_{Kr}. As a result, dofetilide increases the QT interval at clinically effective doses. QT prolongation is intensified by bradycardia, a characteristic known as "reverse use dependence." The main risk of dofetilide is TdP. Dofetilide is contraindicated in patients with a baseline correct QT interval (QT_c) >440 milliseconds, or 500 milliseconds in patients with bundle branch block. Initial dosing of dofetilide is based on the creatinine clearance. A 12-lead ECG should be obtained before the first dose of dofetilide and 1 to 2 hours after each dose. If the QT_c interval after the first dose prolongs by 15% of the baseline or exceeds 500 milliseconds, a 50% dosage reduction is indicated. If the QT_c exceeds 500 milliseconds after the second dose, dofetilide must be discontinued. Several medications block the renal secretion of dofetilide (verapamil, cimetidine, prochlorperazine, trimethoprim, megestrol, ketoconazole) and are contraindicated with dofetilide. The advantages of dofetilide are that it is not associated with increased CHF or mortality in patients with LV dysfunction (*N Engl J Med 1999;341:857*), and dofetilide does not cause sinus node dysfunction or conduction abnormalities.

○ **Amiodarone** has the properties of class I, II, III, and IV drugs, and is arguably the most effective antiarrhythmic agent for maintenance of sinus rhythm. **Because of the extensive toxicity profile of amiodarone, it should not be considered as a first-line agent for rhythm control of AF in patients in whom an alternative antiarrhythmic can be safely used.** Intravenous amiodarone has a low efficacy for acute conversion of AF, although conversion after several days of IV amiodarone has been observed. Given its common use and relative high incidence of side effects, a more detailed discussion of these effects is required.

- Adverse effects of oral amiodarone are partially dose dependent and may occur in up to 75% of patients treated at high doses for 5 years. At lower dosages (200 to 300 mg/d), adverse effects that require discontinuation occur in approximately 5% to 10% of patients per year.

- **Pulmonary toxicity** occurs in 1% to 15% of treated patients but appears less likely in those who receive <300 mg/d (*Circulation 1990;82:580*). Patients characteristically have a dry cough and dyspnea associated with pulmonary infiltrates and rales. The process appears to be reversible if detected early, but undetected cases may result in a mortality of up to 10% of those affected. A chest radiograph and pulmonary function tests should be obtained at baseline and every 12 months or when patients complain of shortness of breath. The presence of interstitial infiltrates on the chest radiograph and a decreased diffusing capacity raise concern of amiodarone pulmonary toxicity.

- **Photosensitivity** is a common adverse reaction, and, in some patients, a violaceous skin discoloration develops in sun-exposed areas. The blue-gray discoloration may not resolve completely with discontinuation of therapy.

- **Thyroid dysfunction** is a common adverse effect. Hypothyroidism and hyperthyroidism have been reported, with an incidence of 2% to 5% per year. Thyroid-stimulating hormone should be obtained at baseline and monitored every 6 months. If hypothyroidism develops, concurrent treatment with levothyroxine may allow continued amiodarone use.
- **Corneal microdeposits,** detectable on slit-lamp examination, develop in virtually all patients. These deposits rarely interfere with vision and are not an indication for discontinuation of the drug. Optic neuritis, leading to blindness, is rare but has been reported in association with amiodarone.
- The most common **ECG changes** are lengthened PR intervals and bradycardia; however, high-grade AV block may occur in patients who have preexisting conduction abnormalities. Amiodarone may prolong QT intervals, although usually not extensively, and **TdP is rare.** Other agents that prolong the QT interval, however, should be avoided in patients who are taking amiodarone.
- **Liver dysfunction** usually manifests in an asymptomatic and transient rise in hepatic transaminases. *If the increase exceeds three times normal or doubles in a patient with an elevated baseline level, amiodarone should be discontinued or the dose should be reduced.* Aspartate transaminase (AST) and alanine transaminase (ALT) should be monitored every 6 months in patients who are receiving amiodarone.
- **Drug interactions.** *Amiodarone may raise the blood levels of warfarin and digoxin;* therefore, these drugs should be reduced routinely by one-half when amiodarone is started, and levels should be followed closely.

Other Nonoperative Therapies

- **DC cardioversion** is the safest and most effective method of acutely restoring sinus rhythm. Prior to cardioversion, consideration of thromboembolic risk and anticoagulation is critical, when possible, to minimize thromboembolic events triggered by the cardioversion process. AF with a rapid ventricular response in the setting of ongoing myocardial ischemia, MI, hypotension, or respiratory distress should receive prompt cardioversion regardless of the anticoagulation status.
  - If the duration of AF is documented to be **<48 hours,** cardioversion may proceed without anticoagulation. If AF has persisted for **>48 hours** (or for an unknown duration), patients should be anticoagulated with warfarin, with an international normalized ratio (INR) of 2.0 to 3.0, for at least 3 weeks before cardioversion, and anticoagulation should be continued in the same therapeutic range following successful cardioversion.
  - An alternative to anticoagulation for 3 weeks before cardioversion is to perform a **transesophageal echocardiogram** to rule out left atrial appendage thrombus before cardioversion. This method is safe and has the advantage of shorter time to cardioversion than warfarin and therefore is indicated in patients who are not able to wait weeks before cardioversion. Therapeutic anticoagulation with warfarin is indicated after the cardioversion for a minimum of 4 weeks (*Am J Cardiol 1998;82:1545*), although the AFFIRM trial (*N Engl J Med 2002;347:1825*) suggests that in patients with high risk for stroke, warfarin should be continued indefinitely.
  - When practical, sedation should be accomplished with *midazolam* (1 to 2 mg IV q2min to a maximum of 5 mg), *methohexital* (25 to 75 mg IV), *etomidate* (0.2 to 0.6 mg/kg IV), or *propofol* (initial dose, 5 mg/kg/hr IV).
  - Proper synchronization to the QRS is critical to avoid induction of ventricular fibrillation (VT) by a cardioversion shock delivered during a vulnerable period.

Synchronization of the external cardioverter-defibrillator should be confirmed by noting the presence of a synchronization marker superimposed on the QRS complex.

- For cardioversion of atrial arrhythmias, the anterior patch electrode should be positioned just right of the sternum at the level of the third or fourth intercostal space, with the second electrode positioned just below the left scapula posteriorly. **Care should be taken to position patch electrodes at least 6 cm from PPM or defibrillator generators.** If electrode paddles are used, firm pressure and conductive gel should be applied to minimize contact impedance. Direct contact with the patient or the bed should be avoided. Atropine (1 mg IV) should be readily available to treat prolonged pauses. Reports of serious arrhythmias, such as VT, VF, or asystole, are rare and are more likely in the setting of improperly synchronized cardioversions, digitalis toxicity, or concomitant antiarrhythmic drug therapy.

- **Curative catheter ablation of AF** has been shown to be highly effective in young patients with structurally normal hearts and a paroxysmal pattern of their AF. Cure rates in this patient category are in the range of 80% to 90%. In patients with structural heart disease, advanced age, and persistent AF, cure rates are diminished. A significant fraction of patients require more than one ablation procedure to achieve cure. The goal of the catheter ablation procedure in paroxysmal AF patients is to achieve electrical isolation of the pulmonary veins. In patients with persistent AF, this goal is frequently combined with substrate modification strategies whereby regions of the atria are targeted for ablation to block reentry or extrapulmonary vein triggers. Because of potential complications and modest success, patients should undergo at least one trial of an antiarrhythmic drug for maintenance of sinus rhythm. If this trial is ineffective or poorly tolerated, curative catheter ablation can be contemplated.

Surgical Management

Surgical techniques for cure of AF have been evaluated since the 1980s. Of these techniques, the Cox Maze III procedure has the highest demonstrated efficacy and the most substantial published follow-up data documenting sustained efficacy. Including patients with persistent AF and structural heart disease, cure rates approach 90%. Because of its highly invasive nature, surgical treatment is usually reserved for patients who have failed a catheter ablation strategy or who have planned concomitant cardiac surgery.

Ventricular Tachyarrhythmias

GENERAL PRINCIPLES

- Ventricular tachyarrhythmias should be initially approached with the assumption that they will have a malignant course until proven otherwise.
- Characterization of the arrhythmia involves consideration of hemodynamic stability, duration, morphology, and the presence or lack of underlying structural heart disease.
- Ultimately, this characterization will aid in determining the patient's risk for **sudden cardiac arrest** and need for device or ablation-based therapy.

Definition

- **Nonsustained VT** is defined as three or more consecutive ventricular complexes (>100 bpm) that terminates spontaneously within 30 seconds without significant hemodynamic consequences or need for intervention.

- **Sustained monomorphic VT** is defined as a tachycardia composed of ventricular complexes of a single QRS morphology that lasts longer than 30 seconds or requires cardioversion due to hemodynamic compromise.
- **Polymorphic VT** is characterized by an ever-changing QRS morphology. **TdP** is a variant of polymorphic VT that is typically preceded by a prolonged QT interval in sinus rhythm. Polymorphic VT is usually associated with hemodynamic collapse or instability.
- **VF** is associated with disorganized mechanical contraction, hemodynamic collapse, and sudden death. The ECG reveals irregular and rapid oscillations (250 to 400 bpm) of highly variable amplitude without uniquely identifiable QRS complexes or T waves.
- Ventricular arrhythmias are the major cause of **sudden cardiac death (SCD). SCD** is defined as the death that occurs within 1 hour of the onset of symptoms. In the United States, 350,000 cases of SCD occur annually. Among patients with aborted SCD, ischemic heart disease is the most common associated cardiac structural abnormality. Most cardiac arrest survivors do not evolve evidence of an acute MI; however, >75% have evidence of previous infarcts. A nonischemic cardiomyopathy is also associated with an elevated risk for SCD.

Etiology

- **VT associated with structural heart disease**
  - Most ventricular arrhythmias are associated with structural heart disease, typically related to active ischemia or history of infarct.
    - Scar and the peri-infarct area provide the substrate for reentry that produces sustained monomorphic VT.
    - Polymorphic VT and VF are commonly associated with ischemia and are the presumed cause of most out-of-hospital SCD.
  - Nonischemic cardiomyopathy typically involves progressive dilation and fibrosis of the ventricular myocardium, providing an arrhythmogenic substrate.
  - Infiltrative cardiomyopathies (sarcoid, hemochromatosis, amyloid) represent a smaller patient population that is at significant risk for ventricular arrhythmias whose management is less clearly defined.
  - Adults with prior repair of congenital heart disease are commonly afflicted with both VT and SVT.
  - Arrhythmogenic right ventricular dysplasia or cardiomyopathy is marked by fibro-fatty replacement of the RV (and sometimes LV) myocardium that gives rise to LBBB (left bundle branch block) morphology VT and is associated with sudden death, particularly in young athletes.
  - Bundle branch reentry VT (BBRT) is a form of VT that utilizes the His-Purkinje system in a reentrant circuit and is typically associated with cardiomyopathy and an abnormal conduction system.
- **VT in the *absence* of structural heart disease**
  - Inherited ion channelopathies, such as those seen in Brugada and long QT syndromes, can lead to polymorphic VT and sudden death in patients without evidence of structural heart disease on imaging.
  - Catecholaminergic polymorphic VT (CPVT) involves familial, exercise-induced VT that is related to irregular calcium processing.
  - **Idiopathic VT** is a diagnosis of exclusion that requires the documented absence of structural heart disease, genetic disorders, and reversible etiologies (i.e., ischemia, electrolyte/metabolic abnormalities).

○ Most idiopathic VTs originate from the right ventricular outflow tract (RVOT) and are amenable to ablation. Less commonly, left ventricular outflow tract VT (LVOT-VT) or fascicular VT (utilizing anterior and posterior divisions of the left bundle branch) may be discovered on EPS.

DIAGNOSIS

Clinical Presentation

• The evaluation of wide-complex tachyarrhythmias should always begin with prompt assessment of vital signs and clinical symptoms. If the arrhythmia is poorly tolerated, postpone further detailed evaluation and proceed to acute management per ACLS guidelines. If stable, there are several important questions to address that can guide one toward the most likely diagnosis. A common mistake is the assumption that hemodynamic stability supports the diagnosis of SVT over VT when VT can often be hemodynamically well tolerated.

• VT represents the vast majority of WCT seen in the inpatient setting with reported prevalence upwards of 80%. With that in mind, one can then proceed to elicit several historical points of emphasis and scrutinize electrocardiographic properties of the arrhythmia to further delineate the mechanism of the underlying rhythm disturbance. Begin with the following questions:

  • *Does the patient have a history of structural heart disease?*
    ○ Patients with structural heart disease are much more likely to have VT rather than SVT as the etiology of a WCT. In one report, 98% of patients with WCT who had prior MI proved to have VT (*Am J Med 1988;84:53*).

  • *Does the patient have a pacemaker, Implantable cardiac defibrillator (ICD), or wide QRS at baseline (i.e., RBBB [right bundle branch block], LBBB, intraventricular conduction delay (IVCD))?*
    ○ The presence of either a pacemaker or an ICD should raise suspicion for a device-mediated WCT.
    ○ **Device-mediated WCT** can be due to ventricular pacing at a rapid rate either due to device tracking of an atrial tachyarrhythmia or an "endless loop tachycardia" created by tracking of the retrograde atrial impulses created by the preceding ventricular paced beat. In either case, the tachycardia rate is a clue to the mechanism as this is typically equal to the programmed upper rate limit (URL) of the device. A commonly programmed URL is 120 paces per minute (ppm). A tachycardia rate above the URL effectively excludes a device-mediated WCT.
    ○ History of device implantation can be confirmed by inspection of the chest wall (usually left chest for right-handed patients), chest x-ray (CXR), or by the presence of pacing spikes seen on ECG. Typically, the wide QRS induced by right ventricular pacing leads has an LBBB pattern and is preceded by a short pacing spike. Modern devices utilize bipolar pacing, in most cases, which is often difficult to recognize on the 12-lead ECG due to the small size of the electrical artifact. Therefore, one should not exclude the presence of a device-mediated tachycardia mechanism by the absence of visible pacing spikes during the tachycardia.
    ○ Patients with known RBBB, LBBB, or IVCD at baseline who present with WCT will have a QRS morphology identical to baseline in the presence of SVT. In addition, some patients with a narrow QRS at baseline will manifest a WCT due to SVT when a rate-related bundle branch block is present. This phenomenon is referred to as SVT with aberrancy and can be distinguished from VT reliably with the criteria described below.

- *What medications is the patient taking?*
  - The medication list should be scanned for any medication with proarrhythmic side effects, especially those that can prolong the baseline QT interval and increase the risk for polymorphic VT or TdP. These medicines include many of the class I and III antiarrhythmics, certain antibiotics, antipsychotics, and many more. The University of Arizona–sponsored Web site, www.qtdrugs.org, provides a comprehensive list of QT-prolonging agents.
  - Medications that can lead to electrolyte abnormalities such as loop and potassium-sparing diuretics, ACEIs, ARBs, etc. should be ascertained. Also, digoxin toxicity is always an important consideration in the setting of any arrhythmia.

Differential Diagnosis

- Diagnosis of VT requires knowledge of the general approach to WCTs.
- WCT may be due to either SVT with aberrant conduction (presence of bundle branch block) or VT. The differentiation between these mechanisms is of the utmost importance. **The pharmacologic agents utilized in the management of SVT (i.e., adenosine, β-blockers, calcium channel blockers) can cause severe hemodynamic instability if used erroneously in the setting of VT.** Therefore, all WCTs are considered to be ventricular in origin until clearly proven otherwise.
- Other, less common mechanisms of WCT include **antidromic AVRT, hyperkalemia-induced arrhythmia, or pacemaker-induced tachycardia.**
- **Telemetry artifact** due to poor lead contact or repetitive patient motion (tremor, shivering, brushing teeth, etc.) can mimic VT or VF.

Diagnostic Testing

Laboratories

Laboratory studies should include basic metabolic panel, magnesium, CBC, and serial troponins.

Electrocardiography

- **Differentiation of SVT with aberrancy from VT** on the basis of analysis of the surface ECG is critical in the determination of appropriate acute and chronic therapy. For acute therapy of SVT, IV medications such as adenosine, calcium channel blockers, or β-adrenergic blockers are used. However, calcium channel blockers and β-adrenergic blockers can produce hemodynamic instability in patients with VT. Chronically, many SVTs are amenable to RFA, whereas most VTs are malignant and require an antiarrhythmic agent and/or ICD implantation.
- Features that are diagnostic of VT are **AV dissociation, capture or fusion beats,** an absence of RS morphology in the precordial leads ($V_1 - V_6$), and **LBBB morphology with right axis deviation.** In the absence of these features, examination of an RS complex in a precordial lead for an RS interval > 100 milliseconds is consistent with VT. In addition, characteristic QRS morphologies that are suggestive of VT may be sought, as shown in Figure 2A and B.
- **ECG pearls**
- **Classic Brugada Pattern:**
  - Baseline: Pseudo-RBBB with ST-segment elevation and T-wave inversion in V_1, V_2.
  - May be unmasked by stress, illness, fever, illicit drug use, etc.

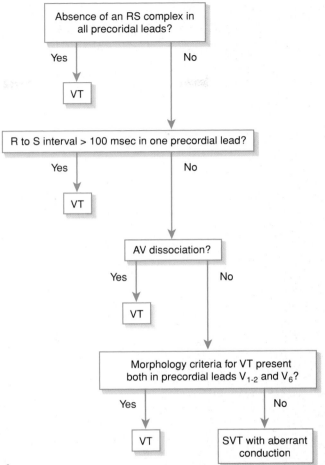

Figure 2. **A and B.** Brugada criteria for distinguishing ventricular tachycardia from supraventricular tachycardia with aberrancy in wide-complex tachycardias. (From Cuculich PS. Advanced electrocardiogram interpretation (ECG 201). In: Cuculich PS, Kates AM, eds. The Washington Manual Cardiology Subspecialty Consult. 2nd Ed. Philadelphia: Lippincott Williams & Wilkins, 2009, with permission.) (*continued*)

- **Arrhythmogenic RV dysplasia:**
  ○ Baseline: Epsilon wave (late potential just after QRS), $+/-$ wide QRS, $+/-$ TWI (V_1, V_2).
  ○ VT: Reflects RV origin, likely LBBB configuration. May present with polymorphic VT.

	LBBB		RBBB	
	VT	SVT	VT	SVT
Lead V_1	In V_1, V_2 any of: (a) r ≥ 0.04 sec (b) Notched S downstroke (c) Delayed S nadir > 0.06 sec	In V_1, V_2 absence of: (a) r ≥ 0.04 sec (b) Notched S downstroke (c) Delayed S nadir > 0.06 sec	Taller left peak Biphasic RS or QR	Triphasic rsR' or rR'
Lead V_6	Monophasic QS 		Biphasic rS 	Triphasic qRs

B

Figure 2. (*Continued*)

- **Bundle branch reentrant VT:**
  - Baseline: Intraventricular conduction delay
  - VT: Left bundle branch morphology typically ("down" the right bundle; "up" the left bundle)
- **Fascicular VT:**
  - VT: Superior axis, RBBB morphology
- **Long QT syndrome:**
  - Baseline: QT > 50% of the RR interval if HR 60 to 100. QTc ≥ 440 milliseconds
  - VT: TdP degenerating into VF.
- **Outflow tract VT:**
  - VT: Inferior axis, LBBB morphology. R/S transition in the precordial leads can aid in localization. Early transition (V_1 or V_2) suggests an LVOT origin; later transition (V_4), RVOT origin.

Imaging
- The presence or absence of structural heart disease should be initially evaluated by transthoracic echocardiography.
- Further imaging (cardiac MRI, noninvasive stress test, coronary angiogram, etc.) should be obtained based on suspected etiology.

TREATMENT

- **Differentiation of SVT with aberrancy from VT** on the basis of analysis of the surface ECG is critical in the determination of appropriate acute and chronic therapy.
  - For acute therapy of SVT, IV medications such as adenosine, calcium channel blockers, or β-blockers are used. However, calcium channel blockers and β-blockers can produce hemodynamic instability in patients with VT.
  - Chronically, many SVTs are amenable to RFA, whereas most VTs are malignant and require an antiarrhythmic agent and/or ICD implantation.
- Immediate unsynchronized DC cardioversion is the primary therapy for pulseless VT and VF.
- **Nonpharmacologic therapy**
  - **ICDs** provide automatic recognition and treatment of ventricular arrhythmias. ICD implantation improves survival in patients resuscitated from ventricular arrhythmias (secondary prevention of SCD) and in individuals without prior symptoms who are at high risk for SCD (primary prevention of SCD).
    - ○ **Secondary prevention of SCD** with ICD implantation is indicated for most patients who survive SCD outside of the peri-MI setting. The superiority of ICD therapy to chronic antiarrhythmic drug therapy has been demonstrated (*AVID trial. N Engl J Med 1997;337:1576*).
    - ○ **Primary prevention of SCD** with ICD implantation is indicated for patients who are at high risk of SCD. The efficacy of ICD implantation for primary prevention of SCD in the setting of cardiomyopathy has been established in multiple prospective clinical trials (see Multicenter Automatic Defibrillator Implantation Trial [**MADIT**], *N Engl J Med 1996;335:1933*; Multicenter UnSustained Tachycardia Trial [**MUSTT**], *N Engl J Med 1999;341:1882*; **MADIT II** Trial, *N Engl J Med 2002;346:877*; and **SCD-HeFT,** *N Engl J Med 2005;352(3):225*). Most patients with an LV ejection fraction (LVEF) of <35% for more than 3 months meet current indications for prophylactic ICD implantation.
    - ○ **Other indications for ICD.**
      - - Phenotypes associated with **HCM, arrhythmogenic right ventricular cardiomyopathy, congenital long QT syndrome, or Brugada syndrome have a high risk of SCD.** ICD implantation is indicated if patients with one of these syndromes have had a resuscitated cardiac arrest or documented ventricular arrhythmias. Prophylactic ICD implantation for asymptomatic patients is generally considered appropriate particularly in patients who have had syncope or with a family history of sudden death.
      - - Patients who are awaiting cardiac transplantation are at high risk for SCD, especially if they are receiving an intravenous inotrope. Prophylactic ICD implantation is reasonable to protect against SCD prior to transplantation.
    - ○ ICDs are **contraindicated** in patients who have incessant VT, recent MI <40 days in the case of primary prevention, significant psychiatric illnesses, or life expectancy of less than 12 to 24 months.
  - **Radiofrequency catheter ablation of VT** is most successfully performed in patients with hemodynamically stable forms of idiopathic VT that is not associated with structural heart disease. Long-term cure rates in these patients are similar to those achieved for catheter ablation of SVT. In the presence of structural heart disease, and particularly with hemodynamically unstable VT, catheter

ablation is generally reserved for drug-refractory VT due to a lower efficacy and a higher morbidity associated with the ablation procedure.

○ **Idiopathic VT is usually associated with a structurally normal heart, but an associated tachycardia-mediated cardiomyopathy has been described.**

- **Right ventricular outflow tract VT (RVOT-VT)** often presents as repetitive, nonsustained bursts of VT that can be exercise induced. RVOT-VT is usually responsive to β-adrenergic blockers, diltiazem or verapamil, and adenosine.
- **LVOT-VT** is frequently responsive to verapamil.
- Both forms of idiopathic VT are thought to be benign in the absence of structural heart disease. Therefore, ICD implantation is not appropriate. All forms of idiopathic VT are amenable to treatment with RFA or drug therapy.

○ **Bundle branch reentry VT (BBRT)** is a form of VT that involves the His–Purkinje system in a reentrant circuit. BBRT can be treated successfully by catheter ablation of the right bundle branch. Because BBRT usually occurs in patients with cardiomyopathy and an abnormal conduction system, an ICD is generally implanted in conjunction with ablation.

○ **VT associated with ischemic heart disease** can also be treated by catheter ablation; however, success rates are significantly lower compared to idiopathic VT. The reasons for the lower success rate include the hemodynamic instability of VT and the multiple different VT circuits (due to multiple areas of scars from prior MIs) that are often present. Catheter ablation of ischemic VT in patients with antiarrhythmic drug-refractory VT and an implanted ICD has been successful in reducing frequent ICD shocks (*Circulation 1997;96: 1525*).

○ **Ablation of VT in nonischemic cardiomyopathy** is possible, but VT circuits may be intramyocardial or epicardial. As a result, success rates are typically lower than those associated with ischemic VT.

Medications

• VF that is resistant to external defibrillation requires the addition of IV antiarrhythmic agents.

  • Intravenous lidocaine is frequently used; however, IV amiodarone appears to be more effective in increasing survival of VF when used in conjunction with defibrillation (*N Engl J Med 2002;346:884*).

  • After successful cardioversion, continuous IV infusion of effective antiarrhythmic therapy should be maintained until any reversible causes have been corrected.

• Chronic antiarrhythmic drug therapy is indicated for the treatment of recurrent symptomatic ventricular arrhythmias. In the setting of hemodynamically unstable ventricular arrhythmias treated with an ICD, antiarrhythmic drug therapy is often necessary to suppress frequent device discharges.

First Line

• **Amiodarone** is safe and well tolerated for the acute management of ventricular arrhythmias. Amiodarone has complex pharmacokinetics and is associated with significant toxicities arising from chronic therapy (*Am Heart J 1993;125: 109*).

  • After oral loading, amiodarone prevents the recurrence of sustained VT or VF in up to 60% of patients. A therapeutic latency of more than 5 days exists before beneficial antiarrhythmic effects are observed with oral dosing, and full suppression of arrhythmias may not occur for 4 to 6 weeks after therapy is initiated.

- Amiodarone has become the most studied antiarrhythmic agent in the treatment of SCD and the main drug against which ICDs are compared, in secondary and in primary prevention trials.
- The balance of multiple prospective clinical trials does not support the prophylactic use of amiodarone for prevention of SCD in cardiomyopathy patients.
- **Class II** agents, the β-adrenergic antagonists, are the only class of antiarrhythmic agents to have consistently shown improved survival in post-MI patients.
  - β-Adrenergic blockers reduce postinfarction total mortality by 25% to 40% and SCD by 32% to 50% (*Lancet 1981;2:823*).
  - After acute therapy of VT/VF and stabilization, β-adrenergic blockers should be initiated and titrated as blood pressure and heart rate allow.
  - Idiopathic VT often responds to AV nodal blocking agents.
- **ACE inhibitors** have also been shown to reduce sudden death and overall mortality in patients with CAD or CHF.

Second Line
- Sotalol is a **class III** agent indicated for the chronic treatment of VT/VF. **Sotalol** prevents the recurrence of sustained VT and VF in 70% of patients (*N Engl J Med 1993;329:452*) but must be used with caution in individuals with CHF.
- **Class I** agents in general have not been shown to reduce mortality in patients with VT/VF. In fact, the class Ic agents, **flecainide** and propafenone, are associated with increased mortality in patients with ventricular arrhythmias (*N Engl J Med 1991;324:781*).
  - **Lidocaine** is a class Ib agent available only in IV form with efficacy in the management of sustained and recurrent VT/VF. The prophylactic use of lidocaine for suppression of PVCs and NSVT in the otherwise uncomplicated post-MI setting is not indicated and may lead to an increase in mortality from bradyarrhythmias (*Arch Intern Med 1989;149:2694*). Toxicities of lidocaine include CNS effects (convulsions, confusion, stupor, and, rarely, respiratory arrest), all of which resolve with discontinuation of therapy. Negative inotropic effects are seen only at high drug levels.
  - **Mexiletine** is similar to lidocaine but is available in oral form. **Mexiletine is most often used in combination with either amiodarone or sotalol for chronic treatment of refractory ventricular arrhythmias.** Mexiletine may have a limited role in the treatment of some patients with congenital long QT syndromes. CNS toxicity includes tremor, dizziness, and blurred vision. Higher levels may result in dysarthria, diplopia, nystagmus, and an impaired level of consciousness. Nausea and vomiting are common.
  - **Phenytoin** is used primarily in the treatment of digitalis-induced ventricular arrhythmias. It may have a limited role in the treatment of ventricular arrhythmias associated with congenital long QT syndromes. The IV loading dose is 250 mg given over 10 minutes (maximum rate of 50 mg/min). Subsequent doses of 100 mg can be given q5min as necessary and as BP tolerates, to a total of 1,000 mg. Frequent monitoring of the ECG, BP, and neurologic status is required. Continuous infusion is not recommended (see Chapter 23, Neurologic Disorders).

SPECIAL CONSIDERATIONS

- **Class IV** agents have no role in the chronic management of VT. Intravenous calcium channel blockers should never be used in the acute management of VT, as

they may cause hemodynamic collapse. Oral calcium channel blockers are not effective in the management of VT. Short-acting nifedipine is associated with a trend toward increasing mortality when used in the post-MI patient (*Arch Intern Med 1993;153:345*).
- Primary VF that occurs within the first 72 hours of an acute MI is not associated with an elevated risk of recurrence and does not require chronic antiarrhythmic therapy.
- In the case of **TdP associated with long QT syndrome,** acute therapy is immediate DC cardioversion.
  - Bolus administration of magnesium sulfate in 1- to 2-g increments up to 4 to 6 g IV is highly effective.
  - In cases of acquired long QT syndrome, identification and treatment of the underlying condition should be undertaken, if possible.
  - Elimination of long–short triggering sequences and shortening of the QT interval can be achieved by increasing the heart rate to the range of 90 to 120 bpm by either intravenous isoproterenol infusion (initial rate at 1 to 2 mcg/min) or temporary transvenous pacing.

BRADYARRHYTHMIAS

GENERAL PRINCIPLES

- Bradyarrhythmias are commonly encountered rhythms in the inpatient setting that result in a ventricular rate of <60 bpm.
- Bradyarrhythmias can be attributed to dysfunction somewhere within the native conduction system; therefore, review of the normal propagation of the wave of depolarization, the respective vascular supply to each section, and the intrinsic and extrinsic influences on the conduction system is useful.
- **Anatomy of the conduction system**
  - The **sinus node** is a collection of specialized pacemaker cells located in the high right atrium. Under normal conditions, it initiates a wave of depolarization that spreads inferiorly and leftward via atrial myocardium and intranodal tracts, producing atrial systole.
    - The typical resting rate of the sinus node is between 50 and 90 bpm, is inversely related to age, and is determined by the relative balance of sympathetic and parasympathetic inputs.
    - Arterial blood is supplied to the sinus node via the sinus node artery, which has variable anatomic origins: right coronary artery (RCA), 65%; circumflex, 25%; or dual (RCA and circumflex), 10%.
  - The wave of depolarization then reaches another grouping of specialized cells, the **AV node,** located in the right atrial side of the interatrial septum. Normally, the AV node should serve as the lone electrical connection between the atria and ventricles.
    - Conduction through the AV node is decremental, producing a delay typically in the range of 55 to 110 milliseconds and accounts for the majority of the PR interval measured on ECG.
    - The AV node consists of slow-response fibers that, like the sinus node, possess inherent pacemaking properties that produce rates of 40 to 50 bpm. Because of its slower rate of depolarization, this only becomes clinically relevant in the setting of sinus node dysfunction or complete AV nodal block.

- ○ Ventricular response to atrial depolarization is modulated by the effects of the autonomic nervous system on the AV node.
  - ○ Blood supply to the AV node is primarily via the AV nodal artery that typically originates from the proximal portion of the posterior descending artery (PDA, 80%), but can also come off the circumflex (10%) or both (10%). In addition, it receives collateral flow from the left anterior descending (LAD) artery. This makes the AV node relatively protected against vascular compromise.
- From the AV node, the wave of depolarization travels down the **His bundle,** located in the membranous septum, and into the **right and left bundle branches** before reaching the **Purkinje fibers** that depolarize the rest of the ventricular myocardium.
  - ○ The His and right bundle receive blood via the AV nodal artery and from septal perforators off the LAD.
  - ○ The left bundle divides further into an anterior fascicle that is supplied by septal perforators and a posterior fascicle, which runs posterior and inferior to the anterior fascicle, which is supplied by branches off the PDA and septal perforators off the LAD.

Etiology

Common causes of bradycardia are listed in Table 7.

DIAGNOSIS

Clinical Presentation

When evaluating a suspected bradyarrhythmia, one should efficiently utilize the history, physical exam, and available data to address the following "five S" approach to an **SSSSS**low heart rate:

- STABLE: Is the patient hemodynamically unstable?
- SYMPTOMS: Does the patient have symptoms and do the symptoms correlate with the bradycardia?
- SHORT-TERM: Are the circumstances surrounding the arrhythmia reversible or transient?
- SOURCE: Where in the conduction system is the dysfunction? Has the bradyarrhythmia been captured on electrocardiographic monitoring?
- SCHEDULE A PACEMAKER: Does the patient require a PPM?

Physical Examination

- If the bradycardia is ongoing, the initial history and physical examination should be truncated, focusing on assessing the hemodynamic stability of the arrhythmia.
  - If the patient is demonstrating signs of poor perfusion (hypotension, confusion, decreased consciousness, cyanosis, etc.) then immediate management per ACLS protocol should be initiated.
  - If stable, a more thorough evaluation can be performed.
- The clinical manifestations of bradyarrhythmias are variable, ranging from asymptomatic to nonspecific (lightheadedness, fatigue, weakness, exercise intolerance) to overt (syncope).
  - Tolerance for bradyarrhythmias is largely dictated by the patient's ability to augment cardiac output in response to the decreased heart rate.

Table 7	Causes of Bradycardia

Intrinsic
Congenital disease (may present later in life)
Idiopathic degeneration (aging)
Infarction or ischemia
Cardiomyopathy
Infiltrative disease: sarcoidosis, amyloidosis, hemochromatosis
Collagen vascular diseases: systemic lupus erythematosus, rheumatoid
  arthritis, scleroderma
Surgical trauma: valve surgery, transplantation
Infectious disease: endocarditis, Lyme disease, Chagas disease
Extrinsic
Autonomically mediated
Neurocardiogenic syncope
Carotid sinus hypersensitivity
Increased vagal tone: coughing, vomiting, micturition, defecation, intubation
Drugs: β-blockers, calcium channel blockers, digoxin, antiarrhythmic agents
Hypothyroidism
Hypothermia
Neurologic disorders: increased intracranial pressure
Electrolyte imbalances: hyperkalemia, hypermagnesemia
Hypercarbia/obstructive sleep apnea
Sepsis

From Cooper DH. Bradyarrhythmias and permanent pacemakers. In: Cuculich PS, Kates AM, eds. The Washington Manual Cardiology Subspecialty Consult. 2nd ed. Philadelphia: Lippincott Williams & Wilkins, 2009, with permission.

- Emphasis should be placed on delineating **whether the presenting symptoms have a direct temporal relationship to underlying bradycardia.** Other historical points of emphasis include the following:
  - Ischemic heart disease, particularly involving the right-sided circulation, can precipitate a number of bradyarrhythmias. Therefore, symptoms of acute coronary syndrome should always be sought.
  - **Precipitating circumstances** (micturition, coughing, defecation, noxious smells) surrounding episodes may help identify a neurocardiogenic etiology.
  - **Tachyarrhythmias,** particularly in patients with underlying sinus node dysfunction, can be followed by long pauses due to sinus node suppression during tachycardia. Therefore, symptoms of palpitations may reveal the presence of an underlying tachy-brady syndrome. Given that the agents used to treat tachyarrhythmias are designed to promote decreased heart rates, this syndrome leads to management dilemmas.
  - History of structural heart disease, hypothyroidism, obstructive sleep apnea, collagen vascular disease, infections (bacteremia, endocarditis, Lyme, Chagas), infiltrative diseases (amyloid, hemochromatosis, and sarcoid), neuromuscular diseases, and prior cardiac surgery (valve replacement, congenital repair) should be sought.
  - **Medications** should be reviewed with particular emphasis on those that affect the sinus and AV nodes (i.e., calcium channel blockers, β-adrenergic blockers, digoxin).

- After hemodynamic stability is confirmed, a more thorough examination with particular emphasis on the cardiovascular exam and any findings consistent with the aforementioned comorbidities is appropriate (Fig. 3).

Diagnostic Testing

Laboratories

Laboratory studies should include serum electrolytes and thyroid function tests in most patients. Digoxin levels and serial troponins should be drawn when clinically appropriate.

Electrocardiography

- The **12-lead ECG** is the cornerstone for diagnosis in any workup where arrhythmia is suspected.
  - Rhythm strips from leads that provide the best view of atrial activity (II, III, AVF, or V_1) should be examined.
  - Emphasis should be placed on identifying evidence of **sinus node dysfunction** (P-wave intervals) or **AV conduction abnormalities** (PR interval).
  - Evidence of both old and acute manifestations of ischemic heart disease should be sought as well.
- The analysis of ECGs in the setting of bradycardia should also focus on localizing the likely site of dysfunction along the conduction system.
  - Along with correlating symptoms to the arrhythmia, localization of the block will help determine if pacemaker implantation is necessary.
- **Sinus node dysfunction. Sinus node dysfunction,** or sick sinus syndrome, represents the most common reason for pacemaker implantation in the United States. Manifestations of sick sinus syndrome include (Fig. 4):
  - **Sinus bradycardia** is defined as a regular rhythm with QRS complexes preceded by "sinus" P waves (upright in II, III, AVF) at a rate <60 bpm. Young patients and athletes often have resting sinus bradycardia that is well tolerated. Nocturnal heart rates are lower in all patients but the elderly tend to have higher resting heart rates and sinus bradycardia is a far less common normal variant.
  - **Sinus arrest** and **sinus pauses** refer to failure of the sinus node to depolarize, which manifest as periods of atrial asystole (no P waves). This may be accompanied by ventricular asystole or escape beats from junctional tissue or ventricular myocardium. Pauses of 2 to 3 seconds can be found in healthy, asymptomatic people, especially during sleep. Pauses >3 seconds, particularly during daytime hours, raise concern for significant sinus node dysfunction.
  - **Sinus exit block** represents the appropriate firing of the sinus node but the wave of depolarization fails to traverse past the perinodal tissue. It is indistinguishable from sinus arrest on surface ECGs except that the R-R interval will be a multiple of the R-R preceding the bradycardia.
  - **Tachy-brady syndrome** occurs when tachyarrhythmias alternate with bradyarrhythmias, especially AF. The rapid atrial rate suppresses sinus node output leading to sinus node dysfunction following termination of the tachyarrhythmia.
  - **Chronotropic incompetence** is the inability to increase the heart rate appropriately in response to metabolic need.
- **AV conduction disturbances**
  - AV conduction can be *diverted* (fascicular or bundle branch blocks), *delayed* (first-degree AV block), *occasionally interrupted* (second-degree AV block), *frequently, but*

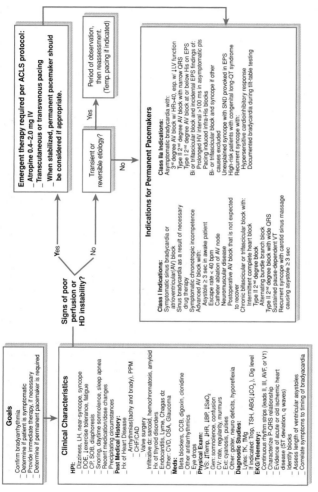

Goals
- Confirm bradyarrhythmia
- Determine if patient is symptomatic
- Provide immediate therapy, if necessary
- Determine if permanent pacemaker is required

Clinical Characteristics

HPI:
- Dizziness, LH, near-syncope, syncope
- DOE, ↓ exercise tolerance, fatigue
- CP, SOB, diaphoresis
- Snoring, daytime somnolence, sleep apnea
- Recent medication/dose changes
- Precipitating circumstances

Past Medical History:
- Hx of Heart Disease
  - Arrhythmias (tachy and brady), PPM
  - CHF/CAD
  - Valve surgery
- Infiltrative dz: sarcoid, hemochromatosis, amyloid
- Hx of thyroid disorders
- Endocarditis, Lyme, Chagas dz
- Other: CVD, OSA, Glaucoma

Meds:
- Beta blockers, CCB, digoxin, clonidine
- Other antiarrhythmics
- Eye drops

Physical Exam:
- VS: ↓Temp, ↓HR, ↓BP, ↓SaO₂
- Gen: somnolence, confusion
- CV: rate, regularity, murmurs
- Other: goiter, neuro deficits, hyporeflexia
- Ext: cyanosis, pulses

Diagnostic Studies:
- Lytes: ↑K, ↑Mg
- If indicated: Trop, TSH, ABG (↓CO₂), Dig level

EKG/Telemetry:
- Continuous rhythm strips (leads II, III, AVF, or V1)
- Characterize P-QRS relationship
- Evidence of acute or old ischemic heart disease (ST deviation, q waves)
- Identify blocks
- Assess length of ventricular asystoles
- Correlate symptoms to timing of bradycardia

Signs of poor perfusion or HD instability?

Yes →

Emergent therapy required per ACLS protocol:
- Atropine 0.4–2.0 mg IV
- Transcutaneous or transvenous pacing
- When stabilized, permanent pacemaker should be considered if appropriate.

No ↓

Transient or reversible etiology?

Yes → **Period of observation, then reassessment. (Temp. pacing if indicated)**

No ↓

Indications for Permanent Pacemakers

Class I Indications:
- Symptomatic sinus bradycardia or atrioventricular (AV) block
- Sinus bradycardia as a result of necessary drug therapy
- Symptomatic chronotropic incompetence
- Advanced AV block with:
  - Asystole ≥ 3 sec in awake patient
  - Escape rate < 40 bpm
  - Catheter ablation of AV node
  - Neuromuscular disease
  - Postoperative AV block that is not expected to recover
- Chronic bifascicular or trifascicular block with:
  - Intermittent complete heart block
  - Type II 2ⁿᵈ degree block
  - Alternating bundle branch block
- Type II 2ⁿᵈ degree block with wide QRS
- Sustained pause-dependent VT
- Recurrent syncope with carotid sinus massage causing asystole ≥ 3 sec

Class IIa Indications:
- Asymptomatic bradycardia with:
  - 3ʳᵈ degree AV block w/ HR>40, esp. w/ ↓LV function
  - Type II 2ⁿᵈ degree AV block with narrow QRS
  - Type I 2ⁿᵈ degree AV block at or below His on EPS
- Bi or trifascicular block and incidental EPS findings of:
  - Prolonged HV interval >100 ms in asymptomatic pts
  - Pacing induced infra-His blocks
- Bi- or trifascicular block and syncope if other causes excluded
- Unexplained syncope with SND provoked in EPS
- High-risk patients with congenital long-QT syndrome
- Recurrent syncope with:
  - Hypersensitive cardioinhibitory response
  - Documented bradycardia during tilt-table testing

Figure 3. Approach to bradyarrhythmias. LH, lightheadedness; DOE, dyspnea on exertion; CP, chest pain; SOB, shortness of breath; PPM, permanent pacemaker; CHF, congestive heart failure; CAD, coronary artery disease; CVD, cerebrovascular disease; OSA, obstructive sleep apnea; CCB, calcium channel blocker; ↓HR, bradycardia; ↓BP, hypotension; ↓SaO₂, hypoxia; ↑K, hyperkalemia; ↑Mg, hypermagnesemia; HD, hemodynamic; VT, ventricular tachycardia; EPS, electrophysiologic study; SND, sinus node dysfunction. (From Cooper DH. Bradyarrhythmias and permanent pacemakers. In: Cuculich PS, Kates AM, eds. The Washington Manual Cardiology Subspecialty Consult. 2nd Ed. Philadelphia: Lippincott Williams & Wilkins, 2009, with permission.)

Sinus Bradycardia

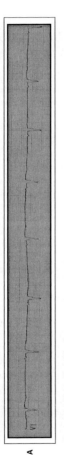

A

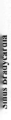

Sinoatrial Node Exit Block

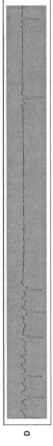

B

Sinus Rhythm with Blocked Premature Atrial Complexes

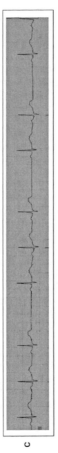

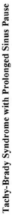

C

Tacky-Brady Syndrome with Prolonged Sinus Pause

D

Figure 4. Examples of sinus node dysfunction. **A.** Sinus bradycardia. The sinus rate is approximately 45 bpm. **B.** Sinoatrial node exit block. Note that the PP interval in which the pause occurs is exactly twice that of the nonpaused PP interval. **C.** Blocked premature atrial complexes. This rhythm is often confused for sinus node dysfunction or AV block. Note the premature, nonconducted P waves inscribed in the T wave that resets the sinus node leading to the observed pauses. **D.** Tachy-brady syndrome. Note the termination of the irregular tachyarrhythmia followed by a prolonged 4.5-second pause prior to the first sinus beat. (From Cooper DH. Bradyarrhythmias and permanent pacemakers. In: Cuculich PS, Kates AM, eds. The Washington Manual Cardiology Subspecialty Consult. 2nd Ed. Philadelphia: Lippincott Williams & Wilkins, 2009, with permission.)

not always, interrupted (advanced or high-degree AV block), or *completely absent* (third-degree AV block). Assignment of the bradyarrhythmia under investigation to one of these categories allows one to better determine prognosis and, therefore, guide therapy.

- **First-degree AV block** describes a conduction delay, usually localized to the AV node, that results in a PR interval >200 milliseconds on the surface ECG. "Block" is a misnomer because, by definition, there are no dropped beats (i.e., there is a P wave for every QRS complex).
- **Second-degree AV block** is present when there are periodic interruptions (i.e., "dropped beats") in AV conduction. Distinction between Mobitz I and II is important because they possess differing natural histories of progression to complete heart block.
  - **Mobitz type I block (Wenckebach)** is represented by a progressive delay in AV conduction with successive atrial impulses until an impulse fails to conduct, followed by reiterations of the sequence. On surface ECG classic Wenckebach block manifests as:
    - Progressive prolongation of the PR interval of each successive beat, before the dropped beat.
    - Shortening of each subsequent RR interval before the dropped beat. Therefore, the RR interval of the dropped beat will equal less than 2× the shortest RR on the tracing.
    - A regularly, irregular grouping of QRS complexes (group beating).
    - Type I block is usually within the AV node and portends a more benign natural history with progression to complete heart block unlikely.
  - **Mobitz type II block** carries a less favorable prognosis and is characterized by abrupt AV conduction block without evidence of progressive conduction delay.
    - On ECG, the PR intervals remained unchanged preceding the nonconducted P wave.
    - The presence of type II block, particularly if a bundle branch block is present, often antedates progression to complete heart block.
  - The presence of **AV 2:1 block** makes the differentiation between Mobitz type I or II mechanisms difficult. Diagnostic clues to the site of block include the following:
    - Concomitant first-degree AV block, periodic AV Wenckebach, or improved conduction (1:1) with enhanced sinus rates or sympathetic input suggests a more proximal interruption of conduction (i.e., Mobitz type 1 mechanism).
    - Concomitant bundle branch block, fascicular block, or worsened conduction (3:1, 4:1, etc.) with enhanced sympathetic input localizes the site of block more distally (Mobitz type II mechanism).
- **Third-degree (complete) AV block** is present when all atrial impulses fail to conduct to the ventricles. There is complete dissociation between the atria and ventricles ("A > V" rates). This should be distinguished from dissociation with competition at the AV node ("V > A" rates).
- **Advanced or high-degree AV block** is present when more than one consecutive atrial depolarization fails to conduct to the ventricles (i.e., 3:1 block or greater). On ECG, consecutive P waves will be seen without associated QRS complexes. However, there will be demonstrable P:QRS conduction somewhere on the record to avoid a "third degree" designation (Fig. 5).

First-Degree AV Block

A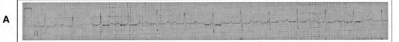

Second-Degree AV Block-Mobitz type I (Wenckebach Block)

B

Second-Degree AV Block-Mobitz type II

C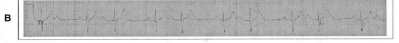

2:1 Second-Degree AV Block

D

Third-Degree (Complete) AV Block

E

Figure 5. Examples of atrioventricular block. **A.** First-degree AVB. There are no dropped beats and the PR interval is >200 milliseconds. **B.** 3:2 Second-degree AVB-Mobitz I. Note the "group beating" and the prolonging PR interval prior to the dropped beat. The third P wave in the sequence is subtly inscribed in the T wave of the preceding beat. **C.** Second-degree AVB-Mobitz II. Note the abrupt AV conduction block without evidence of progressive conduction delay. **D.** 2:1 AVB. This pattern makes it difficult to distinguish between Mobitz I versus II type mechanisms of block. Note the narrow QRS complex which supports a more proximal origin of block (type I mechanism). A wider QRS (concomitant bundle branch or fascicular block) would suggest a type II mechanism. **E.** Complete heart block. Note the independent regularity of both the atrial and ventricular rhythms (junctional escape) with no clear association with each other throughout the rhythm strip. (From Cooper DH. Bradyarrhythmias and permanent pacemakers. In: Cuculich PS, Kates AM, eds. The Washington Manual Cardiology Subspecialty Consult. 2nd Ed. Philadelphia: Lippincott Williams & Wilkins, 2009, with permission.)

Imaging
- The presence or absence of structural heart disease should be initially evaluated by transthoracic echocardiography.
- Further imaging should be obtained based on suspected etiology.

TREATMENT

- **Pharmacologic therapy**
  - Bradyarrhythmias that lead to significant symptoms and hemodynamic instability are considered cardiovascular emergencies and should be managed as outlined in ACLS guidelines (see Appendix C, Advanced Cardiac Life Support-Algorithms).

- **Atropine,** an anticholinergic agent given in doses of 0.5 to 2.0 mg intravenously, is the cornerstone pharmacologic agent for emergent bradycardia treatment.
  - Dysfunction localized more proximally in the conduction system (i.e., symptomatic sinus bradycardia, first-degree AV block, Mobitz I second-degree AV block) tends to be atropine responsive.
  - Distal disease is not responsive and can be worsened by atropine.
- Reversible causes of bradyarrhythmias should be identified as previously described and any agents (digoxin, calcium channel blockers, β-adrenergic blockers) that caused or exacerbated the underlying dysrhythmia should be withheld.
- **Nonpharmacologic therapy**
- For bradyarrhythmias that have irreversible etiologies or that are secondary to medically necessary pharmacologic therapy, pacemaker therapy should be considered.
  - Temporary pacing is indicated for symptomatic second-degree or third-degree heart block caused by transient drug intoxication or electrolyte imbalance and complete heart block or Mobitz II second-degree AV block in the setting of an acute MI.
  - Sinus bradycardia, AF with a slow ventricular response, or Mobitz I second-degree AV block should be treated with temporary pacing only if significant symptoms or hemodynamic instability is present.
  - Temporary pacing is achieved preferably via insertion of a transvenous pacemaker. Transthoracic, external pacing can be utilized although the lack of reliability of capture and patient discomfort clearly makes this a second-line modality.
- Once hemodynamic stability has been established, attention turns to the indications for PPM placement.
  - In symptomatic patients, the key determinants include **potential reversibility of causative factors** and **temporal correlation of symptoms to the arrhythmia.**
  - In asymptomatic patients, the key determinant is based on whether the **discovered conduction abnormality has a natural history of progression to higher degrees of heart block** that portends a poor prognosis.
- **Permanent pacing**
  - Permanent pacing involves the placement of anchored, intracardiac pacing leads for the purpose of maintaining a heart rate sufficient to avoid the aforementioned symptoms and hemodynamic consequences of certain bradyarrhythmias. In addition, advances in pacemaker technology allow contemporary pacers, through maintenance of AV synchrony and rate-adaptive programming, to more closely mimic normal physiologic heart rate behavior.
    - Class I (general agreement/evidence for benefit) and IIa (weight of conflicting opinion/evidence in favor of benefit) indications for permanent pacing are listed in Figure 3.
    - Pacemakers are designed to provide an electrical stimulus to the heart whenever the rate drops below a preprogrammed **lower rate limit.** Therefore, the ECG appearance of a PPM varies depending on the pacer dependence of the individual heart rate.
    - The pacing spike produced by contemporary pacemakers are low-amplitude, sharp, and immediately preceding the generated P wave or QRS complex indicating capture of the chamber.
      - Atrial leads are typically placed in the right atrial appendage and therefore generate P waves of normal (sinus) morphology.
      - However, the QRS complexes generated by a typical right ventricular pacing lead are wide and typically assume an "LBBB-like" morphology.
      - Figure 6 illustrates some common ECG appearances of normally and abnormally functioning pacemakers.

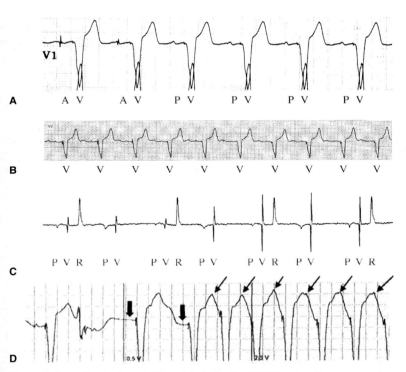

Figure 6. Pacemaker rhythms. **A.** Normal dual-chamber (DDD) pacing. First two complexes are atrioventricular (AV) sequential pacing, followed by sinus with atrial sensing and ventricular pacing. **B.** Normal single-chamber (VVI) pacing. The underlying rhythm is atrial fibrillation (no distinct P waves), with ventricular pacing at 60 bpm. **C.** Pacemaker malfunction. The underlying rhythm is sinus (P) at 80 bpm with 2:1 heart block and first-degree AV block (long PR). Ventricular pacing spikes are seen (V) after each P wave, demonstrating appropriate sensing and tracking of the P waves; however, there is failure to capture. **D.** Pacemaker-mediated tachycardia. A, paced atrial events; V, paced ventricular events; P, sensed atrial events; R, sensed ventricular events. (**A–C.** From Cooper DH, Faddis MN. Cardiac arrhythmias. In: Cooper DH, et al., eds. The Washington Manual of Medical Therapeutics. 32nd Ed. Philadelphia: Lippincott Williams & Wilkins, 2007, with permission; **D:** From Cooper DH. Bradyarrhythmias and permanent pacemakers. In: Cuculich PS, Kates AM, eds. The Washington Manual Cardiology Subspecialty Consult. 2nd Ed. Philadelphia: Lippincott Williams & Wilkins, 2009, with permission.)

- The pacemaker generator is commonly placed subcutaneously in the pectoral region on the side of the nondominant arm. The electronic leads(s) are placed in their cardiac chamber(s) via central veins. Complications of placement include **pneumothorax, device infection, bleeding, and, rarely, cardiac perforation with tamponade.**
  - Before implantation, the patient must be free of any active infections and anticoagulation issues must be carefully considered. Hematomas in the pacemaker pocket develop most commonly in patients who are receiving IV heparin or subcutaneous low-molecular-weight heparin. In severe cases, surgical evacuation is required.

- Following implantation, a **PA and lateral CXR** are obtained to confirm appropriate lead placement. The pacemaker is interrogated at appropriate intervals: typically, before discharge, 2 to 6 weeks following discharge, and every 6 to 12 months thereafter.
- **Pacing modes** are classified by a sequence of three to five letters. Most pacemakers are referred to by the three-letter code alone.
  - **Position I denotes the chamber that is paced:** A for atria, V for ventricle, or D for dual (A + V).
  - **Position II refers to the chamber that is sensed:** A for atria, V for ventricle, D for dual (A + V), or O for none.
  - **Position III denotes the type of response the pacemaker will have to a sensed signal:** I for inhibition, T for triggering, D for dual (I + T), or O for none.
  - **Position IV is utilized to signify the presence of rate-adaptive pacing (R)** in response to increased metabolic need. Almost all contemporary pacers implanted have rate-modulating capabilities.
  - **Position V identifies the presence or absence of multisite pacing:** O for none, A for multiple sites within the atria, V for multiple ventricular sites, or D for both (A + V). Biventricular pacing for resynchronization therapy in heart failure is the most common application of this position.
- The most common pacing systems utilized today include VVIR, DDDR, or AAIR.
  - AAI systems should be utilized only for sinus node dysfunction in the absence of any AV conduction abnormalities.
  - The presence of AV nodal or His–Purkinje disease makes a dual chamber device (i.e., DDD) more appropriate.
  - Patients in chronic AF warrant a single ventricular lead with VVI programming.
  - The 2008 ACC/AHA/HRS guidelines for device-based therapy provide an algorithm to help guide pacing system decisions.
- Modern-day pacemakers also have the capability of **mode-switching.** This is useful in patients with DDD pacers who have paroxysmal tachyarrhythmias. When these patients develop an atrial arrhythmia faster than a programmed mode switch rate, the device will switch to a mode (i.e., VVI) that does not track atrial signals. It will return to DDD when the tachyarrhythmia resolves.
- **Pacemaker malfunction** is a potentially life-threatening situation, particularly for patients who are pacemaker dependent. The workup of suspected malfunction should begin with a 12-lead ECG.
  - If no pacing activity is seen, one can place a magnet over the pacemaker to assess for output failure and ability to capture. **Application of the magnet switches the pacemaker to an asynchronous pacing mode.** For example, VVI mode becomes VOO (ventricular asynchronous pacing), and DDD mode becomes DOO (asynchronous AV pacing).
  - If malfunction is obvious or if the ECG is unrevealing and malfunction is still suspected, then a formal interrogation of the device should be done. **Patients are given a card to carry upon implantation that will identify the make and model of the device to facilitate this evaluation.**
  - **Chest radiograph (two views)** should also be obtained to assess for evidence of overt lead abnormalities (dislodgement, fracture, migration, etc.).
- General categories of pacemaker malfunction include failure to pace (output failure), failure to capture, failure to sense (undersensing), and pacemaker-mediated dysrhythmias.

○ **Failure to pace** refers to situations where a pacemaker does not deliver a stimulus when it should.

  - **Oversensing** of environmental noise, myopotentials, or electrical artifact from a failing lead can cause long pauses in a pacemaker-dependent patient.
  - Also, atrial leads can misinterpret or oversense ventricular depolarizations as atrial activity leading to inhibition of atrial outputs that is referred to as "crosstalk."
  - Lead fracture or dislodgment, battery failure, and generator failure are less common causes of output failure.

○ **Failure to capture** refers to those situations where the pacing stimulus is delivered but fails to generate evidence of myocardial depolarization (i.e., P or QRS complex).

  - Elevation in the threshold voltage required to initiate a wave of depolarization due to changes in the tissue surrounding the electrode is often at fault. This phenomenon is referred to as "exit block."

○ **Undersensing** occurs when the preprogrammed amplitude and/or frequency thresholds for sensing are too high to identify native cardiac activity.

  - This may lead to pacing spikes being identified on top of native P, QRS, or T complexes.

○ **Pacemaker-mediated tachycardias** are wide-complex tachyarrhythmias caused by ventricular pacing at a rapid rate either due to device tracking of an atrial tachyarrhythmia or an "endless loop tachycardia" created by tracking of retrograde atrial impulses created by the previous ventricular paced beat.

  - The rate of the arrhythmia provides a clue to diagnosis because it is typically at or below the programmed URL. A rate exceeding the URL excludes the diagnosis.
  - Similarly, pacemakers with rate-modulation programming can misinterpret febrile illness, external vibrations, hyperventilation, and other external stimuli and cause a **sensor-mediated, paced tachycardia.**

SPECIAL CONSIDERATIONS

• Often episodes of bradycardia are transient and episodic; therefore, a baseline ECG may not be sufficient to capture the bradycardia. Some form of continuous monitoring is often required.

  • In the inpatient setting, **continuous central telemetry monitoring** can be utilized.
  • If further workup is done as an outpatient, **24- to 72-hour Holter monitoring** can be used if the episodes occur somewhat frequently. If infrequent, **an event recorder** or **implantable loop recorder** should be considered.
  • Again, it is vital to correlate symptoms with the rhythm disturbances discovered via continuous monitoring—a task easily accomplished during inpatient care but more difficult as an outpatient. Therefore, the importance of accurate symptom diaries in the ambulatory setting should be emphasized to patients.

• To evaluate the sinus node's response to exertion (chronotropic competence), walking the patient in the hallway or up a flight of stairs under appropriate supervision is easy and inexpensive. A formal **exercise ECG** can be ordered if necessary.

• An **EPS** can also be used to assess sinus node function and AV conduction, but it is rarely necessary if the rhythm is already discovered via noninvasive modalities.

• The role of **tilt-table testing** will be discussed below in the setting of a syncope evaluation.

SYNCOPE

GENERAL PRINCIPLES

Syncope is a common clinical problem and a primary goal of evaluation is to determine whether the patient is at increased risk of death.

Definition

Sudden, self-limited loss of consciousness and postural tone caused by transient global cerebral hypoperfusion and followed by spontaneous, complete, and prompt recovery.

Classification

Syncope can be classified into four major categories based on etiology:

- **Neurocardiogenic** (most common): vasovagal, carotid sinus hypersensitivity, and situational.
- **Orthostatic hypotension:** hypovolemia, medication induced (iatrogenic), and autonomic dysfunction.
- **Cardiovascular:**
  - **Arrhythmia:** sinus node dysfunction, AV nodal block, pacemaker malfunction, VT, SVT, WPW syndrome, and long QT syndrome.
  - **Mechanical:** HVM, valvular stenosis, aortic dissection, myxomas, pulmonary embolism, pulmonary hypertension, acute MI, subclavian steal, etc.
- **Miscellaneous** (not true syncope): seizures, stroke/TIA, hypoglycemia, hypoxia, psychogenic, etc.
  - Atherosclerotic cerebral artery disease is a rare cause of true syncope; exception is severe obstructive four-vessel cerebrovascular disease (expect focal neurologic findings prior to syncope).

Epidemiology

- Common in the general population—**6% of medical admissions and 3% of emergency room visits.**
- Incidence is similar among men and women; one of the largest epidemiologic studies revealed an 11% incidence during an average follow-up for 17 years, with a sharp rise after age 70 years (*N Engl J Med 2002;347:878*).

Pathophysiology

- The two components of **neurocardiogenic syncope** are described as **cardioinhibitory,** in which bradycardia or asystole results from increased vagal outflow to the heart, and **vasodepression,** where the peripheral vasodilation results from sympathetic withdrawal to peripheral arteries. Most patients have a combination of both components as the mechanism of their syncope.
- Specific stimuli may evoke a neurocardiogenic mechanism, leading to **situational syncope** (e.g., micturition, defecation, coughing, swallowing).

Risk Factors

Cardiovascular disease, history of **stroke or TIA,** and **hypertension.** Also, low body mass index, increased alcohol intake and diabetes, or elevated blood glucose concentration are associated with syncope (*N Engl J Med 2002;347:878*; *Am J Cardiol 2000;85:1189*).

DIAGNOSIS

- A syncopal event may herald an otherwise unsuspected, potentially lethal cardiac condition, and therefore, a careful evaluation of the patient with syncope is warranted.
- A meticulous history and physical exam is the key to an accurate diagnosis of the etiology of syncope.
  - In 40% of episodes, the mechanism of syncope remains unexplained (*Ann Intern Med 1997;126:989*).

Clinical Presentation

History

Special attention should be focused on the **events or symptoms** that **precede and follow** the syncopal event, **eyewitness** accounts during the event, the **time course** of loss and resumption of consciousness (abrupt vs. gradual), and the patient's **medical history.**

- A characteristic prodrome of nausea, diaphoresis, visual changes, or flushing suggests neurocardiogenic syncope, as does the identification of a particular emotional or situational trigger and postepisode fatigue.
- Alternatively, an unusual sensory prodrome, incontinence, or a decreased level of consciousness that gradually clears suggests a seizure as a likely diagnosis.
- With transient ventricular arrhythmias, an abrupt loss of consciousness may occur, with a rapid recovery.
- Syncope with exertion is a matter of concern for structural heart disease, pulmonary hypertension, and coronary artery disease.

Physical Examination

The **cardiovascular** and **neurologic** exams should be the primary focus of initial evaluation.

- Orthostatic vital signs are critical in assessing for orthostatic hypotension. All patients should have blood pressure checked in both arms.
- Cardiac exam findings may help detect valvular heart disease, LV dysfunction, pulmonary hypertension, etc.
- Neurologic findings are often absent but if present may point to a possible neurologic etiology of the syncopal event.
- Carotid sinus massage for 5 to 10 seconds with reproduction of symptoms and consequent ventricular pause > 3 seconds is considered positive for carotid sinus hypersensitivity. It is critical to take proper precautions of telemetry monitoring, availability of bradycardia treatments, and avoiding the procedure in patients with known or suspected carotid disease.

Diagnostic Testing

- The presence of known **structural heart disease, abnormal ECG, age older than 65 years, focal neurologic findings,** and **severe orthostatic hypotension** suggest a potentially more ominous etiology. Therefore, these patients should be admitted for their workup to avoid delay and adverse outcomes.
- After the history and physical exam, the ECG is the most important diagnostic tool in the evaluation of the patient. It will be abnormal in 50% of cases but alone will yield a diagnosis in only 5% of these patients.

- If the patient has no history of heart disease or baseline ECG abnormalities, **tilt-table testing** can be used to evaluate a patient's hemodynamic response during transition from supine to upright state for diagnosis of neurally mediated processes. In an unselected population, the predictive value of this test is low.
- Please refer to Figure 7 with regards to the diagnostic approach to syncope.

TREATMENT

In general, therapy is tailored to the underlying etiology of syncope with goals of preventing recurrence and reducing risk of injury or death.

- **Neurocardiogenic syncope:**
  - **Counsel** patients to take precautionary steps to avoid injury by being aware of prodromal symptoms and maintaining a **horizontal position** at those times.
  - Avoid known precipitants and maintain adequate **hydration.**
  - Employ **isometric muscle contraction** during prodrome to abort episode.
  - Evidence suggests that β-adrenergic blockers are probably unhelpful (*Circulation 2006;113:1164*); **SSRI antidepressants** and **fludrocortisone** have a debatable effect; and **midodrine (start at 5 mg PO tid and can be increased to 15 mg tid)** is probably helpful in the treatment of neurocardiogenic syncope (*Am J Cardiol 2001;88:80; Heart Rhythm 2008;5:1609*).
  - In general **PPMs** have no proven benefit (*JAMA 2003;289:2224*); however, permanent dual-chamber pacemakers with a hysteresis function (high-rate pacing in response to a detected sudden drop in heart rate) have been shown to be useful in highly selected patients with recurrent neurocardiogenic syncope with a prominent cardioinhibitory component (*J Am Coll Cardiol 1990;16:165*).
  - **Cardiac pacing** for **carotid sinus hypersensitivity** is appropriate in syncopal patients.
  - In general, neurocardiogenic syncope is not associated with increased risk of mortality.
- **Orthostatic hypotension:**
  - **Adequate hydration** and elimination of offending drugs.
  - Salt supplementation, compressive stockings, and counseling on standing slowly.
  - Midodrine and fludrocortisone can help by increasing systolic blood pressure and expanding plasma volume, respectively.
- **Cardiovascular (arrhythmia or mechanical):**
  - Treatment of **underlying disorder** (valve replacement, antiarrhythmic agent, coronary revascularization, etc.)
  - **Cardiac pacing** for sinus node dysfunction or high-degree AV block.
  - Discontinuation of QT-prolonging drugs.
  - Catheter **ablation** procedures in select patients with syncope associated with SVT.
- **ICD** for documented VT without correctable cause and for syncope with EF <35% even in absence of documented arrhythmia.

CARDIAC RESYNCHRONIZATION THERAPY

GENERAL PRINCIPLES

- CHF is complicated by a significant interventricular conduction delay in about 30% of heart failure patients. In this patient group, dyssynchronous ventricular

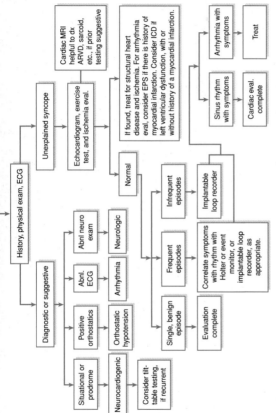

Figure 7. Algorithm for the evaluation of syncope. (Modified from Holley C. Evaluation of syncope. In: Cooper DH, et al., eds. The Washington Manual of Medical Therapeutics. 32nd Ed. Philadelphia: Lippincott Williams & Wilkins, 2007; and AHA/ACCF Scientific Statement on the evaluation of syncope: from the American Heart Association Councils on Clinical Cardiology; Cardiovascular Nursing, Cardiovascular Disease in the Young, and Stroke, and the Quality of Care and Outcomes Research Interdisciplinary Working Group; and the American College of Cardiology Foundation: in collaboration with the Heart Rhythm Society: endorsed by the American Autonomic Society. Strickberger SA, Benson DW, Biaggioni I, et al.; American Heart Association Councils on Clinical Cardiology; Cardiovascular Nursing, Cardiovascular Disease in the Young, and Stroke; Quality of Care and Outcomes Research Interdisciplinary Working Group; American College of Cardiology Foundation; Heart Rhythm Society; American Autonomic Society. *Circulation* 2006 Jan 17;113(2):316–327.)

contraction of the septum and lateral wall complicate systolic dysfunction. The consequences of ventricular dyssynchrony include a loss of mechanical energy for blood ejection due to wasted motion of a partially relaxed opposing wall, an expansion of the isovolumetric phases of the cardiac cycle at the expense of systolic ejection and diastolic filling periods, and excessively high wall strains that can contribute to myopathic changes. The result is a worse prognosis than heart failure uncomplicated by conduction system disease.

- Biventricular pacing was first proposed as a way to restore, to some degree, electrical synchronization of the septum and lateral wall of the left ventricle in the setting of interventricular conduction delay leading to improvement in LV systolic function and heart failure symptoms. Randomized clinical trials have consistently verified these clinical benefits as well as providing evidence for a modification of the natural history of severe heart failure in patients treated with a "state-of-the-art" heart failure medical regimen manifested by a reduction in mortality and incidence of heart failure decompensation (*N Engl J Med 2004;350:2140*; *N Engl J Med 2005;352:1539*).
- As a result, cardiac resynchronization therapy (CRT) has become a standard of care for the treatment of patients with LV conduction delay and concomitant systolic heart failure that has become unresponsive to medical therapy.

Definition

- CRT is indicated for treatment of patients with an LVEF of <35% and QRS duration of >0.12 seconds in the presence of medically refractory advanced heart failure symptoms quantified by NYHA class 3 or 4. Patients who have an indication for ventricular pacing and an LVEF of <35% with NYHA class 1 or 2 heart failure symptoms can also be considered as candidates for implantation of a CRT device.
- CRT can be delivered by a dedicated pacemaker system, or through a combination pacemaker/ICD system. Because most patients who are candidates for CRT also qualify for ICD implantation as primary prevention of SCD, the combination CRT pacemaker/ICD units are usually implanted.

Critical Care
Jennifer Alexander-Brett, Scott T. Micek, and
Marin H. Kollef

Respiratory Failure

GENERAL PRINCIPLES

- **Hypercapnic respiratory failure** occurs with acute carbon dioxide retention (arterial carbon dioxide tension [$PaCO_2$] > 45 to 55 mm Hg) producing a respiratory acidosis (pH < 7.35).
- **Hypoxic respiratory failure** occurs when normal gas exchange is seriously impaired, resulting in hypoxemia (arterial oxygen tension [PaO_2] < 60 mm Hg or arterial oxygen saturation [SaO_2] < 90%). Usually, this type of respiratory failure is associated with tachypnea and hypocapnia; however, its progression can lead to hypercapnia as well. Hypoxic respiratory failure can result from various insults, as shown in Table 1.
  - The **acute respiratory distress syndrome** (ARDS) is a form of hypoxic respiratory failure caused by acute lung injury. The common end result is disruption of the alveolar capillary membrane, leading to increased vascular permeability and accumulation of inflammatory cells and protein-rich edema fluid within the alveolar space.
  - The **American-European Consensus Conference** has defined ARDS as follows: (a) acute bilateral pulmonary infiltrates, (b) ratio of PaO_2 to inspired oxygen concentration (FIO_2) < 200, and (c) no evidence for heart failure or volume overload as the principal cause of the pulmonary infiltrates (*NEJM 2000;342:1334*).

Pathophysiology

- **Hypercapnic respiratory failure** usually involves some combination of the following three processes:
  - **Increased carbon dioxide production** (i.e., respiratory acidosis) can be precipitated by fever, sepsis, seizures, and excessive carbohydrate loads in patients with underlying lung disease. The oxidation of carbohydrate fuels is associated with more carbon dioxide production per molecule of oxygen consumed as compared to the oxidation of fat fuels.
  - **Increased dead space** occurs when areas of the lung are ventilated but not perfused or when decreases in regional perfusion exceed decreases in ventilation. Examples include intrinsic lung diseases (e.g., chronic obstructive pulmonary disease [COPD], asthma, cystic fibrosis, pulmonary fibrosis) and chest wall disorders associated with parenchymal abnormalities (e.g., scoliosis). Usually, these disorders are associated with widened $P(A–a)O_2$ gradients.
  - **Decreased minute ventilation** can result from central nervous system (CNS) disorders (e.g., spinal cord lesions), peripheral nerve diseases (e.g., Guillain-Barré syndrome, botulism, myasthenia gravis, amyotrophic lateral sclerosis), muscle disorders (e.g., polymyositis, muscular dystrophy), chest wall abnormalities (e.g., thoracoplasty, scoliosis), drug overdoses, metabolic abnormalities (e.g., myxedema, hypokalemia), and upper airway obstruction. These disorders are usually associated with a normal $P(A–a)O_2$ gradient unless accompanying lung disease is also present.

Table 1	Causes of Shunts and Hypoxic Respiratory Failure
Clinical Presentation	**Causes**
Cardiogenic pulmonary edema (low permeability, high hydrostatic pressure)	Acute myocardial infarction Left ventricular failure Mitral regurgitation Mitral stenosis Diastolic dysfunction
Noncardiogenic pulmonary edema (high permeability, low hydrostatic pressure)	Aspiration Sepsis Multiple trauma Pancreatitis Near-drowning Pneumonia Reperfusion injury Inhalational injury Drug reaction (aspirin, narcotics, interleukin-2)
Mixed pulmonary edema (high permeability, high hydrostatic pressure)	Myocardial ischemia or volume overload associated with sepsis, aspiration, etc. High-altitude exposure
Pulmonary edema of unclear etiology	Upper airway obstruction Neurogenic cause Lung reexpansion

- **Hypoxic respiratory failure** usually is the result of the lung's reduced ability to deliver oxygen into the bloodstream, owing to one of the following six processes:
  - **Shunt.** This term refers to the fraction of mixed venous blood that passes into the systemic arterial circulation after bypassing functioning lung units. Congenital shunts are due to developmental anomalies of the heart and great vessels. Acquired shunts usually result from diseases that affect lung units, although acquired cardiac and peripheral vascular shunts also can occur (Table 1). Shunts are associated with a widened $P(A–a)O_2$ gradient, and the resultant hypoxemia is resistant to correction with supplemental oxygen alone when the shunt fraction of the cardiac output (CO) is $>30\%$.
  - **Ventilation–perfusion mismatch.** Diseases associated with airflow obstruction (e.g., COPD, asthma), interstitial inflammation (e.g., pneumonia, sarcoidosis), or vascular obstruction (e.g., pulmonary embolism) often produce lung regions with abnormal ventilation-to-perfusion relationships. In ventilation–perfusion mismatch, unlike shunt physiology, increases in FIO_2 result in increases in PaO_2.
  - **Low inspired oxygen.** Usually, FIO_2 is reduced at high altitudes or when toxic gases are inhaled.
  - **Hypoventilation.** This condition is associated with elevated $PaCO_2$ values, and the resultant hypoxemia is due to increased alveolar carbon dioxide, which displaces oxygen. Usually, oxygen therapy improves hypoxemia as a result of hypoventilation but may worsen the overall degree of hypoventilation, especially in patients with

chronic airflow obstruction. Primary treatment is directed at correcting the cause of the hypoventilation.

- **Diffusion impairment.** Hypoxemia due to diffusion impairments usually responds to supplemental oxygen therapy, as is seen in patients with interstitial lung diseases.
- **Low mixed venous oxygenation.** Normally, the lungs fully oxygenate pulmonary arterial blood, and mixed venous oxygen tension (PvO_2) does not affect PaO_2 significantly. However, a decreased PvO_2 can lower the PaO_2 significantly when either intrapulmonary shunting or ventilation–perfusion mismatch is present. Factors that can contribute to low mixed venous oxygenation include anemia, hypoxemia, inadequate CO, and increased oxygen consumption. Improving oxygen delivery to tissues by increasing hemoglobin or CO usually decreases oxygen extraction and improves mixed venous oxygen saturation (SvO_2).
- **Mixed respiratory failure** is seen most commonly after surgery, particularly in patients with underlying lung disease who are undergoing upper abdominal procedures. Abnormalities in oxygenation usually occur on the basis of atelectasis, which often is multifactorial in origin (decreased lung volumes and cough due to the effects of anesthesia, abnormal diaphragmatic function resulting from the surgery or associated pain, and interstitial edema causing small airways to close). Hypoventilation can also result from abnormal diaphragmatic function, particularly when complete paralysis occurs, as with phrenic nerve injury.
- **Blood gas analysis** (see Acid–Base Disturbances in Chapter 9, Fluid and Electrolyte Management).

Noninvasive Oxygen Therapy

GENERAL PRINCIPLES

- **Nasal prongs** allow patients to eat, drink, and speak during oxygen administration. Their disadvantage is that the exact FIO_2 delivered is not known, as it is influenced by the patient's peak inspiratory flow demand. As an approximation, 1 L/min of nasal prong oxygen flow is roughly equivalent to FIO_2 of 24%, with each additional liter of flow increasing the FIO_2 by approximately 4%. Flow rates should be limited to <5 L/min.
- **Venturi masks** allow the precise administration of oxygen. Usual FIO_2 values delivered are 24%, 28%, 31%, 35%, 40%, and 50%. Often, Venturi masks are useful in patients with COPD and hypercapnia because one can titrate the PaO_2 to minimize carbon dioxide retention.
- **Nonrebreathing masks** achieve higher oxygen concentrations (approximately 80% to 90%) than do partial rebreathing systems. A one-way valve prevents exhaled gases from entering the reservoir bag in a nonrebreathing system, thereby maximizing the FIO_2.
- A **continuous positive airway pressure (CPAP) mask** can be used if the PaO_2 is <60 to 65 mm Hg with a nonrebreathing mask and the patient is conscious and cooperative, able to protect the lower airway, and hemodynamically stable (*NEJM 1998;339:429*). CPAP is delivered by a tight-fitting mask equipped with pressure-limiting valves. Many patients cannot tolerate a CPAP mask because of hypoxemia, hemodynamic instability, or feelings of claustrophobia or aerophagia. In these patients, endotracheal intubation should be performed. Initially, 3 to 5 cm H_2O of CPAP should be applied and if the PaO_2 is still <60 mm Hg (SaO_2 < 90%),

the level of CPAP should be increased in steps of 3 to 5 cm H_2O up to a level of 10 to 15 cm H_2O.

- **Bilevel positive airway pressure (BiPAP)** is a method of noninvasive ventilation whereby both inspiratory and expiratory pressures can be applied. The inspiratory support decreases the patient's work of breathing. The expiratory support (CPAP) improves gas exchange by preventing alveolar collapse. Noninvasive ventilation using face or nasal masks has been successfully performed in patients with neuromuscular disease, COPD, and postoperative respiratory insufficiency as a means of decreasing the need for endotracheal intubation and mechanical ventilation (*Crit Care Clin 2007;23:201*). In using BiPAP, an inspiratory pressure of 5 to 10 cm H_2O and an expiratory pressure level of 3 to 5 cm H_2O are reasonable starting points. The inspiratory level can be increased in increments of 3 to 5 cm H_2O, using the patient's respiratory rate as a guide of effectiveness.

Airway Management and Tracheal Intubation

GENERAL PRINCIPLES

- **Airway management**
  - **Head and jaw positioning.** The oropharynx should be inspected, and all foreign bodies should be removed. For patients with inadequate respirations, the jaw thrust or head tilt–chin lift maneuvers should be performed (see Acute Upper Airway Obstruction in Chapter 24, Medical Emergencies).
  - **Oral and nasopharyngeal airways.** When head and jaw positioning fail to establish a patent airway or when more permanent airway maintenance is desired, an oral or nasopharyngeal airway can be used. Initially, oral airways are positioned with the concave curve of the airway facing up into the roof of the mouth. The oral airway then is turned 180 degrees so that the concave curve of the airway follows the natural curve of the tongue. A tongue depressor can also be used to displace the tongue inferiorly and laterally to allow direct positioning of the oral airway. Careful monitoring of airway patency is required, as malpositioning of oral airways can push the tongue posteriorly and can result in obstruction of the oropharynx. Nasopharyngeal airways are made of soft plastic and are passed easily down one of the nasal passages to the posterior pharynx after topical nasal lubrication and anesthesia with viscous lidocaine jelly.
  - **Laryngeal mask airway (LMA).** The LMA is an endotracheal tube with a small mask on one end that can be passed orally over the larynx to provide ventilatory assistance and prevent aspiration. Placement of the LMA is more easily performed than endotracheal intubation. However, it should be considered a temporary airway for patients who require prolonged ventilatory support.
  - **Mask-to-face ventilation.** After an airway is established, respiratory efforts should be evaluated and monitored closely. Ineffective respiratory efforts can be augmented with simple mask-to-face ventilation. Proper fitting and positioning of the mask ensure a tight seal around the mouth and nose, optimizing ventilation. Additionally, proper head positioning and the use of airway adjuncts (e.g., oral or nasopharyngeal airways) optimize ventilation with a mask-to-face system.
- **Endotracheal intubation** (*Int Anesthesiol Clin 2000;38:1*)
  - **Indications** include:
    ○ Initiation of mechanical ventilation
    ○ Airway protection

- ○ Inadequate oxygenation using less invasive methods
- ○ Prevention of aspiration and allowing for the suctioning of pulmonary secretions, and
- ○ Hyperventilation for the treatment of increased intracranial pressure. In an emergency situation, such simple maneuvers as a jaw thrust with mask-to-face ventilation may assist the patient in clearing an obstructed airway and in maintaining adequate ventilation until endotracheal intubation can be performed.
- **Techniques** include:
  - ○ Direct laryngoscopic orotracheal intubation
  - ○ Blind nasotracheal intubation, and
  - ○ Flexible fiberoptically guided orotracheal or nasotracheal intubation depending on the skill of the operator and the urgency.
  - ○ The direct laryngoscopic technique allows for the most rapid intubation of the trachea with the largest endotracheal tube. Nasotracheal intubation often requires smaller endotracheal tubes that are more susceptible to kinking and is associated with a higher incidence of otitis media and sinusitis. Before endotracheal intubation is attempted, a systematic evaluation of the patient's head and neck positioning must be performed. The oral, pharyngeal, and tracheal axes should be aligned before any intubation attempts. This "sniffing" position is achieved by flexing the patient's neck and extending the head. A small pillow or several towels placed under the occiput can assist in maintaining this position. Table 2 offers a step-by-step approach to performing successful orotracheal intubation. After successful intubation of the trachea, the tracheal tube cuff pressures should be monitored at regular intervals and should be maintained below capillary filling pressure (i.e., <25 mm Hg) to prevent ischemic mucosal injury.
- **Verification of correct endotracheal tube positioning.** Proper tube positioning must be ensured by:
  - ○ Direct view of the endotracheal tube entering the trachea through the vocal cords
  - ○ Fiberoptic inspection of the airways through the endotracheal tube, or
  - ○ Use of an end-tidal carbon dioxide monitor. Clinical evaluation of the patient (i.e., listening for bilateral breath sounds over the chest and the absence of ventilation over the stomach) and radiographic evaluation (e.g., standard portable chest radiograph) can be unreliable for establishing correct endotracheal tube positioning.
- **Complications.** Improper endotracheal tube positioning is the most important immediate complication to be recognized and corrected. Ideally, the tip of the endotracheal tube should be 3 to 5 cm above the carina, depending on head and neck positioning. Esophageal or right main-stem intubation should be suspected if hypoxemia, hypoventilation, or cardiac decompensation occurs. Abdominal distention, lack of breath sounds over the thorax, and regurgitation of stomach contents through the endotracheal tube indicate an esophageal intubation. Other complications associated with endotracheal intubation include dislodgment of teeth, trauma to the upper airway, and increased intracranial pressure.
- **Surgical airways**
  - **Tracheostomy**
    - ○ **Indications** include:
      - - The need for prolonged respiratory support
      - - Potentially life-threatening upper airway obstruction (due to epiglottitis, facial burns, or worsening laryngeal edema)
      - - Obstructive sleep apnea that is unresponsive to less invasive therapies, and
      - - Congenital abnormalities (e.g., Pierre Robin syndrome).

Table 2	Procedure for Direct Orotracheal Intubation

Administer oxygen by face mask.

Ensure that basic equipment is present and easily accessible (oxygen source, bag-valve device, suctioning device, endotracheal [ET] tube, blunt stylet, laryngoscope, 20-mL syringe).

Place patient on nonmobile rigid surface.

If patient is in hospital bed, remove backboard and adjust bed height.

Depress patient's tongue with tongue depressor and administer topical anesthesia to patient's pharynx.

Position patient's head in sniffing position.

Administer IV sedation and neuromuscular blocker if necessary.[a]

Have assistant apply Sellick maneuver (compressing cricothyroid cartilage posteriorly against vertebral bodies) to prevent regurgitation and aspiration of stomach contents from esophagus.

Grasp laryngoscope handle in left hand while opening patient's mouth with gloved right hand.

Insert laryngoscope blade on right side of patient's mouth and advance to base of tongue, displacing tongue to the left.

Lift laryngoscope away from patient at a 45-degree angle using arm and shoulder strength. Do not use patient's teeth as a fulcrum.

Suction oropharynx and hypopharynx if necessary.

Grasp ET tube with inserted stylet in right hand and insert it into right corner of patient's mouth, avoiding obscuration of epiglottis and vocal cords.

Advance ET tube through vocal cords until cuff is no longer visible and remove stylet.

Inflate cuff with enough air to prevent significant air leakage.

Verify correct ET tube positioning by auscultation of both lungs and the abdomen.

Obtain a chest radiograph or use end-tidal CO_2 monitor to verify correct position of the ET tube.

---

[a]Neuromuscular blockade can result in complete airway collapse and airway obstruction. Personnel who are skillful in establishment of an emergency surgical airway should be available if paralysis is used.

- ○ Tracheostomy sites usually require at least 72 hours to mature. Tube dislodgment before site maturation, followed by blind attempts at tube reinsertion, can lead to tube malpositioning within a false channel in the pretracheal space. This misplacement can result in complete loss of the airway. If a tracheostomy tube cannot be reinserted easily, standard direct orotracheal intubation should be performed (Table 2), with the exception being after head and neck surgeries that have obliterated the connection between the oral cavity and the trachea (e.g., total laryngectomy). Optimal timing of surgical tracheostomy is controversial but should be considered after 7 to 14 days of mechanical ventilation if prolonged ventilation is anticipated (*CCM 2004;32:1796–1797*).

- **Cricothyrotomy.** This procedure is indicated for the establishment of an emergency airway when direct tracheal intubation cannot be performed owing to upper airway obstruction. A pillow or towel roll should be placed under the patient's shoulders to extend the neck. The thyroid cartilage superiorly and the cricoid

cartilage inferiorly should be located where they border the cricothyroid membrane. The thumb and second finger of the surgeon's nondominant hand should grasp and stabilize the lateral aspects of the cricothyroid membrane. With a scalpel, a transverse skin incision is made over the entire distance of the membrane. The incision then is deepened to the cricothyroid membrane, avoiding injury to surrounding structures. Standard tracheostomy tubes or endotracheal tubes can be inserted into the stoma to ventilate the patient. Alternatively, prepackaged kits using the Seldinger technique with progressive dilation of the stoma can be used.
- **Cricothyroid needle cannulation.** In emergency settings when standard endotracheal intubation cannot be performed and placement of a surgical airway is not immediately possible, needle cannulation of the cricothyroid membrane can be performed as an intermediate procedure until a more definitive airway can be established. The ends of the cricothyroid membrane are grasped with the nondominant hand and a 22-gauge needle is inserted into the airway, aspirating air to confirm positioning. Lidocaine is then injected into the trachea to blunt the patient's cough reflex before the needle is withdrawn. By the same technique, a 14-gauge (or larger) needle-through-cannula device can be passed through the cricothyroid membrane at a 45-degree angle to the skin. When air is aspirated freely, the outer cannula is passed into the airway caudally, and the needle is removed. A 3-mL syringe barrel can then be attached to the catheter and a 7-mm inner-diameter endotracheal tube adapter attached to the syringe to allow bag-valve ventilation. Alternatively, the cannula can be attached directly to high-flow oxygen (i.e., 10 to 15 L/min).

Mechanical Ventilation

GENERAL PRINCIPLES

- **Initiation of mechanical ventilation.** Certain variables should be considered when initiating mechanical ventilation.
  - **Ventilator type.** Often, ventilator selection is dictated by what is available at a particular hospital. A volume-cycled ventilator is used in most clinical circumstances.
- **Mode of ventilation:**
  - **Assist-control ventilation (ACV)** should be the initial mode of ventilation used in most patients with respiratory failure. It produces a ventilator-delivered breath for every patient-initiated inspiratory effort. Controlled ventilator-initiated breaths are delivered automatically when the patient's spontaneous rate falls below the selected backup rate. Respiratory alkalosis is a potential concern when using ACV for patients with tachypnea.
  - **Intermittent mandatory ventilation (IMV)** allows patients to breathe at a spontaneous rate and tidal volume without triggering the ventilator, while the ventilator adds additional mechanical breaths at a preset rate and tidal volume.
  - **Synchronized intermittent mandatory ventilation (SIMV)** allows the ventilator to become sensitized to the patient's respiratory efforts at intervals determined by the frequency setting. This capability allows coordination of the delivery of the ventilator-driven breath with the respiratory cycle of the patient to prevent inadvertent stacking of a mechanical breath on top of a spontaneous inspiration. Potential advantages include less respiratory alkalosis, fewer adverse cardiovascular effects due to lower intrathoracic pressures, less requirement for sedation and paralysis, maintenance of respiratory muscle function, and facilitation of long-term weaning. However, considerable patient-initiated respiratory muscle work

may contribute to respiratory muscle fatigue and failure to wean from mechanical ventilation in some patients. This nonphysiologic work of spontaneous breathing can be alleviated by the addition of low levels of pressure support ventilation (PSV) at 4 to 8 cm H_2O or addition of flow-by, or both.

○ **PSV** augments each patient-triggered respiratory effort by an operator-specified amount of pressure that is usually between 5 and 50 cm H_2O. PSV is used primarily to augment spontaneous respiratory efforts during IMV modes of ventilation or during weaning trials. PSV can also be used as a primary form of ventilation in patients who can trigger the ventilator spontaneously. Increased airway resistance, decreased lung compliance, and decreased patient effort result in diminished tidal volumes and, frequently, in decreased minute ventilation. PSV is not recommended as a primary ventilatory mode in patients in whom any of the aforementioned parameters are expected to fluctuate widely.

○ **Inverse ratio ventilation (IRV)** uses an inspiratory-to-expiratory ratio that is greater than the standard 1:2 to 1:3 ratio (i.e., ≥1:1) to stabilize terminal respiratory units (i.e., alveolar recruitment) and to improve gas exchange primarily for patients with ARDS (*Crit Care Clin 1998;14:707*). The goals of IRV are to decrease peak airway pressures, to maintain adequate alveolar ventilation, and to improve oxygenation. The use of IRV can be considered in patients with a PaO_2 of <60 mm Hg despite an FIO_2 of >60%, peak airway pressures >40 to 45 cm H_2O, or the need for positive end-expiratory pressure (PEEP) of >15 cm H_2O. However, lung strain may be greater in acute lung injury when IRV is employed (*AJRCCM 2004;169:239*).

○ **Lung-protective, pressure-targeted ventilation** (i.e., permissive hypercapnia) is a method whereby controlled hypoventilation is allowed to occur with elevation of the $PaCO_2$ to minimize the detrimental effects of excessive airway pressures. This form of ventilation has been used in patients with respiratory failure due to asthma and ARDS. In patients with ARDS, the application of tidal volumes ≤6 mL/kg has been used as a lung-protective strategy and has been associated with improved outcomes (*CCM 2005;33:S223*). The use of smaller tidal volumes is thought to prevent ventilator-induced lung injury. Additional methods for improving oxygenation while minimizing lung injury during mechanical ventilation in ARDS include prone positioning (*NEJM 2001;345:568*) and the administration of nitric oxide (NO), although these interventions have not been associated with a survival advantage. The administration of corticosteroids for established ARDS is still controversial despite one small randomized trial demonstrating improved survival (*CCM 2003;31:S253*). For patients with asthma, the use of a helium-oxygen mixture may result in improved lung mechanics compared to the use of oxygen alone (*AJRCCM 2002;165:1317*).

○ **Independent lung ventilation** uses two independent ventilators and a double-lumen endotracheal tube. Usually, this modality is reserved for severe unilateral lung disease, such as unilateral pneumonia, respiratory failure associated with hemoptysis, or a bronchopleural fistula.

○ **High-frequency ventilation** uses rates that are substantially faster (60 to 300 breaths/min) than those for conventional ventilation with small tidal volumes (2 to 4 mL/kg). The use of high-frequency ventilation is controversial except during upper airway surgery.

○ **Airway pressure release ventilation (APRV)** uses CPAP with an intermittent pressure release phase. APRV applies CPAP to maintain adequate lung volume and promote alveolar recruitment. A time-cycled release phase to a lower set pressure allows ventilation to occur. APRV allows spontaneous breathing to be integrated independent of the ventilator cycle, making mechanical ventilation more comfortable for some patients (*CCM 2005;33:S228*).

o **Mechanical ventilation with inhaled NO** has been demonstrated to improve gas exchange in adults and children with respiratory failure, including patients with ARDS, primary pulmonary hypertension, cor pulmonale secondary to congenital heart disease, and after cardiac surgery or heart or lung transplantation. Inhaled NO acts as a selective pulmonary artery (PA) vasodilator, decreasing PA pressures (without decreasing systemic blood pressure [BP] or CO) and improving oxygenation by reducing intrapulmonary shunt (*JAMA 2004;291:1603*). Generally, 5 to 20 ppm NO is administered, and the level of methemoglobin is monitored periodically.

- **Ventilator management**
  o **FIO_2.** Hypoxemia is more dangerous than brief exposure to high inspired levels of oxygen. The initial FIO_2 should be 100%. Adjustments in the FIO_2 can be made to achieve a PaO_2 of >60 mm Hg or an SaO_2 of >90%.
  o **Minute ventilation.** Minute ventilation is determined by the respiratory rate and the tidal volume. In general, a respiratory rate of 10 to 15 breaths/min is an appropriate rate with which to begin. Close monitoring of minute ventilation is especially important in ventilating patients with COPD and carbon dioxide retention. In these individuals, the minute ventilation should be adjusted to achieve the patient's baseline $PaCO_2$ and not necessarily a normal $PaCO_2$. Inadvertent hyperventilation with resultant metabolic alkalosis in these patients may be associated with serious serum electrolyte shifts and arrhythmias. Initial tidal volumes usually can be set at 10 to 12 mL/kg. Patients with decreased lung compliance (e.g., ARDS) often need smaller lung volumes (6 to 8 mL/kg) to minimize peak airway pressures and iatrogenic morbidity.
  o **PEEP** is defined as the maintenance of positive airway pressure at the end of expiration. It can be applied to the spontaneously breathing patient in the form of CPAP or to the patient who is receiving mechanical ventilation. The appropriate application of PEEP usually increases lung compliance and oxygenation while decreasing the shunt fraction and the work of breathing. PEEP increases peak and mean airway pressures, which can increase the likelihood of barotrauma and cardiovascular compromise. PEEP is used primarily in patients with hypoxic respiratory failure (e.g., ARDS, cardiogenic pulmonary edema). Low levels of PEEP (3 to 5 cm H_2O) may also be useful in patients with COPD, to prevent dynamic airway collapse during expiration. The main goal of PEEP is to achieve a PaO_2 of >55 to 60 mm Hg with an FIO_2 of $\leq$60% while avoiding significant cardiovascular sequelae. Usually, PEEP is applied in 3 to 5 cm H_2O increments during monitoring of oxygenation, organ perfusion, and hemodynamic parameters. Patients who receive significant levels of PEEP (i.e., >10 cm H_2O) should not have their PEEP removed abruptly, because removal can result in collapse of distal lung units, the worsening of shunt, and potentially life-threatening hypoxemia. PEEP should be weaned in 3 to 5 cm H_2O increments while oxygenation is monitored closely.
  o **Inspiratory flow rate.** Flow rates set inappropriately low can be associated with prolonged inspiratory times that can lead to the development of auto-PEEP. The resultant lung hyperinflation can affect patient hemodynamics adversely by impairing venous return to the heart. Patients with severe airflow obstruction

are at the greatest risk for development of lung hyperinflation when improper flow rates are used. Increasing the inspiratory flow rate usually allows for longer expiratory times that help to reverse this process.

○ **Trigger sensitivity.** Most mechanical ventilators use pressure triggering either to initiate a machine-assisted breath or to permit spontaneous breathing between IMV breaths, or during trials of CPAP. The patient must generate a decrease in the airway circuit pressure equal to the selected pressure sensitivity. Most patients do not tolerate a trigger sensitivity less than −2 cm because of autocycling of the ventilator. Alternatively, excessive trigger sensitivity can increase the patient's work of breathing, contributing to failure to wean from mechanical ventilation. In general, the smallest trigger sensitivity should be selected, allowing the patient to initiate mechanical or spontaneous breaths without causing the ventilator to autocycle.

○ **Flow-by.** To decrease the patient's work of breathing, flow-by can be used as an adjunct to conventional modes of mechanical ventilation. Flow-by refers to triggering of the ventilator by changes in airflow as opposed to changes in airway pressures. A continuous base flow of gas is provided through the ventilator circuit at a preselected flow rate (5 to 20 L/min). A flow sensitivity (i.e., patient rate of inhaled flow that triggers the ventilator to switch from base flow to either a machine-delivered or a spontaneous breath) is selected (usually 2 L/min). Flow-triggered systems are more responsive than are pressure-triggered systems and result in a decreased work of breathing.

• **Management of problems and complications**
  • **Airway malpositioning and occlusion** (see Airway Management and Tracheal Intubation).
  • **Worsening respiratory distress or arterial oxygen desaturation** may develop suddenly as a result of changes in the patient's cardiopulmonary status or secondary to a mechanical malfunction. The first priority is to ensure patency and correct positioning of the patient's airway so that adequate oxygenation and ventilation can be administered during the ensuing evaluation.
    ○ **Note ventilator alarms, airway pressures, and tidal volume.** Low-pressure alarms with decreased exhaled tidal volumes may suggest a leak in the ventilator circuit.
    ○ **Disconnect the patient from the ventilator and manually ventilate with an anesthesia bag using 100% oxygen.** For patients receiving PEEP, manual ventilation with a PEEP valve should be used to prevent atelectasis and hypoxemia.
    ○ **If manual ventilation is difficult:** Check airway patency by passing a suction catheter through the endotracheal tube or tracheostomy. Listen for prolonged expiration continuing up to the point of the next manual breath. This suggests the presence of gas trapping and auto-PEEP.
    ○ **Check vital signs and perform a rapid physical examination with attention to the patient's cardiopulmonary status.** Be attentive to asymmetry in breath sounds or tracheal deviation suggesting tension pneumothorax. Note other parameters, including cardiac rhythm and hemodynamics.
    ○ **Treat appropriately on the basis of the foregoing evaluation.** Treatment should be specific to the identified problems. If the presence of gas trapping and auto-PEEP is suspected, a reduction in the minute ventilation is appropriate. In some circumstances, periods of hypoventilation (4 to 6 breaths/min) or even apnea for 30 to 60 seconds may be necessary to reverse the sequelae of auto-PEEP.

○ **Return the patient to the ventilator only after checking its function.** Increase the level of support provided by the ventilator after an episode of respiratory distress or arterial oxygen desaturation. Usually, this adjustment means increasing the FIO_2 and the delivered minute ventilation unless significant auto-PEEP is present.

- **An acute increase in the peak airway pressure** usually implies either a decrease in lung compliance or an increase in airway resistance. At a minimum, considerations that should be entertained include (a) pneumothorax, hemothorax, or hydropneumothorax; (b) occlusion of the patient's airway; (c) bronchospasm; (d) increased accumulation of condensate in the ventilator circuit tubing; (e) main-stem intubation; (f) worsening pulmonary edema; or (g) the development of gas trapping with auto-PEEP. Some of these possibilities will be addressed in more detail below.

- **Loss of tidal volume,** as evidenced by a difference between the tidal volume setting and the delivered tidal volume, implies a leak in either the ventilator or the inspiratory limb of the circuit tubing. A difference between the delivered tidal volume and the expired tidal volume implies the presence of a leak at the patient's airway due either to cuff malfunction or to malpositioning of the airway (e.g., positioning of the cuff at or above the level of the glottis) or a leak within the patient (e.g., presence of a bronchopleural fistula in a patient with a chest tube).

- **Asynchronous breathing ("fighting" or "bucking" the ventilator)** occurs when a patient's breathing coordinates poorly with the ventilator. This difficulty may indicate unmet respiratory demands. A careful evaluation is mandated, with attention focused at the identification of leaks in the ventilator system or airway, inadequate FIO_2, or inadequate ventilatory support. The problem can be alleviated by adjustments in the mode of mechanical ventilation, rate, tidal volume, inspiratory flow rate, and level of PEEP. The identification of gas trapping with auto-PEEP may require changing multiple settings to allow adequate time for exhalation (e.g., decreasing rate and tidal volume, increasing inspiratory flow rate, switching from assist-control to SIMV in selected cases). Additionally, measures aimed at reducing the work of breathing with mechanical ventilation may resolve the problem (e.g., low levels of PSV to patients taking spontaneous breaths). If these adjustments are unsuccessful, sedation should be attempted. Muscle paralysis should be reserved for patients in whom effective gas exchange and ventilation cannot be achieved with other measures.

- **Organ hypoperfusion or hypotension** can occur. Positive-pressure ventilation can result in decreased CO and BP by decreasing venous return to the right ventricle, increasing pulmonary vascular resistance, and impairing diastolic filling of the left ventricle because of increased right-sided heart pressures. Increasing the preload to the left ventricle with fluid administration should increase stroke volume and CO in most cases. Occasionally, the administration of dobutamine (after appropriate preload replacement) or vasopressors becomes necessary. Under these circumstances, consideration should be given to reducing airway pressures (peak airway pressures < 40 cm H_2O) at the expense of relative hypoventilation (i.e., pressure-targeted ventilation).

- **Auto-PEEP** is the development of end-expiratory pressure caused by airflow limitation in patients with airway disease (emphysema, asthma), excessive minute ventilation, or an inadequate expiratory time. Graphic tracings on modern ventilators can suggest the presence of gas trapping by demonstrating persistent airflow at end expiration. The level of auto-PEEP can be estimated in the spontaneously breathing patient by occluding the expiratory port of the ventilator briefly just before inspiration and measuring the end-expiratory pressure reading on the ventilator's manometer. The presence of auto-PEEP can increase the work of breathing, contribute to barotrauma, and result in organ hypoperfusion by impairing CO. Appropriate adjustments to the ventilator can reduce or eliminate the presence of auto-PEEP.

- **Barotrauma or volutrauma** in the form of subcutaneous emphysema, pneumoperitoneum, pneumomediastinum, pneumopericardium, air embolism, and pneumothorax is associated with high peak airway pressures, PEEP, and auto-PEEP. Subcutaneous emphysema, pneumomediastinum, and pneumoperitoneum seldom threaten the patient's well-being. However, the occurrence of these disorders usually indicates a need to reduce peak airway pressures and the total level of PEEP. The occurrence of a pneumothorax is a potentially life-threatening complication and should be considered whenever airway pressure rises acutely, breath sounds are diminished unilaterally, or BP falls abruptly (for treatment, see Pneumothorax in Chapter 24, Medical Emergencies).
- **Positive fluid balance and hyponatremia** in mechanically ventilated patients often develop from several factors, including applied PEEP, humidification of inspired gases, administration of hypotonic fluids and diuretics, and increased levels of circulating antidiuretic hormone.
- **Cardiac arrhythmias,** particularly multifocal atrial tachycardia and atrial fibrillation, are common in respiratory failure and should be treated as outlined in Chapter 5, Cardiac Arrhythmias.
- **Aspiration** commonly occurs despite the use of a cuffed endotracheal tube, especially in patients who are receiving enteral nutrition. Elevating the head of the bed and avoiding excessive gastric distention help to minimize the occurrence of aspiration. Additionally, pooling of secretions around the cuff of the endotracheal tube requires suctioning of these secretions before deflation or manipulation of the cuff.
- **Ventilator-associated pneumonia** is a frequent complication connected with increased patient morbidity and mortality. Prevention of ventilator-associated pneumonia is aimed at avoiding colonization of pathogenic bacteria in the patient and their subsequent aspiration into the lower airway (*Semin Respir Crit Care Med 2006;27:5*).
- **Upper gastrointestinal (GI) hemorrhage** may develop secondary to gastritis or ulceration. The prevention of stress bleeding requires ensuring hemodynamic stability and, in high-risk patients (e.g., those receiving prolonged mechanical ventilation [>48 to 72 hours] or with a coagulopathy), the administration of proton pump inhibitors, H_2-receptor antagonists, antacids, or sucralfate.
- **Acid–base complications** are common in the critically ill patient:
  - **Nonanion gap metabolic acidosis** may render weaning difficult, as minute ventilation must increase to normalize pH.
  - **Metabolic alkalosis** may compromise weaning by blunting ventilatory drive to maintain a normal pH. In patients with chronic ventilatory insufficiency (e.g., emphysema, cystic fibrosis), correction of metabolic alkalosis usually is inappropriate and can cause an unsustainable minute ventilation requirement. Under these circumstances, a patient should be allowed to adjust minute ventilation gradually to a more appropriate level. This change may be facilitated by switching from ACV to SIMV or PSV.
  - **Respiratory alkalosis** may develop rapidly during mechanical ventilation. When severe, it can lead to arrhythmias, CNS disturbances (including seizures), and a

decrease in CO. Changing the ventilator settings to reduce the minute ventilation or changing the mode of ventilation (ACV to SIMV) usually corrects the alkalosis. However, some patients (such as those with ARDS, interstitial lung disease, pulmonary embolism, asthma) are driven to high respiratory rates by local pulmonary stimuli. In such patients, sedation with or without paralysis may be indicated briefly during the acute phase of the respiratory compromise.

- **Oxygen toxicity** commonly is accepted to occur when an FIO_2 of >0.6 is administered, particularly for more than 48 hours. However, the highest FIO_2 necessary should be used initially to maintain the SaO_2 at >0.9. The application of PEEP or other maneuvers that increase mean airway pressure (e.g., IRV) can be used to reduce FIO_2 requirements. However, an FIO_2 of 0.6 to 0.8 should be accepted before a plateau pressure above 30 cm H_2O is accepted. This cautionary note is due to the greater risk of morbidity associated with plateau pressures above this level (*NEJM 1998;338:347*).

- **Weaning from mechanical ventilation.** Weaning is the gradual withdrawal of mechanical ventilatory support (*Thorax 2005;60:175*). Successful weaning depends on the condition of the patient and on the status of the cardiovascular and respiratory systems. In patients who have had brief periods of mechanical ventilation, the manner in which ventilatory support is discontinued often is not crucial. In patients with marginal respiratory function, chronic underlying lung disease, or incompletely resolved respiratory impairment, the approach to weaning may be critical to obtaining a favorable outcome. In general, the level of supported ventilation (minute ventilation) is decreased gradually, and the patient assumes more of the work of ventilation with each of the techniques described. However, it is important not to fatigue the patient excessively, which can prolong the duration of mechanical ventilation.

- **IMV** allows a progressive change from mechanical ventilation to spontaneous breathing by decreasing the ventilator rate gradually. However, the weaning process may be prolonged if ventilator changes are not made often enough. Prolonged periods at low rates (<6 breaths/min) may promote a state of respiratory muscle fatigue because of the imposed work of breathing through a high-resistance ventilator circuit. The addition of PSV may alleviate this fatigue but can prolong the weaning process if not titrated appropriately. Very often, tachypnea that occurs during weaning of the IMV rate represents a problem related to the imposed work from the ventilator circuit and the endotracheal tube rather than a diagnosis of persistent respiratory failure. In circumstances in which this problem is suspected, a trial of extubation may be appropriate.

- **T-tube technique** intersperses periods of unassisted spontaneous breathing through a T tube (or other continuous-flow circuit) with periods of ventilator support (*NEJM 1995;332:345*). Short daytime periods (5 to 15 minutes two to four times per day) are used initially and then are increased progressively in duration. Small amounts of CPAP (3 to 5 cm H_2O) during these periods may prevent distal airway closure and atelectasis, although the effects on weaning success appear to be negligible (*Chest 1991;100:1655*). Similar to IMV weaning, small amounts of pressure support (4 to 8 cm H_2O) can be used to decrease inspiratory resistance imposed by the ventilator circuit and the endotracheal tube. Extubation may be appropriate when the patient can comfortably tolerate more than 30 to 90 minutes of T-tube ventilation. More prolonged periods of T-tube breathing may produce fatigue, especially when small endotracheal tubes (<8 mm internal diameter) are used.

- **PSV** is preferred by some practitioners when respiratory muscle weakness appears to be compromising weaning success (*AJRCCM 1994;150:896*). PSV can reduce the patient's work of breathing through the endotracheal tube and the ventilator circuit. The optimal level of PSV is selected by increasing the PSV level from a baseline of 15 to 20 cm H_2O in increments of 3 to 5 cm H_2O. A decrease in respiratory rate with achieved tidal volumes of 10 to 12 mL/kg signals that the optimal PSV level has been reached. When the patient is ready to begin weaning, the level of PSV is reduced gradually by 3- to 5-cm H_2O increments. Once a PSV level of 5 to 8 cm H_2O is reached, the patient can be extubated without further decreases in PSV.
- **Protocol-guided weaning of mechanical ventilation** has been safely and successfully used by nonphysicians (*J Trauma 2004;56:943*). The use of protocols or guidelines can reduce the duration of mechanical ventilation by expediting the weaning process.
- **Failure to wean.** Patients who do not wean from mechanical ventilation after 48 to 72 hours of the resolution of their underlying disease process need further investigation. Table 3 lists the factors that should be considered when weaning failure occurs. The acronym "WEANS NOW" has been developed to aid in addressing each of these

Table 3	Factors to be Considered in the Weaning Process

Weaning parameters
See Table 4.
Endotracheal tube
Use largest tube possible.
Consider use of supplemental pressure-support ventilation.
Suction secretions.
Arterial blood gases
Avoid or treat metabolic alkalosis.
Maintain PaO_2 at 60–65 mm Hg to avoid blunting of respiratory drive.
For patients with carbon dioxide retention, keep $PaCO_2$ at or above the baseline level.
Nutrition
Ensure adequate nutritional support.
Avoid electrolyte deficiencies.
Avoid excessive calories.
Secretions
Clear regularly.
Avoid excessive dehydration.
Neuromuscular factors
Avoid neuromuscular-depressing drugs.
Avoid unnecessary corticosteroids.
Obstruction of airways
Use bronchodilators when appropriate.
Exclude foreign bodies within the airway.
Wakefulness
Avoid oversedation.
Wean in morning or when patient is most awake.

Table 4	Guidelines for Assessing Withdrawal of Mechanical Ventilation

Patient's mental status: awake, alert, cooperative
$PaO_2 > 60$ mm Hg with an $FIO_2 < 50\%$
$PEEP \leq 5$ cm H_2O
$PaCO_2$ and pH acceptable
Spontaneous tidal volume > 5 mL/kg
Vital capacity > 10 mL/kg
MV < 10 L/min
Maximum voluntary ventilation double of MV
Maximum negative inspiratory pressure > 25 cm H_2O
Respiratory rate < 30 breaths/min
Static compliance > 30 mL/cm H_2O
Rapid shallow breathing index (ratio of respiratory rate to tidal volume) < 100 breaths/min/L
Stable vital signs after a 1- to 2-hr spontaneous breathing trial

FIO_2, inspired oxygen concentration; MV, minute ventilation; $PaCO_2$, arterial carbon dioxide tension; PaO_2, arterial oxygen tension; PEEP, positive end-expiratory pressure.

factors. Commonly used parameters that can be assessed in predicting weaning success are listed in Table 4.

- **Extubation**
  - Usually, extubation should be performed early in the day, when full ancillary staff are available. The patient should be clearly educated about the procedure, the need to cough, and the possible need for reintubation. Elevation of the head and trunk to more than 30 to 45 degrees improves diaphragmatic function. Equipment for reintubation should be available, and a high-humidity, oxygen-enriched gas source with a higher-than-current FIO_2 setting should be available at the bedside. The patient's airway and the oropharynx above the cuff should be suctioned. The cuff of the endotracheal tube should be deflated partially, and airflow around the outside of the tube—indicating the absence of airway obstruction—should be detected. After the cuff is deflated completely, the patient should be extubated, and high-humidity oxygen should be administered by a face mask. Coughing and deep breathing should be encouraged while the examiner monitors the patient's vital signs and upper airway for stridor. Inspiratory stridor may result from glottic and subglottic edema. If clinical status permits, treatment with nebulized 2.5% racemic epinephrine (0.5 mL in 3 mL normal saline) should be administered. If upper airway obstruction persists or worsens, reintubation should be performed.
  - Extubation should not be reattempted for 24 to 72 hours after reintubation for upper airway obstruction. Otolaryngology consultation may be beneficial to exclude other causes of upper airway obstruction and to perform tracheostomy if upper airway obstruction persists.
- **Medications. Drugs** are commonly used in the ICU to facilitate tracheal intubation and mechanical ventilation (Table 5). Nondepolarizing muscle relaxants have been implicated in muscle dysfunction and prolonged weakness after their use in ICU patients (*Curr Opin Crit Care 2004;10:47*). Some reports suggest a drug interaction between muscle relaxants and glucocorticoids, potentiating this effect. To minimize

| Table 5 | Intensive Care Unit Drugs to Facilitate Endotracheal Intubation and Mechanical Ventilation | | |

Drug	Bolus Dosages (IV)	Continuous-infusion Dosages[a]	Onset	Duration after Single Dose
Succinylcholine[b]	0.3–1 mg/kg	—	45–60 sec	2–10 min
Pancuronium	0.05–0.1 mg/kg	1–2 mcg/kg/min	2–4 min	60–90 min
Vecuronium	0.08–0.1 mg/kg	0.3–1 mcg/kg/min	2–4 min	30–45 min
Atracurium	0.2–0.6 mg/kg	5–15 mcg/kg/min	2–4 min	20–35 min
Lorazepam[a]	0.03–0.1 mg/kg	0.01–0.1 mg/kg/hr, titrate to effect	5–20 min	2–6 hr[c]
Midazolam[a]	0.02–0.08 mg/kg	0.04–0.2 mg/kg/hr, titrate to effect	1–5 min	30–60 min[c]
Morphine	0.01–0.15 mg/kg	0.1–0.5 mg/kg/hr, titrate to effect	2–10 min	2–4 hr[c]
Fentanyl	0.35–1.5 mcg/kg	1–10 mcg/kg/hr, titrate to effect	30–60 sec	30–60 min[c]
Thiopental	50–100 mg; repeat up to 20 mg/kg	—	20 sec	10–20 min
Methohexital	1–1.5 mg/kg	—	15–45 sec	5–20 min
Etomidate[b]	0.3–0.4 mg/kg	—	10–20 sec	4–10 min
Propofol	0.25–0.5 mg/kg	25–80 mcg/kg/min	15–60 sec	3–10 min[c]
Dexmedetomidine	1 mcg/kg	0.2–0.7 mcg/kg/hr	10 min	30 min

[a]A continuous infusion should be started or titrated upward only after the desired level of sedation is achieved with bolus administration.
[b]Use only in the process of rapid sequence intubation.
[c]Duration is prolonged with continuous IV administration. Frequent titration to the minimum effective dose is required to prevent accumulation of drug.

the chances of this complication, the use of muscle relaxants should be limited to as brief a period as possible. Peripheral nerve stimulators should be used to titrate the dose of the muscle relaxant to the lowest effective dose. Finally, glucocorticoids should be avoided in patients who are receiving muscle relaxants unless their use is clearly indicated (e.g., for status asthmaticus, anaphylactic shock).

Shock

GENERAL PRINCIPLES

Circulatory shock is a process in which blood flow and oxygen delivery to tissues are disturbed; this event leads to tissue hypoxia, with resultant compromise of cellular metabolic activity and organ function. Oliguria, diminished mental status, and decreased peripheral pulses represent the major clinical manifestations of circulatory shock. Survival from shock is related to the adequacy of the initial resuscitation and the degree of subsequent organ system dysfunction. The main goal of therapy is rapid cardiovascular resuscitation with the reestablishment of tissue perfusion using fluid therapy and vasoactive drugs. The definitive treatment of shock requires reversal of the underlying etiologic process.

- **Resuscitative principles**
  - **Fluid resuscitation** is usually the first treatment used. All patients in shock should receive an initial IV fluid challenge. The amount of fluid necessary is unpredictable but should be based on changes in clinical parameters, including arterial BP, urine output, cardiac filling pressures, and CO. Crystalloid fluid solutions (0.9% sodium chloride or Ringer lactate) are usually administered, owing to their lower cost and comparable efficacy compared to colloid solutions (5% and 25% albumin, 6% hetastarch, dextran 40, and dextran 70). Blood products should be administered to patients with significant anemia or active hemorrhage. Young, adequately resuscitated patients usually tolerate hematocrits of 20% to 25%. In older patients, individuals with atherosclerosis, and patients who exhibit ongoing anaerobic metabolism, hematocrits of 30% or greater may be required to optimize oxygen transport to tissues.
- **Vasopressors and inotropes** play a crucial role in the management of shock states. Their use usually requires monitoring with intra-arterial and/or PA catheters.
  - **Dopamine** is capable of stimulating cardiac β_1-receptors, peripheral α-receptors, and dopaminergic receptors in renal, splanchnic, and other vascular beds. The effects of dopamine are dose dependent. At dosages of <5 mcg/kg/min, dopamine primarily acts as a vasodilator, increasing renal and splanchnic blood flow. At dosages of 5 to 10 mcg/kg/min, dopamine increases cardiac contractility and CO via the activation of cardiac β_1-receptors. At higher dosages (>10 mcg/kg/min), dopamine increases the BP by activation of peripheral α-receptors.
  - **Dobutamine** is an inotropic agent that is generally considered a selective β_1-agonist. It exerts powerful inotropic effects, reduces afterload by indirect (reflex) peripheral vasodilation, and is a relatively weak chronotropic agent, accounting for its favorable hemodynamic response (increased stroke volume with modest increases in heart rate unless used in high dose or in the setting of hypovolemia).
  - **Epinephrine** has α_1- and nonselective β-adrenergic activity. It is the agent of choice for anaphylactic shock. Like dopamine, its effects are dose dependent.

- ○ **Norepinephrine** also has α_1- and β_1-adrenergic activity but primarily is a potent vasoconstricting agent.
- ○ **Vasopressin** is a vasoconstrictor mediated by three different G-peptide receptors called V_{1a}, V_{1b}, and V_2. The usual dose of vasopressin for hypotension is 0.01 to 0.04 U/min (*Crit Care Med 2008;36:296*).
- ○ **Milrinone** is a noncatecholamine inhibitor of phosphodiesterase III that acts as an inotrope and a direct peripheral vasodilator to increase CO.

Classification

- **Hypovolemic shock** (Table 6) results from a decrease in effective intravascular volume that decreases venous return to the right ventricle. Significant hypovolemic shock (i.e., >40% loss of intravascular volume) that lasts for more than several hours is often associated with a fatal outcome despite resuscitative efforts. Therapy of hypovolemic shock usually is aimed at reestablishing the adequacy of the intravascular volume. At the same time, ongoing sources of volume loss, such as a bleeding vessel, may require surgical intervention. Crystalloid solutions are used initially for the resuscitation of patients in hypovolemic shock. Fluid resuscitation must be prompt and should be given through large-bore catheters placed in large peripheral veins. Rapid infusers can be used to increase the rate of fluid resuscitation. In the absence of overt signs of congestive heart failure (CHF), the patient should receive a 500- to 1000-mL initial bolus of normal saline or Ringer lactate, with further infusions adjusted to achieve adequate BP and tissue perfusion. When shock is due to hemorrhage, packed red blood cells (RBCs) should be given as soon as feasible. When hemorrhage is massive, type-specific unmatched blood can be given safely. Rarely, type O-negative blood is needed.
- **Cardiogenic shock** is seen most commonly after acute myocardial infarction (see Chapter 3, Preventative Cardiology and Ischemic Heart Disease) and usually is the result of pump failure. Other causes of cardiogenic shock include septal wall

Table 6	Hemodynamic Patterns Associated with Specific Shock States							
Type of Shock	CI	SVR	PVR	SvO$_2$	RAP	RVP	PAP	PAOP
Cardiogenic (e.g., MI, cardiac tamponade[a])	↓	↑	N	↓	↑	↑	↑	↑
Hypovolemic (e.g., hemorrhage)	↓	↑	N	↓	↓	↓	↓	↓
Distributive (e.g., septic)	N−↑	↓	N	N−↑	N−↓	N−↓	N−↓	N−↓
Obstructive (e.g., massive pulmonary embolism)	↓	↑−N	↑	N−↓	↑	↑	↑	N−↓

CI, cardiac index; MI, myocardial infarction; N, normal; PAOP, pulmonary artery occlusion pressure; PAP, pulmonary artery pressure; PVR, pulmonary vascular resistance; RAP, right atrial pressure; RVP, right ventricular pressure; SvO$_2$, mixed venous oxygen saturation; SVR, systemic vascular resistance.
[a]Equalization of RAP, PAOP, diastolic PAP, and diastolic RVP establishes a diagnosis of cardiac tamponade.

rupture, acute mitral regurgitation, myocarditis, dilated cardiomyopathy, arrhythmias, pericardial tamponade, and right ventricular failure due to pulmonary embolism. Cardiogenic shock secondary to acute myocardial infarction usually is associated with hypotension (mean arterial BP < 60 mm Hg), decreased cardiac index (<2.0 L/min/m^2), elevated intracardiac pressures (pulmonary artery occlusive pressure [PAOP] > 18 mm Hg), increased peripheral vascular resistance, and organ hypoperfusion (e.g., decreased urine output, altered mentation).

- **Certain general measures should be undertaken.** A PaO$_2$ of >60 mm Hg should be achieved, and the hematocrit should be maintained at ≥30%. Endotracheal intubation and mechanical ventilation should be considered to reduce the work of breathing (and therefore oxygen requirements) and to increase juxtacardiac pressures (P$_{JC}$), which may improve cardiac function. Noninvasive mechanical ventilation with BiPAP can be used to accomplish similar end points in patients who are able to sustain spontaneous breathing. Careful attention to fluid management is necessary to ensure that an adequate preload is present to optimize ventricular function (especially in the presence of right ventricular infarction) and to avoid excessive volume administration with resultant pulmonary edema.

- **Pharmacologic treatment** usually involves two classes of drugs: inotropes and vasopressors. Vasodilators generally are not used in patients with cardiogenic shock due to severe hypotension. The use of vasodilators can be considered after the patient's hemodynamics have stabilized as a means of improving left ventricular function. **Dopamine** usually is administered first in patients with cardiogenic shock because it has inotropic and vasopressor properties. Typically, the dose is titrated to maintain a mean arterial BP of 60 mm Hg or greater. Subsequent guidance using a PA catheter helps to define what further measures are required, including inotropic support (dobutamine, milrinone), afterload reduction (nitroprusside), and changes in intravascular volume (fluid administration vs. diuresis).

- **Mechanical circulatory assist devices** are required in patients who do not respond to medical therapy or who have specific conditions identified as the cause of shock (e.g., acute mitral valve insufficiency, ventricular septal defect). Intra-aortic balloon counterpulsation usually is performed with the device inserted percutaneously. The balloon filling is controlled electronically so that it is synchronized with the patient's electrocardiogram (ECG). The balloon inflates during diastole and deflates during systole, thus reducing afterload and improving CO. Additionally, coronary artery blood flow is improved during diastolic inflation. Intra-aortic balloon pumps should be considered only as an interim step to more definitive therapy.

- **Definitive treatment** must be considered for any patient with cardiogenic shock. This treatment can take the form of relatively noninvasive procedures (e.g., angioplasty) or more invasive surgical procedures (e.g., coronary artery bypass surgery, valve replacement, heart transplantation).

- **Obstructive shock** usually is caused by massive pulmonary embolism. Occasionally, air embolism, amniotic fluid embolism, or tumor embolism also may cause obstructive shock. When shock complicates pulmonary embolism, therapy is directed toward preserving peripheral organ perfusion and removing the vascular obstruction. Fluid administration and the use of vasoconstrictors (e.g., norepinephrine, dopamine) may preserve BP while more definitive measures, such as thrombolytic therapy or surgical embolectomy, are considered.

- **Distributive shock** occurs primarily as septic shock or anaphylactic shock. These two forms are associated with significant decreases in vascular tone.

- **Septic shock** is caused by the systemic release of mediators that is usually triggered by circulating bacteria or their products, although the systemic inflammatory response syndrome can be seen without evidence of infection (e.g., pancreatitis, crush injuries, and certain drug ingestions such as salicylates) (*NEJM 2001;344:759*). Septic shock is characterized primarily by hypotension due to decreased vascular tone. CO also is increased, owing to increased heart rate and end-diastolic volumes despite overall myocardial depression. The main goals of treatment of septic shock include initial fluid resuscitation, adequate treatment of underlying infection, and interruption of the mediator-associated systemic inflammatory response (Fig. 1).
  - **Fluid administration and vasoactive agents.** Using a targeted central venous pressure (CVP) of 8 to 12 cm H_2O during initial resuscitation appears to be important to determine the adequacy of preload and the need for inotropic or vasoconstrictor agents(*NEJM 2001;345:1368*). However, patients with acute lung injury (without evidence of organ hypoperfusion) may actually benefit from a more conservative fluid management strategy (*Chest 2005;128:3098*; *NEJM 2006;354:2564*). Catecholamines remain the first-line vasoconstrictor agents for hypotension refractory to fluid resuscitation, as no mortality benefit has been demonstrated for low-dose vasopressin (*NEJM 2008;358:877*).
  - **Drotrecogin alfa (activated)**, or recombinant human activated protein C, has antithrombotic, anti-inflammatory, and profibrinolytic properties. It has been shown to reduce mortality significantly in patients with severe sepsis when the patient has two or more acute organ failures and/or an APACHE II score of 25 or greater(*NEJM 2005;353:1332*; *NEJM 2001;344:699*). The usual dosage of drotrecogin alfa is a continuous infusion of 24 mcg/kg of body weight per hour for 96 hours. The main contraindication to its use is an increased risk of hemorrhage (e.g., recent invasive procedure, severe thrombocytopenia).
  - **Relative adrenal insufficiency** can be associated with septic shock. Among patients with septic shock who were classified as nonresponders to a corticotropin test (i.e., an increase of <9 mcg/dL in the serum cortisol level), a 7-day course of hydrocortisone (50 mg q6h IV) and fludrocortisone (50 mcg once a day via enteral route) was associated with a significant 28-day survival advantage (*JAMA 2002;288:862*).
  - **Anaphylactic shock** is discussed further in the section Anaphylaxis in Chapter 8, Allergy and Immunology.

Hemodynamic Monitoring

GENERAL PRINCIPLES

- **Pulmonary artery catheterization**
  - **Indications**
    - The PA catheter allows measurement of intravascular and intracardiac pressures, CO, and PvO_2 and SvO_2.
    - A PAC can be placed to differentiate between cardiogenic and noncardiogenic forms of pulmonary edema, to identify the etiology of shock, to evaluate acute renal failure or unexplained acidosis, to evaluate cardiac disorders, or to monitor high-risk surgical patients in the perioperative setting.

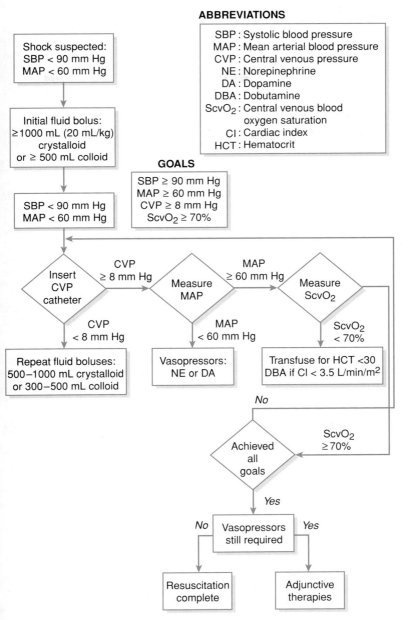

Figure 1. Sepsis protocol.

- **Method**
  - ○ The PA catheter is advanced through a central vein after the distal balloon is inflated. Bedside waveform analysis is used to determine successful passage of the catheter through the right atrium, right ventricle, and PA into a PAOP position. Fluoroscopy should be used when difficulty is encountered in positioning the PA catheter.
  - ○ If, at any time after passage into the PA, the tracing is found to move off the scale of the graph, overwedging of the catheter has occurred. An overwedged catheter should be withdrawn immediately 2 to 3 cm after balloon deflation, and catheter positioning should then be rechecked with re-inflation of the balloon. Overwedging of a PA catheter increases the likelihood of serious complications (e.g., PA rupture).
  - ○ Respiratory variation on the waveform, atrial pressure characteristics (including a and v waves), mean value of the PAOP tracing obtained at end expiration at less than the mean value of the PA pressure measurement, and the aspiration of highly oxygenated blood with the catheter in the PAOP position all indicate an accurate reading.
- **Transmural pressure.** When PEEP is present (applied or auto-PEEP), the positive intra-alveolar pressure at end expiration is transmitted through the lung to the pleural space. In these circumstances, the measured PAOP reflects the sum of the hydrostatic pressure within the vessel and the P_{JC}. When significant levels of total PEEP are present (>10 cm H_2O), it is more appropriate to use the transmural pressure as a measure of left ventricular filling (transmural pressure = PAOP − P_{JC}). For patients with normal lung compliance, one half of the total PEEP can be used as an estimate of P_{JC}. When lung compliance is depressed significantly (e.g., in ARDS), one third of the total PEEP can be used as an estimate for P_{JC}.
- **Cardiac output.** PA catheters are equipped with a thermistor to measure CO. At least two measurements that differ by $<10\%$ to 15% should be obtained. Injections should be synchronized with the respiratory cycle to minimize variability between results. Often, thermodilution measurements of CO are inaccurate at an extremely low CO (e.g., <1.5 L/min) or an extremely high CO (e.g., >7.0 L/min), in the presence of significant valvular disease (e.g., severe tricuspid insufficiency), or when large intracardiac shunts are present. Calculation of the CO using the **Fick formula** may be more accurate in these circumstances.
- **Interpretation of hemodynamic readings.** PAOP can be used as an index of left ventricular filling (preload) and as an index of the patient's propensity for development of pulmonary edema.
  - **Optimizing cardiac function.** Improving cardiac function by optimizing preload is more efficient in terms of myocardial oxygen consumption than similar improvements in cardiac function by use of inotropes when preload is inadequate. As a general rule, preload should be optimized before inotropic agents (which can increase myocardial oxygen consumption) or vasodilators (which can cause hypotension when preload is inadequate) are used. Fluid boluses should be administered in patients who are suspected of having inadequate cardiac filling pressures (i.e., inadequate preload) and should be followed by repeat measurements of PAOP, CO, heart rate, and stroke volume. In low CO states, if the PAOP increases by <5 mm Hg without significant changes in heart rate, CO, and stroke volume, additional fluid boluses may have to be given. An increase in the PAOP by >5 mm Hg usually signals that adequate ventricular filling is being achieved. Once the patient's preload has been optimized, cardiac performance can be reassessed and,

if necessary, further therapy with inotropes or with vasodilators can be initiated to achieve further improvements in cardiac performance and tissue perfusion.

- **Reducing unnecessary lung water.** PAOP is a reflection of the lung's tendency to develop pulmonary edema. Decreased left ventricular compliance results in a "critical pressure" being reached sooner for similar volume changes as compared to a normally compliant left ventricle. This difference is due to the increased stiffness of the noncompliant ventricle that causes higher pressures to be achieved for similar changes in volume. To optimize cardiac performance and to minimize the tendency for pulmonary edema formation, PAOP should be kept at the lowest point at which cardiac performance is acceptable.

- **Differentiating hydrostatic from nonhydrostatic pulmonary edema.** The management of pulmonary edema depends in large part on whether the excessive accumulation of lung water is due to increased hydrostatic pressures (e.g., left ventricular failure, mitral stenosis, acute volume overload), increased permeability of the alveolocapillary barrier (e.g., ARDS due to sepsis, aspiration, or trauma), or a combination of these factors. Clinical and radiographic criteria alone often are insufficient to determine the underlying mechanisms of pulmonary edema. In general, a PAOP of <18 mm Hg suggests that the primary mechanism of pulmonary edema is nonhydrostatic. Values above 18 mm Hg support a hydrostatic cause for the increased lung water.

- **Adequacy of organ perfusion.** Oxygen delivery to tissues depends on (a) an intact respiratory system to provide oxygen for hemoglobin saturation, (b) the concentration of hemoglobin, (c) CO, (d) tissue microcirculation, and (e) the unloading of oxygen from hemoglobin for diffusion into the tissue beds. Oxygen delivery can be measured as the product of CO and arterial oxygen content (CaO_2). CaO_2 is the sum of hemoglobin-bound and dissolved oxygen. Inadequate organ perfusion generally is associated with elevated blood lactate levels and decreased SvO_2 (usually <0.6). Factors that contribute to a low SvO_2 include anemia, hypoxemia, inadequate CO, and increased oxygen consumption. Factors that may elevate measured SvO_2 despite tissue hypoxia include peripheral arteriovenous shunting, the blood flow maldistribution of sepsis or cirrhosis, and cellular poisoning, such as that associated with cyanide toxicity. In general, optimization of gas exchange and CO along with adequate hemoglobin (usually ≥ 10 g/dL) results in improved oxygen delivery to tissues.

- **Noninvasive hemodynamic monitoring.** The PAC remains the reference for hemodynamic monitoring, although the utility of this method is often limited by invasiveness and risks associated with catheter placement. Several noninvasive approaches have emerged as alternatives for cardiac output monitoring, one of which is the esophageal Doppler that has become increasingly utilized in the ICU setting (*Crit Care 2002;6:216*). This method is based upon measurement of aortic blood flow velocity over time via a flexible esophageal probe containing a Doppler transducer (marketed as CardioQ, Deltex Medical Ltd., Chichester, UK). The measured aortic velocity–time integral and estimated aortic cross-sectional area are used to calculate stroke volume, CO, and systemic vascular resistance (SVR). Accuracy and reproducibility of the method is dependent upon proper probe positioning during data acquisition. The esophageal Doppler-derived measurements have been shown to correlate well with thermodilution values, though the method appears to systematically underestimate cardiac output when compared to PA catheter-based measurements (*AJRCCM 1998;158:77*).

7 Pulmonary Diseases

Lee Demertzis, Robert M. Senior, Luke Carlstrom, Mario Castro, Tonya Russell, Meena Murugappan, Murali Chakinala, Devin Sherman, Alexander Chen, Ara Chrissian, Raksha Jain, and Daniel B. Rosenbluth

Chronic Obstructive Pulmonary Disease

GENERAL PRINCIPLES

Definition

Chronic obstructive pulmonary disease (COPD) is a mostly preventable and treatable disorder characterized by expiratory airflow limitation that is not fully reversible. The airflow limitation is usually progressive and associated with an abnormal inflammatory response of the lungs to noxious particles or gases, principally cigarette smoke. The two conditions most commonly associated with COPD are emphysema and chronic bronchitis.

- Emphysema is defined pathologically as enlargement of the distal airways, destruction of the acinus, and absence of associated fibrosis.
- Chronic bronchitis is defined clinically as productive cough on most days for at least 3 consecutive months per year for at least 2 consecutive years, in the absence of other lung disease that could account for this symptom.

Epidemiology

- Although the prevalence of COPD is difficult to determine, it is estimated to affect 10 to 24 million Americans (*MMWR Surveill Summ 2002;51(SS06):1*) and the incidence of this disease is rising.
- COPD and other chronic lower respiratory diseases represent the fourth leading cause of death in the United States, and the age-adjusted death rate is increasing. Death rates for males and females are roughly equivalent (*Nat Vital Stat Rep 2008;56(10)*).

Etiology

- Most cases of COPD are attributable to cigarette smoking. Although only a minority of cigarette smokers develops clinically significant COPD, a much higher proportion develops abnormal lung function.
- Environmental (e.g., wood-burning stove) and occupational dusts, fumes, gases, and chemicals are other etiologic agents of COPD.
- α_1-Antitrypsin deficiency is found in 1% to 2% of COPD patients. Clinical characteristics of affected patients may include (a) a minimal smoking history, (b) early-onset COPD (e.g., younger than 45 years of age), (c) a family history of lung disease, or (d) lower lobe-predominant emphysema. Given the underdiagnosis of this condition, some authorities recommend diagnostic testing in all symptomatic patients with COPD, as well as asymptomatic patients with risk factors for COPD and persistent airflow obstruction on pulmonary function testing (*Am J Respir Crit Care Med 2003;168:818*).

Pathophysiology

- Processes important in the pathogenesis of COPD include inflammation, imbalance of proteinases and antiproteinases in the lung, oxidative stress, and apoptosis.
- Pathologic changes characteristic of COPD are found in the central airways, peripheral airways, lung parenchyma, and pulmonary vasculature. The changes include destruction of alveolar tissue, inflammation, edema, airway mucus, and fibrosis.
- Physiologic changes characteristic of COPD include decreased maximal expiratory airflow, lung hyperinflation, alveolar gas exchange abnormalities, and pulmonary vascular disease.
- An increased incidence of osteoporosis, skeletal muscle dysfunction, and coronary artery disease occur in COPD, perhaps indicating a systemic component of inflammation (*Chest 2005;128:2640*).

Prevention

- Smoking cessation is the most effective preventative measure for COPD.
- In patients with COPD, smoking cessation results in a reduction in the rate of lung function decline (*Am J Respir Crit Care Med 2002;166:675*) and improves survival (*Ann Intern Med 2005;142:233*).
- Tobacco dependence warrants repeated treatment until patients stop smoking. Most smokers fail initial attempts at smoking cessation, and relapse reflects the nature of the dependence and not the failure of the patient or the physician.
- A multimodality approach is recommended to optimize quit rates. Standard interventions include:
  - Counseling (on the preventable health risks of smoking, providing advice to stop smoking, and encouraging patients to make further attempts to stop smoking even after previous failures).
  - Providing smoking cessation materials to patients.
  - Pharmacotherapy (Table 1).
- Formal smoking cessation programs, often administered in a group setting, can be effective (*Cochrane Database Syst Rev 2002;(3):CD001007*).
- The U.S. Department of Health and Human Services has developed a telephone-based support system (1-800-QUIT NOW) with an Internet analog (1800quit-now.cancer.gov).

DIAGNOSIS

Clinical Presentation

History

- The most common symptoms of COPD are dyspnea, cough, sputum production, and wheezing.
- Dyspnea on exertion progresses gradually over time.
- Significant nocturnal symptoms should lead to a search for comorbidities such as gastroesophageal reflux, congestive heart failure, or sleep-disordered breathing.
- Clinicians should obtain a lifelong smoking history and quantify exposure to environmental and occupational risk factors.
- Weight loss often occurs in patients with end-stage COPD, but other etiologies, such as malignancy and depression, should be sought.

Table 1	Pharmacotherapy for Smoking Cessation	
Nicotine Replacement Therapy[a]		
Product	**Dosing**	**Side Effects/Precautions**
Transdermal patch	7, 14, or 21 mg/24 hr Usual regimen = 21 mg qd × 6 wk, 14 mg qd × 2 wk, 7 mg qd × 2 wk[b]	(Apply to all nicotine products) Headache, insomnia, nightmares, nausea, dizziness, blurred vision
Chewing gum, Lozenges	2–4 mg q1–8h Gradually taper use	
Inhaler	4 mg/cartridge 6–16 cartridges/d	
Nasal spray	0.5 mg/spray 1–2 sprays in each nostril q1h	
Non-nicotine Pharmacotherapy		
Bupropion ER (*Zyban*)	150 mg qd × 3 days, then bid × 7–12 wk Start 1 wk before quit date	Dizziness, headache, insomnia, nausea, xerostomia, hypertension, seizure Avoid monoamine oxidase inhibitors
Varenicline (*Chantix*)	0.5 mg qd × 3 days, bid × 4 days, then 1 mg bid × 12–24 wk Start 1 wk before quit date	Nausea, vomiting, headache, insomnia, abnormal dreams Worsening of underlying psychiatric illness

[a]Combination therapy is often employed. A long-acting product (e.g., patch) is used for basal nicotine replacement, with a short-acting product (e.g., inhaler) used for breakthrough cravings.
[b]If patient smokes less than $\frac{1}{2}$ pack per day, start at 14-mg dose.

Physical Examination

- Until significant impairment of lung function occurs (e.g., $FEV_1 < 50\%$ predicted), physical signs of COPD have low sensitivity and specificity.
- Patients with severe COPD may exhibit prolonged (>6 sec) breath sounds on a maximal forced exhalation, decreased breath sounds, use of accessory muscles of respiration, chest hyperresonance to percussion, and enlarged thoracic volume. Expiratory wheezing may or may not be present.
- Signs of pulmonary hypertension (PH) and right heart failure may be present.
- **Clubbing is not a feature of COPD, so its presence should prompt an evaluation for other conditions, especially lung cancer.**

Differential Diagnosis

- Asthma
- Bronchiectasis
- Cystic fibrosis
- Constrictive bronchiolitis
- Diffuse panbronchiolitis
- Mycobacterial infection (tuberculous and nontuberculous)

- Eosinophilic granuloma
- Lymphangioleiomyomatosis
- Airway tumors
- Tracheal stenosis
- Tracheobronchomalacia

Diagnostic Testing

- Consider the diagnosis of COPD in any patient with chronic cough, dyspnea, or sputum production, as well as any patient with a history of exposure to COPD risk factors, especially cigarette smoking (*GOLD Global Strategy for the Diagnosis, Management, and Prevention of Chronic Obstructive Pulmonary Disease [Updated 2008]. Available at www.goldcopd.com*).
- Pulmonary function testing
  - A diagnosis of COPD requires the presence of expiratory airflow limitation on spirometry, defined as a forced expiratory volume in the first second/forced vital capacity ratio (FEV_1/FVC) < 0.70.
  - FEV_1 defines the severity of expiratory airflow obstruction (Table 2) and is a predictor of mortality.
  - The decrement in the FEV_1 is often used to assess the clinical course and response to therapy.
  - Spirometry may assist in the evaluation of worsened symptoms of unclear etiology.
  - Total lung capacity, functional residual capacity, and residual volume often increase to supernormal values in patients with COPD, indicating lung hyperinflation and air trapping.
  - Diffusing capacity of the lungs for carbon monoxide (DLCO) may be reduced.

Laboratories
- A baseline arterial blood gas (ABG) is recommended for patients with severe COPD to assess for the presence and severity of hypoxemia and hypercapnia. Annual monitoring can be considered.

Table 2	GOLD Classification of COPD Severity[a]
Stage I: Mild	FEV_1/FVC < 0.70 $FEV_1 \geq 80\%$ predicted
Stage II: Moderate	FEV_1/FVC < 0.70 FEV_1 50–79% predicted
Stage III: Severe	FEV_1/FVC < 0.70 FEV_1 30–49% predicted
Stage IV: Very severe	FEV_1/FVC < 0.70 FEV_1 < 30% predicted OR FEV_1 < 50% predicted plus chronic respiratory failure[b]

FEV_1, forced expiratory volume in the first second; FVC, forced vital capacity.
[a] Based on post-bronchodilator FEV_1.
[b] Chronic respiratory failure defined as arterial partial pressure of oxygen < 60 mm Hg (8.0 kPa) with or without arterial partial pressure of CO_2 > 50 mm Hg (6.7 kPa) while breathing air at sea level.
From Global Initiative for Chronic Obstructive Lung Disease (GOLD) Global Strategy for the Diagnosis, Management, and Prevention of Chronic Obstructive Pulmonary Disease (Updated 2008). Available at www.goldcopd.com.

- An elevated venous bicarbonate may signify a metabolic response to chronic hypercapnia.
- Polycythemia may reflect a physiologic response to chronic hypoxemia and inadequate supplemental oxygen use.

Imaging
- Chest radiographs are not sensitive for the diagnosis of COPD, but they are useful for evaluating alternative diagnoses. Chest radiographs may also detect other conditions associated with tobacco smoking and COPD, such as lung cancer.
- With increasing severity of COPD, patients often develop thoracic hyperinflation, with flattening of the diaphragm, increased retrosternal/retrocardiac air spaces, and lung hyperlucency with diminished vascular markings. Bullae may be visible.
- Chest CT is not routinely used for diagnosing COPD, though it may help to evaluate for other diagnoses. It is used routinely in assessing patients with severe COPD for lung volume reduction surgery (LVRS) and lung transplantation.

TREATMENT

- Long-term management of patients with COPD aims to improve quality of life, decrease the frequency and the severity of acute exacerbations, slow the progression of disease, and prolong survival.
- Of all chronic medical therapies, only smoking cessation (*Ann Intern Med 2005; 142:233*) and the correction of hypoxemia with supplemental oxygen (*Cochrane Database Syst Rev 2005;(4):CD001744*) have been shown to improve survival. Among surgical interventions, LVRS improves survival in select patients (*Ann Thorac Surg 2006;82:431*).
- A stepwise approach to COPD treatment is presented in Table 3.

Medications
A pharmacotherapeutic treatment plan (Table 4) is based on a patient's disease severity, response to specific medications, drug availability, affordability, and patient compliance.

Table 3	Stepwise Approach to COPD Therapy
GOLD Stage	**Intervention**
Mild	Smoking cessation
	Vaccinations (influenza, pneumococcus)
	Short-acting β-agonist prn
Moderate	All of the above plus:
	Long-acting bronchodilator (one or more)
	Pulmonary rehabilitation
Severe	All of the above plus:
	Inhaled corticosteroid if repeated exacerbations
	Oxygen if needed
Very severe	All of the above plus:
	Consider surgical treatments

Modified from Global Initiative for Chronic Obstructive Lung Disease (GOLD) Global Strategy for the Diagnosis, Management, and Prevention of Chronic Obstructive Pulmonary Disease (Updated 2008). Available at www.goldcopd.com.

Table 4	Inhalational Pharmacotherapy for Stable COPD[a]

Short-acting β-Agonists

Name	Dose	Side Effects[b]
Albuterol	MDI: 2 puffs q4–6h Nebulizer: 2.5 mg q6–8h	Palpitations, tremor, anxiety, nausea/vomiting, throat irritation, dyspepsia, tachycardia, arrhythmia, hypertension. Cardiovascular effects may be less common with Levalbuterol
Levalbuterol (*Xopenex*)	MDI: 2 puffs q4–6h Nebulizer: 0.63–1.25 mg q6–8h	
Pirbuterol (*Maxair*)	MDI: 2 puffs q4–6h	

Long-acting β-Agonists

Name	Dose	Side Effects
Salmeterol (*Serevent*)	DPI: 1 puff (50 mcg) bid	Headache, upper respiratory tract infection, cough, palpitations, fatigue, diarrhea
Formoterol (*Foradil*)	DPI: 1 puff (12 mcg) bid	
Arformoterol (*Brovana*)	Nebulizer: 15 mcg bid	

Anticholinergics[c]

Name	Dose	Side Effects
Ipratropium (*Atrovent*)	MDI: 2 puffs q4–6h Nebulizer: 0.5 mg q6–8h	Xerostomia, cough, nausea/vomiting, diarrhea, urinary retention
Tiotropium (*Spiriva*)	DPI: 1 puff (18 mcg) qd	

Combination Medications

Name	Dose	Side Effects
Albuterol/ Ipratropium (*Combivent, DuoNeb*)	MDI: 2 puffs qid Nebulizer: one 3-mL vial qid (each vial contains 2.5 mg Albuterol and 0.5 mg Ipratropium)	As above
Fluticasone/ Salmeterol (*Advair*)	DPI: 1 puff bid Recommended dose is 250 mcg Fluticasone/50 mcg Salmeterol	As above, plus lower respiratory tract infection and oral candidiasis

MDI, metered-dose inhaler; DPI, dry powder inhaler.
[a]Commonly used medications are listed. This table is not exhaustive.
[b]Only the most common side effects are listed.
[c]Short-acting anticholinergic therapy (e.g., ipratropium) is usually discontinued with initiation of long-acting anticholinergic therapy (e.g., tiotropium), since minimal additional benefit is expected, side effects may increase, and use of two inhaled anticholinergic agents has had limited evaluation.

- **Inhaled bronchodilators**
  - Inhaled bronchodilators, the foundation of COPD pharmacotherapy, work by decreasing or preventing an increase in airway smooth muscle tone. This results in a reduction in expiratory airflow obstruction.
  - Proper use of a metered-dose inhaler (MDI) results in equally effective drug delivery as use of a nebulizer in most patients (*Health Technol Assess 2001;5:1*). Health care providers should routinely assess patient MDI technique and provide training.

- A study of the long-acting inhaled anticholinergic agent **tiotropium** followed about 6,000 COPD patients for 4 years and found that addition of tiotropium to standard COPD therapy resulted in significant improvements in lung function, quality of life, and COPD exacerbations, although the rate of decline of FEV_1 was unaffected (*N Engl J Med 2008;359:1543*).
- **Inhaled corticosteroids**
  - The rationale for using inhaled corticosteroids (ICSs) stems from the central role of inflammation in the pathogenesis of COPD.
  - ICSs may increase the FEV_1 and reduce the frequency of COPD exacerbations, but do not appear to slow the rate of decline of lung function over time (*N Engl J Med 1999;340:1948*; *BMJ 2000;320:1297*; *Eur Respir J 2003;21:68*).
- **Combination therapy:** Compared to single-agent therapy, a combination of medications may yield superior efficacy while reducing the potential for toxicity. Some examples follow:
  - The combination of an ICS and a long-acting β-agonist is effective in reducing the rate of COPD exacerbations, but this benefit must be balanced against an increased risk of pneumonia (*N Engl J Med 2007;356:775*).
  - Combination therapy with a long-acting β-agonist and a long-acting anticholinergic agent sustains improved lung function more than either agent alone (*Eur Respir J 2005;26:214*).
  - Combining a short-acting β-agonist (SABA) with a short-acting anticholinergic agent results in a greater increase in FEV_1 than using either medication alone (*Chest 1994;105:1411*).
- **Theophylline**
  - Theophylline is a xanthine derivative with bronchodilator properties.
  - Patients not responding adequately to inhaled bronchodilator therapy may benefit from the addition of theophylline.
  - Sustained-release theophylline is dosed once or twice a day. Serum levels should be maintained between 8 and 12 mcg/mL to avoid toxicity.
  - Side effects include anxiety, tremor, headache, insomnia, nausea, vomiting, dyspepsia, tachycardia, tachyarrhythmia, and seizure. In the event of toxicity, theophylline should be stopped and a serum level measured.
  - Patients with severe COPD may experience clinical deterioration with discontinuation of theophylline.
- **Systemic corticosteroids are not recommended for the long-term management of COPD,** due to an unfavorable side effect profile. However, they are sometimes used in patients with severe disease who are not responding to other therapies. If used, chronic oral steroid therapy should be administered at the minimum effective dose and discontinued as soon as is feasible.
- **Intravenous α-1 antitrypsin (A1AT)** augmentation therapy may benefit select patients with A1AT deficiency and COPD (*Am J Respir Crit Care Med 2003;168: 818*). Weekly infusion of 60 mg/kg is the standard treatment.
- For the treatment of stable COPD, antibiotics, mucolytics, antioxidants, immunoregulators, antitussives, vasodilators, respiratory stimulants, narcotics, and leukotriene inhibitors have not shown significant benefit.

Other Nonoperative Therapies

- **Supplemental oxygen** decreases mortality and improves physical and mental functioning in hypoxemic patients with COPD.
  - A room air resting ABG is the gold standard test for determining the need for supplemental oxygen. Pulse oximetry may be useful for routine checks after a

baseline oxyhemoglobin saturation is assessed and compared for accuracy with the measured arterial oxyhemoglobin saturation (SaO_2).

- Oxygen therapy is indicated for patients with an arterial partial pressure of oxygen (PaO_2) $\leq$ 55 mm Hg or an SaO_2 $\leq$ 88%. If a patient has a PaO_2 < 60 mm Hg or an SaO_2 < 90% and evidence of pulmonary hypertension (PH), polycythemia (hematocrit > 55%), or heart failure, oxygen therapy is also indicated.
- Supplemental oxygen requirements are typically greatest during exertion and least at rest while awake. Patients who require supplemental oxygen during exertion often need it during sleep as well. Although the exact amount of supplemental oxygen required during sleep can be measured with pulse oximetry, it is reasonable to initially estimate the amount needed by setting the oxygen flow rate at 1 L/min greater than that required during rest while awake.
- The oxygen prescription should include the delivery system (compressed gas, liquid, or concentrator) and the required oxygen flow rates (L/min) for rest, sleep, and exercise.
- Stable patients receiving long-term oxygen therapy should undergo routine reevaluation to assess oxygen requirements at least once a year.
- **Pulmonary rehabilitation** is a multidisciplinary intervention that improves symptoms and quality of life and reduces the frequency of exacerbations in patients with COPD (*Am J Respir Crit Care Med 2006;173:1390*). Components of a rehabilitation program include exercise training, nutritional counseling, and psychosocial support. Pulmonary rehabilitation should be considered for all patients with moderate or more severe COPD (*N Engl J Med 2009;360:1329*).
- **Vaccinations**
  - Annual influenza vaccination reduces the incidence of influenza-related acute respiratory illnesses in COPD patients (*Chest 2004;125:2011*).
  - Although pneumococcal vaccination has not been shown to significantly reduce morbidity and mortality in COPD patients (*Cochrane Database Syst Rev 2006; (4):CD001390*), it is reasonable to give this vaccination every 5 years.

Surgical Management

- **Lung transplantation** for severe COPD can improve quality of life and functional capacity. The data are conflicting regarding survival, and a consistent survival benefit has not been demonstrated to date.
- Selection criteria for COPD patients include a BODE score (see Outcome/Prognosis below) of 7 to 10 or at least one of the following: (a) history of hospitalization for a COPD exacerbation associated with acute hypercapnia ($PaCO_2$ > 50); (b) PH, right heart failure, or both, despite supplemental oxygen therapy; (c) FEV_1 < 20% and either a DLCO < 20% or homogeneous distribution of emphysema (*J Heart Lung Transplant 2006;25:745*).
- **LVRS** may provide quality of life and survival benefits in patients with upper lobe-predominant emphysema and significantly reduced exercise capacity (*Ann Thorac Surg 2006;82:431*).

SPECIAL CONSIDERATIONS

Acute Exacerbation of COPD

- Increased dyspnea, often accompanied by increased cough, sputum production, sputum purulence, wheezing, chest tightness, or other symptoms (and signs) of acutely worsened respiratory status, in the absence of an alternative explanation, define a COPD exacerbation.

- Respiratory infections (viral and bacterial) and air pollution cause most exacerbations (*Thorax 2006;61:250*).
- The differential diagnosis includes pneumothorax, pneumonia, pleural effusion, congestive heart failure, cardiac ischemia, and pulmonary embolism.
- In addition to a history and physical examination, assessment of a patient with a suspected COPD exacerbation includes oxyhemoglobin saturation, ABG testing, an electrocardiogram, and a chest radiograph.
- Criteria for hospital admission include a significant increase in symptom severity, severe underlying COPD, significant comorbidities, failure to respond to initial medical management, diagnostic uncertainty, and insufficient home support (*GOLD Global Strategy for the Diagnosis, Management, and Prevention of Chronic Obstructive Pulmonary Disease [Updated 2008]. Available at www.goldcopd.com*).
- Criteria for admission to an intensive care unit include the need for invasive mechanical ventilation, hemodynamic instability, severe dyspnea that does not adequately respond to therapy, mental status changes, and persistent or worsening hypoxemia, hypercapnia, or respiratory acidosis despite supplemental oxygen and noninvasive ventilation (*GOLD Global Strategy for the Diagnosis, Management, and Prevention of Chronic Obstructive Pulmonary Disease [Updated 2008]. Available at www.goldcopd.com*).
- **Pharmacotherapy** (Table 5)
  - **SABAs are the first-line therapy for COPD exacerbations.** Short-acting anticholinergic agents can be added in the event of inadequate response to SABAs.
  - As many patients experiencing an acute exacerbation of COPD have difficulty performing optimal MDI technique, many clinicians opt to deliver bronchodilators via nebulization.
  - Due to the risk of serious side effects, clinicians typically avoid using methylxanthines (e.g., theophylline) for acute exacerbations. If a patient uses methylxanthines chronically, discontinuation during an exacerbation is discouraged due to the risk of decompensation.
  - **Systemic corticosteroids** produce improvement in hospital length of stay, lung function, and the incidence of relapse, and are recommended for all inpatients and most outpatients experiencing an exacerbation of COPD (*N Engl J Med 2003;348:2618; N Engl J Med 1999;340:1941; Lancet 1999;354:456*).
  - **Antibiotic therapy** most often benefits patients with three cardinal symptoms (increased dyspnea, sputum volume, and sputum purulence), two of three cardinal symptoms if one of the symptoms is sputum purulence, and patients with a need for mechanical ventilation (*Ann Intern Med 1987;106:196; Chest 2000;117:1638; Lancet 2001;358:2020*).
- **Supplemental oxygen** should be administered to maintain oxygen saturation $\geq$ 90%.
- **Noninvasive ventilation** (Table 6) reduces intubation rate, improves respiratory acidosis, decreases respiratory rate, and decreases hospital length of stay (*BMJ 2003; 326:185*).
- **Endotracheal intubation** and invasive mechanical ventilation are required in some patients (Table 7).
- Discharge criteria for patients with acute exacerbations of COPD include use of inhaled bronchodilators less frequently than every 4 hours; clinical and ABG stability for at least 12 to 24 hours; ability to eat, sleep, and ambulate comfortably; adequate patient understanding of home therapy; and adequate home arrangements.

Table 5	Pharmacotherapy for Acute Exacerbations of COPD	
Medication Name	**Dose**	
Albuterol	MDI: 2–4 puffs q1–4h	
	Nebulizer: 2.5 mg q1–4h	
Ipratropium	MDI: 2 puffs q4h	
	Nebulizer: 0.5 mg q4h	
Prednisone	30–40 mg qd × 7–10 days[a]	

Antibiotics

Patient Characteristics	Pathogens to Consider	Antibiotic[b] (One of the Following)
No risk factors for poor outcome or drug-resistant pathogen[c]	*Haemophilus influenza Streptococcus pneumonia Moraxella catarrhalis*	Macrolide, second- or third-generation cephalosporin, Doxycycline, Trimethoprim/ sulfamethoxazole
Risk factors present	As above, plus gram-negative rods, including *Pseudomonas*	Anti-pseudomonal fluoroquinolone or β-lactam

MDI, metered-dose inhaler.
[a]Indicated for all inpatients and most outpatients. Dosing recommendation from Global Initiative for Chronic Obstructive Lung Disease (GOLD) Global Strategy for the Diagnosis, Management, and Prevention of Chronic Obstructive Pulmonary Disease (Updated 2008). Available at www.goldcopd.com.
[b]Treat for 3 to 7 days. If recent antibiotic exposure, select an agent from an alternative class. Take local resistance patterns into account.
[c]Risk factors: age > 65, comorbid conditions (especially cardiac disease), $FEV_1 < 50\%$, > 3 exacerbations/yr, antibiotic therapy within the past 3 months (*Thorax 2006;61:337*).

Table 6	Indications and Contraindications for Noninvasive Ventilation in Acute Exacerbations of COPD
Indications	**Contraindications**
Moderate to severe dyspnea with evidence of increased work of breathing	Respiratory arrest
	Hemodynamic instability
Acute respiratory acidosis with pH ≤ 7.35 and/or $PaCO_2 > 45$ mm Hg (6.0 kPa)	Altered mental status, inability to cooperate
	High risk of aspiration
Respiratory rate > 25	Viscous or copious secretions
	Recent facial or gastroesophageal surgery
	Craniofacial trauma
	Fixed nasopharyngeal abnormalities
	Burns
	Extreme obesity

Modified from Global Initiative for Chronic Obstructive Lung Disease (GOLD) Global Strategy for the Diagnosis, Management, and Prevention of Chronic Obstructive Pulmonary Disease (Updated 2008). Available at www.goldcopd.com.

Table 7	Indications for Invasive Mechanical Ventilation in Acute Exacerbations of COPD

Failure to improve with or not a candidate for noninvasive ventilation (see Table 6)

Severe dyspnea with evidence of increased work of breathing

Acute respiratory acidosis with pH < 7.25 and/or $PaCO_2$ > 60 mm Hg (8.0 kPa)

PaO_2 < 40 mm Hg (5.3 kPa)

Respiratory rate > 35

Coexisting conditions such as cardiovascular disease, metabolic abnormalities, sepsis, pneumonia, pulmonary embolism, pneumothorax, large pleural effusion

Modified from Global Initiative for Chronic Obstructive Lung Disease (GOLD) Global Strategy for the Diagnosis, Management, and Prevention of Chronic Obstructive Pulmonary Disease (Updated 2008). Available at www.goldcopd.com.

- Prior to discharge from the hospital, chronic therapy issues should be readdressed including supplemental oxygen requirements, vaccinations, smoking cessation, assessment of inhaler technique, and pulmonary rehabilitation.

COMPLICATIONS

- Patients with severe COPD and chronic hypoxemia may develop PH and right heart failure.
- COPD patients are at increased risk for lung cancer, pneumothorax, arrhythmias, and psychiatric disorders such as anxiety and depression.
- Sleep disturbances are estimated to affect 50% of patients with COPD (http://aarc. org/resources/confronting_copd/exesum.pdf). Newer non-benzodiazepines medications such as zolpidem appear to be safe for use in patients with less severe COPD (*Proc Am Thorac Soc 2008;5:536*).

OUTCOME/PROGNOSIS

The BODE index (Table 8) is a composite of body mass index, airflow obstruction, dyspnea, and exercise tolerance that has been validated as a more accurate predictor of COPD mortality than FEV_1 alone (*N Engl J Med 2004;350:1005*).

Table 8	BODE Index			
	Points on BODE Index[a]			
Variable	**0**	**1**	**2**	**3**
FEV_1 (% of predicted)	≥65	50–64	36–49	≤35
Distance walked in 6 min (meters)	≥350	250–349	150–249	≤149
MMRC dyspnea scale	0–1	2	3	4
Body mass index	>21	≤21		

FEV_1, forced expiratory volume in the first second; MMRC, modified medical research council.
[a]The total possible cumulative values range from 0 to 10.
From Celli BR, Cote CG, Marin JM, et al. The body mass index, airflow obstruction, dyspnea, and exercise capacity index in chronic obstructive pulmonary disease. *N Engl J Med* 2004 Mar 4;350(10):1005–1012.

Asthma

GENERAL PRINCIPLES

Definition

- Asthma is an airway disease characterized by chronic inflammation, hyperresponsiveness, with exposure to a wide variety of stimuli, and obstruction with variable airflow limitation. As a consequence, patients have **paroxysms of cough, dyspnea, chest tightness, and wheezing.**
- **Asthma is a chronic disease, with episodic acute exacerbations that are interspersed with symptom-free periods.**
  - Exacerbations are characterized by a progressive increase in asthma symptoms that can last minutes to hours. They are associated with viral infections, allergens, and occupational exposures and occur when airway reactivity is increased and lung function becomes unstable.

Classification

- Asthma severity should be classified based on level of impairment (symptoms, lung function, and rescue medication use), risk (exacerbations, lung function decline, medication side effects), and responsiveness to treatment.
- At the initial evaluation, this assessment will determine level of severity in patients not on controller medications (Table 9). The level of severity is based upon the most severe category in which any feature appears. On subsequent visits or if the patient is on a controller medication, this assessment is based on the lowest step of therapy

Table 9		Classification of Severity on Initial Assessment		
	Intermittent	Mild Persistent	Moderate Persistent	Severe Persistent
Daytime symptoms	≤2×/wk	≥2×/wk but not daily	Daily	Continuous
Nighttime symptoms	≤2×/mo	3–4×/mo	≥1×/wk	Nightly
Activity limitations	None	Minor	Some	Extreme
Reliever medicine use	≤2×/wk	≥2×/wk but not daily	Daily	Frequent
FEV$_1$ or PEF	≥80%	≥80%	60–80%	<60%
Exacerbations	0–1×/yr	≥2×/yr	≥2×/yr	≥2×/yr
Management	Step 1	Step 2	Step 3 And consider Short-course OCS	Step 4 or 5 And consider Short-course OCS

OCS, oral corticosteroids; FEV$_1$, forced expiratory volume over 1 second; PEF, peak expiratory flow.
GINA Report, Global Strategy for Asthma Management and Prevention, 2008—www.ginasthma.org and National Asthma Education and Prevention Program-Expert Panel Report 3, 2007—http://www.nhlbi.nih.gov/guidelines/asthma/asthgdln.pdf.

Table 10	Assessment of Asthma Control		
	Well Controlled	Not Well Controlled	Very Poorly Controlled
Daytime symptoms	$\leq 2 \times$/wk	$> 2 \times$/wk	Continuous
Nighttime symptoms	None	$1-3 \times$/wk	$\geq 4 \times$/wk
Activity limitations	None	Some	Extreme
Reliever medicine use	$\leq 2 \times$/wk	$> 2 \times$/wk	Frequent
FEV_1 or PEF	$\geq 80\%$	60–80%	$\leq 60\%$
Validated questionnaire	ACT ≥ 20	ACT 16–19	ACT ≤ 15
Exacerbations	0–1/yr	$\geq 2 \times$/yr	$\geq 2 \times$/yr
Management	Maintain at lowest step possible	Step up one step	Step up one to two steps and consider short-course OCS
Follow-up	1–6 mo	2–6 wk	2 wk

FEV_1, forced expiratory volume over 1 second; PEF, peak expiratory flow; ACT, Asthma Control Test; OCS, oral corticosteroids.
GINA Report, Global Strategy for Asthma Management and Prevention, 2008—www.ginasthma. org and National Asthma Education and Prevention Program-Expert Panel Report 3, 2007—http://www.nhlbi.nih.gov/guidelines/asthma/asthgdln.pdf.

to maintain clinical control (Table 10). Control of asthma is based upon the most severe impairment or risk category.
• During an exacerbation, the acute severity of the attack should be classified based upon symptoms and signs and objective measures of lung function (Table 11).

Epidemiology

In the United States:

• Asthma is the leading chronic illness among children (20% to 30%).
• The prevalence of asthma and asthma-related mortality had been increasing from 1980 to the mid-1990s, but since the 2000s a stabilization in prevalence and decrease in mortality has occurred.
• African Americans are more likely than whites to be hospitalized and have a higher rate of mortality due to asthma.

Etiology

Possible factors for asthma development can be broadly divided into host, genetic and environmental factors.

• There have been multiple genes and chromosomal regions associated with the development of asthma. Racial and ethnic differences have also been reported in asthma but are likely the result of socioeconomic and environmental factors rather than genuine racial predispositions.

Table 11	Classification of Asthma Exacerbation Severity		
	Moderate	**Severe**	**Impending Respiratory Arrest**
FEV₁ or PEF predicted or personal best	40–69%	<40%	<25% or unable to measure
Symptoms	DOE or SOB with talking	SOB at rest	Severe SOB
Exam	Expiratory wheeze	Inspiratory and expiratory wheeze	Wheeze may become absent
	Some accessory muscle use	Accessory muscle use Chest retraction	Accessory muscle use with paradoxical diaphragmatic movement
		Agitation or confusion	Depressed mental status
Vitals	RR < 28/min HR < 110 O₂sat > 91% RA No pulsus paradoxus	RR > 28/min HR > 110 O₂sat < 91% RA Pulsus paradoxus > 25 mm Hg	Same as severe but could develop respiratory depression and/or bradycardia
PaCO₂	Normal to hypocapnic	>42 mm Hg	Hypercapnea is a late sign

RR, respiratory rate; HR, heart rate; SOB, short of breath; DOE, dyspnea on exertions; FEV_1, forced expiratory volume over 1 second; PEF, peak expiratory flow; RA, room air; O_2sat, oxygen saturation
GINA Report, Global Strategy for Asthma Management and Prevention, 2008—www.ginasthma. org and National Asthma Education and Prevention Program-Expert Panel Report 3, 2007—http://www.nhlbi.nih.gov/guidelines/asthma/asthgdln.pdf.

- There are multiple environmental factors that contribute to the development and persistence of asthma. Severe viral infection early in life, particularly respiratory syncytial virus (RSV) and rhinovirus, is associated with the development of asthma in childhood and plays a role in its pathogenesis.
- Childhood exposure and sensitization to a variety of allergens and irritants (e.g., cigarette smoke) may play a role in the development of asthma but the exact nature of this relationship is not yet fully elucidated.

Pathophysiology

Asthma is characterized by airway obstruction, hyperinflation, and airflow limitation resulting from multiple processes:

- Chronic airway inflammation characterized by infiltration of the airway wall, mucosa, and lumen by activated eosinophils, mast cells, macrophages, and T lymphocytes.

- Bronchial smooth muscle contraction resulting from mediators released by a variety of cell types including inflammatory, local neural, and epithelial cells.
- Epithelial damage manifested by denudation and desquamation of the epithelium leading to mucous plugs that obstruct the airway.
- Airway remodeling characterized by the following findings:
  - Subepithelial fibrosis, specifically thickening of the lamina reticularis from collagen deposition
  - Smooth muscle hypertrophy and hyperplasia
  - Goblet cell and submucosal gland hypertrophy and hyperplasia resulting in mucus hypersecretion
  - Airway angiogenesis
  - Airway wall thickening due to edema and cellular infiltration

Risk Factors

A number of factors increase airway hyperresponsiveness and can cause an acute and chronic increase in the severity of the disease:

- Allergens, such as dust mites, cockroaches, pollens, molds, and pet dander in susceptible patients
- Viral upper respiratory tract infections
- Many occupational allergens and irritants such as perfumes or detergents, even in small doses
- Cold air, strong emotional stimuli, and exercise
- Irritants, such as tobacco and wood smoke, can trigger acute bronchospasm and should be avoided by all patients
- Medications such as β-blockers (including ophthalmic preparations), aspirin, and nonsteroidal anti-inflammatory drugs (NSAIDs) can cause the sudden onset of severe airway obstruction

Prevention

- Strict compliance and appropriate follow-up can help prevent worsening of control.
- Identification and avoidance of risk factors (allergens, irritants) that exacerbate symptoms.
- All patients with asthma should receive a yearly influenza vaccination.

Associated Conditions

- Rhinosinusitis, with or without nasal polyps, is frequently present and should be treated with intranasal corticosteroids and/or antihistamines.
- Vocal cord dysfunction (VCD) can coexist or masquerade a severe, uncontrolled asthma. Treatment consists of speech and, if needed, behavioral therapy.
- Symptomatic gastroesophageal reflux disease (GERD) can cause cough and wheezing in some patients and may benefit from treatment with H2 blockers or proton pump inhibitors. Empiric treatment of GERD in asymptomatic patients with uncontrolled asthma is not warranted.
- Obesity is increasingly being recognized as a comorbid condition as well as possibly playing a role in worsening asthma control. Obese patients should be strongly encouraged to focus on weight loss through diet and exercise.
- Smoking prevalence in patients with asthma is the same as the general population. Although no convincing evidence links tobacco use with developing asthma, it may make patients less responsive to ICSs and more difficult to control. Tobacco cessation should be the goal.

- Obstructive sleep apnea (OSA) may make asthma more difficult to control and should be addressed with an overnight polysomnogram if suspected.

DIAGNOSIS

Clinical Presentation

History
- Recurring episodes of cough, dyspnea, chest tightness, and wheezing, most often at night or early morning, in the presence of potential triggers, and/or in a seasonal pattern.
- A personal or family history of atopy can increase the likelihood of asthma.
- Patients presenting for the first time over 50 years old or with >20 pack years of smoking are features that make asthma less likely as the cause of respiratory symptoms.

Physical Examination
- Auscultation of wheezing and possibly a prolonged expiratory phase can be present on exam but a normal chest exam does not exclude asthma.
- Signs of atopy, such as eczema, rhinitis, or nasal polyps, often coexist with asthma.
- During a suspected asthma exacerbation, a rapid assessment should be performed to identify those patients who require immediate intervention (Table 11):
  - Respiratory distress and/or peak flow <25% of predicted.
  - The presence or intensity of wheezing is an unreliable indicator of the severity of an attack.
  - Subcutaneous emphysema should alert the examiner to the presence of a pneumothorax or pneumomediastinum.

Diagnostic Criteria

- In general, the diagnosis is supported by the presence of symptoms consistent with asthma combined with demonstration of variable expiratory airflow obstruction.
- Adequate response to asthma treatment is a valid method to assist with making the diagnosis.

Differential Diagnosis

Other conditions may present with wheezing and must be considered, especially in patients who are not responsive to therapy (Table 12).

Diagnostic Testing

Laboratories
- Routine laboratory tests are not indicated for the diagnosis of asthma and should not delay the initiation of treatment.
- During an exacerbation, monitor oxygen saturation. ABG measurement should be considered in patients in severe distress or with an FEV_1 of <40% of predicted values after initial treatment.
  - A PaO_2 < 60 mm Hg is a sign of severe bronchoconstriction or of a complicating condition, such as pulmonary edema or pneumonia.
  - Initially, the $PaCO_2$ is low, due to an increase in respiratory rate. With a prolonged attack, the $PaCO_2$ may rise as a result of severe airway obstruction, increased dead-space ventilation, and respiratory muscle fatigue. A normal or increased $PaCO_2$ is a sign of impending respiratory failure and necessitates hospitalization.

Table 12	Conditions That Can Present as Refractory Asthma

Upper airway obstruction	**Congestive heart failure**
Tumor	**Gastroesophageal reflux**
Epiglottitis	**Sinusitis**
Vocal cord dysfunction	**Hypersensitivity pneumonitis**
Obstructive sleep apnea	**Churg–Strauss Syndrome**
Lower airway disease	**Eosinophilic pneumonia**
Allergic bronchopulmonary	**Adverse drug reaction**
aspergillosis	Aspirin
Chronic obstructive pulmonary disease	β-Adrenergic antagonist
Cystic fibrosis	Angiotensin-converting enzyme
Bronchiectasis	inhibitors
Bronchiolitis obliterans	Inhaled pentamidine
Tracheomalacia	**Hyperventilation with panic attacks**
Endobronchial lesion	**Dysfunctional breathlessness**
Foreign body	
Herpetic tracheobronchitis	

Imaging
- Obtaining a chest radiograph is not routinely required and is performed only if a complicating pulmonary process, such as pneumonia or pneumothorax, is suspected, or to rule out other causes of respiratory symptoms in patients being evaluated for asthma.
- High-resolution computerized tomography of the chest using a pulmonary embolus evaluation protocol can be considered in patients with severe asthma refractory to treatment to evaluate for alternative diagnosis.

Diagnostic Procedures
- Pulmonary function tests (PFTs) are essential to the diagnosis of asthma. In patients with asthma, PFTs demonstrate an obstructive pattern, the hallmark of which is a decrease in expiratory flow rates:
  - A reduction in FEV_1 and a proportionally smaller reduction in the FVC occur. This produces a decreased FEV_1/FVC ratio (generally <0.75). With mild obstructive disease that involves only the small airways, the FEV_1/FVC ratio may be normal, with the only abnormality being a decrease in airflow at midlung volumes (forced expiratory flow 25% to 75%).
  - The clinical diagnosis of asthma is supported by an obstructive pattern that improves after bronchodilator therapy. Improvement is defined as an increase in FEV_1 of >12% and 200 cc after two to four puffs of a short-acting bronchodilator. Most patients will not demonstrate reversibility at each assessment.
  - In patients with chronic, severe asthma, the airflow obstruction may no longer be completely reversible. In these patients, the most effective way to establish the maximal degree of airway reversibility is to repeat PFTs after a course of oral corticosteroids (usually 40 mg/d for 10 days). The lack of demonstrable airway obstruction or reactivity does not rule out a diagnosis of asthma.
  - In cases in which spirometry is normal, the diagnosis can be made by showing heightened airway responsiveness to a methacholine challenge. A methacholine

challenge is considered positive when a provocative concentration of 8 mg/mL or less causes a drop in FEV_1 of 20% (PC_{20}).

- An objective measurement of airflow obstruction is essential to the evaluation of an exacerbation. The severity of the exacerbation should be classified as:
  - Mild (PEF or FEV_1 > 70% of predicted or personal best),
  - Moderate (PEF or FEV_1 40% to 69%),
  - Severe (PEF or FEV_1 < 40%), or
  - Life-threatening/impending respiratory arrest (PEF or FEV_1 < 25%).

TREATMENT

- Medical management involves chronic management and a plan for acute exacerbations (asthma action plan). Most often it includes the daily use of an anti-inflammatory, disease-modifying medication (long-term-control medications) and as-needed use of a short-acting bronchodilator (quick-relief medications).
- The goals of daily management are to avoid impairment (lack of symptoms while maintaining normal activity and pulmonary function) and to minimize risk (preventing exacerbations, loss of lung function, medication side effects). Successful management requires patient education, objective measurement of airflow obstruction, and a medication plan for daily use and for exacerbations.
- When initiating therapy for a patient not already on controller medicine, one should assess patient's severity and assign the patient to the highest level in which any one feature has occurred over the previous 2 to 4 weeks (Table 9).
- Assessment of control on subsequent visits is used to modify therapy when following patients already on controller medication (Table 10).
- The goal of the stepwise approach is to gain control of symptoms as quickly as possible. At the same time, level of control varies over time, and consequently medication requirements as well, so therapy should be reviewed every 3 months to check whether stepwise reduction is possible (Fig. 1).
- Management of an exacerbation requiring hospital-based care should follow a treatment algorithm to triage patients based on response to treatment (Fig. 2).
  - The response to initial treatment (60 to 90 minutes, three treatments every 20 min with a short-acting bronchodilator) can be a better predictor of the need for hospitalization than is the severity of an exacerbation.
  - Patients at high risk of asthma-related death, including those with history of near-fatal asthma, increased hospitalization or emergency department (ED) care visits, oral corticosteroid use, overdependence on rapid-acting inhaled β_2-agonists, psychiatric or psychosocial difficulties, or noncompliance, should be advised to seek medical attention early in the course of an exacerbation.
  - A low threshold for admission is appropriate for patients with recent hospitalization, a failure of aggressive outpatient management (with oral corticosteroids), or a previous life-threatening attack.

Medications

First Line

- **Short-acting bronchodilators**
  - Quick-relief medications used on an as-needed basis for long-term management of all severities of asthma as well as for rapid treatment of exacerbations given via either MDI or nebulization.

	Step 1	Step 2	Step 3	Step 4	Step 5	Step 6
					If well-controlled for ≥3 mo, step down ⟵⟶ If not well-controlled, step up after addressing avoidance, adherence, comorbidities, and triggers	
Rapid medication	As-needed SABA					
Preferred controller medication	None	Low-dose ICS	Low-dose ICS + LABA or medium-dose ICS	Medium-dose ICS + LABA	High-dose ICS + LABA and evaluation for omalizumab	Add OCS to Step 5 medications
Alternate controller medication		LTRA or Cromolyn or sustained-released theophylline	Low-dose ICS with either LTM or sustained-release theophylline	Consider adding LTM and/or sustained-release theophylline		

Figure 1. Management algorithm based on level of control. ICS, inhaled corticosteroid; LABA, long-acting β_2-agonists; SABA, short-acting β_2-agonists; LTMs, leukotriene modifiers; LTRA, leukotriene receptor antagonists; OCS, oral corticosteroids. (GINA Report, Global Strategy for Asthma Management and Prevention, 2008—www.ginasthma.org and National Asthma Education and Prevention Program-Expert Panel Report 3, 2007—http://www.nhlbi.nih.gov/guidelines/asthma/asthgdln.pdf)

- For long-term management, a short-acting β_2-adrenergic agonist used on an as-needed basis (e.g., albuterol, two to three puffs every 6 hours) is appropriate.
- During an exacerbation, reversal of airflow obstruction is achieved most effectively by frequent administration of inhaled β_2-adrenergic agonists.
  - For a mild to moderate exacerbation, initial treatment starts with two to six puffs of albuterol via MDI or 2.5 mg via nebulizer and is repeated q20min until improvement is obtained or toxicity is noted.
  - For a severe exacerbation, albuterol, 2.5 to 5.0 mg q20min with ipratropium bromide, 0.5 mg q20min, should be administered via nebulizer. Alternatively, albuterol, 10.0 to 15.0 mg, administered continuously over an hour, may be more effective in severely obstructed adults. If used, telemetry monitoring is necessary.
  - Levalbuterol four to eight puffs or nebulized 1.25 to 2.5 mg q20min can be substituted for albuterol but has not been associated with less side effects in adults.
  - The subsequent dosing schedule is adjusted according to the patient's symptoms and clinical presentation. Often, patients require a β_2-adrenergic agonist q2–4h during an acute attack. The use of an MDI with a spacer device under supervision of trained personnel is as effective as aerosolized solution by nebulizer. Cooperation may not be possible in the patient with severe airflow obstruction.
  - Subcutaneous administration of β_2-adrenergic agonist is unnecessary if inhaled medications can be administered quickly with an adequate response. In rare settings, aqueous epinephrine (0.3 to 0.5 mL of a 1:1,000 solution SC q20min) or terbutaline (0.25 mg SC q20min) for up to three doses can be used. Their

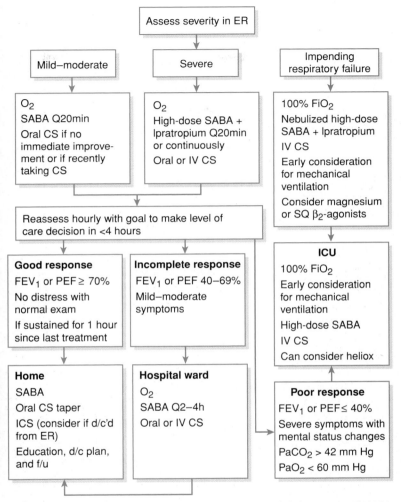

Figure 2. Treatment algorithm for asthma exacerbation. ICS, inhaled corticosteroid; SABA, short-acting β_2-agonists; CS, corticosteroids; d/c, discharge; PEF, peak expiratory flow; FEV$_1$, forced expiratory volume over 1 second. (GINA Report, Global Strategy for Asthma Management and Prevention, 2008—www.ginasthma.org and National Asthma Education and Prevention Program-Expert Panel Report 3, 2007—http://www.nhlbi.nih.gov/guidelines/asthma/asthgdln.pdf).

use is contraindicated if the patient has had an MI within the last 6 months or if having active angina. If used, electrocardiograph monitoring is necessary.

○ All short-acting β_2-adrenergic agonist now use hydrofluoroalkane (HFA) as a propellant. They should be primed with four puffs when first used and again if not used over 2 weeks.

- **Inhaled corticosteroids**
  - Are safe and effective for the treatment of persistent asthma. They are generally administered via a dry powder inhaler (DPI), MDI with a spacing device, or nebulized.
  - Dosing depends on assessment of severity and control (Table 13).

Table 13	Comparative Daily Adult Dosages for Inhaled Corticosteroids		
Drug	**Low Dose**	**Medium Dose**	**High Dose**
Triamcinolone (75 μg/puff)	4–10 puffs	10–20 puffs	>20 puffs
Beclomethasone dipropionate (40, 80 μg/puff)	4–12 puffs: 40 μg 2–6 puffs: 80 μg	12–20 puffs: 40 μg 6–8 puffs: 80 μg	>20 puffs: 40 μg >10 puffs: 80 μg
Budesonide Turbuhaler (DPI: 200 μg/dose)	1–2 inhalations	2–3 inhalations	>3 inhalations
Nebulized respules (250, 500 μg/ respules)	1–2 respules: 500 μg	2–4 respules: 500 μg	>4 respules: 500 μg
Ciclesonide (80, 160 μg/puff)	1–2 puffs: 80 μg	2–4 puffs: 80 μg	4–16 puffs: 80 μg
Flunisolide (250 μg/puff)	2–4 puffs	4–8 puffs	>8 puffs
Fluticasone	2–6 puffs: 44 μg	2–6 puffs: 100 μg	>6 puffs: 100 μg
(MDI: 44, 110, 220 μg/puff)	2 puffs: 110 μg	>3 puffs: 220 μg	
(DPI: 50, 100, 250 μg/dose)	2–6 inhalations: 50 μg	3–6 inhalations: 100 μg	>6 inhalations: 100 μg
Mometasone furoate (110, 220 μg/puff)	1 puff: 220 μg	2 puffs: 220 μg	3–4 puffs: 220 μg
Combination agents			
Budesonide/Formeterol (MDI: 80/4.5, 160/4.5 μg/puff)	1–2 puffs bid: 80/4.5 μg/ puff	2 puffs bid: 80/4.5 to 160/4.5 μg/ puff	2 puffs bid: 160/4.5 μg/ puff
Fluticasone/Salmeterol (MDI: 45/21, 115/21, 230/21 μg/puff) (DPI: 100/50, 250/50, 500/ 50 μg/dose)	1 inhalation bid: 100/ 50 μg	1 inhalation bid: 250/ 50 μg	1 inhalation bid: 500/ 50 μg

DPI, dry powder inhaler; MDI metered-dose inhaler; bid, twice daily.
GINA Report, Global Strategy for Asthma Management and Prevention, 2008—www.ginasthma.org and National Asthma Education and Prevention Program-Expert Panel Report 3, 2007—http://www.nhlbi.nih.gov/guidelines/asthma/asthgdln.pdf.

- Once-daily dosing of ICS may be as effective as twice-daily dosing in the management of mild persistent asthma and may improve adherence.
- Systemic corticosteroid absorption can occur in patients who use high doses of ICS. Consequently, prolonged therapy with high-dose ICS should be reserved for patients with severe disease or for those who otherwise require oral corticosteroids.
- Attempts should be made to decrease the dose of ICS every 2 to 3 months to the lowest possible dose to maintain control.
- **Long-acting inhaled β-agonists (LABA)**
  - Recommended for moderate and severe persistent asthma in patients not adequately controlled with ICS.
  - Salmeterol or the more fast-acting formoterol added to ICS have consistently been shown to improve lung function, both day and nighttime symptoms, reduce exacerbations, and minimize the required dose of ICS.
  - LABA should only be used in combination with ICS in patients with asthma (salmeterol/fluticasone, budesonide/formoterol).
  - The benefits of adding long-acting β_2-adrenergic agonists are more substantial than those achieved by leukotriene modifiers (LTMs), theophylline, or increased doses of ICS.
- **Systemic corticosteroids**
  - May be necessary to gain control of disease quickly via either oral or intravenous route.
  - If chronic symptoms are severe, accompanied by nighttime awakening, or PEF is <70% of predicted values, a short course of oral corticosteroid (prednisone 40 to 60 mg/d for 5 to 7 days) might be necessary.
  - Long-term therapy is occasionally necessary and should be started at prednisone 2 mg/kg/d, not to exceed 60 mg/d, and repeated attempts should be made to reduce the dose while they are receiving high-dose ICS.
  - During an exacerbation, systemic corticosteroids speed the resolution of exacerbations of asthma and should be administered to all patients.
    - *The ideal dose of corticosteroid needed to speed recovery and limit symptoms is not well defined.* Oral corticosteroid administration seems to be as effective as IV if given in equivalent doses (prednisone, 40 to 80 mg PO daily).
    - IV methylprednisolone, 125 mg, given on initial presentation decreases the rate of return to the ED of those patients who are discharged.
    - For maximal therapeutic response, tapering of high-dose corticosteroids should not take place until objective evidence of clinical improvement is observed (usually 36 to 48 hours or when PEF > 70%). Initially, patients are given a daily dose of oral prednisone, which is then reduced slowly.
    - A 7- to 14-day tapering dose of prednisone is usually successful in combination with an ICS instituted at the beginning of the tapering schedule. In patients with severe disease or with a history of respiratory failure, a slower reduction in dose is appropriate.
    - Patients discharged from the ED should receive oral corticosteroids. A dose of prednisone, 40 mg/d for 5 to 7 days, can be substituted for a tapering schedule in selected patients. Either regimen should be accompanied by the initiation of an ICS or an increase in the previous dose of ICS.

Second Line
- **Leukotriene modifiers**
  - **Montelukast** (10 mg PO daily) and **zafirlukast** (20 mg PO bid) are oral leukotriene-receptor antagonists (LTRAs) and zileuton (extended-release 1200 mg

BID) is an oral 5-lipoxygenase inhibitor. The LTRAs are recommended as an alternative medication for mild persistent asthma and all LTMs are recommended as an add-on to ICS for more severe forms of asthma.

- As add-on therapy to ICS, these agents have been shown to improve lung function, lead to improved quality of life, and lead to fewer exacerbations. However, in comparison to ICS + LABA, they are not as effective in improving asthma outcomes.
- **An LTM should be strongly considered for patients with aspirin-induced asthma or for individuals who cannot master the use of an inhaler.**
- **Cromolyn sodium**
  - Anti-inflammatory inhaled medication is an alternative to ICS in children with mild persistent asthma or first-line for exercised-induced asthma. The usual dosage is 8 to 12 puffs/d in three to four divided doses. Maximum improvement may be delayed for 4 to 6 weeks after initiation of therapy.
  - Little additional benefit accrues from using cromolyn with an ICS.
- **Anti-IgE therapy**
  - **Omalizumab** is a monoclonal antibody against IgE that is approved for the management of patients with moderate to severe persistent asthma with a demonstrable sensitivity to a perennial aeroallergen and incomplete control with ICS.
  - It is administered subcutaneously q2–4wk and dosed based upon the patient's baseline IgE level (if between 30 and 700 International Units/mL) and weight.
  - Addition of omalizumab has been shown to reduce exacerbation rates and need for corticosteroids.
- **Methylxanthines:** Sustained-release theophylline at low doses (300 mg/d) may be useful as adjuvant therapy to an anti-inflammatory agent in persistent asthma, especially for controlling nighttime symptoms.
- **Intravenous Magnesium Sulfate:** During a severe exacerbation refractory to standard treatment over 1 hour, one dose of 2 g IV over 20 minutes in the ED should be considered. It has been shown to acutely improve lung function especially in those with severe, life-threatening exacerbations.
- **Inhaled Heliox:** During a severe exacerbation refractory to standard treatment over 1 hour, heliox-driven albuterol nebulization in a mixture with oxygen (70:30) should be considered. It has been shown to acutely improve lung function, especially in those with severe, life-threatening exacerbations.
- **Alternative medications**
  - Add-on therapy to ICS with omalizumab, LTM, or theophylline can be considered.
  - Immunosuppressive medications to reduce the need for chronic oral corticosteroids are rarely used.
- **Antibiotics:** Have not been shown to have any benefit when used to treat exacerbations. They can only be recommended as needed for treatment of comorbid conditions, such as pneumonia or bacterial sinusitis.

Other Nonoperative Therapies

- **Supplemental oxygen** should be administered to the patient who is awaiting an assessment of arterial oxygen tension and should be continued to maintain an O_2 sat > 92% (95% in patients with coexisting cardiac disease or pregnancy).
- **Mechanical ventilation** may be required for respiratory failure.
  - General principles include use of **large ETT ≥ 7.5 mm**, **low tidal volumes**, **prolonged expiratory time with high inspiratory flows** and **low respiratory rate**, and in some patients **permissive hypercapnia,** with goal to avoid

dynamic hyperinflation (elevated plateau pressures and autopositive end expiratory pressures).
- Heavy sedation may be needed and should be maximized before considering using paralytics given their adverse side effects.
- Evidence is lacking to suggest modes of noninvasive ventilation are beneficial.
- Subcutaneous injection allergen immunotherapy can be considered in allergic patients with mild to moderate disease with persistent symptoms despite adherence to allergen avoidance and medication.

Lifestyle/Risk Modification

Diet
There is no general diet that is known to improve asthma control. However, a small percentage of patients may have reproducible deterioration after exposure to dietary sulfites used to prevent discoloration in foods such as beer, wine, processed potatoes, dried fruit, and should be avoided in these patients.

Activity
Patients should be encouraged to lead an active lifestyle. If their asthma is well controlled, they should expect to be as physically active as they desire.

- If exercise is a trigger, patients should be advised to continue physical activity after prophylactic use of LTM or an inhaled β_2-adrenergic agonist (two to four puffs 20 minutes before exposure).

SPECIAL CONSIDERATIONS

- During pregnancy, patients should have more frequent follow-up as the severity often changes and requires medication adjustment. **There is more potential risk to the fetus with poorly controlled asthma compared to asthma medication exposure, most of which are generally considered safe.**
- Occupational asthma requires a detailed history of occupational exposure to a sensitizing agent, lack of asthma symptoms prior to exposure, and a documented relationship with symptoms and the workplace. Beyond standard asthma medical treatment, exposure avoidance is crucial.
- Patients with aspirin sensitivity and nasal polyps typically have the onset of asthma in the third or fourth decade of life. A precipitous onset of symptoms should raise the possibility of reaction to acute ingestion of aspirin or an NSAID.

COMPLICATIONS

Medication side effects

- **SABA:** Sympathomimetic-type (tremor, anxiety, tachycardia), decrease in serum potassium and magnesium, mild lactic acidosis, prolonged QT_c
- **ICS**
  - Increased risk for systemic effects at high doses (equivalent >1,000 μg of beclomethasone per day) including skin bruising, cataracts, elevated intraocular pressure, and accelerated loss of bone mass.
  - Pharyngeal and laryngeal effects are common such as sore throat, hoarse voice, and oral candidiasis. **Patients should be instructed to rinse their mouth after each**

administration to reduce the possibility of thrush and a change in the delivery method and/or use of a valved holding chamber/spacer may alleviate the other side effects.

- **LABA**
  - Minimal sympathomimetic-type effects.
  - Associated with an increased risk of severe asthma exacerbations and asthma-related death, based on the Salmeterol Multi-center Asthma Research Trial (SMART) that showed a very low but significant increase in asthma-related deaths in patients receiving salmeterol (0.01% to 0.04%).
  - Should only be used in combination with ICS.
- **LTM**
  - Cases of newly diagnosed Churg–Strauss vasculitis after exposure to LTRA have been described but it is unclear if it is related to unmasking of a preexisting case with concurrent corticosteroid tapering or if there is a causal relationship.
  - Zileuton can cause a reversible hepatitis so it is recommended that hepatic function be monitored at initiation, once a month during the first 3 months, every 3 months for the first year, and then periodically.
- **Omalizumab (anti-IgE) therapy:** Anaphylaxis occurs in 1 to 2 per 1,000, usually within 2 hours of the first doses. For this reason, patients should be medically observed 2 hours after the initial doses and then 30 minutes for subsequent dosings as well as possess a self-administered epinephrine for 24 hours after each dose.
- **Methylxanthines**
  - Theophylline has a narrow therapeutic range with significant toxicities, such as arrhythmias and seizures, as well as many potential drug interactions, especially with antibiotics.
  - Serum concentrations of theophylline should be monitored on a regular basis, aiming for a level of 5 to 10 μg/mL; however at the lower doses used for asthma, toxicity is much less likely.

REFERRAL

- Patients who require step 4 or higher treatment or if they have had a life-threatening asthma exacerbation.
- Patients being considered for anti-IgE therapy or other alternative treatment.
- Patients with atypical signs or symptoms that make the diagnosis uncertain.
- Patients with comorbidities such as chronic sinusitis, nasal polyposis, allergic bronchopulmonary aspergillosis (ABPA), VCD, severe GERD, severe rhinitis, or significant psychiatric or psychosocial difficulties interfering with treatment.
- Patients requiring additional diagnostic testing, such as rhinoscopy or bronchoscopy, bronchoprovocation testing, or allergy skin testing.
- Patients with a need to be evaluated for allergen immunotherapy.

PATIENT EDUCATION

- Patient education should focus on the chronic and inflammatory nature of asthma, with identification of factors that contribute to increased inflammation.
  - The consequences of ongoing exposure to chronic irritants or allergens and the rationale for therapy should be explained. Patients should be instructed to avoid factors that aggravate their disease, how to manage their daily medications, and

how to recognize and deal with acute exacerbations (known as an asthma action plan).
- The use of a *written* daily management plan as part of the education strategy is recommended for all patients with persistent asthma.
- It is important for patients to recognize signs of poorly controlled disease.
  - These signs include an increased or daily need for bronchodilators, limitation of activity, waking at night because of asthma symptoms, and variability in the PEF.
  - Specific instructions about handling these symptoms, including criteria for seeking emergency care, should be provided.

MONITORING/FOLLOW-UP

- PEF monitoring provides an objective measurement of airflow obstruction and can be considered in patients with moderate to severe persistent asthma. However, symptom-based asthma action plans are equivalent to PEF-based plans in terms of overall self-management and control.
  - The personal-best PEF (the highest PEF obtained when the disease is under control) is identified, and the PEF is checked when symptoms escalate or in the setting of an asthma trigger. This should be incorporated into an asthma action plan, setting 80% to 100% of personal-best PEF as the "green" zone, 50% to 80% as the "yellow" zone, and <50% as the "red" zone.
- Patients should learn to anticipate situations that cause increased symptoms. For most individuals, monitoring symptoms instead of PEF is sufficient (symptom-based asthma action plan).
- Questionnaires can also provide objective monitoring of asthma control. The Asthma Control Test (ACT) or Asthma Control Questionnaire (ACQ) are useful instruments to rapidly assess patient-reported asthma control.

OUTCOME/PROGNOSIS

- Most patients with asthma can be effectively treated and achieve good control of their disease when following the stepwise treatment approach. Goals should be to be free from troublesome symptoms, minimal use of reliever medication, near-normal lung function, absence of serious attacks, and ability to lead a physically, active life.
- Previous exacerbations that have required the use of oral corticosteroids, led to respiratory failure, use of more than two canisters per month of inhaled short-acting bronchodilator, and seizures with asthma attacks have been associated with severe and potentially fatal asthma.

ADDITIONAL RESOURCES

- Global Strategy for Asthma Management and Prevention. Global Initiative for Asthma (GINA). Full text available online at http://www.ginasthma.com.
- National Asthma Education and Prevention Program: Expert Panel Report III: Guidelines for the Diagnosis and Management of Asthma. Bethesda, MD: National Heart, Lung, and Blood Institute, 2007. Full text available online at http://www.nhlbi.nih.gov/guidelines/asthma/asthgdln.htm.
- ACT at http://www.asthmacontrol.com or ACQ at http://www.qoltech.co.uk/acq.html.

Obstructive Sleep Apnea–Hypopnea Syndrome

GENERAL PRINCIPLES

Definition

Obstructive sleep apnea–hypopnea syndrome (OSAHS) is a disorder in which patients experience apneas (cessation of breathing) or hypopneas (shallow breathing) due to upper airway narrowing, and is associated with excessive daytime somnolence (*Sleep 1999;22:667*).

Epidemiology

- Lack of recognition and diagnosis of OSAHS is a significant problem.
- National and international data estimate the prevalence of OSAHS to be 3% to 7% in adult males and 2% to 5% in adult females (*Proc Am Thorac Soc 2008;5:136*).

Pathophysiology

Sleep apnea may be central, obstructive, or a combination of both. In central sleep apnea, the absent central drive to breathe results in no respiratory effort and no airflow, despite adequate airway patency. However, most cases of sleep apnea are OSA and result from decreased or absent respiratory airflow due to narrowing or collapse of the upper airway. The fragmentation of sleep resulting from these abnormal breathing events can cause excessive daytime sleepiness (OSAHS).

Risk Factors

Risk factors commonly associated with OSAHS include obesity, nasal obstruction, adenoidal or tonsillar hypertrophy, micrognathia, retrognathia, macroglossia, acromegaly, hypothyroidism, vocal cord paralysis, and bulbar involvement from neuromuscular disease (*Otolaryngol Clin North Am 1990;23:727*).

Associated Conditions

- Patients with OSAHS often have associated cardiovascular disease, including systemic hypertension, heart failure, arrhythmia, myocardial infarction, and stroke (*Circulation 2008;118:1080*).
- Patients with OSAHS have an increased risk of death, mainly due to cardiovascular events (*Sleep 2008;31:1071; Sleep 2008;31:1079; N Engl J Med 2005;353:2034*).
- An increased prevalence of diabetes has been noted in patients with OSAHS, independent of the effect of obesity (*Am J Respir Crit Care Med 2005;172:1590; J Clin Endocrinol Metab 2000;85:1151*).
- OSAHS is associated with a higher risk of motor vehicle accidents (*Sleep 1997; 20:608*).

DIAGNOSIS

Clinical Presentation

History

- Habitual loud snoring is the most common symptom of OSAHS, although not all people who snore have this syndrome.
- Excessive daytime sleepiness (daytime hypersomnolence) is a classic symptom of OSAHS (Table 14). Patients may describe falling asleep while driving or having difficulty concentrating at work.

Table 14	Symptoms Associated With Obstructive Sleep Apnea–Hypopnea Syndrome
Excessive daytime sleepiness	Enuresis
Snoring	Awakening unrefreshed
Nocturnal arousals	Morning headaches
Nocturnal apneas	Impaired memory and concentration
Nocturnal gasping, grunting, and choking	Irritability and depression
Nocturia	Impotence

- Patients may also complain of personality changes, intellectual deterioration, morning headaches, automatic behavior, loss of libido, and chronic fatigue.
- Subjective sleepiness can be assessed by a validated scale, such as the Epworth Sleepiness Scale (Table 15) (*Sleep 1991;14:540*).

Physical Examination
- All patients should have a thorough nose and throat examination to detect sources of upper airway obstruction that are surgically correctable (e.g., septal deviation, enlarged tonsils, enlarged uvula), especially if continuous positive airway pressure (CPAP; see Other Nonoperative Therapies) is poorly tolerated.
- Increased severity of OSA has been associated with a higher class on the Mallampati score (Table 16) (*Eur Respir J 2003;21:248*).

Differential Diagnosis

In addition to OSAHS and sleep-related hypoventilation, the differential diagnosis for daytime sleepiness includes sleep deprivation, periodic limb movement disorder, narcolepsy, and medication side effects.

Table 15	Epworth Sleepiness Scale

How likely are you to doze off or fall asleep in the following situations, in contrast to just feeling tired? This refers to your usual way of life in recent times. Even if you have not done some of these things recently, try to work out how they would have affected you. Use the following scale to choose the most appropriate number for each situation:

0 = would never doze   2 = moderate chance of dozing
1 = slight chance of dozing   3 = high chance of dozing

Situation
Sitting and reading
Watching TV
Sitting, inactive, in a public place
Sitting as a passenger in a car for an hour
Lying down in the afternoon
Sitting and talking to someone
Sitting quietly after a lunch without alcohol
Sitting in a car, while stopped for a few minutes in traffic

Note: The scores for each situation are summed to obtain the Epworth score. An Epworth score >10 suggests that significant daytime sleepiness is present.
Adapted from *Sleep* 1991;14:541.

Table 16	Mallampati Airway Classification
Class	**Visible Structures with Mouth Maximally Open and Tongue Protruded**
I	Hard palate, soft palate, uvula, tonsillar pillars
II	Hard palate, soft palate, uvula
III	Hard palate, soft palate, base of uvula
IV	Hard palate

From Mallampati SR, Gatt SP, Gugino LD, et al. A clinical sign to predict difficult tracheal intubation: a prospective study. *Can Anaesth Soc J* 1985 Jul;32(4):429–434.

Diagnostic Testing

- The gold standard for the diagnosis of OSAHS is overnight polysomnography (PSG or "sleep study") with direct observation by a qualified technician (*Am Rev Respir Dis 1989;139:559*). Sleep studies are typically performed in the outpatient setting.
- Typical indications for a sleep study include snoring with excessive daytime sleepiness, titration of optimal positive airway pressure therapy, and assessment of objective response to therapeutic interventions.
- PSG involves determination of sleep stages using electroencephalography, electromyography, and electro-oculography, and assessment of respiratory airflow and effort, oxyhemoglobin saturation, cardiac electrical activity (ECG), and body position.
- The sleep study is analyzed for sleep staging, the frequency of respiratory events, limb movements, and abnormal behaviors. Respiratory events are categorized as obstructive or central.
  - **Obstructive:** Airflow is absent or reduced despite continuous respiratory efforts.
  - **Central:** Airflow and respiratory effort are absent.
- The apnea–hypopnea index (AHI) is used to diagnose sleep-disordered breathing and to quantify its severity. All events must have a duration of at least 10 seconds to qualify.
  - Apnea is defined as airflow < 20% of baseline.
  - Hypopnea is defined as a >30% reduction in baseline airflow that must be associated with at least a 4% decrease in oxygen saturation (*Sleep 2001;24:469*).
  - **The AHI is the sum of apneic and hypopneic episodes per hour of sleep.** The respiratory disturbance index (RDI) may also be reported and can include events that do not qualify for the AHI, such as snore arousals or respiratory effort–related arousals.
- OSA is present when a sleep study shows an AHI ≥ 5 in a symptomatic patient. **Mild OSA has an AHI of 5 to 15, moderate OSA has an AHI of 16 to 30, and severe OSA has an AHI > 30** (*Sleep 1999;22:667*).
- The risk of death, hypertension, and poor neuropsychological functioning rises with increasing severity of OSA.
- Most sleep studies are performed as "split studies," where the first few hours of the study are diagnostic and the latter part of the study is used for CPAP titration if the AHI is consistent with moderate to severe OSA. Because some patients only have significant events when lying in certain positions (usually supine) or during rapid eye movement (REM) sleep, these patients may require a complete overnight study for diagnosis and a full second overnight study for initiation of therapy.

• Recognizing the cost, required manpower, and limited availability of PSG, the American Academy of Sleep Medicine supports the use of unattended portable monitoring as an alternative to PSG for patients with a high pretest probability of moderate to severe OSA without significant comorbid medical or sleep disorders (*J Clin Sleep Med 2007;3:737*).

TREATMENT

The therapeutic approach to OSAHS depends on the severity of the disease, the underlying medical conditions, the cardiopulmonary sequelae, and the expected degree of patient compliance. Treatment must be highly individualized, with special attention to correcting potentially reversible exacerbating factors.

Medications

• No pharmacologic agent has sufficient efficacy to warrant replacement of positive airway pressure as the primary therapeutic modality for OSAHS.
• **Modafinil** may improve daytime sleepiness in patients with persistent symptoms despite adequate CPAP use (*Sleep 2006;29:31*).
• Nasal saline and decongestants help with dryness and congestion associated with use of positive airway pressure.

Other Nonoperative Therapies

• **Positive airway pressure**
  • **CPAP** delivers air via a face mask with the goal of pneumatically splinting open the upper airway, thus preventing collapse and airflow obstruction.
  • The benefits of positive airway pressure include consolidated sleep and decreased daytime hypersomnolence in almost all patients. Hypertension, nocturia, peripheral edema, polycythemia, and PH may also improve. Additionally, CPAP is a highly cost-effective intervention (*Can J Physiol Pharmacol 2007;85:179*), appears to reduce the risk of cardiovascular events (*Am J Respir Crit Care Med 2007;176:1274*), and may be associated with increased survival (*Chest 1988;94:9*).
  • **Nasal CPAP (nCPAP) is the current treatment of choice for most patients with OSAHS.** The compliance rate with nCPAP is approximately 50%. Compliance can be improved with education, instruction, follow-up, adjustment of the mask for fit and comfort, humidification of the air to decrease dryness, and treatment of nasal or sinus symptoms. Use of a full face mask (oronasal) has not been shown to improve compliance compared to the use of nCPAP. However, full face masks are frequently used in patients who "mouth breathe" or patients who require higher CPAP pressures, as they will often experience air leak through the mouth when using nCPAP.
  • The PSG determines the positive airway pressure (expressed in cm H_2O) required to optimize airflow. The pressure setting is gradually increased until obstructive events, snoring, and oxygen desaturations are minimized.
  • Autotitrating or "smart" CPAP machines use flow and pressure transducers to sense airflow patterns and then automatically adjust the pressure setting in response. Small studies have shown that autotitrating CPAP may be as effective as traditional CPAP and appears to be preferred by patients (*Respiration 2007;74:279*; *Chest 2006;129:638*).
  • Bilevel positive airway pressure (BiPAP) can be used to treat patients with OSAHS. BiPAP is more expensive than CPAP and does not improve patient compliance.

Patients with intolerance of very high levels of CPAP, a poor response to CPAP, or concomitant alveolar hypoventilation may respond well to noninvasive mechanical ventilation with BiPAP or volume ventilation.

- All noninvasive positive pressure or mechanical ventilation devices may induce dryness of the airway, nasal congestion, rhinorrhea, epistaxis, skin reactions to the mask, nasal bridge abrasions, and aerophagia.
- Some patients, such as those with COPD, require supplemental oxygen to maintain adequate nocturnal oxygen saturations ($SaO_2 \geq 90\%$).
- Oral appliances for mild OSAHS, such as the mandibular repositioning device, aim to increase airway size to improve airflow. The devices can be fixed or adjustable, and most require customized fitting. Many devices have not been well studied.
  - Contraindications include temporomandibular joint disease, bruxism, full dentures, and inability to protrude the mandible.
- Concomitant conditions (e.g., COPD, hypertension, hypothyroidism) should be treated in the standard fashion.

Surgical Management

- **Tracheostomy**
  - Tracheostomy is very effective in treating OSAHS, but is rarely used since the advent of positive airway pressure therapy.
  - Tracheostomy should be reserved for patients with life-threatening disease (cor pulmonale, arrhythmias, or severe hypoxemia) or significant alveolar hypoventilation that cannot be controlled with other measures.
- **Uvulopalatopharyngoplasty**
  - Uvulopalatopharyngoplasty (UPPP) is the most common surgical treatment of mild to moderate OSAHS in patients who do not respond to medical therapy.
  - UPPP enlarges the airway by removing tissue from the tonsils, tonsillar pillars, uvula, and posterior palate. UPPP may be complicated by change in voice, nasopharyngeal stenosis, foreign body sensation, velopharyngeal insufficiency with associated nasal regurgitation during swallowing, and CPAP tolerance problems.
  - The success rate of UPPP for treatment of OSAHS is only approximately 50%, when defined as a 50% reduction of the AHI, and improvements related to UPPP may diminish over time (*Sleep 1996;19:156*). Thus, UPPP is considered a second-line treatment for patients with mild to moderate OSAHS who cannot successfully use CPAP and who have retropalatal obstruction.
- In experienced centers, other staged procedures for OSA can be performed, including mandibular osteotomy with genioglossus advancement, hyoid myotomy with suspension, and maxillomandibular advancement (*Sleep Breath 2000;4:137*).

Lifestyle/Risk Modification

- Weight reduction for the obese is recommended (*Chest 1987;92:631*).
- OSAHS patients should avoid use of alcohol, tobacco, and sedatives.
- Clinicians should counsel patients with OSAHS regarding the increased risk of driving and operating dangerous equipment.

COMPLICATIONS

- When OSAHS is associated with disorders such as obesity and chronic lung disease, patients may develop hypoxemia, hypercapnia, polycythemia, PH, and cor pulmonale (*Mayo Clin Proc 1990;65:1087*).

- Patients with OSAHS are at greater risk for perioperative complications, due to intubation difficulty and/or impaired arousal secondary to the effects of anesthetics, narcotics, and sedatives (*Otolaryngol Clin North Am 2007;40:877*).

REFERRAL

Patients with risk factors and symptoms or sequelae of OSAHS should be referred to a sleep specialist and sleep laboratory for further evaluation.

Pulmonary Hypertension

GENERAL PRINCIPLES

Definition
Pulmonary hypertension (PH) is the sustained elevation of the mean pulmonary artery pressure (≥ 25 mm Hg at rest).

Classification
- PH is subcategorized into five major groups (Table 17):
  - Group I—**Pulmonary arterial hypertension (PAH)**
  - Group II—**PH due to left heart disease**
  - Group III—**PH due to lung diseases and/or hypoxemia**
  - Group IV—**Chronic thromboembolic PH**
  - Group V—**PH with unclear multifactorial mechanisms**
- **PAH** represents a specific group of disorders with similar pathologies and clinical presentation, with a propensity for right heart failure in the absence of elevated left-sided pressures.

Epidemiology
- PH is most often due to left heart disease or parenchymal lung disease.
- **Idiopathic pulmonary arterial hypertension (IPAH)** is a rare disorder with an estimated prevalence of six to nine cases per million compared to an overall PAH prevalence of 15 to 26 cases per million (*Am J Respir Crit Care Med 2006;173:1023; Eur Respir J 2007;30:104*).
  - Average age at diagnosis of PAH is ~50 years (*Am J Respir Crit Care Med 2006;173:1023; Eur Respir J 2007;30:1103*).
- Despite increased awareness, PAH continues to be detected late in its course, with a reported delay of 27 months from symptom onset (*Am J Respir Crit Care Med 2006;173:1023*).
  - Majority display advanced functional and hemodynamic compromise at diagnosis.
- While IPAH has been the most common form of PAH, PAH associated with systemic sclerosis is becoming a more common entity (*Eur Respir J 2007;30:1103*).
- Incidence of **chronic thromboembolic pulmonary hypertension (CTEPH)** may be as high as 4% among survivors of acute pulmonary embolism (*N Engl J Med 2004;350:2257*).
- 1-, 3-, and 5-year survival rates are 84%, 67%, and 58%, respectively, with a median survival of 3.6 years (*Eur Respir J 2007;30:1103*).

Table 17

Clinical Classification of Pulmonary Hypertension: Dana Point (2008) Classification System of Pulmonary Hypertension.

I. Pulmonary arterial hypertension (PAH)
Idiopathic PAH
Heritable:
    BMPR2
    ALK1 or endoglin
    Unknown
Associated with:
    Connective tissue diseases
    HIV infection
    Portal hypertension
    Congenital heart diseases
    Schistosomiasis
    Chronic hemolytic anemia
    Persistent PH of the newborn
Pulmonary veno-occlusive disease and/or pulmonary capillary hemangiomatosis

II. Pulmonary hypertension due to left heart disease
Systolic dysfunction
Diastolic dysfunction
Valvular disease

III. Pulmonary hypertension due to lung diseases and/or hypoxemia
Chronic obstructive lung disease
Interstitial lung disease
Other pulmonary diseases with mixed obstructive and restrictive pattern
Sleep-disordered breathing
Alveolar hypoventilation disorders
Chronic exposure to high altitude
Developmental abnormalities

IV. Chronic thromboembolic pulmonary hypertension (CTEPH)

V. Pulmonary hypertension with unclear multifactorial mechanisms
Hematologic disorders:
    Myeloproliferative disorders
    Post-splenectomy
Systemic diseases:
    Sarcoidosis
    Pulmonary Langerhans cell histiocytosis
    Lymphangioleiomyomatosis
    Neurofibromatosis
    Vasculitis
Metabolic disorders:
    Glycogen storage disease
    Gaucher disease
    Thyroid disorders
Miscellaneous:
    Tumoral obstruction
    Fibrosing mediastinitis
    Chronic renal failure on hemodialysis

From Simonneau G, Robbins IM, Beghetti M, et al. Updated clinical classification of pulmonary hypertension. *J Am Coll Cardiol* 2009 Jun 30;54(1 Suppl):S43–S54, with permission.

Pathophysiology

- The pathogenesis of PAH involves a complex interplay of factors that result in progressive vascular remodeling with endothelial cell and smooth-muscle proliferation, vasoconstriction, as well as thrombosis of small- and medium-sized pulmonary arteries.
- Complex origins of PAH probably include infectious/environmental insults or comorbid conditions in the setting of some form of genetic predisposition.
- Central physiologic abnormality of PH is increased right ventricular (RV) afterload with an elevated pulmonary vascular resistance (PVR).
- Chronically elevated RV afterload affects RV contractility and cardiac output.
- Unlike the left ventricle, the right ventricle has limited ability to overcome high afterload.
  - Initially, cardiac output diminishes during strenuous exercise. As PH severity worsens, maximal cardiac output is achieved at progressively lower workloads; ultimately resting cardiac output is reduced.
- The most common cause of death in patients with PAH is right heart failure.
- In advanced stages, pulmonary artery pressures decline as the right ventricle fails to generate enough blood flow and high pressures.
- Origins of PH in other categories vary and can include hypoxemia-mediated vasoconstriction and remodeling, parenchymal destruction, compression of vasculature, and high postcapillary pressures.

DIAGNOSIS

- Diagnostic testing should **(a) confirm clinical suspicion of PH, (b) determine etiology of PH, and (c) gauge severity of condition, which assists with treatment planning.**
- Acute illnesses (e.g., pulmonary edema, pulmonary embolism, adult respiratory distress syndrome) can cause *acute* **PH** that is *mild* (pulmonary artery systolic pressure [PASP] < 50) or can worsen preexisting PH. Evaluation of *chronic* PH becomes necessary if pulmonary artery pressures remain elevated after resolution of the acute process.
- If chronic PH is considered based on clinical suspicion or during the evaluation of a vulnerable population (e.g., first-degree relative of IPAH patient, liver transplant candidate, or patient with scleroderma or prior veno-thromboembolic event), transthoracic echocardiogram (TTE) should be the initial test. Additional studies, as outlined below and in Figure 3, should be completed if PAH is still a consideration after echocardiography (*Chest 2004;126:14S*).
- **Transthoracic echocardiogram with Doppler and agitated saline injection**
  - Preferred test for initial evaluation of suspected PH.
  - **Estimate PASP** by Doppler interrogation of tricuspid valve regurgitant jet; absence of tricuspid regurgitation does not exclude elevated pulmonary artery pressure. Sensitivity for PH is 80% to 100% and correlation coefficient with invasive measurement is 0.6 to 0.9 (*Chest 2004;126:14S–34S*). **However, invasive measurement is recommended if suspicion of PH remains despite a normal estimation by echocardiogram.**
  - **Assess RV pressure overload and degree of dysfunction** (e.g., RV hypertrophy and/or dilation, RV hypokinesis, displaced intraventricular septum, paradoxical septal motion, left ventricular compression, and pericardial effusion from impaired pericardial drainage).

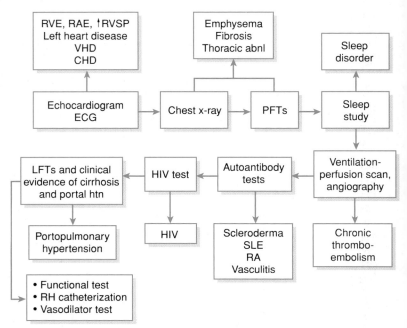

Figure 3. Diagnostic flow-chart for the evaluation of unexplained pulmonary hypertension. RVE, right ventricular enlargement; RAE, right atrial enlargement; RVSP, right ventricular systolic pressure; VHD, valvular heart disease; CHD, congenital heart disease; RH, Right Heart; SLE, systemic lupus erythematosus; RA, rheumatoid arthritis. (From McLaughlin VV, McGoon MD. Pulmonary arterial hypertension. *Circulation* 2006 Sep 26;114(13):1417–1431, with permission.)

- **Identify etiologies for PH** (e.g., left ventricular systolic or diastolic dysfunction, left-sided valvular disease, left atrial structural anomalies, and congenital systemic to pulmonary shunts).
- Transesophageal echocardiogram (TEE) is indicated to exclude intracardiac shunts that may be suspected by TTE, although majority of such shunts are a patent foramen ovale.
- **Pulmonary function testing**
  - Spirometry and lung volumes to assess for obstructive (e.g., **chronic obstructive lung disease**) or restrictive (e.g., interstitial lung disease [ILD]) ventilatory abnormalities.
  - Diffusing capacity for carbon monoxide is usually reduced with parenchymal lung diseases, but isolated mild–moderate reduction is often encountered in PAH.
- **ABG:** Elevated $PaCO_2$ is an important clue for a hypoventilation syndrome.
- **Six-minute walk (6MW) or simple exercise test**
  - Unexplained exercise-induced desaturation could indicate PH.
  - Distance walked correlates with World Health Organization (WHO) **functional classification** (Table 18) and provides intermediate-term **prognostic information** (*Am J Respir Crit Care Med 2000;161:487*).

Table 18	Functional Assessment for Patients with PH
Class I	No limitation of physical activity. Ordinary physical activity does not cause undue dyspnea or fatigue, chest pain, or near syncope.
Class II	Slight limitation of physical activity. Comfortable at rest. Ordinary physical activity causes undue dyspnea or fatigue, chest pain, or near syncope.
Class III	Marked limitation of physical activity. Comfortable at rest. Less than ordinary activity causes undue dyspnea or fatigue, chest pain, or near syncope.
Class IV	Unable to carry out any physical activity without symptoms. Dyspnea and/or fatigue may be present at rest. Discomfort is increased by any physical activity. Signs of right heart failure are present.

Modified after the New York Heart Association Functional Classification; World Health Organization, 1999.

- **Nocturnal oximetry:** Nocturnal desaturations could indicate OSA syndrome. PH patients with symptoms of sleep-disordered breathing should undergo polysomnography. Nocturnal desaturations are also fairly common in PAH and should be treated with nocturnal supplemental oxygen (*Chest 2007;131:109*).

Clinical Presentation

- **Symptoms** include **dyspnea** (most common), exercise intolerance, fatigue, palpitations, exertional dizziness, **syncope**, chest pain, lower extremity swelling, increased abdominal girth (ascites), and hoarseness (impingement of recurrent laryngeal nerve by enlarging pulmonary artery).
- Explore for underlying risk factors (i.e., **anorectic drugs, methamphetamines**) or associated conditions (e.g., connective tissue diseases, left ventricular heart failure [CHF], OSAHS, and venous thromboembolism [VTE]).
- Auscultatory signs of PH include **prominent second heart sound** (loud S_2) with loud P_2 component, right ventricular S_3, and tricuspid regurgitation, and pulmonary insufficiency murmurs.
- Signs of right heart failure include elevated jugular venous pressure, hepatomegaly, pulsatile liver, pedal edema, and ascites.
- Physical examination should focus on identifying underlying conditions linked to PH: skin changes of scleroderma, stigmata of liver disease, clubbing (congenital heart disease), and abnormal breath sounds (parenchymal lung disease).

Diagnostic Testing

Laboratories

- Evaluate for causative conditions and gauge degree of cardiac impairment.
- Tests include complete blood counts, blood urea nitrogen, serum creatinine, hepatic function tests, brain natriuretic peptide (BNP), human immunodeficiency virus (HIV) serology, thyroid-stimulating hormone (TSH), antinuclear antibody (ANA), antitopoisomerase antibodies, and anticentromere antibodies.
- Additional laboratory studies, based on initial findings, could include complete thyroid function studies, hepatitis B and C serologies, hemoglobin electrophoresis,

extractable nuclear antigen (ENA), antiphospholipid antibody, and lupus anticoagulant.

Electrocardiography

Signs of **right heart enlargement** include right ventricular hypertrophy, right atrial enlargement, right bundle branch block, and right ventricular strain pattern (S wave in lead I with Q wave and inverted T wave in lead III) but these findings have low sensitivity in milder PH.

Imaging

- General findings include enlarged central pulmonary arteries as well as RV enlargement with opacification of retrosternal space (best seen on lateral view).
- Clues to specific PH diagnosis include decreased peripheral vascular markings or pruning (PAH), very large pulmonary vasculature throughout lung fields (congenital-to-systemic shunt), regional oligemia of pulmonary vasculature (chronic thromboembolic disease), interstitial infiltrates (ILD), and hyperinflated lungs (chronic obstructive lung disease).
- **Ventilation–Perfusion (V/Q) lung scan**
  - Evaluate for chronic thromboembolic disease but could also be abnormal in pulmonary veno-occlusive disease and fibrosing mediastinitis.
  - Heterogeneous perfusion patterns are associated with PAH.
  - Presence of one or more segmental mismatches raises concern for chronic thromboembolic disease and should be investigated with computed tomography and pulmonary angiography (*N Engl J Med 2001;345:145*).
  - Pulmonary angiography can be done safely in the setting of severe PH and should be performed to (a) confirm chronic thromboembolic disease and (b) determine surgical accessibility of thrombotic material. Inferior vena cava filter can be deployed at the same time.
- **Chest computed tomography (CT) scan**
  - Evaluates lung parenchyma and mediastinum.
  - High-resolution images assess for interstitial or bronchiolar disease.
  - CT angiogram can also identify chronic thromboembolic changes but still warrants a V/Q scan.
- **Cardiac magnetic resonance imaging**
  - MRI investigates cardiac anomalies that lead to the development of PAH, especially if TEE is contraindicated.
  - Provides anatomic and functional information on the RV, including contractility measures.

Diagnostic Procedures

- **Lung biopsy**
  - Lung biopsy is rarely performed but useful if lung disease requires histologic confirmation (e.g., pulmonary vasculitis or veno-occlusive disease).
  - The risk of surgery is usually prohibitive in the setting of severe PH or RV dysfunction.
- **Right heart catheterization:** Essential investigation if PAH is suspected and treatment is being considered.
  - **Confirm noninvasive estimate of PASP,** as echocardiography can under- and overestimate PSAP (*Am J Respir Crit Care Med 2009;179:615*).
  - **Measure cardiac output and mean right atrial pressure (RAP) to gauge severity of condition and predict future course;** increased RAP is an indicator of RV

dysfunction and has greatest odds ratio for predicting mortality (*Ann Intern Med 1987;107:216*).

- **Investigate etiologies of PH,** including left heart disease (by measuring pulmonary artery occlusion pressure [PAOP]) or missed systemic-to-pulmonary shunts (by noting "step-ups" in oxygen saturations).
- Exercise hemodynamics can elicit PH occurring during exercise or also confirm suspicion of diastolic heart failure; but exercise protocols and methods of measurement are not standardized.
- **Acute vasodilator testing** is recommended if PAH is suspected.
- Performed with a *short*-acting vasodilator, such as intravenous adenosine, intravenous epoprostenol, or inhaled nitric oxide; *long*-acting calcium channel blockers (CCBs) should not be used for initial vasodilator testing due to risk of sustained systemic hypotension (*Chest 2004;26:35S*).
- **Not recommended for patients in extreme right heart failure** (mean RAP > 20).
- Definition of a **responder** is **decline in mean pulmonary artery pressure (mPAP) $\geq$ 10 mm Hg *and* concluding mPAP $\leq$ 40 mm Hg** (*Chest 2004;126: 35S*).
- Responders should undergo a CCB trial with pulmonary artery catheter in place. If vasoresponsiveness is recapitulated, chronic CCB therapy can be prescribed (see Treatment section).
- **Left heart catheterization** is only necessary to directly measure **left ventricular end-diastolic pressure** (LVEDP) if PAOP cannot reliably exclude left heart disease.

TREATMENT

- **Management of PH depends on the specific category of PH** (Table 17).
  - Patients with PH due to left heart disease should receive appropriate therapy for underlying causative condition with the goal of minimizing postcapillary pressures.
  - Patients with underlying lung diseases should be treated with bronchodilators (obstructive lung disease), immunomodulators (ILDs), noninvasive ventilation (obstructive sleep apnea syndrome and/or hypoventilation syndrome), and supplemental oxygen, as appropriate for the specific condition.
  - Chronic thromboembolic PH may be treated by **pulmonary thromboendarterectomy** at specialized centers and requires careful screening to determine resectability and expected hemodynamic response (*N Engl J Med 2001;345:1465*).
- Regardless of PH diagnosis, normoxemia should be maintained to avoid hypoxic vasoconstriction and further aggravation of pulmonary artery pressures. **Supplemental oxygen** to maintain adequate arterial saturations (>89%) 24 hours a day is recommended. However, normoxemia may not be possible in the presence of a significant right-to-left shunt (e.g., intracardiac right-to-left shunt).
- **In-line filters** should be used to prevent paradoxical air emboli from intravenous catheters in PH patients with right-to-left shunts.
- **Pneumovax and influenza vaccination** should be given to avoid respiratory tract infections.
- Patients with severe PH and RV dysfunction should minimize behaviors that can acutely decrease RV preload and/or increase RV afterload, which could cause circulatory collapse:
  - **Deep Valsalva** maneuvers can raise intrathoracic pressure and induce syncope through diminished central venous return (e.g., vigorous exercise, severe coughing paroxysm, straining during defecation or micturition).

- **High altitudes** (>5,000 ft) due to low inspired concentration of oxygen.
- **Cigarette smoking,** because of nicotine's vasoactive effects.
- **Pregnancy,** due to hemodynamic alterations that further strain the heart.
- Systemic **sympathomimetic** agents, such as decongestants and cocaine.

Medications

- PAH patients are candidates for **vasomodulator/vasodilator** therapy (Table 19).
  - Three categories of PAH-specific therapies with the unique mechanisms of actions:
    - **Endothelin receptor antagonists** block the binding of endothelin-1 to its receptors on pulmonary artery smooth muscle cells, which would typically cause vasoconstriction and cellular hypertrophy/growth.
    - **Phosphodiesterase-5 inhibitors** block the enzyme that shuts down nitric oxide–mediated vasodilation and platelet inhibition.
    - **Prostanoids** induce vasodilation, inhibit cellular growth, and inhibit platelet aggregation.
  - Initial choice of PAH-specific therapy should be individualized to the severity of one's condition, often relying on the WHO functional classification scheme (Fig. 4). Due to the complexity of some therapies, an individual's comorbid limitations, cognitive abilities, and psychosocial makeup must also be heavily factored.
  - Because current therapies for PAH are palliative and not curative, patients require close follow-up as deterioration often occurs, requiring alternative/additional medical and possibly surgical intervention (Fig. 4). While there is no consensus follow-up strategy, periodic functional (e.g., 6MW and WHO Functional Classification) and cardiac (e.g., echocardiography or right heart catheterization) assessments provide the most sound strategy.
- **Diuretic therapy** (loop diuretic + / − aldosterone antagonist + / − thiazides)
  - Alleviates **right heart failure** and improves symptoms.
  - Overdiuresis or too rapid of a diuresis can be poorly tolerated due to **preload dependency** of the RV and limited ability of the cardiac output to compensate for systemic hypotension.
- **Anticoagulation** (warfarin)
  - Chronic anticoagulation improves survival, based on limited data in IPAH patients (*N Engl J Med 1992;327:76*; *Circulation 1984;70:580*).
  - Warfarin is dosed to **target international normalized ratio (INR) of 1.5 to 2.5** (*Chest 2004;126:35S*).
  - Anticoagulant therapy is not urgent and can be stopped for invasive procedures or active bleeding.
- **Inotropic agents** (dobutamine, milrinone, digoxin)
  - Modestly improves right heart function, cardiac output, and symptoms.
  - Dobutamine and milrinone are best suited for **short-term use** in extremely decompensated states.
  - Digoxin's effects on right ventricular contractility are limited and its use is quite variable (*Chest 1998;114:787*).

Surgical Management

- **Lung transplantation or heart–lung transplantation**
  - Reserved for suitable patients with PAH who **remain in advanced functional class (III–IV) despite maximal medical therapy.**

Table 19	Vasomodulator/Vasodilatory Therapy for Pulmonary Arterial Hypertension					
Drug	Therapeutic Class	Indication	Route of Delivery	Dosing Range	Adverse Effects	Cautions
Nifedipine, Amlodipine, Diltiazem	Calcium channel blockers	Vasoresponders	PO	Varies by patient tolerance	Peripheral edema, hypotension, fatigue	**Use in patients who are vasoresponsive during acute vasodilator challenges;** avoid with low cardiac output or decompensated right heart failure
Sildenafil/ Tadalafil	Phosphodiesterase-5 inhibitor	Functional class II–IV	PO	20 mg T.I.D./ 40 mg Q.D.	Headache, hypotension, dyspepsia, myalgias, visual disturbances	Avoid using with **nitrates** or **protease inhibitors**
Bosentan	Endothelin receptor antagonist	Functional class II–IV	PO	125 mg B.I.D.	Hepatoxicity, teratogen, peripheral edema	**Monthly liver function monitoring;** avoid using with glyburide an glipizide
Ambrisentan	Endothelin receptor antagonist	Functional class II–III	PO	5–10 mg Q.D.	Hepatoxicity, teratogen, peripheral edema, nasal congestion	**Monthly liver function monitoring;** avoid using with glyburide and glipizide
Sitaxsentan	Endothelin receptor antagonist	Functional class II–III	PO	100 mg Q.D.	Hepatoxicity, teratogen, peripheral edema	**Strong interaction with warfarin; monthly liver function monitoring;** not available in United States
Iloprost	Prostanoid	Functional class III–IV	IH	2.5–5.0 mcg 6–8/d	Cough, flushing, headache, trismus	**Suboptimal compliance due to dosing frequency;** overnight drug holiday
Treprostinil	Prostanoid	Functional class II–IV	SQ or IV	Varies by patient tolerance	Headache, jaw pain, diarrhea, extremity pain	**Continuous parenteral agent;** catheter-related complications (IV); **site pain/reaction (SQ)**
Epoprostenol	Prostanoid	Functional class III–IV	IV	Varies by patient tolerance	Headache, jaw pain, diarrhea, extremity pain	**Continuous parenteral agent; very short half-life;** catheter-related complications (IV); **high-output state at higher doses**

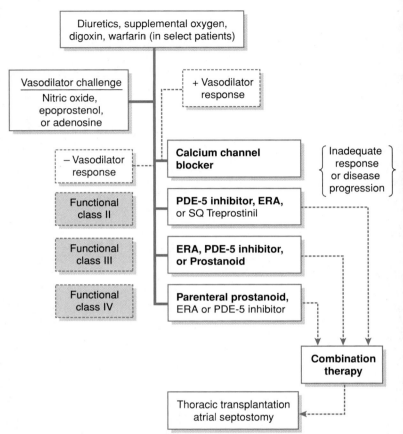

Figure 4. Pulmonary hypertension treatment algorithm. (Bolded drug classes preferred for respective functional class.)

- Because the right ventricle recovers after isolated lung transplantation, heart–lung transplantation is usually reserved for complex congenital heart defects that cannot be repaired.
- Median survival after lung transplantation is ~5 years and **survival for IPAH patients at 5 years is ~50%** (*J Heart Lung Transplant 2005;24:956*).
- **Atrial septostomy**
  - Palliative procedure performed in cases of right heart failure (i.e., syncope, hepatic congestion, prerenal azotemia) refractory to medical therapy.
  - Percutaneous creation of a right-to-left shunt across the interatrial septum in patients whose right atrial pressures are greater than left atrial pressures.
  - Despite arterial oxyhemoglobin desaturation and hypoxemia, oxygen delivery increases from improved left ventricular filling and cardiac output.

- **Septal defect closure**
  - In select cases of intracardiac defects that still have significant left-to-right shunting, closure can be undertaken by **percutaneous or surgical** means.
  - Criteria for closure include net left-to-right shunt with flow ratio (pulmonary flow/systemic flow) ≥ 1.5, resistance ratio (pulmonary vascular resistance/systemic vascular resistance) ≤ 0.6, pressure ratio (pulmonary artery pressure/systemic pressure) ≤ 0.6 (*Circulation 2008;118:2395*).

Interstitial Lung Disease

GENERAL PRINCIPLES

This section focuses on subacute and chronic interstitial lung diseases (ILDs), with emphasis on idiopathic pulmonary fibrosis (IPF) and sarcoidosis.

Definition

ILDs are a heterogeneous group of disorders, pathologically characterized by infiltration of the lung interstitium with cells, fluid, and/or connective tissue.

Etiology

See *Am J Respir Care Med 2002;165:277.*

- ILD of known etiology
  - Medication (e.g., bleomycin, amiodarone, nitrofurantoin, methotrexate)
  - Connective tissue disease (e.g., rheumatoid arthritis, scleroderma)
  - Pneumoconiosis (e.g., coal worker's pneumoconiosis, silicosis, asbestosis)
  - Radiation
  - Toxic inhalation (e.g., cocaine, ammonia)
  - Lymphangitic carcinomatosis
- Idiopathic interstitial pneumonias
  - Idiopathic pulmonary fibrosis (IPF) (usual interstitial pneumonia [UIP])
  - Nonspecific interstitial pneumonia (NSIP)
  - Desquamative interstitial pneumonia (DIP)
  - Respiratory bronchiolitis-interstitial lung disease (RB-ILD)
  - Cryptogenic organizing pneumonia (COP)
  - Lymphocytic interstitial pneumonia (LIP)
  - Acute interstitial pneumonia (AIP)
- Granulomatous ILD (e.g., sarcoidosis, hypersensitivity pneumonitis)
- Other (e.g., lymphangioleiomyomatosis, pulmonary Langerhans cell histiocytosis, eosinophilic pneumonia)

Pathophysiology

- The major pathophysiologic consequence of ILD is **impaired gas exchange,** caused by alteration of the alveolar–capillary interface.
- Interstitial infiltration leads to a **restrictive pulmonary process** characterized by decreased lung compliance.
- Some ILDs (e.g., sarcoidosis, hypersensitivity pneumonitis) can have significant bronchiolar involvement with resulting expiratory airflow obstruction.
- Pulmonary vascular disease in long-standing ILD may lead to the development of pulmonary hypertension (PH).

DIAGNOSIS

Clinical Presentation

History
- Patients typically present with gradually progressive **dyspnea on exertion.** Persistent **cough** is also a frequent complaint. A subset of ILDs have an acute presentation (e.g., acute interstitial pneumonia, acute eosinophilic pneumonia), and urgent evaluation is warranted in these cases.
- The history should focus on possible causes of lung injury, such as medications, occupational exposures, and environmental exposures. Comorbid conditions (e.g., connective tissue disease) may be relevant.
- Taking a smoking history is important given the connection between smoking and certain ILDs (e.g., pulmonary Langerhans cell histiocytosis, DIP, respiratory bronchiolitis-interstitial lung disease).

Physical Examination
The physical examination findings depend on the type of ILD, but may include inspiratory crackles and clubbing. There may be signs of PH and right ventricular failure in end-stage disease.

Diagnostic Testing

- The diagnosis of ILD is often initially suggested by imaging studies (see Imaging, below).
- All stable patients with suspected ILD should undergo (a) pulmonary function testing (spirometry, lung volumes, and diffusing capacity [DLCO]); (b) resting ABG analysis; and (c) exercise assessment of arterial oxygenation.
- Most patients with ILD have abnormal pulmonary function tests. Lung restriction is characterized by a decrease in total lung capacity with preservation of a normal FEV_1/FVC ratio. As previously mentioned, certain ILDs may manifest an obstructive pattern on pulmonary function testing, defined by an FEV_1/FVC ratio < 0.70 (see Pathophysiology, above).
- Gas exchange abnormalities are common with ILD and may be detected by a decrease in DLCO, a widening of the alveolar–arterial oxygen gradient at rest, or a significant decrease in the PaO_2 or SaO_2 with exercise. Hypercapnia may occur in severe ILD.

Laboratories
Blood testing is rarely diagnostic. The laboratory workup should be directed by the history and physical exam, and may provide supportive evidence for certain ILDs. Some examples follow:

- Peripheral eosinophilia may be present in entities such as eosinophilic pneumonia and drug-induced ILD.
- Autoimmune serologies can assist in the diagnosis of connective tissue disease associated with ILD.
- Positive serum precipitating antibody testing indicates host sensitization to certain antigens and may support the diagnosis of hypersensitivity pneumonitis.

Imaging
- ILDs typically result in abnormal imaging (chest radiograph or high-resolution CT [HRCT]), although some patients initially have a normal chest radiograph (Table 20).

Table 20	Imaging Findings in Selected Interstitial Lung Diseases		
ILD	Distribution[a]	CXR Findings[b]	HRCT Findings[b]
IPF/UIP	Lower, subpleural	Reticular infiltrates Honeycombing Decreased lung volume	Reticular infiltrates Honeycombing Traction bronchiectasis Minimal ground-glass opacities (may increase during acute exacerbation)
NSIP	Lower	Reticular infiltrates Ill-defined opacities Consolidation	Reticular infiltrates Ground-glass opacities Patchy consolidation Minimal honeycombing
COP	Usually lower; peripheral, peribronchial	Patchy consolidation Nodular opacities	Patchy consolidation Patchy ground-glass opacities Nodules (small or large)
Sarcoidosis	Upper, middle	Stage 0: Normal Stage 1: Hilar or mediastinal lymphadenopathy Stage 2: Hilar or mediastinal lymphadenopathy with pulmonary infiltrates Stage 3: Pulmonary infiltrates Stage 4: End-stage fibrosis	Perilymphatic nodules Patchy ground-glass opacities Reticular infiltrates Traction bronchiectasis Progressive massive fibrosis Hilar or mediastinal lymphadenopathy

ILD, interstitial lung disease; CXR, chest x-ray; HRCT, high-resolution computed tomography; IPF, idiopathic pulmonary fibrosis; UIP, usual interstitial pneumonia; NSIP, nonspecific interstitial pneumonia; COP, cryptogenic organizing pneumonia.
[a]Refers to the predominant distribution of radiographic abnormalities, for example, upper lung zone, lower lung zone, diffuse.
[b]All findings listed may not be present in a given patient.
From Webb RW. Thoracic Imaging: Pulmonary and Cardiovascular Radiology, 2005.

- **HRCT is the test of choice in patients with suspected ILD.**
- Comparison should be made with prior studies, when available, to assess the radiographic progression of disease.
- Imaging studies are not typically diagnostic; rather, they usually show nonspecific radiographic patterns, which help narrow the differential diagnosis. Additionally,

Table 21	Indications for Lung Biopsy in Interstitial Lung Disease

Atypical clinical features (e.g., age < 50, fever, weight loss, hemoptysis, signs of vasculitis)
Progressive disease course
Normal, atypical, or rapidly changing CXR or HRCT
Unexplained extrapulmonary manifestations
Pulmonary vascular disease of unclear etiology
Assessment of disease activity
Concern for cancer or infection
To identify a more treatable process than originally suspected
To obtain definitive diagnostic and prognostic information before beginning therapy with the potential for significant side effects

CXR, chest x-ray; HRCT, high-resolution computed tomography.
Modified from Raghu G. Interstitial lung disease: a diagnostic approach. Are CT scan and lung biopsy indicated in every patient? *Am J Respir Crit Care Med* 1995 Mar;151(3 Pt 1):909–914.

they may reveal complications of ILD (e.g., infection, malignancy), and provide guidance for biopsy.
• HRCT can be used to make the diagnosis of IPF in some situations (see Table 23).

Diagnostic Procedures
• Bronchoalveolar lavage (BAL) is most often used to evaluate for infection and malignancy, and otherwise has a very limited diagnostic role.
• Lung biopsy (Table 21)
  • Transbronchial lung biopsy has the highest yield in bronchocentric ILDs in which small biopsy samples may suffice for diagnosis, such as sarcoidosis and hypersensitivity pneumonitis (*Thorax 2008;63(Suppl 5):v1*).
  • Surgical lung biopsy can be performed by video-assisted thoracoscopic surgery (VATS) or open thoracotomy. HRCT is used to target areas of active disease and avoid lung regions with end-stage fibrosis.
  • Most patients tolerate lung biopsy well, although certain subgroups of patients are more predisposed to complications. For example, a requirement for mechanical ventilation and an immunocompromised state have been associated with higher mortality after surgical lung biopsy (*Chest 2005;127:1600*). There have also been reports of acute exacerbations of ILD following surgical lung biopsy (*Respir Med 2006;100:1753*).

TREATMENT

• The decision to treat ILD is collaboratively made by the patient and his/her physician based on symptoms, lung function, extrapulmonary manifestations, comorbid conditions, potential treatment side effects, and the potential benefit of the proposed treatment plan.
• Treatment of ILD varies depending on the underlying etiology, but usually involves **immunosuppression and/or avoidance of offending agents** (Table 22).
  • Patients receiving immunosuppressive therapy often require regular laboratory monitoring to assess for the development of common adverse drug effects.

Table 22	Treatment of Selected Interstitial Lung Diseases
ILD	**Potential Therapeutic Interventions[a]**
Medication-induced ILD	Discontinue culprit medication
	Corticosteroids
Connective tissue disease–associated ILD, IPF, NSIP, COP	Corticosteroids
	Cytotoxic therapy (e.g., cyclophosphamide, azathioprine)
DIP, RB-ILD	Smoking cessation
	Corticosteroids
Sarcoidosis[b]	Corticosteroids
	Cytotoxic therapy
	Hydroxychloroquine
	Infliximab
Hypersensitivity pneumonitis	Avoid offending antigens
	Corticosteroids
	Cytotoxic therapy

ILD, interstitial lung disease; IPF, idiopathic pulmonary fibrosis; NSIP, nonspecific interstitial pneumonia; COP, cryptogenic organizing pneumonia; DIP, desquamative interstitial pneumonia; RB-ILD, respiratory bronchiolitis-interstitial lung disease.
[a]Lung transplantation is a consideration for select patients with end-stage interstitial lung disease.
[b]For more detailed information, please see *N Engl J Med* 2007;357:2162, Table 3.

- *Pneumocystis jiroveci* pneumonia prophylaxis should be considered in patients receiving immunosuppressive therapy (*Mayo Clin Proc 1996;71:5*).
- Bone density assessment is recommended for patients receiving chronic systemic corticosteroid therapy (http://www.nof.org/professionals/NOF_Clinicians_Guide.pdf), and periodic reassessment (e.g., every 1 to 2 years) should be performed.
- INH prophylaxis should be considered prior to the initiation of immunosuppressive therapy in patients with a positive PPD.
- All patients with ILD should be offered pulmonary rehabilitation as well as influenza and pneumococcal vaccinations, and patients with severe disease should undergo evaluation for supplemental oxygen.
- Select patients with end-stage ILD may benefit from lung transplantation.

SPECIAL CONSIDERATIONS

- **Idiopathic Pulmonary Fibrosis.** IPF is a **relentlessly progressive** idiopathic interstitial pneumonia associated with the **histologic appearance of UIP on surgical lung biopsy.**
  - Epidemiology
    - IPF is a disease with a worldwide distribution and an estimated prevalence of 14 to 43 cases per 100,000 Americans (*Am J Respir Crit Care Med 2006;174:810*).
    - The mean age at diagnosis is 66 years, and the incidence rises with increasing age. Mean survival from the time of diagnosis is approximately 3 to 5 years (*Am J Respir Crit Care Med 2000;161:646*).
    - Cigarette smoking may be a risk factor for IPF (*Am J Respir Crit Car Med 1997;155:242*), and heritable components have been implicated in disease pathogenesis as well (*N Engl J Med 2007;356:1317*).

Table 23	Diagnostic Criteria for Idiopathic Pulmonary Fibrosis

Major criteria
Exclusion of other known causes of ILD
Abnormal PFTs that include evidence of restriction and/or impaired gas
   exchange
Bibasilar reticular infiltrates with minimal ground-glass opacities on HRCT
TBBx or BAL showing no features to support an alternative diagnosis

Minor criteria
Age > 50 yr
Insidious onset of otherwise unexplained dyspnea on exertion
Duration of illness ≥ 3 mo
Bibasilar inspiratory crackles (dry or "Velcro" type in quality)

Diagnosis
Definite diagnosis = Surgical lung Bx showing UIP plus major criteria 1
   through 3
Probable diagnosis = All major criteria plus at least three out of four minor
   criteria

ILD, interstitial lung disease; PFTs, pulmonary function tests; HRCT, high-resolution computed
tomography; TBBx, transbronchial biopsy; BAL, bronchoalveolar lavage; Bx, biopsy; UIP, usual
interstitial pneumonia.
Modified from American Thoracic Society. Idiopathic pulmonary fibrosis: diagnosis and
treatment. International consensus statement. American Thoracic Society (ATS), and the
European Respiratory Society (ERS). *Am J Respir Crit Care Med* 2000 Feb;161(2 Pt 1):
646–664.

- Patients most commonly present with gradually progressive dyspnea on exertion and persistent, nonproductive cough. Physical examination often demonstrates **bibasilar inspiratory crackles and clubbing.** Signs of PH and right ventricular failure may be seen in advanced disease.
- **Surgical lung biopsy is the diagnostic procedure of choice, but need not be performed in all cases** (Tables 21 and 23).
- Treatment
  - **No treatment has been unequivocally shown to improve survival or quality of life in patients with IPF** (*Am J Respir Crit Care Med 2000;161:646*). Nonetheless, in light of the poor prognosis of IPF, pharmacotherapy is sometimes administered. The goal is to achieve subjective and objective (i.e., radiographic, physiologic) improvement by altering the disease process at an early stage before irreversible fibrosis occurs. Treatment options predominantly include **corticosteroids, cytotoxic agents** (e.g., cyclophosphamide, azathioprine), and the antioxidant **N-acetylcysteine,** often in combination (*Am Rev Respir Dis 1991;144:291*; *N Engl J Med 2005;353:2229*). Long-term use of these medications is associated with significant potential toxicity; this, coupled with the uncertain benefit of treatment, underscores the clinical quandary of deciding which patients to treat and when.
  - Investigational agents include the antifibrotic drug pirfenidone, the endothelin receptor antagonist bosentan, and warfarin. Enrolling patients with IPF in clinical trials, where available, should be considered.
  - **Lung transplantation** should be considered in select patients with IPF (*J Heart Lung Transplant 2006;25:745*).

Table 24	Diagnostic Criteria for Acute Exacerbation of Idiopathic Pulmonary Fibrosis[a]

Previous or concurrent diagnosis of IPF

Unexplained development or worsening of dyspnea within 30 days

HRCT showing new bilateral ground-glass abnormality and/or consolidation superimposed on a background reticular or honeycomb pattern consistent with UIP

No evidence of pulmonary infection by endotracheal aspirate or bronchoalveolar lavage

Exclusion of alternative causes, including left heart failure, pulmonary embolism, and other identifiable causes of acute lung injury

---

IPF, idiopathic pulmonary fibrosis; HRCT, high-resolution computed tomography; UIP, usual interstitial pneumonia.
[a]Patients who do not meet all five criteria should be termed "suspected acute exacerbation."
From *Am J Respir Crit Care Med* 2007;176:636.

- Acute exacerbations of IPF (Table 24) carry a high mortality rate. Systemic corticosteroids are often used to treat acute exacerbations, although their benefit has not been systematically proven (*Chest 2007;132;1652*).
- Patients with IPF are at increased risk for lung cancer (*Curr Opin Pulm Med 2005;11:431*).
- **Sarcoidosis**
  - Sarcoidosis is a granulomatous disease of unknown etiology which can involve any organ system.
  - Patients usually present before 40 years of age, with the highest prevalence rates found in African Americans and persons of Scandinavian descent (*Am J Epidemiol 1997;145:234; Sarcoidosis 1995;12:61*).
  - Clinical manifestations
    - Presenting symptoms are protean, given the systemic nature of sarcoidosis, but may include **constitutional symptoms** (e.g., fever, fatigue, malaise, weight loss), **dyspnea, dry cough, chest pain, rash, or visual complaints.**
    - The pulmonary examination may be normal or may disclose crackles and/or wheezing. Typical extrapulmonary presenting findings include skin and eye lesions, peripheral lymphadenopathy, and hepatosplenomegaly.
    - Cutaneous manifestations of sarcoidosis include **erythema nodosum** (raised, red, tender bumps or nodules on the anterior legs) and lupus pernio (indurated plaques with associated discoloration of the nose, cheeks, lips, and ears).
    - **Uveitis** is the most common eye lesion in sarcoidosis (*Am J Respir Crit Care Med 1999;160:736*).
    - **Löfgren's syndrome** is defined as an acute presentation of sarcoidosis characterized by **arthritis, erythema nodosum, and bilateral hilar lymphadenopathy** (*Acta Med Scand 1953;145:424*).
    - Myocardial involvement is becoming increasingly recognized in patients with sarcoidosis and may result in **cardiomyopathy, arrhythmia, and sudden death** (*Am Heart J 2009;157:9*).
- Diagnosis
  - The diagnosis of sarcoidosis is made in a patient with consistent clinical and radiographic findings (Table 20) and histologic evidence of noncaseating

granulomas, in the absence of an alternate etiology of granulomatous disease (e.g., mycobacterial or fungal infection, berylliosis, granulomatous vasculitis, cancer with a local sarcoid reaction).

- ○ **Biopsy is not required in all patients,** such as patients with stage 1 or stage 2 pulmonary sarcoidosis or patients with Löfgren's syndrome (*Am J Respir Crit Care Med 1999;160:736; N Engl J Med 2007;357:2153*).
- ○ For cases in which a biopsy is indicated, a peripheral, easily accessible biopsy target should be sought. If such a site cannot be found, then transbronchial lung biopsy with or without transbronchial needle aspiration of mediastinal lymph nodes is the diagnostic procedure of choice. **Transbronchial biopsy is approximately 70% accurate in making the diagnosis of sarcoidosis** (*Curr Opin Pulm Med 2008;14:455*).

- The initial evaluation of a patient with sarcoidosis includes a history and physical examination, posteroanterior and lateral chest x-ray, pulmonary function testing (including spirometry and DLCO), complete blood count, comprehensive metabolic panel, urinalysis, electrocardiogram, and ophthalmologic examination. Other studies may be necessary based on clinical suspicion of organ involvement (e.g., central nervous system imaging, cardiac MRI).
- Prognosis
  - ○ The disease course of sarcoidosis is highly variable, but the majority of patients experience spontaneous remission. However, the chance of spontaneous remission decreases with more advanced radiographic stage of disease (see Table 20).
  - ○ In general, patients with an acute disease presentation (e.g., Löfgren's syndrome) have a favorable prognosis, while patients with a chronic presentation are more likely to develop progressive disease and organ dysfunction.
  - ○ Mortality most commonly results from respiratory failure, myocardial involvement, or central nervous system involvement (*Am J Respir Crit Care Med 1999;160:736*).
- Treatment (Table 22) (*N Engl J Med 2007;357:2162*)
  - ○ Given that sarcoidosis regresses in most patients, **treatment is not usually required.** Treatment is typically administered to patients with progressive, severe disease, especially those with extrapulmonary involvement. **Corticosteroids are usually first-line therapy** in patients who require treatment. If chronic steroids are required, second-line agents such as methotrexate and azathioprine can be used as steroid-sparing agents. There are data suggesting that infliximab may improve lung function in chronic sarcoidosis (*Am J Respir Crit Care Med 2006;174:795*).
  - ○ **Lung transplantation** should be considered in select patients with sarcoidosis (*J Heart Lung Transplant 2006;25:745*).

Solitary Pulmonary Nodule

GENERAL PRINCIPLES

- The goal of a careful evaluation of the solitary pulmonary nodule (SPN) is to determine if the lesion is more likely **malignant or benign.**
- **A lesion greater than 3 cm has a high likelihood of malignancy and should be treated as such whereas lesions less than 3 cm need more careful assessment.**
- Benign nodules with low-risk characteristics should be closely followed so that invasive procedures with associated risks can be avoided.

- Identifying early lung cancer is of the utmost importance as there is a >60% survival rate of patients who have a malignant SPN removed (*Chest 1997;111:1710*).

Definition

- **A solitary pulmonary nodule is defined as an asymptomatic rounded lesion less than 3 cm in diameter.** It is completely surrounded by lung parenchyma, unaccompanied by atelectasis, intrathoracic adenopathy, or pleural effusion.
- Pulmonary nodules less than 8 to 10 mm (subcentimeter nodules) remain within this definition; however, there is evidence to suggest that these nodules undergo a less rigorous evaluation due to lower overall malignancy risk (*Chest 2007;132(3 Suppl): 945*).

Epidemiology

- Approximately 150,000 SPNs are identified each year in the United States.
- It has been estimated that such a nodule is noted on 0.09% to 0.20% of all chest radiographs.

Etiology

- Although underlying etiologies for pulmonary nodules are varied, the most important designation clinically is deciphering between a malignant and a nonmalignant process.
- **Malignancy accounts for approximately 40% of SPNs.**
- **Granulomas** (both infectious and noninfectious) account for 50% of undiagnosed SPNs.
- The remaining 10% are composed of **benign neoplasms,** such as **hamartomas** (5%) and a multitude of other causes.

Risk Factors

- **Smoking** is the most important associated risk factor for almost all malignant SPNs.
- For infectious etiologies, an immunocompromised state promotes an increased risk.

DIAGNOSIS

- Diagnosis of the SPN is made radiographically, usually via chest x-ray or CT scan.
- Most frequently, the nodule is noted incidentally on a study performed for other reasons (e.g., chronic cough, chest pain, etc.).

Clinical Presentation

- As stated previously, the majority of SPNs are diagnosed incidentally by radiographic tests done for other reasons so there may not be overt symptoms.
- There are instances when a nodule may precipitate cough, chest pain, hemoptysis, or sputum production depending on the etiology and location of the SPN.

History

- Ask typical screening questions for malignancy including **weight loss and night sweats.**
- Hemoptysis may indicate malignancy, but may also prompt investigations for Wegner's, TB, and Hereditary Hemorrhagic Telangiectasia (HHT).
- Ask about arthritis and arthralgias for possible undiagnosed rheumatoid arthritis or sarcoidosis.

- Take an exposure history including recent travel history related to endemic mycoses (histoplasmosis, coccidioidomycosis, etc.) as well as possible TB exposures.
- A history of previous malignancies increases the risk of metastatic disease of the lung.
- Patients who are immunosuppressed from HIV, organ transplant or chronic steroids have increased risk of infectious causes.
- Smoking is linked to 85% of lung cancers. A patient's risk of lung cancer decreases significantly 5 years after smoking cessation, but it never truly returns to normal.
- An occupational history is important including possible asbestosis exposure (associated with not only mesothelioma, but also nonsmall cell lung cancer), silica, beryllium, radon, ionizing radiation among others.

Physical Examination
- Although there are no specific physical exam findings related to SPNs, evidence for underlying etiologies may be discovered with a thorough exam.
- Note signs of weight loss or cachexia suggestive of malignancy.
- Do a thorough lymph node exam. **A cervical lymph node might provide an easy diagnostic target to determine the etiology of an SPN.**
- Perform breast exam in women and testicular exam in young men.
- A careful skin examination may reveal telangiectasias, erythema nodosum, rheumatoid nodules, or other findings that might suggest a cause.

Diagnostic Criteria
- As mentioned previously, an SPN is identified as a rounded lesion less than 3 cm in circumference. It is completely surrounded by lung parenchyma, unaccompanied by atelectasis, intrathoracic adenopathy, or pleural effusion.
- The first step in managing an SPN is to stratify the patient in terms of malignancy risk: low-, intermediate-, or high-risk categories (see Table 25).
- Risk stratification can be accomplished either qualitatively via clinical judgment or quantitatively using validated risk assessment tools (*Arch Int Med 1997;157:849*).
- Once the risk of malignancy has been established, further management can proceed as outlined in Figure 5.

Table 25	Risk Stratification of a Solitary Pulmonary Nodule		
Variable	Low Risk	Intermediate Risk	High Risk
Lesion diameter (cm)	<1.5	1.5–2.2	>2.2
Patient age	<45	45–60	>60
Smoking status	Never smoked or quit >7 yr ago	Current smoker of <20 cigarettes/d or quit <7 yr ago	Current smoker of >20 cigarettes/d
Lesion margin characteristics	Smooth and rounded	Scalloped	Spiculated or corona radiata
Densitometry in Houndsfield Units (HU)	<15 HU	>15 HU	>15 HU

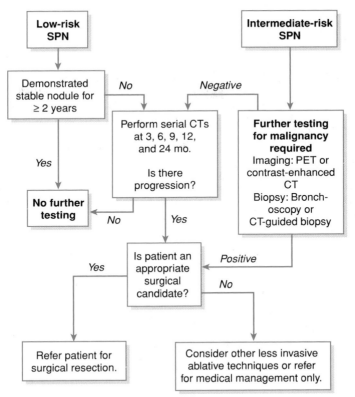

Figure 5. Diagnostic and therapeutic management of low- and intermediate-risk pulmonary nodules.

Differential Diagnosis

Pulmonary nodules are divided here primarily into malignant or benign etiologies, with benign processes further divided into infectious or noninfectious causes (Table 26).

Diagnostic Testing

Laboratories

- Routine laboratory testing is seldom helpful unless the history and physical exam strongly suggest an etiology.
- If connective tissue diseases or vasculitides are suggested, perform appropriate testing.
- Hyponatremia may suggest SIADH associated with primary lung cancer, as well as other pulmonary processes.
- Hypercalcemia might suggest lung cancer as well as sarcoidosis.
- Anemia may indicate chronic pulmonary hemorrhage (e.g., HHT) or a chronic inflammatory disease.

Table 26	Differential Diagnosis of the Solitary Pulmonary Nodule
Malignant (40% of SPNs)	• Primary pulmonary carcinoma (80% of all malignant SPNs) • Primary pulmonary lymphoma • Primary pulmonary carcinoid • Solitary pulmonary metastasis • Melanoma, osteosarcoma, testicular, breast, prostate, colon, and renal cell carcinoma
Benign neoplasms (5% of SPNs)	• Hamartoma (accounts for most benign neoplastic SPNs) • Arteriovenous malformations (consider HHT) • Others including neural tumors (schwannoma, neurofibroma), fibroma, sclerosing hemangioma
Granulomas (50% of SPNs)	Infectious • Mycobacterial disease (most commonly tuberculosis) and fungal infections (histoplasmosis, coccidioidomycosis, blastomycosis, cryptococcus, aspergillosis) Noninfectious granulomas associated with vasculitis • Wegner's granulomatosis, Churg–Strauss syndrome, • Noninfectious granulomas not associated with vasculitis • Sarcoid granulomatosis, hypersensitivity pneumonitis, and berylliosis
Other etiologies (5% of SPNs)	Infectious • Bacterial (nocardia, actinomycosis, round pneumonia), measles, abscess, septic embolus Noninfectious • Lipoid pneumonia, amyloid, subpleural lymph node, rheumatoid nodule, pulmonary scar or infarct, congenital malformations (bronchogenic cyst, sequestration), skin nodule, rib fracture, pleural thickening from mass or fluid

SPN, solitary pulmonary nodule.

- Microbiologic studies, particularly sputum culture, may aid in the diagnosis of an infectious SPN.
- Sputum cytology has limited use as yield is low for peripherally located, small lesions.

Imaging

The mainstay of diagnostic evaluation of the SPN is via radiographic studies, primarily **chest x-ray, chest CT, and PET scan.**

- **Chest x-ray**
  - A previous chest radiograph is an important tool in the initial evaluation of an SPN.
  - If an SPN has been present and unchanged on chest radiograph for more than 2 years, then further evaluation is likely not warranted.
  - If an SPN appears on a new radiograph in less than 30 days, it is certainly not malignant and most likely infectious.

- There are radiographic findings that make it more likely that a lesion is **benign: calcifications, a laminated appearance;** or more likely **malignant: spiculated, irregular border** (see Table 25).
- The chest x-ray is easy to obtain and delivers a low dose of radiation; however, it has limitations in the initial characterization and careful comparisons over time required for SPN evaluation.
- **Computed tomography**
  - Chest CT is now considered the most important radiological exam for SPN evaluation. With few exceptions, an SPN requires assessment by CT.
  - Accurate volumetric measurement of lesion size allows precise comparison to determine stability or growth.
  - Imaging allows a careful examination of mediastinal lymph nodes.
  - Thin cuts through the lesion are more sensitive than chest x-ray for characterizing calcifications and lamination as well as the margins of the lesion.
- **PET scan**
  - 18-Flourodeoxyglucose positron emission tomography (FDG-PET) can help distinguish malignant and benign lesions because cancers are metabolically active and take up FDG avidly.
  - Sensitivity of 80% to 100% and specificity of 79% to 100% of detecting malignancy.
  - False negatives can occur in bronchoalveolar carcinoma, carcinoid, and mucinous neoplasms while false positives are common in nonmalignant "inflammatory" conditions (infectious and autoimmune processes).
  - Higher incidence of both false-positive and false-negative results occurs in nodules < 10 mm (*Lung Cancer 2004;45:19*), thus discouraging the use of PET scan in this situation.
  - PET scan is most commonly utilized in the evaluation of low-to-moderate risk indeterminate nodules for further risk stratification (see Fig. 5).
- **Contrast-enhanced CT**
  - Technique utilizing contrast enhancement and measurement of Hounsfield Units to risk stratify an SPN for malignancy.
  - A multicenter analysis demonstrates high sensitivity but relatively low specificity for identifying malignant nodules (*Radiology 2000;214:73*).
  - This method may be an important tool for risk assessment of an indeterminate SPN in centers that have experience with the technique.

Diagnostic Procedures

- **If a nodule is considered high risk and the patient is an appropriate surgical candidate, then the best approach is to forego biopsy and pursue resection.**
- Any change of an SPN on serial imaging warrants resection or invasive biopsy.
- If a lesion has low-risk characteristics, there is no indication to pursue biopsy and subjecting a patient to unneeded risk.
- Biopsy is most often pursued when there is discordance between clinical risk stratification and imaging tests. For example, when pretest suspicion for malignancy is significant but PET imaging is negative, biopsy may be indicated.
- Also, for patients where surgery represents significant risk secondary to comorbidities, using a less invasive biopsy strategy to determine the presence of malignancy is appropriate.

- There are primarily two options for biopsy of an SPN: transthoracic needle aspiration (TTNA) and fiberoptic flexible bronchoscopy.
  - **Transthoracic needle aspiration**
    - This technique is usually performed under the guidance of fluoroscopy or CT (more common).
    - This approach is most commonly employed for nodules with a peripheral location and without anatomic impediment to a biopsy needle.
    - Specificity for identifying malignancy is high with TTNA; however, there is a significant rate of nondiagnostic biopsies, and sensitivity depends on many factors, including nodule size.
    - A nondiagnostic biopsy does not rule out malignancy.
    - The main complication of TTNA is pneumothorax with 25% incidence of minor pneumothorax and 5% major (requiring chest tube drainage).
  - **Bronchoscopy**
    - Conventional flexible bronchoscopy has traditionally been used to access central airway lesions, mediastinal lymph nodes, and large parenchymal masses, leaving only a limited role in the evaluation of an SPN.
    - However, with the recent use of endobronchial ultrasound (EBUS), evaluating an SPN with bronchoscopy has developed into an important modality, providing diagnostic yields over 80% regardless of lesion size (*Am J Respir Crit Care Med 2007;176:36*).
- Other interventional techniques including electromagnetic navigation and CT virtual bronchoscopy also show promise of improving the use of bronchoscopy in the management of SPN.

TREATMENT

- Management of low- and intermediate-risk SPNs is outlined in Figure 5.
- Overall treatment strategy is to identify lesions with significant malignancy risk and pursue surgical resection when possible.
- If a nodule has low-risk characteristics and has demonstrated stability over a period of 2 years, then no further treatment is warranted.
- If a specific etiology for the SPN is diagnosed (e.g., a connective tissue disease or infection), then treatment is targeted toward the underlying process.

Other Nonoperative Therapies

- Although **surgical resection is preferable in patients with either a high-risk lesion or biopsy proven malignancy,** if surgical resection is not an option, there are other less effective therapies.
- Stereotactic radiation is currently the most widely utilized therapy in this clinical situation. This mode of external beam therapy aims to decrease collateral radiation-induced damage to adjacent lung tissue.
- There are more experimental approaches, including brachytherapy and radiofrequency ablation, that are currently under development.

Surgical Management

- Surgical resection of an indeterminate SPN is indicated in the following situations:
  - The clinical probability of malignancy is moderate to high (>60%).
  - The nodule is hypermetabolic by PET imaging.
  - Biopsy proven malignant nodule.

- A combination of surgical techniques, including video-assisted thoracoscopy (VATS), mediastinoscopy, and thoracotomy, can lead to diagnosis (via intraoperative frozen section), staging, and potential cure during a single induction of anesthesia.

MONITORING/FOLLOW-UP

- For a low- or intermediate-risk pulmonary nodule for which resection is either not warranted (see Fig. 5), desired, or possible, routine follow-up with chest CT is standard practice.
- The typical practice for following an SPN is with serial chest CT performed at intervals of 3, 6, 12, 18, and 24 months from initial detection, assessing for any evidence of growth.
- A pulmonary nodule that has demonstrated stability by lack of growth for a period of 2 years has a very low risk of malignancy and follow-up can be terminated.

Pleural Effusion

GENERAL PRINCIPLES

Definition
The accumulation of fluid in the pleural space.

Classification
Diagnosis and management is based on classifying a pleural effusion as either a **transudate or exudates.**

Etiology
- **Most common causes** (*Pleural Disease. 4th Ed. Lippincott, Williams and Wilkins, 2001*):
  - Left heart failure (36%)
  - Pneumonia (22%)
  - Malignancy (14%): lung, breast, lymphoma
  - Pulmonary embolism (11%)
  - Viral disease (7%)
- **Less common but important causes:** rheumatologic/collagen vascular disease, hepatic cirrhosis, hepatic hydrothorax, pancreatitis, esophageal rupture, lymphatic obstruction, "trapped" lung.

Pathophysiology
- **Normal pleural physiology:**
  - Each pleural space produces and reabsorbs up to 15 mL of fluid per day, and **contains about 10 mL of fluid at any one time;** not apparent on imaging.
  - **Normal pleural fluid chemistries:** LDH < 0.6 of serum, protein < 0.5 of serum, glucose 0.6 to 0.8 of serum, pH 7.60.
- **Transudative effusion: alteration of hydrostatic and/or oncotic factors** that increase the formation and/or decrease reabsorption of pleural fluid.
  - CHF: increased venous pressures and lung edema
  - Hepatic cirrhosis and nephrotic syndrome: hypoalbuminemia

- Malignancy: infiltration/obstruction of pleural capillaries and/or lymphatics (up to 10% of malignant effusions are transudative)
- **Exudative effusion:** either direct or cytokine-induced disruption of normal pleural membranes and/or vasculature leading to **increased capillary permeability.**
  - Infection/pneumonia
  - Malignancy
  - Inflammatory disease (i.e., SLE or RA)
  - Trauma/surgery
  - Pulmonary embolus
- **Fluid markers of pleural infection, inflammation, and/or obstruction** often coexist.
  - **Low glucose and pH levels**
    ○ Byproducts of microorganism and/or inflammatory cell metabolism
    ○ Decreased acid removal due to pleural disruption from inflammation or malignancy
  - **High LDH level**
    ○ Cell turnover and lysis

DIAGNOSIS

The clinical setting, combined with pleural fluid analysis, is crucial to establishing a proper diagnosis.

Clinical Presentation

Symptoms and signs may be directly related to the pleural effusion itself, and/or to any underlying disease process.

History
- **Dyspnea** due to abnormal pulmonary mechanics: most common symptom, usually develops with greater than 500 to 1000 mL of pleural fluid, but may not correlate
- **Often asymptomatic**
- Pleurisy or referred chest/back/shoulder pain from pleural inflammation
- Should include survey of potential underlying causes

Physical Examination
- Vital signs: Assess for fever, hemodynamic instability, hypoxemia.
- Chest exam: **Dullness to percussion, decreased breath sounds, and tactile fremitus.**
  - These signs are more sensitive with larger effusions, but the chest exam is often unreliable and should not be used solely to diagnose and approximate size (*Clev Clin J Med 2008;75:297*).
- A thorough system-based exam should evaluate for CHF, malignancy, pneumonia, hepatic cirrhosis, venous thrombosis, and other potential causes of pleural effusion.

Diagnostic Criteria
- **Analysis of pleural fluid obtained by thoracentesis** is the mainstay of diagnosing an etiology.
- **Transudate: Presence of ALL of Light's criteria** (*Ann Intern Med 1972; 77:507*).
  - Fluid: serum protein ratio < 0.5

- Fluid: serum LDH ratio < 0.6
- Pleural fluid LDH < 0.67 of upper limit of normal for serum LDH
- **Exudate: Presence of ANY of Light's criteria** (*Ann Intern Med 1972;77:507*).
- **Pseudo exudate:** An effusion that meets one or more of Light's criteria, but is actually a transudate.
  - **Usually due to diuretic-treated CHF,** cirrhosis, or nephrotic kidney disease.
  - **Serum to pleural fluid albumin gradient is >1.2**
- **Simple parapneumonic effusion: a sterile, small** (encompassing less than one-half the hemithorax), **free-flowing pleural effusion in the setting of pneumonia,** with pH > 7.20 and glucose > 60 mg/dL
- **Complicated parapneumonic effusion: ANY one of the following** (*Chest 2000; 118:1158*):
  - Large (encompassing more than one-half of the hemithorax), free-flowing
  - Effusion of any size with loculations
  - Thickened parietal pleura on chest CT
  - Positive gram stain or culture
  - pH < 7.20 or glucose < 60 mg/dL
- **Empyema: gross pus in the pleural space or positive gram stain.** Positive culture is NOT required for diagnosis (high false-negative rate).

Differential Diagnosis

See Table 27.

Diagnostic Testing

- Pleural effusion is detected by chest imaging and characterized through sampling by thoracentesis.
- **All parapneumonic effusions, and new, undiagnosed effusions should be sampled.**

Laboratories

- **Pleural fluid** (Table 27):
  - Note color and consistency
  - Chemistries: Protein, albumin, LDH, glucose, pH
  - Cell count with differential
  - Hematocrit if suspicion for hemothorax (> 0.5 of serum is diagnostic)
  - Microbiologic stains and culture per suspicion
  - Cytology (yield approximately 60%)
  - Consider triglyceride, amylase, ADA as indicated
- Serum: CBC, CMP, LDH, urinalysis, coagulation studies, BNP
- Additional labs guided by suggestion of underlying illness

Electrocardiography

Assess for structural heart disease. Otherwise usually nonspecific and noncontributory.

Imaging

- Standard upright **PA/lateral CXR:**
  - Diagnostic for a suspected pleural effusion and approximates size (*Radiology: Diagnosis, Imaging, Intervention. Lippincott, 2000:1*).
    - 75 mL obscures the posterior costophrenic sulcus
    - 175 mL obscures the lateral costophrenic sulcus

Table 27	Clues to Diagnosing the Cause of a Pleural Effusion Based on Fluid Analysis

Gross appearance
- **Clear/serous/light yellow:** Transudate of any etiology (cardiac, liver, kidney disease)
  Urinothorax (consider if smells like ammonia)
- **Bloody/serosanguineous:** Hemothorax (surgery/trauma); PE; malignancy
- **Purulent/turbid/brown:** Infectious/empyema; esophageal rupture
- **Milky/white:** Chylothorax (lymphatic disruption from malignancy, thoracic duct injury, LAM, filariasis, others)

Nucleated cells
- **Total > 50k, neutrophilia:** Infectious/empyema
- **Total < 5k:** Transudate of any etiology; chronic malignant; tuberculous
- **Lymphocytosis (>85%):** Tuberculous; lymphoma; chronic rheumatoid; sarcoid; pseudo exudates
- **Eosinophilia (>10%):** Pneumothorax; hemothorax; fungal; parasitic; meds; malignancy; benign asbestos effusion
- **Mesothelial cells (>5%):** Normal; transudate
  Excludes tuberculous pleurisy

Chemical analysis
- **Elevated protein: >3 g/dL:** Most exudates; pseudo exudates (serum-fluid albumin gradient > 1.2 g/dL)
- **>4:** Tuberculous
- **>7–8:** Blood cell dyscrasias
- **Elevated LDH: >1,000 IU/L:** Empyema; rheumatoid; paragonimiasis; high burden malignant
- **Fluid:serum ratio >1:** Pneumocystis or urinothorax
- **Glucose < 60 mg/dL:** Infectious/empyema; rheumatoid; lupus; tuberculous; esophageal rupture; malignant
- **pH < 7.3:** Infectious/empyema; rheumatoid; lupus; tuberculous; esophageal rupture; high burden malignant
- **Elevated amylase (>serum):** Pancreatitis; esophageal rupture; malignant
- **Adenosine deaminase > 50 U/L:** Tuberculous (unlikely if level < 40)
- **Triglycerides >110 mg/dL:** Chylothorax

- 500 mL obscures the entire diaphragmatic contour
- 1,000 mL reaches the level of the anterior 4th rib
- Helps suggest associated conditions (CHF, pneumonia).
- **Lateral decubitus radiograph:**
  - **Demonstrates fluidity.**
  - Usually amenable for thoracentesis if fluid layers to >1 cm.
- **Thoracic ultrasonography:**
  - Accurate and practical in **detecting loculations.**
  - Provides **real-time guidance for thoracentesis or thoracostomy tube placement,** reducing complication rates.
- **Chest CT with contrast:**
  - Helpful in distinguishing fluid from lung mass, atelectasis, pneumonia, or suggesting hemothorax.

- Defines and characterizes pleural loculations, thickening, nodularity, or other abnormalities.

Diagnostic Procedures
- **Thoracentesis:** can be performed safely at the bedside on effusions layering >1 cm on lateral decubitus CXR.
  - **Complicated/organized effusions should be accessed using real-time ultrasound or CT guidance.**
  - **Optimize hemostasis:** PT/PTT < 2× normal, Platelets > 25k, Cr < 6 (*Transfusion 1991;31:164*).
  - **Microbiologic studies** of a parapneumonic effusion may be falsely negative after antibiotic administration.
  - Repeat thoracentesis increases diagnostic yield.
  - **Cytology for malignancy positive up to 60%,** but probably not dependent on fluid volume obtained (*Chest 2002;122:1913*).
  - **AFB stain and culture sensitivity < 30%** (*Chest 2007;131:880*).
- **Closed pleural biopsy:** performed by transthoracic needle approach.
  - **Indicated for the undiagnosed, suspected tuberculous or rheumatoid effusion.**
    - **Sensitivity > 80% when combined with pleural fluid AFB stain and culture** since tuberculous pleuritis is usually diffuse (*Chest 1997;112:702*).
  - **Consider for the undiagnosed, suspected malignant effusion**
    - Obtaining four to six consecutive samples from a locally thickened pleura (as seen on chest CT), may offer diagnostic yields > 50%, and up to >70% when combined with fluid cytology (*J Bronchol 1998;5:327; Chest 2006;129:1549*).
- **Thoracoscopic pleural biopsy:** performed under direct pleural visualization.
  - **Indicated for the undiagnosed suspected malignant effusion.**
  - **Diagnostic yield is >70% to 90%** (*Ann Intern Med 1991;114:271; ANZ J Surg 2006;76:722*).

TREATMENT

- **Transudates: usually resolve with treatment of the underlying cause** (heart failure, hepatic disease, nephrotic syndrome).
  - Therapeutic thoracentesis as indicated for persistent larger effusions.
  - Uncommonly, more aggressive measures including pleurodesis, shunts, or placement of a chronic indwelling pleural catheter are indicated for comfort or palliation.
- **Simple/uncomplicated parapneumonic effusion: antibiotics and close observation.**
- **Complicated parapneumonic effusion and empyema (Fig. 6): antibiotics and early thoracostomy tube drainage** to avoid inflammatory adhesion and organization (*Chest 2000;118:1158*).
  - **Antibiotics should also target anaerobic organisms** as they often complicate empyema (*Lancet 1974;1:338; Chest 1993;103:1502*).
  - **Intrapleural fibrinolysis for loculated effusions is controversial,** but may improve drainage and decrease the need for surgical intervention (*Chest 2006; 129:783*).
    - Possible **risk of pleural hemorrhage** in patients undergoing concomitant systemic anticoagulation (*Radiology 2008;246:956*).

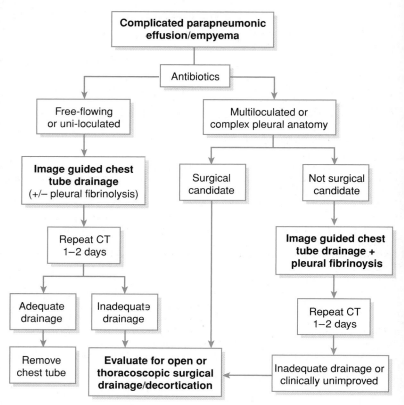

Figure 6. Suggested general approach to managing complicated parapneumonic effusions and empyema.

- Chest tube can be removed when adequate drainage is accomplished (<50 to 100 mL output per day AND resolution documented on follow-up imaging).
- **Surgical decortication (thoracoscopic vs. open) may be required for effusions exhibiting complex anatomy** (extensive pleural thickening, fibrous organization, and/or multiple loculations), or for those unresponsive to tube drainage.
- **Malignant pleural effusion (Fig. 7):** recur in approximately 95% of cases, usually within a week.
  - Observation is appropriate in cases of small, asymptomatic, stable effusions.
  - **Therapeutic (large volume) thoracentesis** (LVT) for comfort.
    - Repeat thoracentesis is reasonable if effusion reaccumulates slowly.
    - **Reexpansion pulmonary edema is very rare,** is unlikely related to rate or volume of fluid removed (*Ann Thorac Surg 2007;84:1656*).
    - **Removal of at least 1.5 L at a time is safe.** However, **LVT should be discontinued with development of chest discomfort,** which may be a surrogate marker for unsafe drop in pleural pressures (*Chest 2006;129:1556*).

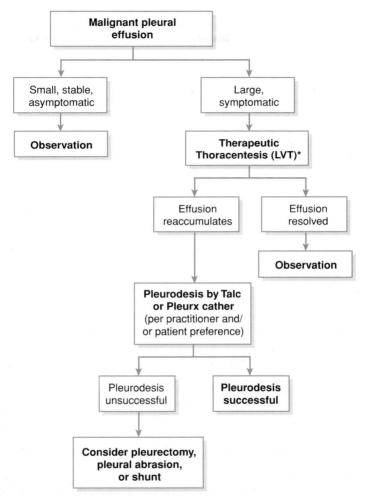

Figure 7. Suggested general approach to managing malignant pleural effusions. *LVT, large-volume thoracentesis.

- **Chemical pleurodesis:** instillation of a pleural sclerosing agent such as talc or doxycycline (*Ann Intern Med 1994;120:56*).
  ○ Recommended when there is **rapid reaccumulation of fluid.**
  ○ **Talc**, instilled either as **"slurry"** through a thoracostomy tube, or through insufflation during thoracoscopy (**"poudrage"**), is very effective and more comfortable than doxycycline (*Chest 2005;127:909*).
  ○ Less effective if lung reexpansion is incomplete after drainage ("trapped lung").
  ○ Often requires hospitalization for approximately 3 to 5 days.

- **Chronic indwelling pleural catheter (Pleurx):** practical, can be performed in the outpatient setting, and maintained easily by the patient and caregiver.
- **Similar indication as chemical pleurodesis,** and preferred if there is "trapped lung."
- 50% pleurodesis rate with repeated drainage, allowing for removal.
- More successful at palliation than doxycycline pleurodesis (*Cancer 1999;86: 1992*).
- Pleurectomy, pleuroperitoneal shunt, chemo/radiation therapy.

Surgical Management

- **Thoracic decortication:** in cases of complicated parapneumonic effusions that have complex pleural anatomy due to fibrous organization and/or not amenable or responsive to pleural drainage.
- **Pleurectomy or pleural abrasion:** for recurring malignant pleural effusion unresponsive to pleurodesis or chronic catheter drainage.

REFERRAL

- Pulmonary (interventional if available)
- Thoracic surgery as needed

OUTCOME/PROGNOSIS

Depends on etiology of the effusion and the extent of pleural disruption

- **Transudate:** depends on management and prognosis of the underlying cause, but **generally a good outcome.**
- **Simple parapneumonic effusion: low morbidity and mortality** if treated appropriately with antibiotics and close observation.
- **Complicated parapneumonic effusion and empyema: with delayed treatment, there is a significantly elevated risk for pleuropulmonary sequelae,** including need for intensive surgical decortication, and possibly death.
- **Malignant pleural effusions** all indicate advanced malignant spread. The **therapeutic options offered** for these patients are **usually successful in achieving desired palliation, and add very little, if any, morbidity or mortality risk.**

Hemoptysis

GENERAL PRINCIPLES

Definition

True hemoptysis is expectoration of blood from the lower respiratory tree (below the glottis).

Classification

- Hemoptysis has been **variably classified in the literature** based on appearance, frequency, rate, volume, and potential for clinical consequences.
  - These characteristics often suggest an underlying etiology and may predict outcome, and therefore help guide diagnostics and management.

- **Massive hemoptysis:** most commonly defined as **greater than 600 mL blood expectorated per 24 hours** (*Flexible Bronchoscopy. 2nd Ed., 2004*).

Epidemiology

Depends on the underlying cause.

Etiology

- According to acuity:
  - **Acute/single or few episodes: bronchitis, pneumonia,** trauma, PE, left heart failure
  - **Subacute/recurrent: malignancy, cavitary lung disease** (TB, aspergilloma, lung abscess), AVM, pulmonary endometriosis
- According to volume:
  - **Nonmassive hemoptysis: bronchitis, malignancy,** bronchiectasis, pneumonias
  - **Massive hemoptysis: bronchiectasis, cavitary lung disease** (TB, aspergilloma, lung abscess), AVM, malignancy
- According to **anatomic location:**
  - **Airway: bronchitis/bronchiectasis, malignancy,** foreign body, trauma
  - **Parenchyma/alveoli: pneumonia, rheumatologic vasculitides and pulmonary hemorrhage syndromes** (ANCA + vasculitis, Goodpasture's, SLE)
  - **Vascular: elevated pulmonary venous pressure** (LV failure, mitral stenosis), PE, AVM, varices/aneurysms, rheumatologic vasculitides, and pulmonary hemorrhage syndromes
- Coagulopathy: thrombocytopenia, DIC
- Meds, drugs: anticoagulants, aspirin, cocaine
- Iatrogenic: lung biopsy, pulmonary arterial trauma (i.e., PA catheter)
- Rare causes: broncholithiasis, pulmonary endometriosis, bronchovascular fistula, bronchopulmonary sequestration, Dieulafoy disease
- **Idiopathic/undiagnosed up to 25%:** prognosis usually favorable (*Ann Intern Med 1985;102:829*)

Pathophysiology

- Specific pathogenesis depends on etiology and location of disease.
- Generally due to **inflammation/irritation of local respiratory tissue and its associated hyperplastic or otherwise abnormal vascular supply.**
- **Bronchial arterial circulation** (branching from the aorta) **supplies high pressure blood to the airways and any associated pathology.**
- **Pulmonary circulation supplies the lung parenchyma** and is under low pressure but receives all of cardiac output.
  - Vascular causes, vascular malformations, Rasmussen's aneurysm (pulmonary artery aneurysm associated with TB).

DIAGNOSIS

Screening for the underlying disease is the basis for diagnosing the cause of hemoptysis and helps guide management.

Clinical Presentation

Hemoptysis may be the only presenting sign or may accompany other manifestations of an underlying disorder (Table 28).

Table 28	Clues to Diagnosing the Cause of Hemoptysis from the History and Physical Exam	
Cause of Hemoptysis	**Historical Clue**	**Physical Exam Finding**
Bronchogenic carcinoma	Smoker, age > 40; recurrent nonmassive hemoptysis, weight loss	Local chest wheezing
Chronic bronchitis/ bronchiectasis	Frequent, copious sputum production; frequent "pneumonias"	Scattered, bilateral coarse chest crackles, wheezes; clubbing
TB, fungal lung disease, lung abscess	Subacute constitutional symptoms; travel and exposure history	Fever, focal coarse chest crackles, cachexia
Acute pneumonia	Acute fever, productive cough, pleurisy, rusty brown hemoptysis	Fever, focal coarse chest crackles, bronchial breath sounds
Vasculitis, hemorrhage syndrome	Subacute constitutional symptoms; hematuria, rash, arthralgias	Diffuse chest crackles, mucosal ulcers, rash
Heart failure	Orthopnea, lower extremity edema, history of valvular disease	Murmurs, diastolic rumble, S_3, loud S_1 or P_2, lower extremity edema
AVM/hereditary hemorrhagic telangiectasia	Platypnea, epistaxis; family history of similar signs and symptoms	Mucosal telangiectasias, orthodeoxia
Pulmonary embolus	Acute dyspnea, pleurisy	Hypoxemia, pleural rub, unilateral lower extremity edema

History
- Most important: age, smoking history, prior lung disease, previous malignancy, risk for coagulopathy.
- Review of systems should focus on symptoms suggesting cardiopulmonary disease, active infection, underlying malignancy, and systemic inflammatory disorders.

Physical Examination
- Most important: vital signs including oxygen saturation, general state of health, lung exam noting focal or diffuse abnormal sounds.
- A thorough exam should always be performed, noting any manifestations suggesting underlying cardiopulmonary, infectious, immunologic, or malignant disease.

Differential Diagnosis

Pseudohemoptysis: Upper airway or GI blood that is expectorated with or without aspiration.

Diagnostic Testing
- Evaluate for adequacy of oxygenation, extent of blood loss, evidence of infection and other underlying systemic disease.
- Localize the source of hemoptysis.

Laboratories
- CBC, CMP, coagulation studies, urinalysis with microscopy
- Type and crossmatch blood if hemoptysis massive
- ABG if indicated
- Sputum studies: routine gram stain and culture. Fungal, AFB, cytology studies as indicated
- Specialized studies as suggested by clinical suspicion
  - CHF: BNP
  - Immunologic disease: ANA/ANCA screen, anti-GBM antibodies, complement levels, cryoglobulins, etc.

Electrocardiography
Assess for underlying structural cardiac disease; otherwise usually noncontributory.

Imaging
- **PA/lateral CXR** should be performed in all cases of hemoptysis.
  - **Normal or nonlocalizing in up to 50% of all cases** (*Chest 1988;92:70*; *Clin Radiol 1996;51:391*).
  - **Normal in up to 10% of cases caused by bronchogenic carcinoma** (*Chest 1988;92:70*).
- **Chest CT:** Indication often depends on clinical suspicion but should be performed if the diagnosis remains in doubt after initial clinical evaluation, or if bronchoscopy is unrevealing (Fig. 8).
  - Advantages:
    - Can visualize parenchyma, vasculature, and airways to varying extent
    - **Especially useful for bronchiectasis, cavitary lung disease, masses, and vascular malformations** (*Chest 1994;105:1155*).
    - High-resolution CT may visualize tumors with efficacy comparable to bronchoscopy (*Radiology 1993;189:677*).
  - Disadvantages:
    - Less efficacious in recognizing subtle bronchial and mucosal lesions (*Chest 1994; 105:1155*).
    - Nonspecific in cases of pulmonary hemorrhage
    - Risky in an unstable patient
- **Echocardiography** if suspect structural or valvular cardiac disease

Diagnostic Procedures
- **Fiberoptic (flexible) bronchoscopy:** Generally **localizes/lateralizes bleeding source** in over two-thirds of cases, depending on the setting (*Ann Thor Surg 1989; 48:272*).
  - **Inspect airways** for mucosal and vascular abnormalities; perform segmental **lavage** for cell count, gram stain, cultures, cytology and to assess for alveolar hemorrhage; brushings, biopsy.
  - **Indications (Fig. 8):**
    - Unclear source after initial evaluation and imaging, or if hemoptysis persists/recurs.

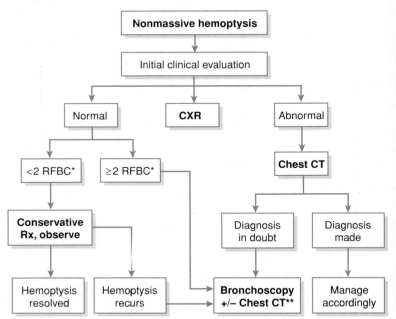

Figure 8. Suggested general approach to diagnosing the cause of nonmassive hemoptysis. *RFBC, risk factors for bronchogenic carcinoma (as outlined in the text). **Consider chest CT if not yet done, as indicated by clinical history.

- ○ Clinical presentation suggests airway abnormality.
- ○ CXR/imaging suggests malignancy.
- ○ CXR/imaging normal or nonlocalizing but with **presence of at least two risk factors for bronchogenic carcinoma:** male sex, age > 40 years, >40 pack-year smoking, duration of hemoptysis > 1 week, volume expectorated > 30 mL (*Chest 1985;87:142; Chest 1988;92:70; Ann Intern Med 1991;151:171*).
- ○ Potential for arterial embolization.
- • Timing: controversial, though increased yield when performed during or within 48 hours of bleeding (*Am Rev Resp Dis 1981;124:221*).
- • **Bronchial and pulmonary arteriography:** perform in **persistent or recurring massive hemoptysis.**
  - • Advantage: **embolization** of the culprit vessel can be simultaneously performed if localized.
  - • Disadvantage: **variable and inexact localization** of bleeding depending on clinical setting (*Ann Thor Surg 1989;48:272*).
    - ○ Anatomic variability.
    - ○ Bleeding usually insufficient for contrast extravasation.
    - ○ Diffuse lung diseases often have associated diffuse vascular abnormalities, making localization difficult (i.e., bronchiectasis).

TREATMENT

- **General approach:**
  - **Distinguish massive from nonmassive hemoptysis.**
  - (a) Stabilize; (b) diagnose and localize; (c) decide on need and type of therapy.
- **Nonmassive hemoptysis:** usually treated conservatively and based on underlying disorder (Fig. 8).
  - Reverse coagulopathy
  - Antitussives and mild sedatives
  - Bronchoscopy if recurrent
- **Massive hemoptysis:** requires urgent action, intensive monitoring, and an early multidisciplinary approach including a pulmonologist and/or thoracic surgeon, and interventional radiologist (Fig. 9).

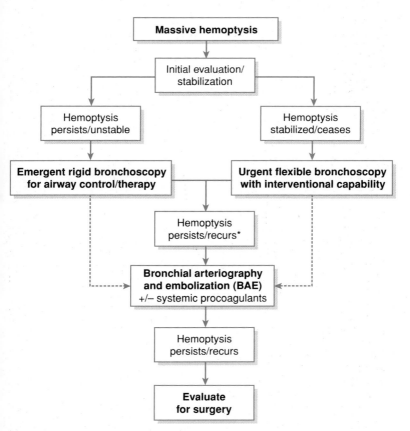

Figure 9. Suggested general approach to managing massive hemoptysis. *Consider BAE in all cases of massive hemoptysis regardless of recurrence.

- **Initial stabilization:**
  - Ensure **airway patency:** very low threshold for intubation, with a large endotracheal tube
  - **Lateral decubitus positioning** (affected lung down) to minimize aspiration into unaffected lung
  - Single-lumen mainstem intubation for selective ventilation of unaffected lung
  - Double-lumen endotracheal intubation for selective ventilation of unaffected lung. Should be performed and managed only under appropriately skilled supervision
- **Bronchoscopy** with directed airway therapy:
  - **Rigid bronchoscopy** favored if available: provides better airway access and ventilatory control, with easier suctioning and manipulation of instruments
  - Direct bronchoscopic tamponade
  - **Balloon tamponade,** left in place for 1 to 2 days. Fogarty, bronchial blocker, PA catheter balloons have all been described. Watch for ischemic mucosal injury or postobstructive pneumonitis (*Thorax 2003;58:814*).
  - **Endobronchial electrocautery, Argon-Plasma coagulation** (*Chest 2001; 119:781*; *Can Resp J 2004;11:305*).
  - **Topical hemostatic agents:** epinephrine, vasopressin, thrombin, cold saline (*Am Rev Resp Dis 1987;135:A108*; *Chest 1989;96:473*; *Thorax 1980;35:901*).
- **Bronchial arteriography and embolization should be performed early** in massive or recurrent hemoptysis
  - **Successful embolization (>85%)** with careful localization (*Chest 2002;121: 789*; *Radiology 2004;233:741*).
  - Particularly useful in **CF patients** (*Am J Resp Crit Care Med 1998;157:1951*; *Chest 2002;121:796*).
  - **Early failure usually due to inadequate or incomplete source vessel identification**
    - Postembolization arteriography may identify additional systemic culprit vessels, most commonly from the intercostal and phrenic arteries (*Am J Roent 2003;180:1577*).
  - **Rebleeding common** (up to 20%) over 1 year (*Chest 1999;115:912*; *Respiration 2000;67:412*).
  - **Risks** include bronchial or partial pulmonary infarct/necrosis and, rarely, ischemic myelopathy due to inadvertent embolization of a spinal artery

Medications

Systemic procoagulants: use only in unstable massive hemoptysis as a temporizing measure, or when conventional bronchoscopic, interventional or surgical therapies are contraindicated and/or unavailable

- Factor VII, vasopressin, aminocaproic acid

Surgical Management

- **Lobectomy/pneumonectomy offers definitive cure**
- **Indications: persistent focal/unilateral massive hemoptysis despite other therapy**
  - Particularly useful for stable patients with hemoptysis due to cavitary lung disease (i.e., aspergilloma), localized bronchogenic carcinoma, AVM, traumatic injuries (*Crit Care Med 2000;28:1642*)

- **Contraindications:** poor pulmonary reserve, advanced malignancy, active TB, diffuse lung disease, diffuse alveolar hemorrhage
- Emergent surgery has high morbidity and mortality compared to elective surgery after stabilization

REFERRAL

- Pulmonary (interventional for massive hemoptysis, if available)
- Thoracic surgery
- Interventional radiology

OUTCOME/PROGNOSIS

Mortality depends on etiology and amount (*Arch Intern Med 1983;143:1343*; *Am J Med Sci 1987;294:301*).

- Up to 80% with massive hemoptysis due to malignancy
- Less than 10% with nonmassive hemoptysis
- Less than 1% in bronchiectasis, lung infections

Cystic Fibrosis

GENERAL PRINCIPLES

Definition
Cystic fibrosis (CF) is a **multisystem autosomal recessive disorder** caused by mutations of the cystic fibrosis transmembrane conductance regulator (CFTR), a gene located on chromosome 7.

Epidemiology
- In the United States, approximately 30,000 people are affected by CF with an incidence of 1 in 3,500 live births (*Clin Chest Med 2007;28:279*).
- CF is the most common lethal genetic disease in Caucasians, but the diagnosis needs to be considered in patients of diverse backgrounds as well.
- Patients are typically diagnosed during childhood, but there is increasing recognition of milder variants that may not present until later in life.

Etiology
- CF is caused by **mutations in the CFTR gene,** a cyclic AMP-regulated chloride channel (*Science 1989;245:1073*).
- CFTR normally maintains hydration of exocrine organ secretions.
- Abnormal CFTR ultimately results in decreased chloride secretion and increased sodium absorption on the surface of epithelial cells resulting in thickened secretions in the airways, pancreatic ducts, biliary tree, intestines, and reproductive tract.

Pathophysiology
- CFTR normally regulates transport of electrolytes across the epithelium (*Curr Opin Pulm Med 2003;9:486–491*).

- The primary pulmonary manifestations of disease are thought to be related to abnormal electrolyte transport in the airway, which results in desiccated airway secretions and impaired mucociliary clearance.
- The airways enter a vicious cycle of infection, inflammation, and chronic airway obstruction, resulting in bronchiectasis, chronic infection, and ultimately premature death (*N Engl J Med 2005;352:1992*).
- Similarly, thickened secretions in the pancreatic and biliary ducts lead to maldigestion, **malabsorption, liver disease, and diabetes.**

DIAGNOSIS

- The diagnosis of CF is typically made during childhood, but approximately 10% of patients are diagnosed after age 10 (*CFF Patient Registry, 2007*).
- Newborn screening leads to increased frequency of early diagnosis (*J Pediatr 2002;141:804*).
- Pulmonary symptoms lead to consideration of the diagnosis in 50% of cases (*J Pediatr 1993;122:1*).
- **At least one criterion** from each set of features must be met to diagnose CF (*J Pediatr 2008;153:S1*):
  - Compatible clinical feature of CF (see clinical features) or
  - A positive family history or
  - A positive newborn screening test
  and
  - Elevated sweat chloride > 60 mmol/L on two occasions or
  - Presence of two disease causing mutations in CFTR or
  - Abnormal nasal potential difference
- Atypical patients may lack classic symptoms and signs or have normal sweat tests (*Curr Opin Pulm Med 2003;9:498*).
- Although genotyping may assist in the diagnosis, it alone cannot establish or rule out the diagnosis of CF, and the **initial test of choice remains the sweat test.**

Clinical Presentation

- **Pulmonary manifestations:**
  - Cough with purulent sputum production
  - Sinopulmonary infection with pathogens typical of CF
  - Progressive dyspnea
  - Acute pulmonary disease exacerbations
  - Recurrent infection and inflammation
  - Bronchiectasis
  - Airflow obstruction
- **Extrapulmonary manifestations**
  - Chronic sinusitis
  - Nasal polyposis
  - Nutritional failure
  - Pancreatic insufficiency—vitamin A, D, E, K deficiency
  - Meconium ileus
  - Distal intestinal obstruction
  - Volvulus, intussusception, and rectal prolapse
  - Diabetes mellitus
  - Liver cirrhosis, portal hypertension

- Cholelithiasis, and cholecystitis
- Nephrolithiasis
- Male infertility (bilateral absence of the vas deferens) and epididymitis
- Growth retardation, osteoarthropathy, osteopenia

History

Presenting symptoms may include (*J Pediatr 1993;122:1*):

- Cough with purulent sputum production (40%)
- Failure to thrive (29%)
- Steatorrhea
- Meconium ileus

Physical Examination

- Malnourished, underweight
- Crackles on lung exam typically anterior and in the apices
- Digital clubbing

Differential Diagnosis

- **Primary ciliary dyskinesia**—bronchiectasis, sinusitis, and infertility, but limited GI symptoms and normal sweat chloride levels
- **Shwachman-Diamond syndrome**—pancreatic insufficiency, cyclic neutropenia and short stature which may lead to lung disease, but normal sweat chloride levels (*Hematol Oncol Clin North Am 2009;23:233*)
- **Young's syndrome**—bronchiectasis, sinusitis, and azoospermia, but mild respiratory symptoms, lacks GI symptoms, and normal sweat chloride levels (*Thorax 1987;42:815–817*)
- **Immunoglobulin deficiency**—recurrent sinus and pulmonary infections but typically no GI symptoms and normal sweat chloride levels
- **Chronic rhinosinusitis**—recurrent sinus infections but limited GI symptoms and normal sweat chloride levels
- **Chronic idiopathic pancreatitis**—recurrent pancreatitis but limited sinopulmonary disease and normal sweat chloride levels

Diagnostic Testing

- **Skin sweat testing** with a standardized quantitative pilocarpine iontophoresis method remains the **gold standard for the diagnosis of CF** (*Am J Respir Crit Care Med 2006;173:475*).
  - A sweat chloride concentration of ≥60 mmol/L on two separate occasions is consistent with the diagnosis of CF.
  - Borderline sweat test results (40 to 59 mmol/L sweat chloride) or nondiagnostic results in the setting of high clinical suspicion should also lead to repeat sweat testing, nasal potential difference testing, or genetic testing.
  - Sweat testing should be performed at a CF care center to ensure reliability of results.
  - Abnormal sweat chloride concentrations are rarely detected in non-CF patients.
- **Genetic tests** have detected more than 1,500 putative CF mutations.
  - Two recessive genes must be abnormal to cause CF.
  - The most commonly encountered CF mutation is the ΔF508 CFTR mutation, which is present in approximately 70% of alleles in affected individuals (*Am J Respir Crit Care Med 2006;173:475*).

- Commercially available probes identify more than 90% of the abnormal genes in a white Northern European population, although they test for only a minority of the known CF genes. Full gene sequencing is available.
- **Nasal potential difference**
  - A test in which the voltage across the epithelium lining the nose is measured at baseline, after inhibiting sodium channels, and after stimulating CFTR (*J Pediatr 1986;108:517; J Cyst Fibros 2004;3:151*).
  - The test should be repeated on two separate days to confirm diagnosis and should be performed at specialized centers.

Laboratories

- Sputum cultures typically identify multiple organisms including *Pseudomonas aeruginosa, Staphylococcus aureus*, nontypeable *Haemophilus influenzae, Stenotrophomonas maltophilia*, and *Burkholderia cepacia*. Sputum sensitivity testing should direct therapy. Isolation of mucoid variants of *P. aeruginosa* from the respiratory tract occurs frequently.
- Testing for malabsorption due to pancreatic exocrine insufficiency is often not formally performed, because clinical evidence (the presence of foul-smelling, bulky, and loose stools; low fat-soluble vitamin levels [vitamins A, D, and E]; and a prolonged prothrombin time [vitamin K dependent]) and a clear response to pancreatic enzyme treatment are usually considered sufficient for the diagnosis.
- Tests that identify chronic sinusitis or infertility, especially obstructive azoospermia in men, would also support the diagnosis of CF.
- Monitoring of electrolytes is indicated in patients with a history of electrolyte abnormalities or renal insufficiency.

Imaging

- Chest radiography ultimately shows enlarged lung volumes with cystic lung disease, bronchiectasis, and mucous plugging especially in the upper lobes.
- High-resolution CT scan may be helpful in evaluating patients with early or mild disease by detecting early airway changes.
- Pulmonary function tests eventually show expiratory airflow obstruction with increased residual volume and total lung capacity.
- Impairment of alveolar gas exchange may be present as well, progressing to hypoxemia and hypercapnia.

TREATMENT

- CF therapy aims to improve quality of life and functioning, decrease the number of exacerbations and hospitalizations, avoid complications associated with therapy, reduce the rate of decline in lung function, and decrease mortality.
- A comprehensive program addressing multiple organ system derangements, as provided at CF care centers, is recommended.
- Most adults with CF have significant lung diseases and a large portion of therapy is focused on clearing pulmonary secretions and controlling infection (*N Engl J Med 1996;335:179*).
- **Pulmonary therapy** (*Am J Respir Crit Care Med 2007;176:957*)
  - Inhaled bronchodilators: β-adrenergic agonists (albuterol MDI, two to four puffs bid–qid; salmeterol or formoterol, one dry powder inhalation bid)

- Used to treat the reversible components of airflow obstruction and facilitate mucus clearance.
- Contraindicated in the rare patient with associated paradoxical deterioration of airflow after their use.
- **Recombinant human deoxyribonuclease:** DNase, dornase-α, Pulmozyme (2.5 mg or one ampule per day inhaled using a jet nebulizer)
  - Digests extracellular DNA, decreasing the viscoelasticity of the sputum.
  - It improves pulmonary function and decreases the incidence of respiratory tract infections that require parenteral antibiotics (*N Engl J Med 1992;326:812*; *American Review of Respiratory Disease 1993;148:145*).
  - Adverse effects may include pharyngitis, laryngitis, rash, chest pain, and conjunctivitis.
- **Hypertonic saline:** (4 mL of inhaled 7% saline twice daily)
  - A recent study showed fewer exacerbations and possible improvement in lung function in patients treated with hypertonic saline (*N Engl J Med 2006;354:229*).
  - Inhaled bronchodilators should be administered prior to treatments to avoid treatment-induced bronchospasm.
- **Antibiotics**
  - **A combination of an IV semisynthetic penicillin, a third- or fourth-generation cephalosporin, or a quinolone and an aminoglycoside is typically recommended during acute exacerbations.**
  - Sputum culture sensitivities should guide therapy. ***P. aeruginosa* is the most frequent pulmonary pathogen.**
  - The duration of antibiotic therapy is dictated by the clinical response. At least 14 days of antibiotics is typically given to treat an exacerbation.
  - Home IV antibiotic therapy is common, but hospitalization may allow better access to comprehensive therapy and diagnostic testing. PO antibiotics are recommended only for mild exacerbations.
  - The use of chronic or intermittent prophylactic antibiotics can be considered, especially in patients with frequent recurrent exacerbations, but antimicrobial resistance may develop.
  - **Inhaled aerosolized tobramycin** (300 mg nebulized bid, 28 days on alternating with 28 days off, using appropriate nebulizer and compressor) improves pulmonary function, decreases the density of *P. aeruginosa,* and decreases the risk of hospitalization (*N Engl J Med 1999;340:23*). Voice alteration (13%) and tinnitus (3%) are potential adverse events associated with long-term inhaled tobramycin (*N Engl J Med 1999;340:23–30*).
  - Patients with CF have atypical pharmacokinetics and often require higher drug doses at more frequent intervals. In adult patients with CF, for example, cefepime is often dosed at 2 g IV q8h and gentamicin or tobramycin is often dosed at 3 mg/kg IV q8h (aiming for peak levels of 10 mg/mL and trough levels of <2 mg/mL).
  - Once-daily aminoglycoside dosing should be guided by pharmacokinetic testing. Monitoring levels (peaks and troughs) of drugs such as aminoglycosides helps to ensure therapeutic levels and decrease the risk of toxicity.
- **Anti-inflammatory therapy**
  - **Azithromycin (500 mg oral Mon, Wed, Fri)** used chronically shows mild improvement in lung function and reduces days in the hospital for treatment of respiratory exacerbations in patients who are chronically infected with *P. aeruginosa* (*JAMA 2003;290:1749*).

- ○ **Glucocorticoids** used in short courses may be helpful to some patients, but long-term therapy should be avoided to minimize the side effects that include glucose intolerance, osteopenia, and growth retardation.
- ○ **Ibuprofen** used in high doses has been used as a chronic anti-inflammatory agent in children with mild impairment of lung function (*Chest 1999;124:689*).
- **Mechanical airway clearance devices:** (flutter valve, acapella device, high-frequency chest oscillation vests, low- and high-pressure positive expiratory pressure devices)
  - ○ Can be used in combination with medical therapy to promote airway clearance.
  - ○ Other alternatives include postural drainage with chest percussion and vibration; and breathing and coughing exercises.
- **Pulmonary rehabilitation:**
  - ○ When done with exercise rehabilitation may improve functional status and promote clearance of airway secretions.
- **Oxygen therapy:**
  - ○ May be indicated based on standard recommendations used for the treatment of COPD.
  - ○ Rest and exercise oxygen assessments should be performed as clinically indicated.
- **Noninvasive ventilation:**
  - ○ Used for chronic respiratory failure due to CF-related bronchiectasis.
  - ○ Has not been clearly demonstrated to provide a survival benefit, although it may provide symptomatic relief or may be used as a bridge to transplantation.
- **Extrapulmonary therapy**
  - **Pancreatic insufficiency (PI):**
    - ○ PI is managed with **pancreatic enzyme supplementation.**
    - ○ Enzyme dose should be titrated to achieve one to two semisolid stools per day, and to maintain adequate growth and nutrition.
    - ○ Enzymes are taken immediately before meals and snacks.
    - ○ Dosing of pancreatic enzymes should be initiated at 500 Units lipase/kg/meal and should not exceed 2,500 Units lipase/kg/meal.
    - ○ **High doses** (6,000 Units lipase/kg/meal) have been associated with **chronic intestinal strictures** (*N Engl J Med 1997;336:1283*).
    - ○ Generic enzyme substitutes may not provide adequate lipase needed for absorption.
    - ○ Gastric acid suppression may enhance enzyme activity.
  - **Vitamin deficiency:**
    - ○ Vitamin supplementation is recommended in extrapulmonary disease, especially with fat-soluble vitamins that are not well absorbed in the setting of pancreatic insufficiency.
    - ○ **Vitamins A, D, E, and K** can all be taken orally on a regular basis.
    - ○ Iron-deficiency anemia requires iron supplementation.
  - **CF-related diabetes mellitus (CFRD):**
    - ○ CFRD is usually managed with **insulin.**
    - ○ Typical diabetic dietary restrictions are liberalized (high-calorie diet with unrestricted fat) to meet the increased energy requirements of patients with CF and to encourage appropriate growth and weight maintenance.
  - **Bowel impaction:**
    - ○ **Laxatives** such as senna, magnesium citrate, or polyethylene glycol can be tried initially.
    - ○ Refractory cases may require a Hypaque enema.

- **Osteopenia:**
  - **Screening** should be routinely performed on patients with CF, and if present may be managed with calcium, vitamin D supplementation, and bisphosphonate therapy as clinically indicated (*Am J Respir Crit Care Med 2004;169:77*).
- **Chronic sinusitis:**
  - Many patients will benefit from chronic **nasal steroid** administration.
  - Nasal saline washes may also be helpful.
  - Patients whose symptoms cannot be controlled with medical management may benefit from functional endoscopic sinus surgery and nasal polypectomy.

Surgical Management
- **Lung transplantation:**
  - The majority of patients with CF die from pulmonary disease.
  - FEV_1 is a strong predictor of mortality (*N Engl J Med 1992;326:1187*) and has been helpful in deciding when to refer patients for lung transplantation.
  - However, other factors such as marked alveolar gas exchange abnormalities (resting hypoxemia or hypercapnia), evidence of PH, or increased frequency or severity of pulmonary exacerbations should also be considered when deciding on referral for transplantation.
- **Massive hemoptysis:**
  - This is usually controlled with antibiotics and bronchial artery embolization. Surgical lung resection is rarely needed.

Lifestyle/Risk Modification
- **Avoidance of irritating inhaled fumes, dusts, or chemicals** including second-hand smoke is recommended.
- **Yearly influenza vaccination** (0.5 mL IM) decreases the incidence of infection and subsequent deterioration (*N Engl J Med 1984;311:1653*).
- **Pneumovax** (0.5 mL IM) may also provide benefit.

Diet
A high-calorie diet with vitamin supplementation is typically recommended.

Activity
- CF patients should maintain as much activity as possible.
- Exercise is an excellent form of airway clearance.

SPECIAL CONSIDERATIONS

- Although fertility may be decreased in women with CF secondary to thickened cervical mucus, many women with CF have tolerated pregnancy well (*N Engl J Med 1984;311:1653*).
- Maternal and fetal outcomes are good for women with adequate pulmonary reserve ($FEV_1 > 50\%$ predicted) and good nutritional status, and pregnancy does not appear to affect these women's survival (*Chest 2000;118:85*).
- Pregnancies should be planned to optimize patient status and coordinate care with obstetrics.

COMPLICATIONS

Other pulmonary complications of CF may include allergic bronchopulmonary aspergillosis, massive hemoptysis, acquisition of atypical mycobacterium, and pneumothorax.

REFERRAL

- CF patients or suspected CF patients should be referred to a national CFF-accredited care center.
- Tests such as sweat chloride testing and nasal potential difference are best done at specialized centers.
- A team of CF specialists including physicians, nutritionists, respiratory therapists, and social workers aid in the routine care of these patients.

PATIENT EDUCATION

Information can be found at the CF Foundation Web site (www.cff.org)

MONITORING/FOLLOW-UP

Recommendations are to follow patients every 3 months with PFTs and yearly lab work including vitamin levels.

OUTCOME/PROGNOSIS

- Predictors of increased mortality include age, female gender, low weight, low forced expiratory volume in 1 second (FEV_1), pancreatic insufficiency, diabetes mellitus, infection with *B. cepacia,* and the number of acute exacerbations (*JAMA 2001;286:2683*).
- With improved therapy, the median survival has been extended to approximately 37 years (CF Foundation www.cff.org).
- New pharmacologic therapies targeting restoration of CFTR function are in various stages of preclinical and clinical development.

Allergy and Immunology
Shirley Joo, Ritu Gupta, and Andrew Kau

Anaphylaxis

GENERAL PRINCIPLES

Definition
Anaphylaxis is a rapidly developing, life-threatening systemic reaction mediated by immunoglobulin E (IgE). The peak severity is seen usually within 5 to 30 minutes.

Classification
- Allergic IgE-mediated anaphylaxis
- Nonallergic anaphylaxis (used to be called anaphylactoid)
- Cytotoxic-mediated anaphylaxis
- Immune complex–complement–mediated anaphylaxis
- Idiopathic

Epidemiology
Incidence of anaphylaxis is approximately 50 to 2,000 episodes per 100,000 person-years with a lifetime prevalence of 0.05% to 2%.

Etiology
- Foods
- Hymenoptera stings (bees, wasps, and fire ants)
- Medications
- Radiocontrast media
- Latex rubber
- Blood products
- Hemodialysis
- Physical factors (cold temperature or exercise)
- Idiopathic

Pathophysiology
- Anaphylaxis is due to sensitization to an antigen and formation of specific IgE to that antigen. On reexposure, the IgE on mast cells and basophils binds the antigen and cross-links the IgE receptor, which causes activation of the cells with subsequent release of preformed mediators, such as histamine.
- The release of mediators ultimately causes capillary leakage, cellular edema, and smooth muscle contractions resulting in the constellation of physical symptoms.

Risk Factors
- IgE-mediated reactions
  - Previous sensitization and formation of antigen-specific IgE with history of anaphylaxis.

- Non-IgE–mediated anaphylaxis
  - Mastocytosis patients are at higher risk for future episodes if not recognized or not premedicated.
  - Radiocontrast sensitivity reactions
    - Age >50 years
    - Preexisting cardiovascular or renal disease
    - History of allergy
    - History of previous reaction to radiocontrast media
    - **Sensitivity to seafood or iodine does not predispose to radiocontrast media reactions.**

Prevention

- **For all types of anaphylaxis, recognition of potential triggers and avoidance is the best prevention.**
- **Self-injectable epinephrine and patient education for all patients with a history of anaphylaxis.**
- Radiocontrast sensitivity reactions
  - Use of low-ionic contrast media is strongly suggested
  - Premedication before procedure
    - Prednisone 50 mg PO given 13, 7, and 1 hour prior to procedure
    - Diphenhydramine 50 mg PO given 1 hour before procedure
    - H2 blocker may also be given 1 hour before procedure
  - **Premedication is not 100% effective and appropriate precautions for handling a reaction should be taken.**
- Red man's syndrome from vancomycin
  - Symptoms can usually be prevented by slowing the rate of infusion and premedicating with diphenhydramine (50 mg PO) 30 minutes prior to start of the infusion.

DIAGNOSIS

Diagnosis is based primarily on history and physical examination with confirmation in some cases provided by the laboratory finding of an elevated serum β-tryptase level. However, the absence of an elevated β-tryptase level does not exclude anaphylaxis.

Clinical Presentation

- The clinical manifestations of allergic and nonallergic anaphylaxis are the same. Most serious reactions occur within minutes after exposure to the antigen. However, the reaction may be delayed for hours. Some patients experience a biphasic reaction characterized by a recurrence of symptoms after 4 to 8 hours. A few patients have a protracted course that requires several hours of continuous supportive treatment.
- Manifestations include pruritus, urticaria, angioedema, respiratory distress (due to laryngeal edema, laryngospasm, or bronchospasm), hypotension, abdominal cramping, and diarrhea.

History

History is taken to help identify the potential trigger, such as new foods, medications, or other commonly known allergens. Also documenting the time of onset of symptoms, that is, minutes to hours or days after a suspected exposure can help to classify the type of anaphylaxis.

Physical Examination

- Pay special attention to vital signs—blood pressure, respiratory rate, oxygen saturation.
- Airway and pulmonary: Assess for any evidence of laryngeal edema or angioedema. Auscultate lung fields to listen for evidence of wheezing. Continue to assess for need to protect the airway.
- Perform a focused cardiovascular exam.
- Skin: urticaria or erythema.

Diagnostic Criteria

- **Mild anaphylaxis** (skin and subcutaneous tissue only): Generalized erythema, urticaria, periorbital edema, or angioedema.
- **Moderate anaphylaxis** (features suggesting respiratory, cardiovascular, or gastrointestinal involvement): Dyspnea, stridor, wheezing, nausea, vomiting, dizziness (presyncope), diaphoresis, chest or throat tightness, and abdominal pain in addition to cutaneous symptoms.
- **Severe anaphylaxis** (hypoxia, hypotension, or neurologic compromise): In addition to the symptoms in the previous two categories, patients may have cyanosis or $PaO_2 \leq 92\%$ at any stage, hypotension (systolic blood pressure < 90 mm Hg), confusion, loss of consciousness, or neurologic compromise.

Differential Diagnosis

- Anaphylaxis due to **preformed IgE and reexposure:** Medications, Hymenoptera sting, and foods are the most common causes of anaphylaxis.
- **Nonallergic anaphylaxis**
  - **Radiocontrast sensitivity reactions** are thought to be from direct degranulation of mast cells in susceptible patients due to osmotic shifts. Reactions can occur in 5% to 10% of the patients with fatal reactions occurring in 1 in 40,000 procedures.
  - **Red man's syndrome** from vancomycin consists of pruritus and flushing of the face and neck.
  - **Mastocytosis** should be considered in patients with recurrent unexplained anaphylaxis or flushing, especially with previous reactions to nonspecific mast cell degranulators such as opiates and radiocontrast media.
  - **Ingestant-related reactions** can mimic anaphylaxis. This is usually due to sulfites or the presence of histamine-like substance in spoiled fish (scombroidosis).
  - **Flushing syndromes** include flushing due to red man's syndrome, carcinoid, vasointestinal peptide (and other vasoactive intestinal peptide-secreting tumors), postmenopausal symptoms, and alcohol use.
- Other forms of shock such as hypoglycemic, cardiogenic, septic, and hemorrhagic
- Miscellaneous syndromes such as C1 esterase (C1 INH) deficiency syndrome, pheochromocytoma, neurologic (seizure, stroke), and capillary leak syndrome
- Idiopathic

Diagnostic Testing

- Serum β-tryptase peaks at 1 hour after symptoms begin and may be present up to 6 hours.
- Epicutaneous skin testing and RAST (radioallergosorbent test) testing when available to identify trigger allergens.

TREATMENT

- Early recognition of signs and symptoms of anaphylaxis is a critical first step in treatment.
- **Maintain recumbent position while assessing and starting therapy.**
- **Airway management is a priority.** Supplemental 100% oxygen therapy should be administered. Endotracheal intubation may be necessary. If laryngeal edema is not rapidly responsive to epinephrine, cricothyroidotomy or tracheotomy may be required.
- **Volume expansion with intravenous (IV) fluids may** be necessary. An initial bolus of 500 to 1,000 mL normal saline should be followed by an infusion at a rate that is titrated to BP and urine output.
- ***α-Adrenergic or mixed adrenergic agonist vasopressors must be avoided in this setting due to resultant unopposed α-mediated vasoconstriction.***

Medications

- **Epinephrine** should be administered immediately.
  - Adult: 0.3 to 0.5 mg (0.3 to 0.5 mL of a 1:1,000 solution) intramuscularly (IM) in the lateral thigh, repeated at 10- to 15-minute intervals if necessary.
  - Child: 1:1,000 dilution at 0.01 mg/kg or 0.1 to 0.3 mL administered IM in the lateral thigh, repeated at 10- to 15-minute interval if necessary.
  - 0.5 mL of 1:1,000 solution sublingually in cases of major airway compromise or hypotension.
  - 3 to 5 mL of 1:10,000 solution via central line.
  - 3 to 5 mL of 1:10,000 solution diluted with 10 mL of normal saline via endotracheal tube.
  - Protracted symptoms that require multiple doses of epinephrine, an IV epinephrine drip may be useful; the infusion is titrated to maintain adequate blood pressure.
- **Glucagon,** given as a 1-mg (1 ampule) bolus and followed by a drip of up to 1 mg/hr can be used to provide inotropic support for patients who are taking β-adrenergic antagonists.
  - β-Adrenergic antagonists therapy increases the risk of anaphylaxis and renders the reaction more difficult to treat (*Ann Intern Med 1991;115:270*).
- **Inhaled β-adrenergic agonists** should be used to treat resistant bronchospasm.
  - Albuterol 0.5 mL (2.5 mg) or metaproterenol 0.3 mL (15 mg) in 2.5 mL of normal saline.
- **Glucocorticoids** have no significant immediate effect. However, they may prevent relapse of severe reactions.
  - Adult: Hydrocortisone 100 mg to 1 g IV or IM.
  - Child: Hydrocortisone 10 to 100 mg IV.
- **Antihistamines** relieve skin symptoms but have no immediate effect on the reaction. They may shorten the duration of the reaction.
  - Adult: Diphenhydramine 25 to 50 mg IM or IV.
  - Child: Diphenhydramine 12.5 to 25 mg IM or IV.

REFERRAL

Referrals to an allergist for further evaluation should be offered to all patients with a history of anaphylaxis. More importantly, patients with *Hymenoptera* sensitivity should be evaluated to determine eligibility for venom immunotherapy.

Eosinophilia

GENERAL PRINCIPLES

- A broad variety of infectious, allergic, neoplastic, and idiopathic diseases are associated with increased blood and/or tissue eosinophilia.
- Accepted upper limits of normal blood eosinophilia vary.
- A value > 600 eosinophils/μL of blood is abnormal in the vast majority of cases.
- The degree of eosinophilia can be categorized as mild (600 to 1,000 cells/μL), moderate (1,500 to 5,000 cells/μL), or severe (>5,000 cells/μL).
- Eosinophils are tissue-dwelling cells and are most abundant in mucosal tissues such as the respiratory and gastrointestinal tracts.

Classification

- Peripheral eosinophilia can be divided into categories as primary, secondary, or idiopathic.
- Primary eosinophilia often occurs in the context of hematologic malignancies, such as chronic myeloid disorders or acute leukemias, when there is clonal expansion of eosinophils.
- The most common causes of secondary eosinophilia include parasites, allergic diseases, autoimmune disorders, toxins, medications, and endocrine disorders, such as Addison's disease.
- Idiopathic eosinophilia is considered when primary and secondary causes are excluded.
- **Eosinophilia associated with atopic disease.** Modest peripheral blood levels of eosinophils are often found in patients with allergic rhinitis, asthma, or atopic dermatitis.
  - In allergic rhinitis, nasal eosinophilia is more common than peripheral blood eosinophilia.
  - Nasal eosinophilia with or without blood eosinophilia may be seen in asthma, nasal polyposis, or nonallergic rhinitis with eosinophilia syndrome (NARES).
  - NARES is a syndrome of marked nasal eosinophilia and nasal polyps. These patients do not have a history of allergies, asthma, aspirin sensitivity, and have negative skin tests and IgE levels.
- **Eosinophilia associated with pulmonary infiltrates.** This classification is inclusive of the pulmonary infiltrates with eosinophilia (PIE) syndromes and the eosinophilic pneumonias.
  - PIE syndromes refer to those diseases with pulmonary infiltrates and blood eosinophilia. The **PIE syndromes** include allergic bronchopulmonary aspergillosis (ABPA), an IgE-dependent immunologic reaction to *Aspergillus fumigatus* consisting of pulmonary infiltrates, proximal bronchiectasis, and asthma- and drug-induced pneumonitis.
  - Eosinophilic pneumonias consist of pulmonary infiltrates with lung eosinophilia. It is important to note that eosinophilic pneumonias are only sometimes associated with blood eosinophilia. The **eosinophilic pneumonias** include acute and chronic eosinophilic pneumonias (idiopathic diseases that present with fever, cough, and dyspnea), Loffler syndrome (combination of blood eosinophilia and transient pulmonary infiltrates due to passage of helminthic larvae, usually *Ascaris lumbricoides*, through the lungs), and tropical pulmonary eosinophilia (a hypersensitivity response in the lung to lymphatic filariae).

- **HIV.** Modest to marked eosinophilia of unknown cause can be seen occasionally in patients with HIV. The eosinophilia is usually due to reactions to medications, adrenal insufficiency due to cytomegalovirus with consequent eosinophilia, or eosinophilic folliculitis (common dermatologic disorder seen in HIV patients).
- **Eosinophilia associated with parasitic infection.** Various multicellular parasites or helminths such as *Ascaris*, hookworm, or *Strongyloides* can induce blood eosinophilia, whereas single-celled protozoan parasites such as *Giardia lamblia* do not. The level of eosinophilia reflects the degree of tissue invasion by the parasite.
  - In cases of blood eosinophilia, ***Strongyloides stercoralis* infection must be excluded** because this helminth can set up a cycle of autoinfection leading to chronic infection with intermittent, sometimes marked, eosinophilia.
  - Tissue eosinophilia may not be accompanied by blood eosinophilia when the organism is sequestered within tissues (e.g., intact echinococcal cysts) or is limited to the intestinal lumen (e.g., tapeworms).
    - Among the helminths, the principal parasites that need to be evaluated are *S. stercoralis*, hookworm, and *Toxocara canis*. The diagnostic consideration can also vary according to geographic region.
    - There are some important caveats that need to be considered when evaluating patients for parasitic diseases and eosinophilia: *Strongyloides* can persist for decades without causing major symptoms and can elicit varying degrees of eosinophilia ranging from minimal to marked eosinophilia.
    - *T. canis* (visceral larva migrans) should be considered in children with a propensity to eat dirt contaminated by dog ascarid eggs.
- **Eosinophilia associated with cutaneous disease**
  - **Atopic dermatitis** is classically associated with blood and skin eosinophilia.
  - **Eosinophilic fasciitis** is characterized by acute erythema, swelling, and induration of the extremities progressing to symmetric induration of the skin that spares the fingers, feet, and face.
  - Antibiotic therapy failure and recurrent swelling of an extremity without tactile warmth is characteristic of **eosinophilic cellulitis.**
  - Patients with HIV are at risk for **eosinophilic pustular folliculitis.**
  - A rare disease, **episodic angioedema with eosinophilia**, leads to recurrent attacks of fever, angioedema, and blood eosinophilia without other organ damage.
- **Eosinophilia associated with multiorgan involvement**
  - **Drug-induced eosinophilia.** Numerous drugs can cause blood and/or tissue eosinophilia. Drug-induced eosinophilia typically responds to cessation of the culprit medication. Asymptomatic drug-induced eosinophilia does not necessitate cessation of therapy.
  - **Churg–Strauss syndrome** (CSS) is a small-vessel vasculitis distinguished from other vasculitides by tissue and blood eosinophilia, intravascular and extravascular eosinophilic granuloma formation, lung involvement with transient infiltrates on chest radiograph, and association with asthma. The onset of asthma and eosinophilia may precede the development of CSS by several years. Other manifestations include sinusitis, mono- or polyneuropathy, and rash.
    - Half the patients have antineutrophil cytoplasmic antibodies directed against myeloperoxidase (p-ANCA). Biopsy of affected tissue reveals a necrotizing vasculitis with extravascular granulomas and tissue eosinophilia.
    - Initial treatment involves high-dose glucocorticoids with the addition of cyclophosphamide if necessary. Leukotriene modifiers, like all systemic steroid-sparing agents (including inhaled steroids), have been associated with unmasking

of CSS due to a decrease in systemic steroid therapy; however, no evidence exists that these drugs *cause* CSS (*Chest 2000;117:708*).

- **Mastocytosis.** Systemic mastocytosis is characterized by infiltration of mast cells into various organs including the skin, liver, lymph nodes, bone marrow, and spleen. Peripheral eosinophilia can be seen in up to 20% of cases of systemic mastocytosis and bone marrow biopsies often show an excess number of eosinophils.
- Idiopathic **hypereosinophilic syndrome** (HES) is a proliferative disorder of eosinophils characterized by infiltration of eosinophils in and consequent damage to organs such as the heart, gastrointestinal tract, kidneys, brain, and lung.
  - HES occurs predominantly in men between the ages of 20 and 50 years and presents with insidious onset of fatigue, cough, and dyspnea and an associated eosinophil count of >1,500 cells/μL.
  - At presentation, patients typically are in the late thrombotic and fibrotic stages of eosinophil-mediated cardiac damage with signs of a restrictive cardiomyopathy and mitral regurgitation. An echocardiogram may detect intracardiac thrombi, endomyocardial fibrosis, or thickening of the posterior mitral valve leaflet. Neurologic manifestations range from peripheral neuropathy to stroke or encephalopathy. Bone marrow examination reveals increased eosinophil precursors.
- **Acute eosinophilic leukemia** is a rare myeloproliferative disorder that is distinguished from HES by several factors: an increased number of immature eosinophils in the blood and/or marrow, >10% blast forms in the marrow, as well as symptoms and signs compatible with an acute leukemia. Treatment is similar to that for other leukemias.
- **Lymphoma.** As many as 5% of patients with non-Hodgkin lymphoma and up to 15% of patients with Hodgkin lymphoma have modest peripheral blood eosinophilia. Eosinophilia in Hodgkin lymphoma has been correlated with IL-5 mRNA expression by Reed–Sternberg cells.
- **Atheroembolic disease.** Cholesterol embolization can lead to eosinophilia, eosinophiluria, renal dysfunction, livedo reticularis, increased erythrocyte sedimentation rate (ESR), and purple toes.
- **Immunodeficiency.** Hyper-IgE syndrome characterized by recurrent infections and dermatitis is often associated with eosinophilia as is Omenn's syndrome (eosinophilia and combined variable immunodeficiency).

Epidemiology

In industrialized nations, peripheral blood eosinophilia is most often due to atopic disease, whereas helminthic infections are the most common cause of eosinophilia in the rest of the world.

Etiology

The etiology of eosinophilia may be classified by associated clinical context as shown in Table 1 or by the level of eosinophilia as shown in Table 2.

Pathophysiology

Activation of eosinophils leads to the release of stored granular components such as major basic proteins, eosinophil peroxidase, and eosinophil cationic protein, which are believed to be responsible for the tissue damage ascribed to these cells. In addition, these activated cells produce cytokines that can exacerbate the immunologic reaction.

Table 1	Causes of Eosinophilia

Eosinophilia associated with atopic disease
Allergic rhinitis
Asthma
Atopic dermatitis

Eosinophilia associated with pulmonary infiltrates
Passage of larvae through the lung (Loffler syndrome)
Chronic eosinophilic pneumonia
Acute eosinophilic pneumonia
Tropical pulmonary eosinophilia
Allergic bronchopulmonary aspergillosis (ABPA)
Coccidiomycosis

Eosinophilia associated with parasitic infection
Helminths (*Ascaris lumbricoides, Strongyloides stercoralis,* hookworm,
    Toxocara canis or cati, Trichinella)
Protozoa (only *Dientamoeba fragilis* and *Isospora belli*)

Eosinophilia associated with primary cutaneous disease
Atopic dermatitis
Eosinophilic fasciitis
Eosinophilic cellulitis
Eosinophilic folliculitis
Episodic angioedema with anaphylaxis

Eosinophilia associated with multiorgan involvement
Drug-induced eosinophilia
Churg–Strauss syndrome
Idiopathic hypereosinophilic syndrome
Eosinophilic leukemia

Miscellaneous causes
Eosinophilic gastroenteritis
Interstitial nephritis
HIV infection
Eosinophilia myalgia syndrome
Transplant rejection
Atheroembolic disease

DIAGNOSIS

There are two approaches that are useful for evaluating eosinophilia, either by associated clinical context (Table 1) or by degree of eosinophilia (Table 2).

Clinical Presentation
History
- The presence of cough, dyspnea, fever, or any symptoms of cancer should be determined, as should any history of rhinitis, wheezing, or rash.
- A complete medication list, including over-the-counter supplements, and a full travel history focused on countries where filariasis may be endemic (e.g., Southeast Asia, Africa, South America, or the Caribbean) should be obtained.
- Any pet exposure should be ascertained for possible exposure to toxocariasis.

Table 2	Classification of Eosinophilia Based on the Peripheral Blood Eosinophil Count		
	Peripheral Blood Eosinophil Count (cells/μL)		
500–2,000	**2,000–5,000**	**>5,000**	
Allergic rhinitis	Intrinsic asthma	Eosinophilia myalgia	
Allergic asthma	Allergic	syndrome	
Food allergy	bronchopulmonary	Idiopathic	
Urticaria	aspergillosis	hypereosinophilic	
Addison disease	Helminthiasis	syndrome	
Pulmonary infiltrates	Churg–Strauss syndrome	Episodic angioedema with	
with eosinophilia	Drug reactions	eosinophilia	
syndromes	Vascular neoplasms	Leukemia	
Solid neoplasms	Eosinophilic fasciitis		
Nasal polyposis	HIV		

Physical Examination

Physical examination should be guided by the history, with a special focus on the skin, upper and lower respiratory tracts, as well as cardiovascular and neurologic systems.

Differential Diagnosis

- Various conditions can result in **eosinophilia associated with pulmonary infiltrates** (Table 1). The presence of asthma should lead to consideration of ABPA, CSS, or tropical pulmonary eosinophilia.
- The etiology of **eosinophilia associated with cutaneous lesions** (Table 1) is guided by the appearance of the lesions and results of the skin biopsy. The diagnosis of CSS cannot be made without a tissue biopsy showing infiltrating eosinophils and granulomas.
- When eosinophilia is marked and all other causes have been ruled out, the diagnosis of **idiopathic HES** should be considered. Diagnosis requires a blood eosinophilia of >1,500/μL for >6 months with associated organ involvement. No specific test exists to identify these patients, and in general this is a diagnosis of exclusion.

Diagnostic Testing

Laboratories

- The differential diagnosis can be narrowed based on the clinical findings and history. Depending on the travel history, stool exam for ova and parasites should be performed.
- Mild **eosinophilia associated with symptoms of rhinitis or asthma** is indicative of underlying atopic disease, which can be confirmed by skin testing.
- **Stool examination** for ova and parasites should be done on three separate occasions. Because only small numbers of helminths may pass in the stool and because tissue- or blood-dwelling helminths will not be found in the stool, **serologic tests** for antiparasite antibodies should also be sent. Such tests are available for strongyloidiasis, toxocariasis, and trichinellosis.
- Diagnosis at the time of presentation with Loffler syndrome can be made by detection of *Ascaris* larvae in respiratory secretions or gastric aspirates, but not stool.

- A history of asthma, significant peripheral blood eosinophilia (>10% of the leukocyte count), and pulmonary infiltrates suggests CSS. In this case, sinus computed tomography, nerve conduction studies, and testing for p-ANCA may aid in diagnosis.

Imaging

Chest x-ray findings may also help to narrow the differential diagnosis. Peripheral infiltrates with central clearing are indicative of chronic eosinophilic pneumonia. Diffuse infiltrates in an interstitial, alveolar, or mixed pattern may be seen in acute eosinophilic pneumonia as well as drug-induced eosinophilia with pulmonary involvement. Transient infiltrates may be seen in Loffler syndrome, CSS, or ABPA. Central bronchiectasis is a major criterion in the diagnosis of ABPA. A diffuse miliary or nodular pattern, consolidation, or cavitation may be found in cases of tropical pulmonary eosinophilia.

Diagnostic Procedures

If no other cause of pulmonary infiltrates has been identified, a **bronchoscopy** may be necessary for analysis of bronchoalveolar lavage (BAL) fluid and lung tissue. The presence of eosinophils in BAL fluid or sputum with eosinophilic infiltration of the parenchyma is most typical of acute or chronic eosinophilic pneumonia.

TREATMENT

- When a drug reaction is suspected, discontinuation of the drug is both diagnostic and therapeutic. Other treatment options depend on the exact cause of eosinophilia because, with the exception of idiopathic HES, eosinophilia itself is a manifestation of an underlying disease.
- **Hypereosinophilic syndrome:** Patients with marked eosinophilia with no organ involvement may have a benign course. In contrast, those with organ involvement and with FIP1L1/PDGFalpha associated disease may have an extremely aggressive course without treatment. Monitoring and early initiation of glucocorticoids should be pursued in all patients except those who have the FIP1L1/PDGFalpha fusion. Patients with the FIP1L1/PDGFalpha fusion mutation should be started on imatinib mesylate (Gleevac), a tyrosine kinase inhibitor. Treatment should be initiated promptly in these patients to prevent progression of cardiac disease and other end organ damage. Imatinib has been shown to induce disease remission and progression (*Blood 2003;101(12):4714*). Hydroxyurea has been the most frequently used effective second-line agent and/or steroid-sparing agent for HES. Interferon-α has been effective in a small number of case series (*Br J Haematol 1996;92:17*). Its mechanism of action is not completely understood but may involve inhibition of eosinophil proliferation and differentiation. Mepolizumab, a humanized anti-IL-5 antibody, has shown promising results in patients who do not have the FIP1L1/PDGFalpha fusion protein (*J Allergy Clin Immunol 2004;113(1):115*). Anti-CD52 antibody (CD52 is expressed on the surface of eosinophils), alemtuzumab, has been shown in a clinical trial to decrease eosinophils counts.
- Primary eosinophilia disorders should be followed by a specialist; any cases of unresolved or unexplained eosinophilia warrant evaluation by an allergist–immunologist.

Urticaria and Angioedema

GENERAL PRINCIPLES

Definition

- **Urticaria** (hives) are raised, flat-topped, well-demarcated pruritic skin lesions with surrounding erythema. Central clearing can cause an annular lesion and is often seen after antihistamine use. An individual lesion usually lasts minutes to hours.
- **Angioedema** is a deeper lesion causing painful areas of skin-colored, localized swelling. It can be found anywhere on the body, but most often involves the tongue, lips, or eyelids. When angioedema occurs without urticaria, specific diagnoses must be entertained (see Differential Diagnosis).

Classification

- **Acute urticaria (with or without angioedema)** is defined as an episode lasting <6 weeks. Usually, it is caused by an allergic reaction to a medication or food, but it may be related to underlying infection, recent insect sting, or exposure (contact or inhalation) to an allergen. A patient can develop a hypersensitivity to a food, medication, or self-care product that previously had been used without difficulty.
- **Chronic urticaria (with or without angioedema)** is defined as episodes that persist for >6 weeks. There are many possible causes of chronic urticaria and angioedema, including medications, autoimmunity, self-care products, and physical triggers. However, the etiology remains unidentified in >80% of cases.

Epidemiology

- Urticaria is a common condition that affects 15% to 24% of the U.S. population at some time in their life. Chronic idiopathic urticaria occurs in 0.1% of the U.S. population, and there does not appear to be an increased risk in persons with atopy.
- Angioedema generally lasts 12 to 48 hours and occurs in 40% to 50% of patients with urticaria.

Etiology

- Allergic: drugs, foods, inhalant, or contact allergen
- Transfusion reactions
- Infections
- Insects
- Autoimmune diseases
- Malignancy
- Physical urticaria: dermographism, cold, cholinergic, pressure, vibratory, solar, and aquagenic
- Mastocytosis
- Hereditary diseases
- Idiopathic

Pathophysiology

Mechanisms for initiation of urticaria and angioedema differ depending on the classification and are not fully understood. However, the final common pathway is the degranulation of mast cells or basophils and the release of inflammatory mediators. Histamine is the primary mediator and elicits edema (wheal) and erythema (flare).

DIAGNOSIS

Diagnosis is based upon complete history and physical examination, which should elicit identifiable triggers.

Clinical Presentation
- Patients with acute urticaria episode will present with history of pruritus, erythematous cutaneous lesions with less than 6 weeks duration and usually after exposure to an antigen. Chronic patients will have relapsing symptoms interspersed with symptom-free periods.
- Angioedema patients usually present without symptoms of pruritus and the lesions are described as swollen and painful.
- Urticaria and angioedema can occur together.

History
- A detailed history should elicit identifiable triggers and rule out any systemic causes. This also includes determining whether an individual lesion lasts >24 hours, in which case, the diagnosis of urticarial vasculitis must be investigated by a skin biopsy.
- Any changes in environmental exposures, foods, medications, personal care products, etc. should be determined.

Physical Examination
- Complete examination of the affected and nonaffected skin.
- Urticaria appears as erythematous, raised lesions that blanch with pressure.
- Angioedema often involves the face, tongue, extremities, or genitalia, and may be asymmetric.

Differential Diagnosis
- Allergic reaction to drugs, foods, insects, inhalant, or contact allergen.
- Physical urticaria.
- Mast cell releasability syndromes such as systemic mastocytosis and cutaneous mastocytosis, including urticaria pigmentosa, should be considered.
- **Urticarial vasculitis** presents with urticaria-like lesions that do not fade within 24 hours. It is a systemic vasculitis characterized by vascular damage with findings of fragmentation of neutrophils, red cell extravasation, and swelling of endothelial cells on biopsy.
- **Angioedema without urticaria** should lead to consideration of specific entities.
  - Use of **angiotensin-converting enzyme inhibitors** (ACEIs) or **angiotensin II receptor blockers** (ARBs) can be associated with angioedema at any point in the course of therapy.
  - **Hereditary angioedema (HAE), or C1 esterase inhibitor (C1 INH) deficiency,** is inherited in an autosomal dominant pattern.
  - **Acquired C1 INH deficiency** presents similarly to HAE but is typically associated with an underlying lymphoproliferative disorder or connective tissue disease.

Diagnostic Testing
Epicutaneous skin testing and patch testing when indicated.

Laboratories
- A complete blood count (CBC), ESR, urinalysis, and liver function tests should be obtained to screen for systemic etiologies of chronic urticaria, such as hematologic malignancies, autoimmune diseases, and occult infections, including hepatitis.
- All patients with **angioedema without urticaria** *should be screened with a C4 level, which is reduced during and between attacks of HAE.* If the C4 level is reduced, a quantitative and functional C1 INH assay should be performed. Measuring C1 INH levels alone is not sufficient because 15% of patients have normal levels of a dysfunctional C1 INH protein; therefore, it is important to also obtain the functional assay.
- Acquired C1 INH deficiency patients have reduced C1q, C1 INH, and C4 levels. Other patients with the acquired form have an autoantibody to C1 INH with low C4 and C1 INH levels but a normal C1 level.

Diagnostic Procedures
- A skin biopsy should be performed if individual lesions persist for >24 hours to rule out urticarial vasculitis.
- Biopsy of acute urticarial lesions reveals dilation of small venules and capillaries located in the superficial dermis with widening of the dermal papillae, flattening of the rete pegs, and swelling of collagen fibers.
- Chronic urticaria is characterized by a dense, non-necrotizing, perivascular infiltrate consisting of T lymphocytes, mast cells, eosinophils, basophils, and neutrophils.
- Angioedema shows similar pathologic alterations in the deep, rather than superficial, dermis and subcutaneous tissue.

TREATMENT

- The ideal treatment of acute urticaria with or without angioedema is identification and avoidance of specific causes. **All potential causes should be eliminated.** Most cases resolve within 1 week. In some instances, it is possible to reintroduce an agent cautiously if it is believed not to be the etiologic agent. This trial should be done in the presence of a physician with epinephrine readily available.
- Careful consideration should be given to the **elimination or substitution of each prescription or over-the-counter medication** or supplement. If a patient reacts to one medication in a class, the reaction likely will be triggered by all medications in that class. Exacerbating agents (such as nonsteroidal anti-inflammatory drugs [NSAIDs], including aspirin, opiates, vancomycin, and alcohol) should be avoided because they may induce nonspecific mast cell degranulation and exacerbate urticaria caused by other agents.
- **Elimination of all self-care products,** with the exception of those that contain no methylparaben, fragrance, or preservative, is useful when sensitivity to these products is a possibility.
- In patients presenting with hereditary and acquired angioedema, a prompt assessment of airway is critical in especially those presenting with a laryngeal attack.

Medications
In acute urticaria in the presence of anaphylaxis, which consists of systemic symptoms such as hypotension, laryngeal edema, or bronchospasm, treatment with **epinephrine** (0.3 to 0.5 mL of a 1:1,000 solution IM) should be administered immediately. See Anaphylaxis section for additional information.

First Line
- **Acute urticaria**
  - **A second-generation oral antihistamine** such as cetirizine, levocetirizine, fexofenadine, desloratadine, or loratadine should be administered to patients until the hives have cleared. A first-generation antihistamine such as hydroxyzine may be added as an evening dose if needed to obtain control in refractory cases.
  - **Oral corticosteroids** should be reserved for patients with laryngeal edema or systemic symptoms of anaphylaxis after treatment with epinephrine. Corticosteroids will not have an immediate effect but may prevent relapse. They may also be helpful for patients with severe symptoms who have not responded to antihistamines.
  - If a patient presents with systemic symptoms, self-administered epinephrine should be prescribed for use in the case of accidental exposure to the same trigger in the future.
- **Chronic urticaria**
  - **Antihistamines** for symptom control are the mainstay of treatment. Treatment should be continued for a period of 6 months, and then lowered to the level needed to maintain symptom control.
  - Second-generation H_1 antihistamines, such as cetirizine, levocetirizine, fexofenadine, loratadine, and desloratadine, are well tolerated and should be used as first-line agents. Cetirizine, the breakdown product of hydroxyzine, is often used for chronic urticaria treatment because it is thought to concentrate in the skin; however, it is minimally sedating. Several drugs in this class are now available over the counter.
  - Classic H_1 antihistamines, such as hydroxyzine, 25 mg PO q4–6h or prn, can be added for better control of lesions or for breakthrough lesions. The dose is usually limited by sedation.
- **Hereditary and Acquired Angioedema (Disorder of C1-inhibitor)**
  - Laryngeal attacks or severe abdominal attacks: C1-inhibitor replacement (C1INHRP) is first-line agent. Other options include fresh frozen plasma and tranexamic acid. Also pursue symptomatic therapy and rehydration.

Second Line
Chronic urticaria

- Doxepin, an antidepressant with H_1- and H_2-blocking effects, is a useful addition and often is less sedating than hydroxyzine.
- H2-blocking agents may be helpful in addition to H_1 antihistamines to control breakthrough hives.
- Oral corticosteroids should be reserved for those patients in whom adequate control cannot be achieved with a combination of the aforementioned agents. Steroids should be used only for short periods of time.
- Cyclosporine may be used in cases where patients require chronic systemic steroids for symptom control.

REFERRAL

All patients with chronic urticaria or a history of anaphylaxis should be referred to an allergy specialist for evaluation to identify potential allergic and autoimmune triggers, including the presence of antithyroid antibodies or antibodies against the Fc portion of the IgE receptor.

Immunodeficiency

GENERAL PRINCIPLES

Definition

- Primary immunodeficiencies (PIDs) are disorders of the immune system that result in an increased susceptibility to infection.
- Secondary immunodeficiencies are also disorders of increased susceptibility to infection but are attributable to an external source.

Classification

PIDs can be organized by the defective immune components.

- Humoral immunodeficiency: the defect is primarily in the ability to make antibodies.
  - Common variable immune deficiency
  - X-linked (Bruton's) agammaglobulinemia
  - IgG subclass deficiency
  - IgA deficiency
  - Hyper-IgE (Job) syndrome
- Cell-mediated immunodeficiency: the defect is primarily with cell-mediated (T-cell) immune response.
- Combined immunodeficiency: the defect results in deficiencies in both cellular and humoral immune responses.
- Innate immune system defects:
  - Chronic granulomatous disease (CGD)
  - Complement deficiencies

Epidemiology

- Secondary immunodeficiency syndromes, particularly HIV/AIDS, are the most common immunodeficiency disorders.
- Most PIDs presenting in adulthood are humoral immune defects.
- CVID is the most common symptomatic PID, occurring with a frequency of 1/10,000.

Etiology

- CVID is largely idiopathic, though there are genetic mutations (such as TACI, ICOS and CD19) with some forms of the disorder.
- Humoral immune deficiencies are generally thought to be caused by defects in B-cell maturation.
- A variety of genetic mutations have been associated with specific PID syndromes.
- Secondary immunodeficiencies can be caused by medications (chemotherapy, immunomodulatory agents, corticosteroids), infectious agents (HIV), malignancy, antibody loss (nephrotic syndrome, protein losing enteropathy, or consumption during a severe underlying infection), autoimmune disease (SLE, RA, etc.), malnutrition (vitamin D), and other underlying diseases (DM, cirrhosis, uremia, etc.).

DIAGNOSIS

Clinical Presentation

- The hallmark of PID is recurrent infections. Clinical suspicion should be increased by recurrent sinopulmonary infection, deep-seated infections, or disseminated infections in an otherwise healthy patient.
- Recurrent urinary tract infections are only rarely associated with PID.
- **Immunoglobulin A (IgA) deficiency** is the most common immune deficiency, with a prevalence of 1 in 500 people.
  - Patients may be asymptomatic or present with recurrent sinus and pulmonary infections. Therapy is directed at early treatment with antibiotics because IgA replacement is not available.
  - In 15% of cases, an associated immunoglobulin G (IgG) subclass deficiency is present.
  - Truly IgA-deficient patients (rather than those with very low levels) are at risk for developing a severe transfusion reaction because of the presence in some individuals of IgE anti-IgA antibodies; therefore, these patients should be transfused with washed red blood cells or receive blood products only from IgA-deficient donors.
- **Common variable immunodeficiency (CVID)** includes a heterogeneous group of disorders in which patients present in the second to fourth decade of life with recurrent sinus and pulmonary infections and are discovered to have *low or dysfunctional IgG, IgA, and IgM antibodies.*
  - Patients with CVID are particularly susceptible to infection with encapsulated organisms.
  - B-cell numbers are usually normal, but there is decreased ability to produce immunoglobulin after immunization. Some patients may also exhibit T-cell dysfunction and be anergic.
  - Patients may have associated gastrointestinal disease or autoimmune abnormalities (most commonly autoimmune hemolytic anemia, idiopathic thrombocytopenic purpura, pernicious anemia, and rheumatoid arthritis).
  - There is an increased incidence of malignancy, especially lymphoid and gastrointestinal malignancy.
  - Therapy consists of IV immunoglobulin (IVIG) replacement therapy as well as prompt treatment of infections with antibiotics.
- **X-linked (Bruton's) agammaglobulinemia** clinically manifests very similarly to severe CVID and is typically diagnosed in childhood but can present in adulthood.
  - Patients usually have low levels of all immunoglobulin types and very low levels of B cells.
  - Specific genetic defect is in Bruton's tyrosine kinase, which is involved in B-cell maturation.
- **Subclass deficiency.** Deficiencies of each of the IgG subclasses (IgG1, IgG2, IgG3, and IgG4) have been described.
  - These patients present with similar complaints as the CVID patients.
  - Total IgG levels may be normal. A strong association with IgA deficiency exists. There is disagreement as to whether this is a separate entity from CVID.
  - In most cases, there is no need to evaluate IgG subclass levels.
- **Hyper-IgE syndrome (Job syndrome)** is characterized by recurrent pyogenic infections of the skin and lower respiratory tract. This infection can result in severe abscess and empyema formation.

- The most common organism involved is *Staphylococcus aureus*, but other bacteria and fungi have been reported.
- Patients present with recurrent infections and have associated pruritic dermatitis, coarse (lion-like) facies, growth retardation, and hyperkeratotic nails. Laboratory data reveal the presence of normal levels of IgG, IgA, and IgM, but markedly elevated levels of IgE. A marked increase in tissue and blood eosinophils may also be observed.
- Mutations in STAT3 have been linked to development of this disease (*N Engl J Med 2007;357(16):1608*).
- No specific therapy exists except for early treatment of infection with antibiotics.
- **Complement deficiencies** are a broad category of PID characterized recurrent infections to a range of pathogens.
  - Recurrent disseminated neisserial infections are associated with a deficiency in the terminal complement system (C5–C9).
  - Systemic lupus-like disorders and recurrent infection with encapsulated organisms have been associated with deficiencies in other components of complement.
- **CGD** is characterized by defective killing of intracellular pathogens by neutrophils.
  - Patients usually present with frequent infection, often with abscesses, from *S. aureus* and other catalase-positive organisms. *Aspergillus* is a particularly troublesome pathogen for patients with CGD.
  - Diagnosis is made by demonstration of defective respiratory burst with nitroblue tetrazolium or using flow cytometry assay using dihydrorhodamine.

Diagnostic Testing

- Initial evaluation should focus on identifying possible secondary causes of recurrent infection such as allergy, medications,and anatomic abnormalities.
- Workup begins with a CBC with differential, HIV test, quantitative immunoglobulin levels, and complement levels. Often the evaluation will need to include enumeration of B and T cells in the peripheral blood.
- If clinical suspicion is high foran underlying humoral PID, B-cell function can be assessed by measuring immunoglobulin response to vaccinations. Pre- and postimmunization titers for both a protein antigen (i.e., tetanus) and a polysaccharide antigen (i.e., Pneumovax, the unconjugated 23-valent vaccine) are measured because proteins and polysaccharide antigens are handled differently by the immune system.
- Titers of specific antibodies are measured before and at least 4 weeks after immunization, with a good response defined as a fourfold increase in the antibody titer of at least 70% of the tested serotypes (*Ann Allergy Asthma Immunol 2005; 94(5 Suppl 1):S1*).
- A patient with normal or low IgG and a poor response to immunization is classified as having CVID.

TREATMENT

- IgA deficiency: No specific treatment is available. However, these patients should be promptly treated at the first sign of infection with an antibiotic that covers *Streptococcus pneumoniae* or *Haemophilus influenzae*.
- CVID should be treated with IVIG. Numerous preparations of IVIG are available, all of which undergo viral inactivation steps.
  - Replacement should be initiated with 400 mg/kg and infused slowly according to the manufacturer's suggestions (for most preparations, begin at 30 mL/hr

Table 3	Immunologically Mediated Drug Reactions	
Type of Reaction	**Representative Examples**	**Mechanism**
Anaphylactic (type 1)	Anaphylaxis Urticaria Angioedema	IgE-mediated degranulation of mast cell with resultant mediator release
Cytotoxic (type 2)	Autoimmune hemolytic anemia Interstitial nephritis	IgG or IgM antibodies against cell antigens and complement activation
Immune complex (type 3)	Serum sickness Vasculitis	Immune complex deposition and subsequent complement activation
Cell mediated (type 4)	Contact dermatitis Photosensitivity dermatitis	Activated T cells against cell surface—bound antigens

and increase by 30 mL/hr every 15 minutes as tolerated to a maximum rate of 210 mL/hr).
- Possible side effects include myalgias, vomiting, chills, and lingering headache (due to immune complex–mediated aseptic meningitis).
- Patients, especially those with no detectable IgA, need to have vital signs monitored q15min initially because anaphylaxis from IgE anti-IgA antibodies can develop in these patients. For these patients, it is best to use IVIG preparations that have very low IgA.

Adverse Drug Reactions

GENERAL PRINCIPLES

Adverse drug reactions (ADRs) are a very common problem. Only a subset of reactions are mediated immunologically; other drug reactions may be toxic or idiosyncratic.

Classification
- **Type A drug reactions** are due to toxicities associated with the medication's mechanism of action or metabolism and are dose dependent and predictable.
- **Type B drug reactions** include idiosyncratic drug reactions and immune-mediated reactions that occur in a small portion of the population and are unpredictable and not dose dependent.
  - Many different mechanisms can account for immunologically mediated drug reactions (Table 3). These reactions can occur with relatively low doses of the drug, usually on reexposure after an initial sensitization to the drug.
  - **Pseudoallergic reactions** (formerly called anaphylactoid reactions) clinically appear as IgE-mediated allergy but are the result of non-IgE–mediated mast cells degranulation.

Epidemiology
- ADRs are very common with some estimates placing the frequency between 10% and 20% of hospitalized patients.

- The majority of ADR are type A drug reactions.
- Type B reactions account for 10% to 15% of all ADRs.
- Factors that predispose to ADRs include prior drug reaction, history of atopy, type of medication used, and comorbid conditions.

Etiology

- β-Lactam sensitivity. Penicillins and other β-lactam antibiotics are commonly associated with immunologically mediated drug reactions.
- Penicillins have a high incidence of immunologic reactivity as a result of their chemical structure.
  - The core structure consists of a reactive bicyclic β-lactam ring that serves as a hapten by covalently binding to tissue carrier proteins. Ninety-five percent of tissue-bound penicillin is found to be haptenated as the benzylpenicilloyl form and is called the major determinant.
  - Five percent of tissue-bound penicillin consists of three non–cross-reactive metabolites, termed the minor determinants.
  - Immediate allergic reactions are most often related to the major determinant.
  - In addition, some modified penicillins, such as ampicillin, can produce allergic reactions in which the antigenic determinant is the side chain.
- Cephalosporins share cross-reactivity with penicillins because of their related structure.
  - Studies report a fourfold increased risk of hypersensitivity reactions to cephalosporins in penicillin-allergic patients as compared to the general population (8% vs. 2%) (*J Infect Dis 1978;137:S74*). The degree of cross-reactivity is related to the generation of the cephalosporin (first generation > second generation > third generation).
  - Although many of the reactions to second- and third-generation cephalosporins are directed at the side chains, skin testing to penicillin in these patients can be helpful because most severe anaphylactic reactions are directed against the reactive bicyclic core.
  - Patients with a history of a severe reaction to penicillin should be considered sensitive to cephalosporin unless they are skin test negative. Although patients with a history of a nonanaphylactic reaction to penicillin can often be given a second- or third-generation cephalosporin safely, it is advisable to precede the dose with an oral provocation challenge.
- Other related antibiotics
  - Monobactams. Aztreonam is the prototype antibiotic of this group with a monocyclic structure. No significant cross-reactivity is found between this group and the β-lactams.
  - Carbapenems. Skin test cross-reactivity has been documented. However, most patients with documented penicillin allergy by skin testing tolerate graded dose challenge with a carbapenem.
  - Carbacephems (e.g., loracarbef) are structurally related to cephalosporins. Few data exist in regard to cross-reactivity, but they are assumed to be related antigenically and should be avoided in severely penicillin-sensitive patients.
- **NSAIDs** (including aspirin) can induce pseudoallergic reactions through shunting of prostaglandin production to leukotriene synthesis in susceptible individuals.
  - **Samter's triad** is the combination of asthma, NSAID sensitivity, and nasal polyposis.

DIAGNOSIS

Clinical Presentation

- Urticaria, angioedema, wheezing, and anaphylaxis are all characteristics of IgE-mediated (type 1) reactions.
  - Symptoms do not typically occur on the first exposure to the medication unless the patient has been exposed to structurally related medication. On reexposure, however, symptoms tend to manifest acutely (often <1 hour).
  - IgE-mediated reactions tend to worsen with repeated exposure to offending medication.
  - Pseudoallergic reactions (non-IgE mediated) can be clinically indistinguishable from IgE-mediated reactions because the final common pathway for their reaction is mast cell degranulation.
- **Maculopapular exanthems** are the most common cutaneous manifestation of drug allergy.
  - These reactions are mediated by T cells and typically delayed in onset, first occurring between 2 and 14 days of exposure to culprit medications. Lesions typically begin on the trunk, especially in dependent areas, and spread to the extremities.
  - Rarely, these rashes can progress to DRESS (Drug reaction with eosinophilia and systemic symptoms) or SJS (Stevens–Johnson Syndrome).
- **Drug reaction with eosinophilia and systemic symptoms (DRESS)** or hypersensitivity syndrome is a serious ADR often presenting with rash and fever (*Expert Opin Drug Saf 2005;4(3):571*).
  - Systemic involvement can manifest as hepatitis, eosinophilia, pneumonitis, lymphadenopathy, and nephritis.
  - Symptoms tend to present 2 to 6 weeks after introduction of medication.
  - First described with antiepileptic agents but has also been reported to occur with allopurinol, NSAIDs, some antibiotics and β-blockers.
- **Erythema multiforme (EM), SJS, and toxic epidermal necrolysis (TEN)** are all serious drug reactions involving primarily the skin.
  - EM is characterized most typically by target lesions.
  - SJS and TEN manifest with varying degrees of sloughing of the skin and mucous membranes (<10% of the epidermis in SJS and >30% in TEN).
  - Readministration or future skin testing with the offending drug is absolutely contraindicated.

TREATMENT

- **Discontinuation** of the suspected drug or drugs is the most important initial approach in managing an allergic drug reaction.
- Other therapeutic maneuvers are directed at limiting further exacerbation of ADR and may include management of anaphylaxis (see above) as well as other supportive measures. Care in ICU may be required for severe adverse reactions.
- Future use of the drug in question should **always be avoided** unless there is no therapeutic alternative available.
- If use of the drug must be considered, a careful history of the reaction is helpful in defining the potential risk. The date of a reaction is useful, given that patients may lose their sensitivity to a drug over time. Timing of symptoms is important; symptoms occurring with the start of a drug course are more likely to be IgE mediated than are symptoms that develop several days after the completion of a course.

- On occasion, a history of an unrecognized, inadvertent reexposure to a drug that had previously caused a reaction may be elicited. If this reexposure was not associated with any reaction, it is due to lack of true IgE-mediated hypersensitivity or potentially a loss of sensitivity that may have developed.
- The type of symptoms must be detailed. Toxic reactions (e.g., nausea secondary to macrolide antibiotics or codeine) are not immunologic reactions and do not necessarily predict problems with other members in their respective class.
- If the patient is taking the drug for a life-threatening illness (e.g., meningitis with penicillin allergy) and the reaction is a mild skin reaction, it may be reasonable to continue the medication and treat the reaction symptomatically. **If the rash is progressive, however, the drug must be discontinued to avoid a desquamative process such as SJS.**

REFERRAL

- If no alternative drug is available and the patient has a history of an IgE-mediated reaction, the patient should be referred to an allergist for further evaluation.
- The allergist may perform one of several procedures if indicated depending on the medication, type of reaction, and availability of testing reagents.
  - **Skin testing** may be performed to assess for the presence of IgE to the medication.
    - While skin testing may be performed to nearly any medication, sensitivity and specificity of the skin test results have only been established for penicillin. No case of penicillin-induced anaphylaxis has been reported in a patient who is skin test negative.
    - Results of testing to drugs other than penicillin must be interpreted within the clinical context of the case.
  - **Graded dose challenge** assesses how the patient tolerates progressively larger doses of medication (e.g., 1/1,000, 1/10 and full dose given 20 minutes apart).
  - **Drug desensitization** is performed when patient has an identified IgE-mediated reaction, but still requires the medications.
    - The exact mechanism by which desensitization prevents anaphylaxis is unclear.
    - The drug must be taken daily at a specified dose to maintain the "desensitized state."
    - If a dose of drug is missed for >48 hour period following a desensitization procedure, the patient will often need to undergo a repeat desensitization.

Successful desensitization or graded challenge does not preclude the development of a non–IgE-mediated, delayed reaction (e.g., rash).

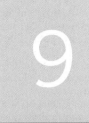

Fluid and Electrolyte Management

Bala Sankarpandian and Steven Cheng

FLUID MANAGEMENT AND PERTURBATIONS IN VOLUME STATUS

Evaluation of Volume Status

GENERAL PRINCIPLES

- **Total body water (TBW).** Water comprises approximately 60% of lean body weight in men and 50% in women. TBW is distributed in two major compartments: two-thirds are **intracellular fluid** (ICF) and one-third is **extracellular fluid** (ECF). The latter is further subdivided into intravascular and interstitial spaces in a ratio of 1:4. This proportional distribution of water enables us to approximate the amount of water in each compartment under normal circumstances.
  - **Example:** For a healthy 70-kg man:

$$TBW = 0.6 \times 70 = 42 \text{ L}$$

   - ICF = 2/3 TBW = $0.66 \times 42 = 28$ L
   - ECF = 1/3 TBW = $0.33 \times 42 = 14$ L
   - Intravascular compartment = $0.25 \times 14 = 3.5$ L
   - Interstitial compartment = $0.75 \times 14 = 10.5$ L
- The distribution of water between intravascular and interstitial spaces can also be affected by changes to the Starling balance of forces. Low oncotic pressure (i.e., low albumin states) and high hydrostatic pressure (i.e., Na-retentive states) increase the movement of fluid from vascular to interstitial compartments. This is an important step in the development of edema.
- Because the majority of water is contained in the intracellular space, the loss of water alone (without Na) does not typically result in the hemodynamic changes associated with volume depletion. Instead, disturbances in TBW change serum **osmolality** and electrolyte concentrations.
- The intact kidney adapts to changes in TBW by increasing water excretion or reabsorption. This is mediated by the **antidiuretic hormone (ADH; vasopressin),** which permits water movement across the distal nephron. Although vasopressin release is predominately responsive to osmotic cues, volume contraction can cause a nonosmotic release of vasopressin, resulting in a reduction of renal water excretion.
- **Total body Na^+.** Eighty-five to ninety percent of **total body Na^+** is extracellular and constitutes the predominate solute in the ECF. Changes to the body's total Na^+ content typically result from a loss or gain of this Na-rich fluid, leading to contraction

or expansion of the ECF space. Clinically, this manifests as volume depletion (hypotension, tachycardia) and volume expansion (peripheral or pulmonary edema), respectively.

- Na^+ *concentration* is distinct from Na^+ *content*. Na^+ concentration reflects the amount of Na^+ distributed in a fixed quantity of water. As such, an increase in TBW can decrease the Na^+ concentration even if the body's total Na^+ content remains unchanged.
- The intact kidney can respond to altered Na^+ content in the ECF space by increasing or decreasing Na^+ reabsorption. This response is mediated by cardiovascular, renal, hepatic, and central nervous system sensors of the effective circulating volume.

The Euvolemic Patient

GENERAL PRINCIPLES

Maintenance Fluids

- In the euvolemic patient, the goal of fluid and electrolyte administration is to maintain homeostasis. The best way to accomplish this is to allow free access to food and drink rather than providing intravenous (IV) therapy. However, patients who are unable to tolerate oral input require maintenance fluids to replace renal, gastrointestinal (GI), and insensible fluid losses.
- The decision to provide maintenance IV fluid should be thoughtfully considered and not administered by rote. Fluid administration should therefore be reassessed *at least* daily and patient weight, which may indicate net fluid balance, should be monitored carefully.
- Consider the **water** and **electrolyte** needs of the patient separately when prescribing IVF therapy.
  - Minimum **water** requirements for daily fluid balance can be approximated from the sum of the required urine output, stool water loss, and insensible losses.
    - The minimum urine output necessary to excrete the daily solute load is simply the amount of solute consumed each day (roughly 600 to 800 mOsm/d in the average individual) divided by the maximum amount of solute that can be excreted per liter of urine (maximum urine-concentrating capacity is 1,200 mOsm/L in healthy kidneys). The result is an obligate urine output of *at least* 0.5 L/d.
    - The water lost in stool is typically 200 mL/d.
    - **Insensible water losses** from the skin and respiratory tract amount to roughly 400 to 500 mL/d. The volume of water produced from endogenous metabolism ($\sim$250 to 350 mL/d) should be considered as well. The degree of insensible loss may vary tremendously depending on respiratory rate, metabolic state, and temperature (water losses increase by 100 to 150 mL/d for each degree of body temperature over 37°C).
    - Fluid from drain losses must be factored in as well.
    - After adding each of these components, the minimum amount of water needed to maintain homeostasis is roughly 1,400 mL/d or 60 mL/hr.
  - The **electrolytes** that are usually administered during maintenance fluid therapy are Na^+ and K^+ salts. Requirements depend on minimum obligatory and ongoing losses.

					HCO_3^-
IV solution	Osmolality (mOsm/L)	[Glucose] (g/L)	[Na$^+$] (mEq/L)	[Cl$^-$] (mEq/L)	Equivalents (mEq/L)
D$_5$W	278	50	0	0	0
0.45% NaCl^a	154	—^{b}	77	77	0
0.9% NaCl^a	308	—^{b}	154	154	0
3% NaCl	1,026	—	513	513	0
Lactated Ringer's^c	274	—^{b}	130	109	28

Table 1 Commonly Used Parenteral Solutions

D$_5$W, 5% dextrose in water; D$_{5C}$W, 50% dextrose in water.
^{a}NaCl 0.45% and 0.9% are half-normal and normal saline, respectively.
^{b}Also available with 5% dextrose.
^{c}Also contains 4 mEq/L K$^+$, 1.5 mEq/L Ca^{2+}, and 28 mEq/L lactate.

- ○ It is customary to provide **75 to 175 mEq Na$^+$/d** as NaCl. (A typical 2-g Na$^+$ diet provides 86 mEq Na$^+$/d.)
- ○ Generally, **20 to 60 mEq K$^+$/d** is included if renal function is normal.
- ○ Carbohydrate in the form of **dextrose, 100 to 150 g/d,** is given to minimize protein catabolism and prevent starvation ketoacidosis.
- Table 1 provides a list of common IV solutions and their contents. By combining the necessary components, one can derive an appropriate maintenance fluid regimen tailored for each patient.
- **Example:** A patient is admitted for a GI procedure and is made NPO. To maintain homeostasis, you desire to replace 2 L of water, 154 mEq Na$^+$, 40 mEq K$^+$, and 100 g dextrose over the next 24 hours (values are within **water** and **electrolyte** requirements described above).
  - ○ 2 L of water: Dose fluid at 85 mL/hr (2,000 mL ÷ 24 hours).
  - ○ 154 mEq of Na$^+$: Use 0.45% NS (77 mEq Na/L).
  - ○ 40 mEq of K$^+$: Add 20 mEq/L KCl to each liter of IVF.
  - ○ 100 g dextrose: Use D$_5$ (50 g of dextrose per liter).
  - ○ Order: D$_5$ 0.45% NaCl with 20 mEq/L KCl at 85 mL/hr.

The Hypovolemic Patient

GENERAL PRINCIPLES

Etiology

- Volume depletion generally results from a deficit in **total body Na$^+$** content. This may result from **renal** or **extrarenal losses** of Na from the ECF. **Water** losses alone can also cause volume depletion, but the quantity required to do so is large, as water is lost mainly from the ICF and not the ECF, where volume contraction can be assessed.
- **Renal losses** may be secondary to enhanced diuresis, salt-wasting nephropathies, mineralocorticoid deficiency, or the resolution of obstructive renal disease.
- **Extrarenal losses** include fluid loss from the GI tract (vomiting, nasogastric suction, fistula drainage, and diarrhea), respiratory losses, skin losses (especially with burns), hemorrhage, and severe third spacing of fluid in critical illness.

DIAGNOSIS

Clinical Presentation

- **Symptoms** include complaints of thirst, fatigue, weakness, muscle cramps, and postural dizziness. Sometimes syncope and coma can result with severe volume depletion.
- **Signs** of hypovolemia include low jugular venous pressure, postural hypotension, postural tachycardia, and the absence of axillary sweat. Diminished skin turgor and dry mucous membranes are poor markers of decreased interstitial fluid. Mild degrees of volume depletion are often not clinically detectable, while larger fluid losses can lead to mental status changes, oliguria, and hypovolemic shock.

Diagnostic Testing
Laboratories
Laboratory studies are often helpful but must be used in conjunction with the clinical picture.

- **Urine sodium** is a marker for Na avidity in the kidney.
  - Urine Na^+ < 15 mEq is consistent with volume depletion, as is the fractional excretion of sodium (FeNa) < 1%. The latter can be calculated as [(Urine Na × Serum Cr) ÷ (Urine Cr × Serum Na)] × 100.
  - Concomitant metabolic alkalosis may increase urine Na excretion despite volume depletion due to obligate excretion of Na to accompany the bicarbonate anion. In such cases, a urine chloride of <20 mEq is often helpful to confirm volume contraction.
- **Urine osmolality** and **serum bicarbonate** levels may also be elevated.
- **Hematocrit** and **serum albumin** may be increased from hemoconcentration.

TREATMENT

- It is often difficult to estimate the **volume deficit** present and therapy is thus largely empiric, requiring frequent reassessments of volume status while resuscitation is under way.
- Mild volume contraction can usually be corrected via the oral route. However, the presence of hemodynamic instability, symptomatic fluid loss, or intolerance to oral administration requires IV therapy.
- The primary therapeutic goal is to protect hemodynamic stability and replenish **intravascular volume** with fluid that will preferentially expand the ECF compartment. This can be accomplished with Na-based solutions, since the Na will be retained in the ECF.
  - **Isotonic fluid,** such as normal saline (0.9% NaCl), contains a Na^+ content similar to that of plasma fluid in the ECF, and thus remains entirely in the ECF space. It is the initial fluid of choice for replenishing **intravascular volume.**
    - The administration of solute-free water is largely ineffective, since the majority of water will distribute to the ICF space.
    - Half-normal saline (0.45% NS) has 77 mEq Na^+/L, roughly half the Na^+ content of an equal volume in the ECF. Thus, half of this solution will stay in the ECF, and half will follow the predicted distribution of water.
  - Fluids can be administered as a bolus or at a steady maintenance rate. In patients with symptomatic volume depletion, a 1 to 2 L bolus is often preferable to acutely expand the intravascular space. This should be followed by a careful reassessment of

the patient's volume status. The bolus can be repeated if necessary, although close attention should be directed toward possible signs of volume overload. Smaller boluses should be used for patients with poor cardiac reserve or significant edema. Once the patient is stable, fluids can be administered at a maintenance rate to replace ongoing losses.
  ○ In patients with hemorrhage or GI bleeding, blood transfusion can accomplish both volume expansion and concomitant correction of anemia.

The Hypervolemic Patient

GENERAL PRINCIPLES

Etiology

The clinical manifestations of hypervolemia result from a surplus of **total body Na^+.** Na^+ retention can be caused by a primary disorder of renal Na^+ retention. Alternatively, it may be secondary to decreased **effective circulating volume,** as in heart failure, cirrhosis, or profound hypoalbuminemia.

DIAGNOSIS

Clinical Presentation

* Expansion of the **interstitial compartment** may result in edema and effusions. Expansion of the **intravascular compartment** may result in pulmonary rales, elevated jugular venous pressure, hepatojugular reflux, an S_3 gallop, and elevated blood pressures.
* As overt signs of hypervolemia may not manifest until 3 to 4 L of fluid retention, a gradual rise in water weight is often the earliest indication of Na^+ retention.
* **Symptoms** may include dyspnea, abdominal distention, or swelling of the extremities.

Diagnostic Testing

Laboratories
* Laboratory studies are generally not needed and hypervolemia is primarily a bedside diagnosis.
* **The urine [Na^+]** may be low (<15 mEq/L) with decreased **effective circulating volume** reflecting renal sodium retention.

Imaging
A chest radiograph may show pulmonary edema or pleural effusions, but clear lung fields do not exclude volume overload.

TREATMENT

Treatment must address not only the ECF volume excess, but also the underlying pathologic process. Alleviating the Na^+ excess can be accomplished by the judicious use of diuretics and by limiting Na^+ intake.

Medications

* Diuretics enhance the renal excretion of Na^+ by blocking the various sites of Na^+ reabsorption along the nephron.

- Thiazide diuretics block the NaCl transporters in the distal convoluted tubule. They are often used for mild states of chronic Na^+ retention. Because of their specific site of action, thiazide diuretics impair urinary dilutional capacity (the ability to excrete water) and often stimulate a responsive increase in proximal tubule reabsorption.
- Loop diuretics block the Na–K–2Cl transporter in the ascending loop of Henle. They are often used in circumstances requiring a brisk and immediate diuresis, such as acute volume overload. Loop diuretics impair urinary concentration (increase renal free water excretion) and enhance the excretion of divalent cations (Ca^{2+} and Mg^{2+}).
- Potassium-sparing diuretics act by decreasing Na reabsorption in the collecting duct. While the overall diuretic of these agents is comparatively small, they serve as useful adjunctive agents. Furthermore, as aldosterone antagonists do not require tubular secretion, they can be particularly useful in those with decreased renal perfusion or impaired tubular function.
- Treatment of the underlying disease process is critical to prevent continued Na^+ reabsorption in the kidney. Nephrotic syndrome is discussed in Chapter 10, Renal Diseases; treatment of heart failure is discussed in Chapter 4, Heart Failure, Cardiomyopathy, and Valvular Heart Disease, and cirrhosis is addressed in Chapter 16, Liver Diseases.

DISORDERS OF WATER BALANCE

Hyponatremia

GENERAL PRINCIPLES

Hyponatremia and **hypernatremia** are primarily disorders of *water balance* or *water distribution*. The body is designed to withstand both drought and deluge with adaptations to renal water handling and the thirst mechanism. A persistent abnormality in $[Na^+]$ thus requires both an initial challenge to water balance, as well as a disturbance of the adaptive response.

Definition
Hyponatremia is defined as a plasma $[Na^+]$ < **135 mEq/L.**

Etiology
- To maintain a normal $[Na^+]$, the ingestion of water must be matched with an equal volume of water excretion. Any process that limits the elimination of water or expands the volume around a fixed Na^+ content may lead to a decrease in Na^+ concentration.
- Expansion of the space surrounding the Na^+ content can occur in a variety of ways:
  - **Pseudohyponatremia** refers to a laboratory phenomenon by which a high content of plasma proteins and lipids expands the nonaqueous portion of the plasma sample, leading to an errant report of a low ECF $[Na^+]$. This can be averted with Na^+-sensitive electrodes and the normal ECF $[Na^+]$ can be confirmed with a normal serum osmolality.
  - **Hyperosmolar hyponatremia** refers to circumstances in which an osmotically active solute other than Na accumulates in the ECF, drawing water into the ECF

and diluting the Na^+ content. This is most commonly caused by **hyperglycemia,** resulting in a fall in plasma $[Na^+]$ of 1.6 to 2.4 mEq/L for every 100 mg/dL rise in plasma glucose (*Am J Med 1999;106:399*). Other solutes, such as glycine, mannitol, or sorbitol, can be absorbed into the ECF during bladder irrigation, leading to the transient hyponatremia seen in **post-transurethral resection of the prostate (post-TURP) syndrome.** Prompt renal excretion and metabolism of the absorbed fluid usually corrects the hyponatremia rapidly, although symptomatic hyponatremia can occasionally be seen in the setting of renal insufficiency.

- Rarely, the ECF water content rises simply because the ingested quantity of water exceeds the physiologic capacity of water excretion in the kidney. This is seen in psychogenic polydipsia, water intoxication from poorly conceived drinking games, beer potomania, and the so-called "tea and toast" diet. Underlying each of these circumstances is the fact that there is a limit to renal water clearance. Urine cannot be diluted to an osmolality less than ~50 mOsm/L, meaning that a small amount of solute is required in even the most dilute urine. Ingestion of a high volume of water can thus exceed the capacity for excretion, particularly in those with a solute-poor diet, since the solute load required to generate urinary water loss is quickly depleted. The excess water is retained, Na^+ concentrations falls, and hyponatremia results.

- Decreased clearance of water from the kidney can also occur through a variety of processes. As mentioned previously, renal water handling is largely controlled by the antidiuretic hormone (ADH or vasopressin). Nonosmotic stimulation of this hormone occurs with volume contraction. Although this seems counterintuitive from an osmotic standpoint (it further reduces renal water clearance and increases water retention), it is an "appropriate" adaptive response to the threat of volume loss, tissue hypoperfusion, and impending hemodynamic collapse. Other conditions are characterized by secretion of the ADH, which is "inappropriate"—stimulated by neither osmotic nor volume-related changes.

- **"Appropriate"** ADH secretion occurs with a fall in effective circulating volume. In these conditions, thirst and water retention is stimulated, protecting volume status at the cost of the osmolar status. This category is classically subdivided based on the associated assessment of ECF status.
  - **Hypovolemic hyponatremia** may result from **any** causes of net Na^+ loss.
  - **Hypervolemic hyponatremia** occurs in edematous states such as congestive heart failure (CHF), hepatic cirrhosis, and severe nephrotic syndrome. Despite the expanded interstitial space, the circulating volume is reduced. Alterations in Starling forces contribute to this apparent paradox, shifting fluid from the intravascular to interstitial space.

- **"Inappropriate"** secretion of ADH is characterized by the activation of water-conserving mechanisms despite the absence of osmotic or volume-related stimuli. Because the renal response to volume expansion remains intact, these patients are typically **euvolemic.** However, because of the rise in TBW, serum concentrations of Na are decreased.
  - The most common form of this is the well-named **Syndrome of Inappropriate ADH (SIADH).** This disorder is caused by the nonphysiologic release of vasopressin from the posterior pituitary or an ectopic source. Common causes of SIADH include neuropsychiatric disorders (e.g., meningitis, encephalitis, acute psychosis, cerebrovascular accident, head trauma), pulmonary diseases (e.g., pneumonia, tuberculosis, positive pressure ventilation, acute respiratory failure), and malignant tumors (most commonly small cell lung cancer).

- **SIADH** is diagnosed by the following:
  - Hypo-osmotic hyponatremia
  - Urine osmolality > 100 mOsm/L
  - Euvolemia
  - The absence of conditions that stimulate ADH secretion, including volume contraction, nausea, adrenal dysfunction, and hypothyroidism
- **Pharmacologic agents** may also stimulate inappropriate ADH secretion. Common culprits include antidepressants (particularly selective serotonin reuptake inhibitors [SSRIs]), narcotics, antipsychotic agents, chlorpropamide, and nonsteroidal anti-inflammatory drugs (NSAIDs).
- **Reset osmostat** is a phenomenon in which the set point for plasma osmolality is reduced. Thus, ADH and thirst responses, though functional, maintain plasma osmolality at this new, lower level. This phenomenon occurs in almost all pregnant women (perhaps in response to changes in the hormonal milieu), and occasionally in those with a chronic decreased effective circulating volume.

DIAGNOSIS

Clinical Presentation

- The clinical features of hyponatremia are related to the osmotic intracellular water shift leading to cerebral edema. Therefore, the symptoms are primarily neurologic, and their severity is dependent on both the magnitude of the fall in plasma [Na^+] and the rapidity of the decrease. In **acute hyponatremia** (i.e., developing in <2 days), patients may complain of nausea and malaise with [Na^+] ~125 mEq/L. As the plasma [Na^+] falls further, symptoms may progress to include headache, lethargy, confusion, and obtundation. Stupor, seizures, and coma do not usually occur unless the plasma [Na^+] falls acutely below 115 mEq/L. In **chronic hyponatremia** (>3 days' duration), adaptive mechanisms designed to defend cell volume occur and tend to minimize the increase in ICF volume and its symptoms.
- The underlying cause of hyponatremia can often be ascertained from an accurate history and physical examination, including an assessment of **ECF volume status** and the **effective circulating volume.**

Diagnostic Testing

Laboratories

Three laboratory analyses, when used with a clinical assessment of volume status, can narrow the differential diagnosis of hyponatremia: (a) the **plasma osmolality,** (b) the **urine osmolality,** and (c) the **urine [Na^+]** (Fig. 1).

- **Plasma osmolality.** Most patients with hyponatremia have a low plasma osmolality (<275 mOsm/L). If the plasma osmolality is not low, **pseudohyponatremia** and **hyperosmolar hyponatremia** must be ruled out.
- **Urine osmolality.** The appropriate renal response to hypo-osmolality is to excrete a maximally dilute urine (urine osmolality < 100 mOsm/L and specific gravity < 1.003). A urine sample which is not dilute suggests impaired free water excretion due to appropriate or inappropriate secretion of the ADH.
- **Urine [Na^+]** adds laboratory corroboration to the bedside assessment of effective circulating volume and can discriminate between **extrarenal** and **renal losses** of Na^+. The appropriate response to decreased effective circulating volume is to enhance tubular Na^+ reabsorption such that urine [Na^+] is <10 mEq/L. A urine [Na^+] of

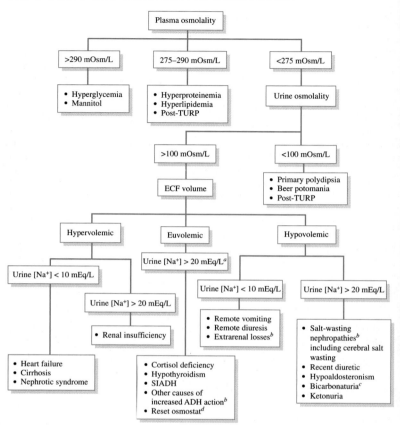

Figure 1. Algorithm depicting the diagnostic approach to hyponatremia. ECF, extracellular fluid; SIADH, syndrome of inappropriate antidiuretic hormone; post-TURP, post-transurethral resection of the prostate syndrome. [a]Urine [Na$^+$] may be <20 mEq/L with low Na$^+$ intake. [b]See text for details. [c]From vomiting-induced contraction alkalosis or proximal renal tubular acidosis. [d]Urine osmolality may be <100 mOsm/L after a water load.

>20 mEq/L suggests a normal effective circulating volume or a Na-wasting defect. Occasionally, the excretion of a nonreabsorbed anion obligates the loss of the Na$^+$ cation despite volume depletion (ketonuria, bicarbonaturia).

TREATMENT

- Management requires one to determine:
  - **The rate of correction**
  - **The appropriate intervention**
  - **The presence of other underlying disorders**

- **The rate of correction** of hyponatremia depends on the acuity of its development and the presence of neurologic dysfunction.
- **Acute symptomatic hyponatremia**
  - **Fluid administration.** Severe symptomatic hyponatremia, with evidence of neurologic dysfunction, should generally be treated promptly with hypertonic saline; however, any saline solution that is hypertonic to the urine (if the urine osmolality is known at the start of therapy) can increase the [Na$^+$] when oral water intake is restricted.
    - The risks of correcting hyponatremia too rapidly are volume overload and the development of **central pontine myelinolysis** (CPM). CPM is thought to result from damage to neurons resulting from rapid osmotic shifts. In its most overt form, it is characterized by flaccid paralysis, dysarthria, and dysphagia, and in more subtle presentations, it can be confirmed by computed tomography (CT) scan or magnetic resonance imaging (MRI) of the brain. The risk of precipitating CPM is increased with correction of the [Na$^+$] by > 12 mEq/L in a 24-hour period (*J Am Soc Nephrol 1994;4:1522*). In addition to overaggressive correction, other risk factors for developing CPM include preexisting hypokalemia, malnutrition, and alcoholism.
    - In patients with severe hyponatremia, in which an immediate rise in [Na$^+$] is necessary, [Na$^+$] should be corrected 1 to 2 mEq/L/hr for 3 to 4 hours. However, this initial rate of correction should be tapered off once the patient is safe, such that the rise in [Na$^+$] does not exceed 10 to 12 mEq/L over the 24-hour period.
- **Severe symptomatic hyponatremia**
  - **Fluid administration.** In patients with symptomatic hyponatremia, hypertonic saline provides an immediate and titratable intervention necessary to acutely raise serum Na levels while avoiding the disastrous complications of overcorrection.
    - The most accurate way to correct hyponatremia entails a detailed registry matching total solute and water output with desired input. In clinical practice, this is often impractical.
    - In lieu of this, the following equation is often used to approximate the change in [Na$^+$] in mEq/L from the infusion of 1 L of fluid:

$$\Delta[Na^+] = \{[Na^+_i] + [K^+_i] - [Na^+_s]\} \div \{TBW + 1\}$$

[Na^+_i] and [K^+_i] are the sodium and potassium concentrations in the infused fluid and [Na^+_s] is the starting serum sodium (*Intensive Care Med 1997;23:309*). Recall that TBW is estimated by multiplying the lean weight (kg) by 0.6 in men (and by 0.5 in women). This formula does not account for ongoing electrolyte or water losses and is only a rough guide.
    - Dividing the desired rate of correction (mEq/L/hr) by Δ[Na$^+$] (mEq/L/L of fluid) gives you the appropriate rate of administration (liters of fluid per hour).
    - Because this equation does not account for ongoing losses, one must recheck laboratory data and adjust fluid rates to make sure the patient is improving appropriately.
    - **Example:** An 80-kg woman is seizing. Her [Na$^+$] is 103 mEq/L.
      - Rate of correction: She has symptomatic hyponatremia requiring an acute correction (1 to 2 mEq/L/hr for the first 3 to 4 hours), but no more than 12 mEq/L corrected over 24 hours.
      - Means of correction:
      - Given the acuity, the patient should be given hypertonic saline, which has 513 mEq Na$^+$/L.

- One liter of this fluid would increase $[Na^+]$ by $+10$ mEq/L

$$\Delta[Na^+] = \{513 - 108\} \div \{80 \times 0.5 + 1\} = 10 \text{ mEq/L}$$

- Dose hypertonic saline at 200 mL/hr until symptoms improve

$$\text{Rate} = [2 \text{ mEq/L/hr}] \div [10 \text{ mEq/L/L of saline}])$$

- To prevent a change of >10 to 12 mEq/L over 24 hours, no more than 1 L of fluid should be given.
- **Chronic asymptomatic hyponatremia.** The risk of iatrogenic injury is actually increased in patients with chronic hyponatremia. Because cells gradually adapt to the hypo-osmolar state, an abrupt normalization presents a dramatic change from the accommodated osmotic milieu. As such, we suggest a more modest rate of correction, on the order of 5 to 8 mEq/L over a 24-hour period.
- **Asymptomatic hypovolemic hyponatremia**
  - **Fluid administration**
    - In patients with asymptomatic hypovolemic hyponatremia, isotonic saline can be used to restore the intravascular volume. Restoration of a euvolemic state will reduce the impetus toward renal water retention, leading to normalization of $[Na^+]$. If the duration of hyponatremia is unknown, the process described above can be used to calculate the expected change from 1 L of 0.9% NS, the rate of administration, and the maximal amount that can be given to avoid overcorrection.
    - Asymptomatic hypervolemic hyponatremia. Hyponatremia in CHF and cirrhosis often reflects the severity of the underlying disease. However, the hyponatremia itself is typically asymptomatic. Although *effective* circulating volume is decreased, the administration of fluid may worsen the volume-overloaded state. Definitive treatment requires management of the underlying condition, although restriction of water intake and increasing water diuresis may help to attenuate the degree of hyponatremia.

Medications

- Loop diuretics promote urinary excretion of water by reducing the concentration gradient necessary to reabsorb water in the distal nephron and impair the ability to excrete concentrated urine.
- Vasopressin antagonists are also being evaluated and may be helpful in both euvolemic (SIADH) and hypervolemic hyponatremia (particularly CHF). At present, only IV formulations are approved in the United States. When using medications to promote water loss, laboratory data and volume status must be followed extremely closely, as the effect on water and electrolyte loss cannot be accurately predicted.
- Lithium and demeclocycline interfere with the collecting tubule's ability to respond to ADH, but are rarely used because of significant side effects. They should only be considered in severe hyponatremia that is unresponsive to more conservative measures.
- Vasopressin antagonists promote a water diuresis and may be useful in the therapy of SIADH. As of yet, the only formulation approved in the United States is conivaptan, which is an IV preparation and thus not applicable to chronic outpatient management of euvolemic hyponatremia.

Lifestyle/Risk Modification

Diet

- Oral fluid intake should be less than daily urine output.
- **SIADH** should first be distinguished from the previously listed conditions, which stimulate vasopressin secretion. The standard first-line therapy is water restriction and correction of any contributing factors (nausea, pneumonia, drugs, etc.). If this fails or if the patient is symptomatic, the following can be attempted to promote water excretion.
- **Water restriction.** The amount of fluid restriction necessary depends on the extent of water elimination. A useful guide to the necessary degree of fluid restriction is as follows:
  - If (Urine Na + Urine K)/Serum Na < 0.5, restrict to 1 L/d.
  - If (Urine Na + Urine K)/Serum Na is 0.5 to 1.0, restrict to 500 mL/d.
  - If (Urine Na + Urine K)/Serum Na is >1, the patient has a negative renal free water clearance and is actively reabsorbing water. Any amount of water given may be retained and clinicians should consider the options below to enhance free water excretion.
- **High dietary solute load.** As the volume of water excreted as urine is governed by a relatively fixed urine osmolality, increasing solute intake with a high-salt, high-protein diet or administration of oral urea (30 to 60 g) may increase the capacity for water excretion and improve the hyponatremia.

Hypernatremia

GENERAL PRINCIPLES

Definition

Hypernatremia is defined as a plasma $[Na^+]$ > **145 mEq/L** and represents a state of **hyperosmolality.**

Etiology

- Hypernatremia may be caused by a primary **Na^+ gain** or a **water deficit,** the latter being much more common. Normally, this hyperosmolar state stimulates thirst and the excretion of a maximally concentrated urine. For hypernatremia to persist, one or both of these compensatory mechanisms must also be impaired.
- **Impaired thirst response** may occur in situations where access to water is limited. This is often due to physical restrictions (institutionalized, handicapped, postoperative, or intubated patients) or to conditions of mental impairment (delirium, dementia).
- **Hypernatremia due to water loss.** The loss of water must occur in excess of electrolyte losses in order to raise $[Na^+]$.
  - **Nonrenal water loss** may be due to evaporation from the skin and respiratory tract (insensible losses) or loss from the GI tract. Diarrhea is the most common GI cause of hypernatremia. Osmotic diarrheas (induced by lactulose, sorbitol, or malabsorption of carbohydrate) and viral gastroenteritides in particular result in disproportional water loss.
  - **Renal water loss** results from either **osmotic diuresis** or **diabetes insipidus (DI).**
    - **Osmotic diuresis** is frequently associated with glucosuria and high osmolar feeds. In addition, increased urea generation from accelerated catabolism, high-protein feeds, and stress dose steroids can also result in an osmotic diuresis.

- Hypernatremia secondary to nonosmotic urinary water loss is usually caused by (a) impaired vasopressin secretion (**central diabetes insipidus [CDI]**) or (b) resistance to the actions of vasopressin (**nephrogenic diabetes insipidus [NDI]**). Partial defects occur more commonly than complete defects in both types.
  - The most common cause of CDI is destruction of the neurohypophysis from trauma, neurosurgery, granulomatous disease, neoplasms, vascular accidents, or infection. In many cases, CDI is idiopathic.
  - NDI may either be inherited or acquired. The latter often results from a disruption to the renal concentrating mechanism due to drugs (lithium, demeclocycline, amphotericin), electrolyte disorders (hypercalcemia, hypokalemia), medullary washout (loop diuretics), and intrinsic renal diseases.
- **Hypernatremia due to primary Na$^+$ gain** occurs infrequently due to the kidney's capacity to excrete the retained Na$^+$. However, it can rarely occur after repetitive **hypertonic saline** administration or chronic **mineralocorticoid excess.**
- **Transcellular water shift** from ECF to ICF can occur in circumstances of transient intracellular hyperosmolality, as in seizures or rhabdomyolysis.

DIAGNOSIS

Clinical Presentation

- Hypernatremia results in contraction of brain cells as water shifts to attenuate the rising ECF osmolality. Thus, the most severe symptoms of hypernatremia are neurologic, including altered mental status, weakness, neuromuscular irritability, focal neurologic deficits, and occasionally coma or seizures. As with hyponatremia, the severity of the clinical manifestations is related to the *acuity* and *magnitude* of the rise in plasma [Na$^+$]. **Chronic hypernatremia** is generally less symptomatic as a result of adaptive mechanisms designed to defend cell volume.
- **CDI** and **NDI** generally present with complaints of polyuria and thirst. Signs of volume depletion or neurologic dysfunction are generally absent unless the patient has an associated thirst abnormality.

Diagnostic Testing

Laboratories

Urine osmolality and the **response to dDAVP** can help narrow the differential diagnosis for hypernatremia (Fig. 2).

- The appropriate renal response to hypernatremia is a small volume of concentrated (urine osmolality > 800 mOsm/L) urine. Submaximal **urine osmolality** (<800 mOsm/L) suggests a defect in renal water conservation.
  - A urine osmolality < 300 mOsm in the setting of hypernatremia suggests complete forms of CDI and NDI.
  - Urine osmolality between 300 and 800 mOsm/L can occur from partial forms of DI as well as osmotic diuresis. The two can be differentiated by quantifying the daily solute excretion (estimated by the urine osmolality × urine volume in 24 hours). A daily solute excretion > 900 mOsm defines an osmotic diuresis.
- **Response to dDAVP.** Complete forms of CDI and NDI can be distinguished by administering the vasopressin analog dDAVP (10 mcg intranasally) after careful water restriction. The urine osmolality should increase by at least 50% in complete CDI and does not change in NDI. The diagnosis is sometimes difficult when partial defects are present.

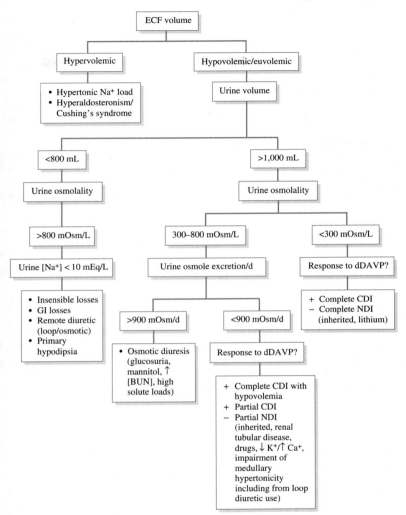

Figure 2. Algorithm depicting the diagnostic approach to hypernatremia. BUN, blood urea nitrogen; CDI, central diabetes insipidus; dDAVP, desmopressin acetate; ECF, extracellular fluid; GI, gastrointestinal; NDI, nephrogenic diabetes insipidus; ↓K^+, hypokalemia; ↑Ca^+, hypercalcemia; (+), conditions with increase in urine osmolality in response to desmopressin acetate; (–), conditions with little increase in urine osmolality in response to desmopressin acetate.

TREATMENT

- Management requires one to determine:
  - The rate of correction
  - The appropriate intervention
  - The presence of other underlying disorders

- **The rate of correction** of hypernatremia depends on the acuity of its development and the presence of neurologic dysfunction.
- **Symptomatic hypernatremia.** As in hyponatremia, aggressive correction of hypernatremia is potentially dangerous. The rapid shift of water into brain cells increases the risk of seizures or permanent neurologic damage. Therefore, the water deficit should be reduced gradually, by roughly **10 to 12 mEq/L/d.**
- In **chronic asymptomatic hypernatremia,** the risk of treatment-related complication is increased due to the cerebral adaptation to the chronic hyperosmolar state, and the plasma $[Na^+]$ should be lowered at a more moderate rate (between 5 and 8 mEq/L/d).
- **Fluid administration**
  - The mainstay of management is the administration of water, preferably by mouth or nasogastric tube. Alternatively, D_5W or quarter normal saline can be given intravenously.
  - Traditionally, correction of hypernatremia has been accomplished by calculating **free water deficit** by the equation:

$$\text{Free water deficit} = \{([Na] - 140)/140\} \times (TBW)$$

While this is helpful in approximating the total water deficit, it does not provide sufficient guidance regarding the rate and content of infusate. Alternatively, we suggest approaching treatment in a manner similar to that used in the treatment of hyponatremia. The change in $[Na^+]$ from the administration of fluids can be estimated as follows:

$$\Delta[Na^+] = \{[Na^+_i] + [K^+_i] - [Na^+_s]\} \div \{TBW + 1\}$$

$[Na^+_i]$ and $[K^+_i]$ are the sodium and potassium concentrations in the infused fluid and $[Na^+_s]$ is the starting serum sodium (*Intensive Care Med 1997;23:309*). Because hypernatremia suggests a contraction in water content, TBW is estimated by multiplying lean weight (kg) by 0.5 in men (rather than 0.6) and 0.4 in women.
  - **Example.** A 70-kg man with diarrhea (2 L/d) from laxative abuse presents with obtundation and $[Na^+] = 164$ mEq/L, $[K^+] = 3.0$. A replacement fluid of D_5W with 20 mEq KCl/L is chosen.
    - The $\Delta[Na^+]$ with 1 L of this fluid would be –4 mEq/L.

$$\{0 + 20 - 164\} \div \{(70 \times 0.5) + 1\}$$

3 L is necessary for a $\Delta[Na^+]$ − 12 mEq/L/24 hr

$$(-12 \text{ mEq/L/d}) \div (-4 \text{ mEq/L/L of solution})$$

    - The hourly rate of infusion is 125 cc/hr (3 L/d ÷ 24 hr/d = 0.125 L/hr). However, this should be followed closely as it does not account for ongoing GI or insensible losses, which may account for another 1.4 L/d of water required to keep $[Na^+]$ stable.
- **Specific therapies for the underlying cause**
- **Hypovolemic hypernatremia.** In patients with mild volume depletion, Na-containing solutions, such as 0.45% NS, can be used to replenish the ECF as well as the water deficit. If patients have severe or symptomatic volume depletion, correction of volume status with **isotonic fluid** should take precedence over correction of the hyperosmolar state. Once the patient is hemodynamically stable, administration of hypotonic fluid can be given to replace the free water deficit.

- **Hypernatremia from primary Na^+ gain** is unusual. Cessation of iatrogenic Na is typically sufficient.
- **Diabetes insipidus without hypernatremia.** Diabetes insipidus is best treated by removing the underlying cause. Despite the renal water loss, DI should not result in hypernatremia if the thirst mechanism remains intact. Therefore therapy, if required at all, is directed toward symptomatic polyuria.
  - **CDI.** Because the polyuria is the result of impaired secretion of vasopressin, treatment is best accomplished with the administration of dDAVP, a vasopressin analog.
  - **NDI.** A low-Na^+ diet combined with *thiazide* diuretics will decrease polyuria through inducing mild volume depletion. This enhances proximal reabsorption of salt and water, decreasing excess water loss. Decreasing protein intake will further decrease urine output by minimizing the solute load that must be excreted.

DISORDERS OF POTASSIUM BALANCE

Potassium Homeostasis

GENERAL PRINCIPLES

- Potassium is the major **intracellular** cation. Of the 3,000 to 4,000 mEq of K^+ found in the average human, 98% is sequestered within cells. Thus, while ECF $[K^+]$ is normally 3.5 to 5.0 mEq/L, the intracellular concentration is roughly 150 mEq/L. This difference in ICF and ECF K^+ content is maintained by the **Na^+ K^+-adenosine triphosphatase pump.**
- The K^+ intake of individuals in an average Western diet is approximately 1 mEq/kg/d, 90% of which is absorbed by the GI tract. Maintenance of the steady state necessitates matching K^+ excretion with ingestion.
- The elimination of potassium occurs predominately through **renal excretion** at the distal nephron. K^+ secretion is enhanced by distal Na^+ reabsorption, which generates a **lumen-negative gradient,** and **distal urine flow rate.**
- Renal potassium handling is responsive to **aldosterone,** which stimulates the expression of distal luminal Na^+ channels, and the **serum potassium concentration.** Aldosterone secretion is, in turn, responsive to angiotensin II and hyperkalemia.

Hypokalemia

GENERAL PRINCIPLES

Definition
Hypokalemia is defined as a plasma $[K^+] < 3.5$ mEq/L.

Etiology
- **Spurious hypokalemia** may be seen in situations in which high numbers of metabolically active cells present in the blood sample absorb the ECF potassium.
- True hypokalemia may result from one or more of the following: (a) **decreased net intake,** (b) **shift into cells,** or (c) **increased net loss.**
  - **Diminished intake** is seldom the sole cause of K^+ depletion because urinary excretion can be effectively decreased to <15 mEq/d. However, dietary K^+ restriction may exacerbate the hypokalemia from GI or renal loss.

- **Transcellular shift.** Movement of K^+ into cells may transiently decrease the plasma $[K^+]$ without altering total body K^+ content. These shifts can result from alkalemia, insulin, and catecholamine release. Periodic paralysis is a rare disorder that predisposes patients to transcellular K^+ shifts that result in episodic muscle weakness. Both hypokalemic and hyperkalemic forms have been described.
- **Nonrenal K^+ loss.** Hypokalemia may result from the loss of potassium-rich fluids from the lower GI tract. Hypokalemia from the loss of upper GI contents is typically more attributable to renal K secretion from secondary hyperaldosteronism. Rarely, in excessive sweating, loss of K^+ through the integument can provoke hypokalemia.
- **Renal K^+ loss** accounts for most cases of *chronic* hypokalemia. This may be caused by factors that increase the lumen-negative gradient, thus enhancing K^+ secretion, or that augment distal urine flow rate.
  - **Augmented distal urine flow** rate occurs commonly with diuretic use and osmotic diuresis (e.g., glucosuria). Bartter's and Gitelman's syndromes mimic diuretic use and promote renal K^+ loss by the same mechanism.
  - A variety of disorders promote K^+ loss by increasing the **lumen-negative gradient,** which drives K^+ secretion. This can be achieved with the reabsorption of a cation (Na^+) or presence of a nonreabsorbed anion.
    - Distal Na^+ reabsorption is largely influenced by mineralocorticoid activity.
    - **Primary mineralocorticoid excess** can be seen in primary hyperaldosteronism due to an adrenal adenoma or adrenocortical hyperplasia.
    - Cortisol also has an affinity for mineralocorticoid receptors, but is typically converted quickly to cortisone, which has markedly less mineralocorticoid activity. Still, if cortisol is present in abundance (Cushing's syndrome) or fails to be converted to cortisone (syndrome of mineralocorticoid excess), it may mimic hyperaldosteronism.
    - **Secondary hyperaldosteronism** can be seen in any situation with a decreased effective circulating volume.
    - Constitutive activation of the distal renal epithelial Na^+ channel, independent of aldosterone, occurs in **Liddle's syndrome.**
  - The increased distal delivery of a nonreabsorbable anion can also potentiate the lumen-negative gradient that drives K^+ secretion. Examples include bicarbonate (metabolic alkalosis or type 2 RTA [renal tubular acidosis]), ketones, and hippurate (from toluene intoxication or glue sniffing).

DIAGNOSIS

Clinical Presentation

- The clinical features of K^+ depletion vary greatly, and their severity depends in part on the degree of hypokalemia. Symptoms seldom occur unless the plasma $[K^+]$ is <3.0 mEq/L.
- Fatigue, myalgias, and muscular weakness or cramps of the lower extremities are common. Smooth muscle function may also be affected and may manifest with complaints of constipation or frank paralytic ileus. Severe hypokalemia may lead to complete paralysis, hypoventilation, or rhabdomyolysis.

Diagnostic Testing

Laboratories

- When the etiology is not immediately apparent, **renal K^+ excretion** and the **acid–base status** can help identify the cause (Table 2).

Table 2	Approach to Dyskalemias	
	Hypokalemia	**Hyperkalemia**
Transcellular shift	Insulin, alkalemia, catecholamines, hypokalemic periodic paralysis	Cell lysis, ↓ insulin, metabolic acidosis, β-blockers, hyperkalemic periodic paralysis
Change in K⁺ content (nonrenal causes)	Dx: $[K^+]$ < 25 mEq/d or TTKG < 2 Examples: Poor intake or GI loss	Dx: TTKG > 10 Examples: Salt substitutes, tomatoes, potatoes, bananas, oranges
Change in K⁺ content (renal causes)	Dx: TTKG > 4 Examples: Enhanced diuresis, increased luminal gradient (hyperaldosteronism, Liddle's syndrome, nonreabsorbed anion)	Dx: TTKG < 7 Examples: Acute/chronic kidney disease, hypoaldosteronism, type 4 RTA

- **Urine K^+.** The appropriate response to hypokalemia is to excrete <25 mEq/d of K^+ in the urine. The patient's urinary K^+ excretion can be measured with a 24-hour urine collection or estimated by multiplying the spot urine $[K^+]$ by the total daily urine output. A spot urine $[K^+]$ may also be helpful (urine $[K^+]$ < 15 mEq/L suggests appropriate K^+ conservation), but the results can be confounded by a variety of factors. Alternatively, a transtubular potassium gradient (TTKG) can be calculated as follows:
  ○ TTKG = (Urine K/Serum K) ÷ (Urine Osmolality/Serum Osmolality)
  ○ A TTKG < 2 suggests a nonrenal source, while a TTKG > 4 suggests inappropriate renal K^+ secretion.
- **Acid–Base status.** Intracellular shifting and renal excretion of K^+ are often closely linked with the acid–base status. Hypokalemia is generally associated with metabolic alkalosis and can play a critical role in the maintenance of metabolic alkalosis. The finding of metabolic acidosis in a patient with hypokalemia thus narrows the differential significantly, implying lower GI loss, distal RTA, or the excretion of a nonreabsorbable anion from an organic acid (DKA, hippurate from toluene intoxication).

Electrocardiography

Electrocardiogram (ECG) changes associated with hypokalemia include flattening or inversion of the T wave, a prominent U wave, ST-segment depression, and a prolonged QT interval. Severe K^+ depletion may result in a prolonged PR interval, decreased voltage, and widening of the QRS complex.

TREATMENT

The **therapeutic goals** are to safely correct the K^+ deficit and to minimize ongoing losses through treatment of the underlying cause. Hypomagnesemia should also be sought in all hypokalemic patients and corrected to allow effective K^+ repletion.

Medications

- Correction of the K^+ deficit can be accomplished with either oral or IV therapy. It is generally safer to correct the K^+ deficit via the oral route when hypokalemia is mild and the patient can tolerate oral administration. Oral doses of 40 mEq are generally well tolerated and can be given as often as every 4 hours. Traditionally, 10 mEq of potassium salts are given for each 0.10-mEq/L decrement in serum $[K^+]$. However, with increasing severity of hypokalemia, this grossly underestimates the K^+ necessary to normalize *total* K content. Furthermore, as the K^+ shifts back to the intracellular space, it may appear as though K^+ supplementation is doing very little to correct ECF $[K^+]$. Although this may appear discouraging, it simply reflects the true extent of hypokalemia. In such cases, potassium supplementation should be increased and continued until serum levels rise.
- Patients with imminently life-threatening hypokalemia and those who are unable to take anything by mouth require IV replacement therapy with KCl. The maximum concentration of administered K^+ should be no more than 40 mEq/L via a peripheral vein or 100 mEq/L via a central vein. The rate of infusion should not exceed 20 mEq/hr unless paralysis or malignant ventricular arrhythmias are present. Ideally, KCl should be mixed in normal saline because dextrose solutions may initially exacerbate hypokalemia (as a result of insulin-mediated movement of K^+). Rapid IV administration of K^+ should be used judiciously and requires close observation.

Hyperkalemia

GENERAL PRINCIPLES

Definition

Hyperkalemia is defined as a plasma $[K^+]$ > **5.0 mEq/L.**

Etiology

- **Pseudohyperkalemia** represents an artificially elevated plasma $[K^+]$ due to K^+ movement out of cells immediately before or following venipuncture. Contributing factors include repeated fist clenching, hemolysis, and marked leukocytosis or thrombocytosis.
- True hyperkalemia occurs as a result of (a) **transcellular shift,** (b) **increased exposure to K^+,** and most commonly, (c) **decreased renal K^+ excretion.** Combinations of these mechanisms often underlie cases of hyperkalemia in clinical practice, and decreased renal excretion is nearly always some component of the pathophysiology.
  - **Transcellular shift.** Insulin deficiency, hyperosmolality, nonselective β-blockers, digitalis, metabolic acidosis (excluding those from organic acids), and depolarizing muscle relaxants, such as succinylcholine, release K^+ from predominate ICF stores into the ECF compartment. Familial periodic paralysis, mentioned previously, may result in hyperkalemia, particularly following exercise or fasting. Massive cellular destruction, as seen in tumor lysis syndrome, also liberates cellular K stores and releases them into the ECF.
  - **Increased exposure to K^+** is rarely the sole cause of hyperkalemia unless there is an impairment in renal excretion. Foods with a high content of K^+ include salt substitutes, dried fruits, nuts, tomatoes, potatoes, spinach, bananas, and oranges. Juices derived from these foods may be especially rich sources.

- **Decreased renal K$^+$ excretion.** In the setting of hyperkalemia, the kidney is capable of generating a significant urinary excretion of K$^+$. This process can be impaired by a number of processes, including intrinsic renal disease, decreased delivery of filtrate to the distal nephron, adrenal insufficiency, and hyporeninemic hypoaldosteronism (type 4 RTA).
- **Drugs** may also be implicated in the genesis of hyperkalemia through a variety of mechanisms. Common culprits include angiotensin-converting enzyme inhibitors and angiotensin receptor blockers, potassium-sparing diuretics, NSAIDs, and cyclosporine. Heparin and ketoconazole can also contribute to hyperkalemia through the decreased production of aldosterone, although these agents alone are typically insufficient to sustain a clinically significant hyperkalemia.

DIAGNOSIS

Clinical Presentation

- The most serious effect of hyperkalemia is cardiac arrhythmogenesis secondary to potassium's pivotal role in membrane potentials. Patients may present with palpitations, syncope, or even sudden cardiac death.
- Severe hyperkalemia causes partial depolarization of the skeletal muscle cell membrane and may manifest as weakness potentially progressing to flaccid paralysis and hypoventilation if the respiratory muscles are involved.

Diagnostic Testing

Laboratories

- If the etiology is not readily apparent and the patient is asymptomatic, **pseudohyperkalemia** should be excluded by rechecking laboratory data.
- An assessment of **renal [K$^+$]** excretion and the **renin–angiotensin–aldosterone axis** can help narrow the differential diagnosis when the etiology is not immediately apparent.
  - Renal [K$^+$] excretion can be assessed using the TTKG previously described.
    - A TTKG > 10 suggests that renal tubular mechanisms for K$^+$ secretion are intact. The persistence of hyperkalemia despite an intact renal response suggests poor filtrate delivery to the distal mechanisms of K$^+$ regulation, as occurs with a decreased effective circulating volume.
    - A TTKG < 7 implies impaired K$^+$ secretion caused by hypoaldosteronism, aldosterone resistance, or hyporeninemic hypoaldosteronism. An evaluation of the renin–aldosterone axis may help to differentiate these entities.
      - Low aldosterone levels suggest either adrenal disease (renin levels elevated; TTKG improves with fludrocortisone) or hyporeninemic hypoaldosteronism (renin levels low; occurs with type 4 RTA as well as chloride shunting, or Gordon's syndrome).
      - High aldosterone levels, typically accompanied by high renin levels, suggest aldosterone resistance (pseudohypoaldosteronism), but can also be seen in K$^+$-sparing diuretics.

Electrocardiography

ECG changes include increased T-wave amplitude, or peaked T waves. More severe degrees of hyperkalemia result in a prolonged PR interval and QRS duration, atrioventricular conduction delay, and loss of P waves. Progressive widening of the QRS complex and its merging with the T wave produce a sine wave pattern. The terminal event is usually ventricular fibrillation or asystole.

TREATMENT

Severe hyperkalemia with ECG changes is a medical emergency and requires immediate treatment directed at minimizing membrane depolarization and acutely reducing the ECF [K^+]. **Acute therapy** may consist of some or all of the following (the hypokalemic effect is additive).

Medications

- **Administration of calcium gluconate** decreases membrane excitability but does not lower [K^+]. The usual dose is 10 mL of a 10% solution infused over 2 to 3 minutes. The effect begins within minutes but is short-lived (30 to 60 minutes), and the dose can be repeated if no improvement in the ECG is seen after 5 to 10 minutes.
- **Insulin** causes K^+ to shift into cells and temporarily lowers the plasma [K^+]. A commonly used combination is 10 to 20 units of regular insulin and 25 to 50 g glucose administered intravenously. Hyperglycemic patients should be given the insulin alone.
- **NaHCO$_3$** is effective for severe hyperkalemia associated with metabolic acidosis. In the acute setting, it can be given as an IV isotonic solution (three ampules of NaHCO$_3$ in 1 L of 5% dextrose).
- **β_2-Adrenergic agonists** promote cellular uptake of K^+. The onset of action is 30 minutes, lowering the plasma [K^+] by 0.5 to 1.5 mEq/L, and the effect lasts for 2 to 4 hours. Albuterol can be administered in a dose of 10 to 20 mg as a continuous nebulized treatment over 30 to 60 minutes.
- **Longer-term** means for [K^+] removal
  - Increasing distal Na delivery in the kidney enhances renal K^+ clearance. This can be achieved with the administration of saline in patients who appear volume depleted. Otherwise, diuretics can be used if renal function is adequate.
  - **Cation exchange resins,** such as sodium polystyrene sulfonate (Kayexalate), promote the exchange of Na$^+$ for K^+ in the GI tract. When given by mouth, the usual dose is 25 to 50 g mixed with 100 mL of 20% sorbitol to prevent constipation. This generally lowers the plasma [K^+] by 0.5 to 1.0 mEq/L within 1 to 2 hours and lasts for 4 to 6 hours. Sodium polystyrene sulfonate can also be administered as a retention enema consisting of 50 g resin in 150 mL tap water. Enemas should be avoided in postoperative patients because of the increased incidence of colonic necrosis, especially following renal transplantation.
- **Dialysis.** Dialysis should be reserved for patients with renal failure and those with severe life-threatening hyperkalemia that is unresponsive to more conservative measures.
- **Chronic management** of hyperkalemia
  - **Chronic therapy** may involve dietary modifications to avoid high K^+ foods (see Potassium, Hyperkalemia, General Principles, Etiology), correction of metabolic acidosis with oral alkali, promoting kaliuresis with diuretics, and/or administration of exogenous mineralocorticoid in states of hypoaldosteronism.

DISORDERS OF CALCIUM METABOLISM

Calcium Homeostasis

GENERAL PRINCIPLES

- Calcium is essential for bone formation and neuromuscular function.
- Approximately 99% of body calcium is in bone; most of the remaining 1% is in the ECF. Nearly 50% of serum calcium is ionized (free), whereas the remainder is complexed to albumin (40%) and anions such as phosphate (10%).
- **Calcium balance** is regulated by **parathyroid hormone** (PTH) and **calcitriol.**
  - **PTH** increases serum calcium by stimulating bone resorption, increasing calcium reclamation in the kidney, and promoting renal conversion of vitamin D to calcitriol. Serum calcium regulates PTH secretion by a negative feedback mechanism: hypocalcemia stimulates and hypercalcemia suppresses PTH release.
  - **Calcitriol** (1,25-dihydroxycholecalciferol, 1,25-dihydroxyvitamin D_3, or $1,25(OH)_2D_3$) is the active form of vitamin D. It stimulates intestinal absorption of calcium and is one of many factors that provide feedback to the parathyroid gland.

Hypercalcemia

GENERAL PRINCIPLES

Definition

A serum calcium > **10.3 mg/dL** with a normal serum albumin or an ionized calcium > **5.2 mg/dL** defines hypercalcemia.

Etiology

- Clinically significant hypercalcemia typically requires both an increase in ECF calcium and decrease in renal calcium clearance. Underlying disturbances to calcium metabolism are thus often masked by compensatory mechanisms until the patient develops a concomitant disorder, such as decreased renal clearance from volume depletion. More than 90% of cases are due to **primary hyperparathyroidism** or **malignancy.**
- **Primary hyperparathyroidism** causes most cases of hypercalcemia in *ambulatory* patients. It is a common disorder, especially in elderly women, in whom the annual incidence is approximately 2 in 1,000. Nearly 85% of cases are due to an **adenoma** of a single gland, 15% due to **hyperplasia** of all four glands, and 1% due to **parathyroid carcinoma.**
- **Malignancy** is responsible for most cases of hypercalcemia among *hospitalized* patients. Patients usually have advanced, clinically obvious disease. In these patients, hypercalcemia may develop from stimulation of osteoclast bone resorption from tumor cell products, tumor-derived **PTH-related peptide** (PTHrP), and tumor calcitriol production.
- Less common causes account for about 10% of cases of hypercalcemia:
  - **Increased vitamin D activity** occurs with exogenous exposure to vitamin D or increased generation of calcitriol in chronic granulomatous diseases (e.g., sarcoidosis, tuberculosis).

- The **milk-alkali syndrome** describes the acute or chronic development of hypercalcemia, alkalosis, and renal failure that may result from the ingestion of large quantities of calcium-containing antacids.
- **Other.** Hyperthyroidism, adrenal insufficiency, prolonged immobilization, Paget's disease, and acromegaly may be associated with hypercalcemia. **Familial hypocalciuric hypercalcemia** is a rare, autosomal dominant disorder of the calcium-sensing receptor, which is characterized by asymptomatic hypercalcemia from childhood and a family history of hypercalcemia.

DIAGNOSIS

Clinical Presentation

Clinical manifestations are generally present only if serum calcium exceeds 12 mg/dL and tend to be more severe if hypercalcemia develops rapidly. Most patients with **primary hyperparathyroidism** have asymptomatic hypercalcemia that is found incidentally.

- Renal manifestations include polyuria and nephrolithiasis. If serum calcium rises above 13 mg/dL, renal failure with nephrocalcinosis and ectopic soft tissue calcifications are possible.
- GI symptoms include anorexia, vomiting, constipation, and, rarely, signs of pancreatitis.
- Neurologic findings include weakness, fatigue, confusion, stupor, and coma.
- Osteopenia and frequent fractures may occur from the disproportional resorption of bone in hyperparathyroidism. Rarely, **osteitis fibrosa cystica** can develop when hyperparathyroidism is profound and prolonged, resulting in "brown tumors" and marrow replacement.

History

The history and physical examination should focus on (a) the duration of symptoms of hypercalcemia, (b) clinical evidence of any of the unusual causes of hypercalcemia, and (c) symptoms and signs of malignancy (which almost always precede **malignant hypercalcemia**). If hypercalcemia has been present for more than 6 months without an obvious etiology, primary hyperparathyroidism is almost certainly the cause.

Diagnostic Testing

Laboratories

- In most patients, the diagnosis can be made with the history and physical and a limited laboratory workup.
- The **serum calcium** should be interpreted with knowledge of the serum albumin, or an ionized calcium should be measured. **Corrected [Ca^{2+}]** = [Ca^{2+}] + {0.8 × (4.0 − [Albumin])}. Many patients with primary hyperparathyroidism will have a calcium level that is chronically within the high-normal range.
- The **serum PTH** level is mandatory for the evaluation of hypercalcemia. Assays measuring intact PTH should be used, as these are independent of renal function.
  - Elevations in ECF calcium typically result in suppression of PTH. Thus, the finding of a normal or elevated intact PTH in the setting of hypercalcemia is suggestive of primary hyperparathyroidism.
  - When the intact PTH is appropriately suppressed, **PTHrP** can be measured to investigate possible humoral hypercalcemia of malignancy. Causes of vitamin D

disorders should also be considered. **1,25(OH)$_2$D$_3$** levels are elevated in granulomatous disorders, primary hyperparathyroidism, calcitriol overdose, and acromegaly. **25(OH)D$_3$** levels are elevated with non-calcitriol vitamin D intoxication.

- The **serum phosphorus** may help to identify the underlying disturbance in calcium homeostasis. Hyperparathyroidism often decreases phosphorus levels by stimulating phosphaturia, while Paget's disease and vitamin D intoxication both tend to increase phosphorus levels.
- **Urine calcium** may be elevated in primary hyperparathyroidism due to a filtered load of calcium that exceeds the capacity for renal reabsorption. If the family history and clinical picture is suggestive, patients with **familial hypocalciuric hypercalcemia** can be distinguished from primary hyperparathyroidism by documenting a low calcium clearance by 24-hour urine collection (<200 mg calcium/d) or fractional excretion of calcium (<1%).

Electrocardiography
The **ECG** may reveal a shortened QT interval and, with very severe hypercalcemia, variable degrees of atrioventricular block.

TREATMENT

- **Acute management** of hypercalcemia is warranted if severe symptoms are present or with serum calcium > 12 mg/dL. The following regimen is presented in the order that therapy should be given.
- **Fluid Administration. Correction of hypovolemia** with 0.9% saline fluid is mandatory in patients who demonstrate volume depletion, since hypovolemia prevents effective calciuresis. Maintenance fluids can be continued after achieving euvolemia to sustain a urine output of 100 to 150 mL/hr. The patient should be monitored closely for signs of volume overload.

Medications
- Loop diuretics can be used if further saline administration is limited by signs of volume overload while hypercalcemia persists. These agents reduce paracellular reabsorption of calcium in the loop of Henle and thus may slightly enhance calcium excretion. However, they should not be used in euvolemic or hypervolemic patients as they may further contract the ECF volume and prevent adequate restoration of the volume status.
- **IV bisphosphonates** can be used to decrease the liberation of calcium from bone in persistent hypercalcemia. Pamidronate 60 mg is infused over 2 to 4 hours; for severe hypercalcemia (>13.5 mg/dL), 90 mg can be given over the same duration. A hypocalcemic response is typically seen within 2 days and may persist for 2 weeks or longer. Treatment can be repeated after 7 days if hypercalcemia recurs. Zoledronate is a more potent bisphosphonate that is given as a 4-mg dose infused over at least 15 minutes. Hydration should precede their use and renal insufficiency is a relative contraindication.
- **Calcitonin** inhibits bone resorption and increases renal calcium excretion. Salmon calcitonin 4 to 8 International Units/kg IM or SC q6–12h, lowers serum calcium 1 to 2 mg/dL within several hours in 60% to 70% of patients. Although it is less potent than other inhibitors of bone resorption, it has no serious toxicity, is safe in renal failure, and may have an analgesic effect in patients with skeletal metastases.

- **Glucocorticoids** are effective in hypercalcemia due to hematologic malignancies and granulomatous production of calcitriol. The initial dose is 20 to 60 mg/d of prednisone or its equivalent. After serum calcium stabilizes, the dose should be gradually reduced to the minimum needed to control symptoms of hypercalcemia. Toxicity (see Chapter 22, Arthritis and Rheumatologic Diseases) limits the usefulness of glucocorticoids for long-term therapy.
- **Gallium nitrate** inhibits bone resorption as effectively as the IV bisphosphonates and has a similar delayed onset of 2 days. It is given as a 100 to 200-mg/m^2/d continuous infusion for up to 5 days, unless normocalcemia is achieved sooner. There is, however, a significant risk of nephrotoxicity and it is contraindicated if the serum creatinine is >2.5 mg/dL.
- **Dialysis.** Hemodialysis and peritoneal dialysis using low-calcium dialysate are effective for patients with very severe hypercalcemia (>16 mg/dL) and CHF or renal insufficiency.
- **Chronic management** of hypercalcemia
  - **Primary hyperparathyroidism.** In many patients this disorder has a benign course, with minimal fluctuation in serum calcium concentration and no obvious clinical sequelae. Parathyroidectomy is indicated in patients with (a) corrected serum calcium > 1 mg/dL over the upper limit of normal, (b) calciuria > 400 mg/d, (c) renal insufficiency, (d) reduced bone mass (T score ≤ 2.5 by dual-energy absorptiometry), (e) age < 50 years, and (f) unfeasibility of long-term follow-up (*J Bone Miner Res 2002;17(Suppl 2):N2*). Surgical intervention typically has a high success rate (95%), with low morbidity and mortality.
  - **Medical therapy** may be a reasonable option in asymptomatic patients who are not surgical candidates. Management consists of liberal oral hydration with a high-salt diet, daily physical activity to lessen bone resorption, and avoidance of thiazide diuretics. Oral bisphosphonates and estrogen replacement therapy or raloxifene in postmenopausal women can be considered in the appropriate clinical context. Cinacalcet, an activator of the calcium-sensing receptor, has also been shown to reduce PTH secretion and serum calcium levels, although it is not approved for use in primary hyperparathyroidism at this time.
  - **Malignant hypercalcemia.** Bisphosphonate, glucocorticoid, and a calcium-restricted diet (<400 mg/d) can be tried, although these maneuvers rarely succeed for a long period of time unless the cancer responds to treatment.

Hypocalcemia

GENERAL PRINCIPLES

Definition

A serum calcium < **8.4 mg/dL** with a normal serum albumin or an ionized calcium < **4.2 mg/dL** defines hypocalcemia.

Etiology

- **Pseudohypocalcemia** describes the situation in which the total calcium is reduced due to hypoalbuminemia but the **corrected [Ca^{2+}]** (see Calcium, Hypercalcemia, Diagnosis, Laboratory Studies) and ionized calcium remain within the normal ranges.
- **Effective hypoparathyroidism.** Reduced PTH activity can result from decreased PTH release from autoimmune, infiltrative, or iatrogenic (e.g., post-thyroidectomy)

destruction of parathyroid tissue. In rare patients the hypoparathyroidism is congenital, as in DiGeorge's syndrome or **familial hypocalcemia.** Release of PTH is also impaired with both hypomagnesemia (<1 mg/dL) and severe hypermagnesemia (>6 mg/dL).

- **Vitamin D deficiency** lowers total body calcium but does not usually affect serum calcium levels unless the deficiency is severe, since the resultant secondary hyperparathyroidism often corrects serum calcium levels. Significant vitamin D deficiency can occur in the elderly or those with limited sun exposure, in advanced liver disease (due to decreased synthesis of precursors), and in nephrotic syndrome. Reduced activity in vitamin D activation via 1-α-hydroxylase activity can be seen with vitamin D–Dependent rickets and chronic renal insufficiency.

- Serum calcium levels may also be reduced by profound elevations in serum phosphorus, which binds with the calcium and deposits in a variety of tissues. Calcium can also be bound by citrate (during transfusion of citrate-containing blood products or with continual renal replacement using citrate anticoagulation) as well as drugs such as foscarnet and fluoroquinolones. Increased binding to albumin can also be seen in the context of alkalemia, which increases the exposure of negatively charged binding sites on albumin.

- A low serum free calcium level is common in critically ill patients perhaps due to a cytokine-mediated decrease in PTH and calcitriol release with target organ resistance to their effects.

DIAGNOSIS

Clinical Presentation

- Clinical manifestations vary with the *degree of hypocalcemia* and *rate of onset.*
- Acute, moderate hypocalcemia may cause increased excitability of nerves and muscles leading to circumoral or distal paresthesias and tetany.
- Acute, severe hypocalcemia may cause laryngospasm, confusion, seizures, or vascular collapse with bradycardia and decompensated heart failure.

History

Clues to the diagnosis may be provided by a bedside evaluation for (a) previous neck surgery (postoperative hypoparathyroidism), (b) systemic diseases (autoimmune, infiltrative disorders), (c) family history of hypocalcemia, (d) drug-induced hypocalcemia, and (e) conditions associated with vitamin D deficiency (e.g., uremia).

Physical Examination

Trousseau's sign is the development of carpal spasm when a blood pressure cuff is inflated above systolic pressure for 3 minutes. **Chvostek's sign** refers to twitching of the facial muscles when the facial nerve is tapped anterior to the ear. The presence of these signs is known as **latent tetany.**

Diagnostic Testing

Laboratories

- Laboratory data should be used to evaluate the calcium–PTH axis as well concurrent mineral abnormalities.
- **Albumin** should be measured anytime there is an abnormality in serum calcium levels to rule out pseudo hypocalcemia. As mentioned previously, calcium can be corrected by adding $\{0.8 \times (4 - [\text{Albumin}])\}$ to the total serum calcium level.

- **Serum PTH** that is low or inappropriately normal in the setting of hypocalcemia is indicative of hypoparathyroidism. A high PTH is often found with vitamin D deficiency, PTH resistance, and hyperphosphatemia.
- **Serum phosphorus** is often helpful in identifying vitamin D deficiency (low calcium, low phosphorus) or intravascular chelation of calcium (low calcium, high phosphorus).
- **Vitamin D** stores are usually assessed by measuring only 25(OH)D$_3$ since calcitriol (1,25(OH)$_2$D$_3$) levels can be normalized through the compensatory increase of 1-α-hydroxylase activity.
- **Magnesium** deficiency should always be ruled out during management of hypocalcemia.

Electrocardiography
The **ECG** may show a prolonged QT interval and bradycardia.

TREATMENT

Acute management of symptomatic hypocalcemia requires prompt and aggressive therapy.

Medications

- **Phosphorus** must first be checked. In severe hyperphosphatemia, administration of calcium will increase the calcium–phosphorus product and may exacerbate the formation of ectopic calcifications. In acute, symptomatic hypocalcemia with severe hyperphosphatemia, dialysis may be needed to acutely manage the mineral abnormalities. If the hypocalcemia is asymptomatic, reduction of phosphorus should precede aggressive calcium supplementation.
- **Hypomagnesemia,** if present, must be treated first in order to effectively correct the hypocalcemia. Two grams of magnesium sulfate can be given IV over 15 minutes followed by an infusion (see Magnesium, Hypomagnesemia, Treatment) and may even be given empirically if renal failure is not present.
- **Calcium supplementation.** IV calcium should be reserved for severe or symptomatic hypocalcemia and can be administered as calcium chloride or calcium gluconate. Calcium gluconate is typically favored due to reduced risk of tissue toxicity with extravasation. Calcium gluconate is often prepared as a 10% solution (100 mg of calcium gluconate per milliliter). One ampule (10 mL) of calcium gluconate thus contains 1,000 mg of calcium gluconate and ~90 mg of elemental calcium.
  - When necessary to treat severe or symptomatic hypocalcemia, an initial dose of 90 to 180 mg of elemental calcium can be achieved with 1 to 2 g of **calcium gluconate** (equal to 10 to 20 mL or one to two ampules of 10% calcium gluconate) mixed in 50 to 100 mL of D$_5$W administered over 10 to 20 minutes.
  - The effect of initial treatment is only transient and maintenance of calcium levels typically requires a continuous infusion of 0.5 to 1.5 mg/kg/hr of elemental calcium. A solution comprised of 1 L of D$_5$W with 100 mL of 10% calcium gluconate contains ~900 mg of elemental calcium per liter, approximating 1 mg of elemental calcium per milliliter of fluid. Infusion is typically begun at a rate of 50 mL/hr (~50 mg of elemental calcium per hour) and titrated up as needed.
- **Chronic management.** Treatment requires calcium supplements and vitamin D or its active metabolite to increase intestinal calcium absorption.

- **Oral calcium supplements.** Calcium carbonate (40% elemental calcium) or calcium acetate (25% elemental calcium) can be given with the goal administration of 1 to 2 g of *elemental* calcium PO tid. Calcium supplementation should be given apart from meals, to minimize binding with phosphorus and maximize enteric absorption. Serum levels should be checked once to twice per week to guide ongoing therapy.
- **Vitamin D.** Simple dietary deficiency can be corrected by the use of ergocalciferol 400 to 1,000 International Units/d. However, in conjunction with other hypocalcemic disorders, larger doses may be required. A 6- to 8-week regimen of 50,000 International Units should be dosed weekly in those with underlying impairments in vitamin D metabolism (i.e., renal insufficiency), and daily in patients with severe malnutrition or malabsorption.
- In comparison, **calcitriol** has a much more rapid onset of action. The initial dosage is 0.25 mcg daily, and most patients are maintained on 0.5 to 2.0 mcg daily. The dose can be increased at 2- to 4-week intervals. Because calcitriol increases enteric absorption of phosphorus as well as calcium, phosphorus levels should be monitored and oral phosphate binders initiated if phosphorus exceeds the normal range.

COMPLICATIONS

Development of hypercalcemia. In the event that hypercalcemia develops, vitamin D and calcium supplements should be stopped until serum calcium falls to normal, then both should be restarted at lower doses. Hypercalcemia due to calcitriol usually resolves within 1 week.

DISORDERS OF PHOSPHORUS METABOLISM

Phosphorus Homeostatis

GENERAL PRINCIPLES

- Phosphorus is critical for bone formation and cellular energy metabolism.
- Approximately 85% of **total body phosphorus** is in bone, and most of the remainder is within cells. Thus, serum phosphorus levels may not reflect total body phosphorus stores.
- **Phosphorus balance** is determined primarily by four factors:
  - **PTH** regulates the incorporation and release of minerals from bone stores and decreases proximal tubular reabsorption of phosphate, causing urinary wasting.
  - The **phosphate concentration** itself regulates renal proximal reabsorption.
  - **Insulin** lowers serum levels by shifting phosphate into cells.
  - **Calcitriol** $(1,25[OH]_2D_3)$ increases serum phosphate by enhancing intestinal phosphorus absorption.

Hyperphosphatemia

GENERAL PRINCIPLES

Definition

A serum phosphate > **4.5 mg/dL** defines hyperphosphatemia.

Etiology

- **Hyperphosphatemia** is caused by (a) **transcellular shift,** (b) **increased intake,** and most commonly (c) **decreased renal excretion.** In clinical practice, renal insufficiency is usually present and serves as the major predisposing factor toward the development of hyperphosphatemia.
- **Transcellular shift** occurs in rhabdomyolysis, tumor lysis syndrome, and massive hemolysis as phosphorus is released from cells into the ECF. Metabolic acidosis and hypoinsulinemia reduce phosphorus flux into cells and contribute to the hyperphosphatemia sometimes seen in DKA.
- **Increased intake** leading to hyperphosphatemia usually occurs in the setting of renal insufficiency, either with dietary indiscretion in chronic kidney disease or as an iatrogenic complication. The latter can be seen when phosphosoda enemas (e.g., Fleets) or active vitamin D analogs are given to patients with renal insufficiency.
- **Decreased renal excretion** occurs most commonly in the setting of renal failure. Occasionally, hypoparathyroidism and pseudohypoparathyroidism reduce renal phosphorus clearance as well.

DIAGNOSIS

Clinical Presentation

- Signs and symptoms are typically attributable to hypocalcemia and the metastatic calcification of soft tissues. Occasionally, skin deposition can result in severe pruritus. **Calciphylaxis** describes the tissue ischemia that may result from the calcification of smaller blood vessels and their subsequent thrombosis.
- Chronic hyperphosphatemia contributes to the development of renal osteodystrophy (see Chapter 10, Renal Diseases).

Diagnostic Testing

Laboratories

Elevated serum phosphorus can be accompanied by hypocalcemia as a result of **intravascular chelation** of calcium by phosphorus.

TREATMENT

- **Acute hyperphosphatemia** is treated by increasing renal excretion of phosphorus and, as such, is limited when renal insufficiency is present.
  - **Recovery of renal function** will often correct the hyperphosphatemia in the patient within 12 hours. Saline and/or acetazolamide (15 mg/kg q4h) can be given to further encourage phosphaturia, if needed.
  - **Hemodialysis** may be required, especially if irreversible renal insufficiency or symptomatic hypocalcemia is present.
- **Chronic hyperphosphatemia** is almost always associated with chronic renal insufficiency. Its management consists of reducing phosphorus intake through dietary modification and the use of phosphate binders. This is discussed more fully in Chapter 10, Renal Diseases.

Hypophosphatemia

GENERAL PRINCIPLES

Definition

A serum phosphate < **2.8 mg/dL** defines hypophosphatemia.

Etiology

Hypophosphatemia may be caused by (a) **impaired intestinal absorption,** (b) **increased renal excretion,** or (c) **transcellular shift** into cells. Often there are several mechanisms that work in concert to lower serum phosphate.

* **Impaired intestinal absorption** occurs with the malabsorption syndromes, the use of oral phosphate binders, or vitamin D deficiency from any cause (see Calcium, Hypocalcemia, General Principles, Etiology). *Chronic alcoholism* is often associated with poor intake of both phosphate and vitamin D resulting in total body phosphorus depletion.

* **Increased renal excretion** occurs with high levels of PTH, as seen in hyperparathyroidism. This can be particularly pronounced in patients with secondary or tertiary hyperparathyroidism who undergo renal transplantation, as the high PTH causes exerts a profound phosphaturic effect on the functional allograft. Hypophosphatemia may also occur from osmotic diuresis and disorders of proximal tubular transport such as familial X-linked hypophosphatemic rickets and Fanconi syndrome.

* **Transcellular shift** is stimulated by respiratory alkalosis as well as insulin. The latter is responsible for the paradoxical reduction in phosphorus during treatment of malnutrition with hyperalimentation (the refeeding syndrome). The endogenous increase in insulin during treatment shifts phosphorus intracellularly, further reducing serum phosphorus in the malnourished individual. Phosphorus can also be rapidly absorbed into bone following parathyroidectomy for severe hyperparathyroidism (hungry-bone syndrome).

DIAGNOSIS

Clinical Presentation

Signs and symptoms typically occur only if total body phosphate depletion is present and the serum phosphorus level is <1 mg/dL. These end-organ effects are due to the inability to form ATP and the impaired tissue oxygen delivery that occurs with a decrease in red blood cell 2,3-diphosphoglycerate. These include muscle injury (rhabdomyolysis, impaired diaphragmatic function, and heart failure), neurologic abnormalities (paresthesias, dysarthria, confusion, stupor, seizures, and coma) and, rarely, hemolysis and platelet dysfunction.

Diagnostic Testing

Laboratories

* The cause is usually apparent from the clinical situation in which the hypophosphatemia occurs. If not, measurement of **urine phosphorus excretion** helps define the mechanism.
  * Renal excretion of >100 mg by 24-hour urine collection or a fractional excretion of phosphate >5% during hypophosphatemia indicates excessive renal loss.

- Low serum **25(OH)D₃** suggests dietary vitamin D deficiency or malabsorption. An elevated **intact PTH** may occur in primary or secondary hyperparathyroidism.

TREATMENT

- **Acute moderate hypophosphatemia** (1.0 to 2.5 mg/dL) is common in the hospitalized patient and is often due simply to **transcellular shifts,** requiring no treatment if asymptomatic except correction of the underlying cause.
- **Acute severe hypophosphatemia** (<1.0 mg/dL) may require IV phosphate therapy when associated with serious clinical manifestations.

Medications

- IV preparations include potassium phosphate (1.5 mEq potassium/mmol phosphate) and sodium phosphate (1.3 mEq sodium/mmol phosphate).
  - An infusion of phosphate, 0.08 to 0.16 mmol/kg in 500 mL of 0.45% saline, is given intravenously over 6 hours (1 mmol phosphate = 31 mg phosphorus). IV repletion should be stopped when the serum phosphorus level is >1.5 mg/dL and when oral therapy (see below) is possible. Because of the need to replenish intracellular stores, 24 to 36 hours of phosphate administration may be required.
  - Extreme care must be used to avoid hyperphosphatemia, which may lead to hypocalcemia. If hypotension occurs, acute hypocalcemia should be suspected and the infusion should be stopped or slowed. Further doses should be based on symptoms and on the serum calcium and phosphorus levels, which should be measured every 8 hours.
- **Chronic hypophosphatemia.** Vitamin D deficiency, if present, should be treated first (see Calcium, Hypocalcemia, Treatment) followed by oral supplementation of 0.5 to 1.0 g elemental phosphorus PO bid–tid. Preparations include Neutra-Phos (250 mg elemental phosphorus and 7 mEq of Na⁺ and K⁺ per capsule) and Neutra-Phos K (250 mg elemental phosphorus and 14 mEq K⁺ per capsule). Contents of the capsules should be dissolved in water. Fleet Phospho-soda (815 mg phosphorus and 33 mEq sodium per 5 mL) is an alternative oral agent. Limiting side effects include nausea and diarrhea.

DISORDERS OF MAGNESIUM BALANCE

Magnesium Homeostasis

GENERAL PRINCIPLES

- **Magnesium** plays an important role in neuromuscular function.
- Approximately 60% of body magnesium is stored in bone, and most of the remainder is found in cells. Only 1% is in the ECF. As a result, the serum magnesium is a poor predictor of intracellular and total body stores and may grossly underestimate total magnesium deficits.
- The main determinant of magnesium balance is the **magnesium concentration** itself, which directly influences renal excretion. Hypomagnesemia stimulates tubular reabsorption of magnesium, whereas hypermagnesemia inhibits this.

Hypermagnesemia

GENERAL PRINCIPLES

Definition
A serum magnesium > **2.2 mEq/L** defines hypermagnesemia.

Etiology
- Most cases of clinically significant hypermagnesemia are **iatrogenic,** occurring with large doses of magnesium-containing antacids or laxatives and during treatment of preeclampsia with IV magnesium. Since renal excretion is the only means of lowering serum magnesium levels, the presence of significant renal insufficiency can lead to magnesium toxicity with even therapeutic doses of these antacids and laxatives.
- Mild, insignificant elevations in magnesium can occur in end-stage renal disease patients, theophylline intoxication, DKA, and the tumor lysis syndrome.

DIAGNOSIS

Clinical Presentation
- Signs and symptoms are seen only if the serum magnesium level is >4 mEq/L.
- Neuromuscular abnormalities usually include hyporeflexia (usually the first sign of magnesium toxicity), lethargy, and weakness that can progress to somnolence and paralysis. With diaphragmatic involvement, this can lead to respiratory failure.
- Cardiac findings include hypotension, bradycardia, and cardiac arrest.

Diagnostic Testing
Laboratories
Hypocalcemia may be seen with hypermagnesemia due to diminished PTH release.

Electrocardiography
The **ECG** may reveal bradycardia and prolonged PR, QRS, and QT intervals with magnesium levels of 5 to 10 mEq/L. Complete heart block or asystole may eventually ensue with levels > 15 mEq/L.

TREATMENT

- **Prevention.** In the setting of significant renal insufficiency, the inadvertent administration of magnesium-containing medications (e.g., Maalox, magnesium citrate) should be avoided.
- **Asymptomatic hypermagnesemia.** In the setting of normal renal function, normal magnesium levels will be quickly attained with removal of the magnesium load.
- **Symptomatic hypermagnesemia**
  - Prompt supportive therapy is critical, including mechanical ventilation for respiratory failure and a temporary pacemaker for significant bradyarrhythmias.
  - The effects of hypermagnesemia can be antagonized quickly by the administration of 10% calcium gluconate, 10 to 20 mL IV (1 to 2 g) over 10 minutes.
  - Renal excretion can be encouraged with saline administration.
  - With significant renal insufficiency, hemodialysis is required for definitive therapy.

Hypomagnesemia

GENERAL PRINCIPLES

Definition

A serum magnesium < **1.3 mEq/L** defines hypomagnesemia.

Etiology

- Hypomagnesemia is most commonly caused by impaired intestinal absorption and increased renal excretion.
  - **Decreased intestinal absorption** occurs in malnutrition, as is common in chronic alcoholics or any malabsorption syndrome. Magnesium can also be lost through prolonged diarrhea and nasogastric aspiration.
  - **Increased renal excretion** of magnesium can occur from increased renal tubular flow (as occurs with osmotic diuresis) as well as impaired tubular function (as seen with resolving Acute Tubular Necrosis (ATN), loop diuretics, and Bartter's and Gitelman's syndromes).
- **Drugs.** Several medications similarly induce defects in tubular magnesium transport including aminoglycosides, amphotericin B, cisplatin, pentamidine, and cyclosporine.

DIAGNOSIS

Clinical Presentation

- Neurologic manifestations include lethargy, confusion, tremor, fasciculation, ataxia, nystagmus, tetany, and seizures.
- Atrial and ventricular arrhythmias may occur, especially in patients treated with digoxin.

Diagnostic Testing

Laboratories
- Low serum [Mg] in conjunction with an appropriate clinical scenario is sufficient to establish the diagnosis of **magnesium deficiency.** However, due to the slow exchange of magnesium between the bone and intracellular pools (see Magnesium, General Principles), a normal serum level does not exclude total body **magnesium deficiency.**
- The etiology of hypomagnesemia is usually evident from the clinical context, but if there is uncertainty, measurement of **urine magnesium excretion** is helpful. A 24-hour urine magnesium of >2 mEq (or >24 mg) or a fractional excretion of magnesium of >2% during hypomagnesemia suggests **increased renal excretion.** The fractional excretion of magnesium is calculated by

$$(Urine\ Mg/Urine\ Cr) \div \{(Serum\ Mg \times 0.7)/Serum\ Cr\} \times 100$$

- Hypocalcemia (see Calcium, Hypocalcemia, General Principles, Etiology) and/or hypokalemia (see Potassium, Hypokalemia, General Principles, Etiology) can often be found as a result of hypomagnesemia-induced derangements in mineral homeostasis.
- **ECG** abnormalities may include a prolonged PR and QT interval with a widened QRS. **Torsades de pointes** is the classically associated arrhythmia.

TREATMENT

In patients with normal renal function, excess magnesium is readily excreted, and there is little risk of causing hypermagnesemia with recommended doses. However, *magnesium must be given with extreme care in the presence of renal insufficiency.*

Medications

The route of administration depends on whether clinical manifestations from magnesium deficiency are present.

- **Asymptomatic hypomagnesemia** can be treated orally. Numerous preparations exist, including Mag-Ox 400 (240-mg elemental magnesium per 400-mg tablet), Uro-Mag (84 mg per 140-mg tablet), and sustained-release Slow-Mag (64 mg per tablet). Typically, ~240 mg of elemental magnesium is administered daily for mild deficiency, while more severe hypomagnesemia may require up to 720 mg/d of elemental magnesium. The major side effect is diarrhea. Normalization of serum magnesium levels can be deceiving, since the administered magnesium slowly shifts to replete intracellular and bone stores. Furthermore, abrupt increases in serum levels stimulate renal excretion. Thus, serum levels should be followed closely and replacement should be maintained until patients demonstrate stable normalization of serum magnesium concentrations.
- **Severe symptomatic hypomagnesemia** should be treated with 1 to 2 g magnesium sulfate (1 g magnesium sulfate = 96 mg elemental magnesium) IV over 15 minutes. Again, to account for gradual redistribution to severely depleted intracellular stores, replacement therapy may need to be maintained, often for 3 to 7 days. Serum magnesium should be measured q24h and the infusion rate adjusted to maintain a serum magnesium level of <2.5 mEq/L. Tendon reflexes should be tested frequently, as hyporeflexia suggests hypermagnesemia. Reduced doses and more frequent monitoring must be used even in mild renal insufficiency.

ACID–BASE DISTURBANCES

Acid–Base Homeostasis

GENERAL PRINCIPLES

- The normal ECF **pH is 7.40 ± 0.03.** Perturbations in pH can occur with changes in the ratio of $[HCO_3^-]$ to pCO_2 as described by the **Henderson–Hasselbalch equation:**

$$pH = 6.1 + \log\{[HCO_3^-] \div (pCO_2 \times 0.3)\}$$

- Maintenance of pH is essential for normal cellular function. Three general mechanisms exist to keep it within a narrow window:
  - **Chemical buffering** is mediated by HCO_3^- in the ECF and by protein and phosphate buffers in the ICF. The normal $[HCO_3^-]$ is 24 ± 2 mEq/L.
  - **Alveolar ventilation** minimizes variations in the pH by altering the partial pressure of carbon dioxide (pCO_2). The normal pCO_2 is 40 ± 5 mm Hg.
  - **Renal H^+ handling** allows the kidney to adapt to changes in acid–base status via HCO_3^- reabsorption and excretion of titratable acid (e.g., $H_2PO_4^-$) and NH_4^+.

Definition

Acidemia and **alkalemia** refer to processes that lower and raise pH regardless of mechanism. They can be caused by metabolic or respiratory disturbances:

- **Metabolic acidosis** is characterized by a decrease in the plasma $[HCO_3{}^-]$ due to either $HCO_3{}^-$ loss or the accumulation of acid.
- **Metabolic alkalosis** is characterized by an elevation in the plasma $[HCO_3{}^-]$ due to either H^+ loss or $HCO_3{}^-$ gain.
- **Respiratory acidosis** is characterized by an elevation in pCO_2 resulting from alveolar hypoventilation.
- **Respiratory alkalosis** is characterized by a decrease in pCO_2 resulting from hyperventilation.

DIAGNOSIS

Differential Diagnosis

Analysis should be systematic so that accurate conclusions are drawn and appropriate therapy initiated. Once the acid–base process is correctly identified, further diagnostic studies may be undertaken to determine the precise etiologies at play. The systematic approach to acid–base conditions follows five steps: checking an ABG, establishing a primary disorder, assessing compensation, calculating an anion gap (AG), and evaluating the delta gap.

- **Step 1.** Check an arterial blood gas (ABG). Acidemia is present when pH is <7.37 and alkalemia when pH is >7.43.
- **Step 2.** Establish the primary disturbance by determining whether the change in $[HCO_3{}^-]$ or pCO_2 can account for the observed deflection in pH. In alkalemia, an elevated $[HCO_3{}^-]$ suggests metabolic alkalosis while a decreased pCO_2 suggests respiratory alkalosis. In academia, a decreased $[HCO_3{}^-]$ suggests metabolic acidosis and an elevated pCO_2 suggests respiratory acidosis.
  - A **combined disorder** is present when:
    - pH is normal but the pCO_2 and $[HCO_3{}^-]$ are both abnormal
    - Changes in both pCO_2 and $[HCO_3{}^-]$ can cause the change in pH
- **Step 3.** Determine whether compensation is appropriate. The **compensatory mechanism** is an adaptation to the primary acid–base disturbance intended to stabilize the changing pH. A respiratory process that shifts the pH in one direction will be compensated by a metabolic process that shifts the pH in the other, and vice versa.
  - The effect of compensation is to attenuate, but not completely correct, the primary change in pH.
  - The expected compensations for the various primary acid–base derangements are given in Table 3.
  - An inappropriate compensatory response suggests the presence of a combined disorder.
  - **Example:** In a patient with metabolic acidosis, respiratory compensation attenuates the metabolic disturbance to pH by lowering pCO_2. However, if the pCO_2 is higher than expected, respiratory compensation is insufficient, revealing a respiratory acidosis with the primary metabolic acidosis. If pCO_2 is lower than expected, compensation is excessive, revealing a concomitant respiratory alkalosis.

Table 3		Expected Compensatory Responses to Primary Acid–Base Disorders
Disorder	**Primary Change**	**Compensatory Response**
Metabolic acidosis	↓ [HCO$_3^-$]	↓ pCO$_2$ 1.2 mm Hg for every 1 mEq/L ↓ [HCO$_3^-$] OR pCO$_2$ = last two digits of pH
Metabolic alkalosis	↑ [HCO$_3^-$]	↑ pCO$_2$ 0.7 mm Hg for every 1 mEq/L ↑ [HCO$_3^-$]
Respiratory acidosis	↑ pCO$_2$	
Acute		↑ [HCO$_3^-$] 1.0 mEq/L for every 10 mm Hg ↑ pCO$_2$
Chronic		↑ [HCO$_3^-$] 3.5 mEq/L for every 10 mm Hg ↑ pCO$_2$
Respiratory alkalosis	↓ pCO$_2$	
Acute		↓ [HCO$_3^-$] 2.0 mEq/L for every 10 mm Hg ↓ pCO$_2$
Chronic		↓ [HCO$_3^-$] 5.0 mEq/L for every 10 mm Hg ↓ pCO$_2$

- **Step 4.** Determine the **AG.** What is an AG? In normal individuals, the total serum cations are balanced with the total serum anions. Total cations are comprised of measured cations (MC) and unmeasured cations (UC), while total anions are comprised of measured anions (MA) and unmeasured anions (UA). Certain forms of acidosis are characterized by an increase in the pool of UA. The AG is merely a way of demonstrating the accumulation of this unmeasured anion.
- $AG = [Na^+] - ([Cl^-] + [HCO_3^-])$. The normal AG is 10 ± 2 mEq/L.
- How did we get this equation?:

$$AG = \text{the excess of UA (vs. UC)}$$
$$= UA - UC$$

Since total cations = total anions:

$$MC + UC = MA + UA$$

Rearranging the equation:

$$UA - UC = MC - MA$$

MC are Na^+; MA are Cl^- and HCO_3^-

Since albumin is the principal unmeasured anion, the AG should be corrected if there are gross changes in serum albumin levels:

$$\textbf{AG}_{\textbf{correct}} = \textbf{AG} + \{(4 - [\textbf{albumin}]) \times \textbf{2.5}\}$$

- An elevated AG suggests the presence of metabolic acidosis with a circulating anion (see Table 2).
- **Step 5.** Assess the delta gap. To maintain a stable total anion content, every increase in an unmeasured anion should be met with a decrease in [HCO$_3^-$]. Comparing the change in the AG (ΔAG) with the change in the [HCO$_3^-$] (Δ[HCO$_3$]) is a simple way of making sure that each change in the AG is accounted for.

- If the $\Delta AG = \Delta[HCO_3]$, this is a simple AG metabolic acidosis.
- If the $\Delta AG > \Delta[HCO_3]$
  - The $[HCO_3^-]$ did not decrease as much as expected.
  - This is a metabolic alkalosis **and** AG metabolic acidosis.
  - **Example:** A patient with DKA has been vomiting prior to admit. He has an AG of 20 and a $[HCO_3]$ of 18. His $\Delta AG = 10$ and $\Delta[HCO_3] = 6$, reveal an AG metabolic acidosis (DKA) with a metabolic alkalosis (vomiting).
  - If the $\Delta AG < \Delta[HCO_3]$, the $[HCO_3]$ decreases more than expected.
  - This is a nongap metabolic acidosis **and** AG metabolic acidosis.
  - **Example:** A patient is admitted with fever and hypotension after a prolonged course of diarrhea. She has an AG of 15 and a $[HCO_3]$ of 12. Her ΔAG is 5 and her $\Delta[HCO_3]$ is 12, revealing a nongap metabolic acidosis (diarrhea) and an AG metabolic acidosis (lactic acidosis).

Metabolic Acidosis

GENERAL PRINCIPLES

Etiology

- The causes of a metabolic acidosis can be divided into those that cause an **elevated anion gap** and those with a **normal anion gap.** Many of the causes seen in clinical practice can be found in Table 4.

Table 4	The Four Primary Acid–Base Disorders and Their Common Etiologies			
	Acidosis			**Alkalosis**
Metabolic	Gap: • Ketoacids (starvation, alcoholic, diabetic) • Exposures (methanol, ethylene glycol, salicylates) • Lactic acid (shock, drug related) • Profound uremia			Generation: • Loss of H^+-rich fluids (GI loss) • Contraction alkalosis • Alkali administration
	Nongap: • Nonrenal HCO_3^- loss (diarrhea) • Renal HCO_3^- loss/RTA2 • ↓ H+ secretion/RTA1 • Hypoaldosterone related/RTA4			Maintenance: • Volume contraction • Chloride depletion • Hypokalemia
		RTA1	**RTA2**	**RTA4**	
	Serum $[K^+]$	↓ or nl	↓ or nl	↑	
	Serum $[HCO_3]$	<10	15–20	>15	
	U pH	>5.3	Varies	<5.3	
Respira-tory	Depression of respiratory Center Neuromuscular failure Lung disease			CNS stimulation Hypoxemia Anxiety

- Anion gap acidosis results from exposure to acids, which contribute an unmeasured anion to the ECF. Common causes are diabetic ketoacidosis, lactic acidosis, and toxic alcohol ingestions.
- Nonanion gap acidosis can result from the loss of $[HCO_3]$ from the GI tract. Enteric $[HCO_3]$ loss occurs most commonly in the setting of severe diarrhea. Renal causes due to renal excretion of $[HCO_3]$ or disorders of renal acid handling are referred to collectively as **renal tubular acidoses (RTAs).**
- The three forms of RTA correlate with the three mechanisms that facilitate renal acid handling: proximal bicarbonate reabsorption, distal H^+ secretion, and generation of NH_3, the principal urinary buffer. Urinary buffers reduce the concentration of free H^+ in the filtrate, thus attenuating the backleak of H^+, which occurs at low urinary pH.
  - **Proximal (type 2) RTA** is caused by impaired proximal tubular HCO_3^- reabsorption. Causes include inherited disorders (Wilson's disease), toxins (heavy metals, ifosfamide), multiple myeloma, autoimmune diseases (Sjögren's syndrome), and acetazolamide use.
  - **Distal (type 1) RTA** results from impaired distal H^+ secretion. This may occur due to an impairment in H^+ secretion, as seen with a variety of autoimmune (Sjögren's syndrome, lupus, rheumatoid arthritis) or renal disorders. It can also be caused by a backleak of H^+ due to increased membrane permeability, as seen with amphotericin B.
  - **Distal Hyperkalemic (type 4) RTA** may result from either low aldosterone levels or from aldosterone resistance. The resulting hyperkalemia reduces the availability of NH_3 to buffer urinary H^+. Hyporeninemic hypoaldosteronism is seen with some frequency in patients with diabetes. Certain drugs including NSAIDs, β-blockers, and cyclosporine have also been implicated.
- Occasionally, the kidney is unable to secrete sufficient H^+ due to an impaired luminal gradient. In these situations, poor filtrate delivery or impaired Na reabsorption in the distal nephron are responsible for decreasing the voltage gradient, which augments H^+ secretion. This can be seen with marked volume depletion, urinary tract obstruction, sickle cell nephropathy, and amiloride or triamterene use.

DIAGNOSIS

Diagnostic Testing

Laboratories

- The first step in narrowing the differential diagnosis for a metabolic acidosis is to calculate the **AG.**
  - The specific cause of an **elevated AG** can usually be determined by clinical history. However, specific laboratory studies are available to identify certain anions such as lactate, acetoacetate, acetone, and β-hydroxybutyrate. (It should be noted that the use of nitroprusside to detect ketones may fail to identify ketoacidosis due to β-hydroxybutyrate.) The presence of an alcohol (methanol, ethanol, ethylene glycol) can also be determined with laboratory assays. Clinical suspicion for toxic alcohol ingestion is corroborated by an increased **osmolal gap.** This gap is the difference between measured and calculated serum osmolality:

$$[Osm]_{meas} - \{([Na^+] \times 2) + ([glucose] \div 18) + ([BUN] \div 2.8)\}$$

- If a **normal anion gap** is present, the GI HCO_3^- losses can be differentiated from RTAs via the **urine anion gap** (UAG).

- The **UAG** is the difference between the major measured anions and cations in urine: $[Na^+]_u + [K^+]_u - [Cl^-]_u$. Because NH_4^+ is the major unmeasured urinary cation, a negative UAG reflects high NH_4^+ excretion, an appropriate response to a metabolic acidosis. Conversely, a positive UAG signifies low NH_4^+ excretion, which, in the face of a metabolic acidosis, suggests a renal tubular defect.
- Serum $[K^+]$ and urine pH can be helpful in distinguishing between the RTAs.
  - Types 1 and 2 are typically associated with hypokalemia, while type 4 is characterized by hyperkalemia.
  - Urine pH is low (usually <5.3) in type 4 RTA since the mechanism for H^+ secretion is intact (recall that the defect is in the generation of the NH_3 buffer). In contrast, urine pH is inappropriately high in type 1 RTA (urine pH > 5.3). In type 2 RTA, the urine pH is variable. It is elevated during the initial bicarbonaturia, when filtered bicarbonate exceeds the threshold for reabsorption, and low when the filtered load is below this threshold.

TREATMENT

- **Ketoacidosis** attributable to ethanol abuse and starvation can be corrected with the resumption of caloric intake through PO intake or dextrose-containing fluids, and by correction of any volume depletion that may be present. The treatment of *diabetic* ketoacidosis is described in Chapter 20, Diabetes Mellitus and Related Disorders.
- **Lactic acidosis** will resolve once the underlying cause is treated and tissue perfusion is restored. Often this involves aggressive therapeutic maneuvers for the treatment of shock as described in Chapter 6, Critical Care. The administration of alkali does not appear to have clear benefit in lactic acidosis, and it may lead to a rebound metabolic alkalosis once the underlying cause is managed. Its use in dire circumstances or severe acidosis remains controversial.
- Management of toxic ingestions is described in Chapter 24, Medical Emergencies.
- **Normal AG metabolic acidosis.** Treatment with $NaHCO_3$ is appropriate for patients with a normal AG metabolic acidosis. The HCO_3^- deficit can be calculated in mEq:

$$HCO_3 \text{ deficit} = (0.5 \times \text{Lean Wt} \times [24 - (HCO_3^-)])$$

However, this assumes a volume of distribution equal to 50% of total body weight. In reality, the distribution of HCO_3 increases with the severity of the acidosis and may exceed 100% of total body weight in very severe acidosis. It should be noted that the standard 650-mg tablet of oral $NaHCO_3$ provides only 7 mEq of HCO_3^-, while one ampule of IV $NaHCO_3$ contains 50 mEq. Still, parenteral $NaHCO_3$ should always be prescribed with caution because of the potential adverse effects, including pulmonary edema, hypokalemia, and hypocalcemia.
- **Treatment of the RTAs.** Correction of the chronic acidemia with alkali administration is warranted to prevent its catabolic effect on bone and muscle.
  - In *Distal (type 1) RTA* correction of the metabolic acidosis requires oral HCO_3^- replacement on the order of 1 to 2 mEq/kg/d with $NaHCO_3$ or sodium citrate. Potassium citrate replacement may be necessary for patients with hypokalemia, nephrolithiasis, or nephrocalcinosis. Underlying conditions should be sought and treated.
  - In *Proximal (type 2) RTA* much larger amounts of alkali (10 to 15 mEq/kg/d) are required to reverse the acidosis. Administration of potassium salts minimizes the degree of hypokalemia associated with alkali therapy.

- Management of *Type 4 RTA* requires correction of the underlying hyperkalemia. This consists of dietary K^+ restriction (40 to 60 mEq/d) and possibly a loop diuretic with or without oral $NaHCO_3$ (0.5 to 1 mEq/kg/d). Chronic sodium polystyrene sulfonate therapy may also be necessary. Mineralocorticoid administration (fludrocortisone, 50 to 200 mcg PO daily) should be used in patients with primary adrenal insufficiency and may be considered in other causes of hypoaldosteronism.

Metabolic Alkalosis

GENERAL PRINCIPLES

Etiology

- Development of a persistent metabolic alkalosis requires both generation (an inciting cause) and maintenance (a persistent impairment of the corrective renal response).
- Generation often occurs with a primary increase in the plasma $[HCO_3^-]$ and may be due to either **HCO_3^- gain** from alkali administration or, more commonly, **excessive H^+ loss.** The latter results may result from the loss of H^+-rich fluids, including upper GI secretions. **Contraction alkalosis** refers to the contraction of volume around a fixed content of bicarbonate.
- Maintenance requires a concomitant impairment in renal HCO_3^- excretion, since the kidney normally has a large capacity to excrete HCO_3^-. This occurs as a result of a **decreased GFR** (glomerular filtration rate) or enhanced tubular HCO_3^- reabsorption from **chloride depletion, volume contraction,** and **hypokalemia.**
  - A decrease in filtered chloride is sensed by the macula densa and, as a result of tubuloglomerular feedback, reduces filtered HCO_3 and stimulates aldosterone release. It also limits adaptive distal HCO_3 secretion. Metabolic alkalosis is often described as being **chloride responsive** or **chloride unresponsive.**

DIAGNOSIS

Clinical Presentation

As key causes of metabolic alkalosis are related to volume contraction (vomiting and diuretic use), patients may present with signs of volume depletion. Occasionally, patients demonstrate hypertension or mild ECF expansion as a result of mineralocorticoid excess.

History

Discovery of the specific cause of metabolic alkalosis is often obvious from the history. Common causes include loss of upper GI secretions through vomiting, or excessive urinary H^+ loss from diuretics.

Diagnostic Testing

Laboratories

- Urine electrolytes are generally useful in identifying the etiology of a metabolic alkalosis when the history and physical are unrevealing.
  - A **urine $[Cl^-]$** < 20 mEq/L is consistent with **chloride-responsive** metabolic alkalosis and usually indicates volume depletion. A urine $[Cl^-]$ > 20 mEq/L indicates a chloride-unresponsive cause (see Table 4).

- Urine $[Na^+]$ is not reliable in predicting the effective circulating volume in these conditions, since bicarbonaturia obligates renal Na^+ loss even in volume depletion.
- **Serum potassium** levels are often low in metabolic alkalosis. Hypokalemia contributes to alkalosis by increasing tubular H^+ secretion and Cl^- wasting. Hypokalemia is also a result of alkalosis due to transcellular shifts.

TREATMENT

- **Chloride-responsive** metabolic alkaloses are most effectively treated with saline resuscitation until euvolemia is achieved. The increase in filtered chloride leads to improved renal handling of the bicarbonate load.
- **Chloride-unresponsive** metabolic alkaloses do not respond to saline administration and are often associated with a normal or expanded ECF volume.
  - Mineralocorticoid excess can be managed with a K^+-sparing diuretic (amiloride or spironolactone) and repletion of the K^+ deficit.
  - Alkalosis from excessive alkali administration will quickly resolve once the HCO_3^- load is withdrawn, assuming normal renal function.
- The presence of hypokalemia will continue to perpetuate some degree of alkalosis regardless of other interventions. Potassium must, therefore, be repleted in all cases of metabolic alkalosis.
- Acetazolamide may be useful if the alkalosis persists despite the above interventions, or if saline administration is limited by a patient's volume overload. This therapy promotes bicarbonaturia, although renal K^+ loss is enhanced as well. Acetazolamide can be dosed at 250 mg q6h × 4, or with a single dose of 500 mg.
- Severe alkalemia (pH > 7.70) with ECF volume excess and/or renal failure can be treated with isotonic (150 mEq/L) HCl administered via a central vein. The amount of HCl required can be calculated as: $\{(0.5 \times \text{lean weight in kg}) \times ([HCO_3^-] - 24)\}$. Correction should occur over 8 to 24 hours.

Respiratory Acidosis

GENERAL PRINCIPLES

Etiology

The causes of respiratory acidosis can be divided into hypoventilation from (a) **respiratory center depression,** (b) **neuromuscular failure,** (c) **decreased respiratory system compliance,** (d) **increased airway resistance,** and (e) **increased dead space** (see Table 4).

DIAGNOSIS

Clinical Presentation

- Symptoms of respiratory acidosis result from changes in the cerebrospinal fluid (CSF) pH. A very severe hypercapnia may be well tolerated if it is accompanied by renal compensation and a relatively normal pH. Conversely, a modest rise in pCO_2 can be very symptomatic if acute.
- Initial signs and symptoms may include headache and restlessness, which may progress to generalized hyperreflexia/asterixis and coma.

TREATMENT

- Treatment is directed at correcting the underlying disorder and improving ventilation (see Chapter 7, Pulmonary Diseases).
- Administration of $NaHCO_3$ to improve the acidemia may paradoxically worsen the pH in situations of limiting ventilation. The administered HCO_3^- will combine with H^+ in the tissues and form pCO_2 and water. If ventilation is fixed, this extra CO_2 generated cannot be blown off and worsening hypercapnia will result. Therefore, HCO_3^- should, in general, be avoided in *pure* respiratory acidoses.

Respiratory Alkalosis

GENERAL PRINCIPLES

Etiology

Common causes of hyperventilation resulting in respiratory alkalosis are given in Table 4.

DIAGNOSIS

Clinical Presentation

- The rise in CSF pH that occurs with **acute respiratory alkalosis** is associated with a significant reduction in cerebral blood flow that may lead to lightheadedness and impaired consciousness. Generalized membrane excitability can result in seizures and arrhythmias. Symptoms and signs of acute hypocalcemia (see Calcium, Hypocalcemia, Diagnosis, Clinical Presentation) may be evident from the abrupt fall in ionized calcium that can occur.
- **Chronic respiratory alkalosis** is usually asymptomatic since a normal pH is well defended by compensation.

Diagnostic Testing

Laboratories

The rise in pH from **acute respiratory alkalosis** can cause a reduced ionized calcium (see Calcium, Hypocalcemia, General Principles, Etiology), a profound hypophosphatemia (see Phosphorus, Hypophosphatemia, General Principles, Etiology), and hypokalemia (see Potassium, Hypokalemia, General Principles, Etiology).

TREATMENT

- Treatment of respiratory alkalosis should focus on identifying and treating the underlying disease.
- In ICU patients, this may involve changing the ventilator settings to decrease ventilation (see Chapter 6, Critical Care).

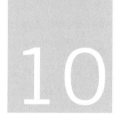

Renal Diseases

Seth Goldberg and Daniel Coyne

Evaluation of the Patient with Renal Disease

DIAGNOSIS

Clinical Presentation

- Renal disease is often asymptomatic or presents with nonspecific complaints. Its presence is frequently first noted on abnormal routine laboratory data, generally as an elevated serum creatinine (Cr) level. An abnormal urinalysis or sediment, with proteinuria, hematuria, or pyuria, may also indicate renal disease.
- When the decline in renal function is acute or advanced, a variety of nonspecific symptoms may be present. Generalized malaise, worsening hypertension, dependent or generalized edema, or decreasing urine output may accompany more severe renal insufficiency.
- The focus of the initial evaluation of the patient with renal disease is to determine the need for emergent dialysis. Then, investigations to identify the etiology are undertaken, while differentiating components of acute and chronic disease.

Diagnostic Testing

Laboratories

- **Serum chemistries**
  - A basic evaluation includes electrolytes (with calcium and phosphorus), Cr, blood urea nitrogen (BUN), and albumin. When stable, the creatinine is a serviceable marker of the glomerular filtration rate (GFR), which can be calculated by the Cockcroft–Gault formula for creatinine clearance:

  $$[(140 - age) \times (ideal\ body\ weight\ in\ kg) \times 0.85\ (for\ women)]/[72 \times Cr\ in\ mg/dL]$$

  - However, as creatinine is secreted by the tubules, particularly as renal function worsens, this formula has the tendency to overestimate the GFR.
  - The Modification of Diet in Renal Disease (MDRD) formulas can calculate the GFR and can take into account BUN, albumin, and race in addition to age and gender (http://mdrd.com). When the MDRD GFR is >60 mL/min/1.73 m^2, chronic kidney disease (CKD) should not be diagnosed unless other evidence of renal damage (e.g., proteinuria) is present.
    - When a glomerular process is suspected, it may be useful to check the erythrocyte sedimentation rate (ESR), antinuclear antibodies (ANA), antiglomerular basement membrane (anti-GBM) antibodies, anti-neutrophil cytoplasmic antibodies (ANCA), complement levels (C3, C4), cryoglobulins, antistreptolysin-O (ASO) titers, and viral (HIV, hepatitis B and C) serologies. A serum protein electrophoresis (SPEP) can be performed in proteinuric patients to evaluate for monoclonal gammopathy, and may be suspected by a large protein–albumin gap.
- **Urine studies**
  - Routine urine studies include a urine dipstick (for protein, blood, glucose, leukocyte esterase, nitrites, pH, and specific gravity) as well as a freshly voided specimen

for microscopic examination (for cells, casts, and crystals). The urine sample is centrifuged at 2,100 rpm for 5 minutes, and then most of the supernatant is poured off. The pellet is resuspended by gently tapping the side of the tube.

- o Proteinuria can be estimated from a spot urine protein-to-creatinine ratio, where the serum creatinine must be stable to ensure a steady state in the urine. A normal ratio is <250 mg of protein per gram of creatinine. A 24-hour urine collection for protein can be obtained when the serum creatinine is not at a stable baseline.
- o Hematuria (>3 red blood cells [RBCs] per high-power field) can represent an infectious, inflammatory, or malignant process anywhere along the urinary tract. Dysmorphic RBCs suggest a glomerular source of bleeding and can be accompanied by RBC casts formed within the tubules. The absence of RBCs in a patient with a positive dipstick for blood suggests hemolysis or rhabdomyolysis (forms of pigment nephropathy).
- o White blood cells (WBCs) in the urine represent an infectious or inflammatory process. This may be seen with a urinary tract infection (UTI), parenchymal infections such as pyelonephritis or abscess, or acute interstitial nephritis (AIN). Urine eosinophils can be identified with the Giemsa stain when evaluating for AIN, atheroembolic disease, or prostatitis.
- Supplemental urine studies can be ordered in specific circumstances. When differentiating between oliguric prerenal azotemia and acute tubular necrosis (ATN), a urine sodium, urea, and creatinine can be obtained with simultaneous serum measurements to calculate the fractional excretions of sodium and urea (see below). Urine sodium, potassium, and chloride can be helpful in evaluating acid–base disturbances while a urine osmolality can be useful in disorders of water handling (hyponatremia and hypernatremia, see Chapter 9, Fluid and Electrolyte Management). A urine protein electrophoresis (UPEP) can help identify dysproteinemic disorders. Routine dipstick is less sensitive to nonalbumin proteins and may not detect heavy and light immunoglobulin chains.

Imaging

- Renal ultrasonography can document the presence of two kidneys, assess size, and identify hydronephrosis or renal cysts. Small kidneys (<9 cm) generally reflect chronic disease, although kidneys may be large in diabetes, HIV, deposition disorders, and polycystic kidney disease. A discrepancy in kidney size of >2 cm suggests unilateral renal artery stenosis with atrophy of the affected kidney. The presence of hydronephrosis suggests obstructive nephropathy. Retroperitoneal fibrosis can encase the ureters and prevent dilation despite the presence of an obstruction.
- Intravenous urography is useful in the evaluation of nonglomerular hematuria, stone disease, and voiding disorders. It should be reserved for patients with normal renal function as the iodinated contrast dye has the potential to adversely affect kidney function.
- Radionuclide scanning uses technetium isotopes to assess the contribution of each kidney to the overall renal function, providing important information if unilateral nephrectomy is being considered for malignancy or living donation. Renal scanning is also useful in transplantation, where renal perfusion and excretion of the tracer can be followed.
- Magnetic resonance imaging (MRI) and magnetic resonance angiography (MRA) can be helpful in evaluating renal masses, detecting renal artery stenosis, and diagnosing renal vein thrombosis. Unlike standard arteriography, MRA does not require the administration of nephrotoxic contrast agents, but does employ gadolinium-based

contrast agents, which are associated with development of nephrogenic fibrosing dermopathy in patients with advanced renal failure or dialysis dependence (*Am J Kidney Dis 2008;51:966*).

- Computed tomography (CT) has less utility in the evaluation of kidney disease as the iodinated contrast dye can be nephrotoxic and cause worsening renal function. However, noncontrast helical CT scanning has become the test of choice in evaluating nephrolithiasis.

Diagnostic Procedures

- Kidney biopsy can determine diagnosis, guide therapy, and provide prognostic information in many settings, particularly in the evaluation of glomerular or deposition diseases. Biopsy of a renal transplant allograft may be necessary to distinguish acute rejection from medication toxicity and other causes of renal dysfunction.
- Biopsy of a native kidney may be indicated in adults with unexplained proteinuria or hematuria. In systemic lupus erythematosus (SLE) with renal involvement, biopsy results may help classify disease and guide therapy. Shrunken fibrotic kidneys are unlikely to yield useful diagnostic information; they also have an increased risk of postprocedural bleeding and biopsy should generally be avoided in these cases.
- Preparative measures for native kidney biopsy include ultrasonography (to document the presence of two kidneys, assess size, and location), urinalysis or urine culture to exclude infection, blood pressure control, and correction of coagulation parameters. If uremic platelet dysfunction is suspected by an elevated bleeding time (>10 minutes) or abnormal platelet function assays, intravenous desmopressin acetate (ddAVP at 0.3 mcg/kg) can be infused 30 minutes prior to biopsy. Aspirin and other antiplatelet agents should be avoided for several days before and immediately after the biopsy. Patients on dialysis should not receive heparin immediately after the biopsy.
- Serial blood counts should be obtained at 6-hour intervals overnight. A hemoglobin drop of approximately 10% is common postprocedurally. Difficulty voiding after the procedure may represent urethral clot obstructing the flow of urine.

Acute Renal Failure

GENERAL PRINCIPLES

Definition

There is no precise definition for acute renal failure (ARF), which may be characterized by an abrupt increase in serum creatinine ≥ 0.3 mg/dL within 48 hours, or a similar increase over a few weeks or months. ARF has multiple etiologies, which are usually revealed by careful history, physical exam, and laboratory testing.

Classification

Renal failure can be classified as oliguric or nonoliguric based on the amount of urine output. Cutoffs of approximately 500 mL/d or 25 mL/hr for 4 hours are frequently used in clinical practice.

Etiology

Etiologies of ARF are classically divided according to the anatomic location of the physiologic defect. Prerenal disease involves a disturbance of renal perfusion, while

Table 1	Causes of Acute Renal Failure

Prerenal
Hypovolemia
Hypotension (including sepsis)
Loss of autoregulation (NSAIDs, RAAS blockers)
Abdominal compartment syndrome
Heart failure
Hepatic cirrhosis

Intrinsic renal
Tubular: ischemic ATN, toxic ATN (contrast, pigment, uric acid)
Vascular: glomerulonephritis, dysproteinemia, thrombotic microangiopathy
   (HUS, TTP), atheroembolic disease
Interstitial: acute interstitial nephritis, pyelonephritis

Postrenal
Urethral obstruction
Ureteral obstruction (bilateral, or unilateral if solitary kidney)

ATN, acute tubular necrosis; HUS, hemolytic–uremic syndrome; NSAIDs, nonsteroidal anti-inflammatory drugs; RAAS, renin–angiotensin–aldosterone system; TTP, thrombotic thrombocytopenic purpura.

postrenal disease involves obstruction of the urinary collecting system. Intrinsic renal disease involves the glomeruli, microvasculature, tubules, or interstitium of the kidneys. Table 1 lists some of the common causes of ARF.

DIAGNOSIS

- Uncovering the cause of ARF requires careful attention to the events preceding the rise in creatinine. In the hospitalized patient, blood pressure patterns, hydration status, medications, and radiocontrast use must be investigated. Antibiotic dose and duration as well as PRN medications should not be overlooked.
- Evidence of ongoing hypovolemia or hypoperfusion is suggestive of prerenal disease. Most causes of postrenal disease are identified on ultrasound by dilation of the collecting system or by massive urine output on placement of a bladder catheter. When promptly corrected, prerenal and postrenal disorders can show a rapid decrease in the serum creatinine and failure of this to occur can suggest an alternative diagnosis.
- Urinary casts point toward an intrinsic cause of ARF. Granular casts suggest ATN, WBC casts suggest an inflammatory or infectious interstitial process, and RBC casts strongly suggest glomerular disease.
- Various laboratory parameters can be used to differentiate prerenal states from ATN and are summarized in Table 2. The basis for these tests is to evaluate tubular integrity, which is preserved in prerenal disease and lost in ATN. In states of hypoperfusion, the kidney avidly reabsorbs sodium, resulting in a low fractional excretion (FE_{Na}): $FE_{Na} = [(U_{Na} \times P_{Cr})/(P_{Na} \times U_{Cr})] \times 100$, where U is urine and P is plasma.
  - A value $< 1\%$ suggests renal hypoperfusion with intact tubular function. Loop diuretics and metabolic alkalosis can induce natriuresis, which may falsely increase the FE_{Na}. The fractional excretion of urea (FE_{Urea}) can instead be calculated in these settings, where a value of $<35\%$ suggests a prerenal process.

Table 2			Laboratory Findings in Oliguric Acute Renal Failure			
Diagnosis	BUN:Cr	FE_{Na} (%)	Urine osmolality (mOsm/kg)	Urine Na	Urine SG	Sediment
Prerenal azotemia	>20:1	<1%	>500	<20	>1.020	Bland
Oliguric ATN	<20:1	>1%	<350	>40	Variable	Granular casts

ATN, acute tubular necrosis; BUN, blood urea nitrogen; Cr, creatinine; FE_{Na}, fractional excretion of sodium; SG, specific gravity.

- Contrast and pigment nephropathy can result in a low FE_{Na}, as can glomerular diseases due to intact tubular function. The FE_{Na} also has limited utility when ARF is superimposed on CKD.
- With hypoperfusion, the urine is typically concentrated, containing an osmolality > 500 mOsm/kg and a high specific gravity (>1.020). In ATN, concentrating ability is lost and the urine is usually isosmolar to the serum. In the blood, the ratio of BUN to creatinine is normally <20:1 and an elevation is consistent with hypovolemia.

Differential Diagnosis
Identifying whether the defect is prerenal, postrenal, or intrinsic to the kidney is useful in arriving at the diagnosis.

- **Prerenal**
  - The term prerenal azotemia implies preserved intrinsic renal function in the setting of renal hypoperfusion and reduced GFR. The effective circulating volume is decreased, resulting from intravascular volume depletion, low cardiac output, or disordered vasodilation (hepatic cirrhosis).
  - When the cause is true volume depletion, presentation involves a history or excessive fluid loss, reduced intake, or orthostatic symptoms. The physical exam may reveal dry mucous membranes, poor skin turgor, and orthostatic vital signs (drop in blood pressure by at least 20/10 mm Hg or an increase in heart rate by 10 beats per minute after standing from a seated position). The central venous pressure is typically < 8 cm H_2O.
  - Low cardiac output causes prerenal azotemia via a drop in the effective circulating volume, despite total body volume overload. In heart failure, diuresis may paradoxically improve the prerenal azotemia by unloading the ventricles and improving cardiac function (see Chapter 4, Heart Failure, Cardiomyopathy, and Valvular Heart Disease).
  - Hepatic failure leads to splanchnic vasodilation and venous pooling, which diminishes the effective circulating volume despite total body volume overload. This can progress to the hepatorenal syndrome (HRS), which is characterized by a rising creatinine in the setting of low systolic blood pressures (90 to 100 mm Hg), mild to moderate hyponatremia (120 to 130 mEq/L), and very low urine sodium excretion (<10 mEq/L). Spontaneous bacterial peritonitis, overdiuresis, gastrointestinal bleeding, or large-volume paracentesis can precipitate HRS in a cirrhotic patient. Management of the renal disease is supportive and if definitive treatment of the liver

disorder (either through recovery or via transplantation) can occur, renal recovery is common. Temporizing measures include treatment of the underlying precipitating factor (e.g., peritonitis, gastrointestinal bleeding) and withholding diuretics. Dialytic support can be used as a bridge to transplantation in appropriate candidates. Additional treatment options are discussed further in Chapter 16, Liver Diseases.

- In the volume-depleted patient, certain medications can block the ability of the kidney to autoregulate blood flow and GFR. Nonsteroidal anti-inflammatory drugs (NSAIDs) inhibit the counterbalancing vasodilatory effects of prostaglandins and can induce ARF in volume-depleted patients. Angiotensin-converting enzyme (ACE) inhibitors and angiotensin receptor blockers (ARBs) can cause efferent arteriolar vasodilation and a drop in the GFR.
- Abdominal compartment syndrome, from intestinal ischemia, obstruction, or massive ascites, can compromise flow through the renal vasculature via increased intra-abdominal pressure (IAP). An IAP > 20 mm Hg, measured via a pressure transducer attached to the bladder catheter, suggests the diagnosis.

- **Postrenal**
  - Postrenal failure occurs when the flow of urine is obstructed anywhere within the urinary collecting system. Common causes include prostatic enlargement, bilateral kidney stones, or malignancy. The increased intratubular hydrostatic pressure leads to the diminished GFR. Bilateral involvement (or unilateral obstruction to a solitary kidney) is required to produce a significant change in the creatinine level. When the diagnosis is suspected, a renal ultrasound should be performed early to evaluate for hydronephrosis. However, hydronephrosis may be less pronounced when there is concomitant volume depletion or if retroperitoneal fibrosis has encased the ureters, preventing their expansion.
  - Treatment depends on the level of obstruction. When urethral flow is impeded (usually by prostatic enlargement in men), placement of a bladder catheter can be both diagnostic and therapeutic; a postvoid residual urine volume >300 mL strongly suggests the diagnosis. When the upper urinary tract is involved, urologic or radiologic decompression is necessary, with stenting or placement of percutaneous nephrostomy tubes.
  - Relief of bilateral obstruction is frequently followed by a postobstructive diuresis. Serum electrolytes need to be closely monitored if polyuria ensues, and replacement of approximately half of the urinary volume with 0.45% saline is recommended.
  - Crystals may cause micro-obstructive uropathy within the tubules. Intravenous acyclovir and the protease inhibitor indinavir can induce ARF by this mechanism. The urine may show evidence of crystals, although sometimes not until urine flow is reestablished. Treatment is typically supportive after the offending agent is discontinued. As with relief of other forms of obstructive uropathy, a polyuric phase may occur.
- **Intrinsic renal.** Causes of intrinsic renal failure can be divided anatomically into tubular, glomerular/vascular, and interstitial categories. Disease can be primarily renal in nature, or part of a systemic process.
- **Tubular**
  - Ischemic ATN is the most common cause of renal failure in the intensive care setting, and is the end result of any process that leads to significant hypoperfusion of the kidneys, including sepsis, hemorrhage, or any prolonged prerenal insult.
  - The injury results in the sloughing of renal tubular cells, which can congeal with cellular debris in a matrix of Tamm–Horsfall protein to form granular casts. These have a "muddy brown" appearance and are strongly suggestive of ATN in the

proper context. The FE_{Na} (>1%) and FE_{Urea} (>50%) are typically elevated as the tubules lose their ability to concentrate the urine.

- Management of ATN is supportive, with avoidance of further nephrotoxic insults. Fluid management is aimed at maintaining euvolemia. Volume deficits, if present, should be corrected. If volume overload and oliguria become evident, a diuretic challenge is reasonable, typically with intravenous furosemide (40 to 120 mg boluses or a continuous drip at 10 to 20 mg/hr). This has not been shown to hasten recovery but can simplify overall management.

- Recovery from ATN may take days to weeks to occur, but can be expected in over 85% of patients with a previously normal creatinine. Dialysis may be necessary to bridge the time to recovery.

- Toxic ATN can result from endogenous chemicals (e.g., hemoglobin, myoglobin) or exogenous medications (e.g., iodinated contrast, aminoglycosides). These forms share many of the diagnostic features of ischemic ATN.

- Iodinated contrast is a potent renal vasoconstrictor and is toxic to renal tubules. When renal injury occurs, the creatinine typically rises 24 hours after exposure and peaks in 3 to 5 days. Risk factors for contrast nephropathy include CKD, diabetes, volume depletion, heart failure, higher contrast volumes, and use of hyperosmolar contrast. Preventative measures include peri-procedure hydration and discontinuation of diuretics. Sodium bicarbonate at 154 mEq/L (three ampules in D_5W) can be given at 3 mL/kg/hr for 1 hour prior to exposure, then at 1 mL/kg/hr for 6 hours after the procedure (*JAMA 2004;291:2328*). Acetylcysteine may reduce the incidence of contrast nephropathy and is given as four oral doses of 1,200 mg 12 hours apart, with two doses given prior to the contrast study.

- Aminoglycoside nephrotoxicity is typically nonoliguric, occurs from direct toxicity to the proximal tubules, and results in the renal wasting of potassium and magnesium. Replacement of these electrolytes may become necessary. A similar pattern of potassium and magnesium loss is seen in cisplatin toxicity. A prolonged exposure to the aminoglycoside of at least 5 days is required. Peak and trough levels correlate poorly with the risk of developing renal injury. Risk may be minimized by avoiding volume depletion and by using the extended-interval dosing method (see Chapter 12, Antimicrobials).

- Pigment nephropathy results from direct tubular toxicity by hemoglobin and myoglobin. Vasoconstriction may also play a role. The diagnosis may be suspected by a positive urine dipstick test for blood but an absence of RBCs on microscopic examination. In rhabdomyolysis, the creatine phosphokinase (CPK) level is elevated to at least 10 times the upper limit of normal with a disproportionate rise in creatinine, potassium, and phosphorus. Aggressive intravenous fluid administration should be initiated immediately, and large quantities are generally required to replace the fluid lost into necrotic muscle tissue. If urine flow is established, alkalinization with sodium bicarbonate (154 mEq/L, approximately three ampules) can increase the solubility of these pigments and hasten recovery.

- In the treatment of hematologic malignancies, acute uric acid nephropathy can result as part of the tumor lysis syndrome. In addition to the elevated creatinine, there is typically hyperuricemia, hyperphosphatemia, and hypocalcemia. A ratio of urine uric acid to urine creatinine that is >1 is consistent with this diagnosis. Prophylaxis with allopurinol 600 mg can decrease uric acid production. Rasburicase (15 mg/kg intravenously) is highly effective at depleting uric acid levels and can be given as prophylaxis or as treatment. Alkalinization of the urine should be avoided if hyperphosphatemia is present as this could increase the risk of calcium phosphate precipitation in the urine.

- **Glomerular/vascular**
  - The finding of dysmorphic urinary RBCs, RBC casts, or proteinuria in the nephrotic range (>3.5 g/d) strongly suggests the presence of a glomerular disease. This group encompasses a large variety of primary renal or systemic disorders. Glomerular diseases are described individually in further detail later in this chapter.
  - A small subgroup of glomerular diseases can present with rapidly deteriorating renal function, termed rapidly progressive glomerulonephritis (RPGN). A nephritic picture is common, with RBC casts, edema, and hypertension. A renal biopsy may reveal the specific underlying disease, but crescent formation in >50% of glomeruli is usually present. For those deemed to have salvageable renal function, management is with high-dose pulse glucocorticoid therapy (intravenous methylprednisolone 7 to 15 mg/kg/d for 3 days) followed by a course of oral prednisone (1 mg/kg/d for 1 month, then tapered over the next 6 to 12 months). Addition of oral cyclophosphamide at 2 mg/kg/d may be beneficial.
  - Thrombotic microangiopathy (TMA) includes both hemolytic–uremic syndrome (HUS) and thrombotic thrombocytopenic purpura (TTP). These diseases share many of the same characteristics. Causes include bacterial toxins (diarrheal forms) and medications (mitomycin-C, clopidogrel, cyclosporine, tacrolimus), and may be associated with pregnancy or malignancies of the gastrointestinal tract. Diagnosis and therapy are discussed in Chapter 17, Disorders of Hemostasis and Thrombosis.
  - Atheroembolic disease can be seen in patients with diffuse atherosclerosis after undergoing an invasive aortic or other large artery manipulation, including cardiac catheterization, coronary bypass surgery, aortic aneurysm repair, and placement of an intra-aortic balloon pump. Physical findings may include retinal arteriolar plaques, lower extremity livedo reticularis, and areas of digital necrosis. Eosinophilia, eosinophiluria, and hypocomplementemia may be present, and WBC casts may be found in the urine sediment. However, in many cases, the only laboratory abnormality is a rising creatinine that follows a stepwise progression. Renal biopsy shows cholesterol clefts in the small arteries. Anticoagulation may worsen embolic disease and should be avoided if possible. No specific treatment is available. Many patients progress to CKD, and even to end-stage renal disease (ESRD).

- **Interstitial**
  - AIN involves inflammation of the renal parenchyma, typically caused by medications or infections. The classic triad of fever, rash, and eosinophilia is seen in less than one-third of patients. Pyuria, WBC casts, and eosinophiluria are all also suggestive of AIN. Beta-lactam antibiotics are the most frequently cited causative agents, but nearly all antibiotics can be implicated. The time course typically requires exposure for at least 5 to 10 days before renal impairment occurs. Other medications, such as proton pump inhibitors and allopurinol, have been associated with AIN. NSAIDs can produce AIN with nephrotic range proteinuria. Streptococcal infections, leptospirosis, and sarcoidosis have all been implicated in AIN.
  - Treatment is principally the withdrawal of the offending agent. Renal recovery typically ensues, although the time course is variable, and temporary dialytic support

may be necessary in severe cases. A short course of prednisone at 1 mg/kg/d may hasten recovery.

- Parenchymal infections with pyelonephritis or renal abscesses are uncommon causes of ARF. Bilateral involvement is usually necessary to induce a rise in creatinine. Urine findings include pyuria and WBC casts, and antibiotic therapy is guided by culture results.

TREATMENT

- Disease-specific therapies are covered above. With advanced renal failure, general complications can be anticipated and addressed.
- Hyperkalemia, when mild (<6 mEq/L), can be treated with dietary potassium restriction and potassium-binding resins (e.g., sodium polystyrene sulfonate). When further elevated or accompanied by electrocardiogram abnormalities, immediate medical therapy is indicated, with calcium gluconate, insulin and glucose, and bicarbonate (see Chapter 9, Fluid and Electrolyte Management). Severe hyperkalemia that is refractory to medical management is an indication for urgent dialysis.
- Mild metabolic acidosis can be treated with oral sodium bicarbonate, 650 to 1,300 mg thrice daily. Severe acidosis (pH < 7.2) can be temporized with intravenous sodium bicarbonate, but requires monitoring for volume overload, rebound alkalosis, and hypocalcemia. Acidosis that is refractory to medical management is an indication for urgent dialysis.
- Volume overload can complicate ARF. After volume deficits are corrected, the goal of fluid management should be to keep input equal to output. In the oliguric setting, a trial of diuretics (usually high-dose loop diuretics in a bolus or as a continuous drip) may simplify management. Volume overload causing respiratory compromise that is refractory to medical management is an indication for urgent dialysis.
- Anemia is common in ARF and is usually caused by decreased RBC production and increased blood loss. Gastrointestinal bleeding may be exacerbated by uremic platelet dysfunction and may respond to ddAVP 0.3 mcg/kg. Transfusion is appropriate for patients with symptoms attributable to anemia. Erythropoiesis stimulating agents (e.g., epoetin) are not effective for short-term correction of anemia.

SPECIAL CONSIDERATIONS

Dialysis

- All patients with ARF require daily assessment to determine the need for renal replacement therapy. It is preferable to initiate dialytic support before significant uremia develops or a life-threatening complication becomes evident. Patients suffering from oliguric renal failure who are not expected to recover promptly likely benefit from earlier initiation of dialysis.
- Severe acidosis, hyperkalemia, or volume overload refractory to medical management mandates the initiation of dialysis. Certain drug and alcohol intoxications (methanol, ethylene glycol, or salicylates) should be treated with hemodialysis. Uremic pericarditis (with a friction rub) or encephalopathy should also be treated promptly with renal replacement therapy. Issues specific to dialysis techniques are discussed later in this chapter.

Glomerulopathies

GENERAL PRINCIPLES

Classification

- The presentation of glomerular diseases can be thought of as existing on a continuum. On one end is the nephrotic syndrome, characterized by proteinuria >3.5 g/d, and accompanied by hypoalbuminemia, hyperlipidemia, and edema. On the other end of the spectrum is the nephritic syndrome, characterized by hematuria, hypertension, edema, and renal insufficiency. Most specific disease entities present somewhere in between, with overlapping features, but with a tendency to produce one syndrome over the other.
- Biopsy findings also correlate with these syndromes. Nephrotic diseases typically show injury along the filtration barrier, with thickening of the glomerular basement membrane or fusion of the podocyte foot processes. Nephritic diseases generally show varying degrees of mesangial cell proliferation.

TREATMENT

- Specific therapies for individual glomerular diseases are discussed below. However, many disorders share the same features and general therapeutic maneuvers can be addressed as a group.
- Glomerular disease presenting with proteinuria should rely on treatment with ACE inhibitors or ARBs to reduce the intraglomerular pressure. Efficacy can be monitored by serial urine protein-to-creatinine ratios. Electrolytes and creatinine should be checked within 1 to 2 weeks of initiation of therapy or an increase in dose to document stability of renal function and potassium. Modest dietary protein restriction to 0.8 g/kg/d may slow progression, but this remains controversial.
- Edema and volume overload can usually be effectively managed with diuretics combined with salt restriction. Aggressive treatment of hypertension can also slow progression of renal disease.
- The hyperlipidemia associated with the nephrotic syndrome responds to dietary modification and HMG-CoA reductase inhibitors. They are effective at improving the lipoprotein profile and may slow renal decline.
- The nephrotic syndrome produces a hypercoagulable state and can predispose to thromboembolic complications. Deep venous thrombi and renal vein thrombosis may occur and should be treated with heparin anticoagulation followed by long-term warfarin therapy. Prophylactic anticoagulation is controversial and may be beneficial in severely nephrotic patients, particularly with membranous nephropathy (MN).
- When immunosuppression is considered, the risk of therapy should always be weighed against the potential benefit. Renal salvageability should be addressed and patients with advanced disease on presentation who are unlikely to benefit from such treatment may be better served by avoiding the risks of high-dose immunosuppression. Cytotoxic agents (e.g., cyclophosphamide, chlorambucil) require close monitoring of WBC counts, checked at least weekly at the initiation of therapy. Dose adjustments may be needed to maintain the WBC count above 3,000 to 3,500 cells/μL. Rituximab, a monoclonal antibody directed against CD20, has shown promise in a variety of immune-mediated disorders, particularly in severe lupus

nephritis and MN, where it has been given intravenously as four weekly doses of 375 mg/m^2 (*Clin J Am Soc Nephrol 2009;4:579*).

PRIMARY GLOMERULOPATHIES

Minimal Change Disease

GENERAL PRINCIPLES

Epidemiology

Minimal change disease (MCD) is the most common cause of the nephrotic syndrome in children but has a second peak in adults aged 50 to 60. Typically, there is sudden onset of proteinuria with hypertension and edema as well as the full nephrotic syndrome, although renal insufficiency is unusual.

Associated Conditions

Secondary forms of MCD may accompany certain malignancies (Hodgkin disease and solid tumors being the most common). A form of interstitial nephritis associated with NSAID use may also be associated with MCD.

DIAGNOSIS

The kidney biopsy reveals normal glomeruli on light microscopy and negative immunofluorescence. Electron microscopy shows effacement of the foot processes as the only histological abnormality.

TREATMENT

- In adults, treatment with oral prednisone at 1 mg/kg/d may induce remission (decrease in proteinuria) in 8 to 16 weeks. Once in remission, the steroids can be tapered over 3 months then discontinued. The urine protein excretion should be followed during this taper.
- Relapse may occur in up to 75% of adults. Reinstitution of prednisone is often effective. If the patient is steroid dependent or steroid resistant, cytotoxic agents may be needed, with cyclophosphamide 2 mg/kg/d or chlorambucil 0.2 mg/kg/d. Cyclosporine 5 mg/kg/d is an alternative therapy.

Focal Segmental Glomerulosclerosis

GENERAL PRINCIPLES

Focal segmental glomerulosclerosis (FSGS) is not a single disease but rather a descriptive classification for diseases with shared histopathology. Presentation is with the nephrotic syndrome, hypertension, and renal insufficiency.

Associated Conditions

Secondary forms of FSGS are associated with obesity, HIV (collapsing variant), and intravenous drug abuse.

DIAGNOSIS

The kidney biopsy reveals focal and segmental sclerosis of glomeruli under light microscopy. The degree of interstitial fibrosis and tubular atrophy (rather than glomerular scarring) correlates with prognosis. Immunofluorescence shows staining for C3 and IgM in areas of sclerosis, representing areas of trapped immune deposits. Electron microscopy shows effacement of the podocyte foot processes.

TREATMENT

For patients with nephrotic range proteinuria, a trial of prednisone 1 mg/kg/d can be attempted for 16 weeks. Patients who relapse after a period of apparent responsiveness may benefit from a repeat course of steroids. Nonresponders and relapsers may respond to treatment with cyclosporine 5 mg/kg/d. Cyclophosphamide and mycophenolate mofetil can also be used.

Membranous Nephropathy

GENERAL PRINCIPLES

Membranous nephropathy (MN) usually presents with the nephrotic syndrome or heavy proteinuria, while renal function is often normal or near-normal. Disease progression is variable, with one-third remitting spontaneously, one-third progressing to ESRD, and one-third with an intermediate course.

Associated Conditions
Secondary forms of MN are associated with SLE, viral hepatitis, syphilis, or solid organ malignancies. Medications such as gold and penicillamine can also induce this process.

DIAGNOSIS

Kidney biopsy shows thickening of the glomerular basement membrane on light microscopy, with "spikes" on silver stain, representing areas of normal basement membrane interposed between subepithelial deposits. These deposits correlate with IgG and C3 on immunofluorescence and are also seen on electron microscopy.

TREATMENT

Because of the generally good prognosis, specific therapy should be reserved for patients at higher risk for progression (reduced GFR, male gender, age > 50, hypertension), or severe nephrotic syndrome (proteinuria > 10 g/d). Treatment options include regimens with prednisone 0.5 mg/kg/d and cytotoxic agents (chlorambucil 0.2 mg/kg/d or cyclophosphamide 2.5 mg/kg/d) on alternating months for 6 to 12 months.

Membranoproliferative Glomerulonephropathy

GENERAL PRINCIPLES

Associated Conditions
Primary idiopathic membranoproliferative glomerulonephropathy (MPGN) is uncommon. Hepatitis C accounts for most cases of secondary MPGN, frequently

in association with cryoglobulinemia. Other secondary causes include SLE, chronic infections, and various malignancies.

DIAGNOSIS

Clinical Presentation

MPGN can present with the nephrotic syndrome, nephritic syndrome, or a combination of both. Complement levels (C3, C4) are frequently low and a C3-nephritic factor may also interfere with the complement cascade.

Diagnostic Testing

Diagnostic Procedures

The kidney biopsy shows mesangial proliferation and hypercellularity on light microscopy, with "lobulization" of the glomerular tuft. Mesangial interpositioning within the glomerular basement membrane can give a double-contour or "tram-track" appearance on silver stain. Immunofluorescence and electron microscopy can show subendothelial (type I) or intramembranous (type II) deposits.

TREATMENT

In adult idiopathic MPGN, treatment has not been shown to improve disease-free survival, although the use of corticosteroids may stabilize disease in children. Treatment of the secondary forms is targeted at the underlying disease. If renal function is rapidly declining in the presence of cryoglobulins, plasmapheresis may help stabilize disease.

IgA Nephropathy/Henoch–Schönlein Purpura

DIAGNOSIS

Clinical Presentation

- IgA nephropathy is typically idiopathic, characterized by a nephritic picture with microscopic (and less commonly macroscopic) hematuria, and mild proteinuria. Presentation is most commonly in the second or third decade of life, generally following a slowly progressive course. However, some patients may experience a rapid decline in renal function resulting in ESRD.
- Henoch–Schönlein purpura is a related disorder that may represent a systemic form of the same disease, with vasculitic involvement of the skin (palpable purpura of the lower trunk and extremities), gastrointestinal tract, and joints.

Diagnostic Testing

Diagnostic Procedures

Kidney biopsy shows increased mesangial cellularity on light microscopy, with IgA and C3 deposition on immunofluorescence. Although many patients have elevated serum IgA levels, this is not a specific finding and the levels do not correlate with disease severity.

TREATMENT

Aggressiveness of therapy depends on severity of disease. For patients with a benign course, conservative management with ACE inhibitors, ARBs, or fish oil (omega-3 fatty acids) may prevent deterioration of renal function, although the benefit of fish oil remains controversial. Progressive disease may benefit from a course of prednisone 1 mg/kg/d with or without cytotoxic agents.

Pulmonary–Renal Syndromes

DIAGNOSIS

Clinical Presentation

Several distinct clinical entities make up the pulmonary–renal syndromes where there is vasculitic involvement of the alveolar and glomerular capillaries. Typically, this results in rapidly progressive renal failure often with concurrent pulmonary involvement in the form of alveolar hemorrhage. A nephritic picture predominates, with dysmorphic RBCs and RBC casts in the urine. Arthralgias and fever may represent other systemic symptoms.

Differential Diagnosis

- In anti-GBM antibody disease, circulating antibody to the alpha-3 chain of type IV collagen is deposited in the basement membrane of alveoli and glomeruli, resulting in linear staining on immunofluorescence. Goodpasture's syndrome includes pulmonary involvement and can present with life-threatening alveolar hemorrhage. The presence of anti-GBM antibody in the serum supports the diagnosis, and 10% to 30% of patients will have a positive ANCA serology.
- In Wegener's granulomatosis, vasculitic lesions involve the small vessels of the kidneys and may also involve the lungs, skin, and gastrointestinal tract. As in anti-GBM antibody disease, pulmonary hemorrhage may be severe. Biopsy findings include a small vessel vasculitis with noncaseating granuloma formation in the kidneys, lungs, or sinuses. Wegener's granulomatosis is part of a group of diseases known as pauci-immune glomerulonephritis, including Churg–Strauss syndrome (asthma and eosinophilia) and microscopic polyangiitis. This name refers to the general absence of immune deposits on immunofluorescence, although they all exhibit circulating ANCA. In Wegener's granulomatosis and Churg–Strauss syndrome, there is a positive cytoplasmic ANCA directed against serine proteinase-3, while in microscopic polyangiitis, there is a positive perinuclear ANCA directed against myeloperoxidase.

TREATMENT

- In anti-GBM antibody disease, the goal of therapy is to clear the pathogenic antibody while suppressing new production. Treatment is with daily total volume plasmapheresis for approximately 14 days in conjunction with cyclophosphamide 2 mg/kg/d and glucocorticoids (intravenous methylprednisolone 7 to 15 mg/kg/d for 3 days, followed by oral prednisone 1 mg/kg/d). Immunosuppression is tapered over 8 weeks. Serial measurement of the anti-GBM antibody level is useful to monitor therapy with plasmapheresis and immunosuppression continuing until it is undetectable. Poor response to therapy is predicted by the presence of oliguria, creatinine > 5.7 mg/dL, or dialysis dependence on presentation. Even if the likelihood of renal recovery is low, evidence of pulmonary involvement warrants aggressive therapy.

- Treatment of Wegener's granulomatosis is with combined prednisone 1 mg/kg/d (with taper) and cyclophosphamide 2 mg/kg/d for at least 3 months to induce remission. Therapy should then continue with oral steroids for 1 year to prevent relapse. Double-strength sulfamethoxazole–trimethoprim given twice daily has been shown to reduce extrarenal relapses. More aggressive management with plasmapheresis and pulse intravenous steroids may be beneficial for patients presenting with pulmonary hemorrhage or dialysis dependence.

SECONDARY GLOMERULOPATHIES

Diabetic Nephropathy

DIAGNOSIS

Diagnostic Criteria

Diabetic nephropathy (DN) is the most common cause of ESRD in the United States. Albuminuria is "microscopic" when levels are 30 to 300 mg/gram creatinine. Overt nephropathy is characterized by albuminuria > 300 mg/gram creatinine. Early disease has glomerular hyperfiltration with an elevated GFR, followed by a linear decline that may progress to ESRD.

Diagnostic Testing

Diagnostic Procedures

Kidney biopsy is not usually performed, unless the rate of renal decline is more rapid than would be anticipated, suggesting another possible diagnosis. Histology for DN shows glomerular sclerosis with nodular mesangial expansion (Kimmelstiel–Wilson nodules) on light microscopy. Immunofluorescence does not reveal immune deposition. Electron microscopy may show GBM thickening.

TREATMENT

Treatment is centered on aggressive control of glucose and blood pressure. Specific hyperglycemic therapy is discussed further in Chapter 20, Diabetes Mellitus and Related Disorders. ACE inhibitors and ARBs are considered first-line agents in the treatment of hypertension in diabetic patients and should be used for control of proteinuria even in the absence of hypertension.

Lupus Nephritis

DIAGNOSIS

Diagnostic Testing

Laboratories

Lupus nephritis (LN) can manifest as proteinuria of varying degrees with dysmorphic RBCs and RBC casts, and renal insufficiency. Positive lupus serology (e.g., ANA, anti-double-stranded DNA antibodies) and hypocomplementemia are often present during acute flares.

Diagnostic Procedures

Renal biopsy can provide useful information on disease activity and prognosis. The World Health Organization classification has five major categories based on histologic appearance. Class I has normal glomeruli, classes II to IV have increasing degrees of mesangial proliferation, and class V has an appearance similar to MN. Immunofluorescence is usually positive for IgG, IgA, IgM, C3, and C4, for the "full-house" fluorescence pattern.

TREATMENT

Aggressiveness of therapy considers the renal and extrarenal manifestations of the disease. Classes I and II LN rarely require specific treatment and therapy is directed at the extrarenal manifestations. Class III LN, when mild or moderate, can generally be treated with a short course of high-dose steroids (prednisone 1 mg/kg/d). Patients with more severe class III or class IV LN should undergo pulse intravenous methylprednisolone (7 to 15 mg/kg/d for 3 days) followed by oral prednisone at 0.5 to 1 mg/kg/d. A second agent should be used and can be monthly intravenous cyclophosphamide 0.5 to 1 g/m² or oral mycophenolate mofetil 1,000 mg thrice daily for a course of 6 months. As the prognosis of class V LN is better as compared to classes III or IV, treatment is reserved primarily for patients with severe nephrotic syndrome, with a short course of high-dose steroids (prednisone 1 mg/kg/d).

Postinfectious Glomerulonephropathy

DIAGNOSIS

Clinical Presentation

Postinfectious GN classically presents with the nephritic syndrome of hematuria, hypertension, edema, and renal insufficiency. Proteinuria may be present and is usually in subnephrotic range. Streptococcal infection typically affects children under the age of 10, after a latent period of 2 to 4 weeks from onset of pharyngitis or skin infection. Bacterial endocarditis, visceral abscesses, and ventriculoperitoneal shunt infections can also lead to this immune complex–mediated disease. Low complement levels are usually seen. Antistreptolysin-O (ASO) titers may be elevated serially as may anti-DNaseB antibodies in streptococcal-associated disease.

Diagnostic Testing

Diagnostic Procedures

Kidney biopsy reveals subepithelial humps on light and electron microscopy corresponding to the deposits on immunofluorescence (IgG, C3). There is widespread mesangial proliferation as well as an infiltration of polymorphonuclear cells.

TREATMENT

Treatment of the renal disease is primarily supportive. Resolution of the underlying infection typically leads to renal recovery in 2 to 4 weeks, even in cases where dialytic support was needed. A brisk diuresis should be anticipated in the recovery period.

Deposition Disorders/Dysproteinemias

DIAGNOSIS

Differential Diagnosis

Dysproteinemias include amyloidosis, light chain deposition disease (LCDD), heavy chain deposition disease (HCDD), and fibrillary/immunotactoid glomerulopathy. Multiple myeloma may be associated with amyloidosis or LCDD. These disorders can affect the kidney in a variety of ways, including glomerular or tubular deposition, formation of insoluble protein casts in the tubules (micro-obstructive cast nephropathy), or through hypercalcemia. Glomerular involvement is typically associated with heavy proteinuria.

Diagnostic Testing

Laboratories

Diagnosis is suggested by an abnormal monoclonal protein found in the SPEP or UPEP. Immunoglobulin chains are not detected by routine urine dipstick and may be missed unless glomerular involvement has led to general protein leakage.

Diagnostic Procedures

- Biopsy of the kidney can show characteristic deposits. For amyloidosis, this appears as Congo Red positive beta-pleated fibrils of 10 nm in diameter under electron microscopy. Immunofluorescence can identify the specific immunoglobulin chains for LCDD (more likely to occur with kappa light chains) and HCDD. Fibrillary/immunotactoid deposits are Congo Red negative and the fibrils (20 to 50 nm) are typically thicker than those for amyloid.
- When cast nephropathy is implicated in a dysproteinemic disorder, the biopsy shows enlarged tubules filled with proteinaceous material. Immunofluorescence can identify the specific components of these casts.

TREATMENT

Melphalan and prednisone are beneficial in the treatment of amyloidosis and LCDD. Chemotherapy aimed at the underlying disease can be effective in reversing or stabilizing renal disease. There is no known specific treatment for fibrillary/immunotactoid glomerulopathy, although addressing an underlying malignancy, if present, may slow progression.

HIV-Associated Nephropathy

DIAGNOSIS

- HIV-associated nephropathy (HIVAN) is characterized by nephrotic range proteinuria, edema, and hypertension with or without an elevated creatinine. Kidneys are typically enlarged (>12 cm) on ultrasonography.
- On biopsy, HIVAN has an appearance similar to the collapsing variant of FSGS, with proliferative podocytes. However, it should be mentioned that HIV can produce secondary forms of other glomerular diseases, including MPGN and MN.

TREATMENT

The widespread use of antiretroviral therapy has improved the overall outcomes of HIVAN, allowing stabilization of renal function and proteinuria. Use of ACE inhibitors and ARBs can also help reduce the degree of proteinuria.

Polycystic Kidney Disease

GENERAL PRINCIPLES

Epidemiology

Autosomal dominant polycystic kidney disease (ADPKD) is a hereditary disorder resulting in cystic enlargement of the kidney. Prevalence is approximately 1/1,000. There are two known mutations in the polycystin genes, with PKD1 being the most common (85%). PKD2 is associated with a later onset of disease.

Pathophysiology

The polycystin gene products primarily localize to the cilia of the tubular apical membrane where they are thought to sense flow. Disordered regulation of cell division may lead to overgrowth of the tubular segment, eventually pinching off from the rest of the collecting system. A defect in cell adhesion to the basement membrane may also be involved as the polycystin gene products have been shown to localize to the basolateral membrane as well.

Associated Conditions

- Onset of kidney failure is highly variable, with half of patients reaching ESRD by the age of 65.
- Hypertension is an early feature of ADPKD. As the affected tubules enlarge, they impinge upon the blood flow to neighboring glomeruli, rendering them ischemic. This is turn activates the renin–angiotensin–aldosterone system leading to systemic hypertension.
- Cerebral aneurysms, hepatic cysts, and colonic diverticula are features found in association with ADPKD. Patients with a family history of cerebral aneurysms or with symptoms attributable to a cerebral aneurysm should undergo evaluation with brain MRI/MRA.
- As cysts enlarge, they may result in a palpable flank mass. Gross hematuria and pain may indicate cysts hemorrhage into the collecting system. Flank pain may also be caused by cyst infection.

DIAGNOSIS

Ultrasonography reveals multiple cysts. In the setting of a positive family history, a diagnosis of ADPKD can be made from ultrasound findings, with criteria differing according to age. At least three cysts are required in patients under the age of 40. In patients aged 40 to 59, at least two cysts in each kidney are needed. For patients 60 and older, the diagnosis requires at least four cysts in each kidney.

TREATMENT

- There is currently no specific treatment to prevent cysts formation. Aggressive control of hypertension should be practiced and blockade of the renin–angiotensin-aldosterone system with an ACE inhibitor or ARB is recommended as first-line therapy.
- Gross hematuria can usually be managed with bedrest and hydration. Resolution may take several days.
- Cyst infections are generally treated with antibiotics that achieve good penetration into the cysts. Sulfamethoxazole-trimethoprim or ciprofloxacin are the antibiotics of choice. The absence of bacterial growth in the urine does not rule out infection since the cystic fluid does not generally communicate with the rest of the collecting system.

PROGRESSIVE LOSS OF RENAL FUNCTION

Chronic Kidney Disease

GENERAL PRINCIPLES

Classification

- Chronic kidney disease (CKD) is divided into five stages based on the estimated GFR (Table 3). To be classified as stage 1 or stage 2, there must be an accompanying structural or functional defect (e.g., proteinuria, hematuria) as the GFR is normal or near-normal in these stages. Treatment goals are frequently guided by CKD stage.
- Patients are usually asymptomatic until significant renal function is lost (late stage 4 and stage 5). However, complications including hypertension, anemia, and bone mineral disease (renal osteodystrophy and secondary hyperparathyroidism) often develop during stage 3 and thus must be investigated and addressed before patients become symptomatic.
- The decline in GFR may be followed by plotting the reciprocal of creatinine versus time; revealing a linear decrement. This can be useful in end-stage planning and in predicting when renal replacement therapy will be needed. In the absence of another metabolic or nutritional indication, dialysis is typically started when the GFR is <10 mL/min in individuals without diabetes and <15 mL/min in patients with diabetes. A steeper than anticipated decline in GFR suggests a superimposed renal insult.

Table 3	Stages of Chronic Kidney Disease
CKD Stage	**Glomerular Filtration Rate**
1	>90 mL/min
2	60–89 mL/min
3	30–59 mL/min
4	15–29 mL/min
5	<15 mL/min or dialysis

CKD, chronic kidney disease.

Risk Factors

- Decreased renal perfusion can lead to a decline in GFR. This can occur with true volume depletion or diminished effective circulating volume (e.g., congestive heart failure, hepatic cirrhosis). The use of NSAIDs can be particularly deleterious in this setting as they block the renal autoregulatory mechanisms to preserve GFR. ACE inhibitors or ARBs can also produce a reversible decrement in GFR.
- Uncontrolled hypertension can also be harmful to kidneys. Hyperfiltration may lead to worsening proteinuria and further damage to the glomeruli.
- Nephrotoxic agents, such as iodinated contrast agents and aminoglycosides, should be avoided when possible. Careful attention to drug dosing is mandatory, frequently guided by the estimated GFR or CKD stage. Drug levels should be monitored where appropriate.
- Patients undergoing coronary angiography are at particular risk for worsening CKD. Contrast nephropathy and atheroembolic disease are potential complications and the risks and benefits of the procedure must be weighed with the patient prior to proceeding.
- UTI or obstruction should be considered in all patients with an unexplained drop in renal function. Worsening renal artery stenosis may also lead to a more rapid decline in GFR as well as sudden worsening in previously controlled hypertension.
- Renal vein thrombosis may occur as a complication of the nephrotic syndrome and can exacerbate CKD. Hematuria and flank pain may occur.

TREATMENT

- Treatment of CKD is focused on avoidance of risk factors (listed above), dietary modification, blood pressure control, adequate treatment of the associated conditions (listed below) and ultimately, preparation for renal replacement therapy.
- **Dietary restrictions**
  - Sodium restriction to less than 3 g/d is usually adequate for most CKD patients. Restriction to less than 2 g/d should be employed if heart failure or refractory hypertension is present. A 24-hour urine sodium level of 100 mEq correlates with a 2 g/d diet.
  - Fluid restrictions are generally not required in CKD patients, and if excessive may lead to volume depletion and hypernatremia. Restriction is appropriate in patients with dilutional hyponatremia, or if ARF occurs.
  - Potassium should be restricted to 60 mEq/d in individuals with hyperkalemia. Tomato-based products, bananas, potatoes, and citrus drinks are high in potassium and should be avoided in these patients.
  - Dietary phosphate restriction should be to 800 to 1,000 mg/d. Dairy products and nuts should be avoided in hyperphosphatemia. Oral binders can be used if dietary restrictions are unable to control phosphate levels.
- **Hypertension**
  - Uncontrolled hypertension accelerates the rate of decline of renal function. Adequate control of blood pressure in patients with CKD is <130/80.
  - ACE inhibitors and ARBs should be used preferentially in the CKD population. They lower intraglomerular pressure and possess renoprotective properties beyond the antihypertensive effect, particularly in proteinuric states. Due to their effects on intrarenal hemodynamics, a 30% rise in serum creatinine should be anticipated and tolerated; a further rise should prompt a search for possible renal artery stenosis.

The creatinine and serum potassium should be checked approximately 1 to 2 weeks after a dose adjustment.

- Diuretics are also beneficial in achieving euvolemia in hypertensive CKD patients. Thiazide diuretics become less effective as the GFR falls below 30 mL/min, while loop diuretics retain their efficacy although higher doses may be required for the desired effect.

- **Anemia**
  - A normocytic anemia is common in CKD, and should be searched for once the GFR falls below 60 mL/min (stage 3).
  - Alternate causes for an anemia should be entertained in the appropriate setting and iron stores assessed. If the transferrin saturation is <20% or the ferritin level is <200 mg/dL, consideration should be given to iron repletion with 1 g of an intravenous preparation of iron dextran (1,000 mg, once with test dose of 25 mg), ferric gluconate (125 mg, 8 doses), or iron sucrose (100 mg, 10 doses).
  - Erythropoietic hormones such as epoetin and darbepoetin can be effective in treating anemia. The minimum dose that maintains the hemoglobin at 10 to 12 g/dL should be used, and the correction of iron deficiency frequently decreases the dose requirement. Raising the hemoglobin to higher levels with these hormones has been associated with increased cardiovascular mortality (*N Engl J Med 2006;355:2085*).

- **Renal osteodystrophy and secondary hyperparathyroidism**
  - Renal osteodystrophy (ROD) refers to a variety of bone mineral disorders encountered in CKD and ESRD. Prevalence increases as the GFR declines, through stage III and more advanced disease.
  - Osteitis fibrosa is commonly associated with secondary hyperparathyroidism and increased bone turnover, resulting in bone pain and fractures. Adynamic bone disease is a low-turnover state with suppressed PTH levels. Osteomalacia can involve deposition of aluminum into bone and is less commonly seen today with the decreased use of aluminum-based phosphate binders.
  - In CKD, starting in stage 3, vitamin D deficiency, low calcium, and elevated phosphate can all contribute to hyperparathyroidism. The general goal of therapy is to suppress PTH toward normal while maintaining normal serum calcium and phosphorus. This can be addressed in three steps: repletion of vitamin D stores (25-OH vitamin D), control of dietary phosphate with binders, and administration of active vitamin D (1,25-dihydroxyvitamin D or an analog).
    - Deficient stores (25-OH vitamin D < 30 ng/mL) should be corrected with oral ergocalciferol 50,000 IU capsule weekly, or cholecalciferol 2,000 to 4,000 IU daily. The duration of treatment depends on severity of the deficiency, with levels <5 ng/dL warranting at least 12 weeks of treatment.
    - Phosphate control can be difficult as GFR declines, even with appropriate dietary restriction. Phosphate binders inhibit gastrointestinal absorption. Calcium-based binders are effective when given with meals, as calcium carbonate (200 mg of elemental calcium per 500 mg tablet) or calcium acetate (169 mg of elemental calcium per 667 mg tablet). In general, the total daily elemental calcium administered should be <1,500 mg. Lanthanum carbonate and sevelamer carbonate are non–calcium-based alternatives.
    - Active vitamin D (1,25-dihydroxyvitamin D) and analogs are potent suppressors of PTH, and can be administered if serum PTH is elevated. Options include daily calcitriol (0.25 to 1 mcg), paricalcitol (1 to 5 mcg), or doxercalciferol (1 to 5 mcg). Calcium levels need to be monitored regularly and doses adjusted to avoid hypercalcemia.

○ Cinacalcet is a calcimimetic that acts on the parathyroid gland to suppress PTH release. It should be used only in dialysis patients, and usually in conjunction with active vitamin D, as it may induce significant hypocalcemia and is relatively ineffective as monotherapy.

- **Metabolic acidosis.** As renal function deteriorates, the kidney is unable to appropriately excrete sufficient acid resulting in metabolic acidosis (mixed high and normal anion gap). To compensate, alkaline buffer is released from the skeleton, but can worsen bone mineral disease.
  - Treatment with sodium bicarbonate 650 to 1,300 mg thrice daily can help maintain the serum bicarbonate level at 22 mEq/L or greater. Such therapy, however, can increase the sodium load and contribute to edema or hypertension.
  - Citrate, another alkaline source, should not be used in the CKD or ESRD population as it can dramatically enhance gastrointestinal absorption of aluminum and lead to aluminum toxicity or osteomalacia.
- **Preparation for renal replacement therapy**
  - Patients should be counseled at an early stage to determine preferences for renal replacement therapies, including hemodialysis, peritoneal dialysis, and eligibility for renal transplantation.
  - Preparation for the creation of a permanent vascular access for hemodialysis should be initiated by protecting the nondominant forearm from intravenous catheters and blood draws. Timely referral to an access surgeon can facilitate the creation and maturation of an AV access.

RENAL REPLACEMENT THERAPIES

Approach to Dialysis

TREATMENT

- **Modalities**
  - Renal replacement therapy is indicated when conservative medical management is unable to control the metabolic derangements of kidney disease. This applies to the acute and chronic settings. Common acute indications include hyperkalemia, metabolic acidosis, and volume overload that are refractory to medical management. Uremic encephalopathy or pericarditis, as well as certain intoxications (methanol, ethylene glycol, or salicylates), can all be indications to initiate dialytic therapy acutely. In the chronic setting, renal replacement therapy is typically begun when the creatinine clearance falls below 10 mL/min in individuals without diabetes or below 15 mL/min in diabetic patients. A deteriorating nutritional status is also an indication to start dialytic therapy in advanced CKD.
  - Dialysis modalities work by solute diffusion and water transport across a selectively permeable membrane. In hemodialysis, blood is pumped countercurrently to a dialysis solution within an extracorporeal membrane. This can be performed intermittently (3 to 4 hours during the day) or in a continuous 24-hour fashion depending on hemodynamic stability or goals of therapy. Peritoneal dialysis utilizes the patient's peritoneal membrane as the selective filter and dialysis fluid is instilled into the peritoneal cavity. Transplantation offers the best long-term survival and most completely replaces the filtrative and endocrine functions of the kidney. However, it carries the risks that accompany long-term immunosuppression.

- **Diffusion**
  - The semipermeable membrane contains pores that allow electrolytes and small molecules to pass by diffusion while holding back larger molecules and cellular components of the blood. Movement relies on the molecular size and the concentration gradient, where creatinine, urea, potassium, and other waste products of metabolism pass into the dialysis solution while alkaline buffers (bicarbonate or lactate) enter the blood from the dialysis solution.
- **Ultrafiltration/convection**
  - Removal of water is termed ultrafiltration (UF). It can be achieved in hemodialysis via a transmembrane hydrostatic pressure that removes excess fluid from of the blood compartment. In peritoneal dialysis, water follows its osmotic gradient into the relatively hyperosmolar dialysis solution (usually with dextrose providing the osmotic driving force).
  - As water is removed from the vascular compartment, it drags along solute. This is termed convective clearance. This usually accounts for only a small fraction of the total clearance, but can be significantly increased if a physiologic "replacement fluid" is infused into the patient concurrently to prevent hypovolemia. This strategy is frequently employed by continuous hemodialysis modalities (see below).

Hemodialysis

GENERAL PRINCIPLES

- **Modalities**
  - Hemodialysis is by far the most commonly used form of renal replacement therapy in the United States. Intermittent hemodialysis (IHD) typically runs for 3 to 4 hours per session, and is performed three times weekly. Outpatient, in-center hemodialysis for ESRD generally employs this modality, although variations are available for patients undergoing home treatments.
  - Continuous renal replacement therapy (CRRT) can be used in specialized circumstances, particularly when the patient's hemodynamic status would not tolerate the rapid fluid shifts of IHD. Although less efficient (with slower blood flows) and utilizing slower ultrafiltration rates, CRRT can achieve equivalent clearances of both solute and fluid as compared to IHD due to its continuous, 24-hour nature. The slower blood flows necessitate anticoagulation (with systemic heparin or regional citrate) in order to prevent the filter from clotting. Continuous modalities generally require specialized nursing and an intensive care setting.
  - The most frequently employed form of CRRT is continuous veno-venous hemodiafiltration (CVVHDF) where blood is slowly pumped countercurrently to a dialysis solution (diffusion) and a replacement fluid is infused into the circuit to balance most of the ultrafiltrate (convection); the difference between the rates of total UF and the replacement fluid is the net fluid removal.
  - Sustained low efficiency dialysis (SLED) is essentially a hybrid form of IHD and CRRT. Intermediate blood flows lower the clotting risk if anticoagulation is not used, while intermediate treatment lengths (8 to 10 hours) still allow for adequate clearances. Patients also spend a significant portion of the day off the machine to allow for nonbedside testing, procedures, and physical therapy.
- **Prescription and adequacy**
  - IHD typically runs for 3 to 4 hours and can ultrafiltrate 3 to 4 L safely in hemodynamically stable patients. It can be used in ESRD as well as ARF. In the chronic

setting, IHD is generally performed three times weekly. In the acute setting, the appropriate dose is not clearly known, although a thrice-weekly schedule is likely adequate; daily assessment should be performed to reevaluate dialytic needs.
- Adequacy is assessed by calculating the clearance of BUN, which serves as a surrogate marker of the "uremic factors." The urea reduction ratio (URR) can be calculated by the following:

$$URR = [(predialysis\ BUN\ -\ postdialysis\ BUN)/(predialysis\ BUN)] \times 100$$

  ○ A reduction rate of >65% is considered adequate in the chronic setting (*N Engl J Med 2002;347:2010*). An adequacy target is less well defined for ARF. Intensive daily hemodialysis was not shown to be superior to standard thrice-weekly treatments (*N Engl J Med 2008;359:7*).
- Clearance is measured differently in CRRT where dialytic therapy is taking place around the clock, effectively serving as an extracorporeal "GFR." Drug dosing needs to be adjusted accordingly. An estimate of this clearance can be calculated by the sum of the dialysis fluid, replacement fluid, and net ultrafiltration rates and expressed in the number of milliliters per minute. For most circumstances, this approximates a clearance of 20 to 50 mL/min.
  ○ With CRRT, the net UF rate can be adjusted as needed, according to the patient's hemodynamic status. One must be vigilant in checking electrolyte levels (particularly ionized calcium and phosphorus) to ensure they remain within the desired ranges. Calcium levels are especially important to follow when regional citrate anticoagulation is being used.

COMPLICATIONS

- Nontunneled catheters are typically placed in the internal jugular or femoral vein and carry the same risks as other central venous catheters (infection, bleeding, pneumothorax). They are almost exclusively used in the inpatient setting and are generally used for 1 to 2 weeks. Tunneled catheters have lower rates of infection and can be used for 6 months while a more definitive access is maturing (AV fistula or graft).
  - Fevers and rigors, particularly during dialysis, should prompt a search for an infectious cause and empiric antibiotic coverage for *Staphylococci* and gram-negative bacteria should be administered. The catheter should then be replaced after a period of defervescence and sterilization of the blood (at least 48 hours). Documented bacteremia should be treated with antibiotics for at least 3 weeks.
- Thrombosis of an AV fistula or graft can frequently be recanalized by thrombolysis or thrombectomy. Stenotic regions can be evaluated by a fistulogram and treatment may encompass angioplasty or stent deployment.
- Intradialytic hypotension is most commonly due to intravascular volume depletion from rapid ultrafiltration. Antihypertensive medications may also contribute. Infectious causes should be sought in the appropriate setting. Acute treatment of the drop in blood pressure includes infusion of normal saline (as 200 mL boluses) and reduction of the ultrafiltration rate.
- Dialysis disequilibrium is an uncommon syndrome that may occur in severely uremic patients undergoing their first few treatments. Rapid clearance of toxins is thought to induce cerebral edema by osmolar shifts and can present as nausea, emesis, headache, confusion, or seizures. Occurrence can be prevented or ameliorated by initiating patients on dialysis with slower blood flows and shorter treatments.

Peritoneal Dialysis

GENERAL PRINCIPLES

- **Modalities**
  - Historically, peritoneal dialysis (PD) has been used in the acute setting for hemodynamically unstable patients. However, with the development and availability of safe and effective continuous hemodialysis, use of PD in the treatment of ARF in adults has been mostly abandoned in the United States. Currently, its use is primarily in the treatment of ESRD.
  - There are two modalities in use: manual exchanges and automated cycler exchanges.
    - The manual modality, also called continuous ambulatory peritoneal dialysis (CAPD), has the patient instill dialysis fluid into the peritoneum for a specified length of time after which the dialysate is drained and replaced by another dwell.
    - The automated modality, also called continuous cycling peritoneal dialysis (CCPD), typically operates overnight where a machine runs a preprogrammed set of exchanges while the patient sleeps. A final fill usually remains in the peritoneum and is carried during the daytime for continued solute exchange.
  - Either PD modality requires strict adherence to sterile technique and careful patient selection is necessary. Generally, PD should not be used if there is a history of recent abdominal surgery or if multiple peritoneal adhesions are present.
- **Prescription and adequacy**
  - The choice between CAPD and CCPD usually depends on patient preference and on the transport characteristics of the peritoneal membrane. Manual exchanges (CAPD) can be used as a backup modality, particularly in the hospital where nurse staffing or machine availability may be limited.
  - In writing PD orders, the following variables must be specified: dwell volume, dwell time, number of exchanges, and dextrose concentration of the dialysis solution. The dwell volume is typically between 2 and 3 L. The dextrose concentration can be 1.5%, 2.5%, or 4.25%, providing the osmotic gradient for fluid removal. Higher concentrations allow for greater ultrafiltration, but also lead to more glucose absorption and worsening control of diabetes. Icodextrin is a glucose polymer preparation that is minimally absorbed and thus maintains an effective osmotic gradient up to 18 hours. Commercially available PD solutions may have color-coded tabs and patients may know these better than the actual concentrations (yellow for 1.5%, green for 2.5%, red for 4.25%). A sample order set for CAPD would be 2.5 L, four exchanges, 6 hours each, with 2.5% dextrose.
  - Peritoneal dialysis is less efficient than conventional hemodialysis. However, given its continuous nature, solute clearance and ultrafiltration can approximate that of other modalities. Larger volumes and more frequent exchanges can assist with solute exchange. Increasing the concentration of dextrose can promote greater ultrafiltration in volume overloaded patients. Residual renal function is very important in the PD population and avoidance of nephrotoxins should be practiced (*J Am Soc Nephrol 2002;13:1307*).

COMPLICATIONS

- Peritonitis typically presents with diffuse abdominal pain and cloudy peritoneal fluid. A sample should be sent for cell count, differential, Gram stain, and culture.

A WBC count of >100 cells/mm^3, of which at least 50% are neutrophils, supports the diagnosis.

- Empiric therapy should cover for both gram-positive and gram-negative organisms, with a first-generation cephalosporin (cefazolin or cephalothin) and ceftazidime at 15 to 20 mg/kg of each in the longest dwell of the day (*Perit Dial Int 2005;25:107*). The intraperitoneal route is the preferred method of administration, unless the patient is overtly septic in which case intravenous antibiotics should be employed. Antibiotics can be tailored once culture results are known and should be continued for 2 to 3 weeks. Multiple organisms, particularly if gram negative, should prompt a search for intestinal perforation.

- Tunnel or exit site infections may present with local erythema, tenderness, or purulent drainage, although crusting at the exit site alone does not necessarily indicate infection. Treatment can be with oral cephalosporins (gram positive) or fluoroquinolones (gram negative). Infections can be difficult to eradicate, however, and catheter removal may be required with a temporary transition to hemodialysis.

- Failure of PD fluid to drain is termed outflow failure. This may result from kinking of the catheter, constipation, or plugging of the catheter with fibrin strands. Conservative treatment should aim at resolving constipation if present and instilling heparin into the PD fluid at 500 units/L.

- Small hernias are at particularly higher risk for incarceration and should be corrected surgically while the patient is temporarily treated with hemodialysis. Fluid leaks can lead to abdominal wall and genital edema and typically result from anatomic defects. Hydrothorax usually occurs on the right side, and can be diagnosed by a markedly elevated glucose concentration in the pleural fluid. Pleurodesis can eliminate the potential space and permit continuation of peritoneal dialysis.

- Sclerosing encapsulating peritonitis is a complication of long-term peritoneal dialysis. The peritoneal membrane becomes thickened and entraps loops of bowel leading to symptoms of bowel obstruction. A bloody drainage may be present. Treatment is supportive with the focus on bowel rest and surgical lysis of adhesions. A trial of immunosuppression with prednisone 10 to 40 mg/d may have limited benefit.

- Hyperglycemia results from the systemic absorption of glucose from the dialysis fluid. Since peritoneal uptake of insulin is unpredictable, treatment with subcutaneous insulin is preferred. Hyperlipidemia is common in the PD population and treatment should be for a goal LDL of <100 mg/dL, with HMG-CoA reductase inhibitors as the first-line agents.

- Unlike hemodialysis, patients on PD tend to experience hypokalemia, likely due to a continuous potassium exodus in the dialysate as well as from an intracellular shift from the increased endogenous insulin production. Oral replacement is usually sufficient, either with relaxation of prior dietary restrictions or with low-dose supplementation (10 to 20 mEq/d of potassium chloride).

- Protein loss can be high and the dietary protein intake should be 1.2 to 1.3 g/kg/d. Episodes of peritonitis can make the membrane even more susceptible to protein losses.

Transplantation

GENERAL PRINCIPLES

- Renal transplantation offers patients an improved quality of life and survival as compared to other renal replacement modalities.

- The pretransplant evaluation focuses on cardiopulmonary status, vascular sufficiency, and human lymphocyte antigen typing. Structural abnormalities of the urinary tract need to be addressed. Contraindications include most malignancies, active infection, or significant cardiopulmonary disease.
- In adult recipients, the renal allograft is placed in the extraperitoneal space, in the anterior lower abdomen. Vascular anastomosis is typically to the iliac vessels while the ureter is attached to the bladder through a muscular tunnel to approximate sphincter function.
- Immunosuppression protocols vary among institutions. A typical regimen would include prednisone along with a combination of a calcineurin inhibitor (cyclosporine or tacrolimus) and an antimetabolite (mycophenolate derivative, azathioprine, or rapamycin).
- Evaluation of allograft dysfunction frequently requires kidney biopsy. Current laboratory and radiologic tests cannot reliably distinguish acute rejection from drug toxicity, the two most common causes of a rising creatinine in the transplant population.
- Complications and long-term management of transplant recipients are discussed further in Chapter 14, Solid Organ Transplant Medicine.

NEPHROLITHIASIS

Approach to Kidney Stones

GENERAL PRINCIPLES

Classification

- Overall, calcium-based stones are the most common and appear predominantly as calcium oxalate or calcium phosphate salts. These stones are radiopaque. Calcium phosphate stones can appear as elongated, blunt crystals and form in alkaline urine. Calcium oxalate stones can be found in acidic urine and can be dumbbell-shaped or appear as paired pyramids (giving them an envelope appearance when viewed on end).
- Uric acid stones can be idiopathic or develop as part of hyperuricosuric states such as gout and myeloproliferative disorders. These stones are radiolucent and are found in acidic urine. Uric acid crystals exhibit a variety of shapes, with needles and rhomboid forms being the most common.
- Struvite stones contain magnesium, ammonium, and phosphate. They develop in alkaline urine associated with urea-splitting organisms (e.g., *Proteus*, *Klebsiella*). They are radiopaque and can extend to fill the renal pelvis, taking on a staghorn configuration. On microscopy, struvite crystals have a characteristic coffin-lid shape.
- Cystine stones are uncommon and can form as the result of an autosomal recessive disorder. These stones have an intermediate radiolucency and appear as hexagonal crystals in the urine.

DIAGNOSIS

Clinical Presentation

Clinical presentation is with costovertebral angle or flank pain which can radiate to the scrotum or labia. Hematuria with nondysmorphic RBCs may be noted. Oliguria and ARF are uncommon but can result if there is bilateral obstruction or if a solitary functioning kidney is affected.

Diagnostic Testing

Laboratories

- Metabolic evaluation should include urine culture, pH, and microscopy. Serum calcium, phosphate, parathyroid hormone, and uric acid levels complement routine studies. Urine should be strained and passed stones analyzed for composition.
- Recurrent stone formers should undergo a more extensive evaluation, with 24-hour urine collections for calcium, phosphate, uric acid, citrate, oxalate, and cystine. This collection should not be done during an acute episode in a hospitalized patient but rather reserved for when the patient is on his or her normal outpatient diet.

Imaging

A plain abdominal film may reveal the radiopaque stones composed of calcium salts, struvite, or cystine. However, noncontrast CT scanning has replaced other imaging modalities as the study of choice for suspected nephrolithiasis.

TREATMENT

- General treatment of nephrolithiasis is with hydration to increase urine output and with analgesia (ketorolac or narcotics such as meperidine). If the stone is obstructing outflow or is accompanied by infection, removal is indicated with urgent urologic or radiologic intervention.
- After passage of a stone, treatment is directed at prevention of recurrent stone formation. Regardless of stone type, the foundation of therapy is maintenance of high urine output (2 to 3 L/d) with oral hydration and a low-salt diet (<2 g/d).
- For calcium oxalate stones, a low-calcium diet is no longer recommended given the risks of osteoporosis. A normal-calcium diet with no added calcium supplements is now in favor. Patients should avoid oxalate-rich foods (e.g., spinach, rhubarb). Thiazide diuretics may reduce calciuria and potassium citrate may be added in patients with hypocitraturia.
- Uric acid stones can be prevented or reduced in size by allopurinol. A low-protein diet may be helpful as can urinary alkalinization with citrate, bicarbonate, or acetazolamide.
- Struvite calculi frequently require surgical intervention for their removal. Extracorporeal shock-wave lithotripsy can be used as adjunctive therapy. Aggressive antibiotic treatment is indicated if monthly urine cultures become positive.
- Cystine stones require extensive urinary alkalinization to a pH of 7 to 7.5 to induce solubility. D-penicillamine and mercaptopropionylglycine can further increase solubility through breakage and exchange of disulfide bonds.

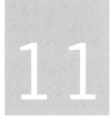

Treatment of Infectious Diseases

José E. Hagan, Hilary M. Babcock, and Nigar Kirmani

Principles of Therapy

GENERAL PRINCIPLES

- The decision to initiate, continue, and stop antimicrobial therapy should be carefully made. Indiscriminate use of antibiotics is associated with adverse effects, the development of drug resistance, and excess costs.
- When antimicrobial therapy is indicated, a number of factors reviewed in this chapter must be considered. In case of industry-related shortages of antibiotics, consultation with an infectious disease expert for alternative options is prudent.

DIAGNOSIS

- **During the initial evaluation,** a Gram stain of potentially infected material often permits a rapid presumptive diagnosis and helps in antibiotic selection.
- **Local susceptibility patterns** must be considered in selecting empiric therapy because patterns vary widely among communities and individual hospitals.
- **Cultures** are usually necessary for precise diagnosis and are required for susceptibility testing. Whenever organisms with special growth requirements are suspected, the microbiology laboratory should be consulted to ensure appropriate transport and processing of cultures.
- **Antimicrobial susceptibility testing** facilitates a rational selection of antimicrobial agents and should be performed on most positive bacterial cultures.
- **Rapid diagnostic testing,** such as use of polymerase chain reaction (PCR) and antigen detection, may also provide early confirmation of an infectious etiologic agent.

TREATMENT

- **Choice of initial antimicrobial therapy**
  - Empiric therapy should be directed against the most likely pathogens and possess the narrowest spectrum that adequately covers the predicted organisms.
  - Therapy should then be altered in accordance with the patient's course and culture results.
- **Timing of the initiation of antimicrobial therapy**
  - In acute clinical scenarios, empiric therapy is usually begun immediately after appropriate cultures have been obtained. However, if the patient's condition is stable, delaying the empiric use of antimicrobials allows for specific therapy based on the results of initial tests and avoids the use of unnecessary drugs.
  - Urgent therapy is indicated in febrile patients who are neutropenic or asplenic; however, in other immunosuppressed patients, fever alone seldom warrants urgent

therapy. Sepsis, meningitis, and rapidly progressive anaerobic or necrotizing infections should also be treated promptly with antimicrobials.

- **Route of administration.** Patients with serious infections should be given antimicrobial agents intravenously (IV). In less urgent circumstances, intramuscular (IM) or oral (PO) therapy often is sufficient. Oral therapy is acceptable when it is tolerated and can achieve adequate drug concentrations at the site of infection.
- **Type of therapy.** Bactericidal therapy is preferred over bacteriostatic regimens for patients with immunologic compromise or life-threatening infection. It is also preferred for infections characterized by impaired regional host defenses, such as endocarditis, meningitis, and osteomyelitis. Examples of bactericidal antibiotics include β-lactams and fluoroquinolones.
- **Assessment of antimicrobial therapy**
  - When therapy is reviewed from the perspective of potential treatment failure, one should consider the following questions:
    - Is the isolated organism the etiologic agent?
    - Is adequate antimicrobial therapy being provided?
    - Is the concentration of antimicrobial agent adequate at the site of infection?
    - Have resistant pathogens emerged?
    - Is a persistent fever due to underlying disease, abscess formation, an iatrogenic complication, a drug reaction, or another process?
- **Duration of therapy**
  - The duration of therapy depends on the nature of infection and the severity of clinical presentation.
  - Treatment of acute uncomplicated infections should be continued until the patient has been afebrile and clinically well, usually for a minimum of 72 hours.
  - Infections at certain sites (e.g., endocarditis, septic arthritis, osteomyelitis) require prolonged therapy.

SPECIAL CONSIDERATIONS

- **Status of the host**
  - The clinical status of the patient guides the speed with which therapy must be instituted, the route of administration, and the type of therapy.
  - Patients should be evaluated promptly for hemodynamic stability, rapidly progressive or life-threatening infections, and immune defects.
- **Pregnancy and the postpartum patient.** Although no antimicrobial agent is known to be completely safe in pregnancy, the penicillins and cephalosporins are used most often. **Tetracyclines and fluoroquinolones are among the agents specifically contraindicated,** and the sulfonamides and aminoglycosides should not be used if alternative agents are available. Most adequately dosed antibiotics appear in breast milk and should be used with caution in patients who are breast-feeding.

TOXIN-MEDIATED INFECTIONS

Clostridium Difficile-Associated Diarrhea

GENERAL PRINCIPLES

Frequently seen after systemic antimicrobial therapy.

DIAGNOSIS

Diagnosis is made by detection of *Clostridium difficile* toxin in stool or by colonoscopic visualization of pseudomembranes.

Differential Diagnosis

Diarrhea directly due to antibiotic use without *C. difficile* infection should be first considered, which will resolve with withdrawal of the antibiotic.

TREATMENT

- For **mild episodes:** Metronidazole, 500 mg PO (preferred over IV) tid for 10 to 14 days, and discontinuation of the offending antibiotic, if possible. Vancomycin, 125 to 500 mg PO qid (IV is not effective), is superior for **severe disease** or debilitated patients, but is otherwise reserved for refractory disease (*Clin Infect Dis 2007;45:302*). Intracolonic vancomycin is sometimes used in severe cases in which gut motility is altered and surgical intervention is imminent (*Clin Infect Dis 2002;35:690*).
- Endpoint of therapy is cessation of diarrhea; *do not retest stool for toxin clearance.* Avoid antimotility agents in severe disease.
- Recurrence is common and is treated with metronidazole or vancomycin in extended duration, pulsed, or tapered regimens. Adjunctive therapy with oral rifampin or bacitracin is sometimes used.

Tetanus

GENERAL PRINCIPLES

Caused by intoxication with *Clostridium tetani* toxin from wound contamination with spores.

Prevention

Tetanus is best prevented by immunization. For high-risk wounds, human tetanus immunoglobulin, 250 units IM, is used.

DIAGNOSIS

Clinical Presentation

Classically presents with muscle weakness and intensely painful rigidity, and spasms frequently precipitated by sensory stimuli, followed by autonomic dysfunction. Initial symptoms are in the face and neck muscles, such as masseter spasm (trismus). Delirium and high fever are usually absent. Diagnosis is clinical.

TREATMENT

Human tetanus immunoglobulin, 3,000 to 5,000 units IM. Benzodiazepines or paralytics can be used to control spasms. Surgical debridement is critical. Antibiotics, usually metronidazole 2 g/d IV or PO, are controversial. Care is otherwise supportive.

TOXIC SHOCK SYNDROME

Toxic shock syndrome (TSS) is a life-threatening systemic disease caused by exotoxin super antigens produced by *Staphylococcus aureus* or group A beta-hemolytic *Streptococcus* (GABHS) tissue infections. (See Table 1 for detailed treatment recommendations.)

Staphylococcal Toxic Shock Syndrome

GENERAL PRINCIPLES

Definition

Most often associated with colonization of surgical wounds, burns, vaginitis, or tampon use in young women; cases are also seen after nasal packing for epistaxis.

DIAGNOSIS

Clinical Presentation

Typical findings are fever, hypotension, mucosal hyperemia, macular desquamating erythroderma of the palms and soles, and multisystem involvement, such as vomiting, diarrhea, or multiorgan failure.

Table 1	Treatment of Toxic Shock Syndromes		
Etiology	Antibiotic Therapy	Adjunctive Therapy	Notes
Group A β-hemolytic Streptococcus (GABHS)	Penicillin G 4 million units IV q4h + Clindamycin 900 mg IV q8h for 10–14 d	IVIG 1 g/kg on day 1, then 0.5 g/kg on days 2 and 3 (*Clin Infect Dis 2003; 37:333*)	Surgical intervention almost always indicated for necrotizing infections. Clindamycin is added to decrease toxin production.
Staphylococcus	Oxacillin 2 g IV q4h or vancomycin 1 g IV q12h for 10–14 d	IVIG as per GABHS may be useful in severe cases, but higher doses may be needed (*Clin Infect Dis 2004;38:836*)	Treatment is primarily supportive. Tampons must be removed and avoided in future, especially if TSST-1 antibody titers are negative. Antibiotics decrease the risk of relapse.

Diagnostic Testing
Laboratories
Blood cultures are usually negative. Creatine phosphokinase (CPK) is often elevated. Detection of antibodies against Toxic Shock Syndrome Toxin-1 (TSST-1) is helpful in that it indicates protection against recurrence.

OUTCOME/PROGNOSIS

Mortality is relatively low.

Streptococcal Toxic Shock Syndrome

GENERAL PRINCIPLES

Associated with invasive GABHS infections, particularly necrotizing fasciitis or myositis (80% of cases).

DIAGNOSIS

Clinical Presentation
Initial presentation is typically abrupt onset of severe diffuse or localized pain. The systemic manifestations are otherwise similar to Staph TSS, but the desquamating erythroderma is much less common.

Diagnostic Testing
Laboratories
Blood cultures are usually positive and ASO titers are elevated.

TREATMENT

See Table 1.

OUTCOME/PROGNOSIS

Mortality is much higher than in Staphylococcal TSS.

SKIN AND SOFT-TISSUE INFECTIONS

Infections of intact skin are usually treated empirically; however, surgical sampling with culture should be pursued whenever possible.

Because of the rising incidence of community-associated methicillin-resistant *S. aureus* (CA-MRSA) and nosocomial MRSA, severe infections in which *S. aureus* is the likely primary pathogen should be treated empirically with vancomycin, 1 g IV q12h, until susceptibilities are available. Therapy should be switched to oxacillin or cefazolin if the strain proves susceptible. Linezolid and daptomycin should be reserved for severe infections that have not responded to treatment.

CA-MRSA has emerged in patients with no risk factors. It can cause necrotizing skin infections (often associated with the Panton-Valentine leukocidin virulence factor), recurrent boils, or indurated skin lesions mistaken for spider bites. The organism is sensitive to vancomycin and usually to trimethoprim/sulfamethoxazole and clindamycin. Surgical drainage is necessary for most lesions(*N Engl J Med 2007;357: 380*).

Erysipelas

GENERAL PRINCIPLES

Erysipelas appears as painful, superficial, erythematous, sharply demarcated lesion that is usually found on lower extremities and is caused by GABHS in the normal host.

TREATMENT

- Penicillin V, 250 to 1,000 mg PO qid or penicillin G, 1 to 2.0 million units IV q6h, depending on the severity of illness.
- In patients who are penicillin allergic, macrolides or clindamycin are alternatives.

Cellulitis

GENERAL PRINCIPLES

- Cellulitis involves the skin and underlying soft tissue superficial to fascia, with less distinct margins than erysipelas (*Clin Infect Dis 2005;41:1373*).
- GABHS and *S. aureus* are the usual pathogens and are clinically indistinguishable.

TREATMENT

- Initial therapy is oxacillin, 1 to 2 g IV q4h or cefazolin, 1 to 2 g IV q8h; consider vancomycin, 1 g IV q12h in sick patients (see CA-MRSA above). Alternatives for the severely penicillin-allergic patient include macrolides or clindamycin. Mild disease can be treated with oral equivalents of the above. If present, coexisting tinea pedis should be treated with topical antifungals to prevent recurrence of lower extremity cellulitis.
- **Diabetic patients** with cellulitis often require broader-spectrum coverage (see diabetic foot ulcers below).
- **Water-borne pathogens:** Severe cellulitis is sometimes seen after exposure to fresh (*Aeromonas hydrophila*) or salt water (*Vibrio vulnificus*). Initial therapy should include ceftazidime, 2 g IV q8h; cefepime, 2 g IV q8h; or ciprofloxacin, 750 mg PO bid. Doxycycline, 100 mg IV/PO q12h should be added for *Vibrio* infections, which have a strong predilection for patients with cirrhosis.

Infected Decubitus Ulcers and Limb-Threatening Diabetic Foot Ulcers

GENERAL PRINCIPLES

Usually polymicrobial; *superficial swab cultures are unreliable.* Osteomyelitis is a frequent complication and should be excluded.

TREATMENT

- Wound care and debridement is the primary therapy.
- **Moderately severe infections** require systemic antibiotics covering *S. aureus*, anaerobes, and enteric gram-negative organisms. Options include clindamycin, 450 to 900 mg IV q8h plus either a third-generation cephalosporin or ciprofloxacin, 500 to 750 mg PO bid; a β-lactam/β-lactamase inhibitor combination, or a carbapenem (ertapenem, or meropenem) depending on the severity of illness.
- **Less severe diabetic foot infections** are usually due to *S. aureus* and *Streptococci* and can be treated with cephalexin, dicloxacillin, or clindamycin, unless MRSA is isolated, in which case vancomycin may be necessary (*Clin Infect Dis 2004;39:885*).

Necrotizing Fasciitis

GENERAL PRINCIPLES

- This is an infectious disease emergency with high mortality manifested by extensive soft-tissue infection and thrombosis of the microcirculation with resulting necrosis (*Clin Infect Dis 2007;44:705*).
- Infection spreads quickly along fascial planes and may be associated with sepsis or TSS.
- Fournier's gangrene is necrotizing fasciitis of the perineum.

DIAGNOSIS

- Diagnosis is mostly clinical. High suspicion should prompt *immediate surgical exploration* where lack of resistance to probing is diagnostic.
- Bacterial etiology is either mixed (aerobic and anaerobic organisms) or monomicrobial (GABHS or *S. aureus*, including CA-MRSA).

Clinical Presentation

It may present initially like simple cellulitis, with rapid progression to necrosis with dusky, hypoesthetic skin and bulla formation in association with severe pain.

Diagnostic Testing
Laboratories
Cultures of operative specimens and blood should be obtained.

Imaging
Early in the disease process, computed tomography (CT) scans and plain films may demonstrate gas and fascial edema.

TREATMENT

- Aggressive surgical debridement is critical, along with IV antibiotics and volume support.
- Initial empiric antibiotic therapy should be broad spectrum and include a carbapenem or β-lactam/β-lactamase inhibitor or high-dose penicillin, or clindamycin with a fluoroquinolone. Vancomycin should be added until MRSA can be excluded.
- Adjunctive hyperbaric oxygen may be useful.

Anaerobic Myonecrosis (Gas Gangrene)

GENERAL PRINCIPLES

This is usually due to *Clostridium perfringens*, *Clostridium septicum*, *S. aureus*, GABHS, or other anaerobes. Distinguishing this condition from necrotizing fasciitis requires gross inspection of the involved muscle at the time of surgery.

TREATMENT

Treatment requires prompt surgical debridement and combination antimicrobial therapy with intravenous penicillin and clindamycin. A third-generation cephalosporin, ciprofloxacin, or an aminoglycoside should be added until the Gram stain excludes gram-negative involvement.

Osteomyelitis

GENERAL PRINCIPLES

Osteomyelitis is an inflammatory process caused by an infecting organism that can lead to bone destruction. It should be considered when skin or soft-tissue infections overlie bone and when localized bone pain accompanies fever or sepsis (*Lancet 2004;364:369*).

Etiology

- **Acute hematogenous osteomyelitis** is caused most frequently by *S. aureus*.
- **Vertebral osteomyelitis** may be due to *S. aureus*, gram-negative bacilli, or *Mycobacterium tuberculosis*.
- **Osteomyelitis associated with a contiguous focus of infection** may be due to *S. aureus*, gram-negative bacilli, coagulase-negative staphylococci (surgical-site infections), or anaerobes (infected sacral decubitus ulcers).
- **Osteomyelitis in the presence of orthopedic devices** is most often caused by *S. aureus* or coagulase-negative *Staphylococcus* species.
- **Osteomyelitis associated with hemoglobinopathies** is caused by *S. aureus* or *Salmonella* species.
- **Chronic osteomyelitis** is usually associated with a sequestrum of necrotic bone and may involve gram-negative pathogens as well as *S. aureus*.

DIAGNOSIS

- Diagnosis is made by detection of exposed bone through a skin ulcer or by imaging with plain films, bone scintigraphy, or magnetic resonance imaging (*Clin Infect Dis 2008;47:519*). Biopsy and cultures of the affected bone should be performed (before initiation of antimicrobials, if possible) for pathogen-directed therapy.
- Erythrocyte sedimentation rate and C-reactive protein are usually markedly elevated and can be used to monitor the response to therapy.

TREATMENT

- If a causative organism is not identified, empiric therapy should be selected to cover *S. aureus* (oxacillin or vancomycin) and any other likely pathogens (as listed above).

- Cure typically requires at least 4 to 6 weeks of high-dose antimicrobial therapy. Parenteral therapy should be given initially; oral regimens may be considered after 2 to 3 weeks only if the pathogen is susceptible and adequate bactericidal levels can be achieved.
- **Acute hematogenous osteomyelitis.** In the absence of vascular insufficiency or a foreign body, this disease can be treated with antimicrobial therapy alone.
- **Osteomyelitis associated with vascular insufficiency** (e.g., in diabetic patients) is seldom cured by drug therapy alone; revascularization, debridement, or amputation is often required. Infections are generally polymicrobial, including anaerobes.
- **Osteomyelitis in the presence of orthopedic devices** is rarely eradicated by antimicrobials alone. Cure typically requires removal of the device. When removal is impossible, the addition of rifampin, 300 mg PO tid, is recommended. Long-term, suppressive antimicrobial therapy may be needed.
- **Salmonella osteomyelitis** may require surgical treatment and administration of a third-generation cephalosporin or ciprofloxacin.
- **Chronic osteomyelitis.** Eradication requires a combination of medical and surgical treatment to remove the persistent nidus of infection. Long-term, suppressive antimicrobial therapy can be used if surgery is not feasible. Hyperbaric oxygen may be a useful adjunctive therapy.

CENTRAL NERVOUS SYSTEM INFECTIONS

Meningitis

GENERAL PRINCIPLES

- Meningitis is the inflammation of the meninges around the brain and/or spinal cord. It can be caused by bacterial or viral infections, or by noninfectious causes such as medications.
- Meningitis should be considered in any patient with fever and stiff neck or neurologic symptoms, especially if another concurrent infection or head trauma is present.
  - **Aseptic meningitis** is usually milder than bacterial meningitis and may be preceded by upper respiratory symptoms or pharyngitis. Viruses are common causes, as is drug-induced inflammation (e.g., nonsteroidal anti-inflammatory drugs, TMP/SMX). The distinction between bacterial, viral, and noninfectious etiologies cannot be made clinically.
  - **Bacterial meningitis** is a medical emergency. Therapy should not be delayed for diagnostic measures because prognosis depends on rapid initiation of antimicrobial treatment.

DIAGNOSIS

Diagnosis requires a lumbar puncture with measurement of opening pressure, examination of CSF protein, glucose, cell count with differential, and Gram stain with culture. Blood cultures should always be obtained.

- Typical CSF findings in **bacterial meningitis** include a neutrophilic pleocytosis, markedly elevated CSF protein, and decreased glucose level.

- In **aseptic meningitis,** a lymphocytic CSF pleocytosis is common (although neutrophils may predominate very early in the disease course), and CSF PCR can detect enteroviruses, herpes simplex virus (HSV), and HIV.
- Depending on the clinical scenario, other potentially useful CSF studies include rapid plasma reagin (RPR), acid-fast stain, latex agglutination antigen detection, cryptococcal antigen, arbovirus antibodies, and PCR for HSV and enteroviruses.
- A head CT scan before lumbar puncture is controversial but is generally not required for nonelderly, immunocompetent patients who present without focal neurologic abnormalities, seizures, or diminished level of consciousness (*N Engl J Med 2001;345:1727*).

TREATMENT

- Treatment consists of supportive measures and antimicrobial therapy. Whenever acute bacterial meningitis is suspected, high-dose parenteral antimicrobial therapy should be started as soon as possible. Until the etiology of the meningitis is known, an empiric regimen should be based on the CSF Gram stain and patient risk factors:
  - **If no organisms are seen,** high-dose third-generation cephalosporins (ceftriaxone, 2 g IV q12h) and vancomycin, 1 g IV q8–12h, are recommended while culture results are pending.
  - Ampicillin, 2 g IV q4h, should be added for **immunocompromised and older (>50 years of age) patients** for coverage of *Listeria.*
  - In the **postneurosurgical setting, or after head or spinal trauma,** broad-spectrum coverage with high-dose vancomycin and ceftazidime or cefepime, 2 g IV q8h, is indicated. Empiric regimens should be altered once culture and sensitivity data are known.
  - **Dexamethasone,** 10 mg IV q6h, started just before or during initial antibiotics and given for 4 days, reduces the risk of a poor neurologic outcome in patients with meningitis caused by ***Streptococcus pneumoniae.*** Steroids have not proven to be of benefit for bacterial meningitis caused by other organisms, and thus should be discontinued if a different pathogen is isolated (*N Engl J Med 2002;347:1549*).
- **Therapy for specific infections**
  - For ***S. pneumoniae,*** IV penicillin G, 4 million units q4h, for 14 days, is appropriate when the isolate is fully susceptible to penicillin. High-dose ceftriaxone or cefotaxime (as described above) is used for susceptible or intermediate penicillin-resistant isolates, and vancomycin is added if there is ceftriaxone resistance or high-level penicillin resistance. Options for severely penicillin-allergic patients are vancomycin plus rifampin, 300 mg PO tid; or chloramphenicol, 1 g IV q6h. Vancomycin should not be used alone. Dexamethasone, as described above, is a useful adjunct early in treatment.
  - For ***N. meningitidis,*** high-dose ceftriaxone or cefotaxime is continued for at least 5 days after the patient has become afebrile, usually a 7-day total course. Chloramphenicol is an option for the penicillin-allergic patient. Patients should be placed in a private room on respiratory isolation for at least the first 24 hours of treatment. Close contacts (e.g., persons living in the same household and health care workers having close contact with secretions, e.g., intubation) should receive prophylaxis with either ciprofloxacin, 500 mg PO once; rifampin, 600 mg PO bid for 2 days; or ceftriaxone, 250 mg IM. Terminal component complement deficiency (C5–C9) should be ruled out in patients with recurrent meningococcal infections.

- ***Listeria monocytogenes*** meningitis is seen in immunosuppressed adults and the elderly. Treatment is with ampicillin, 2 g IV q4h, in combination with a systemically administered aminoglycoside, for at least 3 to 4 weeks. Trimethoprim/sulfamethoxazole (TMP/SMX; TMP, 5 mg/kg IV q6h) is an alternative for the penicillin-allergic patient.
- **Gram-negative bacillary meningitis** is usually a complication of head trauma or neurosurgical procedures. High-dose ceftazidime or cefepime, 2 g IV q8h, is used for most pathogens, including *Pseudomonas aeruginosa*. High-dose ceftriaxone or cefotaxime may be used for susceptible pathogens. Alternatives include meropenem and ciprofloxacin.
- ***S. aureus*** **meningitis** is usually a result of high-grade bacteremia, direct extension from a parameningeal focus, or neurosurgical procedures. Oxacillin and nafcillin, 2 g IV q4h, are the drugs of choice. First-generation cephalosporins do not reliably penetrate into the CSF. Vancomycin should be used for penicillin-allergic patients, and when methicillin resistance is likely or confirmed. RIF may also be necessary.
- For **enteroviral** meningitis, the treatment is supportive care. Acyclovir, 10 mg/kg IV q8h, is used for moderate to severe **HSV meningitis.**

Ventriculitis and Ventriculoperitoneal Shunt Infections

GENERAL PRINCIPLES

Typically seen in neurosurgical patients.

Etiology
Caused by coagulase-negative staphylococci, *S. aureus*, and *Propionibacter* species.

TREATMENT

Treated with IV vancomycin with or without rifampin or intraventricular vancomycin. Removal of an infected shunt is often necessary for cure.

Encephalitis

GENERAL PRINCIPLES

Definition
Encephalitis is the inflammation of the brain parenchyma, usually associated with viral infections.

Etiology
- **HSV-1** is the most common and most important cause of sporadic infectious encephalitis.
- Other important causes include **Dengue** and the arboviral meningoencephalitides such as **West Nile Virus (WNV)** (see the Mosquito-Borne Infections section).

DIAGNOSIS

Clinical Presentation

Presenting complaints include fever and neurologic abnormalities, particularly with personality change or seizures, and usually without meningeal signs.

Diagnostic Testing

Laboratories

Diagnosis is confirmed by detection of HSV-1 in the CSF by PCR; however, a negative PCR does not rule out HSV encephalitis.

Imaging

Temporal lobe enhancement is typically seen on brain MRI.

TREATMENT

Treatment is acyclovir, 10 mg/kg IV q8h infused over 1 hour with adequate hydration, which should be initiated at first suspicion and continued for 14 to 21 days, unless diagnosis is ruled out. Delayed initiation of therapy greatly increases the risk of poor neurologic outcomes.

Brain Abscess

GENERAL PRINCIPLES

Etiology

Brain abscess in the immunocompetent host is usually bacterial in origin and a result of spread from a contiguous focus or from septic emboli from endocarditis. Infection is often mixed, with oral streptococci, *S. aureus*, and anaerobes being the most common pathogens.

DIAGNOSIS

Diagnostic Testing

Imaging

Diagnosis is radiographic, with ring-enhancing lesions seen on MRI or contrast CT scans. A microbiologic etiology must be determined by aspiration, biopsy, or at the time of surgery.

TREATMENT

Empiric therapy should be chosen to cover the most likely pathogens based on the primary infection site.

Medications

When no preceding infection can be found, a third-generation cephalosporin combined with metronidazole and vancomycin is a reasonable regimen until culture data are available.

Surgical Management

Therapy is often surgical with the addition of systemic antimicrobials.

Neurocysticercosis

GENERAL PRINCIPLES

Etiology

This disease is caused by cyst forms of *Taenia solium* in the brain. Infection is acquired from eating undercooked pork that contains the eggs of *T. solium*, which is endemic in Mexico and Central America.

DIAGNOSIS

Diagnosis should be suspected in patients with new-onset seizures of unknown etiology and exposure to endemic areas. Brain imaging reveals characteristic multiple unilocular cysts that may or may not enhance. Serologic tests are available at the Centers for Disease Control and Prevention (CDC).

Clinical Presentation

It can present as new-onset seizures, hydrocephalus, or focal neurologic abnormalities.

TREATMENT

Treatment may require surgery and/or high-dose albendazole or praziquantel, depending on the location of cysts and severity. Anticonvulsants, intracranial pressure monitoring, and steroids can be needed to control symptoms.

CARDIOVASCULAR INFECTIONS

Infective Endocarditis

GENERAL PRINCIPLES

Epidemiology

- The incidence of acute bacterial endocarditis (ABE) and health care–associated endocarditis is rising (*Arch Int Med 2009;109:463*).
- **Prosthetic valve endocarditis (PVE)** occurs in 1% to 4% of patients with prosthetic valves.

Etiology

- Infective endocarditis (IE) is usually caused by gram-positive cocci. *S. aureus* is the most common pathogen and is often associated with intravascular devices and injection drug use.
- Gram-negative and fungal IE occur infrequently and are usually associated with injection drug use or prosthetic valves.
- **Acute bacterial endocarditis or ABE.** Causative organisms are usually *S. aureus* and gram-negative bacilli.

- **Subacute bacterial endocarditis or SBE.** Causative organisms are usually *Strepto-coccus* species. A deformed or previously damaged valve is the usual focus of infection in SBE.
- Dental procedures and bacteremia from distant foci of infection are frequent seeding events.
- **Prosthetic valve endocarditis or PVE.** Early infections (within 2 months of surgery) are caused by *S. aureus*, coagulase-negative staphylococci, gram-negative bacilli, and *Candida* species. S. aureus, coagulase-negative staphylococci, enterococci, and virid-ians strep are the most common causes of late-onset PVE.

DIAGNOSIS

Clinical Presentation

- Patients with **ABE** may present within 3 to 10 days with critical illness.
- **SBE** presents over weeks to months with constitutional symptoms (fever, malaise, anorexia), immune complex disease (nephritis, arthralgias), and emboli (renal, splenic, and cerebral infarcts; petechiae; Osler nodes; Janeway lesions).

Diagnostic Testing

Laboratories

- The most reliable diagnostic criterion is continuous bacteremia in a compatible clinical setting. Blood cultures are positive in at least 90% of patients, but may be negative if the patient has received prior antimicrobial therapy.
- Three blood cultures should be taken from separate sites over at least a 1-hour period before empiric therapy is begun in patients who are critically ill. In patients with SBE, repeat blood cultures and observation is a reasonable option.

Imaging

- Patients with IE and vegetations seen by transthoracic echocardiography are at higher risk of embolism, heart failure, and valvular disruption; however, a negative transthoracic echocardiogram does not exclude the diagnosis of IE.
- When clinical evidence of IE exists, **transesophageal echocardiography (TEE)** improves the sensitivity of the Duke criteria to diagnose IE, especially in patients with prosthetic valves (*Clin Infect Dis 2000;30:633*).
- Echocardiography helps define potential need for surgical intervention (see indications for surgery below).

TREATMENT

- *High doses of intravenous antimicrobials for extended periods are required.*
- Quantitative susceptibility testing of the responsible organism(s) to multiple antibiotics is more reliable than disk diffusion testing and is essential for optimal treatment.
- Baseline audiometry is recommended for patients who will receive 7 or more days of aminoglycoside therapy, with repeat testing weekly while on treatment or if symptoms develop.
- **ABE** often requires empiric antimicrobial treatment before culture results become available. Initial treatment for *S. aureus* should include vancomycin, 15 mg/kg IV q12h, plus gentamicin or tobramycin, 1.0 mg/kg IV q8h. Therapy should then be modified on the basis of culture and susceptibility data. For methicillin-sensitive isolates, oxacillin, 2 g IV q4h, is superior to vancomycin and should be substituted.

- **SBE** caused by susceptible organisms should be treated with penicillin, as this typically results in cure rates of >90%. Therapy can usually be delayed until culture data confirm specific organism and susceptibilities.
- **PVE** should be treated aggressively for extended periods because of the increased risk for treatment failure and relapse. See below for indications for surgical replacement.
- **Therapy for specific infections** (see table for details)
  - For **viridians streptococci** that are penicillin-susceptible, penicillin G or ceftriaxone for 4 weeks should be given. An abbreviated 2-week course in combination with gentamicin can be given, but carries the risk of nephro- and ototoxicity and should not be used for PVE or serious disease. Streptococci with intermediate or high resistance to penicillin should receive combination and often extended therapy. Penicillin desensitization is preferable to vancomycin for penicillin allergy.
  - ***S. pyogenes*** and ***S. pneumoniae*** should be treated with penicillin G, 2 to 4 million units IV q4h, for 4 to 6 weeks. Penicillin-resistant pneumococci should be treated with ceftriaxone, 2 g IV q24h for 4 to 6 weeks. *Streptococcus bovis* bacteremia and endocarditis are associated with lower GI tract disease, including neoplasms. Groups B and G streptococcal endocarditis may also be associated with lower intestinal pathology.
  - ***Enterococcus* species** cause 5% to 20% of cases of SBE. Isolates from patients with enterococcal endocarditis should be screened for β-lactamase production and susceptibility to vancomycin, quinupristin/dalfopristin, linezolid, and gentamicin. Vancomycin-resistant enterococcus (VRE) IE is difficult to treat, and infectious disease consult is recommended.
  - ***S. aureus*** should be treated with oxacillin. Penicillins are superior to vancomycin, and desensitization is preferred when possible (*Medicine (Baltimore) 2003;82:333*). Cefazolin can be substituted in penicillin-allergic patients with no history of anaphylaxis. Right-sided IE in intravenous drug users can be treated with 2 weeks of oxacillin plus an aminoglycoside. Vancomycin, linezolid, and daptomycin can be used for MRSA. Initial low-dose gentamicin for synergy in native valve IE risks renal impairment without demonstrated benefit (*Clin Infect Dis 2009;48:713*).
  - ***Coagulase-negative staphylococcus* (e.g., *Staphylococcus epidermidis*)** IE primarily occurs in patients with valvular prostheses although native valve endocarditis is increasing, especially in health care settings. *Staphylococcus lugdunensis* IE is associated with a high rate of perivalvular extension and metastatic spread. These organisms are increasingly resistant to β-lactam agents.
  - **PVE** requires aggressive combination therapy for at least 6 weeks. Initial empiric therapy pending culture data includes rifampin, which is added to vancomycin and gentamicin to improve biofilm penetration. Oxacillin should be substituted for vancomycin if supported by culture and sensitivity data. Treatment failure or relapse is common.
  - **HACEK** is an acronym for a group of fastidious, slow-growing gram-negative bacteria (*Haemophilus*, *Actinobacillus*, *Cardiobacterium*, *Eikenella*, and *Kingella* species) that have a predilection for infecting heart valves.
  - **Blood culture–negative IE** is usually encountered when prior antimicrobial therapy has been given, or, rarely, with fastidious pathogens, such as nutritionally deficient streptococci, HACEK organisms, *Coxiella burnetii* (Q fever), *Bartonella*, *Brucella*, *Tropheryma whippelii* (Whipple's disease), and fungi. Empiric therapy as for HACEK can be initiated despite negative cultures (Table 2).
- **Response to antimicrobial therapy**
  - Frequently, clinical improvement is seen within 3 to 10 days.

Table 2   Treatment of Endocarditis Caused by Specific Organisms[a]

Organism	Antibiotic Regimen	Duration	Notes
Viridians streptococci			
MIC < 0.12 mcg/mL	• [Penicillin G 12–18 million units IV q24h or Ceftriaxone] + gentamicin • Vancomycin if PCN allergic	• 4 wk (2 wks total if in combination with gentamicin)	• 2-wk course not indicated for prosthetics valves, major embolic or extended symptoms.
MIC 0.12–0.5 mcg/mL	• [Penicillin G 4 million units IV q4h or ceftriaxone] + gentamicin • Vancomycin if PCN allergic	• 4 wk total with 2 wk of gentamicin	
MIC > 0.5 mcg/mL	• Ampicillin/sulbactam + gentamicin • Vancomycin + gentamicin	• 4–6 wk	
Enterococcus species			
Penicillin-susceptible	• Ampicillin + gentamicin • Vancomycin	• 4–6 wk	• Substitute streptomycin 7 mg/kg q12h for high-level gentamicin resistance.
Penicillin-resistant	• *β-Lactamase:* Ampicillin/sulbactam + gentamicin • *Intrinsically resistant:* Vancomycin + gentamicin	• 6 wk	
Vancomycin- and ampicillin-resistant	• Linezolid or daptomycin • Quinupristin/dalfopristin ± doxycycline	• ≥8 wk	• Consult infectious diseases specialist.

(continued)

Table 2   Treatment of Endocarditis Caused by Specific Organisms[a] *(Continued)*

Organism	Antibiotic Regimen	Duration	Notes
Staphylococcus species (prosthetic valve) MSSA/MSSE MRSA/MRSE	• Oxacillin + rifampin + gentamicin • Vancomycin + rifampin + gentamicin	• ≥6 wk total (2 wk of gentamicin)	
Staphylococcus species (native valve)	• Oxacillin • Cefazolin if penicillin allergy without anaphylaxis • Oxacillin + gentamicin for right-sided IE in IV drug users* • Vancomycin or daptomycin or linezolid if anaphylactic allergy or methicillin-resistant	• 4–6 wk • *2 wk for combination therapy in right-sided IE	• Initial low-dose gentamicin for synergy in native-valve S. aureus IE may not be beneficial.
HACEK organisms and culture-negative IE	• Ceftriaxone or ampicillin-sulbactam or ciprofloxacin	• 4 wk	• HACEK stands for *Haemophilus, Actinobacillus, Cardiobacterium, Eikenella, Kingella.*

Dosing: Ceftriaxone, 2 g IV q24h; gentamicin, 2 g qd or 1 mg/kg q8h; vancomycin, 1 g IV q24h; ampicillin-sulbactam, 3 g IV q6h; ampicillin, 2 g IV q4h; oxacillin, 2 g IV q4h; rifampin, 300 mg PO q8h; cefazolin, 2 g IV q8h; daptomycin, 6 mg/kg/d; linezolid, 600 mg IV q12h; ciprofloxacin, 400 mg IV q12h. Baseline and weekly audiometry recommended for patients receiving aminoglycosides for >7 days. Monitor aminoglycoside and vancomycin levels. Goal vancomycin trough levels are near 15 mcg/mL.
[a] See *Circulation 2005;11:e393.*

- Daily blood cultures should be obtained until sterility is documented.
- Persistent or recurrent fever usually represents extensive cardiac infection but also might be due to septic emboli, drug hypersensitivity, or subsequent nosocomial infection (*Circulation 2005;111:e393*). (See Table 2 for detailed treatment recommendations.)

Surgical Management
Prosthetic valve endocarditis

- Late PVE occurs >2 months after surgery; the organisms causing late PVE are similar to those seen on native valves (staphylococci, streptococci, and enterococci).
- PVE must be considered in any patient with sustained bacteremia after valve surgery.
- For native valve endocarditis, indications for surgery include refractory heart failure, aortic or mitral regurgitation with hemodynamic evidence of elevated left ventricular end-diastolic pressure, complications such as heart block, annular or aortic abscess, fistula or perforation, and infection with fungi or other highly resistant organisms. Recurrent emboli and sustained bacteremia on appropriate therapy are other indications.
- For PVE, indications include heart failure, valve dehiscence, increasing valve obstruction or worsening regurgitation, complications such as abscess formation, persistent bacteremia or recurrent emboli, and relapsing infection.

SPECIAL CONSIDERATIONS

The American Heart Association recommendations for prophylaxis for IE have been changed recently and are outlined in Table 3.

Myocarditis

GENERAL PRINCIPLES

- When the heart is involved in an inflammatory process, the cause is often an infectious agent. Myocarditis may occur during and after viral, rickettsial, bacterial, and parasitic infection.
- Viruses are the most frequent cause, and include entero viruses (Coxsackie B and echovirus), adenovirus, human herpes virus 6, parvovirus B-19, and many others. It is also a rare complication of smallpox vaccination.

DIAGNOSIS

Diagnostic Testing
Laboratories
- Nasopharyngeal swab testing, serology, and PCR studies may be performed for viruses.
- Tissue diagnoses via endomyocardial biopsies may be helpful.

TREATMENT

Therapeutic regimen should be targeted to the identified agent. The role of IV immunoglobulin and antiviral agents in viral-mediated myocarditis remains anecdotal.

Table 3	Endocarditis Prophylaxis[a]
Clinical Scenario	**Drug and Dosage**

I. Endocarditis prophylaxis is recommended for the following cardiac conditions: prosthetic valves, previous endocarditis, unrepaired congenital heart disease, including palliative shunts or conduits, repaired congenital heart disease with prosthetic material during the first 6 mo after procedure, or with residual defects at or adjacent to the site of the prosthetic device, cardiac valvulopathy in transplant recipients.

II. Regimens for dental, oral, or respiratory tract procedures (including dental extractions, periodontal or endodontal procedures, professional teeth cleaning, bronchoscopy with biopsy, rigid bronchoscopy, surgery on respiratory mucosa, tonsillectomy).

Standard prophylaxis	Amoxicillin, 2 g PO 1 h before procedure
Unable to take PO	Ampicillin, 2 g IM or IV, or cefazolin or ceftriaxone, 1 g IM or IV within 30 min before procedure
Penicillin-allergic patient	Clindamycin, 600 mg PO, or cephalexin, 2 g PO, or clarithromycin or azithromycin, 500 mg PO 1 h before procedure
Penicillin-allergic and unable to take PO	Clindamycin, 600 mg IV, or cefazolin or ceftriaxone, 1 g IV within 30 min before procedure

III. Gastrointestinal and genitourinary procedures do not require routine use of prophylaxis. High-risk patients infected or colonized with enterococci should receive amoxicillin, ampicillin, or vancomycin to eradicate the organism prior to urinary tract manipulation.

IV. Prophylaxis is recommended for procedures on infected skin, skin structures, or musculoskeletal tissue ONLY for patients with cardiac conditions outlined above. An antistaphylococcal penicillin or cephalosporin should be used.

[a]See *Circulation 2007;116:1736*

Pericarditis

GENERAL PRINCIPLES

Definition

Acute pericarditis is a syndrome caused by inflammation of the pericardium and characterized by chest pain, a pericardial friction rub, and diffuse ST-segment elevations on ECG.

Etiology

- In most cases, viruses are implicated as the infectious etiologies of pericarditis.
- TB or histoplasmosis are occasional causes (see the Tuberculosis section).

TREATMENT

The role of antiviral therapies in viral pericarditis remains unclear. NSAIDS can be used for pain.

UPPER RESPIRATORY TRACT INFECTIONS

Pharyngitis

GENERAL PRINCIPLES

Etiology

Pharyngitis is usually caused by viruses, although distinction from streptococcal (GABHS) and gonococcal pharyngitis is difficult on clinical grounds.

DIAGNOSIS

- Diagnostic testing is usually reserved for symptomatic patients exposed to streptococcal pharyngitis, individuals with signs of significant infection (i.e., fever, pharyngeal exudate, and cervical adenopathy), patients whose symptoms fail to clear despite symptomatic therapy, and patients with a history of rheumatic fever.
- Rapid antigen detection testing (RADT) is useful for identifying **GABHS,** which requires therapy to prevent acute pyogenic complications and rheumatic fever. A negative test does not reliably exclude GABHS, making a culture necessary when RADT is negative.
- Serology for **Epstein–Barr virus** (e.g., heterophile agglutinin or monospot) and examination of a peripheral blood smear for atypical lymphocytes should be performed when infectious mononucleosis is suspected.

Differential Diagnosis

- **Acute HIV infection** should be considered in the differential diagnosis of pharyngitis with atypical lymphocytosis and negative streptococcus and Epstein–Barr virus testing.
- **Epiglottitis** should be considered in the febrile patient who complains of severe sore throat, odynophagia, new-onset drooling, and dysphagia but in whom minimal findings are noted on inspection of the pharynx. Diagnosis relies on clinical suspicion.

TREATMENT

- Most cases of pharyngitis are self-limited and do not require antimicrobial therapy.
- Treatment for **GABHS** is needed with a positive culture or RADT, if the patient is at high risk for development of rheumatic fever, or if the diagnosis is strongly suspected, pending the results of culture. Treatment schedules include penicillin V, 250 mg PO qid or 500 mg PO bid for 10 days, erythromycin, 250 mg PO qid for 10 days, or benzathine penicillin G, 1.2 million units IM as a one-time dose.
- Gonococcal pharyngitis is treated with ceftriaxone 125 mg IM as a single dose.

Epiglottitis

GENERAL PRINCIPLES

Epiglottitis should be considered in the febrile patient who complains of severe sore throat, odynophagia, new-onset drooling, and dysphagia but in whom minimal findings are noted on inspection of the pharynx.

DIAGNOSIS

Diagnosis relies on clinical suspicion.

Diagnostic Testing

Laboratories
Throat and blood cultures are useful in determining the etiology.

Imaging
Lateral soft-tissue radiograph of the neck should be obtained to assess airway occlusion.

TREATMENT

Prompt treatment including hospitalization and otolaryngologic consultation for airway management is suggested in all suspected cases. Antimicrobial therapy should include an agent that is active against *Haemophilus influenzae*, such as ceftriaxone, 1 to 2 g IV q24h, or cefotaxime, 1 to 2 g IV q6–8h.

Sinusitis

GENERAL PRINCIPLES

Sinusitis is caused by obstruction of the osteomeatal complex. The goals of medical therapy for acute and chronic sinusitis are to control infection, reduce tissue edema, facilitate drainage, maintain patency of the sinus ostia, and break the pathologic cycle that leads to chronic sinusitis.

Etiology

- **Acute rhinosinusitis.** The etiology is usually upper respiratory viruses. Bacterial pathogens, such as *S. pneumoniae, H. influenzae, Moraxella catarrhalis*, and anaerobes are involved in less than 2% of cases and should be considered only if symptoms are severe or if they persist for more than 10 days (*Ann Intern Med 2001;134:479*).
- **Chronic rhinosinusitis.** Possible contributing factors include asthma, nasal polyps, allergies, or immune deficiency. The etiologic agents include those for acute sinusitis, as well as *S. aureus, Corynebacterium diphtheriae, Prevotella* species, and *Veillonella* species.

DIAGNOSIS

The diagnosis requires objective evidence of mucosal disease, usually with a sinus CT; plain films are not recommended. Nasal endoscopy may complement CT scan by permitting direct inspection of the mucosa of the ethmoid air cells. Cultures can be obtained from endoscopy or sinus puncture. Nasal swabs are not helpful.

Clinical Presentation

- **Acute rhinosinusitis** is a clinical diagnosis that presents with cough, purulent nasal discharge, and sinus tenderness with or without fever, lasting for less than 4 weeks.
- **Chronic rhinosinusitis.** With chronic rhinosinusitis, patients experience nasal congestion or obstruction with symptoms lasting more than 12 weeks. Secondary complaints include pain, pressure, anterior or posterior nasal discharge, and decreased sense of smell.

TREATMENT

- **Acute rhinosinusitis**
  - **Symptomatic treatment** is the mainstay of therapy, including systemic decongestants and analgesics with or without a short course of topical decongestant.
  - **Empiric antibiotic therapy** is indicated only for severe persistent symptoms or failure of symptomatic therapy. First-line antibiotics include a 10-day regimen of amoxicillin, 500 mg PO tid, or TMP/SMX, one double-strength (DS) tablet PO bid. Second-generation cephalosporins, amoxicillin-clavulanate, and macrolides are good second-line agents in case of primary treatment failure.
- **Chronic rhinosinusitis.** Treatment usually includes topical and/or systemic glucocorticoids; the role of antimicrobial agents is unclear. If they are used, amoxicillin-clavulanate is the first-line treatment, with clindamycin for penicillin-allergic patients. Some chronic cases require endoscopic surgery.

Influenza Virus Infection

GENERAL PRiNCIPLES

Definition

Influenza virus infection causes an acute, self-limited febrile illness with myalgias, cough, and malaise. The virus is readily transmissible and associated with outbreaks of varying severity during the winter months.

DIAGNOSIS

Diagnosis of influenza is usually made clinically during influenza season, with confirmation by nasopharyngeal swab for rapid antigen testing, PCR, or direct fluorescent antibody test and culture.

TREATMENT

- Treatment is usually symptomatic. Antiviral medications may shorten the duration of illness but must be initiated within 24 to 48 hours of the onset of symptoms to be effective in immunocompetent patients.
  - The **neuraminidase inhibitors** (oseltamivir, 75 mg PO bid or zanamivir, 10 mg inhaled twice a day; each for 5 days) are used in treatment and prophylaxis of influenza A and B.
  - **Adamantanes** (amantadine and rimantadine, each 100 mg PO bid) are *not* effective for the treatment and prophylaxis of influenza B.
  - Circulating strains change annually with varying resistance patterns to both classes of antivirals. *Treatment decisions must be based on annual resistance data*, usually available from the CDC Web site http://www.cdc.gov.
- **Vaccination** is the most reliable prevention strategy. Annual vaccination is recommended for all children aged 6 months to 18 years, and for any adult who wants to avoid influenza infection. Those over age 50, women who are or will be pregnant during influenza season, and anyone with underlying medical conditions are specifically encouraged to be vaccinated, as are their contacts, including health care workers.

COMPLICATIONS

Complications of influenza virus infection include viral pneumonia and secondary bacterial pneumonia. Viral antigenic drift and shift can cause emergence of strains with enhanced virulence or the potential for pandemic spread, requiring modified therapy or heightened infection control measures (see the Emerging Infections and Bioterrorism section).

LOWER RESPIRATORY TRACT INFECTIONS

Acute Bronchitis

GENERAL PRINCIPLES

Acute bronchitis involves inflammation of the bronchi causing acute onset of cough, sputum production, and symptoms of upper respiratory tract infection.

Etiology

The usual etiologies are viral agents, such as coronavirus, rhinovirus, influenza, or parainfluenza. Uncommon causes include *Mycoplasma pneumoniae*, *Chlamydophila pneumoniae*, and *Bordetella pertussis*.

DIAGNOSIS

Diagnosis is usually made clinically. Pneumonia should be routinely ruled out either clinically or radiographically, and diagnostic tests for influenza should be performed if it is suspected. Cough that lasts for >2 weeks in an adult should be evaluated for pertussis with a nasopharyngeal swab for culture or PCR.

TREATMENT

Treatment is symptomatic and is directed most often at controlling cough (dextromethorphan, 15 mg PO q6h). Routine antimicrobial use is not recommended unless pertussis is confirmed (*Ann Intern Med 2001;134:521*).

- **Pertussis** treatment is clarithromycin 500 mg PO bid for 14 days or azithromycin, 500 mg PO single dose, followed by 250 mg PO daily for 4 more days.
- Pertussis cases should be reported to the local health department for contact tracing and administration of postexposure prophylaxis with azithromycin when indicated.

Community-Acquired Pneumonia

GENERAL PRINCIPLES

Etiology

The predominant etiologic agent is *S. pneumoniae*, in which multidrug resistance is rapidly increasing. Pneumonia caused by atypical agents, such as *Legionella pneumophila*, *C. pneumoniae*, or *M. pneumoniae*, cannot be reliably determined clinically.

DIAGNOSIS

Diagnosis is based on clinical, laboratory, and radiographic findings. Fever and respiratory symptoms, including cough with sputum production, dyspnea, and pleurisy, are common presenting features in immunocompetent patients. Signs include tachypnea, rales, or consolidation on auscultation.

Diagnostic Testing

Laboratories
- Assessment of etiologic agents in all hospitalized patients should include pretreatment expectorated sputum examination for Gram stain and culture and blood cultures.
- If an atypical agent is suspected, urinary *Legionella* antigen should be sent. PCR assays for detecting other atypical pathogens may be available in some areas. Acute and convalescent serologic testing can retrospectively identify several atypical pathogens including *C. pneumoniae*, *C. burnetii* (Q fever), and *Hantavirus*.

Imaging
Chest radiograph reveals a new pulmonary infiltrate.

Diagnostic Procedures
Fiberoptic bronchoscopy is used for detection of less common infections, especially in immunocompromised hosts, associated anatomic lesions, biopsy for histopathologic workup, or quantitative cultures.

TREATMENT

- Most patients can be treated as outpatients, although all should be evaluated for severity of illness, comorbid factors, and oxygenation. Guidelines giving detailed empiric treatment regimens have been published, with an emphasis on targeting the most likely pathogens within specific risk groups (*Clin Infect Dis 2003;37:1405*). Antibiotic therapy should be narrowed if a specific microbiological etiology is obtained.
- **Immunocompetent outpatients** with no recent antibiotic exposure and no comorbidities should receive doxycycline or a macrolide.
- **Patients with recent antibiotic exposure or comorbidities** should receive a respiratory fluoroquinolone (e.g., moxifloxacin) monotherapy or advanced macrolide (azithromycin or clarithromycin) with or without high-dose amoxicillin.
- **Hospitalized patients** should be treated with ceftriaxone, 1 g IV daily, or cefotaxime, 1 g IV q8h, plus azithromycin or clarithromycin, or monotherapy with a respiratory fluoroquinolone.
- In **critically ill patients,** the addition of azithromycin or clarithromycin or a respiratory fluoroquinolone to a β-lactam regimen is necessary to provide coverage for *L. pneumophila*. MRSA coverage with vancomycin or linezolid should also be considered. Intravenously administered penicillin G, which reaches high concentrations in lung tissue, remains an effective treatment for sensitive *S. pneumoniae* isolates (*Clin Infect Dis 2003;37:230*).
- **Thoracentesis** of pleural effusions should be performed, with analysis of pH, cell count, Gram stain and bacterial culture, protein, and lactate dehydrogenase (see Chapter 7, Pulmonary Diseases). Empyemas should be drained.

Lung Abscess

GENERAL PRINCIPLES

Epidemiology
Polymicrobial infection is common.

Etiology
Lung abscess typically results from macro aspiration of oral flora. Bacterial causes of lung abscess include oral anaerobes (*Prevotella* spp., *Actinomyces* spp., and anaerobic and microaerophilic streptococci), enteric gram-negative bacilli, *S. aureus*, and *S. pneumoniae* serotype III.

Risk Factors
Risk factors include periodontal disease and conditions that predispose patients to aspiration of oropharyngeal contents.

DIAGNOSIS

Diagnosis is straightforward as chest radiography is very sensitive and typically reveals infiltrates with cavitation and air–fluid levels in dependent areas of the lung, such as lower lobes or the posterior segments of the upper lobes.

Clinical Presentation
Clinical presentation of lung abscess is indolent and reminiscent of pulmonary tuberculosis, with dyspnea, fever, chills, night sweats, weight loss, and cough productive of putrid or blood-streaked sputum.

TREATMENT

Treatment may require drainage, either postural or surgical. Antibiotic treatment should include an antipneumococcal fluoroquinolone plus clindamycin or a β-lactam/β-lactamase inhibitor. MRSA can cause cavitary lung lesions similar to abscesses too, in which case vancomycin or linezolid could be used.

Tuberculosis

GENERAL PRINCIPLES

Epidemiology
The prevalence of TB, particularly multidrug-resistant forms (MDR-TB), has increased among immigrants from Southeast Asia, Sub-Saharan Africa, the Indian subcontinent, and Central America. Extensively drug resistant TB (XDR-TB) is becoming increasingly prevalent in Sub-Saharan Africa.

Etiology
Tuberculosis is a systemic disease caused by *M. tuberculosis*. Most cases are the result of reactivation of prior infection.

Risk Factors

Persons at highest risk include those with HIV infection, silicosis, diabetes mellitus, chronic renal insufficiency, malignancy, malnutrition, and other forms of immuno-suppression, especially therapy with tumor necrosis factor (TNF) antagonists like infliximab and etanercept (*Clin Infect Dis 2004;39:300*).

DIAGNOSIS

Drug susceptibility testing should be performed on all initial isolates as well as on follow-up isolates from patients who do not respond to standard therapy.

Clinical Presentation

The most frequent clinical presentation is pulmonary disease, with either a focal infiltrate or a disseminated, "miliary" pattern. Focal infiltrates are classically in the upper lobes for reactivation disease. Lower lobe disease can be seen in primary infection.

Differential Diagnosis

Extrapulmonary disease may present as cervical lymphadenitis, genitourinary disease, osteomyelitis, miliary dissemination, meningitis, peritonitis, or pericarditis.

Diagnostic Testing

Laboratories
- The diagnosis is usually made with positive fluorochrome or acid-fast bacteria (AFB) smears of sputum, which are presumptive evidence of active TB, although nontuber-culous mycobacteria and some *Nocardia* species may give positive results with these techniques.
- TB can take several weeks to grow in culture so if the clinical suspicion is high, presumptive therapy even with negative smears may be indicated until cultures are negative. Use of radiometric culture systems and species-specific DNA probes can provide results faster than traditional methods.

TREATMENT

Treatment (*Clin Infect Dis 2000;31(3):633*) does not have to take place in a hospital setting, but hospitalization to initiate therapy provides an opportunity for intensive patient education. If a patient is hospitalized, proper isolation in a **negative-pressure room** is essential.

- The local health department should be notified of all cases of TB so that contacts can be identified and adherence to the regimen can be ensured by directly observed therapy.
- At least two drugs to which the organism is susceptible must be used because of the high frequency with which primary drug resistance to a single drug develops. Extended therapy is necessary because of the prolonged generation time of mycobac-teria. Because adherence to multidrug regimens for prolonged periods is difficult, directly observed therapy should be used for all patients.
- **Initial therapy** of uncomplicated pulmonary TB should usually include four drugs: INH (5 mg/kg; maximum, 300 mg PO daily), rifampin (RIF, 10 mg/kg; maximum, 600 mg PO daily), pyrazinamide (PZA, 15 to 30 mg/kg; maximum, 2 g PO daily),

and either ethambutol (EMB, 15 to 25 mg/kg PO daily) or streptomycin (15 mg/kg; maximum, 1.5 g IM daily). Pyridoxine (vitamin B_6), 25 to 50 mg PO daily, should be used with INH to prevent neuropathy.

- If the isolate proves to be **fully susceptible** to INH and RIF, then EMB (or streptomycin) can be dropped and INH, RIF, and PZA continued to finish 8 weeks, followed by 16 weeks of INH and RIF. Patients at high risk for relapse (cavitary pulmonary disease or positive TB cultures after 2 months of therapy) should be treated for 9 months. After at least 2 weeks of daily therapy, the drugs can be administered two or three times per week at adjusted doses.
- When **INH resistance** is documented, the INH should be discontinued, and the remaining three drugs should be continued for the duration of therapy. Organisms that are resistant only to INH can be effectively treated with a 6-month regimen if a standard four-drug regimen consisting of INH, RIF, PZA, and EMB or streptomycin was started initially. Therapy for multidrug-resistant TB has been less well studied, and consultation with an expert in the treatment of TB should be considered.

- **Extrapulmonary disease** in adults can be treated in the same manner as pulmonary disease, with 6- to 9-month regimens. TB meningitis should be treated for 9 to 12 months.
- **Glucocorticoid administration.** In TB, the administration of glucocorticoids is controversial. Prednisone, 1 mg/kg PO daily initially, has been used *in combination with* antituberculous drugs for life-threatening complications such as meningitis (*NEJM 2004;351:1741*; *Pediatrics 1997;99:226*) and pericarditis (*MMWR 2003;52(RR-11):1*).
- **Monitoring response to therapy.** Patients with pulmonary TB whose sputum AFB smears are positive before treatment should submit sputum for AFB smear and culture every 1 to 2 weeks until AFB smears become negative. Sputum should then be obtained monthly until two consecutive negative cultures are documented. Conversion of cultures from positive to negative is the most reliable indicator of a response to treatment. Continued symptoms or persistently positive AFB smears or cultures after 3 months of treatment should raise the suspicion of drug resistance or nonadherence and prompt referral to an expert in the treatment of TB.
- **Monitoring for adverse reactions.** Most patients should have a baseline laboratory evaluation at the start of therapy that includes hepatic enzymes, bilirubin, CBC, and serum creatinine. Routine laboratory monitoring for patients with normal baseline values is probably unnecessary except in patients with HIV, concerns for alcohol consumption, chronic liver disease, and in pregnant women. Monthly clinical evaluations with specific inquiries about symptoms of drug toxicity are essential. Patients who are taking EMB should be tested monthly for visual acuity and red–green color perception.
- **Pregnant patients** should not receive PZA or streptomycin, and thus a 9-month course of therapy is recommended. Pregnancy-related TB should be treated with INH, RIF, EMB, and pyridoxine for the first 2 months, after which the EMB can be stopped if the isolate proves to be drug sensitive.
- **Latent tuberculosis infection.**
  - Latent TB infection (LTBI) occurs when someone has been exposed to tuberculosis, as demonstrated by a positive TST or QuantiFERON-TB blood test, but has no signs or symptoms of current active disease. Criteria for a **positive TST** are based on the **maximum diameter of induration** (not erythema).

- ○ A **5-mm induration** is considered positive in patients with HIV infection or another defect in cell-mediated immunity, close contacts of a known case of TB, patients with chest radiographs that are typical for healed TB, and individuals with organ transplantation or other immunosuppression.
- ○ A **10-mm induration** is considered positive in immigrants from high-prevalence areas (Asia, Africa, Latin America, Eastern Europe), prisoners, the homeless, parenteral drug abusers, nursing home residents, low-income populations, patients with chronic medical illnesses or health and economic disparities, and those people who have frequent contact with these groups (e.g., health care workers, prison guards).
- ○ A **15-mm induration** is a positive TST for otherwise healthy individuals who are not in a high-prevalence group.
- Untreated, approximately 5% of persons with LTBI develop active TB disease within 2 years of infection. TB disease develops in an additional 5% of persons over the life span. Adequate prophylactic treatment can substantially reduce the risk of disease.
- **Chemoprophylaxis for latent tuberculosis infection**
- Chemoprophylaxis for LTBI should be administered only after active disease has been ruled out by a proper evaluation (chest radiography, sputum collection, or both). INH, 300 mg PO daily for 9 months, should be administered to persons with LTBI who have risk factors for progression to active TB disease, regardless of age.
  - ○ Risk factors for progression include a TST conversion within 2 years of a previously negative TST; a history of untreated TB or chest radiographic evidence of previous disease; HIV infection, diabetes mellitus, end-stage renal disease, hematologic or lymphoreticular malignancy, conditions associated with rapid weight loss, chronic malnutrition, silicosis, or patients who are receiving immunosuppressive therapy; household members and other close contacts of patients with active disease who have a reactive TST.
- Persons with **HIV** infection who have had *known contact with a patient with active TB should be treated for LTBI regardless of tuberculin status.*
- Contacts with a nonreactive TST should undergo a repeat TST 3 months after the last exposure to the infectious person.
- A 9-month course of INH is adequate for all patients with LTBI even among those with HIV infection. Alternative regimens of shorter duration but higher toxicity can be considered in consultation with a TB expert. Referral to the health department for chemoprophylaxis is recommended to ensure adherence and to monitor for medication-related complications.

GASTROINTESTINAL AND ABDOMINAL INFECTIONS

Peritonitis

GENERAL PRINCIPLES

- **Primary** or **spontaneous bacterial peritonitis (SBP)** is a common complication of cirrhosis and ascites and should be ruled out in any patients with ascites and fever

or other clinical decompensation including encephalopathy, renal failure, and GI bleed.
- *M. tuberculosis* and *Neisseria gonorrhoeae* (Fitz-Hugh–Curtis syndrome in women) also occasionally cause primary peritonitis in patients at risk.
- **Secondary peritonitis** is caused by a perforated viscus in the GI or genitourinary tract, or contiguous spread from a visceral infection, usually resulting in an *acute* surgical abdomen. Pathogens are virtually always mixed.
- Peritonitis related to **peritoneal dialysis** is addressed in Chapter 10, Renal Diseases.

DIAGNOSIS

Diagnosis of **secondary peritonitis** is made clinically, supplemented by blood culture (positive 20% to 30%) and imaging to evaluate for free air (perforation) or other source of infection.

Diagnostic Testing
Laboratories
Diagnosis of **SBP** is made by sending paracentesis fluid for culture (directly inoculate blood culture bottles at bedside), cell count, and differential. Blood cultures are often positive. SBP is diagnosed when ascites fluid has >250 neutrophils.

TREATMENT

- Initial broad IV coverage for SBP, culture-negative neutrophilic ascites (CNNA), and *symptomatic* non-neutrophilic bacterascites (Culture-positive ascites with <250 PMNs) should be narrowed if a causative organism is isolated. Treatment duration is 7 days but should be extended to 2 weeks if bacteremia is present. Administration of IV albumin on days 1 and 3 of treatment may improve survival (*N Engl J Med 1999;341(6):403*). If a repeat paracentesis reveals <250 PMNs and cultures remain negative, treatment may be shortened to 5 days.
  - **SBP prophylaxis** should be initiated after the first episode of SBP or after variceal bleeding.
- **Secondary peritonitis** primarily requires surgical intervention. Empiric antimicrobial therapy must be broad spectrum and tailored for severity and the presumed source while awaiting cultures. Empiric antifungal coverage is not usually indicated. Intra-abdominal abscess formation is a complication of secondary peritonitis that usually requires drainage; antibiotics often must be continued until imaging demonstrates resolution of the fluid collection (Table 4).

Hepatobiliary Infections

GENERAL PRINCIPLES

- **Acute cholecystitis** is typically preceded by biliary colic associated with cholelithiasis and characteristically presents with fever, right upper quadrant tenderness with Murphy's sign, and vomiting. Acalculous cholecystitis occurs in 5% to 10% of cases. Organisms usually consist of normal gut flora. Leukocytosis and mild elevations of bilirubin, transaminases, and alkaline phosphatase are possible.

Table 4	Empiric Therapy for Peritonitis		
Disease	Common Pathogens	Empiric IV Therapy	Notes
Secondary peritonitis (acute abdomen)	Mixed gut flora (enteric gram negatives, gram positives, anaerobes)	β-Lactam/β-lactamase inhibitor[a] or third-/fourth-generation cephalosporin + metronidazole/clindamycin [b] or carbapenem[c]	Always look for and address source of infection. Treat for 5–7 d post-operatively
Fungal peritonitis or abscess	*Candida* spp.	Anidulafungin or voriconazole or itraconazole[d]	Treat for 2 wk
Chronic TB peritonitis	*M. tuberculosis*	Treat the same as pulmonary TB	
Primary or spontaneous bacterial peritonitis	See Chapter 16, Liver diseases		
Peritoneal dialysis-related peritonitis	See Chapter 10, Renal Diseases		
Fitz-Hugh–Curtis	See Sexually Transmitted Diseases section for treatment of disseminated *N. gonorrhea*.		

[a]Ticarcillin-clavulanate, 3.1 g q6h; piperacillin-tazobactam, 3.375 g q6h or 4.5 g q8h; ampicillin-sulbactam, 3 g q6h.
[b]For example, ceftriaxone, 1 g q24h plus either metronidazole, 500 mg q8h or clindamycin, 600 to 900 mg q8h.
[c]Ertapenem, 1 g q24h; imipenem, 500 mg q6h; meropenem, 1 g q8h; doripenem, 500 mg q8h.
[d]Anidulafungin, 200 mg × 1, then 100 mg IV q24h; voriconazole, 6 mg/kg IV q12h × 1 d, then 4 mg/kg IV q12h; itraconazole, 200 mg PO q12h.

- **Ascending cholangitis** is a sometimes fulminant infectious complication of an obstructed common bile duct, often following pancreatitis or cholecystis.

DIAGNOSIS

Clinical Presentation

The classic presentation is the Charcot triad of fever, right upper quadrant pain, and jaundice; the additional symptoms of confusion and hypotension (Reynold's pentad) warrant rapid intervention. Bacteremia and shock are common.

Diagnostic Testing

Laboratories

Hepatic function panel abnormalities are usually severe.

Imaging

Diagnosis of biliary tract infections is usually made by imaging, with ultrasonography being the primary modality. Technetium-99m-hydroxy iminodiacetic acid scanning and CT scanning may also be useful.

Diagnostic Procedures

Endoscopic retrograde cholangiopancreatography (ERCP) allows for diagnosis as well as therapeutic intervention in the case of common bile duct obstruction and should be considered in patients with common bile duct dilation, jaundice, or LFT abnormalities.

TREATMENT

- Management of **acute cholecystitis** includes parenteral fluids, restricted PO intake, analgesia, and surgery. Consider perioperative antibiotics in mild disease as they may reduce the risk of postsurgical infections, but advanced age, severe disease, or complications such as gallbladder ischemia or perforation, peritonitis, or bacteremia mandate broad-spectrum antibiotics. Immediate surgery is usually necessary

Table 5	Empiric Therapy for Cholangitis and Cholecystitis[a]		
Disease	**Common Pathogens**	**Empiric IV Therapy**	**Notes**
Cholecystitis	E. coli Klebsiella Enterococcus Enterobacter	β-Lactam/β-lactamase inhibitor[b] or fluoroquinolone[c] or third-generation cephalosporin + metronidazole/ clindamycin[d] or Carbapenem[e] if severe or risk of resistant organisms.	Treat for 3–4 d post-op or 5–7 d if no cholecystec- tomy.
Cholangitis	E. coli Klebsiella Enterococcus Enterobacter	β-Lactam/β-lactamase inhibitor or carbapenem or tigecycline (100 mg × 1, then 50 mg q12h).	Requires biliary decompression. Treat 4–7 d after relief of obstruction.

[a] *Clin Infect Dis* 2003;37:997
[b] Ticarcillin-clavulanate, 3.1 g q6h; piperacillin-tazobactam, 3.375 g q6h or 4.5 g q8h; ampicillin-sulbactam, 3 g q6h.
[c] Ciprofloxacin, 400 mg q24h; levofloxacin, 500 mg q24h; moxifloxacin, 400 mg q24h.
[d] For example, ceftriaxone, 1 g q24h plus either metronidazole, 500 mg q8h or clindamycin, 600 to 900 mg q8h.
[e] Ertapenem, 1 g q24h; imipenem, 500 mg q6h; meropenem, 1 g q8h; doripenem, 500 mg q8h.

for severe disease, but surgery can be otherwise delayed up to 6 weeks if there is an initial response to medical therapy.

- The mainstay of therapy for **ascending cholangitis** is aggressive supportive care and surgical or endoscopic decompression and drainage. Broad-spectrum antibiotics are mandatory. Development of abscess is a complication requiring surgical drainage (Table 5).

OTHER INFECTIONS

Infectious diarrhea (see Chapter 15, Gastrointestinal Diseases).
Viral hepatitis (see Chapter 16, Liver Diseases).
Helicobacter pylori–associated disease (see Chapter 15, Gastrointestinal Diseases).

Diverticulitis

GENERAL PRINCIPLES

Etiology

Enteric gram-negative bacilli and gut anaerobes are the causative organisms.

DIAGNOSIS

Diagnosis is frequently clinical but abdominal/pelvic CT scan can be helpful to rule out pericolic abscess.

Clinical Presentation

Diverticulitis presents initially with left lower quadrant abdominal pain and fever.

TREATMENT

The standard treatment regimen for mild diverticulitis is TMP/SMX, 160 mg/800 mg (DS) PO bid, or ciprofloxacin, 500 mg PO bid, and metronidazole, 500 mg PO bid, for 7 to 10 days. Broader antimicrobial coverage (as for secondary peritonitis) and surgical intervention are warranted for more severe cases.

Appendicitis

DIAGNOSIS

As with diverticulitis, diagnosis is frequently clinical.

Clinical Presentation

Presents classically with vague abdominal pain followed by more localizing right lower quadrant (RLQ) pain and signs and symptoms of secondary peritonitis.

TREATMENT

Treatment is surgical, usually with adjuvant antimicrobial therapy as for secondary peritonitis.

GENITOURINARY INFECTIONS

The diagnostic and therapeutic approaches to adult genitourinary infections are determined by gender-specific anatomic differences, prior antimicrobial exposures, and the presence of medical devices.

Lower Urinary Tract Infections

GENERAL PRINCIPLES

Definition

Lower urinary tract infections (UTIs) are characterized by pyuria and bacteriuria, often with dysuria, urgency, or frequency. Fever is usually absent unless pyelonephritis is present.

DIAGNOSIS

- A rapid presumptive diagnosis can be made by urinalysis (UA) or microscopic examination of a fresh, unspun, clean-voided urine specimen suggesting pyuria (positive leukocyte esterase or >8 leukocytes per high-power field) or bacteriuria (positive nitrites or >1 organism per oil-immersion field). A urine Gram stain can be helpful in guiding initial antimicrobial choices. Quantitative culture often yields $>10^5$ bacteria/mL, but colony counts as low as 10^2 to 10^4 bacteria/mL may indicate infection in women with acute dysuria.
- An incidental finding of **asymptomatic bacteriuria** is of limited clinical significance except in pregnant women or patients planned for urologic surgery (*Clin Infect Dis 2005;40:643*).
- Dysuria without pyuria in sexually active patients warrants consideration of sexually transmitted infection.
- **Acute uncomplicated cystitis in women.** A pretreatment urine culture is recommended for diabetics, patients who are symptomatic for >7 days, individuals with recurrent UTI, women who use a contraceptive diaphragm, and individuals older than 65 years. Therapy should be extended to 7 days in this subset of patients. Caused primarily by *E. coli* (80%) and *Staphylococcus saprophyticus* (5% to 15%).
- **Recurrent cystitis in women.** Repeat infections are usually reinfections rather than recurrences, due to host-dependent risk factors, which vary for young women, healthy postmenopausal women, and older women who are institutionalized.
- **Complicated UTIs.** UTIs associated with anatomic abnormalities, functional, metabolic, or immunological abnormalities, pregnancy, indwelling catheters, or unusual pathogens are termed "complicated." Pre- and posttreatment urine cultures are needed, and initial broad coverage pending culture data for 10 to 14 days of therapy is appropriate. Foreign bodies must be removed.
- **UTIs in men.** Cystitis is uncommon in young men. It does not necessarily indicate a urologic abnormality, but sexually transmitted infections should be considered as an alternate diagnosis. Risk factors include anal intercourse and lack of circumcision. Chronic prostatitis is a frequent cause of recurrent UTI in men.

- **Catheter-associated bacteriuria.** Catheter-associated bacteriuria is a common source of gram-negative bacteremia in hospitalized patients. Duration of catheterization is the biggest risk factor. This is often polymicrobial.
- **Acute urethral syndrome** is a condition occurs in women who have lower UTI symptoms and pyuria with <10^5 bacteria/mL urine. These patients may have bacterial cystitis or urethritis caused by *Chlamydia trachomatis*, *Ureaplasma urealyticum*, or, less frequently, *N. gonorrhoeae*. Specific cultures of the endocervix for sexually transmitted diseases should be performed (see the Sexually Transmitted Diseases section). If no specific etiology is found, **empiric treatment** with doxycycline, 100 mg PO bid for 7 days or azithromycin, 1 g PO in a single dose, is recommended.
- **Acute prostatitis** is often a severe systemic illness characterized by fever, chills, dysuria, and a boggy, tender prostate on examination. Diagnosis is usually obvious by physical exam and urine Gram stain and culture. Prostatic massage is not necessary or recommended to diagnose acute prostatitis. Enteric gram negatives are the usual causative organisms.
- **Chronic prostatitis** can manifest vaguely as low back pain, perineal, testicular, or penile pain, dysuria, ejaculatory pain, recurrent UTIs with the same organism, or hematospermia. Physical exam is usually unrevealing. Prostatitis is frequently abacterial; diagnosis requires identification of organisms by quantitative urine cultures before and after prostatic massage (*Tech Urol 1997;3:38*). Causative organisms are the same as for acute prostatitis. Transrectal ultrasound is only helpful if abscess is suspected.
- **Epididymitis** presents as a unilateral scrotal ache with swollen and tender epididymis on exam. Causative organisms are usually *N. gonorrhoeae* or *C. trachomatis* in sexually active young men and by gram-negative enteric organisms in older men. Diagnosis and therapy should be directed according to this epidemiology, with ceftriaxone and doxycycline in young men and TMP/SMX or ciprofloxacin in men older than 35 years.

TREATMENT

See Table 6 for details

- **Acute uncomplicated cystitis** in women. A 3-day course of empiric antibiotic therapy is recommended for symptomatic women with pyuria.
- **Recurrent cystitis in women**
  - Treatment regimens for simple cystitis are successful for most recurrences. Relapses with the original infecting organism that occur within 2 weeks of cessation of therapy should be treated for 2 weeks and may indicate a urologic abnormality.
  - **Prophylactic therapy** for patients with frequent reinfection should be initiated only after sterilization of the urine with a standard treatment regimen. An alternative method of contraception might decrease the frequency of reinfection in women who use a diaphragm and/or spermicide. Prophylaxis regimens can be continuous, postcoital, or self-initiated.
- **UTIs in men.** Treatment with a typical antibiotic regimen as for cystitis in women should be continued for a full 7-day course. If the response to therapy is prompt, a urologic evaluation is unlikely to be useful. Urologic studies are appropriate when no underlying risk factor is identified, when treatment fails, in the event of recurrent infections, or when pyelonephritis occurs.

Table 6	Empiric Therapy for Urinary Tract Infections	
Disease	**Empiric Therapy**	**Notes**
Simple cystitis	*First line:* TMP-SMX DS PO bid or TMP (if sulfa-allergic) 100 mg PO bid or nitrofurantoin sustained release 100 mg PO bid (× 3–7 d therapy only). *Alternate:* Ciprofloxacin 250 mg PO bid or norfloxacin 400 mg PO bid for *severe symptoms* or based on local resistance patterns.	Choose antibiotics based on local susceptibility patterns. Usually treat for 3 d. Extend therapy to 7 d for diabetics and older patients, avoid TMP/SMX in older women.
Cystitis in men (*N Engl J Med* 1993;329:1328)	As per simple cystitis in women. Treat × 7 d.	Consider urologic evaluation for recurrent disease or pyelonephritis.
Recurrent cystitis (*N Engl J Med* 2003;349:259)	*Postcoital prophylaxis:* TMP-SMX SS × 1 or ciprofloxacin 125 mg × 1 or nitrofurantoin 100 mg × 1. *Continuous prophylaxis:* TMP-SMX ½ SS qd or qod. *Self-treatment:* TMP-SMX ½ SS PO qhs × 3 d or nitrofurantoin 100 mg PO qd × 3 d or ciprofloxacin 125 mg PO qd × 3 d.	Cranberry juice, topical vaginal estrogen in postmenopausal women, and voiding after intercourse *may* have a role in preventing recurrent UTI.
Pregnancy (*N Engl J Med* 2003;349:259)	Nitrofurantoin 100 mg PO qid × 7 d or Cephalexin 250–500 mg PO qid × 7 d or Cefuroxime axetil 250 mg PO qid × 7 d.	Treat all asymptomatic bacteriuria in pregnancy. Screen pregnant women near end of first trimester with urine culture (*Clin Infect Dis 2005;40: 643–654*).
Complicated UTI (*N Engl J Med 2003; 349:259*)	*Mild–moderate illness:* second-generation FQ[a]. *Severe illness, recent FQ, or institutionalized:* cefepime 2 g IV q12h or third-generation cephalosporin[b] or carbapenem[c] or piperacillin-tazobactam 3.375–4.5 g IV q6h. Consider adding vancomycin empirically for gram-positive cocci on urine Gram stain.	Base empiric coverage on local sensitivity patterns, and narrow therapy when organism identified. Continue therapy for 10–14 d but can consider shortening if complicating factor is resolved (i.e., removal of indwelling device or stone).

(*continued*)

Table 6	Empiric Therapy for Urinary Tract Infections (*Continued*)	
Disease	**Empiric Therapy**	**Notes**
Candiduria (*Clin Infect Dis 2004; 38:161*)	*Candida albicans:* fluconazole 100–200 mg PO qd × 5 d. *Critically ill or non-albicans species:* Amphotericin B × 5 d.	Remove catheter if present. *Indications to treat:* symptoms with pyuria, hardware, pregnancy, prior to GU surgery, or risk of dissemination.
Pyelonephritis (*Clin Infect Dis 1999; 29:745*)	*Outpatient:* second-generation FQ.[a] *Inpatient:* second-generation FQ[a] or aminoglycoside[d] or Ampicillin-sulbactam 1–2 g IV q6h or third-generation cephalosporin.[b] *Pregnancy:* Cefazolin 1 g IV q8h or Ceftriaxone 1 g IV or IM q24h or Piperacillin 4 g IV q8h.	Treat IV until afebrile × 48 h, then change to PO to complete 14 d. Consider single dose IV followed by outpatient oral therapy in stable patients. Do not use fluoroquinolones in pregnancy.

[a]Oral: Ciprofloxacin, 500 mg PO bid; ofloxacin, 200 mg PO bid; levofloxacin, 500 mg PO qd; norfloxacin, 400 mg PO bid. Parenteral: levofloxacin, 500 mg IV qd; ciprofloxacin, 400 mg IV q12h.
[b]Cefotaxime, 1 or 2 g IV q8h; ceftriaxone, 1 g IV qd; ceftazidime, 1 to 2 g IV q8–12h.
[c]Imipenem, 500 mg IV q6h; meropenem, 1 g IV q8h.
[d]Gentamicin or tobramycin 2 mg/kg loading dose IV, then 1.5 to 3.0 mg/kg/d or divided dose.

- **Catheter-associated bacteriuria**
  - Treatment is generally not indicated for asymptomatic bacteriuria in the absence of pregnancy, immunocompromise, or planned urologic procedure.
  - Symptomatic catheter-associated UTIs should prompt removal or exchange of the catheter, blood and urine cultures, and treatment with 7 to 10 days of antibiotic therapy appropriate for complicated UTI.
  - Candiduria should not be treated unless there is immunocompromise and high risk for candidemia, or there are symptoms and pyuria with no bacterial source. Otherwise, host status optimization (glucose control in diabetics, removal or change of Foley catheter) is sufficient.
  - **Prevention** measures include aseptic technique for urinary catheter insertion, use of a closed drainage system, and removal of the catheter as soon as possible.
  - In patients with chronic indwelling catheters, the development of bacteriuria is inevitable, and long-term antimicrobial suppression simply selects for multidrug-resistant bacteria. Such patients should be treated with systemic antimicrobials only when symptomatic infection with pyuria is evident.
- Treatment of **acute bacterial prostatitis** is a 2- to 4-week course of either ciprofloxacin, 500 mg PO bid, or TMP/SMX, 160 mg/800 mg (DS) PO bid. Culture-positive chronic bacterial prostatitis should receive prolonged therapy (for at least 6 weeks with the fluoroquinolones or 3 months with TMP/SMX).

Pyelonephritis

DIAGNOSIS

Clinical Presentation

Patients present with fever, flank pain, and lower UTI symptoms due to ascending infection from the lower urinary tract.

Diagnostic Testing

Laboratories

- Urine specimens characteristically demonstrate significant bacteriuria, pyuria, RBCs, and occasional leukocyte casts.
- Diagnosis should include urine culture in all patients, and blood cultures should be obtained in those who are hospitalized because bacteremia will be detected in 15% to 20%. The causative agents usually are *E. coli*, *S. saprophyticus*, and rarely, *Proteus* sp. No further tests are usually needed for initial workup, but the presence of other organisms suggests an anatomic abnormality or immune compromise.

TREATMENT

Treatment of patients with **mild to moderate illness** who are able to take oral medication can be safely initiated in the outpatient setting. Patients with more **severe illness,** those who are nauseated and vomiting, and pregnant patients should be treated initially with parenteral therapy.

SPECIAL CONSIDERATIONS

Evaluation for anatomic abnormalities should be done for patients who do not respond to initial empiric treatment within 48 hours. Presence of an anatomic abnormality such as intrarenal abscess or renal calculi should be evaluated by ultrasonography, CT scan, or intravenous pyelogram (IVP) (Table 6).

SEXUALLY TRANSMITTED INFECTIONS, ULCERATIVE DISEASES

Genital Herpes

GENERAL PRINCIPLES

Etiology

Genital herpes is caused by **HSV,** usually type 2.

Pathophysiology

Characterized by painful grouped vesicles in the genital and perianal regions that rapidly ulcerate and form shallow tender lesions.

Associated Conditions

The initial episode may be associated with inguinal adenopathy, fever, headache, myalgias, and aseptic (Mollaret) meningitis; recurrences are usually less severe.

DIAGNOSIS

The confirmation of HSV infection requires culture or PCR; however, clinical presentation is usually adequate for diagnosis.

TREATMENT

For treatment options, see Table 7.

Syphilis

GENERAL PRINCIPLES

- **Primary syphilis** may develop within several weeks of exposure and manifests as one or more painless, indurated, superficial ulcerations (chancre).
- **Secondary syphilis** develops 4 to 10 weeks after the chancre resolves and may produce a rash, mucocutaneous lesions, adenopathy, and constitutional symptoms.
- **Tertiary syphilis** follows between 1 and 20 years after infection, and includes cardiovascular, gummatous, and neurologic disease (general paresis, tabes dorsalis, or meningovascular syphilis).

Etiology

Syphilis is caused by the *Treponema pallidum* spirochete.

Associated Conditions

There is a high degree of HIV coinfection in patients with syphilis, and HIV infection should be excluded with appropriate testing (*JAMA 2003;290(11):1510*).

DIAGNOSIS

Diagnosis of **tertiary disease** requires clinical correlation with cardiovascular, neurologic, or systemic symptoms.

Diagnostic Testing

Laboratories
- In **primary syphilis,** dark-field microscopy of the lesion exudates may show organisms. A nontreponemal serologic test (e.g., RPR or Venereal Disease Research Laboratory [VDRL]) should be confirmed with a treponemal specific test (e.g., fluorescent treponemal antibody absorption or *T. pallidum* particle agglutination).
- Diagnosis of **secondary syphilis** is made on the basis of positive serologic studies and the presence of a compatible clinical illness.
- **Latent syphilis** is a serologic diagnosis in the absence of symptoms—early latent syphilis is serologically positive for <1 year, and late latent syphilis is serologically positive for >1 year.

Diagnostic Procedures
To exclude **neurosyphilis,** a lumbar puncture should be performed in the presence of neurologic or ophthalmic signs or symptoms, evidence of tertiary disease, treatment

Table 7	Treatment of Sexually Transmitted Diseases[a]	
Disease	**Recommended Regimen**	**Alternative Regimen**
Genital ulcer disease		
Herpes simplex		
First episode	• Acyclovir 200 mg 5 × /d × 7–10 d or 400 mg PO tid × 7–10 d. • Valacyclovir 1 g PO bid × 7–10 d. • Famciclovir 250 mg PO tid × 7–10 d.	
Recurrent episodes	• Acyclovir 400 mg PO tid × 5 d or 800 mg PO tid × 2 d. • Valacyclovir 1 g PO qd × 5 d or 1 g PO bid × 1 d or 500 mg PO bid × 3 d. • Famciclovir 1 g PO bid × 1 d or 125 mg PO bid × 5 d.	
Suppressive therapy	• Acyclovir 400 mg PO bid. • Valacyclovir 500 mg or 1 g orally once a day. • Famciclovir 250 mg orally twice a day.	
Syphilis		
Primary, secondary, or early latent < 1 yr	• Benzathine penicillin G 2.4 million units IM single dose.	(Penicillin-allergic, nonpregnant): • Doxycycline: 100 mg orally twice daily × 14 d. • Tetracycline: 500 mg orally four times daily × 14 d.
Latent >1 yr, latent unknown duration	• Benzathine penicillin G 2.4 million units IM × 3 doses.	• Doxycycline: 100 mg orally twice daily × 28 d. • Tetracycline: 500 mg orally four times daily × 28 d.
Neurosyphilis	• Aqueous crystalline penicillin G 18–24 million units a day × 10–14 d.	• Procaine penicillin 2.4 million units IM once daily + probenecid 500 mg orally four times daily × 10–14 d.
Pregnancy	• Penicillin only recommended treatment—desensitize if necessary.	

(*continued*)

Table 7	Treatment of Sexually Transmitted Diseases[a] (Continued)	
Disease	Recommended Regimen	Alternative Regimen
Chancroid	• Azithromycin 1 g orally single dose. • Ceftriaxone 250 mg IM single dose.	• Ciprofloxacin 500 mg orally twice daily × 3 d. • Erythromycin base 500 mg orally twice daily × 7 d.
Lymphogranuloma venereum	• Doxycycline 100 mg twice a day × 21 d.	• Erythromycin base 500 mg orally four times a day × 21 d.
Urethritis/cervicitis		
Gonorrhea (GC)	• Ceftriaxone 125 mg IM once or Cefixime 400 mg orally once, + Azithromycin/doxycycline (see below) if chlamydia not ruled out.	• If allergy, use spectinomycin 2 g IM once (not for pharyngeal GC). • Fluoroquinolones are not recommended for GC.
Disseminated gonococcal infection	• Ceftriaxone 1 g IV daily or • Cefotaxime 1 g IV every 8 h × 7 d (can switch to oral cefixime to complete treatment).	• Spectinomycin 2 g IM every 12 h (switch to cefixime to finish course).
Chlamydia	• Azithromycin 1 g orally single dose. • Doxycycline 100 mg orally twice daily × 7 d.	• Erythromycin base 500 mg orally four times a day × 7 d.
Pelvic inflammatory disease		
Outpatient	• Ceftriaxone 250 mg IM once + Doxycycline 100 mg orally twice daily × 14 d + Metronidazole 500 mg orally twice daily × 14 d.	
Inpatient	• Cefoxitin 2 g IV every 6 h or cefotetan 2 g IV every 12 h + Doxycycline 100 mg orally twice daily × 14 d + Metronidazole 500 mg orally twice daily × 14 d.	• Ampicillin-sulbactam 3 g IV every 6 h + doxycycline. • Clindamycin 900 mg IV every 8 h + gentamicin 2 mg/kg loading dose, then 1.5 mg/kg every 8 h + doxycycline 100 mg orally twice daily × 14 d.

(continued)

Table 7	Treatment of Sexually Transmitted Diseases[a] (*Continued*)	
Disease	**Recommended Regimen**	**Alternative Regimen**
Vaginitis/vaginosis		
Trichomonas	• Metronidazole 2 g orally single dose. • Tinidazole 2 g orally single dose.	• Metronidazole: 500 mg orally twice daily × 7 d.
Pregnancy	• Metronidazole 2 g orally × 1, as adverse outcomes associated with trichomoniasis during pregnancy.	
Bacterial vaginosis	• Metronidazole 500 mg orally twice daily × 7 d. • Clindamycin cream 2% intravaginal at bedtime × 7 d. • Metronidazole gel 0.75% intravaginal once a day for 5 d.	• Clindamycin 300 mg orally twice daily for 7 d. • Clindamycin ovules 100 mg intravaginal at bedtime for 3 d.
Candidiasis	• Fluconazole 150 mg orally × 1. • Itraconazole 200 mg orally twice daily × 1 d.	• Intravaginal azoles in variety of strengths for 1–14 d.
Recurrent candidiasis	• Fluconazole 100, 150, or 200 mg once weekly for 6 mo.	

[a] *MMWR 2006;55(RR-11).*

failure, or serum RPR or VDRL of 1:32 or greater (unless the duration of infection is <1 year). VDRL should be performed on CSF. Patients with HIV and syphilis of >1 year's duration also should usually undergo a lumbar puncture.

Chancroid

GENERAL PRINCIPLES

Etiology

Chancroid is caused by *Hemophilus ducreyi* and produces a painful genital ulcer and tender suppurative inguinal lymphadenopathy. Identification of the organism is difficult and requires special culture media.

TREATMENT

For treatment options, see Table 7

Lymphogranuloma Venereum

GENERAL PRINCIPLES

Etiology

Lymphogranuloma venereum (LGV) is caused by *C. trachomatis* (serovars L_1, L_2, or L_3).

DIAGNOSIS

Diagnosis is based on clinical suspicion and *C. trachomatis* antibody testing, if available.

Clinical Presentation

Manifests as a painless genital ulcer, followed by heaped up, matted inguinal lymphadenopathy.

TREATMENT

For treatment options, see Table 7

SEXUALLY TRANSMITTED INFECTIONS, VAGINITIS AND VAGINOSIS

Trichomoniasis

DIAGNOSIS

Clinical Presentation

Clinical symptoms of infection by *Trichomonas vaginalis* include malodorous purulent vaginal discharge, dysuria, and genital inflammation.

Physical Examination
Physical examination reveals profuse frothy discharge and cervical petechiae.

Diagnostic Testing

Laboratories
Diagnosis requires visualization of motile trichomonads on a saline wet mount of discharge. The pH of vaginal fluid usually is ≥ 4.5.

Bacterial Vaginosis

GENERAL PRINCIPLES

Results from replacement of normal lactobacillus in the vagina with high concentrations of anaerobic bacteria.

DIAGNOSIS

Diagnosis requires three of the following criteria:

- A homogenous, thin, white discharge
- Presence of clue cells on microscopic examination
- pH of vaginal fluid is usually ≥ 4.5
- A fishy odor of vaginal discharge before or after addition of 10% KOH (the whiff test)

TREATMENT

For treatment options, see Table 7

Vulvovaginal Candidiasis

GENERAL PRINCIPLES

Vulvovaginal candidiasis (VVC) ("yeast infection") is generally not a sexually transmitted disease but commonly develops in relation to oral contraceptive use or antibiotic therapy. If recurrent, it may be a presenting manifestation of unrecognized HIV infection.

DIAGNOSIS

- Definitive diagnosis requires visualization of fungal elements on a potassium hydroxide preparation of vaginal discharge fluid.
- Fluconazole failure could indicate the presence of a **non-*albicans Candida* species**.

Clinical Presentation

It presents with thick, cottage cheese–like vaginal discharge in conjunction with intense vulvar inflammation, pruritus, and dysuria.

TREATMENT

Therapy is often initiated on the basis of the clinical presentation (Table 7).

Cervicitis/Urethritis

GENERAL PRINCIPLES

This is a frequent presentation of infection with ***N. gonorrhoeae* or *C. trachomatis*** and occasionally *Mycoplasma hominis*, *U. urealyticum*, and *T. vaginalis*. These infections frequently coexist, and the clinical presentations may be identical (*N Engl J Med 2003; 349:2424*).

DIAGNOSIS

Clinical Presentation

Women with urethritis or cervicitis, or both, complain of mucopurulent vaginal discharge, dyspareunia, and dysuria. Men with urethritis complain of dysuria and a purulent penile discharge.

Diagnostic Testing

Laboratories

A positive endocervical or urethral culture, endocervical DNA probe test, or urinary PCR is required for diagnosis. For gonorrhea, a Gram stain of endocervical or urethral discharge with gram-negative diplococci can also establish the diagnosis.

TREATMENT

Because of increasing resistance, fluoroquinolones *should not be used* to treat gonorrhea (*Morb Mortal Wkly Rep 2007;56(14);332*). (See Table 7 for treatment options.)

Pelvic Inflammatory Disease

GENERAL PRINCIPLES

Pelvic inflammatory disease (PID) is an upper genital tract infection in women, usually preceded by cervicitis that ranges from mild illness with lower abdominal pain and dyspareunia to peritonitis and tubo-ovarian abscess. Long-term consequences of untreated PID include chronic pain, infertility, and ectopic pregnancy.

DIAGNOSIS

Diagnosis is clinical, supported by microbiological studies.

Diagnostic Testing

Laboratories

Cervical motion tenderness and the presence of at least 10 white blood cells per low-power field on endocervical smear Gram stain are consistent with PID. Endocervical cultures or probes for chlamydia and gonorrhea should be obtained.

TREATMENT

See Table 7 for treatment options.

SPECIAL CONSIDERATIONS

Severely ill, pregnant, HIV-infected, and severely nauseated patients should be hospitalized.

SYSTEMIC MYCOSES AND ATYPICALS

Clinical presentations are protean and not pathogen specific. The systemic mycoses should be considered in normal hosts with unexplained chronic pulmonary pathology, chronic meningitis, lytic bone lesions, chronic skin lesions, FUO, or cytopenias. In immunocompromised patients, the development of new pulmonary, cutaneous, funduscopic, or head-and-neck signs and symptoms, or persistent unexplained fever should prompt consideration of these pathogens.

The mycoses can often be identified by taking into account epidemiological clues (many are geographically restricted), site of infection, inflammatory response, and microscopic fungal appearance. These infections can be complex and difficult to treat, and specialist consultation is recommended. For details on treatment of fungal pathogens, Nocardia, and Actinomyces, see Table 8.

Candidiasis

GENERAL PRINCIPLES

Infection with *Candida* species is often associated with concurrent antibiotic use, contraceptive use, immunosuppressant and cytotoxic therapy, and indwelling foreign bodies. Mucocutaneous disease may resolve after elimination of the causative condition (e.g., antibiotic therapy) or may persist and progress in the setting of immunosuppressive conditions. Serious complications, such as candidemia leading to skin lesions, ocular disease, and osteomyelitis, can occur.

DIAGNOSIS

Diagnostic Testing
Laboratories
Diagnosis of **mucocutaneous candidiasis** is usually based on clinical findings, but can be confirmed by a potassium hydroxide preparation of exudates. Cultures can be obtained in refractory cases to exclude the presence of non-*albican Candida* species. **Invasive candidiasis** is diagnosed by positive cultures of blood or tissue.

TREATMENT (Table 8)

- **Mucocutaneous candidiasis** usually responds to topical therapy but oral and even parenteral therapy can be required based on severity and other host factors. **Candidemia and other invasive candidiasis** require a more prolonged course of therapy.
- **Isolated catheter-related candidemia** (see the Nosocomial Infections section).

Cryptococcosis

GENERAL PRINCIPLES

Cryptococcus neoformans is a ubiquitous yeast associated with soil and pigeon excrement. Disease is principally meningeal (headache and mental status changes) and pulmonary (ranging from asymptomatic nodular disease to fulminant respiratory failure). Significant infections are usually opportunistic.

DIAGNOSIS

Diagnostic Testing
Laboratories
Diagnosis requires detection of encapsulated yeast in tissue or body fluids (India ink stain) with confirmation by culture. The latex agglutination test for cryptococcal antigen in serum or CSF is helpful, and a positive serum antigen titer is highly suggestive of disseminated disease.

Table 8   Treatment of Fungal Infections, *Nocardia*, and *Actinomyces*

Pathogen	Primary Therapy	Suppressive Rx	Notes
***Candida* spp.** Mucosal (*Clin Infect Dis 2004;38:161*)	Topical clotrimazole troches, 10 mg dissolved PO 5 × /d × 14 d. *Esophageal:* fluconazole 100–200 mg PO qd × 14 d. *Vaginal:* topical azole × 1–14 d or fluconazole 150 mg PO × 1.	Generally not indicated in *HIV* unless frequent severe recurrences. *Neutropenia:* Fluconazole 400 mg PO qd or itraconazole 200 mg PO q12h. Continue prophylaxis until ANC > 500 or 3 mo post solid organ transplant.	
Invasive (*Clin Infect Dis 2006;42:244*)	Fluconazole, 800 mg loading dose, then 400 mg IV/PO qd × 7 d, then PO × 14 d. *Severe dz, recent azole exposure, suspicion of non-albicans species:* echinocandin, for example, Amphotericin B* or anidulafungin 200 mg IV × 1, then 100 mg qd See Nosocomial Infections section		Treat all positive blood cultures as invasive disease, with at least 14-d therapy. Catheters must be removed. Treat for 14 d beyond last positive blood Cx. *C. parapsilosis* should not be initially treated with an echinocandin.
Catheter-associated			
Cryptococcus neoformans Nonmeningeal disease (*Clin Infect Dis 2000;30:710*)	Fluconazole 400 mg PO or IV qd × 8 wk–6 mo.	Immunosuppressed: Fluconazole 200 mg PO qd.	Isolated pulmonary disease in immunocompetent patients can be followed expectantly. *(continued)*

485

Table 8   Treatment of Fungal Infections, *Nocardia*, and *Actinomyces* (*Continued*)

Pathogen	Primary Therapy	Suppressive Rx	Notes
C. neoformans Meningitis (*Clin Infect Dis* 2000;30:710)			
Immunocompetent	Amphotericin B* + flucytosine 25 mg/kg q6h IV × 2 wk, then fluconazole 400 mg PO qd × 8 wk.	Not indicated.	Always check opening pressure, and reduce by 50% if elevated above 25 cm H_2O by removing up to 30 cc CSF. Serial LPs to reduce pressure are required as long as CSF is elevated.
Immunosuppressed	Amphotericin B* + flucytosine 25 mg/kg q6h IV × 2 wk, then fluconazole 400 mg PO qd × 8 wk.	Fluconazole 200 mg PO qd.	Continue prophylaxis until immunocompetent or CD4 count sustained >200 for 6 mo.
Histoplasma capsulatum (*Clin Infect Dis* 2007;45:807)			
Chronic forms, mild disease, immuno-competent	Itraconazole 200–400 mg/d PO for ≥6 mo.	Not indicated.	Goal serum itraconazole level >1 mcg/mL.
Acute dissemination; severe disease; immunocompromised	Amphotericin B* for 2 weeks or until clinically improved, then itraconazole 200 mg PO bid >12 mo.	Itraconazole 200 mg PO qd.	Continue prophylaxis until sustained CD4 count >200 for 6 mo.

Condition	Primary therapy	Suppressive/maintenance	Comments
(Clin Infect Dis 2000;30:679) Nonmeningeal disease; mild to moderate disease; immunocompetent	Itraconazole 200–400 mg/d PO for 6 mo.	Not indicated.	Follow serum CF titers after treatment. Rising titers suggest recurrence.
Acute dissemination; severe disease; immunocompromised	Amphotericin B* for 2 weeks or until clinically improved, then itraconazole 200–400 mg PO qd × 6 mo.	Itraconazole 200–400 mg PO qd.	
Coccidioides immitis (Clin Infect Dis 2005;41:1217) Nonmeningeal disease	Itraconazole 200 mg PO bid or fluconazole 400 mg PO qd × 12 mo.	Fluconazole 400 mg PO qd (lifelong suppression required if disseminated).	For pulmonary nodules and asymptomatic cavitary disease, no therapy indicated. Consider surgery if cavitary disease persists >2 yr, progresses >1 yr, or is located near pleura.
Meningitis	Fluconazole 400–800 mg IV/PO q24h. Intrathecal Amphotericin B deoxycholate 0.1–1.5 mg qd to qwk may be added to azole therapy for severe meningeal disease.	Fluconazole 400 mg PO qd indefinitely.	
Aspergillus Aspergilloma	Surgical resection in case of severe hemoptysis.	Not indicated.	Use liposomal
Invasive aspergillosis (Clin Infect Dis 2008;46:327)	Voriconazole 6 mg/kg q12h PO/IV × 2 doses, then 4 mg/kg q12h, then 200 mg bid. Continue for at least 6–12 wk, as long as immunosuppression continues, and until lesions resolve.	Continue or restart therapy if immunosuppression recurs.	Amphotericin B* to cover mucormycosis as initial therapy for sinus disease pending confirmation of diagnosis.

(continued)

Table 8	Treatment of Fungal Infections, *Nocardia*, and *Actinomyces* (*Continued*)		
Pathogen	Primary Therapy	Suppressive Rx	Notes
Sporothrix	Itraconazole, 100–200 mg PO qd × 3–12 mo. *Alt:* saturated solution of K Iodide, 5 drops PO tid, increased to 40 drops tid as tolerated.	Not indicated.	Severe and meningeal disease: Amphotericin B* for initial 6 weeks of therapy Follow levels of itraconazole.
Mucormycosis	Amphotericin B* at upper dose range × 6 mo.	Not indicated.	
Nocardia (*Clin Infect Dis* 1996;22:891) Pulmonary	TMP/SMX 5–10 mg/kg/d IV (TMP) in div. doses × 3–6 wk, then 1–2 DS PO bid. *Less serious:* TMP/SMX 1–2 DS bid up to 2 DS tid or minocycline 100 mg PO bid.	TMP/SMX 1–2 DS bid or dapsone 100 mg PO qd or minocycline 100 mg PO bid.	Treat initially for 6 mo if immunocompetent or ≥12 mo if immunocompromised.
CNS	TMP/SMX 15 mg/kg/d IV (TMP) × 3–6 wk, then 3 DS PO bid.		
Actinomyces	(Penicillin G 18–24 million units IV/d or clindamycin 600 mg IV q8h) × 2–6 wk, then doxycycline 100 mg PO bid for 6–12 mo.	Not indicated.	

*Amphotericin dosing: amphotericin B deoxycholate 0.7–1 mg/kg. Liposomal amphotericin B 3–5 mg/kg.

Diagnostic Procedures
Lumbar puncture is necessary in persons with systemic disease to exclude coexistent CNS involvement. Always measure opening pressure, as elevated opening pressure (>25 cm H$_2$O) has poor prognostic implications and must be managed, usually with serial LPs, sometimes with a lumbar drain.

TREATMENT (Table 8)

- Treatment depends on the patient's immune function and the site of infection.
- *Management of elevated intracranial pressure is critical.* CSF opening pressure above 25 cm H$_2$O should be reduced by 50% if possible by removal of up to 30 cc of fluid, repeating daily as needed. If initial opening pressure is not elevated, repeat LP is only needed if new symptoms arise.
- HIV patients need suppressive therapy until immune function is improved by antiretrovirals.

Histoplasmosis

GENERAL PRINCIPLES

Clinical manifestations are extremely varied, including acute flulike or chronic granulomatous pulmonary disease, or fulminant multiorgan failure in the immunocompromised patient.

Epidemiology
Histoplasma capsulatum is more prevalent in the Ohio and Mississippi River Valleys of the United States and in Latin America, and grows best in soil contaminated by bat or bird droppings.

DIAGNOSIS

Diagnostic Testing
Laboratories
Diagnosis is based on culture or histopathology, antigen assay (urine, blood, or CSF), or complement fixation assay ($\geq$1:16 or 4-fold rise). Urine antigen assay is good for detecting disseminated disease and is helpful in following response to therapy.

TREATMENT (Table 8)

Treatment for most symptomatic infections is an extended course of itraconazole. Mild pulmonary disease can be observed without specific therapy.

Blastomycosis

GENERAL PRINCIPLES

This organism commonly disseminates, even in immunocompetent patients, and tends to affect the lungs, skin, bone, and genitourinary tract. Aggressive pulmonary and CNS disease can occur in immunocompromised patients.

Epidemiology

Blastomyces dermatitidis is endemic in the upper midwestern, south-central, and south-eastern United States.

DIAGNOSIS

Diagnostic Testing

Laboratories

Diagnosis requires isolation of the organism by culture or histopathology. Serologic studies cross-react with tests for *Histoplasma* and *Cryptococcus* species and are unreliable for diagnosis, but can be used to assess early response to therapy if positive.

TREATMENT (Table 8)

Treatment is usually a 6-month course of itraconazole but requires an initial course of Amphotericin B for life-threatening or CNS disease.

Coccidioidomycosis

GENERAL PRINCIPLES

Disease is usually a self-limited pulmonary syndrome. Less common are chronic pulmonary illness and disseminated disease, which can affect the meninges, bones, joints, and skin.

Epidemiology

Coccidioides immitis is endemic to the southwestern United States and Central America.

DIAGNOSIS

Diagnostic Testing

Laboratories

- Diagnosis requires culture or histopathology, or positive complement fixation serology.
- Serum CF titer of 1:16 or greater suggests extrathoracic dissemination.

Diagnostic Procedures

- **Lumbar puncture** should be performed for culture and complement fixation (CF) to rule out CNS involvement in persons with severe, rapidly progressive, or disseminated disease.
- **Skin test** should be used for epidemiologic purposes to evaluate exposure only.

TREATMENT (Table 8)

Treatment can be avoided for most forms of **acute pulmonary disease,** as it resolves spontaneously. For **disseminated disease,** immunocompromised patients, or pulmonary disease that persists beyond 6 weeks, treatment is typically 1 year of oral azole therapy. CF titers can be followed after therapy, as rising titers suggest recurrence.

Aspergillosis

GENERAL PRINCIPLES

Definition

- **Pulmonary aspergilloma.** Pulmonary aspergilloma occurs in the setting of preexisting bullous lung disease and can be easily recognized by characteristic radiographic presentation and *Aspergillus* serology.
- **Invasive aspergillosis.** Invasive aspergillosis (IA) is a serious condition associated with vascular invasion, thrombosis, and ischemic infarction of involved tissues and progressive disease after hematogenous dissemination. IA is usually seen in severely immunocompromised patients and clinical features vary by predisposing host characteristics.
- **Allergic bronchopulmonary aspergillosis (ABPA).** ABPA is a chronic relapsing and remitting respiratory syndrome associated with colonization with *Aspergillus*.

Classification

Aspergillus species are ubiquitous environmental fungi that cause a broad spectrum of disease, usually affecting the respiratory system and sinuses.

DIAGNOSIS

Invasive aspergillosis

- Diagnosis can be very difficult given the varied manifestations of IA, and a high index of suspicion should be applied to patients with prolonged severe immunosuppression.
- Radiographic findings can be highly suggestive, if not diagnostic of pulmonary IA, particularly the halo-crescent sign on CT in immunosuppressed patients.
- The diagnosis can be confirmed with characteristic histologic evidence of involved tissue. Fungal culture has a low yield.
- The galactomannan assay can support a diagnosis of IA and can be followed prospectively in at-risk patients (*Clin Infect Dis 2004;39:797*). Sensitivity is higher when performed on respiratory secretions as compared to serum (*Am J Respir Crit Care Med 2008;177:27*).

TREATMENT (Table 8)

- **Pulmonary aspergilloma.** Treatment by surgical resection or arterial embolization is indicated only in the setting of severe hemoptysis.
- **Invasive aspergillosis.** Treatment of locally IA requires surgical excision of affected tissue. Empiric therapy of head and neck disease should include Amphotericin B in order to also cover the zygomycoses, while awaiting final speciation (*NEJM 2009;360:1870*).
- **Allergic bronchopulmonary aspergillosis.** Intermittent steroids are the primary therapy; a course of itraconazole may decrease exacerbations.

Sporotrichosis

GENERAL PRINCIPLES

Untreated disease can persist and slowly progress over time; hematogenous dissemination can rarely occur in immunocompromised hosts, causing severe pneumonia, arthritis, or meningitis.

Etiology

Sporothrix schenckii is a globally endemic fungus and causes disease following traumatic inoculation after contact with soil or plant material; most cases are vocational. Lymphocutaneous disease is the usual manifestation.

DIAGNOSIS

Diagnosis requires culture or histopathologic demonstration of yeast in tissue or body fluids. Serology has a limited role.

TREATMENT (Table 8)

Treatment for lymphocutaneous disease is itraconazole elixir or saturated solution of potassium iodide. Severe and meningeal disease should be treated with Amphotericin B.

Mucormycosis

GENERAL PRINCIPLES

Etiology

Caused by class of fungi called Zygomycetes that includes *Mucor*, though most disease is caused by others in the class, such as *Rhizopus*. This group causes head and neck, pulmonary, GI, cutaneous, and disseminated disease with angioinvasion and multiorgan infarction.

Risk Factors

Risk factors include immunosuppression, iron overload, and ketoacidosis.

DIAGNOSIS

Diagnostic Testing

Laboratories

Diagnosis requires tissue culture and silver stain with care to avoid disrupting fungal architecture.

Imaging

MRI with contrast is helpful in head and neck disease to identify involved structures.

TREATMENT (Table 8)

Treatment requires aggressive surgical resection and debridement with clean margins, followed by liposomal amphotericin B 5 mg/kg qd for 6 months.

Non-desferrioxamine iron chelators can be tried as salvage adjuncts (*Antimicrob Agents Chemother 2006;50:3768*).

OUTCOME/PROGNOSIS

Mortality is very high in immunosuppressed patients and disseminated disease.

Nocardiasis

GENERAL PRINCIPLES

Typical infection tends to be pulmonary infiltrate, abscess, or empyema, but dissemination is common and tends to favor CNS infection, causing abscess.

Etiology

Nocardia is a ubiquitous group of aerobic gram-positive branching filamentous bacteria that causes severe local and disseminated disease in the setting of impaired cell-mediated immunity.

DIAGNOSIS

Diagnosis requires sputum or tissue culture, Gram stain, and AFB, often needing multiple samples as yield is low.

Diagnostic Testing

Imaging

Look for CNS disease with brain MRI in patients with pulmonary disease.

TREATMENT (Table 8)

Treatment with high-dose sulfonamides is preferred, with duration of treatment of 6 to 12 months, depending on immune status. Suppressive treatment is necessary as long as immunocompromise continues.

Actinomycosis

GENERAL PRINCIPLES

Classic infections are chronic, indurated soft-tissue lesions associated with draining fistulae that pass through tissue planes, and microscopic "sulfur granules." Unlike *Nocardia*, infection is not limited to immunosuppressed hosts.

Etiology

Actinomyces is a microaerophilic gram-positive bacillus that usually causes oropharyngeal, pulmonary, and GI disease.

DIAGNOSIS

Diagnosis is made by histopathology or observation of "sulfur granules" in drainage.

TREATMENT (Table 8)

Treatment requires an extended course of amoxicillin, doxycycline, or clindamycin, with an initial 2- to 6-week course of high-dose IV penicillin or clindamycin. Surgery is occasionally required.

Atypical Mycobacteria

GENERAL PRINCIPLES

Nontuberculous mycobacteria

- Nontuberculous mycobacteria (NTM) are ubiquitous environmental organisms that cause a spectrum of disease involving the lungs, skin, soft tissue, and lymph nodes. Susceptibility testing and specialist consultation is recommended to guide treatment.
- *M. avium (MAI)*, *M. Kansasii* (see Chapter HIV Infection and AIDS)
- *M. fortuitum, M. marinum, M. ulcerans, M. haemophilum,* and *M. scrofulaceum* cause a spectrum of chronic progressive disease of soft tissue and bone. *M. leprae* is typically classified separately from the other NTM because of its human–human transmission potential.

TICK-BORNE INFECTIONS

Tick-borne infections (TBIs) are common during the summer months in many areas of the United States; prevalence of specific diseases depends on the local population of vector ticks and animal reservoirs.

Coinfection with multiple TBIs is common and should be considered when patients present with overlapping syndromes. Risk should be assessed by outdoor activity in endemic regions rather than known tick bite or attachment, which often go unnoticed.

Lyme Borreliosis (Lyme Disease)

GENERAL PRINCIPLES

Lyme borreliosis is the most common vector-borne disease in the United States and is a systemic illness of variable severity caused by the spirochete *Borrelia burgdorferi*. It has three distinct clinical stages, which start after an incubation period of 7 to 10 days:

- Stage 1 (early local disease) is characterized by erythema migrans, a slowly expanding macular rash >5 cm in diameter, often with central clearing, and by mild constitutional symptoms.
- Stage 2 (early disseminated disease) occurs within several weeks to months and includes multiple erythema migrans lesions, neurologic symptoms (e.g., seventh cranial nerve palsy, meningoencephalitis), cardiac symptoms (atrioventricular block, myopericarditis), and asymmetric oligoarticular arthritis.
- Stage 3 (late disease) occurs after months to years and includes chronic dermatitis, neurologic disease, and asymmetric monoarticular or oligoarticular arthritis. Chronic fatigue is not seen more frequently in patients with Lyme borreliosis than in control subjects.

Epidemiology

It is seen in endemic regions, including northeastern coastal states, the upper Midwest, and northern California.

Prevention

Prophylactic doxycycline, 200 mg PO single dose, may reduce the risk of Lyme disease in endemic areas following a bite by a nymph-stage deer tick (*N Engl J Med 2001;345:79*).

DIAGNOSIS

Diagnostic Testing

Diagnosis rests on clinical suspicion in the appropriate setting but can be supported by two-tiered serologic testing (screening enzyme-linked immunosorbent assay [ELISA] followed by Western blot) with acute and convalescent serologies.

TREATMENT

- Treatment depends on stage and severity of disease (*Clin Infect Dis 2006;43:1089*). Oral therapy (doxycycline, 100 mg PO bid; amoxicillin, 500 mg PO tid; or cefuroxime axetil, 500 mg PO bid for 10 to 21 days) is used for early localized or disseminated disease without neurologic or cardiac involvement. The same agents, given for 28 days, are recommended for late Lyme disease. Doxycycline has the added benefit of covering potential coinfection with ehrlichiosis.
- Parenteral therapy (ceftriaxone, 2 g IV daily; cefotaxime, 2 g IV q8h; penicillin G, 3 to 4 million units IV q4h) for 14 to 28 days should be used for severe neurologic or cardiac disease, regardless of stage.

Rocky Mountain Spotted Fever

GENERAL PRINCIPLES

Epidemiology

Endemic regions are east of the Rocky Mountains.

Etiology

Rocky Mountain Spotted Fever (RMSF) is caused by *Rickettsia rickettsii* after a tick bite, which may go unrecognized.

DIAGNOSIS

Initial diagnosis leading to presumptive treatment should be based on the clinical syndrome, but skin biopsy and acute and convalescent serologies can provide additional support.

Clinical Presentation

Clinical signs include fever, headache, and myalgias, followed 1 to 5 days later with a petechial rash starting on the distal extremities that may be faint and difficult to detect.

TREATMENT

Antibiotic treatment of choice is doxycycline, 100 mg q12h IV or PO for 7 days, or for 2 days after becoming afebrile. Chloramphenicol is an alternative.

OUTCOME/PROGNOSIS

Death can occur when treatment is delayed.

Ehrlichiosis and Anaplasmosis

GENERAL PRINCIPLES

- Ehrlichiosis and Anaplasmosis are systemic TBIs caused by intracellular pathogens of the closely related *Ehrlichia* and *Anaplasma* genera. Two similar syndromes are recognized:
  - **Human monocytic ehrlichiosis** (HME), caused by *Ehrlichia chaffeensis*, is endemic in the south and south-central United States.
  - **Human granulocytic anaplasmosis** (HGA, formerly HGE), caused by *Anaplasma phagocytophilum*, is found in the same regions as Lyme borreliosis due to a shared tick vector.
- Clinical onset of illness usually occurs 1 week after tick exposure, with fever, headache, and myalgias. Rash is only occasionally seen. Severe disease can result in respiratory failure, renal insufficiency, and neurologic decompensation.
- Leukopenia, thrombocytopenia, and elevated liver transaminases are the hallmarks of moderately severe disease.

DIAGNOSIS

Diagnostic Testing

Laboratories

Diagnosis can be made by identification of morulae in circulating monocytes (HME) or granulocytes (HGA), which is uncommon but diagnostic in the appropriate clinical setting. Confirmation is by acute and convalescent serologies or PCR of blood or other fluids.

TREATMENT

Prompt initiation of treatment with antimicrobials is likely to improve prognosis in severe disease. The drugs of choice are doxycycline, 100 mg PO or IV q12h, or tetracycline, 25 mg/kg/d PO divided qid, for 7 to 14 days.

Tularemia

GENERAL PRINCIPLES

- Tularemia is caused by the gram-negative *Francisella tularensis* and is endemic to the south-central United States. It is transmitted by tick bite, by exposure to infected animals (particularly rabbits), or by exposure to infectious aerosol.

- Fever and malaise occurs 2 to 5 days after exposure. The clinical presentation depends on the inoculation site and route of exposure. Painful regional lymphadenitis with (ulceroglandular) or without (glandular) a skin ulcer is the most common finding. Oculoglandular disease can occur. Systemic (typhoidal) and pneumonic diseases are more likely to be severe, with high mortality if not treated promptly.

DIAGNOSIS

Diagnostic Testing

Laboratories

Diagnosis can be confirmed by culture of blood, sputum, or pleural fluid but it is insensitive. The microbiology laboratory must be alerted promptly of culture specimens from patients with suspected tularemia to allow for use of advanced biohazard precautions. Acute and convalescent serologic studies provide a retrospective diagnosis.

TREATMENT

Treatment of choice is Streptomycin, 1 g IM q12h for 10 days; however, gentamicin, 5 mg/kg IV divided q8h, is nearly as effective and easier to administer. Doxycycline, 100 mg PO for 14 to 21 days, is an oral alternative but is more likely to result in relapse. Ciprofloxacin, 500 to 750 mg PO bid for 14 to 21 days, may also be effective.

Babesiosis

GENERAL PRINCIPLES

Clinical disease ranges from subclinical to severe, with fever, chills, myalgias, and headache. Hemolytic anemia may also be present.

Epidemiology

It is endemic in the same regions as Lyme borreliosis, with which patients may be coinfected.

Etiology

Babesiosis is a malaria-like illness is caused by the intraerythrocytic parasite *Babesia microti* after a tick bite.

DIAGNOSIS

Diagnostic Testing

Laboratories

Diagnosis is made by visualization of the parasite in erythrocytes on thick or thin blood smears. A serologic test is also available at the CDC.

TREATMENT

Treatment may be necessary for moderate or severe disease, especially in asplenic patients. Atovaquone, 750 mg PO bid, plus azithromycin, 600 mg PO daily, for 7 to 10 days is the first choice. Clindamycin, 600 mg PO/IV q8h, plus quinine, 650 mg PO tid, for 7 to 10 days should be considered for life-threatening disease.

MOSQUITO-BORNE INFECTIONS

Arboviral Meningoencephalitis

GENERAL PRINCIPLES

- Arboviral meningoencephalitis can be caused by multiple viral agents, which vary by geographic area (WNV, Eastern and Western equine encephalitis, La Crosse encephalitis, St. Louis encephalitis). In addition to mosquitoes, transmission can occur from blood transfusion, organ transplant, and breast-feeding. Infections usually occur in the summer months, and most are subclinical.
- Symptomatic cases of WNV infection range from a mild febrile illness to aseptic meningitis, fulminant encephalitis, or a poliomyelitis-like presentation with flaccid paralysis. Long-term neurologic sequelae are common with severe disease.

DIAGNOSIS

Diagnostic Testing

Laboratories

Diagnosis is usually clinical or by acute and convalescent serologic studies. Specific IgM antibody detection in CSF is diagnostic for acute WNV.

TREATMENT

Treatment for all arboviral meningoencephalitides is supportive.

Malaria

GENERAL PRINCIPLES

- Malaria is a systemic parasitic disease that is endemic to most of the tropical and subtropical world. Several species of the parasite exist.
- The onset of illness occurs within weeks or up to 6 to 12 months after infection with fever, headache, myalgias, and fatigue. Malaria is sometimes characterized by triphasic, periodic (every 48 hours for *Plasmodium ovale* and *Plasmodium vivax*) paroxysms of rigors followed by high fever with headache, cough, and nausea, then culminating in profuse sweating.
- *Plasmodium falciparum* malaria, the most severe form of the disease, is a potential medical emergency. Complicated, or severe, falciparum malaria is diagnosed in the setting of hyperparasitemia (>5%), cerebral malaria, hypoglycemia, lactic acidosis, renal failure, acute respiratory distress syndrome, or coagulopathy.

Prevention

Travel advice and appropriate chemoprophylaxis regimens are available at the CDC Web site, http://www.cdc.gov/travel/.

DIAGNOSIS

Diagnosis is by visualization of parasites on examination of Giemsa-stained thick blood smears. Smears should be obtained prior to febrile episodes to maximize parasite yield.

Malaria should be suspected and excluded in all persons with fever who have been in an endemic area within the previous year.

TREATMENT

- Treatment is dependent on the type of malaria, severity, and risk of chloroquine resistance where the infection occurred. Updated information on geographic locations of chloroquine resistance and recommended treatment regimens can be found on the CDC Web sites, www.cdc.gov/travel/ and www.cdc.gov/malaria/pdf/treatmenttable.pdf.
- **Uncomplicated *P. falciparum* from chloroquine-sensitive areas and *P. malariae*:** chloroquine, 600-mg base (1,000 mg chloroquine phosphate) PO single dose, followed by 300-mg base PO 6, 24, and 48 hours later.
- ***P. ovale* and most *P. vivax* from chloroquine-sensitive areas:** same as preceding, plus primaquine phosphate, 15.3-mg base (26.5 mg salt) PO daily, for 14 days to prevent relapse. Glucose 6-phosphate dehydrogenase deficiency must be ruled out before primaquine is initiated.
- **Uncomplicated *P. falciparum* from chloroquine-resistant areas and *P. vivax* from Australia, Indonesia, or South America:** quinine sulfate, 650 mg PO tid, plus doxycycline, 100 mg PO bid for 7 days. Alternatives are atovaquone, 1 g PO daily, plus proguanil, 400 mg PO daily, both for 3 days; mefloquine; or halofantrine.
- **Complicated or severe *P. falciparum*:** quinidine gluconate, 10 mg salt/kg (maximum, 600 mg) IV over 1 to 2 hours, followed by 0.02 mg/kg/min as a continuous infusion for 72 hours or until parasitemia is <1%, at which time the 72-hour course can be completed with oral quinine sulfate as previously described. Exchange transfusion can be considered when P. falciparum parasitemia exceeds 15%, although the benefit has not been proven.

ZOONOSES

Avian and Swine Influenza (see the Emerging Infections and Bioterrorism section).
Anthrax (see the Emerging Infections and Bioterrorism section).
Plague (see the Emerging Infections and Bioterrorism section).

Cat-Scratch Disease (Bartonellosis)

GENERAL PRINCIPLES

Etiology
Bartonellosis is caused by the bacterium *Bartonella henselae*. It is usually self-limiting.

DIAGNOSIS

Diagnosis is made by exclusion of other causes of lymphadenitis and by detection of antibodies to *B. henselae* or PCR of infected tissue, skin, or pus.

Clinical Presentation
- Clinically, a single or a few papulopustular lesions appear 3 to 10 days after a cat bite or scratch, followed by regional lymphadenitis (usually cervical or axillary) and mild constitutional symptoms.

- Atypical presentations include oculoglandular disease, encephalopathy, arthritis, and severe systemic disease.

TREATMENT

Treatment of localized disease is usually unnecessary because spontaneous resolution usually occurs in 2 to 4 months. If antimicrobial therapy is prescribed, azithromycin, 500 mg PO single dose followed by 250 mg PO for 4 more days, is recommended. Needle aspiration of suppurative lymph nodes may provide symptomatic relief.

Leptospirosis

GENERAL PRINCIPLES

- Leptospirosis is an acute febrile illness with varying presentations caused by *Leptospira interrogans*, a ubiquitous pathogen of wild and domestic mammals, reptiles, and amphibians. Symptom onset is 5 to 14 days after contact with infected animals or water contaminated with their urine.
- **Anicteric leptospirosis,** which accounts for most cases, is a biphasic illness that starts with influenza-like symptoms and proceeds to conjunctival suffusion and aseptic meningitis after a brief defervescent period.
- A minority of cases progress directly to **Weil's disease (icteric leptospirosis),** with multiorgan failure manifested by severe jaundice, uremia, and hemorrhagic pneumonitis.

DIAGNOSIS

Diagnosis is confirmed by specific cultures of urine or blood, PCR, or paired serologic studies.

TREATMENT

Therapy for anicteric disease, which can shorten the duration of illness, is doxycycline, 100 mg PO bid, or amoxicillin, 500 mg PO q6h, for 7 days. Penicillin G, 1.5 million U IV q4–6h, or a third-generation cephalosporin, is used for treatment of severe disease, during which a Jarisch–Herxheimer reaction is possible.

Brucellosis

GENERAL PRINCIPLES

Brucellosis is usually preceded by direct contact with body fluids of livestock animals or by eating unpasteurized dairy foods.

Etiology

Brucellosis is a protean systemic infection caused by members of the *Brucella* genus of gram-negative coccobacilli.

DIAGNOSIS

Clinical Presentation

Symptoms are initially nonspecific, but complications within every organ system can occur (diarrhea, arthritis, meningitis, endocarditis, pneumonia).

Diagnostic Testing

Laboratories

Diagnosis is confirmed by blood or tissue culture.

TREATMENT

Antimicrobial treatment with doxycycline, 100 mg PO bid, for 6 weeks with or without gentamicin for 2 to 3 weeks, or RIF for 6 weeks, reduces duration and complications of the disease. Audiometry should be performed weekly while gentamicin therapy is administered.

BITE WOUNDS

Animal Bites

GENERAL PRINCIPLES

- Management includes copious irrigation, obtaining cultures only from visibly infected wounds, and radiographic studies to exclude fracture, foreign body, or joint space involvement.
- Most wounds should not be sutured unless they are on the face and have been copiously irrigated. Wound elevation should be encouraged.

TREATMENT

- Antimicrobial therapy is given to treat overt infection and as prophylaxis for high-risk bite wounds based on severity (moderate to severe), location (on hands, genitalia, or near joints), bite source (cats), immune status, and type of injury (puncture or crush). Tetanus booster should be given if none has been administered to the patient in the last 5 years.
- Prophylactic antibiotic therapy with amoxicillin-clavulanate, 875 mg-125 mg PO bid, for 3 to 5 days should usually be administered, unless the bite is trivial. Antibiotics are most effective for patients presenting >8 hours after the injury (*Arch Emerg Med 1989;6:251*).

SPECIAL CONSIDERATIONS

- **Dog bites:** The normal oral flora includes *Pasteurella multocida*, streptococci, staphylococci, and *Capnocytophaga canimorsus*. Dog bites comprise 80% of animal bites, but only 5% of such bites become infected. For infected dog-bite wounds, amoxicillin-clavulanate, or clindamycin plus ciprofloxacin, is effective.
- **Cat bites:** Normal oral flora includes *P. multocida* and *S. aureus*. Because more than 80% of cat bites become infected, prophylaxis with amoxicillin-clavulanate should

be routinely provided. Cephalosporins should not be used. Bartonellosis can also occur after bites.

- **Wild animal bites:** Need for rabies vaccination should be determined (see below). For most animal bites, amoxicillin-clavulanate is a good choice for prophylaxis and empiric treatment. Monkey bites should be treated with acyclovir because of the risk of *Herpesvirus simiae.*
- *Rabies*
  - Rabies causes an invariably fatal neurologic disease manifested by hydrophobia, pharyngeal spasm, seizures, and coma.
  - The need for rabies vaccination and immunoglobulin prophylaxis (see Appendix A, Immunizations and Postexposure Therapies) should be determined after any animal bite. Risk of rabies depends on the animal species and the geographic location; disease is endemic in bats in particular.
  - Regardless of species, if the animal is rabid or suspected to be rabid, the human diploid vaccine and rabies immunoglobulin should be administered immediately. Bites by domestic animals rarely require prophylaxis unless the animal's condition is unknown. Public health authorities should be consulted to determine whether prophylaxis is recommended for other animals.
  - A single case of survival after symptom onset by an aggressive coma-inducing regimen has been reported.

Human Bites

GENERAL PRINCIPLES

- Human bites, particularly clenched-fist injuries, are prone to infection and other complications. The normal oral flora of humans includes viridans streptococci, staphylococci, *Bacteroides* species, *Fusobacterium* species, peptostreptococci, and *Eikenella corrodens.*
- **Prophylaxis** with amoxicillin-clavulanate, 875 mg-125 mg PO bid for 5 days is recommended for uninfected wounds.
- Infected wounds may require **parenteral therapy,** such as ampicillin-sulbactam, 1.5 g IV q6h; cefoxitin, 2 g IV q8h; or ticarcillin-clavulanate, 3.1 g IV q6h, for 1 to 2 weeks. Therapy should be extended to 4 to 6 weeks if osteomyelitis is present.

NOSOCOMIAL INFECTIONS

Nosocomial infections substantially contribute to morbidity, mortality, and excess health care costs. Efforts to control and prevent the spread of nosocomial infections require an institutional assessment of resources, priorities, and commitment to infection control practices (see Appendix B, Infection Control and Isolation Recommendations).

Catheter-Related Bloodstream Infections

GENERAL PRINCIPLES

- Catheter-related bloodstream infections (CR-BSIs) should be suspected in any febrile patient with a central catheter.

- Clinical findings that increase the suspicion of CR-BSIs are local inflammation or phlebitis at the central venous catheter (CVC) insertion site, sepsis, endophthalmitis, lack of another source of bacteremia, and resolution of fever after catheter removal.
- **CVC removal** is preferred but may involve complex decision making with consideration of host status, need for and type of vascular access, and the identified pathogen. Remove CVCs in the following settings:
  - Insertion-site or tunnel-site infection (i.e., pus or significant inflammation at the site).
  - *Candida*, *S. aureus*, and most gram-negative CR-BSIs.
  - Immunosuppressed patients who have fever, neutropenia, and hemodynamic instability.
  - Nontunneled CVCs should generally be removed for CR-BSI caused by organisms other than coagulase-negative staphylococci.
  - Antibiotic lock therapy is an option that may be used to help salvage CVCs.

Etiology

S. aureus, *S. epidermidis* (coagulase-negative staphylococci), aerobic gram-negative species, and *Candida* species are most commonly associated with CR-BSIs (*Clin Infect Dis 2001;32:1249*).

Prevention

- Subclavian vein CVCs are associated with lower CR-BSI rates than internal jugular CVCs, whereas femoral CVCs have the highest rates of CR-BSIs and should be removed within 72 hours of placement.
- Strategies for decreasing the incidence of CR-BSIs include the use of full sterile barrier precautions during insertion, transparent dressings, skin preparation with chlorhexidine-based product, strict adherence to aseptic technique and hand washing, topical antiseptic solutions, and removing nonessential catheters as soon as possible (*ICHE 2008;29(Suppl 1):S22*). Subcutaneous tunneling and use of antiseptic-impregnated CVCs may further reduce the incidence of CR-BSIs. Routine exchange of CVCs over guidewire is not recommended.

DIAGNOSIS

Diagnosis is made by blood cultures, drawn before the initiation of antibiotics. When notified of positive blood cultures, repeat cultures before initiating antibiotics are recommended.

TREATMENT

- Host factors, such as comorbidities, severity of illness, multidrug-resistant colonization, prior infections, and current antimicrobial agents, are important considerations when selecting the initial antimicrobial regimen. Documentation of clearance of bacteremia after initiation of antibiotics is critical.
- Vancomycin, 1 g IV q12h, is usually appropriate for empiric therapy because the majority of CR-BSIs are caused by staphylococci.
- **Gram-negative bacilli** should be treated broadly, for example, cefepime 1 g IV q12h, to cover nosocomial pathogens such as *Pseudomonas* until species identification and susceptibilities are known.

- Duration of treatment depends on whether the infection is complicated or uncomplicated. Duration of therapy is counted from the date of the first negative blood culture. Duration of treatment should be longer if the CVC remains in situ.
- **Pathogen-specific therapy:** Once the pathogen has been identified, antimicrobial therapy should be narrowed to the most effective regimen.
  - **S. aureus: Methicillin-sensitive S. aureus** CR-BSI should be treated with oxacillin, 2 g IV q4h, or alternatively with cefazolin, 1 to 2 g IV q8h. First-line therapy for **MRSA** is vancomycin, 1 g IV q12h. Linezolid, 600 mg PO or IV q12h, or daptomycin, 6 mg/kg IV daily, are alternatives. Routine use of gentamycin for synergy in S. aureus bacteremia is not recommended (*Clin Infect Dis 2009;48:722*). TEE should be considered to exclude endocarditis. Duration of therapy is 2 to 4 weeks if TEE is negative, another source is identified, and cultures clear quickly. Four to six weeks of treatment is required for suspected endovascular or complicated infections (prolonged bacteremia, suspected catheter-related clot or venous stenosis) (*Clin Infect Dis 2001;32:1249*).
  - **S. epidermidis (coagulase-negative staphylococci)** CR-BSI is treated similarly to MRSA, with vancomycin being the drug of choice in most cases. Duration of therapy is 5 to 7 days after CVC removal or 10 to 14 days if the CVC is retained.
- **Catheter-related candidemia** in hosts who are hemodynamically unstable or have had prolonged fluconazole therapy should be treated with caspofungin, 70 mg IV single dose, followed by 50 mg IV daily while awaiting identification of the species. Patients who are hemodynamically stable and have had low fluconazole exposure, have a *Candida* species that is usually sensitive to fluconazole and can be treated with fluconazole, 400 mg IV or PO daily. Duration of antifungal treatment for candidemia should be for 14 days after the last positive blood culture result and when signs and symptoms of infection have resolved (*Clin Infect Dis 2009;48:503*).
- Updated guidelines for management of catheter related blood stream infections will be published soon by the Infectious Diseases Society of America.

Hospital and Ventilator-Associated Pneumonia

GENERAL PRINCIPLES

Etiology
The most frequent pathogens are gram-negative bacilli and *S. aureus*.

DIAGNOSIS

Clinical Presentation
The clinical presentation includes a new pulmonary infiltrate or increasing oxygen requirement in patients with fever, with or without cough, that occurs >48 hours after admission.

Diagnostic Testing
Laboratories
Diagnosis is made by clinical criteria as well as microbiologic testing. Optimal specimens are uncontaminated sterile body fluids (pleural or blood), bronchoscopy aspirates (cultured quantitatively), or aspirates from endotracheal tubes.

Diagnostic Procedures
Fiberoptic bronchoscopy may be diagnostic (quantitative cultures) and therapeutic (reexpansion of lung segment) in these patients.

TREATMENT

Initial empiric antimicrobial therapy should target treatment of nosocomially acquired pathogens, particularly *P. aeruginosa* and MRSA. Targeted therapy should be based on culture results and in vitro sensitivity testing. Empyemas require drainage.

Methicillin-resistant *Staphylococcus Aureus* Infections

GENERAL PRINCIPLES

- MRSA infection should be distinguished from MRSA colonization, especially when found from nonsterile sites such as sputum.
- Contact precautions are indicated.

TREATMENT

- First-line therapy for most MRSA infections is vancomycin (dosed to therapeutic trough levels). Linezolid, 600 mg IV or PO q12h, is an alternative.
- Eradication of MRSA nasal carriage can sometimes be achieved with a 5-day course of twice-daily intranasal mupirocin. Other regimens include chlorhexidine soap products, bleach baths, oral antibiotic treatment with Bactrim with or without rifampin. However, mupirocin resistance can develop and carriage often recurs. Eradication efforts should be targeted at patients with recurrent clinical infections with MRSA.

Vancomycin-Resistant Enterococcus Infections

GENERAL PRINCIPLES

- VRE infection should be distinguished from VRE colonization.
- Most VRE-related lower UTIs can be treated with nitrofurantoin, ampicillin, ciprofloxacin, or other agents that achieve high urinary concentrations.
- Contact precautions are indicated. Eradication of enteric VRE colonization has been attempted without success.

TREATMENT

The majority of patients with VRE bloodstream infections are treated with linezolid, daptomycin, or quinupristin/dalfopristin.

Multidrug-Resistant Gram-Negative Infections

GENERAL PRINCIPLES

Etiology
Highly resistant gram-negative organisms (e.g., *Acinetobacter*, *Klebsiella*, and *Pseudomonas* species) are becoming increasingly common causes of nosocomial infections.

TREATMENT

Antimicrobial choices are often limited. In addition to broad-spectrum agents such as β-lactam/β-lactamase inhibitor combinations and carbapenems, tigecycline, and colistin may occasionally be useful.

REFERRAL

Infectious diseases consultation is recommended for such complicated multidrug-resistant infections.

EMERGING INFECTIONS AND BIOTERRORISM

Changing patterns in human behavior and demographics, natural phenomena, and microbial evolution continually introduce new pathogens to human contact, leading to the introduction and spread of new or previously rare diseases. Included in this category are several highly fatal and easily produced microorganisms, which have the potential to be used as agents of bioterrorism and produce substantial illness in large populations via an aerosol route of exposure. Most of the likely diseases are rare, so a high index of suspicion is necessary to identify the first few cases. A bioterrorism-related outbreak should be considered if an unusually large number of patients present simultaneously with a respiratory, GI, or febrile rash syndrome; if several otherwise healthy patients present with unusually severe disease; or if an unusual pathogen for the region is isolated.

Anthrax

GENERAL PRINCIPLES

- Natural transmission can occur through butchering and eating infected animals, usually leading to cutaneous ("Woolsorters disease") and gastrointestinal disease.
- Inhalational anthrax (45% case-fatality rate) presents initially with influenza-like illness, GI symptoms, or both, followed by fulminant respiratory distress and multiorgan failure. Cutaneous anthrax is characterized by a painless black eschar with surrounding edema.

Etiology

Spores from the gram-positive *Bacillus anthracis* germinate at the site of entry into the body, causing inhalational, cutaneous, or gastrointestinal anthrax.

DIAGNOSIS

Diagnosis of inhalational disease is suggested by a widened mediastinum without infiltrates on chest radiography and confirmed by blood culture. Notify local infection control and Public Health department immediately for confirmed cases.

TREATMENT

- Treatment with immediate antibiotic initiation on first suspicion of inhalational anthrax reduces mortality. Empiric therapy is ciprofloxacin, 400 mg IV q12h, *or* doxycycline, 100 mg IV q12h, *and* one or two other antibiotics that are active against *B. anthracis* (e.g., penicillin, clindamycin, vancomycin) (*JAMA 2002;287:2236*). Oral therapy with ciprofloxacin, 500 mg PO bid, *or* doxycycline, 100 mg PO bid, *and* one other active agent should be started after improvement and continued for 60 days to reduce the risk of delayed spore germination.
  - Uncomplicated cutaneous anthrax can be treated with oral ciprofloxacin, 500 mg bid, *or* doxycycline, 100 mg bid, for the same duration.
- Postexposure prophylaxis consists of oral ciprofloxacin, 500 mg bid for 60 days after exposure. Doxycycline or amoxicillin is an alternative if the strain proves susceptible.

Smallpox

GENERAL PRINCIPLES

The variola virus that causes smallpox is easily transmitted person to person through respiratory droplets and carries a case-fatality ratio of 25% to 30%. It was declared eradicated as a naturally occurring disease in 1979; however, remaining viral stocks pose a potential bioterrorism threat to an unimmunized population.

DIAGNOSIS

Diagnosis is primarily clinical but can be confirmed by electron microscopy and PCR of pustule fluid at reference laboratories. Notify local infection control, Public Health departments, and CDC immediately. Treat all diagnostic samples as highly infectious.

Clinical Presentation

- High fever, myalgias, low back pain, and headache appear 7 to 17 days after exposure, followed by the distinctive rash 3 to 5 days later.
- Lesions progress through stages of macules, deep vesicles, pustules, scabs, and permanent pitting scars. The rash starts on the face and distal extremities, including palms and soles, with relative sparing of the trunk, and all lesions in one area are in the same stage of development. *These features help to distinguish smallpox from chickenpox(varicella).*

TREATMENT

- Treatment consists of supportive care; no specific antiviral treatment is available. All suspected cases must be placed in contact and airborne isolation; patients remain infectious until all scabs have separated from the skin.
- Postexposure prophylaxis with live vaccinia virus vaccine within 3 days of exposure offers near-complete protection for responders but is associated with uncommon severe adverse reactions. Progressive vaccinia, eczema vaccinatum, and severe cases of generalized vaccinia can be treated with vaccinia immunoglobulin.

Plague

GENERAL PRINCIPLES

Plague is caused by the gram-negative bacillus *Yersinia pestis* and takes one of three forms:

- **Bubonic:** Local painful lymphadenitis (bubo) and fever (14% case-fatality ratio).
- **Septicemic:** Can cause peripheral necrosis and DIC ("black death"). Usually from progression of bubonic disease (30% to 50% case-fatality ratio).
- **Pneumonic:** Severe pneumonia with hemoptysis preceded by initial influenza-like illness (57% case-fatality ratio, nearing 100% when treatment is delayed). Pneumonic disease can be transmitted from person to person and would be expected after inhalation of aerosolized *Y. pestis*.

Epidemiology

Naturally acquired plague occurs rarely in the southwestern United States after exposure to infected animals.

DIAGNOSIS

Diagnosis is confirmed by isolation of *Y. pestis* from blood, sputum, or CSF. Notify local infection control and Public Health departments immediately.

TREATMENT

- Treatment should start at first suspicion of plague because rapid initiation of antibiotics improves survival. Agents of choice are streptomycin, 1 g IM q12h; gentamicin, 5 mg/kg IV/IM q24h *or* a 2 mg/kg loading dose, then 1.7 mg/kg IV/IM q8h, with appropriate monitoring of drug levels; or doxycycline, 100 mg PO/IV bid. Alternatives include ciprofloxacin and chloramphenicol. Oral therapy can be started after clinical improvement, for a total course of 10 to 14 days.
- Postexposure prophylaxis is doxycycline, 100 mg PO bid, or ciprofloxacin, 500 mg PO bid, for 7 days after exposure.

Botulism

GENERAL PRINCIPLES

Botulism can occur from ingestion of toxin from improperly canned food, or contamination of wounds with soil.

Etiology

Botulism is the result of intoxication with botulinum toxin, produced by the anaerobic gram-positive bacillus *Clostridium botulinum*.

DIAGNOSIS

Diagnosis is confirmed by detection of toxin in serum. Notify local infection control and Public Health departments.

Clinical Presentation

The classic symptom triad is lack of fever, clear sensorium, and symmetric descending flaccid paralysis with cranial nerve involvement, beginning with ptosis, diplopia, and dysarthria and progressing to loss of gag reflex and diaphragmatic function followed by diffuse skeletal muscle paralysis. Sensation remains intact. Paralysis lasts for weeks to months.

TREATMENT

Treatment is primarily supportive, particularly ventilatory support. Wound botulism requires debridement. Further progression of paralysis can be halted by administration of botulinum antitoxin, which is available from the local health department. Postexposure prophylaxis with antitoxin is not recommended because of the high incidence (10%) of hypersensitivity reactions and limited supply.

OUTCOME/PROGNOSIS

Mortality is low when it is recognized early but may be very high in the setting of mass exposure if supportive care equipment supplies (i.e., ventilators) are exhausted.

Viral Hemorrhagic Fever

GENERAL PRINCIPLES

Etiology

This syndrome is caused by many different RNA viruses, including filoviruses (Ebola and Marburg), flaviviruses (dengue, yellow fever), bunyaviruses (Hanta viruses, Congo-Crimean hemorrhagic fever [CCHF], Rift Valley Fever), and arenaviruses (South American hemorrhagic fevers, Lassa fever). All cause sporadic disease in endemic areas, and most can be transmitted as an aerosol or contact with infected body fluids.

DIAGNOSIS

Diagnosis requires consideration of epidemiology and patient risk factors, especially travel to endemic areas. Serology performed by reference laboratories can confirm diagnosis. Notify local infection control and Public Health departments immediately.

Clinical Presentation

Early symptoms are fevers, myalgias, and malaise, with varying severity and symptomatology depending on the virus, but all can severely disrupt vascular permeability and cause DIC. Thrombocytopenia, leukopenia, and hepatitis are common.

TREATMENT

- Treatment is primarily supportive with attention to infection control. Ribavirin (2 g IV × 1, then 1 g/d × 6 d, then 500 mg/d) can be used for CCHF, Lassa, and Rift Valley Fevers (*JAMA 2002;287:2391*; *Clin Infect Dis 2003;36:1613*).

- Exposed contacts should monitor temperature twice daily for 3 weeks. Postexposure prophylaxis with oral ribavirin can be administered to febrile CCHF, Lassa, and RVF contacts.

OUTCOME/PROGNOSIS

Case-fatality ratios are variable but can be as high as 90% for severe Ebola cases.

Severe Acute Respiratory Syndrome

GENERAL PRINCIPLES

Severe acute respiratory syndrome (SARS) is a fulminant febrile influenza-like respiratory illness that progresses to pneumonia and ARDS, caused by SARS-associated coronavirus (SARS-CoV). SARS should be considered in clusters of cases of undiagnosed atypical, especially in the setting travel to Mainland China, Hong Kong, or Taiwan within 10 days of symptom onset.

DIAGNOSIS

Diagnosis is confirmed by acute or convalescent SARS-CoV antibodies or PCR by the CDC.

TREATMENT

Treatment is primarily supportive. Interferon and high-dose steroids have been used.

Pandemic, Avian, and Swine Influenza

GENERAL PRINCIPLES

- Genetic reassortment can result in influenza strains that were previously confined to avian and swine hosts gaining human infectivity, causing severe disease and/or rapid spread through human populations.
- Infection control measures and close communication with public health authorities are critical when pandemic strains are circulating.
- Each new strain may have different virulence, affected age ranges, clinical presentation, and antiviral susceptibilities. Following updated, local data during an outbreak is essential.

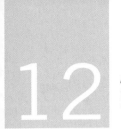

12 Antimicrobials

David J. Ritchie and Bernard C. Camins

Empiric antimicrobial therapy should be initiated based on expected pathogens for a given infection. As microbial resistance is increasing among many pathogens, a review of institutional as well as local, regional, national, and global susceptibility trends can assist in the development of empiric therapy regimens. In addition, an accurate allergy history and pregnancy/lactation status should be elicited from patients. Antimicrobial therapy should be modified, if possible, based on results of culture and sensitivity testing to agent(s) that have the narrowest spectrum possible. Attention should be paid to the possibility of switching from parenteral to oral therapy where possible, as many oral agents have excellent bioavailability. Several antibiotics have major drug interactions or require alternate dosing in renal or hepatic insufficiency, or both. For antiretroviral and antiparasitic agents, see Chapter 13, Human Immunodeficiency Virus and Acquired Immunodeficiency Syndrome, and Chapter 11, Treatment of Infectious Diseases, respectively.

ANTIBACTERIAL AGENTS

Penicillins

GENERAL PRINCIPLES

- Penicillins (PCNs) irreversibly bind PCN-binding proteins in the bacterial cell wall, causing osmotic rupture and death. These agents have a somewhat diminished role today because of acquired resistance in many bacterial species through alterations in PCN-binding proteins or expression of hydrolytic enzymes.
- PCNs remain among the drugs of choice for syphilis, group A streptococci, *Listeria monocytogenes*, *Pasteurella multocida*, *Actinomyces*, and some anaerobic infections.

TREATMENT

Medications

- **Aqueous penicillin G** (2 to 5 million units intravenous [IV] q4h or 12 to 30 million units daily by continuous infusion) is the IV preparation of PCN and the drug of choice for most penicillin-susceptible streptococcal infections and neurosyphilis.
- **Procaine penicillin G** is an IM repository form of penicillin G that can be used as an alternative treatment for neurosyphilis at a dose of 2.4 million units IM daily in combination with probenecid, 500 mg PO qid for 10 to 14 days.
- **Benzathine PCN** is a long-acting IM repository form of penicillin G that is commonly used for treating early latent syphilis (<1 year duration [1 dose, 2.4 million units IM]) and late latent syphilis (unknown duration or >1 year [2.4 million units IM weekly for three doses]). It is occasionally given for group A streptococcal pharyngitis and prophylaxis after acute rheumatic fever.

- **Penicillin V** (250 to 500 mg PO q6h) is an oral formulation of PCN that is typically used to treat group A streptococcal pharyngitis.
- **Ampicillin** (1 to 3 g IV q4–6h) is the drug of choice for treatment of infections caused by susceptible enterococcus species, or *L. monocytogenes*. Oral ampicillin (250 to 500 mg PO q6h) may be used for uncomplicated sinusitis, pharyngitis, otitis media, and urinary tract infections (UTIs), but amoxicillin is generally preferred.
- **Ampicillin/sulbactam** (1.5 to 3.0 g IV q6h) combines ampicillin with the β-lactamase inhibitor sulbactam, thereby extending its spectrum to include methicillin-sensitive *Staphylococcus aureus* (MSSA), anaerobes, and many Enterobacteriaceae. The sulbactam component also has unique activity against some strains of *Acinetobacter*. The agent is effective for infections of the upper and lower respiratory tract, genitourinary tract, and abdominal, pelvic, and polymicrobial soft tissue infections, including those due to human or animal bites.
- **Amoxicillin** (250 to 1,000 mg PO q8h or 775 mg extended-release q24h) is an oral antibiotic similar to ampicillin that is commonly used for uncomplicated sinusitis, pharyngitis, otitis media, community-acquired pneumonia and UTIs.
- **Amoxicillin/clavulanic acid** (875 mg PO q12h, or 500 mg PO q8h, or 90 mg/kg/d divided q12h [Augmentin ES-600 suspension], or 2,000 mg PO q12h [Augmentin XR]) is an oral antibiotic similar to ampicillin/sulbactam that combines amoxicillin with the β-lactamase inhibitor clavulanate. It is useful for treating complicated sinusitis and otitis media and for prophylaxis of human or animal bites after appropriate local treatment.
- **Nafcillin and oxacillin** (1 to 2 g IV q4–6h) are penicillinase-resistant synthetic PCNs that are the drugs of choice for treating MSSA infections. Dose reduction should be considered in decompensated liver disease.
- **Dicloxacillin and cloxacillin** (250 to 500 mg PO q6h) are oral antibiotics with a spectrum of activity similar to that of nafcillin and oxacillin, which are typically used to treat localized skin infections.
- **Piperacillin** (3 g IV q4h or 4 g IV q6h) is an extended-spectrum PCN with enhanced gram-negative activity as well as enterococcal activity. This agent has reasonable antipseudomonal activity but generally requires coadministration of an aminoglycoside for treatment of serious infections.
- **Ticarcillin/clavulanic acid** (3.1 g IV q4–6h) combines ticarcillin with the β-lactamase inhibitor clavulanic acid. This combination extends the spectrum to include most Enterobacteriaceae, MSSA, and anaerobes, making it useful for intra-abdominal and complicated soft tissue infections. Ticarcillin/clavulanic acid also has a unique role in treatment of *Stenotrophomonas* infections. This agent has a high sodium content and should be used cautiously in patients at risk for fluid overload.
- **Piperacillin/tazobactam** (3.375 g IV q6h or the higher dose of 4.5 g IV q6h for *Pseudomonas*) combines piperacillin with the β-lactamase inhibitor tazobactam. It has a similar spectrum and indications as ticarcillin/clavulanic acid but enhanced has activity against ampicillin-sensitive enterococci. The addition of an aminoglycoside should be considered for treatment of serious infections caused by *Pseudomonas aeruginosa* or for nosocomial pneumonia.

SPECIAL CONSIDERATIONS

All PCN derivatives have been rarely associated with anaphylaxis, interstitial nephritis, anemia, and leukopenia. Prolonged high-dose therapy (>2 weeks) is typically monitored with weekly serum creatinine and complete blood cell counts. Liver function tests (LFTs) are also monitored with oxacillin/nafcillin as these agents can cause hepatitis. Ticarcillin/clavulanic acid can aggravate bleeding by interfering with platelet adenosine diphosphate receptors. All patients should be asked about PCN, cephalosporin, or carbapenem allergy. These agents should not be used in patients with a reported serious PCN allergy without prior skin testing or desensitization, or both.

Cephalosporins

GENERAL PRINCIPLES

- Cephalosporins exert their bactericidal effect by interfering with cell wall synthesis by the same mechanism as PCNs.
- They are clinically useful because of their low toxicity and broad spectrum of activity. However, all currently available first- to fourth-generation cephalosporins are devoid of activity against enterococci and methicillin-resistant *S. aureus* (MRSA).

TREATMENT

Medications

- **First-generation cephalosporins** have activity against staphylococci, streptococci, and some *Escherichia coli*, *Klebsiella*, and *Proteus* species. These agents have limited activity against other enteric gram-negative bacilli and anaerobes. **Cefazolin** (1 to 2 g IV/IM q8h) is the most commonly used parenteral preparation, and **cephalexin** (250 to 500 mg PO q6h) and **cefadroxil** (500 mg to 1 g PO q12h) are oral preparations. These limited-activity agents are commonly used for treating skin/soft tissue infections, UTIs, minor MSSA infections, and for surgical prophylaxis (cefazolin).
- **Second-generation cephalosporins** have expanded coverage against enteric gram-negative rods and can be divided into above-the-diaphragm and below-the-diaphragm agents.
- **Cefuroxime** (1.5 g IV/IM q8h) is useful for treatment of infections above the diaphragm. This agent has reasonable antistaphylococcal and antistreptococcal activity in addition to an extended spectrum against gram-negative aerobes and can be used for skin/soft tissue infections, complicated UTIs, and some community-acquired respiratory tract infections. It does not reliably cover *Bacteroides fragilis*.
- **Cefuroxime axetil** (250 to 500 mg PO q12h), **cefprozil** (250 to 500 mg PO q12h), and **cefaclor** (250 to 500 mg PO q12h) are oral second-generation cephalosporins typically used for bronchitis, sinusitis, otitis media, UTIs, local soft tissue infections, and oral step-down therapy for pneumonia or cellulitis responsive to parenteral cephalosporins.
- **Cefoxitin** (1 to 2 g IV q4–8h) and **cefotetan** (1 to 2 g IV q12h) are useful for treatment of infections below the diaphragm. These agents have reasonable activity against gram-negatives and aerobes, including *B. fragilis*, and are commonly used for intra-abdominal or gynecologic surgical prophylaxis and infections, including diverticulitis and pelvic inflammatory disease.
- **Third-generation cephalosporins** have broad coverage against aerobic gram-negative bacilli and retain significant activity against streptococci and MSSA. They have moderate anaerobic activity but generally not against *B. fragilis*. Ceftazidime is the only third-generation cephalosporin that is useful for treating serious *P. aeruginosa*

infections. Some of these agents have substantial central nervous system (CNS) penetration and are useful in treating meningitis (see Chapter 11, Treatment of Infectious Diseases). Third-generation cephalosporins are not reliable for the treatment of serious infections caused by organisms producing AmpC β-lactamases regardless of the results of susceptibility testing. These pathogens should be treated empirically with carbapenems, cefepime, or fluoroquinolones.

- **Ceftriaxone** (1 to 2 g IV/IM q12–24h) and **cefotaxime** (1 to 2 g IV/IM q4–12h) are very similar to one another in spectrum and efficacy. They can be used as empiric therapy for pyelonephritis, urosepsis, pneumonia, intra-abdominal infections (combined with metronidazole), gonorrhea, and meningitis. They can also be used for osteomyelitis, septic arthritis, endocarditis, and soft tissue infections caused by susceptible organisms.
- **Cefpodoxime proxetil** (100 to 400 mg PO q12h), **cefdinir** (300 mg PO q12h), **ceftibuten** (400 mg PO q24h), and **cefditoren pivoxil** (200 to 400 mg PO q12h) are oral third-generation cephalosporins useful for the treatment of bronchitis and complicated sinusitis, otitis media, and UTIs. These agents can also be used as step-down therapy for community-acquired pneumonia. Cefpodoxime can be used as single-dose therapy for uncomplicated gonorrhea.
- **Ceftazidime** (1 to 2 g IV/IM q8h) may be used for treatment of infections caused by susceptible strains of *P. aeruginosa*.
- **The fourth-generation cephalosporin cefepime** (500 mg to 2 g IV/IM q8–12h) has excellent aerobic gram-negative coverage, including *P. aeruginosa* and other bacteria producing AmpC β-lactamases. Its gram-positive activity is similar to that of the ceftriaxone and cefotaxime. **Cefepime** is routinely used for empiric therapy in febrile neutropenic patients. It also has a prominent role in treating infections caused by antibiotic-resistant gram-negative bacteria and some infections involving both gram-negative and gram-positive aerobes in most sites, although clinical experience for treatment of meningitis is more limited. Anti-anaerobic coverage should be added where anaerobes are suspected.

SPECIAL CONSIDERATIONS

All cephalosporins have been rarely associated with anaphylaxis, interstitial nephritis, anemia, and leukopenia. **PCN-allergic patients have a 5% to 10% incidence of a cross-hypersensitivity reaction to cephalosporins.** These agents should not be used in a patient with a reported severe PCN allergy (i.e., anaphylaxis, hives) without prior skin testing or desensitization, or both. Prolonged therapy (>2 weeks) is typically monitored with a weekly serum creatinine and complete blood count. Ceftriaxone can cause biliary sludging requiring discontinuation of the medication.

Monobactams

GENERAL PRINCIPLES

Definition

- **Aztreonam** (1 to 2 g IV/IM q6–12h) is a monobactam that is active only against aerobic gram-negative bacteria, including *P. aeruginosa*.
- It is useful in patients with known β-lactam allergy, as no apparent cross-reactivity is present.

Carbapenems

GENERAL PRINCIPLES

- **Imipenem** (500 mg to 1 g IV/IM q6–8), **meropenem** (1 to 2 g IV q8h or 500 mg IV q6h), **doripenem** (500 mg IV q8h), and **ertapenem** (1 g IV q24h) are the currently available carbapenems.
- Carbapenems exert their bactericidal effect by interfering with cell wall synthesis, similar to PCNs and cephalosporins and are active against most gram-positive and gram-negative bacteria, including anaerobes. They are among the antibiotics of choice for infections caused by organisms producing AmpC or extended-spectrum β-lactamases (ESBLs).

TREATMENT

- Carbapenems are important agents for treatment of many antibiotic-resistant bacterial infections at most body sites. These agents are commonly used for severe polymicrobial infections, including Fournier's gangrene, intra-abdominal catastrophes, and sepsis in immunocompromised hosts.
- Notable bacteria that are **resistant** to carbapenems include ampicillin-resistant enterococci, MRSA, *Stenotrophomonas*, *Burkholderia*, and *Klebsiella pneumoniae* carbapenemase- (KPC-) producing gram-negative organisms. In addition, ertapenem does not provide reliable coverage against *P. aeruginosa*, *Acinetobacter*, or enterococci; therefore, imipenem, doripenem, or meropenem would be preferred for empiric treatment of nosocomial infections when these pathogens are suspected. **Meropenem** is the preferred carbapenem for treatment of CNS infections.

SPECIAL CONSIDERATIONS

- Carbapenems can precipitate seizure activity, especially in older patients, individuals with renal insufficiency, and patients with preexisting seizure disorders or CNS pathology. Carbapenems should be avoided in these patients unless no reasonable alternative therapy is available. Like cephalosporins, carbapenems have been rarely associated with anaphylaxis, interstitial nephritis, anemia, and leukopenia.
- **Patients who are allergic to PCNs/cephalosporins may have a cross-hypersensitivity reaction to carbapenems,** and these agents should not be used in a patient with a reported severe PCN allergy without prior skin testing, desensitization, or both. Prolonged therapy (>2 weeks) is typically monitored with a weekly serum creatinine, LFTs, and CBC.

Aminoglycosides

GENERAL PRINCIPLES

- Aminoglycosides exert their bactericidal effect by binding to the bacterial ribosome, causing misreading during translation of bacterial messenger RNA into proteins. These drugs are often used in combination with cell wall–active agents (i.e., β-lactams and vancomycin) for treatment of severe infections caused by gram-positive and gram-negative aerobes.

- Aminoglycosides tend to be synergistic with cell wall–active antibiotics such as PCNs, cephalosporins, and vancomycin. However, they do not have activity against anaerobes, and their activity is impaired in the low pH/low oxygen environment of abscesses. Cross-resistance among aminoglycosides is common and in cases of serious infections, susceptibility testing with each aminoglycoside is recommended. Use of these antibiotics is limited by significant nephrotoxicity and ototoxicity.

TREATMENT

Medications

- Traditional dosing of aminoglycosides involves daily divided dosing with the upper end of the dosing range reserved for life-threatening infections. Peak and trough concentrations should be obtained with the third or fourth dose and then every 3 to 4 days, along with regular serum creatinine monitoring. **Increasing serum creatinine or peak/troughs out of the acceptable range require immediate attention.**
- **Extended-interval dosing of aminoglycosides** is an alternative method of administration and is more convenient than traditional dosing for most indications. Extended-interval doses are provided in the following specific drug sections. A drug concentration is obtained 6 to 14 hours after the first dose, and a nomogram (Fig. 1) is consulted to determine the subsequent dosing interval. Monitoring includes obtaining a drug concentration 6 to 14 hours after the dosage at least every week and a serum creatinine at least three times a week. In patients who are not responding to therapy, a 12-hour concentration should be checked, and if that concentration is undetectable, extended-interval dosing should be abandoned in favor of traditional dosing.
- For **obese patients** (actual weight >20% above ideal body weight [IBW]), an obese dosing weight (IBW + 0.4 × [actual body weight − IBW]) should be used for determining doses for both traditional and extended-interval methods. Traditional dosing, rather than extended-interval dosing, should be used for pregnant patients, patients with endocarditis, burns that cover more than 20% of the body, cystic fibrosis, anasarca, and creatinine clearance (CrCl) of <20 mL/min.
- **Specific agents**
  - **Gentamicin and tobramycin** traditional dosing is an initial loading dose of 2 mg/kg IV (2 to 3 mg/kg in the critically ill), followed by 1.0 to 1.7 mg/kg IV q8h (peak, 4 to 10 mcg/mL; trough, <1 to 2 mcg/mL). Extended-interval dosing is an initial 5 mg/kg, with the subsequent dosing interval determined by a nomogram (Fig. 1). Tobramycin is also available as an inhaled agent for adjunctive therapy for patients with cystic fibrosis or bronchiectasis complicated by *P. aeruginosa* infection (300 mg inhalation q12h).
  - **Amikacin** has an additional unique role for mycobacterial and *Nocardia* infections. Traditional dosing is an initial loading dose of 5.0 to 7.5 mg/kg IV (7.5 to 9.0 mg/kg in the critically ill), followed by 5 mg/kg IV q8h or 7.5 mg/kg IV q12h (peak, 20 to 35 mcg/mL; trough, <10 mcg/mL). Extended-interval dosing is 15 mg/kg, with the subsequent dosing interval determined by a nomogram (Fig. 1).

SPECIAL CONSIDERATIONS

- **Nephrotoxicity** is the major adverse effect of aminoglycosides. Nephrotoxicity is reversible when detected early but can be permanent, especially in patients with tenuous renal function due to other medical conditions. Aminoglycosides should be used cautiously or avoided, if possible, in patients with decompensated kidney disease.

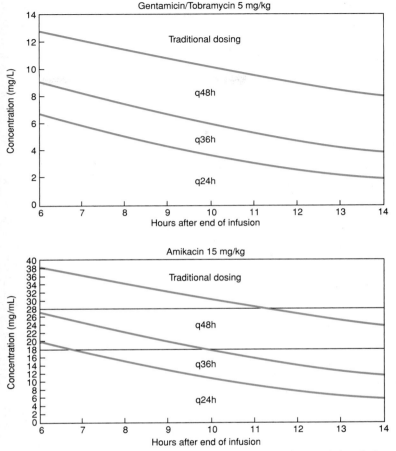

Figure 1. Nomograms for extended-interval aminoglycoside dosing. (Adapted from Reichley RM, Little JR, Bailey TC. Barnes-Jewish Hospital and Washington University School of Medicine.)

- **Ototoxicity** (vestibular or cochlear) is another possible adverse event that necessitates baseline and weekly hearing tests with extended therapy (>14 days). Concomitant administration of aminoglycosides with other known nephrotoxic agents (i.e., amphotericin B formulations, foscarnet, nonsteroidal anti-inflammatory drugs, pentamidine, polymyxins, cidofovir, and cisplatin) should be avoided if possible.

Vancomycin

GENERAL PRINCIPLES

- Vancomycin (15 mg/kg IV q12h; up to 30 mg/kg IV q12h for meningitis) is a glycopeptide antibiotic that interferes with cell wall synthesis by binding to

Table 1	Indications for Vancomycin Use

Treatment of serious infections caused by methicillin-resistant *Staphylococcus aureus* (MRSA)

Treatment of serious infections caused by ampicillin-resistant, vancomycin-sensitive enterococci

Treatment of serious infections caused by gram-positive bacteria in patients who are allergic to other appropriate therapies

Oral treatment of severe *Clostridium difficile* colitis

Surgical prophylaxis for placement of prosthetic devices at institutions with known high rates of MRSA or in patients who are known to be colonized with MRSA

Empiric use in suspected gram-positive meningitis until an organism has been identified and sensitivities confirmed

Life-threatening sepsis syndrome in patients with known methicillin-resistant *S. aureus* colonization or extended hospitalization until pathogen(s) are identified

Documented coagulase-negative staphylococcal endocarditis or catheter-related bloodstream infection

Empiric use for serious dialysis catheter–related bloodstream infections until the results of blood culture data are available

D-alanyl-D-alanine precursors that are critical for peptidoglycan cross-linking in most gram-positive bacterial cell walls. Vancomycin is bactericidal for staphylococci, but bacteriostatic for enterococci.

- Today, most hospitals have serious problems with vancomycin-resistant *Enterococcus faecium* (VRE), and there are now reports of clinical isolates of *S. aureus* that are intermediately resistant (VISA) and resistant to vancomycin (VRSA).

TREATMENT

- Indications for use are listed in Table 1.
- The **goal trough** concentration is 10 to 20 mcg/mL and perhaps up to 15 to 20 mcg/mL or more for other serious infections. Patients with advanced renal disease should receive a single 15 mg/kg dose and then be re-dosed when the concentration drops below 10 to 20 mcg/mL.

SPECIAL CONSIDERATIONS

Vancomycin is typically administered by slow IV infusion over at least 1 hour. More rapid infusion rates can cause the **red man syndrome,** which is a histamine-mediated reaction that is typically manifested by flushing and redness of the upper body. Nephrotoxicity, ototoxicity, neutropenia, thrombocytopenia, and rash may also occur.

Fluoroquinolones

GENERAL PRINCIPLES

- Fluoroquinolones exert their bactericidal effect by inhibiting bacterial DNA gyrase and topoisomerase, which are critical for DNA replication. In general, these antibiotics are well absorbed orally, with serum concentrations that approach those of parenteral administration.

- These agents typically have poor activity against enterococci, although they may have some efficacy for enterococcal UTIs when other agents are inactive or contraindicated. Concomitant administration with aluminum- or magnesium-containing antacids, sucralfate, bismuth, oral iron, oral calcium, and oral zinc preparations can markedly impair absorption of all orally administered fluoroquinolones.

TREATMENT

Medications

- **Norfloxacin** (400 mg PO q12h) is useful for the treatment of UTIs caused by gram-negative bacilli; however, other fluoroquinolones are preferred in this setting. This agent should not be used to treat systemic infections.
- **Ciprofloxacin** (250 to 750 mg PO q12h or 500 mg PO q24h [Cipro XR] or 200 to 400 mg IV q8–12h) and **ofloxacin** (200 to 400 mg IV or PO q12h) are active against gram-negative aerobes including many AmpC β-lactamase–producing pathogens. These agents are commonly used for UTIs, pyelonephritis, infectious diarrhea, prostatitis, and intra-abdominal infections (with metronidazole). Ciprofloxacin is the most active quinolone against *P. aeruginosa* and is the quinolone of choice for serious infections with that pathogen. However, ciprofloxacin has relatively poor activity against gram-positive cocci and anaerobes and should not be used as empiric monotherapy for community-acquired pneumonia, skin and soft tissue infections, or intra-abdominal infections. Oral and IV ciprofloxacin give similar maximum serum levels; thus, oral therapy is appropriate unless contraindicated. If given orally, fluoroquinolones should not be taken with milk products, multivitamins, antacids, liquid nutritional supplements or any other product with polyvalent metallic cations (e.g. iron).
- **Levofloxacin** (250 to 750 mg PO or IV q24h), **moxifloxacin** (400 mg PO/IV q24h daily), and **gemifloxacin** (320 mg PO q24h daily) are newer fluoroquinolones with improved coverage of streptococci, but less gram-negative activity (especially against *P. aeruginosa*) than ciprofloxacin. Moxifloxacin may be used as monotherapy of complicated intra-abdominal or skin and soft tissue infections due to its anti-anaerobic activity. Each of these agents is useful for treatment of sinusitis, bronchitis, community-acquired pneumonia, and UTIs (except moxifloxacin, which is only minimally eliminated in the urine). Some of these agents have activity against mycobacteria and have a potential role in treating drug-resistant TB and atypical mycobacterial infections. Levofloxacin may be used as an alternative for treatment of chlamydial urethritis.

SPECIAL CONSIDERATIONS

- Adverse reactions include nausea, CNS disturbances (headache, restlessness, and dizziness, especially in the elderly), rash, and phototoxicity. These agents can cause prolongation of the QT_c interval and should not be used in patients who are receiving class I or class III antiarrhythmics, in patients with known electrolyte or conduction abnormalities, or in those who are taking other medications that prolong the QT_c interval or induce bradycardia. These agents should also be used cautiously in the elderly, in whom asymptomatic conduction disturbances are more common.

Fluoroquinolones should not be routinely used in patients younger than 18 years or in pregnant or lactating women due to the risk of arthropathy in pediatric patients. They may also cause tendinitis or tendon rupture, especially the Achilles tendon particularly in elderly patients.

- **This class of antibiotics has major drug interactions,** necessitating that concomitant medication and patient's other medications should be checked for safety of concurrent fluoroquinolone use.

Macrolide and Lincosamide Antibiotics

GENERAL PRINCIPLES

- Macrolide and lincosamide antibiotics are bacteriostatic agents that block protein synthesis in bacteria by binding to the 50S subunit of the bacterial ribosome.
- This class of antibiotics has activity against gram-positive cocci, including streptococci and staphylococci, and some upper respiratory gram-negative bacteria, but minimal activity against enteric gram-negative rods.

TREATMENT

Medications

- Macrolides are commonly used to treat pharyngitis, otitis media, sinusitis, and bronchitis, especially in PCN-allergic patients, and are among the drugs of choice for treating *Legionella*, *Chlamydia*, and *Mycoplasma* infections. Azithromycin and clarithromycin can be used as monotherapy for outpatient community-acquired pneumonia and have a unique role in the treatment and prophylaxis of *Mycobacterium avium* complex (MAC) infections in patients with HIV. Many PCN-resistant strains of pneumococci are also resistant to macrolides.
- **Erythromycin** (250 to 500 mg PO q6h or 0.5 to 1.0 g IV q6h) possesses activity against gram-positive cocci (except enterococci) and can be used to treat bronchitis, pharyngitis, sinusitis, otitis media, and soft tissue infections in PCN-allergic patients. It is effective for treatment of atypical respiratory tract infections due to *Legionella pneumophila* (1 g IV q6h), *Chlamydophila pneumoniae*, and *Mycoplasma pneumoniae*. However, there is significant resistance to erythromycin among *Haemophilus influenzae* species and therefore, efficacy of this drug for upper and lower respiratory tract infections is limited. It can also be used for treatment of *Chlamydia trachomatis* infections (500 mg PO q6h for 7 days) and as an alternate therapy for syphilis in PCN-allergic patients. Use is limited by poor tolerability and drug interactions.
- **Clarithromycin** (250 to 500 mg PO q12h or 1,000 mg XL PO q24h) has a spectrum of activity similar to that of erythromycin but with enhanced activity against some respiratory pathogens (especially *Haemophilus*). It is commonly used to treat bronchitis, sinusitis, otitis media, pharyngitis, soft tissue infections, and community-acquired pneumonia. It has a prominent role in treating MAC infection in HIV patients and is an important component of regimens used to eradicate *Helicobacter pylori* (see Chapter 15, Gastrointestinal Diseases).
- **Azithromycin** (500 mg PO for 1 day, then 250 mg PO q24h for 4 days; 500 mg PO q24h for 3 days; 2,000 mg microspheres PO for one dose; 500 mg IV q24h) has a similar spectrum of activity to clarithromycin and is commonly used to treat bronchitis, otitis media, pharyngitis, soft tissue infections, and community-acquired pneumonia. It has a prominent role in MAC prophylaxis (1,200 mg PO

every week) and treatment (500 to 600 mg PO q24h) in HIV patients. It is also commonly used to treat *C. trachomatis* infections (1 g PO single dose). A major advantage of azithromycin is that it does not have the numerous drug interactions seen with erythromycin and clarithromycin.

- **Clindamycin** (150 to 450 mg PO q6–8h or 600 to 900 mg IV q8h) is chemically classified as a lincosamide (related to macrolides), with a predominantly gram-positive spectrum similar to that of erythromycin with additional activity against most anaerobes, including *B. fragilis*. It has excellent oral bioavailability (90%) and penetrates well into bone and abscess cavities. It is also used for treatment of aspiration pneumonia and lung abscesses. Clindamycin is often active against community-acquired strains of methicillin-resistant *S. aureus* (MRSA), and the agent has emerged as a treatment option for skin and soft tissue infections caused by this organism. Clindamycin may be used as a second agent in combination therapy for invasive streptococcal and clostridial infections to decrease toxin production. The agent may also be used for treatment of suspected anaerobic infections (peritonsillar/retropharyngeal abscesses, necrotizing fasciitis), although metronidazole is used more commonly for intra-abdominal infections (clindamycin has less reliable activity against *B. fragilis*). Clindamycin has additional uses, including treatment of babesiosis (in combination with quinine), toxoplasmosis (in combination with pyrimethamine), and *Pneumocystis jiroveci* pneumonia (in combination with primaquine).

SPECIAL CONSIDERATIONS

Macrolides and clindamycin are associated with nausea, abdominal cramping, and LFT abnormalities (particularly erythromycin). Liver function profiles should be checked intermittently during extended therapy. Hypersensitivity reactions with prominent skin rash are more common with clindamycin, as is pseudomembranous colitis secondary to *Clostridium difficile*. **Erythromycin and clarithromycin have major drug interactions** caused by inhibition of the cytochrome P-450 system.

Sulfonamides and Trimethoprim

GENERAL PRINCIPLES

Sulfadiazine, sulfisoxazole, trimetrexate, and trimethoprim slowly kill bacteria by inhibiting folic acid metabolism. This class of antibiotics is most commonly used for uncomplicated UTIs, sinusitis, and otitis media. Some sulfonamide-containing agents also have unique roles in the treatment of *P. jiroveci*, *Nocardia*, *Toxoplasma*, and *Stenotrophomonas* infections.

TREATMENT

Medications

- **Sulfisoxazole** (1 g PO q6h) and **trimethoprim** (100 mg PO q12h) are occasionally used as monotherapy for treatment of UTIs. Trimethoprim is more often used in the combination preparations outlined in the following sections. Trimethoprim in combination with dapsone is an alternate therapy for mild *P. jiroveci* pneumonia.
- **Trimethoprim/sulfamethoxazole** is a combination antibiotic (IV or PO) with a 1:5 ratio of trimethoprim to sulfamethoxazole. The IV preparation is dosed at 5 mg/kg

IV q8h (based on the trimethoprim component) for serious infections. The oral preparations (160 mg trimethoprim/800 mg sulfamethoxazole per double-strength [DS] tablet) are extensively bioavailable, with similar drug concentrations obtained with IV and PO formulations. Both components have excellent tissue penetration, including bone, prostate, and CNS. The combination has a broad spectrum of activity but typically does not inhibit *P. aeruginosa*, anaerobes, or group A streptococci. It is the therapy of choice for *P. jiroveci* pneumonia, *Stenotrophomonas maltophilia*, *Tropheryma whippelii*, and *Nocardia* infections. It is commonly used for treating sinusitis, otitis media, bronchitis, prostatitis, and UTIs (1 DS PO q12h). Trimethoprim/sulfamethoxazole is active against the majority of community-acquired strains of MRSA, and the agent has emerged as a viable treatment for uncomplicated cases of skin and soft tissue infections caused by this organism (2 to 3 DS tabs PO q12h). It is used as *P. jiroveci* pneumonia prophylaxis (1 DS PO twice a week, three times a week, or single strength or DS daily) in HIV-infected patients, solid organ transplant patients, bone marrow transplant patients, and patients receiving fludarabine. IV therapy is routinely converted to the PO equivalent for patients who require prolonged therapy.
- For serious infections, such as *Nocardia* brain abscesses, it may be useful to monitor trimethoprim/sulfamethoxazole with sulfamethoxazole peaks (100 to 150 mcg/mL) and troughs (50 to 100 mcg/mL) occasionally during the course of therapy and adjust dosing accordingly. In patients with renal insufficiency, doses can be adjusted by following trimethoprim peaks (5 to 10 mcg/mL). Prolonged therapy can cause bone marrow suppression, possibly requiring treatment with leucovorin (5 to 10 mg PO q24h) until cell counts normalize.
- **Sulfadiazine** (1.0 to 1.5 g PO q6h) in combination with pyrimethamine (200 mg PO followed by 50 to 75 mg PO q24h) and leucovorin (10 to 20 mg PO q24h) is the therapy of choice for toxoplasmosis. Sulfadiazine is also occasionally used to treat *Nocardia* infections.

SPECIAL CONSIDERATIONS

These drugs are associated with cholestatic jaundice, bone marrow suppression, hyperkalemia (with Trimethoprim/sulfamethoxazole) interstitial nephritis, "false" elevations in serum creatinine, and severe hypersensitivity reactions (Stevens–Johnson syndrome/erythema multiforme). Nausea is common with higher doses. **All patients should be asked whether they are allergic to "sulfa drugs,"** and specific commercial names should be mentioned (i.e., Bactrim or Septra).

Tetracyclines

GENERAL PRINCIPLES

- Tetracyclines are bacteriostatic antibiotics that bind to the 30S ribosomal subunit and block protein synthesis.
- These agents have unique roles in the treatment of *Rickettsia*, *Ehrlichia*, *Chlamydia*, and *Mycoplasma* infections. They are used as therapy for most tick-borne infections, lyme disease–related arthritis, alternate therapy for syphilis, and for *P. multocida* infections in PCN-allergic patients. Their general use is limited because of widespread resistance among more common bacterial pathogens.

TREATMENT

Medications

- **Tetracycline** (250 to 500 mg PO q6h) is commonly used for severe acne and in some *H. pylori* eradication regimens. It can also be used for treatment of acute Lyme borreliosis, Rocky Mountain spotted fever, ehrlichiosis, psittacosis, *Mycoplasma* pneumonia, *Chlamydia* pneumonia, and chlamydial infections of the eye or genitourinary tract, but these infections are generally treated with doxycycline or other antibiotics. Aluminum- and magnesium-containing antacids and preparations that contain oral calcium, oral iron, or other cations can significantly impair oral absorption of tetracycline and should be avoided within 2 hours of each dose.
- **Doxycycline** (100 mg PO/IV q12h) is the most commonly used tetracycline and is standard therapy for *C. trachomatis*, Rocky Mountain spotted fever, ehrlichiosis, and psittacosis. This agent also has a role for malaria prophylaxis and for treatment of community-acquired pneumonia.
- **Minocycline** (200 mg PO, then 100 mg PO q12h) is similar to doxycycline in its spectrum of activity and clinical indications. It is second-line therapy for pulmonary nocardiosis and cervicofacial actinomycosis. Both minocycline and doxycycline also have activity against some multidrug-resistant gram-negative pathogens and may be used as adjunctive agents in this setting as per results of susceptibility testing.

SPECIAL CONSIDERATIONS

Nausea and photosensitivity are common side effects. Patients should be warned about sun exposure. Rarely, these medications are associated with pseudotumor cerebri. **They should not routinely be given to children or to pregnant or lactating women** because they can cause tooth enamel discoloration in young children. Minocycline is associated with vestibular disturbances.

ANTIMICROBIAL AGENTS, MISCELLANEOUS

Chloramphenicol

GENERAL PRINCIPLES

Definition

Chloramphenicol (12.5 to 25 mg/kg IV q6h; maximum, 1 g IV q6h) is a bacteriostatic antibiotic that binds to the 50S ribosomal subunit, blocking protein synthesis in susceptible bacteria. It has broad-spectrum activity against aerobic and anaerobic gram-positive and gram-negative bacteria, including *S. aureus*, enterococci, and enteric gram-negative rods. It is also active against spirochetes, *Rickettsia*, *Mycoplasma*, and *Chlamydia*. The drug may also be used for some serious VRE infections and for treatment of meningitis caused by *Francisella tularensis* or *Yersinia pestis*.

SPECIAL CONSIDERATIONS

Adverse events include idiosyncratic aplastic anemia (~1/30,000) and dose-related bone marrow suppression. Peak drug levels (1 hour postinfusion) should be checked every 3 to 4 days (goal peak <25 mcg/mL) and doses adjusted accordingly. Dosage adjustment is necessary in the presence of significant liver disease. **This class of antibiotics has major drug interactions.**

Colistin and Polymyxin B

GENERAL PRINCIPLES

- Colistimethate sodium (2.5 to 5 mg/kg/d IV divided q12h) and polymyxin B (15,000 to 25,000 units/kg/d IV divided q12 hours) are bactericidal polypeptide antibiotics that kill gram-negative bacteria by disrupting the cell membrane. These drugs have roles in the treatment of multiple drug–resistant gram-negative bacilli, but are inactive against *Proteus, Providencia,* and *Serratia.*
- **These medications should only be given under the guidance of an experienced clinician,** as parenteral therapy has significant CNS side effects and potential nephrotoxicity. Inhaled colistin (75 to 150 mg q12h given by nebulizer) is better tolerated, with only mild upper airway irritation, and has some efficacy as adjunctive therapy for *P. aeruginosa* or *Acinetobacter* pulmonary infections.

SPECIAL CONSIDERATIONS

Adverse events with parenteral therapy include paresthesias, slurred speech, peripheral numbness, tingling, and significant dose-dependent nephrotoxicity. The dosage should be carefully reduced in patients with renal insufficiency, as overdosage in this setting can result in neuromuscular blockade and apnea. Serum creatinine should be monitored daily early in therapy and then at a regular interval for the duration of therapy. **Concomitant use with aminoglycosides, other known nephrotoxins, or neuromuscular blockers should be avoided if at all possible.**

Daptomycin

GENERAL PRINCIPLES

Daptomycin (4 mg/kg IV q24h for skin and skin structure infections; 6 mg/kg IV q24h for bloodstream infections) is a cyclic lipopeptide. The drug exhibits rapid bactericidal activity against a wide variety of gram-positive bacteria, including enterococci, staphylococci, and streptococci. Daptomycin also maintains activity against many antibiotic-resistant gram-positive bacteria and is currently U.S. FDA-approved for treatment of complicated skin and skin structure infections as well as *Staphylococcus aureus* bacteremia and right-sided endocarditis. The drug should not be used to treat primary lung infections due to its decreased activity in the presence of pulmonary surfactant. Resistance can develop and it is imperative that organism susceptibility be verified.

SPECIAL CONSIDERATIONS

Adverse events include GI disturbances, injection site reactions, elevated LFTs, and elevated creatine phosphokinase. Serum creatine phosphokinase should be monitored at baseline and weekly, as daptomycin has been associated with skeletal muscle effects, including rhabdomyolysis, patients should also be monitored for signs of muscle weakness and pain, and the drug should be discontinued if these symptoms develop in conjunction with marked creatine phosphokinase elevations (5 to 10 times the upper limit of normal with symptoms or 10 times the upper limit of normal without symptoms). Consideration should also be given to avoiding concomitant use of daptomycin and HMG-CoA reductase inhibitors due to the potential increased risk of myopathy.

Fosfomycin

GENERAL PRINCIPLES

- **Fosfomycin** (3-g sachet dissolved in cold water PO once) is a bactericidal oral antibiotic that kills bacteria by inhibiting an early step in cell wall synthesis. It has a spectrum of activity that includes most urinary tract pathogens, including *P. aeruginosa*, *Enterobacter* species, and enterococci (including VRE), and some multidrug-resistant gram-negative bacteria.
- It is most useful for treating uncomplicated UTIs in women with susceptible strains of *E. coli* or *Enterococcus faecalis*. It should not be used to treat pyelonephritis or systemic infections.

SPECIAL CONSIDERATIONS

Adverse events include diarrhea. It should not be taken with metoclopramide, as that drug interferes with fosfomycin absorption.

Linezolid

GENERAL PRINCIPLES

- Oxazolidinones are a new class of antibiotics that block assembly of bacterial ribosomes and inhibit protein synthesis. **Linezolid** (600 mg IV/PO q12h) is the first FDA-approved drug in this class. IV and oral formulations produce equivalent serum concentrations, and the drug has potent activity against gram-positive bacteria, including drug-resistant enterococci, staphylococci, and streptococci. However, it has no meaningful activity against Enterobacteriaceae and borderline activity against *Moraxella* and *H. influenzae*.
- Linezolid is useful for serious infections with VRE, as an alternative to vancomycin for treatment of MRSA infections, for patients with an indication for vancomycin therapy who are intolerant of that medication, and as oral therapy of MRSA infections when IV access is unavailable. Limited data support use for treatment of osteomyelitis, endocarditis, and meningitis and routine use for these infections should be carefully undertaken. In addition, linezolid is not U.S. FDA-approved for catheter-related bloodstream or catheter-site infections. Resistance can develop to this antibiotic, and it is imperative that organism susceptibility is verified.

SPECIAL CONSIDERATIONS

- **Adverse events** include diarrhea, nausea, and headache. Thrombocytopenia occurs frequently in patients who receive more than 2 weeks of therapy, and serial platelet count monitoring is indicated. A CBC, should be checked every week during prolonged therapy with this agent. Extremely prolonged therapy (typically longer than 6 months) has been associated with peripheral and optic neuropathy. Lactic acidosis may also rarely occur.

- Linezolid has **several important drug interactions.** It is a mild monoamine oxidase inhibitor, and patients should be advised not to take selective serotonin reuptake inhibitors (SSRIs), triptans, or meperidine while on linezolid to avoid the serotonin syndrome. Ideally, patients should be off the SSRI for at least a week before initiating linezolid. Over-the-counter cold remedies that contain pseudoephedrine or phenylpropanolamine should also be avoided, as coadministration with linezolid can elevate blood pressure. Linezolid does not require dose adjustments for renal or hepatic dysfunction.

Methenamine

GENERAL PRINCIPLES

- Methenamine hippurate or methenamine mandelate (one or two tablets [depending on the specific preparation] PO q6h) is a urine/bladder antiseptic that is converted into formaldehyde in the urine when the pH is <6.0.
- This agent has a limited role in treating uncomplicated UTI caused by multiple drug-resistant bacteria or yeast.

SPECIAL CONSIDERATIONS

Adverse events include bladder irritation, dysuria, and hematuria with prolonged use. Therapy should be limited to a maximum of 3 weeks at a time, and urine pH should be obtained once early during therapy to ensure an appropriately acidic pH. Vitamin C can be used to assist in urine acidification. It is contraindicated in the setting of glaucoma, significant renal insufficiency, and acidosis. It should not be given concomitantly with sulfonamides, as these drugs form an insoluble precipitate in the urine.

Metronidazole

GENERAL PRINCIPLES

- Metronidazole (250 to 750 mg PO/IV q6–12h) is only active against anaerobic bacteria and some protozoa. The drug exerts its bactericidal effect though accumulation of toxic metabolites that interfere with multiple biologic processes. It has excellent tissue penetration, including abscess cavities, bone, and CNS.
- It has greater activity against gram-negative than gram-positive anaerobes but is active against *Clostridium perfringens* and *C. difficile*. It is the treatment of choice as monotherapy for mild–moderate *C. difficile* colitis as well as bacterial vaginosis, and can be used in combination with other antibiotics to treat intra-abdominal infections and brain abscesses. Protozoal infections that are routinely treated with metronidazole include *Giardia*, *Entamoeba histolytica*, and *Trichomonas*

vaginalis. A dose reduction may be warranted for patients with decompensated liver disease.

SPECIAL CONSIDERATIONS

Adverse events include nausea, dysgeusia, disulfiram-like reactions to alcohol, and mild CNS disturbances (headache, restlessness). Rarely, metronidazole causes peripheral neuropathy and seizures.

Nitrofurantoin

GENERAL PRINCIPLES

- **Nitrofurantoin** (50 to 100 mg PO macrocrystals q6h or 100 mg PO dual-release formulation q12h for 5 to 7 days) is a bactericidal oral antibiotic that is useful for uncomplicated UTIs except those caused by *Proteus, P. aeruginosa,* or *Serratia.* The drug is metabolized by bacteria into toxic intermediates that inhibit multiple bacterial processes. It has had a modest resurgence in use, as it is frequently effective for uncomplicated VRE UTIs.
- Although it was commonly used in the past for UTI prophylaxis, this practice should be avoided, as prolonged therapy is associated with chronic pulmonary syndromes that can be fatal. Nitrofurantoin should not be used for pyelonephritis or any other systemic infections.

SPECIAL CONSIDERATIONS

Adverse events. Nausea is the most common adverse effect, and the drug should be taken with food to minimize this problem. Patients should be warned that their urine may become brown secondary to the medication. Neurotoxicity, hepatotoxicity, and pulmonary fibrosis may also rarely occur with nitrofurantion. Furthermore, it should not be used in patients with creatinine clearance <60 mL/min as the risk for development of treatment-associated adverse effects is increased. It should not be given with probenecid, as this combination decreases the concentration of nitrofurantoin in the urine.

Quinupristin/Dalfopristin

GENERAL PRINCIPLES

- **Quinupristin/dalfopristin** (7.5 mg/kg IV q8h) is the first U.S. FDA-approved drug in the streptogramin class.
- This agent has activity against antibiotic-resistant gram-positive organisms, especially VRE, MRSA, VISA, VRSA, and antibiotic-resistant strains of *Streptococcus pneumoniae.* It has some activity against gram-negative upper respiratory pathogens (*Haemophilus* and *Moraxella*) and anaerobes, but more appropriate antibiotics are available to treat these infections. Quinupristin/dalfopristin is bacteriostatic for enterococci and can be used for treatment of serious infections with VRE

(however, it is inactive against *E. faecalis*). It can also be used for treatment of serious infections with MRSA or *S. pneumoniae* when other agents are not feasible.

SPECIAL CONSIDERATIONS

Adverse events include arthralgias and myalgias, which occur frequently and can necessitate discontinuation of therapy. IV site pain and thrombophlebitis are common when the drug is administered through a peripheral vein. It has also been associated with elevated LFTs and, as it is primarily cleared by hepatic metabolism, patients with significant hepatic impairment require a dose adjustment. Quinupristin/dalfopristin is similar to erythromycin with regard to drug interactions.

Telavancin

GENERAL PRINCIPLES

Telavancin (7.5 to 10 mg/kg q24–48h, based on creatinine clearance) is a new lipoglycopeptide antibiotic that is U.S. FDA-approved for treatment of complicated skin and skin structure infections. The drug has also been shown to be effective for treatment of hospital-associated pneumonia and is currently under U.S. FDA review for this indication. Telavancin is broadly active against gram-positive bacteria, including MRSA, VISA, hVISA, daptomycin- and linezolid-resistant *Staphylococcus aureus*, streptococci, vancomycin-sensitive enterococci, and some gram-positive anaerobes. The agent is not active against gram-negative bacteria and most VRE.

Adverse effects include nausea, vomiting, metallic or soapy taste, foamy urine, and nephrotoxicity (which necessitates serial monitoring of serum creatinine). Telavancin can also cause a minor (4.1 to 4.6 milliseconds) prolongation of the QT_c interval and should be avoided in patients with underlying cardiac conditions associated with QT_c prolongation. Women of childbearing potential require a negative serum pregnancy test prior to receiving telavancin, due to teratogenic effects noted in animals.

Tigecycline

GENERAL PRINCIPLES

Tigecycline (100 mg IV loading dose, then 50 mg IV q12h) is the only U.S. Food and Drug Administration (FDA)-approved antibiotic in the class of glycylcyclines. Its mechanism of action is similar to that of tetracyclines by inhibiting the translation of bacterial proteins through binding to the 30S ribosome. The addition of the glycyl side chain expands its activity against bacterial pathogens that are normally resistant to tetracycline and minocycline. It has a broad spectrum of bactericidal activity against gram-positive, gram-negative, and anaerobic bacteria except *P. aeruginosa* and some *Proteus* isolates. It is currently U.S. FDA-approved for treatment of complicated skin and skin structure infections, complicated intra-abdominal infections, and community-acquired pneumonia, but may be used for treatment of some other tissue infections due to susceptible strains of VRE and some multidrug-resistant gram-negative bacteria. Until more data are available, it should not be used to treat primary bacteremia.

SPECIAL CONSIDERATIONS

Adverse events. Nausea and vomiting are the most common adverse events. Tigecycline has not been studied in patients younger than 18 years and is contraindicated in pregnant and lactating women. Since it has a similar structure to tetracyclines, photosensitivity, tooth discoloration, and rarely pseudotumor cerebri may occur.

ANTIMYCOBACTERIAL AGENTS

Effective therapy of *Mycobacterium tuberculosis* (MTB) infections requires combination chemotherapy designed to prevent the emergence of resistant organisms and maximize efficacy. Increased resistance to conventional antituberculous agents has led to the use of more complex regimens and has made susceptibility testing an integral part of TB management (see Chapter 11, Treatment of Infectious Diseases).

Isoniazid

GENERAL PRINCIPLES

Isoniazid (INH, 300 mg PO q24h) exerts bactericidal effects on susceptible mycobacteria by interfering with the synthesis of lipid components of the mycobacterial cell wall. INH is a component of nearly all treatment regimens and can be given twice a week in directly observed therapy (15 mg/kg/dose; 900 mg maximum). INH remains the drug of choice for treatment of latent tuberculosis infection (300 mg PO q24h for 9 months).

SPECIAL CONSIDERATIONS

Adverse events include elevations in liver transaminases (20%). This effect can be idiosyncratic but is usually seen in the setting of advanced age, underlying liver disease, or concomitant consumption of alcohol, and may be potentiated by rifampin. Transaminase elevations to greater than threefold the upper limit of the normal range necessitate holding therapy. Patients with known liver dysfunction should have weekly LFTs during the initial stage of therapy. INH also antagonizes vitamin B_6 metabolism and potentially can cause a peripheral neuropathy. This can be avoided or minimized by coadministration of pyridoxine, 25 to 50 mg PO daily, especially in the elderly, in pregnant women, and in patients with diabetes, renal failure, alcoholism, and seizure disorders.

Rifamycins

GENERAL PRINCIPLES

Rifamycins exert bactericidal activity on susceptible mycobacteria by inhibiting DNA-dependent RNA polymerase, thereby halting transcription.

- **Rifampin** (600 mg PO q24h or twice a week) is an integral component of most TB treatment regimens. It is also active against many gram-positive and gram-negative bacteria. Rifampin is used as adjunctive therapy in staphylococcal prosthetic valve endocarditis (300 mg PO q8h), for prophylaxis of close contacts of patients with infection caused by *Neisseria meningitidis* (600 mg PO q12h), and as adjunctive treatment of bone and joint infections associated with prosthetic material or devices. The drug is well absorbed orally and is widely distributed throughout the body including the cerebrospinal fluid (CSF).

- **Rifabutin** (300 mg PO q24h) is primarily used to treat TB and MAC infections in HIV-positive patients who are receiving highly active antiretroviral therapy, as it has less deleterious effects on protease inhibitor metabolism than does rifampin (see Chapter 13, Human Immunodeficiency Virus and Acquired Immunodeficiency Syndrome).

SPECIAL CONSIDERATIONS

Adverse events. Patients should be warned about reddish-orange discoloration of body fluids, and contact lenses should not be worn during treatment. Rash, GI disturbances, hematologic disturbances, hepatitis, and interstitial nephritis can occur. Uveitis has also been associated with rifabutin. **This class of antibiotics has major drug interactions.**

Pyrazinamide

GENERAL PRINCIPLES

- **Pyrazinamide** (15 to 30 mg/kg PO q24h; maximum, 2 g or 50 to 75 mg/kg PO twice a week; maximum, 4 g/dose) kills mycobacteria replicating in macrophages by an unknown mechanism.
- It is well absorbed orally and widely distributed throughout the body including the CSF. Pyrazinamide is typically used for the first 2 months of therapy.

SPECIAL CONSIDERATIONS

Adverse events include hyperuricemia and hepatitis.

Ethambutol

GENERAL PRINCIPLES

- **Ethambutol** (15 to 25 mg/kg PO q24h or 50 to 75 mg/kg PO twice a week; maximum, 2.4 g/dose) is bacteriostatic with an unknown mechanism of action.
- Doses should be reduced in the presence of renal dysfunction.

SPECIAL CONSIDERATIONS

Adverse events. These may include optic neuritis, which manifests as decreased red-green color perception, decreased visual acuity, or visual field deficits. Baseline and monthly visual examinations should be performed during therapy. Renal function should also be carefully monitored as drug accumulation in the setting of renal insufficiency can increase risk of ocular effects.

Streptomycin

GENERAL PRINCIPLES

Streptomycin is an aminoglycoside that can be used as a substitute for ethambutol and for drug-resistant MTB. It does not adequately penetrate the CNS and should not be used for TB meningitis.

ANTIVIRAL AGENTS

Current antiviral agents only suppress viral replication. Viral containment or elimination requires an intact host immune response. Anti-HIV agents will be discussed in Chapter 13, Human Immunodeficiency Virus and Acquired Immunodeficiency Syndrome.

Anti-Influenza Agents

GENERAL PRINCIPLES

Anti-influenza drugs include not only **amantadine** and **rimantadine,** but also two newer drugs, **zanamivir** and **oseltamivir,** which block influenza A and B neuraminidases. This enzymatic activity is necessary for successful viral egress and release from infected cells. These drugs have shown modest activity in clinical trials, with a 1- to 2-day improvement in symptoms in patients who are treated within 48 hours of the onset of influenza symptoms. At the onset of each influenza season, a consultation with the local health department officials is recommended to determine the most effective antiviral agent. Although there are data showing that these agents are effective for prophylaxis of influenza, annual influenza vaccination remains the intervention of choice in all high-risk patients and health care workers (see Appendix A, Immunizations and Post-Exposure Therapies).

- **Amantadine and rimantadine** (100 mg PO q12h for both; 100 mg PO q24h in elderly patients, dialysis patients, or those with decompensated liver disease) prevent influenza A entry into cells by blocking endosomal acidification, which is necessary for fusion of the viral envelope with the host cell membrane. **These agents have no activity against influenza B.** They are effective when therapy is initiated within 48 hours of initial symptoms and continued for 7 to 10 days. These drugs can also be used for influenza prophylaxis in nonimmune individuals who have been exposed to the virus and in patients and staff members of nursing homes or hospitals during an epidemic.
  - **Adverse events.** GI disturbances and CNS dysfunction, including dizziness, nervousness, confusion, slurring of speech, blurred vision, and sleep disturbances, may be experienced with use of these antivirals. Rimantadine has fewer side effects than amantadine.

- **Zanamivir** (10 mg [two inhalations] q12h for 5 days, started within 48 hours of the onset of symptoms) is an inhaled neuraminidase inhibitor that is active against influenza A and B. It is indicated for treatment of uncomplicated acute influenza infection in adults and children 7 years of age or older who have been symptomatic for <48 hours. The drug is also indicated for influenza prophylaxis in patients age 5 and older.
  - **Adverse events.** Headache, GI disturbances, dizziness, and upper respiratory symptoms are sometimes reported. Bronchospasms or declines in lung function, or both, may occur in patients with underlying respiratory disorders and may require a rapid-acting bronchodilator for control.
- **Oseltamivir** (75 mg PO q12h for 5 days) is an orally administered neuraminidase inhibitor that is active against influenza A and B.
  - It is indicated for treatment of uncomplicated acute influenza in adults and children 1 year of age or older who have been symptomatic for up to 2 days. This agent is also indicated for prophylaxis of influenza A and B in adults and children 1 year of age or older.
  - **Adverse events** include nausea, vomiting, and diarrhea. Dizziness and headache may also occur.

Antiherpetic Agents

GENERAL PRINCIPLES

Antiherpetic agents are nucleotide analogs that inhibit viral DNA synthesis.

- **Acyclovir** is active against herpes simplex virus (HSV) and varicella–zoster virus (VZV) (400 mg PO q8h for HSV, 800 mg PO five times a day for localized VZV infections, 5 mg/kg IV q8h for severe HSV infections, and 10 mg/kg IV q8h for severe VZV infections and HSV encephalitis).
  - It is indicated for treatment of primary and recurrent genital herpes, severe herpetic stomatitis, and herpes simplex encephalitis. It can be used as prophylaxis in patients who have frequent HSV recurrences (400 mg PO q12h). It is also used for herpes zoster ophthalmicus, disseminated primary VZV in adults (significant morbidity compared to the childhood illness), and severe disseminated primary VZV in children.
  - **Adverse events.** Reversible crystalline nephropathy may occur; preexisting renal failure, dehydration, and IV bolus dosing increase the risk of this effect. Rare cases of CNS disturbances, including delirium, tremors, and seizures, may also occur, particularly with high doses, in patients with renal failure and in the elderly.
- **Valacyclovir** (1,000 mg PO q8h for herpes zoster, 1,000 mg PO q12h for initial episode of genital HSV infection, and 500 mg PO q12h or 1,000 mg PO q24h for recurrent episodes of HSV) is an orally administered prodrug of acyclovir used for the treatment of acute herpes zoster infections and for treatment or suppression of genital HSV infection.
  - The most common **adverse event** is nausea. Valacyclovir can rarely cause CNS disturbances, and high doses (8 g/d) have been associated with development of hemolytic–uremic syndrome/thrombotic thrombocytopenic purpura in immunocompromised patients, including those with HIV and bone marrow and solid organ transplants.

- **Famciclovir** (500 mg PO q8h for herpes zoster, 250 mg PO q8h for the initial episode of genital HSV infection, and 125 mg PO q12h for recurrent episodes of genital HSV infection) is an orally administered antiviral agent used for the treatment of acute herpes zoster reactivation and for treatment or suppression of genital HSV infections.
  - **Adverse events** include headache, nausea, and diarrhea.

Anti-CMV Agents

GENERAL PRINCIPLES

- **Ganciclovir** (5 mg/kg IV q12h for 14 to 21 days for induction therapy of cytomegalovirus [CMV] retinitis, followed by 6 mg/kg IV for 5 days every week or 5 mg/kg IV q24h; the oral dose is 1,000 mg PO q8h with food) is used to treat CMV.
  - It has activity against HSV and VZV, but safer drugs are available to treat those infections. The drug is widely distributed in the body, including the CSF.
  - It is indicated for treatment of CMV retinitis and other serious CMV infections in immunocompromised patients (e.g., transplant and AIDS patients). Chronic maintenance therapy is generally required to suppress CMV disease in patients with AIDS.
  - **Adverse events.** Neutropenia, which may require treatment with granulocyte colony-stimulating factor for management (300 mcg SC daily–qwk), is the main therapy-limiting adverse effect. Thrombocytopenia, rash, confusion, headache, nephrotoxicity, and GI disturbances may also occur. Blood counts and electrolytes should be monitored weekly while the patient is receiving therapy. Other agents with nephrotoxic or bone marrow suppressive effects may enhance the adverse effects of ganciclovir.
- **Valganciclovir** (900 mg PO q12–24h) is the oral prodrug of ganciclovir. This agent has excellent bioavailability and can be used for treatment of CMV retinitis and, thus, has supplanted the use of oral ganciclovir, which has poor oral bioavailability. Adverse events are the same as those for ganciclovir.
- **Foscarnet** (60 mg/kg IV q8h or 90 mg/kg IV q12h for 14 to 21 days as induction therapy, followed by 90 to 120 mg/kg IV q24h as maintenance therapy for CMV; 40 mg/kg IV q8h for acyclovir-resistant HSV and VZV) is used to treat CMV retinitis in patients with AIDS. It is typically considered for use in patients who are not tolerating or not responding to ganciclovir.
  - It is occasionally used for CMV disease in bone marrow transplant patients to avoid the bone marrow–suppressive effects of ganciclovir. It also has a role in treatment of acyclovir-resistant HSV/VZV infections or ganciclovir-resistant CMV infections.
  - **Adverse events.** Risk for nephrotoxicity is a major concern. Creatinine clearance should be determined at baseline and electrolytes (PO_4, Ca^{2+}, Mg^{2+}, K^+) and serum creatinine checked at least twice a week. Normal saline (500 to 1,000 mL) should be given before and during infusions to minimize nephrotoxicity. Foscarnet should be avoided in patients with a serum creatinine of >2.8 mg/dL or baseline CrCl of <50 mL/min. Concomitant use of other nephrotoxins (e.g., amphotericin, aminoglycosides, pentamidine, nonsteroidal anti-inflammatory drugs, cisplatin, or cidofovir) should also be avoided. Foscarnet chelates divalent cations

and can cause tetany even with normal serum calcium levels. Use of foscarnet with pentamidine can cause severe hypocalcemia. Other side effects include seizures, phlebitis, rash, and genital ulcers. **Prolonged therapy with foscarnet should be monitored by physicians who are experienced with administration of home IV therapy and can systematically monitor patients' laboratory results.**

- **Cidofovir** (5 mg/kg IV qwk for 2 weeks as induction therapy, followed by 5 mg/kg IV q14d chronically as maintenance therapy) is used primarily to treat CMV retinitis in patients with AIDS. It can be administered through a peripheral IV line.
  - **Adverse events.** The most common is nephrotoxicity. It should be avoided in patients with a CrCl of <55 mL/min, a serum creatinine >1.5 mg/dL, significant proteinuria, or a recent history of receipt of other nephrotoxic medications.
  - **Each cidofovir dose should be administered with probenecid** (2 g PO 3 hours before the infusion and then 1 g at 2 and 8 hours after the infusion) along with 1 L normal saline IV 1 to 2 hours before the infusion to minimize nephrotoxicity. Patients should have a serum creatinine and urine protein check before each dose of cidofovir is given. These patients should be followed by a physician regularly, as administration of this drug requires systematic monitoring of laboratory studies.

ANTIFUNGAL AGENTS

Amphotericin B

GENERAL PRINCIPLES

Amphotericin B is fungicidal by interacting with ergosterol and disrupting the fungal cell membrane. Reformulation of this agent in various lipid vehicles has decreased some of its adverse side effects.

- **Amphotericin B deoxycholate** (0.3 to 1.5 mg/kg q24h as a single infusion over 2 to 6 hours) was once the mainstay of antifungal therapy, but has now been supplanted by lipid-based formulations of the drug as a result of their improved tolerability.
  - It is not effective for *Pseudallescheria boydii* or *Candida lusitaniae* infections.
- **Lipid complexed preparations** of amphotericin B, including amphotericin B lipid complex (5 mg/kg IV q24h), liposomal amphotericin B (3 to 6 mg/kg IV q24h), and amphotericin B colloidal dispersion (3 to 4 mg/kg IV q24h), have decreased nephrotoxicity and are generally associated with fewer infusion-related reactions than amphotericin B deoxycholate. Liposomal amphotericin B has the most U.S. FDA-approved uses and also appears to be the best tolerated lipid formulation.

SPECIAL CONSIDERATIONS

- The major **adverse event** of all amphotericin B formulations, including the lipid formulations, is **nephrotoxicity.** Patients should receive 500 mL of normal saline before and after each infusion to minimize nephrotoxicity. Irreversible renal failure appears to be related to cumulative doses. Therefore, concomitant administration of other known nephrotoxins should be avoided if possible.

- Common **infusion-related effects** include fever/chills, nausea, headache, and myalgias. Premedication with 500 to 1,000 mg of acetaminophen and 50 mg of diphenhydramine may control many of these symptoms. More severe reactions may be prevented by premedication with hydrocortisone, 25 to 50 mg IV. Intolerable infusion-related chills can be managed with meperidine, 25 to 50 mg IV.
- Amphotericin B therapy is associated with **potassium and magnesium wasting** that generally requires supplementation. Serum creatinine and electrolytes (including Mg^{2+} and K^+) should be monitored at least two to three times a week.

Azoles

GENERAL PRINCIPLES

Azoles are fungistatic agents that inhibit ergosterol synthesis.

- **Fluconazole** (100 to 800 mg PO/IV q24h) is the drug of choice for many localized candidal infections, such as UTIs, thrush, vaginal candidiasis (150-mg single dose), esophagitis, peritonitis, and hepatosplenic infection. It is also a viable agent for severe disseminated candidal infections (e.g., candidemia) and the treatment of choice for consolidation therapy of cryptococcal meningitis following an initial 14-day course of an amphotericin B product, or as a second-line agent for primary treatment of cryptococcal meningitis (400 to 800 mg PO q24h for 8 weeks, followed by 200 mg PO q24h thereafter for chronic maintenance treatment).
  - Fluconazole does not have activity against *Aspergillus* species or *Candida krusei* and therefore should not be used for treatment of those infections. *Candida glabrata* may also be resistant to fluconazole. Its absorption is not dependent on gastric acid.
- **Itraconazole** (200 to 400 mg PO q24h) is a triazole with broad-spectrum antifungal activity.
  - It is commonly used to treat histoplasmosis, blastomycosis, and sporotrichosis.
  - It is an alternative therapy for *Aspergillus* and can also be used to treat infections caused by dermatophytes, including onychomycosis of the toenails (200 mg PO q24h for 12 weeks) and fingernails (200 mg PO q12h for 1 week, with a 3-week interruption, and then a second course of 200 mg PO q12h for 1 week).
  - The capsules require adequate gastric acidity for absorption and, therefore, should be taken with food or carbonated beverage, whereas the liquid is not significantly affected by gastric acidity and is better absorbed on an empty stomach.
- **Posaconazole** (200 mg PO q8h for prophylaxis of invasive fungal infections; 100 to 400 mg PO q12–24 for oropharyngeal candidiasis) is an oral azole agent that is U.S. FDA-approved for prophylaxis of invasive aspergillosis and candidiasis in hematopoietic stem cell transplant patients with graft-versus-host disease or in patients with hematologic malignancies experiencing prolonged neutropenia from chemotherapy, as well as oropharyngeal candidiasis. This drug has also been shown to be a useful agent for treatment of mucormycosis.

- Each dose should be administered with a full meal, liquid supplement, or acidic carbonated beverage (e.g., ginger ale).
- Rifabutin, phenytoin, and cimetidine significantly reduce posaconazole concentrations and should not routinely be used concomitantly.
- Posaconazole significantly increases bioavailability of cyclosporine, tacrolimus, and midazolam necessitating dosage reductions of these agents when used with posaconazole. Dosage reduction of vinca alkaloids, statins, and calcium channel blockers should also be considered.
- Terfenadine, astemizole, pimozide, cisapride, quinidine, and ergot alkaloids are contraindicated with posaconazole.
- **Voriconazole** (loading dose of 6 mg/kg IV [2 doses 12 hours apart], followed by a maintenance dose of 4 mg/kg IV q12h or 200 mg PO q12h [100 mg PO q12h if <40 kg]) is a triazole antifungal with a spectrum of activity against a wide range of pathogenic fungi. It has enhanced in vitro activity against all clinically important species of *Aspergillus*, as well as *Candida* (including most non-albicans), *Scedosporium apiospermum*, and *Fusarium* species.
  - It is the treatment of choice for most forms of invasive aspergillosis, for which it demonstrates typical response rates of 40% to 50% and superiority over conventional amphotericin B. It is also effective in treating candidemia, esophageal candidiasis, and *Scedosporium* and *Fusarium* infections.
  - An advantage of voriconazole is the easy transition from IV to PO therapy because of excellent bioavailability. For refractory fungal infections a dose increase of 50% may be useful. The maintenance dose is reduced by 50% for patients with moderate hepatic failure.
  - Because of its metabolism through the **cytochrome P-450 system** (enzymes 2C19, 2C9, and 3A4), there are several **clinically significant drug interactions** that must be considered. Rifampin, rifabutin, carbamazepine (markedly reduced voriconazole levels), sirolimus (increased drug concentrations), and astemizole (prolonged QT_c) are contraindicated with voriconazole. Concomitantly administered cyclosporine, tacrolimus, and warfarin require more careful monitoring.

SPECIAL CONSIDERATIONS

Nausea, diarrhea, and rash are mild side effects of the azoles. Hepatitis is a rare but serious complication. Therapy must be monitored closely in the setting of compromised liver function, and LFTs should be monitored regularly with chronic use. Itraconazole levels should be checked after 1 week of therapy to confirm absorption. The IV formulation of voriconazole should not be used in patients with a CrCl of <50 mL/min because of the potential for accumulation and toxicity from the cyclodextrin vehicle. Transient visual disturbance is a common adverse effect (30%) of voriconazole. **This class of antibiotics has major drug interactions.**

Echinocandins

GENERAL PRINCIPLES

This class of antifungals inhibit the enzyme $(1,3)$-β-D-glucan synthase that is essential in fungal cell wall synthesis.

- **Caspofungin acetate** (70 mg IV loading dose, followed by 50 mg IV q24h) has fungicidal activity against most *Aspergillus* and *Candida* species, including azole-resistant *Candida* strains. However, *Candida guilliermondii* and *Candida parapsilosis* may be relatively resistant.Caspofungin does not have appreciable activity against *Cryptococcus*, *Histoplasma*, *Blastomyces*, *Coccidioides*, or *Mucor* species. It is U.S. FDA-approved for treatment of candidemia, refractory invasive aspergillosis, and as empiric therapy in febrile neutropenic.
  - Metabolism is primarily hepatic, although the cytochrome P-450 system is not significantly involved. An increased maintenance dosage is necessary with the use of drugs that induce hepatic metabolism (e.g., efavirenz, nelfinavir, phenytoin, rifampin, carbamazepine, dexamethasone). The maintenance dose should be reduced to 35 mg for patients with moderate hepatic impairment; however, no dose adjustment is necessary for renal failure.
  - In vitro and limited clinical data suggest a synergistic effect when caspofungin is given in conjunction with itraconazole, voriconazole, or amphotericin B for *Aspergillus* infections.
  - **Adverse events.** Fever, rash, nausea, and phlebitis at the injection site are infrequent.
- **Micafungin sodium** is used for candidemia (100 mg IV daily), esophageal candidiasis (150 mg IV q24h), and as fungal prophylaxis for patients undergoing hematopoietic stem cell transplantation (50 mg IV q24h).The spectrum of activity is similar to that of anidulafungin and caspofungin. Although micafungin increases serum concentrations of sirolimus and nifedipine, these increases may not be clinically significant. Micafungin may increase cyclosporine concentrations in about 20% of patients. No change in dosing is necessary in renal or hepatic dysfunction.
  - **Adverse events** include rash and delirium. Some patients may have elevated LFTs while on therapy.
- **Anidulafungin** (200-mg IV loading dose, followed by 100 mg IV q24h) is useful for treatment of candidemia and other systemic *Candida* infections (intra-abdominal abscess and peritonitis) as well as esophageal candidiasis (100-mg loading dose, followed by 50 mg daily). The spectrum of activity is similar to that of caspofungin and micafungin. Anidulafungin is not a substrate, inhibitor, or inducer of cytochrome P-450 isoenzymes and does not have clinically relevant drug interactions. No dosage change is necessary in renal or hepatic insufficiency.
  - **Adverse events** include possible histamine-mediated reactions, elevations in LFTs, and rarely hypokalemia.

Miscellaneous

GENERAL PRINCIPLES

- **Flucytosine** (25 mg/kg PO q6h) exerts its fungicidal effects on susceptible *Candida* and *Cryptococcus* species by interfering with DNA synthesis.
  - Main clinical uses are for the treatment of cryptococcal meningitis and severe *Candida* infections in combination with amphotericin B.
  - **Adverse events** include dose-related bone marrow suppression and bloody diarrhea due to intestinal flora conversion of flucytosine to 5-fluorouracil.
  - Peak drug concentrations should be kept between 50 and 100 mcg/mL. Close monitoring of serum concentrations and dose adjustments are critical in the setting of renal insufficiency. LFTs should be obtained at least once a week.

- **Terbinafine** (250 mg PO c24h for 6 to 12 weeks) is an allylamine antifungal agent that kills fungi by inhibiting ergosterol synthesis. It is U.S. FDA approved for the treatment of onychomycosis of the fingernail (6 weeks of treatment) or toenail (12 weeks of treatment). It is not generally used for systemic infections.
  - **Adverse events** include headache, GI disturbances, rash, LFT abnormalities, and taste disturbances. This drug should not be used in patients with hepatic cirrhosis or a CrCl of <50 mL/min because of inadequate data. It has only moderate affinity for cytochrome P-450 hepatic enzymes and does not significantly inhibit the metabolism of cyclosporine (15% decrease) or warfarin.

13 Human Immunodeficiency Virus and Acquired Immunodeficiency Syndrome

Diana Nurutdinova and E. Turner Overton

HIV Type 1

GENERAL PRINCIPLES

Definition

Human immunodeficiency virus (HIV) type 1 is a retrovirus that infects predominantly lymphocytes that bear the CD4 surface protein as well as coreceptors belonging to the chemokine receptor family (CCR5 or CXCR4) and causes acquired immunodeficiency syndrome (AIDS).

Classification

CDC classification is based on the CD4 count and presence of AIDS-associated conditions. Diagnosis of AIDS is made on the basis of CD4 cell count < 200, CD4 percentage <14%, or development of one of the 25 AIDS-defining conditions (*MMWR 1992;41(RR-17)*).

Epidemiology

- HIV type 1 is common throughout the world. By the most recent estimates, over 33 million people worldwide are living with HIV or AIDS with a significant burden of disease in Sub-Saharan Africa (http://www.who.int/hiv/data/en/index.html).
- In the United States, 1.2 million people are estimated to be infected with HIV with one-fourth of these persons unaware of their infection. The CDC estimates that as many as 70% of the 56,000 new infections in the United States are transmitted by persons who are unaware of their HIV status.
- Despite comprising only 13% of the population in the United States, African Americans are disproportionately affected by HIV, accounting for nearly 50% of all new cases of HIV in this country. Hispanics are also disproportionately affected by HIV. Women comprise approximately 30% to 35% of the US epidemic.
- HIV type 2 is endemic to regions in West Africa. It is characterized by much slower progression to AIDS and resistance to nonnucleoside reverse transcriptase inhibitors (NNRTIs).

Etiology

HIV utilizes reverse transcriptase, transcribing viral RNA into DNA, which integrates into the host DNA. The host cell machinery is then used to produce the relevant viral proteins, which are appropriately truncated by a viral protease. Infectious viral particles bud away to infect other CD4 lymphocytes before the infected cell is destroyed by the immune system. Infection usually leads to CD4 T-cell depletion, and impaired cell-mediated immunity.

Pathophysiology

Without highly active antiretroviral therapy (HAART), the immune dysfunction progresses to AIDS, which is characterized by development of opportunistic infections (OIs), malignancies, and wasting. The time from acute HIV infection to development of AIDS varies from months to years (depending on host and viral factors), with a median *latency* period of 10 years.

Risk Factors

The virus is primarily transmitted sexually but also parenterally and perinatally.

DIAGNOSIS

Clinical Presentation

- Acute retroviral syndrome is experienced by up to 75% of patients and is similar to other acute viral illnesses such as infectious mononucleosis due to Epstein–Barr virus (EBV) or cytomegalovirus (CMV) infection. As the acute illness resolves spontaneously, most people do not present for evaluation unless diagnosed by subsequent routine screening. A larger proportion of persons are presenting to care late (CD4 count < 200 cells/mm^3) within the first year after diagnosis.
- Common presenting symptoms of acute retroviral syndrome are sore throat, exanthema, myalgias, headache, and fatigue.

History

- **Initial evaluation** of persons with a confirmed HIV infection should include the following measures:
  - Complete history with emphasis on previous OIs, viral coinfections, and other complications.
  - Psychological and psychiatric history. Depression and substance use are common and should be identified and treated as necessary.
  - Family and social support assessment.
  - Assessment of knowledge and perceptions regarding HIV is also crucial to initiate ongoing education regarding the nature and ramifications of HIV infection.

Physical Examination

Complete physical exam is important to evaluate for manifestations of immune compromise. Initial findings may include the following:

- Oral findings: hairy leukoplakia, aphthous ulcers, thrush
- Lymphatic system: generalized lymphadenopathy
- Skin: molluscum contagiosum, Cryptococcus, psoriasis, eosinophilic folliculitis, Kaposi's Sarcoma
- Abdominal exam: evidence of hepatosplenomegaly
- Genital exam: presence of ulcers, genital warts, vaginal discharge, and rectal discharge
- Neurologic exam: note presence of sensory deficits and cognitive testing

Diagnostic Criteria

The CDC recommends that all persons aged 13 to 64 be offered HIV testing in all health care settings using an opt-out format (*MMWR Recomm Rep 2006;55:1–17*). These recommendations are based on the following considerations: significant individual health benefits if HAART is initiated earlier in the course of illness; significant public health benefits with knowledge of HIV status leading to changes in risk behaviors; and the availability of inexpensive, reliable, and rapid testing technology. Barriers, however, still exist in certain settings and include inadequate infrastructure to provide testing and linkage to care, legally mandated counseling, and the requirement for a separate, signed informed consent.

Diagnostic Testing

Serology. HIV serology should be checked in all persons at risk when on an opt-out basis (assent is inferred unless the patient declines testing).

- **Persons at high risk,** including IV drug users, homosexual and bisexual men, hemophiliacs, sexual partners of the aforementioned patients, sexual partners of a known HIV patient, persons involved in sex trading and their sexual partners, persons with sexually transmitted diseases, persons who received blood products between 1977 and 1985, persons who have multiple sexual partners or who engage in unprotected intercourse, persons who consider themselves at risk, and patients with findings that are suggestive of HIV infection, should be screened least at least annually.
  - Other categories that require HIV testing:
    - Pregnant women (opt-out screening)
    - Patients with active tuberculosis (TB)
    - Donors of blood, semen, and organs
    - Health care workers who perform invasive procedures (depending on the policy of the institution in which they work)
    - Persons with occupational exposures (e.g., needlesticks) and source patients of the exposures
- Screening is performed with an **enzyme-linked immunosorbent assay (ELISA) or rapid HIV test.** The current HIV ELISA used in the United States is a combination HIV-1/HIV-2 enzyme immunoassay test kit that is also sensitive to antibodies to HIV-2.
- A positive screening test is confirmed by a repeat positive ELISA and a positive **Western blot** (presence of at least two of the following bands: p24, gp41, gp120/160).
- **An isolated positive ELISA result should not be reported to the patient until this result is confirmed by a Western blot.** In settings where the rapid HIV test is used for screening, preliminary positive results may be given to the patient with scheduled follow-up to give the results of the confirmatory Western Blot testing. An indeterminate test is one for which the ELISA is positive but the criteria for a positive Western blot are not fulfilled. Repeat testing should be considered for these patients to confirm whether they have a false-positive ELISA or have recent/acute HIV infection.

Laboratories

- **Complete blood cell (CBC) count, comprehensive metabolic panel with assessment of liver and kidney parameters including urinalysis to evaluate for proteinuria and glucosuria.**

- **CD4 cell count** (normal range, 600–1,500 cells/mm^3) and CD4 percentage. CD4 cell count should be checked periodically (three to four times a year) to assess the immune status of the patient and to determine the need for OI prophylaxis.
- **Virologic markers.** Plasma HIV RNA is used for monitoring of HAART efficacy. The goal is to achieve maximal virologic suppression, that is, to reduce the viral load level to undetectable by currently available assays. Several quantitative HIV RNA viral load assays are currently in use, including a branched DNA assay and a nucleic acid sequence amplification assay. The reverse transcriptase polymerase chain reaction (PCR) assay is the most widely used with a lower limit of detection of 40 to 50 copies/mL.
- **Tuberculin skin test**
- **Rapid plasma reagin (RPR) test**
- **Toxoplasma immunoglobulin (Ig) G and hepatitis A, B (HBsAg, HBsAb, HBcAb), and C serologies**
- **Chlamydia/gonococcal urine/cervical probe**
- **Cervical Papanicolaou smear** (most commonly using the thin prep method)
- **HIV resistance testing** at baseline, with treatment failure, and particularly for pregnant women
- **HLA B5701** for patients in whom one is considering the use of abacavir
- **CCR5** Tropism testing for patients in whom one is considering the use of maraviroc

TREATMENT

Immunizations

- **Pneumococcal vaccine.** HIV infection is an indication for polysaccharide pneumococcal vaccination. Some experts recommend deferring the vaccine until the CD4 cell counts are >200 cells/mm^3, as responses are poor when vaccination occurs with low CD4 cell counts. Revaccination after 5 years is recommended (http://www.cdc.gov/vaccines/recs/schedules/downloads/adult/06-07/adult-schedule.pdf).
- **Hepatitis A and B virus (HAV and HBV).** Vaccination for HAV is recommended for certain high-risk HIV-positive subjects without HAV antibodies, although some experts recommend HAV vaccination for all. HIV-positive patients are at higher risk of becoming chronic carriers of HBV after having an acute HBV infection. Therefore, if antibodies against hepatitis B core and hepatitis B surface antigens are negative, HBV vaccination is indicated. Coinfection with HCV is very prevalent in this population (especially among IV drug abusers); no vaccine for HCV currently exists. Antibody response is improved with undetectable HIV viral load and higher CD4 count.
- **Influenza.** Annual inactivated influenza vaccination is recommended for all HIV-infected patients regardless of CD4 cell count. Use of the intranasally administered, live, attenuated vaccine is not currently recommended for HIV-infected persons.
- **Varicella.** The live, attenuated varicella vaccine can be safely given to persons with CD4 cell counts > 200 cells/mm^3 but is contraindicated for persons with CD4 counts < 200 cells/mm^3. There are currently no data on the safety or efficacy of the use of the zoster vaccine in HIV-infected adults.
- **Measles/mumps/rubella.** MMR is a vaccine that can be safely given to persons with CD4 cell counts > 200 cells/mm^3 but is contraindicated for persons with CD4 counts < 200 cells/mm^3.

- **Tetanus/diphtheria/pertussis.** All adults should receive tetanus/diphtheria (Td) booster every 10 years with a one-time substitution with tetanus/diphtheria/acellular pertussis vaccine (Tdap).
- **HPV (human papilloma virus) vaccine.** There are ongoing studies evaluating the safety and efficacy of HPV vaccination in HIV-infected men and women.

Medications

Antiretroviral therapy

- Treatment decisions should be individualized by patient readiness, drug interactions, adherence issues, drug toxicities, comorbidities, and the level of risk indicated by CD4 T-cell counts.
- Maximal and durable suppression of HIV replications is the goal of therapy once it is initiated. Reductions in plasma viremia correlate with increased CD4 cell counts and prolonged AIDS-free survival. Isolated viral "blips" are not indicative of virologic failure, but confirmed virologic rebound should trigger an evaluation of adherence, drug interactions, and viral resistance.
- Women, especially if pregnant, should receive optimal antiretroviral therapy (ART) to reduce the risk of vertical transmission.
- **HAART** should be individualized and closely monitored by measuring plasma HIV viral load. Reductions in plasma viremia correlate with increased CD4 cell counts and prolonged AIDS-free survival.
- Any change in ART increases future therapeutic constraints and potential drug resistance.
- **Current Recommendations from the IAS/USA (http://www.iasusa.org/guidelines/)** for the initiation of ART include the following:
  - All patients with clinical AIDS or immunologic AIDS (CD4 count <200 cells/mm^3) to prevent progression of disease and incident or recurrent opportunistic disease.
  - Patients with symptomatic HIV disease, regardless of CD4 cell count.
  - Patients with CD4 cell count <350 cells/mm^3 with asymptomatic disease.
  - Other indications include the presence of HIV-associated nephropathy, hepatitis B virus coinfection, and pregnancy.
  - **In the asymptomatic patient, if the CD4 count is >350 cells/mm^3,** the decision regarding treatment initiation should be determined on case-by-case basis.
  - Initiation of ART depends on the patient's readiness, comorbidities, and drug toxicities.
- **Antiretroviral drugs.** Specific drug information is summarized in Tables 1 through 5. Approved antiretroviral drugs are grouped into five categories. Experts currently recommend using three active drugs from two different classes to maximally and durably suppress HIV viremia.
- **Nucleotide and nucleoside reverse transcriptase inhibitors (NRTIs)** constrain HIV replication by incorporating into the elongating strand of DNA, causing chain termination. All nucleoside analogs have been associated with **lactic acidosis,** presumably related to mitochondrial toxicity.
- **NNRTIs** inhibit HIV by binding noncompetitively to the reverse transcriptase. A single dosage of nevirapine at the time of labor has been shown to decrease perinatal transmission of the virus. Side effects of NNRTIs include rash, hepatotoxicity, and Stevens–Johnson syndrome (more likely with nevirapine). Central nervous system (CNS) side effects are commonly experienced with the use of efavirenz.

Table 1	Nucleoside Analog Reverse Transcriptase Inhibitors		
NRTIs	Dosage[a]	Food Restrictions	Common Side Effects
Abacavir (ABC) baseline testing for HLA B5701 is needed prior to initiating ABC	300 mg PO bid or combination tablets: ABC 300 mg + 3TC 150 mg + AZT 300 mg (Trizivir) one tablet bid or ABC 600 mg + 3TC 300 mg (Epzicom) one tablet daily	No	Hypersensitivity reaction; rechallenge in the setting of hyper-sensitivity can be fatal[b]
Didanosine (ddI)	Preferred as an enter ccoated formula (Videx EC); >60 kg: 400 mg PO daily, <60 kg: 250 mg PO daily When coadministered with ⁻DF decrease ddI dose to 250 mg	On empty stomach	Pancreatitis, peripheral neuropathy, diarrhea
Emtricitabine (FTC)[c]	Closely related to 3TC (cross-resistance possible); 200 mg PO daily	No	No common severe side effects; may have gastrointestinal (GI) intolerance
Lamivudine (3TC)	150 mg PO bid 300 mg PO daily	No	Rare
Stavudine (d4T)	>60 kg: 40 mg PO bid, <60 kg: 30 mg PO bid; extended-release form: >60 kg: 100 mg PO daily, <60 kg: 75 mg PO daily	No	Peripheral neuropathy, pancreatitis, lipoatrophy
Zidovudine (ZDV, AZT)	300 mg PO bid or combination tablet AZT + 3TC (Combivir) one tablet bid or AZT + 3TC + ABC (Trizivir) one tablet bid	No	Bone marrow suppression, GI intolerance

(*continued*)

Table 1	Nucleoside Analog Reverse Transcriptase Inhibitors (*Continued*)		
NRTIs	**Dosage**[a]	**Food Restrictions**	**Common Side Effects**
Tenofovir (TDF)[d]	300 mg PO daily or combination tablet TDF 300 mg + FTC 200 mg one tablet daily or combination tablet TDF 300 mg + FTC 200 mg + Efavirenz 600 mg one tablet daily	No	Rare cases of renal toxicity, rare GI intolerance

[a]Dose adjustment required in patients with renal failure for most NRTIs.
[b]ABC-related hypersensitivity reaction: flulike symptoms, fever, rash, upper respiratory symptoms, GI intolerance.
[c]Zalcitabine (ddC) belongs to this class of NRTIs; however, it is rarely used in clinical practice.
[d]Tenofovir (TDF) is a nucleotide that is available as tenofovir disoproxil fumarate.

Table 2	Nonnucleoside Reverse Transcriptase Inhibitors		
NNRTI[a]	**Dosage**	**Food Restrictions**	**Side Effects**
Efavirenz (EFV)	600 mg PO daily	On empty stomach; avoid taking after high-fat meals because of increased peak concentration	Central nervous system symptoms (dizziness, somnolence, insomnia, abnormal dreams), teratogenicity; false-positive urine cannabinoid test[b]
Nevirapine (NVP)[c]	200 mg PO daily for 2 wk, then 200 mg PO bid or 400 mg daily	No	Skin rash; hepatitis; severe life-threatening hepatotoxicity observed when used with initial CD4 count > 250 cells/mm^3 in women and >400 cells/mm^3 in men
Etravirine (ETV)	100 mg PO BID	Take with food	Skin rash

[a]See Table 5 for interactions with other antiretrovirals.
[b]Use of gas chromatography or mass spectroscopy is recommended if screening for cannabis is desired.
[c]Delavirdine is rarely used in clinical practice in the United States.

Table 3	Protease Inhibitors		
PI	**Dosage**[a]	**Food Restrictions**	**Side Effects**
Fosamprenavir (fAPV)[b]	1,400 mg PO bid; combined with RTV(r): fAPV/r, 700/100 mg bid or fAPV/r, 1,400/200 mg daily	No	Rash, diarrhea, nausea
Atazanavir (ATV)	400 mg PO daily; combined with RTV(r): ATZ/r, 300/100 mg daily if prior experience with PIs or taken with tenofovir (TDF)	Take with food	Increased indirect bilirubin, fewer metabolic effects
Indinavir (IDV)	800 mg PO tid usually with RTV(r): IDV/r, 800/100 mg bid; IDV/r, 800/200 mg bid	No food if taken alone, can be taken with or without food if combined with RTV(r)	Nephrolithiasis, increased indirect bilirubin, headache
Lopinavir (LPV)	Available only in fixed combination with RTV(r): LPV/r, 400/100 mg PO bid (Kaletra) 200/50 mg tablet, four tablets qd may be used in treatment-naïve patients only	Take with food; new formulation can be taken with or without food	Diarrhea, hyperlipidemia, hyperglycemia
Nelfinavir (NFV)	750 mg PO tid or 1,250 mg PO bid	Take with food	Diarrhea, nausea
Ritonavir (RTV)[c]	Usually added to achieve booster effect in combination with other PIs; not longer used in full dose	Take with food	Nausea and vomiting, paresthesias, hepatitis, taste perversion
Saquinavir (SQV)	SQV/r, 1,000/100 mg PO bid or used only with RTV boosting	Take with food	Headache, diarrhea
Tipranavir (TPV)	Used only with RTV boosting: TPV/r, 500/200 mg PO bid	Take with food	Hepatitis, skin rash, hyperlipidemia, hyperglycemia
Darunavir (DRV)	DRV/r 800 mg PO qd with 100 mg RTV boosting may be used in treatment-naïve patients only or 600 mg po BID with RTV boosting	Take with food	Diarrhea, nausea, headache

[a]See Tables 5 and 6 for interactions with antiretrovirals and other medications.
[b]fAPV is the prodrug of amprenavir; amprenavir is no longer available in United States.
[c]RTV is usually added using a lower dose to achieve a booster effect, especially with LPV, SQV, fAPV, and IDV.

Table 4	Entry Inhibitors		
EI	Dosage	Food Restrictions	Side Effects
Enfuvirtide (T-20)	90 mg SQ bid	No	Injection site reactions
Maraviroc (MVC)[a]	300 mg po bid 150 mg po bid with all PIs except TPV/r 600 mg po bid if used with EFV	No	Abnormal liver function tests

[a]MVC is a CCR5 receptor antagonist; it is indicated for use only if evidence of CCR5 tropic virus.

- **Protease inhibitors (PIs)** block the action of the viral protease required for protein processing late in the viral cycle. Gastrointestinal (GI) intolerance is one of the most commonly encountered adverse effects. All PIs can produce increased bleeding in hemophiliacs; these agents have also been associated with metabolic abnormalities such as glucose intolerance, increased cholesterol and triglycerides, and body fat redistribution. Due to their metabolism via cytochrome P-450, **PIs have important drug interactions** and concomitant medications should be reviewed carefully (Table 6). Boosting with ritonavir is a common practice to achieve better therapeutic concentrations.
- **HIV entry inhibitors** target different stages of the HIV entry process. Two drugs are available in this class: **T-20 (enfuvirtide)** is a fusion inhibitor that prevents the fusion of the virus into the host cell; maraviroc is a CCR5 receptor blocker. T-20 is only available for use as a subcutaneous injection, 90 mg bid; the most frequent side effect for T-20 is a significant local site reaction after the injection. Initiation of CCR5 inhibitor requires baseline determination of HIV coreceptor tropism (CCR5 or CXCR4). Both of these medications are indicated for treatment-experienced individuals.
- **Integrase inhibitors** are a new class of antiretroviral agents that target DNA strand transfer and integration into a human genome. There is one drug currently available for use—raltegravir, which demonstrated excellent potency and a low side effect profile.
- **Initial therapy.** ART should be started in an outpatient setting by a physician with expertise in the management of HIV infection. Adherence is the key factor for success. Treatment should be individualized and adapted to the patient's lifestyle and comorbidities. Any treatment decision influences future therapeutic options because of the possibility of drug cross-resistance. Potent initial ART generally consists of a combination of two NRTIs plus one or two PIs or an NNRTI.

Table 5	Integrase Inhibitors		
II	Dosage[a]	Food Restrictions	Side Effects
Raltegravir	400 mg po BID	No	Rare, headache, depression

Table 6	Selected Interactions between Antiretrovirals and Other Medications

ARV	Interactions

Protease inhibitors

Do not coadminister with simvastatin, lovastatin: levels increased; can cause myopathy and rhabdomyolysis. Atorvastatin or pravastatin can be administered with PIs with close monitoring

Rifampin and rifapentine cannot be coadministered with PIs due to decreased plasma concentrations

St. John's Wort should not be used with any PIs: reduces PI plasma concentration

Decrease in methadone levels observed with most of the PIs

Caution when coadministered with sildenafil: increased concentration with all PIs

Lopinavir/ritonavir (LPV/r)	Inhibitor of P-450 system
	Fluticasone use can result in suppressed adrenal function
	Decrease rifabutin to 150 mg every other day or three times per week
Atazanavir (ATV)	Decreases clarithromycin dose by 50%
	PPIs significantly decrease ATV concentration: should not be coadministered
	When coadministered with H_2 blockers, should be given 12 hours apart
	Caution due to increased levels of antiarrhythmics
	Decrease rifabutin to 150 mg every other day or three times per week
	Monitor anticonvulsant levels
Nelfinavir (NFV)	Monitor anticonvulsant levels
	Decrease rifabutin to 150 mg every other day or three times per week
Tipranavir (TPV)	Inhibitor of P-450 system
	Fluticasone use can result in suppressed adrenal function
	Do not coadminister with amiodarone, quinidine, flecainide
	Do not coadminister with oral contraceptives
	Decrease rifabutin to 150 mg every other day or three times per week
Darunavir (DRV)	Use the lowest dose of pravastatin with close monitoring

Nonnucleoside reverse transcriptase inhibitors

St. John's Wort should not be coadministered due to suboptimal levels of NNRTIs

Decreased levels of oral contraceptives when coadministered

Efavirenz (EFV)	Inducer/inhibitor of the P-450 system
	Do not coadminister with voriconazole: decreases voriconazole levels
	Decreases methadone levels; can cause opiate withdrawal

(*continued*)

Table 6	Selected Interactions between Antiretrovirals and Other Medications (*Continued*)
ARV	Interactions
Nevirapine (NVP)	Inducer of the P-450 system
	Rifabutin lowers NVP levels; do not coadminister with rifampin
	Decreases methadone levels; can cause opiate withdrawal
Nucleoside reverse transcriptase inhibitors	
Tenofovir (TDF)	Coadministration with cidofovir, acyclovir, valacyclovir, ganciclovir, and valganciclovir may increase serum concentrations of either tenofovir or the coadministered drug
Didanosine (ddI)	Do not coadminister with allopurinol (decreased didanosine concentrations), ribavirin (hepatic failure)
	Monitor for didanosine toxicity when coadministered with ganciclovir or valganciclovir
Zidovudine (AZT)	Avoid concomitant ribavirin and interferon use
	Increased hematologic toxicity with ganciclovir, valganciclovir, cidofovir

Complete updated HIV clinical guidelines available at: http://www.aidsinfo.nih.gov/Guidelines/Default.aspx? Menuitem=Guidelines.
From U.S. Food and Drug Administration. Available at: http://www.fda.gov/cder/drug/default.htm and National Institutes of Health. Available at: http://www.aidsinfo.nih.gov/.

- **Treatment monitoring.** After starting or changing ART, the viral load should be checked at 4 to 6 weeks with an expected 10-fold reduction ($1.0 \log_{10}$) and suppression to <50 copies/mL by 24 weeks of therapy. The regimen should be then reassessed if response to treatment is inadequate. When the HIV RNA becomes undetectable and the patient is on a stable regimen, monitoring can be done every 3 months.
- **Treatment failure** is defined as (a) less than a log (10-fold) reduction of the viral load 4 to 6 weeks after starting a new antiretroviral regimen; (b) failure to reach an undetectable viral load after 6 months of treatment; (c) detection of the virus after initial complete suppression of viral load, which suggests development of resistance; or (d) persistent decline of CD4 cell count or clinical deterioration. Confirmed treatment failure should prompt changes in HAART based on results of genotype testing. In this situation, at least two of the drugs should be substituted with other drugs that have no expected cross-resistance.
- **HIV resistance testing** at this stage may help determine a salvage regimen in the patients with prior ART. The importance of adherence should be stressed. Referral to an HIV specialist is highly recommended in this situation.
- **Drug interactions.** Antiretroviral medications, especially PIs, have multiple drug interactions. **PIs both inhibit and induce the P-450 system,** and thus interactions are frequent with other inhibitors of the P-450 system, including macrolides (erythromycin, clarithromycin) and antifungals (ketoconazole, itraconazole), as well as other inducers such as rifamycins (rifampin, rifabutin) and anticonvulsants

(phenobarbital, phenytoin, carbamazepine). **Drugs with narrow therapeutic indexes that should be avoided or used with extreme caution** include antihistamines (although loratadine is safe), antiarrhythmics (flecainide, encainide, quinidine), long-acting opiates (fentanyl, meperidine), long-acting benzodiazepines (midazolam, triazolam), warfarin, 3-hydroxy-3-methylglutaryl coenzyme A (HMG-CoA) reductase inhibitors (pravastatin is the safest), and oral contraceptives. Sildenafil concentrations are increased, while methadone and theophylline concentrations are decreased with concomitant administration of certain PIs and NNRTIs. Grapefruit juice can increase levels of saquinavir and decrease levels of indinavir. See Table 6 for common interactions between antiretrovirals and other medications.

SPECIAL CONSIDERATIONS

With the success of ART, HIV-related mortality is decreasing and HIV-infected persons are experiencing prolonged survival. The CDC estimates that in 2015, one-half of all HIV-infected persons will be over the age of 50. With the recognition that HIV induces premature end-organ disease, many of the comorbidities associated with aging may be exacerbated in this growing population including cardiovascular disease, insulin resistance and diabetes, osteoporosis, neurocognitive impairment, and physical frailty.

COMPLICATIONS

Complications of ART. The long-term use of antiretrovirals has been associated with toxicity, the pathogenesis of which is only partially understood at this time.

- **Lipodystrophy syndrome** is an alteration in body fat distribution and can be stigmatizing to individuals. Changes consist of the accumulation of visceral fat in the abdomen, neck (buffalo hump), and pelvic areas, and/or the depletion of subcutaneous fat, causing facial or peripheral wasting. Lipodystrophy has been associated in particular with PIs and NRTIs, but other factors may also be important. Changes in the patient's ART regimen and lifestyle modifications such as exercise may improve morphologic changes. Other supplemental therapies such as rosiglitazone and cosmetic surgery are currently under investigation.
- **Hyperlipidemia,** especially hypertriglyceridemia, is associated mainly with PIs (especially ritonavir). Improvement has been seen after treatment with atorvastatin, pravastatin, and/or gemfibrozil.
- **Peripheral insulin resistance, impaired glucose tolerance, and hyperglycemia** have been associated with the use of PI-based regimens, mainly indinavir and ritonavir. Lifestyle changes or changing ART can be considered in these cases.
- **Lactic acidosis** with liver steatosis is a rare but sometimes fatal complication associated with NRTIs. The mechanism appears to be part of mitochondrial toxicity. Higher rates of lactic acidosis have been reported with the use of stavudine and didanosine. The clinical picture can range from asymptomatic hyperlactatemia to severe lactic acidosis with hepatomegaly and steatosis. Suspected drugs should be discontinued and supportive care given as needed.
- **Osteopenia and osteoporosis** are well described in HIV-infected individuals. The pathogenic mechanism of this problem is likely related to the inflammatory milieu of HIV itself. The role of ART is being further studied.
- **Osteonecrosis,** particularly of the hip, has been increasingly associated with HIV disease.

REFERRAL

- To HIV specialist
- **Contraception, safer sex practices,** counseling on medication adherence, and proper health maintenance
- **Social worker referral** to ensure adequate social support system including housing, mental health assistance, and substance abuse treatment

MONITORING/FOLLOW-UP

- Plasma HIV RNA is used for monitoring of ART efficacy. The goal is to reduce the viral load levels to undetectable. CD4 cell count should be checked periodically (three to four times a year) to assess the immune status of the patient and to determine the need for OI prophylaxis. After starting or changing ART, the viral load should be checked at 4 to 6 weeks, and the regimen should be then reassessed if response to treatment is inadequate. When the HIV RNA becomes undetectable and the patient is on a stable regimen, monitoring can be done every 3 months.
- **HIV resistance testing** is done using two different types of assays: genotypic (in which the reverse transcriptase and the polymerase genes are sequenced using different techniques) and phenotypic (in which the HIV replication in vitro in the presence of antiretroviral drugs is examined). Results of resistance testing should be used to guide ART.

OUTCOME/PROGNOSIS

With the advent of potent HAART that causes durable virologic suppression and reconstitution of the immune system, the mortality among HIV-infected persons continues to decline. In the modern era of HAART, the noninfectious conditions start to play a much more important role in the mortality among persons with HIV (*AIDS 2007;21(15):2093–2100*).

ASSOCIATED CONDITIONS

Opportunistic Infections

GENERAL PRINCIPLES

Definition

- Potent ART has decreased the incidence, changed the manifestations, and improved the outcome of OIs.
- A clinical syndrome associated with the immune enhancement induced by potent ART, **immune reconstitution syndrome (IRIS),** has been described and generally presents as local inflammatory reactions. Examples include paradoxical reactions with TB reactivation, localized *Mycobacterium avium* complex adenitis, and CMV vitreitis immediately after the initiation of potent ART. Hepatitis virus infections can be aggravated with the immune reconstitution associated with ART.

Table 7	Opportunistic Infection Prophylaxis	
Opportunistic Infection	Indications for Prophylaxis	Medications
PCP	Primary: CD4 < 200 cells/mm³	TMP/SMX DS PO daily or three times per week Alternatives: Dapsone[a], Atovaquone, aerosolized pentamidine
Tuberculosis[b]	PPD test >5 mm or a history of a previous untreated PPD test, or recent contact with an individual with active TB	Isoniazid (INH) + pyridoxine, for 9 months. Alternatives: Rifampin or Rifabutin for 4 months[c]
Toxoplasmosis	CD4 < 100 cells/mm³, one tablet daily, is the preferred regimen	TMP/SMX DS PO daily Alternatives: combination of dapsone, + pyrimethamine and leucovorin; atovaquone
Mycobacterium avium complex prophylaxis	CD4 cell count < 50 cells/mm³	Azithromycin 1,200 mg PO weekly Alternatives: Clarithromycin or Rifabutin

[a]G6PD testing should be done for Dapsone.
[b]If Toxo IgG is positive.
[c]Potential for drug interactions.

TREATMENT

Medications

- **Prophylaxis for OIs** can be divided into primary and secondary prophylaxis.
- **Primary prophylaxis** is established before an episode of OI occurs. Institution of primary prophylaxis depends on the level of immunosuppression as judged by the patient's CD4 cell count and percentage. The interventions considered as a standard of care in every patient are listed in Table 7.
  - **Primary prophylaxis is not routinely recommended** for the following OIs: recurrent bacterial pneumonia, mucosal candidiasis, CMV retinitis, cryptococcosis, and endemic fungal infections such as histoplasmosis and coccidioidomycosis.
- **Secondary prophylaxis** is instituted after an episode of infection has been adequately treated. Most OIs will require extended therapy.
- **Withdrawal of prophylaxis.** Recommendations suggest withdrawing primary and secondary prophylaxis for most OIs if sustained immunologic recovery has occurred (CD4 cell counts consistently above 150 to 200 cells/mm³) (*MMWR Recomm Rep 2009;58(RR-4):1–207*).

SPECIAL CONSIDERATIONS

- Careful monitoring is important after starting ART.
- In the case of IRIS, ART is usually continued, and the addition of low-dose steroids might decrease the degree of inflammation.

VIRAL INFECTIONS

Cytomegalovirus Infection

GENERAL PRINCIPLES

CMV retinitis accounts for 85% of CMV disease in patients with AIDS. It commonly develops in a setting of profound CD4 depletions (CD4 cell count < 50 cells/mm^3).

TREATMENT

- **Treatment of CMV retinitis** can be local or systemic and is administered in two phases, induction and maintenance.
- **Valganciclovir,** a ganciclovir prodrug, has been approved for use in CMV retinitis. Drug levels are equivalent to those of IV ganciclovir. For induction 900 mg PO bid for 21 days is given, followed by 900 mg once a day. **Treatment is indefinite unless immunologic recovery occurs.** Adverse effects are similar to those of ganciclovir.
- **Ganciclovir** is given at an induction dosage of 5 mg/kg IV bid for 14 to 21 days and a maintenance dosage of 5 mg/kg IV daily indefinitely (unless immune reconstitution occurs). The most common side effect of ganciclovir is myelotoxicity resulting in neutropenia. The neutropenia may respond to granulocyte colony-stimulating factor therapy. An intraocular ganciclovir implant is effective but does not provide systemic CMV therapy.
- Alternatives include **IV Foscarnet, IV Cidofovir, and intraocular Fomivirsen** (which does not provide systemic therapy). **Both IV Foscarnet and Cidofovir** administrations carry a significant risk of nephrotoxicity; therefore, adequate hydration and electrolyte monitoring (including calcium) are required.
- **For other invasive CMV disease,** the optimal therapy is with IV ganciclovir, PO valganciclovir, IV foscarnet, or a combination of two drugs (in persons with prior anti-CMV therapy), for at least 3 to 6 weeks. Foscarnet has the best cerebrospinal fluid (CSF) penetration and is the drug of choice for CMV encephalitis and myelopathy. Long-term maintenance therapy is indicated.

MYCOBACTERIAL INFECTIONS

Mycobacterium Tuberculosis

GENERAL PRINCIPLES

M. tuberculosis is more frequent among HIV-infected patients, particularly IV drug abusers. Primary or reactivated disease is common (*MMWR Recomm Rep 2009; 58(RR-4):1–207*).

DIAGNOSIS

- Clinical manifestations depend on the level of immunosuppression. Patients with higher CD4 cell counts tend to exhibit classic presentations with **apical cavitary disease.**

- Profoundly immunosuppressed patients may demonstrate atypical presentations that can resemble disseminated primary infection, with diffuse or localized pulmonary infiltrates and hilar lymphadenopathy.
- Extrapulmonary dissemination is common.

TREATMENT

For treatment recommendations, see Chapter 11, Treatment of Infectious Diseases.

- Current recommendations suggest the **substitution of rifabutin for rifampin** in patients who are receiving concomitant ART, especially PIs.
- The dosage for rifabutin needs readjustment due to many significant interactions (http://www.hivmedicationguide.com/); it should be reduced to 150 mg daily if the patient is receiving ritonavir, indinavir, nelfinavir, or fosamprenavir, whereas it should be increased to 450 mg daily when combined with nevirapine or efavirenz.
- In subjects who are ART-naïve, ART can be delayed for a few weeks after TB-specific therapy is started.

M. Avium Complex (MAC) Infection

GENERAL PRINCIPLES

M. avium complex (MAC) infection is the most commonly occurring mycobacterial infection in AIDS patients and is responsible for significant morbidity in patients with advanced disease (CD4 cell count < 100cells/mm^3).

DIAGNOSIS

- Disseminated infection with fever, weight loss, and night sweats is the most frequent presentation.
- MAC infection can result in bacteremia in AIDS patients.

Diagnostic Testing
Laboratories
- Anemia and an elevated alkaline phosphatase level are the usual laboratory abnormalities.
- Mycobacterial blood cultures should be sent in suspected cases.

TREATMENT

- Initial therapy should include a macrolide (clarithromycin, 500 mg PO bid) and ethambutol, 15 mg/kg PO daily.
- Rifabutin, 300 mg PO daily, or ciprofloxacin, 500 mg PO bid, can be added in severe cases.
- Secondary prophylaxis for disseminated MAC can be discontinued if the CD count had a sustained increase >100 cells/mm^3 for 6 months or longer in response to ART, and if 12 months of therapy for MAC is completed and there are no symptoms or signs attributable to MAC.

FUNGAL INFECTIONS

Pneumocystis Jiroveci Pneumonia

GENERAL PRINCIPLES

P. jiroveci pneumonia (PCP) is the most common infection in patients with AIDS and is the leading cause of death in this population.

TREATMENT

- TMP/SMX is the treatment of choice. The dosage is 5 mg/kg of the TMP component IV q6–8h for severe cases, with a switch to oral therapy when the patient's condition improves. Total duration of therapy is 21 days. Prednisone should be added if the patient has an arterial oxygen tension (PaO_2) of <70 mm Hg or an alveolar arterial oxygen gradient ($P[A - a]O_2$) in excess of 35 mm Hg. The most frequently prescribed prednisone regimen is 40 mg PO bid on days 1 to 5 and 20 mg bid on days 6 to 10, followed by 10 mg on days 11 to 21. For patients who cannot receive TMP/SMX, the following alternatives are available:
  - For mild to moderately severe disease (PaO_2 > 70 mm Hg or $P[A - a]O_2$ < 35 mm Hg)
    - Trimethoprim, 20 mg/kg/d PO, and dapsone, 100 mg PO daily. Glucose-6-phosphate dehydrogenase deficiency should be ruled out before dapsone is used.
    - Clindamycin, 600 mg IV or PO tid, plus primaquine, 15 mg PO daily. Glucose-6-phosphate dehydrogenase deficiency should be ruled out before primaquine is used.
    - Atovaquone, 750 mg PO tid. This drug should be administered with meals to increase absorption.
  - For severe disease (PaO_2 < 70 mm Hg or $P[A - a]O_2$ > 35 mm Hg)
    - Prednisone taper should be added.
    - IV Pentamidine or Trimetixate are used in cases when all other options are exhausted. Both drugs require close monitoring for side effects.
- Prophylaxis is indicated as described in Table 7. Secondary PCP prophylaxis can be discontinued if the CD4 count is >200 cells/mm^3 for more than 3 months as a result of ART treatment.

Candidiasis

GENERAL PRINCIPLES

- The severity of infection depends on the degree of the patient's immunosuppression.
- Candidiasis is common in the HIV-infected host.

DIAGNOSIS

Location of infection can be oral, esophageal, or vaginal.

TREATMENT

- Oral and vaginal candidiasis usually respond to local therapy with troches or creams (**nystatin** or **clotrimazole**).

- For patients who do not respond or who have esophageal candidiasis, **fluconazole,** 100 to 200 mg PO daily, is the treatment of choice.

SPECIAL CONSIDERATIONS

- **Fluconazole-resistant candidiasis** is increasing especially in patients with advanced disease who have been receiving antifungal agents for prolonged periods.
- **Caspofungin,** an echinocandin, can be considered for refractory cases using an induction dose of 70 mg IV the first day and then 50 mg IV daily for mainte-nance.
- **Itraconazole** oral suspension (200 mg bid) is occasionally effective. Many patients require amphotericin B, either as an oral suspension (100 mg/mL swish and swallow qid) or parenterally.
- **Voriconazole** may also be useful.

Cryptococcus Neoformans

GENERAL PRINCIPLES

- The severity of infection depends on the degree of the patient's immunosuppres-sion.
- Cryptococcal meningitis is the most frequent CNS fungal infection in AIDS patients.

DIAGNOSIS

- Patients with CNS infection usually present with headaches, fever, and possibly mental status changes, but presentation can be more subtle.
- Cryptococcal infection can present as pulmonary or cutaneous disease.

Diagnostic Testing
Laboratories
- Diagnosis is based on **lumbar puncture** results and on the determination of latex cryptococcal antigen, which is usually positive in the serum and in the CSF.
- CSF opening pressure should always be measured to assess the possibility of elevated intracranial pressure.

TREATMENT

- Initial treatment is with **amphotericin B,** 0.7 mg/kg/d IV, and **5-flucytosine,** 25 mg/kg PO q6h for 2 to 3 weeks, followed by **fluconazole,** 400 mg PO daily for 8 to 10 weeks and then 200 mg PO daily indefinitely.
- The 5-flucytosine level should be monitored during therapy to avoid toxicity. A lipid preparation of **amphotericin** can be used in patients with renal insufficiency.
- Repeat lumbar punctures (removing up to 30 mL CSF until the pressure is below 20 to 25 cm H_2O) may be required to relieve elevated intracranial pressure.
- In persons who have persistent elevation of intracranial pressure, a temporary lumbar drain is indicated.

Histoplasma Capsulatum Infections

GENERAL PRINCIPLES

- The severity of infection depends on the degree of the patient's immunosuppression.
- Histoplasmosis often occurs in AIDS patients who live in endemic areas such as the Mississippi and Ohio River Valleys.
- Such infections are usually disseminated at the time of diagnosis.

DIAGNOSIS

- Suspect histoplasmosis in patients with fever, hepatosplenomegaly, and weight loss.
- Pancytopenia develops due to bone marrow involvement.

Diagnostic Testing
Laboratories
Diagnosis is made by a positive culture, but the urine *Histoplasma* antigen can also be used for diagnosis and to monitor treatment.

TREATMENT

- Treatment is with **amphotericin B,** 0.5 mg/kg IV daily for a total dose of 0.5 to 1.0 g, followed by **itraconazole,** 300 mg PO bid for 3 days for induction therapy, followed by 200 mg PO bid indefinitely.
- **Itraconazole absorption** should be documented by a serum drug level.
- Discontinuation of itraconazole is possible if sustained increase in CD4 count is observed >100 to 200 cells/mm^3 for more than 6 months.

PROTOZOAL INFECTIONS

Toxoplasma Gondii

DIAGNOSIS

Toxoplasmosis typically causes multiple CNS lesions and presents with encephalopathy and focal neurologic findings.

Diagnostic Testing
Laboratories
Disease represents reactivation of a previous infection, and the serologic workup is usually positive.

Imaging
- MRI of the brain is the best radiographic technique for diagnosis.
- Often the diagnosis relies on response to empiric treatment, as seen by a reduction in the size of the mass lesions.

TREATMENT

- Sulfadiazine, 25 mg/kg PO q6h, plus pyrimethamine, 100 mg PO on day 1, followed by 75 mg PO daily, is the therapy of choice.
- Leucovorin, 5 to 10 mg PO daily, should be added to prevent hematologic toxicity. For patients who are allergic to sulfonamides, clindamycin (600 mg IV or PO q8h) can be used instead of sulfadiazine.
- Doses are reduced after 3 to 6 weeks of therapy.
- Secondary prophylaxis can be discontinued among patients with a sustained increase in CD4 count > 200 cells/mm^3 for more than 6 months as a result of response to ART and if the initial therapy is complete and there are no symptoms or signs attributable to *Pneumocystis.*

Cryptosporidium

DIAGNOSIS

Cryptosporidium causes chronic watery diarrhea with malabsorption in HIV-infected patients.

Diagnostic Testing
Laboratories
Diagnosis is based on the visualization of the parasite in an acid-fast stain of stool.

TREATMENT

- No effective specific therapy has been developed.
- **Nitazoxanide,** 500 mg PO bid, may be effective.
- Potent **ART** also has been reported to be effective.

Cyclospora

DIAGNOSIS

Cyclospora causes chronic diarrhea.

TREATMENT

TMP/SMX, one DS tablet PO bid for 7 to 10 days, is usually effective.

Isospora Belli

DIAGNOSIS

Isospora causes chronic diarrhea.

TREATMENT

Treatment with TMP/SMX, one DS tablet PO qid for 10 days, followed by chronic suppression with TMP/SMX, one DS tablet PO daily, is effective.

Microsporidia

DIAGNOSIS

Microsporidia can produce diarrhea and biliary tree disease in patients with advanced infection.

Diagnostic Testing
Laboratories
Diagnosis is difficult and requires special staining of the stool. *Enterocytozoon bieneusi* and *Encephalitozoon intestinalis* are the microsporidia most commonly found. *E. intestinalis* can cause disseminated disease.

TREATMENT

Conventional therapy is with albendazole, 400 mg PO bid, but this regimen has only modest success for *E. bieneusi* infections. Relapses are common when therapy is stopped.

Strongyloides

GENERAL PRINCIPLES

Strongyloides presents as disseminated infection in AIDS patients from endemic areas (southeastern United States, immigrants from tropical and subtropical countries).

TREATMENT

Thiabendazole, 22 mg/kg (maximum, 1.5 g) PO daily for 7 to 14 days, is the drug of choice for disseminated strongyloidiasis.

ASSOCIATED NEOPLASMS

Kaposi Sarcoma

GENERAL PRINCIPLES

- Kaposi sarcoma is caused by coinfection with human herpes virus 8 (HHV8), also called KSHV.
- It usually presents as a cutaneous lesion; the GI tract and lungs are the usual visceral organs involved.

DIAGNOSIS

In AIDS patients, it commonly presents as skin lesions but can be disseminated, even visceral.

TREATMENT

- Local therapy with liquid **nitrogen** or intralesional injection with alitretinoin or vinblastine has been used. Cryotherapy or radiation may be useful as well.

- Systemic therapy involves chemotherapy (e.g., liposomal doxorubicin, paclitaxel, liposomal daunorubicin, thalidomide, retinoids), radiation, and interferon-α.

Lymphoma

GENERAL PRINCIPLES

- Lymphomas commonly associated with AIDS are non-Hodgkin lymphoma, CNS and systemic lymphoma, and lymphomas of B-cell origin.
- **EBV** appears to be the associated pathogen.

DIAGNOSIS

- Primary CNS lymphomas are common and can be multicentric.
- Diagnosis is based on clinical symptoms, the presence of enhancing brain lesions, brain biopsy, and a positive EBV-PCR of the CSF.
- Other OIs need to be ruled out.
- Other potential extranodal sites of involvement including bone marrow, GI tract, and liver require tissue biopsy to confirm the diagnosis.

TREATMENT

Treatment involves **chemotherapy** and **radiation.**

Cervical and Perianal Neoplasias

GENERAL PRINCIPLES

- Both HIV-infected men and women are at high risk for HPV-related disease.
- Certain HPV subtypes such as 16 and 18 are oncogenic.
- Cancer can also arise from perianal condyloma acuminata.

DIAGNOSIS

- Screening for vaginal dysplasia with a Papanicolaou smear is indicated every 6 months during the first year and, if results are normal, annually afterwards.
- Screening for anal intraepithelial neoplasms is currently under evaluation.

SEXUALLY TRANSMITTED DISEASES

Genital Herpes

GENERAL PRINCIPLES

Herpes simplex virus 2 (HSV-2) (less frequently herpes simplex virus 1 [HSV-1]) causes recurrent genital and perirectal lesions. HIV-infected individuals are more likely to have prolonged and severe disease as well as treatment failures due to the development of resistance.

DIAGNOSIS

Type-specific HSV serology, HSV-PCR from the genital fluid; viral culture.

TREATMENT

- Acyclovir (400 mg PO tid), famciclovir (250 mg PO tid), or valacyclovir (500 mg PO tid) for 1 week is usually effective. For more severe disease, IV acyclovir, 5 mg/kg q8h, is recommended.
- Relapses are frequent, and prophylactic acyclovir, 400 mg PO bid, may prevent recurrence as a part of a suppressive or episodic treatment strategy.
- **If resistant HSV, foscarnet, 40 mg/kg IV q8h for 10 to 14 days, or one dose of cidofovir, 5 mg/kg IV, should be used.**

Genital Warts

GENERAL PRINCIPLES

Genital warts are caused by HPV. Different serotypes have been associated with the lesions, notably types 6 and 11. Other common HPV types (16, 18, 31, and 33) are associated with malignant transformation in different anatomic sites. Genital warts in HIV-infected persons are typically more resistant to treatment in addition to a higher chance of recurrence (http://www.cdc.gov/STD/treatment/2006/genital-warts.htm).

DIAGNOSIS

Diagnosis is made on the basis of physical exam and history. In some situations, biopsy of the lesions may be necessary.

TREATMENT

Local therapy aimed at the removal of the warts.

Syphilis

GENERAL PRINCIPLES

Syphilis can have an atypical course in HIV-infected patients, and treatment failures are more frequent in this population.

DIAGNOSIS

A lumbar puncture should be performed in HIV-infected patients with latent syphilis to rule out neurosyphilis.

TREATMENT

- **Benzathine penicillin,** 2.4 million units IM one time for primary syphilis or weekly for 3 weeks for secondary or latent syphilis (of >1 year in duration), is the regimen of choice.

Table 8 HIV-Associated Conditions

Disease	Definitions	Treatment Strategy	Medications
Viral infections			
Varicella–Zoster virus	VZV may cause typical dermatomal lesions or disseminated infection	May cause encephalitis, which is more common with ophthalmic distribution of facial nerve	Acyclovir, 10 mg/kg IV q8h for 7 to 14 days, is the recommended therapy. For milder cases, administration of acyclovir (800 mg PO five times a day), famciclovir (500 mg PO tid), or valacyclovir (1 g PO tid) for 1 week is usually effective
JC virus	Associated with progressive multifocal leukoen-cephalopathy. Symptoms include mental status changes, weakness, and disorders of gait	Characteristic periventricular and subcortical white matter lesions are seen on magnetic resonance imaging	Potent ART has improved the survival of patients with progressive multifocal leukoencephalo-pathy
Parvovirus B19	Chronic parvovirus infections can cause pure red blood cell (RBC) aplasia	Relapses are frequent	Treatment is with IV immunoglobulin, 0.4 g/kg IV daily for 10 days
Chronic hepatitis C	Chronic hepatitis C has a significant impact on morbidity and mortality in HIV-infected patients	Sustained virologic response rates are lower, specifically in genotype 1	Combination of pegylated interferon-α and ribavirin. New antiviral drugs against the hepatitis C virus are in development
Chronic hepatitis B	Chronic hepatitis B has a significant impact on morbidity and mortality in HIV infection	Determine the need for HIV treatment	Antiretroviral combination of TDF/FTC (or 3TC) as part of a HAART. If HIV does not require treatment can use pegylated interferon-α, adefovir or telbivudine

Bacterial infections

Bacillary angiomatosis	Rare condition caused by *Bartonella henselae*	Characterized by multiple nodular, purplish lesions on the skin and other organs	Erythromycin, 500 mg PO q6h Alternatives: Doxycycline, 100 mg PO bid; other macrolides and ciprofloxacin, 500 mg PO bid
Campylobacter jejuni *Rhodococcus equi*	*C. jejuni* can cause GI or disseminated infections *R. equi* can cause necrotizing cavitary pneumonia	Either erythromycin, 500 mg PO qid, or ciprofloxacin, 500 mg PO bid, can be used Vancomycin, 1 g IV q12h, followed by chronic suppression with erythromycin, 500 mg PO qid, plus rifampin, 600 mg PO daily, or with ciprofloxacin, 500 mg PO bid
Salmonella species	Can result in recurrent bacteremia in AIDS. It occurs more commonly in men who have sex with men	Antibacterial therapy should be based on susceptibility pattern	Ceftriaxone, 1 g IV daily; or ampicillin, 1 g IV q6h; or TMP/SMX, 1 DS tablet PO bid; or ciprofloxacin, 500 mg PO bid
Bacterial pneumonias	Risk for bacterial pneumonia is several times higher in HIV-infected individuals	*Streptococcus pneumoniae* or *Haemophilus influenzae.* Gram-negative rods (especially *Pseudomonas aeruginosa*)	Third-generation cephalosporin, oral fluoroquinolones or antipseudomonal agent if indicated

(continued)

Table 8	HIV-Associated Conditions (*Continued*)		
Disease	**Definitions**	**Treatment Strategy**	**Medications**
Mycobacterial			
M. kansasii	Frequently occurs in HIV; should always be considered when identified in clinical samples	Clinically, the infection appears similar to TB	A combination of rifampin, 600 mg PO daily, ethambutol, 15 mg/kg/d PO, and INH, 300 mg PO daily, is the recommended therapy
Mycobacterium haemophilum infection	M. haemophilum causes ulcerative skin lesions		It requires treatment with a macrolide, rifampin, and two other drugs active against the organism
Fungal			
Coccidioides immitis	Frequent in AIDS patients in endemic areas of the southwestern United States. Extensive disease with extra-pulmonary spread is common	Diagnosis is made by a positive culture, serum detection of IgM and IgG by immunodiffusion, and complement fixation	Amphotericin B therapy initially, followed by lifelong suppression with fluconazole, 400 mg PO daily, or itraconazole, 200 mg bid. Coccidioidal meningitis requires intracisternal or intraventricular therapy with amphotericin B. Fluconazole may also be effective

Adapted from Soriano V, Puoti M, Peters M, et al. Care of HIV patients with chronic hepatitis B: updated recommendations from the HIV-Hepatitis B Virus International Panel. *AIDS.* 2008 Jul 31;22(12):1399–1410.

- **Doxycycline,** 100 mg PO bid for 14 days, is an alternative.
- If neurosyphilis is present, penicillin G, 12 to 24 million units IV daily for 14 days, is the only approved treatment of choice. Patients who are allergic to penicillin should be desensitized. Data regarding the use of ceftriaxone, 1 to 2 g IV daily for 14 days, are limited.

SPECIAL CONSIDERATIONS

Other sexually transmitted diseases are treated as they would be in non–HIV-infected patients (see Chapter 13, Treatment of Infectious Diseases). Other commonly encountered conditions in HIV-infected persons are listed in Table 8.

MONITORING/FOLLOW-UP

- Close monitoring and follow-up using the nontreponemal test at 3, 6, and 12 months are necessary in all cases.
- Persons with a sustained positive nontreponemal titer should receive retreatment and be considered for CSF evaluation to rule out neurosyphilis (*MMWR Recomm Rep 2006;55(RR-11)*).

ADDITIONAL RESOURCES

- www.aifsinfo.org
- www.aidsmeds.com
- www.thebody.com
- www.hivmedicine.com

Solid Organ Transplant Medicine

Brent W. Miller

Solid Organ Transplant Basics

GENERAL PRINCIPLES

- Solid organ transplantation is a **treatment, not a cure,** for end-stage organ failure of the kidney, liver, pancreas, heart, and lung. The benefits of organ replacement coexist with the risks of chronic immunosuppression. Thus, not all patients with organ failure are transplant candidates.
- All organs remain in short supply with increasing waiting times for potential recipients. **Living-donor transplants** are increasingly common in kidney transplantation and are being evaluated in liver and lung transplantation as a partial solution to this shortage. Xenotransplantation is **not** a viable option in the near future.
- **Immunologic considerations** prior to the transplant must be fully evaluated including ABO compatibility with the donor, human leukocyte antigen (HLA) typing, and some degree of immune response testing to the proposed donor. Newer protocols using desensitization techniques have had some success in overcoming these immunologic barriers (*Primer on Transplantation. 2nd Ed., 2001*).

DIAGNOSIS

For indications and contraindications of heart, lung, kidney, and liver transplantations, see sections devoted to cardiology, pulmonology, nephrology, and hepatology.

- **Evaluation of the transplant patient with medical problems.** The evaluation of the transplant recipient with general medical or surgical problems should always encompass the details of the patient's organ transplant and treatment. Thus, the following should always be reviewed when taking a history from an organ transplant recipient:
  - Cause of organ failure
  - Treatment for organ failure prior to transplantation
  - Type and date of transplant
  - CMV status of donor and recipient
  - Initial immunosuppression, particularly use of antibody-based induction therapy
  - Initial function of transplant (e.g., nadir creatinine, FEV_1, ejection fraction, synthetic function and transaminases, etc.)
  - Current function of allograft
  - Complications of transplantation (surgical problems, acute rejection, infections, chronic organ dysfunction, etc.)
  - Current immunosuppression regimen and recent drug levels

TREATMENT

- **Immunosuppression.** Immunosuppressive medications are used to promote acceptance of a graft (induction therapy), to reverse episodes of acute rejection (rejection therapy), and to prevent rejection (maintenance therapy). These agents are associated with immunosuppressive effects, immunodeficiency toxicity (e.g., infection and malignancy), and nonimmune toxicity (e.g., nephrotoxicity, diabetes mellitus, bone disease, gout, hyperlipidemia, cardiovascular disease, or neurotoxicity) (*N Engl J Med 2004;351:2715*; *Rose BD, ed. UpToDate, 2006*). Immunosuppressive medications should only be prescribed and administered by physicians and nurses who have appropriate knowledge and expertise. Many variables factor into the choice and dose of drug, and the guidelines for each specific organ are different.
- **Glucocorticoids.** Glucocorticoids are immunosuppressive and anti-inflammatory. Their mechanisms of action include inhibition of cytokine transcription, induction of lymphocyte apoptosis, downregulation of adhesion molecule and major histocompatibility complex expression, and modification of leukocyte trafficking (*N Engl J Med 2005;353:1711*).
  - The side effects of chronic glucocorticoid therapy are well known. As a result of the associated morbidity, steroids are tapered rapidly in the immediate posttransplant period to achieve maintenance doses of 0.1 mg/kg or less. Four further strategies are developing to minimize side effects: steroid-free immunosuppression, steroid avoidance, rapid steroid tapering, and steroid withdrawal. Although most long-term transplant recipients have abnormalities in the adrenal axis, increases in glucocorticoid therapy are not indicated for routine surgery or illness (*Rose BD, ed. UptoDate, 2006*).
- **Antiproliferative agents**
  - **Azathioprine** is a purine analog that is metabolized by the liver to 6-mercaptopurine (active drug), which in turn is catabolized by xanthine oxidase. Azathioprine inhibits the synthesis of DNA and thereby suppresses the proliferation of activated lymphocytes. The major dose-limiting toxicity of this agent is myelosuppression, which is usually reversible after dose reduction or discontinuation of the drug. The usual maintenance dose is 1.5 to 2.5 mg/kg/d in a single dose. Drug levels are generally not obtained.
  - **Mycophenolic Acid (MPA)** is available in two forms: mycophenolic acid or its precursor, mycophenolate mofetil (which is converted to the active metabolite, MPA). MPA inhibits the rate-limiting step in de novo purine synthesis. Because lymphocytes are relatively dependent on the de novo pathway for purine synthesis, lymphocyte proliferation is selectively inhibited by MPA.
    - The major adverse effects of MPA are gastrointestinal disturbances (including nausea, diarrhea, and abdominal pain) and hematologic disturbances (leukopenia and thrombocytopenia). Antacids that contain magnesium and aluminum interfere with the absorption of MPA and should not be given concurrently. The usual dose is 1 to 2 g daily in divided doses, although lesser doses may be used with concomitant tacrolimus than cyclosporine because of enterohepatic circulation affecting MPA levels. Additionally, the dosage of MPA should be reduced in the presence of renal impairment. Drug levels can be obtained to verify absorption or compliance, but the clinical utility of MPA levels has not been determined.
  - **Sirolimus** is a macrocyclic antibiotic produced by *Streptomyces hygroscopicus*. Sirolimus forms a complex with the same receptor-binding protein as tacrolimus; this complex inhibits the activation of a regulatory kinase, mammalian target of

rapamycin (mTOR), and thus prohibits T-cell progression from the G1 to the S phase of the cell cycle. Unlike the calcineurin inhibitors, sirolimus does not affect cytokine transcription but inhibits cytokine and growth factor–induced cell proliferation.

○ The major adverse effects of this drug include hyperlipidemia, anemia, proteinuria, difficulty with wound healing, cytopenias, peripheral edema, oral ulcers, and gastrointestinal symptoms, although other less common side effects are present. Sirolimus is not nephrotoxic, although it may compound the vasoconstriction of calcineurin inhibitors and potentiate their nephrotoxicity. Thus, sirolimus is best utilized alone or with steroids and/or other antiproliferative agents. Sirolimus interacts with cyclosporine metabolism, making monitoring of both drugs difficult. The typical dose is 2 to 5 mg daily in a single dose. Therapeutic drug monitoring is being perfected, with current trough levels between 5 and 15 ng/mL most commonly being used. Sirolimus should be avoided in moderate-to-advanced chronic kidney disease and immediately postoperatively.

○ Calcineurin inhibitors bind to immunophilins (intracellular binding proteins). The calcineurin inhibitor–immunophilin complex inhibits a key phosphatase that is involved in transducing the signal from the T-cell receptor to the nucleus. The net effect is blockade of interleukin-2 and other cytokine transcription, leading to inhibition of T-lymphocyte activation and proliferation. Current strategies are being developed for calcineurin withdrawal and avoidance in solid organ transplantation. Intravenous calcineurin inhibitors should be avoided because of their extreme toxicity and must never be given as a bolus under any circumstance.

- **Cyclosporine** (CsA) is a cyclic 11-amino acid peptide derived from a fungus. Its major nonimmune side effect is nephrotoxicity due to glomerular afferent arteriolar vasoconstriction. This action leads to an immediate decline in glomerular filtration rate of up to 30% and a long-term vaso-occlusive fibrotic renal disease that often results in chronic kidney disease in recipients of all organ transplants. Angiotensin-converting enzyme inhibitors, sirolimus, volume depletion, and other nephrotoxins may potentiate this toxicity. Acute nephrotoxicity is reversible with dose reduction; chronic nephrotoxicity is generally irreversible and nearly universally present in all patients after 8 to 10 years of therapy.

  ○ Other **adverse effects** include gingival hyperplasia, hirsutism, tremor, hypertension, glucose intolerance, hyperlipidemia, hyperkalemia, and, rarely, thrombotic microangiopathy. CsA has a narrow therapeutic window, and doses are adjusted based on blood levels (recommended maintenance trough levels of 100 to 300 ng/mL and 2-hour levels <800 to 1,200 ng/mL). Usual doses are 6 to 8 mg/kg/d in divided doses, with careful attention to levels and toxicities.

- **Tacrolimus** is a macrolide antibiotic and, like CsA, is nephrotoxic. Tacrolimus is more neurotoxic and diabetogenic than CsA, but it is associated with less hirsutism, hypertension, and gingival hyperplasia. Tacrolimus dosing is based on trough blood levels (recommended maintenance levels of 5 to 10 ng/mL). Usual starting dose is 0.15 mg/kg/d in divided doses.

- **Biologic agents**
  - **Polyclonal antibodies**
    ○ Antithymocyte globulin is produced by injecting human thymocytes into animals and collecting sera. This process generates antibodies against a wide variety of human immune system antigens. When subsequently infused into human patients, T lymphocytes are depleted as a result of complement-mediated lysis and clearance of antibody-coated cells by the reticuloendothelial system.

Lymphocyte function is also disrupted by blocking and modulating the expression of cell surface molecules by the antibodies. Infusion is through a central vein over 4 to 6 hours. The most common side effects are fever, chills, and arthralgias.
- ○ Other important adverse effects include myelosuppression, serum sickness, and, rare anaphylaxis. Two preparations are available: horse antithymocyte globulin (ATGAM) and rabbit antithymocyte globulin (Thymoglobulin). Current literature suggests that rabbit antithymocyte globulin is more efficacious. These drugs can be utilized at the time of transplantation to promote engraftment ("induction") or as a subsequent treatment for acute rejection. The long-term risk of increased malignancy, particularly lymphoma, remains a concern with these agents. These drugs have largely replaced **OKT3**, a murine monoclonal antibody directed against the CD E chain of the T-cell receptor, in clinical transplantation.

- **Monoclonal antibodies**
  - ○ **Anti-interleukin-2 receptor monoclonal antibodies.** Daclizumab (humanized) and basiliximab (chimeric) are monoclonal antibodies that competitively inhibit the alpha subunit of the interleukin-2 receptor (CD25) and thereby inhibit activation of T cells. Humanization and chimerization result in antiobidies with an extended half-life and minimize the chance of developing antimurine antibodies. These modifications result in antibodies with an extended half-life and minimize the chances of developing human antimurine antibodies. These drugs are administered by a peripheral vein perioperatively at the time of transplantation and are associated with few side effects.
  - ○ Other biological agents in development for transplantation include **Alemtuzumab,** a monoclonal antibody against CD52, a molecule present on B and T cells; **Belatacept,** a fusion protein combining the extracellular portion of cytotoxic T lymphocyte–associated antigen 4 (CTLA4) with the constant portion of human IgG; **Eculizumab,** a humanized monoclonal antibody blocking activation of complement protein C5; and **Rituximab,** a chimeric monoclonal antibody against the B-cell protein CD20.

- **Infection prophylaxis**
  - **Immunization.** Pneumococcal and hepatitis B vaccination should be given at the time of pretransplant evaluation. Influenza A vaccination should be administered yearly. Live vaccines should be avoided after transplantation (*Am J Transplant 2004;4(Suppl 10):160*).
  - **Trimethoprim/sulfamethoxazole** prevents urinary tract infections, *Pneumocystis jiroveci* pneumonia, and *Nocardia* infections. The optimal dose and duration of prophylaxis have not been determined though a minimum of 1 year is recommended. In sulfa allergic patients, dapsone, aerosolized pentamidine, or atovaquone are alternatives.
  - **Acyclovir** prevents reactivation of herpes simplex virus (HSV) and varicella–zoster but is ineffective in cytomegalovirus (CMV) prophylaxis. HSV can be a serious infection in immunosuppressed individuals, and some form of prophylaxis should be utilized during the first year. Patients with recurrent HSV infections (oral or genital) should be considered candidates for long-term prophylaxis. Lifetime acyclovir should also be used in Epstein–Barr virus (EBV)-seronegative patients who receive an EBV-positive organ.
  - **Ganciclovir** or **valganciclovir** prevents reactivation of CMV infection when administered to patients who were previously CMV seropositive or received a CMV-positive organ, or both. Typically, they are administered from 3 to 12 months

following transplantation. CMV hyperimmune globulin or IV ganciclovir can also be used for this purpose. Alternatively, patients can be monitored for the presence of CMV replication in the bloodstream by polymerase chain reaction before symptoms develop and treated preemptively.

- **Fluconazole** or **ketoconazole** can be given to patients with a high risk of systemic fungal infections or recurrent localized fungal infections. Both medications increase cyclosporine and tacrolimus levels (see Immunosuppressive Medications). **Nystatin suspension, clotrimazole** troches, or weekly fluconazole are used to prevent oropharyngeal candidiasis (thrush).

GRAFT REJECTION

Acute Rejection, Kidney

GENERAL PRINCIPLES

Most episodes of acute rejection occur in the first year after transplantation. The low incidence of acute rejection today usually entails a careful search for inadequate drug levels, noncompliance, or less common forms of rejection (such as antibody-mediated rejection or plasma cell rejection). Late acute rejection (>1 year after transplantation) usually results from inadequate immunosuppression or patient nonadherence.

Definition

An immunologically mediated, acute deterioration in renal function associated with specific pathologic changes on renal biopsy including lymphocytic interstitial infiltrates, tubulitis, and arteritis. The pathophysiology of this form of rejection is mediated by the cellular immune system and T lymphocytes.

Epidemiology

Kidney allograft rejection currently occurs in only 10% of patients. Patients who do not receive induction therapy have a 20% to 30% incidence of acute rejection.

Associated Conditions

Diagnosis of acute renal allograft rejection is made by percutaneous renal biopsy after excluding prerenal azotemia via hydration and repeating laboratory tests. Further workup includes evaluation for calcineurin inhibitor nephrotoxicity (trough and/or peak levels and associated signs), infection (urinalysis and culture), and obstruction (renal ultrasound). Newer techniques evaluating early markers of acute rejection in the blood and urine are being developed.

DIAGNOSIS

Clinical Presentation

Manifestations include an elevated serum creatinine, decreased urine output, increased edema, or worsening hypertension. Initial symptoms are often absent except for the rise in creatinine. Constitutional symptoms (fever, malaise, arthralgia, painful or swollen allograft) are uncommon in current practice.

Table 1	Differential Diagnosis of Renal Allograft Dysfunction	
< 1 wk Posttransplant	< 3 mo Posttransplant	> 3 mo Posttransplant
Acute tubular necrosis	Acute rejection	Prerenal azotemia
Hyperacute rejection	Calcineurin inhibitor toxicity	Calcineurin inhibitor toxicity
Accelerated rejection	Prerenal azotemia	Acute rejection (nonadherence, low levels)
Obstruction	Obstruction	Obstruction
Urine leak (ureteral necrosis)	Infection	Recurrent renal disease
Arterial or venous thrombosis	Interstitial nephritis	De novo renal disease
Atheroemboli	Recurrent renal disease	Renal artery stenosis (anastomotic or atherosclerotic)

Differential Diagnosis

Differential diagnosis varies with duration after transplantation (Table 1).

Acute Rejection, Lung

GENERAL PRINCIPLES

Of the solid organ transplants, the lung is the most immunogenic organ. The majority of patients have at least one episode of acute rejection. Multiple episodes of acute rejection predispose to the development of chronic rejection (bronchiolitis obliterans syndrome).

Epidemiology

Lung transplant rejection occurs frequently and most commonly in the first few months after transplantation.

DIAGNOSIS

Diagnosis is generally made by fiberoptic bronchoscopy with bronchoalveolar lavage and transbronchial biopsies.

Clinical Presentation

Manifestations are nonspecific and include fever, dyspnea, and a nonproductive cough. The chest radiograph is usually unchanged, and is generally nondiagnostic even when abnormal (perihilar infiltrates, interstitial edema, pleural effusions). Change in pulmonary function testing is not specific for rejection, but a 10% or greater decline in forced vital capacity or forced expiratory volume in 1 second, or both, is usually clinically significant.

Differential Diagnosis

It is important to attempt to distinguish rejection from infection, because although the symptoms are similar, the treatments are markedly different.

Acute Rejection, Heart

Epidemiology

Heart transplant recipients typically have two to three episodes of acute rejection in the first year after transplantation with a 50% to 80% chance of having at least one rejection episode, most commonly in the first 6 months.

DIAGNOSIS

Diagnosis is established by endomyocardial biopsy performed during routine surveillance or as prompted by symptoms. None of the noninvasive techniques has demonstrated sufficient sensitivity and specificity to replace the endomyocardial biopsy.

Repeated endomyocardial biopsies predispose to severe tricuspid regurgitation.

Clinical Presentation

Manifestations may include symptoms and signs of left ventricular dysfunction, such as dyspnea, paroxysmal nocturnal dyspnea, orthopnea, syncope, palpitations, new gallops, and elevated jugular venous pressure. Many patients are asymptomatic. Acute rejection may also be associated with a variety of tachyarrhythmias, atrial more often than ventricular.

Acute Rejection, Liver

GENERAL PRINCIPLES

Many **liver transplant recipients** may be maintained on minimal immunosuppression. Acute rejection typically occurs within the first 3 months after transplant and often in the first 2 weeks after the operation. Acute rejection in the liver is generally reversible and does not portend a potentially serious adverse outcome as in other organs. Recurrent viral hepatitis is a much more frequent and morbid problem.

Epidemiology

Liver transplant recipients commonly experience acute allograft rejection, with at least 60% having one episode.

DIAGNOSIS

Diagnosis is made by liver biopsy after technical complications are excluded.

Clinical Presentation

Manifestations may be absent with only a slight elevation in transaminases, or the patients may have signs and symptoms of liver failure including fever, malaise, anorexia, abdominal pain, ascites, decreased bile output, elevated bilirubin, and elevated transaminases.

Differential Diagnosis
Differential diagnosis of early liver allograft dysfunction includes primary graft nonfunction, preservation injury, vascular thrombosis, biliary anastomotic leak, or stenosis. These disorders should be excluded clinically or by Doppler ultrasonography. Late allograft dysfunction may be due to rejection, recurrent hepatitis B or C, CMV infection, EBV infection, cholestasis, or drug toxicity.

Chronic Allograft Dysfunction

GENERAL PRINCIPLES

Chronic allograft dysfunction accounts for the vast majority of late graft losses and is the major obstacle to long-term graft survival.

Definition
Chronic allograft dysfunction (formerly chronic rejection) is a slowly progressive, insidious decline in function of the allograft characterized by gradual vascular and ductal obliteration, parenchymal atrophy, and interstitial fibrosis.

DIAGNOSIS

Diagnosis is often difficult and generally requires a biopsy. The process is mediated by immune and nonimmune factors.

Clinical Presentation
The manifestations of chronic rejection are unique to each organ system.

TREATMENT

To date, no effective therapy is available for established immune-mediated chronic allograft dysfunction. Some patients, particularly those with renal transplants, will require a second solid organ transplant. Current investigational strategies are aimed at prevention.

Complications

GENERAL PRINCIPLES

- **Infections**
  - **CMV infection** (*N Engl J Med 1998;338:1741*) (Table 2) from reactivation of CMV in a seropositive recipient or new infection from a CMV-positive organ can lead to a wide range of presentations from a mild viral syndrome to allograft dysfunction, invasive disease in multiple organ systems, and even death. CMV-seronegative patients who receive a CMV-seropositive organ are at substantial risk, particularly in the first year. Because of the potential progression and severity of untreated disease, treatment is usually indicated in the transplant patient without

Table 2	Timing and Etiology of Posttransplant Infections	
Time Period	**Infectious Complication**	**Etiology**
<1 mo posttransplant	Nosocomial pneumonia, wound infection, urinary tract infection, catheter-related sepsis	Bacterial or fungal infections
1–6 mo posttransplant	Opportunistic infections	Cytomegalovirus *Pneumocystis jiroveci* *Aspergillus* spp. *Toxoplasma gondii* *Listeria monocytogenes* *Strongyloides stercoralis* West Nile virus Varicella–zoster virus
	Reactivation of preexisting infections	*Mycobacteria* spp. Endemic mycoses
>6 mo posttransplant	Community-acquired infections	Bacterial Tick-borne disease
	Chronic progressive infection	Hepatitis B Hepatitis C Cytomegalovirus Epstein–Barr virus Papillomavirus Polyoma virus (BK)
	Opportunistic infections	*P. jiroveci* *L. monocytogenes* *Nocardia asteroides* *Cryptococcus neoformans* *Aspergillus* spp. West Nile virus

tissue diagnosis of invasive disease. Shell-vial culture of the buffy coat is accurate only when plated within 24 hours of sample collection. Seroconversion with a positive immunoglobulin (Ig) M titer or a fourfold increase in IgM or IgG titer suggests acute infection; however, many centers now use polymerase chain reaction–based diagnostic techniques from blood samples, and treatment is usually administered in the patient with evidence of viral replication (*J Am Soc Nephrol 2001;12:848*).

○ Treatment is with oral valganciclovir, 450 to 900 mg PO bid (adjusted for renal function) or IV ganciclovir, 2.5 to 5.0 mg/kg bid (adjusted for renal function), for 3 to 4 weeks. Hyperimmune globulin is often used in combination with ganciclovir for patients with organ involvement.

○ Foscarnet and cidofovir are more toxic alternatives and should be reserved for ganciclovir-resistant cases.

• **Hepatitis B and C.** Patients with active hepatitis or cirrhosis are not considered for nonhepatic transplantation. Immunosuppression increases viral replication in organ transplant recipients with either hepatitis B or C.

○ **Hepatitis B** can recur as fulminant hepatic failure even in patients with no evidence of viral DNA replication before transplantation. In liver transplantation, the risk of recurrent hepatitis B virus infection can be reduced by the administration of hepatitis B immunoglobulin during and after transplantation. Experience with lamivudine therapy initiated before transplantation to lower viral load has shown decreased likelihood of recurrent hepatitis B virus.

- o **Hepatitis C** typically progresses slowly in nonhepatic transplants, and the effect of immunosuppression on mortality due to liver disease remains to be determined. Treatment protocols for hepatitis C in the nonhepatic transplant population are not yet established. Hepatitis C nearly always recurs in liver transplant recipients whose original disease was due to hepatitis C. Therapy for recurrent hepatitis C virus with a combination of ribavirin and interferon results in histopathologic improvement of disease, although dosage and duration of therapy remain controversial.

- **EBV** plays a role in the development of posttransplant lymphoproliferative disease. This life-threatening lymphoma is treated by withdrawal or reduction in immunosuppression and often aggressive chemotherapy (see Long-Term Complications of Transplantation).

- o The role of newly discovered viral agents such as HHV-6, HHV-7, HHV-8, and polyoma (BK and JC) virus after transplantation remains to be established, although BK virus is known to cause interstitial nephritis resulting in renal allograft loss and occasionally ureteral stricture resulting in obstruction.

- **Fungal and parasitic infections,** such as *Cryptococcus, Mucor,* aspergillosis, and *Candida* species, result in increased mortality after transplantation and should be aggressively diagnosed and treated. The role of prophylaxis with oral fluconazole has not been established.

- **Renal disease.** Chronic allograft dysfunction is the leading cause of allograft loss in renal transplant recipients. Calcineurin inhibitor (CsA or tacrolimus) nephrotoxicity or recurrent native disease may also develop in these patients. Chronic calcineurin inhibitor nephrotoxicity may also lead to chronic renal insufficiency and end-stage renal disease (ESRD), requiring dialysis or transplantation in recipients of lung, heart, liver, or pancreas transplants. The incidence of ESRD secondary to calcineurin inhibitor toxicity in recipients of solid organ transplants is at least 10%, and the incidence of significant chronic kidney disease approaches 50% (*N Engl J Med 2003;349:931*).

- **Malignancy** occurs in transplant patients with an overall incidence that is three- to fourfold higher than that seen in the general population (age matched). Some cancers occur at the same rate, whereas other neoplasms have a much higher frequency than normal. The spontaneous malignancies that occur most frequently in transplant recipients include cancers of the skin and lips, lymphoproliferative disease, bronchogenic carcinoma, Kaposi sarcoma, uterine/cervical carcinoma, renal cell carcinoma, and anogenital neoplasms (*N Engl J Med 1990;323:1767*).

- **Skin and lip cancers** are the most common malignancies (40% to 50%) seen in transplant recipients, with an incidence 10 to 250 times that of the general population. Risk factors include immunosuppression, ultraviolet radiation, and human papillomavirus infection. These cancers develop at a younger age, and they are more aggressive in transplant patients than in the general population. Using protective clothing and sunscreens and avoiding sun exposure are recommended. Examination of the skin is the principal screening test, and early diagnosis offers the best prognosis.

- **Posttransplant lymphoproliferative disease** accounts for one-fifth of all malignancies after transplantation, with an incidence of approximately 1%. This is

30- to 50-fold higher than in the general population, and the risk increases with the use of antilymphocyte therapy for induction or rejection. The majority of these neoplasms are large-cell non-Hodgkin lymphomas of the B-cell type. Posttransplant lymphoproliferative disease results from EBV-induced B-cell proliferation in the setting of chronic immunosuppression. The presentation is often atypical and should always be considered in the patient with new symptoms. Diagnosis requires a high index of suspicion followed by a tissue biopsy. Treatment includes reduction or withdrawal of immunosuppression and chemotherapy.

SPECIAL CONSIDERATIONS

Important drug interactions are always a concern given the polypharmacy associated with transplant patients. Before prescribing a new medication to a transplant recipient, always investigate drug interactions.

- The combination of allopurinol and azathioprine should be avoided or used cautiously due to the risk of profound myelosuppression.
- CsA and tacrolimus are metabolized by cytochrome P-450 (3A4). Therefore, CsA and tacrolimus levels are decreased by drugs that induce cytochrome P-450 activity, such as rifampin, isoniazid, barbiturates, phenytoin, and carbamazepine. Conversely, CsA and tacrolimus levels are increased by drugs that compete for cytochrome P-450, such as verapamil, diltiazem, nicardipine, azole antifungals, erythromycin, and clarithromycin. Similar effects are seen with tacrolimus and sirolimus.
- Tacrolimus and CsA should not be taken together because of the increased risk of severe nephrotoxicity.
- Lower doses of MPA should be used when either tacrolimus or sirolimus is taken concurrently.
- Concomitant administration of CsA and sirolimus may result in a twofold increase in sirolimus levels; to avoid this drug interaction, CsA and sirolimus should be dosed 4 hours apart.

Gastrointestinal Diseases

C. Prakash Gyawali and Ahmad Manasra

Gastrointestinal Bleeding

GENERAL PRINCIPLES

Definition

- Gastrointestinal (GI) bleeding may manifest as passage of bright or altered blood with emesis or bowel movements. Acute GI bleeding typically presents with overt blood loss that can be readily recognized by the patient or the treating physician.
- **Overt GI bleeding** is the passage of fresh or altered blood in emesis or in the stool.
- **Occult bleeding** refers to a positive fecal occult blood test (stool guaiac) or iron-deficiency anemia without visible blood in the stool.
- **Obscure bleeding** consists of GI blood loss of unknown origin that persists or recurs after negative initial endoscopic evaluation; obscure bleeding can be either overt or occult (*Gastroenterology 2007;133:1697*).
- The following segments refer primarily to overt bleeding.

DIAGNOSIS

Clinical Presentation

- Hematemesis, coffee-ground emesis, and aspiration of blood or coffee-ground material from a nasogastric (NG) tube suggest an upper GI source of blood loss.
- **Melena,** black sticky stool with a characteristic odor, usually indicates an upper GI source of blood loss, although small-bowel and sometimes right colonic bleeds can result in melena.
- Various shades of **bloody stool (hematochezia)** are seen with distal small-bowel or colonic bleeding, depending on the rate of blood loss and colonic transit. Patients with rapid upper GI bleeding can also present with bloody stool, but this is invariably associated with hemodynamic compromise or circulatory shock.
- **Bleeding from the anorectal area** typically results in bright blood coating the exterior of formed stool, sometimes associated with distal colonic symptoms (e.g., rectal urgency, straining, or pain with defecation).
- Other symptoms may include fatigue, weakness, abdominal pain, pallor, or dyspnea.
- Estimation of **amount of blood lost** can be attempted, but is often inaccurate. If the baseline hematocrit is known, the drop in hematocrit provides a rough estimate of blood loss. In general, patients with lower GI bleeding have less hemodynamic compromise compared to those with upper GI bleeding.
- **Coagulation abnormalities** can propagate bleeding from a preexisting lesion in the GI tract. Disorders of coagulation, such as liver disease, von Willebrand disease, vitamin K deficiency, and disseminated intravascular coagulation, can influence the course of GI bleeding (see Chapter 17, Disorders of Hemostasis and Thrombosis).

- **Medications** known to affect the coagulation process include warfarin, heparin, aspirin, nonsteroidal anti-inflammatory drugs (NSAIDs), clopidogrel (Plavix), thrombolytic agents, antithrombotic agents such as glycoprotein IIb/IIIa receptor antagonists (abciximab [ReoPro], eptifibatide [Integrilin], tirofiban [Aggrastat]), and direct thrombin inhibitors (argatroban, bivalirudin). NSAIDs and aspirin can result in mucosal damage anywhere in the GI tract.

Physical Examination
- **Color of stool.** Direct examination of spontaneously passed stool or stool obtained during a digital rectal examination can provide important clues to the level of bleeding (*Dig Dis Sci 1995;40:1614*). Further, a digital rectal examination may identify a potential source of bleeding in the anorectum. Anal fissures, typically seen in the posterior midline, can result in extreme pain during a rectal examination.
- **NG aspirate.** Fresh blood on an NG aspirate may indicate ongoing upper GI bleeding that requires urgent endoscopic attention (*GIE 2004;59:172*). The aspirate should be considered positive only if blood or dark particulate matter ("coffee grounds") is seen, and hemoccult testing of a normal-appearing NG aspirate has no clinical utility. A bleeding source in the duodenum can result in a negative NG aspirate. Gastric lavage with water or saline may be useful in assessing the activity and severity of upper GI bleeding and in clearing the stomach of blood and clots before endoscopy (*NEJM 2008;359:928*). After a diagnosis of upper GI bleeding is made, the NG tube is not required further in a stable patient, especially if endoscopy is to follow.
- **Intravascular volume and hemodynamic status.** Constant monitoring or frequent assessment of vital signs is necessary early in the evaluation, as a sudden increase in pulse rate or decrease in blood pressure (BP) may be an early indicator of recurrent or ongoing blood loss.
- If the baseline BP and pulse are within normal limits, sitting the patient up or having the patient stand may result in **orthostatic hemodynamic changes** (drop in systolic BP of > 10 mm Hg, rise in pulse rate of > 15 beats/min [bpm]). Orthostatic changes in pulse and BP are seen with loss of 10% to 20% of the circulatory volume; supine hypotension suggests a > 20% loss. Hypotension with a systolic blood pressure of < 100 mm Hg or baseline tachycardia > 100 bpm suggests significant hemodynamic compromise that requires urgent volume resuscitation (*NEJM 2008;359:92*).

Diagnostic Testing

Laboratories
- Complete blood cell count
- Coagulation parameters (prothrombin time, partial thromboplastin time)
- Blood group, cross-matching of two to four units of blood
- Comprehensive chemical profile (including liver function tests, serum creatinine)

Diagnostic Procedures
- **Endoscopy**
  - **Esophagogastroduodenoscopy (EGD)** is the preferred method of investigation and therapy of upper GI bleeding and is associated with high diagnostic accuracy, therapeutic capability, and low morbidity. Volume resuscitation or blood transfusion should precede endoscopy in hemodynamically unstable patients. Patients with ongoing bleeding or at risk for an adverse outcome (Table 1) benefit most from urgent EGD, while stable patients with minimal bleeding (e.g., "coffee-ground" emesis with stable hematocrit) can have the procedure performed electively during the hospitalization.

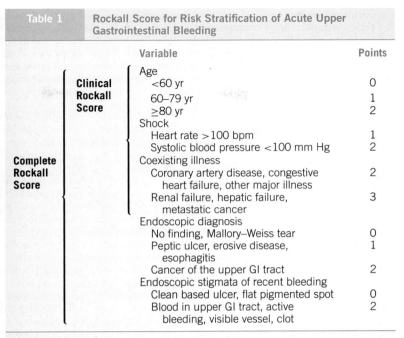

Table 1		Rockall Score for Risk Stratification of Acute Upper Gastrointestinal Bleeding	
		Variable	Points
Complete Rockall Score	**Clinical Rockall Score**	Age	
		<60 yr	0
		60–79 yr	1
		≥80 yr	2
		Shock	
		Heart rate >100 bpm	1
		Systolic blood pressure <100 mm Hg	2
		Coexisting illness	
		Coronary artery disease, congestive heart failure, other major illness	2
		Renal failure, hepatic failure, metastatic cancer	3
		Endoscopic diagnosis	
		No finding, Mallory–Weiss tear	0
		Peptic ulcer, erosive disease, esophagitis	1
		Cancer of the upper GI tract	2
		Endoscopic stigmata of recent bleeding	
		Clean based ulcer, flat pigmented spot	0
		Blood in upper GI tract, active bleeding, visible vessel, clot	2

Adapted from Gralnek et al. *N Engl J Med* 2008;359:928, with permission.

- **Colonoscopy** can be performed after a rapid bowel purge in patients whose condition has clinically stabilized and who can tolerate an adequate bowel purge. The yield of finding a potential bleeding source in the colon is greatest if colonoscopy is performed within the initial 24 hours of presentation (*AJG 2005;100:2395*).
  - Patients unable to drink adequate amounts of the balanced electrolyte solution can have an NG tube placed for infusion of the bowel purge. All patients with acute lower GI bleeding from an unknown source should eventually undergo endoscopic evaluation of the colon during the initial hospitalization, regardless of the initial mode of investigation. Although early diagnostic endoscopy does not reduce mortality, therapeutic endoscopy reduces transfusion requirements, need for surgery, and length of hospital stay.
- **Anoscopy** may be useful in the detection of internal hemorrhoids and anal fissures. In an outpatient or emergency room setting, anoscopy and sigmoidoscopy may be useful in rapid diagnosis of the level of bleeding before patient triage, but is usually followed by colonoscopy after bowel preparation.
- **Push enteroscopy** allows evaluation of the proximal small bowel if a bleeding source is not seen within reach of a standard upper endoscope, especially if the colon has been excluded as a bleeding source by careful colonoscopy.
- **Capsule endoscopy.** This technique is most useful after the upper gut and the colon have been thoroughly examined, and the bleeding source is expected in the small bowel (*Gastroenterology 2007;133:1697*). Disadvantages are that the images

cannot be viewed in real time, exact localization within the small bowel cannot be pinpointed, and therapy cannot be administered.

- **Single- and double-balloon enteroscopy.** This allows visualization of most of the small bowel, using a special endoscope with an overtube. Balloons at the endoscope tip and the overtube can be consecutively inflated and deflated while inserting and pulling out the endoscope to allow bowel to pleat over the overtube, thus allowing deep endoscope insertion into the small bowel, either through the mouth or the anus. This procedure is only available in advanced centers.
- **Intraoperative enteroscopy.** When an actively bleeding source is identified within the small bowel, endoscopic therapy or surgical intervention can be facilitated by performing intraoperative enteroscopy. The surgeon, through an abdominal incision, advances the endoscope (inserted either through the mouth, the anus, or an enterotomy) by pleating bowel over the instrument.
- **Tagged red blood cell (TRBC) scanning.** RBCs labeled with technetium-99m remain in circulation for as long as 48 hours and extravasate into the bowel lumen with active bleeding. This extravasation can be detected as pooling of the radioactive tracer on gamma camera scanning. The pattern of peristaltic movement of the pooled tracer can help identify the potential site of bleeding (*Dis Colon Rectum 1997;40:471*).
  - A positive TRBC scan identifies patients likely to require invasive intervention and with high in-hospital morbidity, while a negative test may imply a better short-term prognosis. Therefore, the clinical utility of this test is for assessing location and intensity of bleeding before more invasive tests are performed, especially in patients with evidence of ongoing active bleeding precluding urgent colonoscopy.
- **Arteriography** allows rapid localization and potential therapy of GI bleeding by demonstrating extravasation of the dye into the intestine when bleeding rates exceed 0.5 mL/min.
  - When an actively bleeding lesion is found, intra-arterial infusion of vasopressin can cause vasoconstriction and stop bleeding. Superselective cannulation and embolization of the bleeding artery can also be performed (*AJG 2005;100:2395*).
  - In upper GI bleeding, arteriography is reserved for situations where brisk bleeding makes endoscopy difficult.
  - In small-bowel or lower GI bleeding, arteriography is utilized for both diagnosis and therapy of the acutely bleeding lesion, typically after initial localization with TRBC scanning or capsule endoscopy. Immediate or early extravasation on TRBC scanning carries the greatest likelihood of a positive arteriogram.

TREATMENT

- **Restoration of intravascular volume.** Two large-bore IV lines with 16- to 18-gauge catheters or a central venous line should be urgently placed. Isotonic saline, lactated Ringer solution, or 5% hetastarch can be initiated; patients in shock may require volume administration using pressure infusion devices or hand infused using large syringes and stopcocks. **Packed red blood cell (RBC) transfusion** should be used for volume replacement whenever possible; O-negative blood or simultaneous multiple-unit transfusions may be indicated if bleeding is massive. Transfusion should be continued until hemodynamic stability is achieved and the hematocrit reaches $\geq 25\%$; patients with cardiac or pulmonary disease may require transfusion to a hematocrit of $\geq 30\%$. The rate of volume infusion should be guided by the patient's condition and the rate and degree of volume loss (*NEJM 2008;359:928*).

Vasopressors are generally not indicated, although transient IV pressor therapy is sometimes beneficial until enough volume is infused.

- **Oxygen administration.** Supplemental oxygen may enhance oxygen-carrying capacity of blood, and should be administered, particularly in patients with comorbid cardiopulmonary illnesses.

- **Correction of coagulopathy.** Discontinuation of the anticoagulant, if possible, followed by infusion of fresh frozen plasma (FFP) can be used to correct prolonged coagulation parameters from warfarin. An initial infusion of two to four units of FFP can be supplemented with further infusion based on reassessment of the coagulation parameters. Parenteral vitamin K (10 mg SC or IM) may be indicated for prolonged prothrombin time from warfarin therapy or hepatobiliary disease but takes several hours to days for adequate reversal. It should be repeated daily for a total of three doses in hepatobiliary disease. Protamine infusion (1 mg antagonizes ~100 units of heparin) can be used for immediate reversal of anticoagulation from heparin infusion. Platelet infusion may be indicated when the platelet count is $<50,000/mm^3$.

- **Airway protection.** Endotracheal intubation to prevent aspiration should be considered in the presence of altered mental status (shock, hepatic encephalopathy), massive hematemesis, or active variceal hemorrhage.

- **Risk stratification.** Validated risk stratification tools are available to identify patients at highest risk for an adverse outcome. The Rockall score (Table 1) has a clinical component that can be rapidly calculated at presentation, and a complete final score that takes endoscopic findings into account. A clinical score of 0 or a complete score of 2 or less indicate low risk for rebleeding or death (*Gut 1996;38:316*).

Medications

- **Nonvariceal upper GI bleeding.** Intravenous proton pump inhibitors (PPIs) or high-dose PPIs administered orally (e.g., omeprazole, 40 mg PO bid) reduce the rate of recurrent bleeding and the need for surgery in patients with upper GI bleeding awaiting endoscopic treatment or if endoscopy is contraindicated or postponed. Mortality is reduced in peptic ulcer bleeding, but not other causes of upper GI bleeding with high dose oral or IV PPI (*AJG 2004;99:1238; APT 2005;21:677*). Conventional oral doses of PPIs may suffice after endoscopic therapy has been administered. PPI therapy, oral or IV, is better than IV histamine-2 receptor antagonist (H$_2$RA) therapy in bleeding peptic ulcers.

- **Variceal bleeding**
  - When variceal bleeding is suspected, **octreotide** infusion should be initiated immediately (50- to 100-mcg bolus, followed by infusion at 25 to 50 mcg/hr), and continued for 3 to 5 days after the diagnosis is confirmed (*Hepatology 2007;46:922*). Octreotide acutely reduces portal pressures and controls variceal bleeding with very few side effects, improving the diagnostic yield and therapeutic success of subsequent endoscopy.
  - **Vasopressin** (0.3 units/min IV, titrated by increments of 0.1 units/min q30 min until hemostasis is achieved, side effects develop, or the maximum dose of 0.9 units/min is reached) is an alternative agent, rarely used because of significant cardiovascular complications including cardiac arrest and myocardial infarction. Concomitant infusion of **nitroglycerin** may reduce undesirable cardiovascular side effects and provide more effective control of bleeding. Nitroglycerin is administered only if the systolic BP is >100 mm Hg, at a dose of 10 mcg/min IV, increased by 10 mcg/min q10–15 min until the systolic BP falls to 100 mm Hg or a maximum dose of 400 mcg/min is reached.

• Antibiotic prophylaxis with a fluoroquinolone (**norfloxacin** or **ciprofloxacin**) is recommended in any patient with cirrhosis and variceal bleeding. Intravenous **ceftriaxone** (1 g/d) is a substitute in patients with advanced cirrhosis or when quinolone-resistant organisms are suspected (*Hepatology 2007;46:922*).

Other Nonoperative Therapies

• **Endoscopic therapy**
  • **Therapeutic endoscopy** offers the advantage of immediate treatment in acute upper GI bleeding, and should be implemented early in the hospital course (within 12 to 24 hours) if possible. Fluid resuscitation and hemodynamic stability are essential before endoscopy. A single dose of erythromycin (250 mg IV) administered 30 to 60 minutes prior to upper endoscopy may induce gastric emptying of clots and debris, and improve visualization (*NEJM 2008;359:928*).
  • **Variceal ligation** or **banding** is the endoscopic therapy of choice for esophageal varices. This is effective in controlling active hemorrhage and achieves variceal eradication rapidly, with lower rates of rebleeding and fewer complications compared to sclerotherapy (*Hepatology 2007;46:922*). Intensive care unit (ICU) admission and endotracheal intubation for airway protection should be considered when active variceal bleeding is suspected. Complications of banding include superficial ulceration, dysphagia, transient chest discomfort, and, rarely, esophageal strictures.
  • **Sclerotherapy** is also effective but is used less frequently because of complications (ulcerations, strictures, perforation, pleural effusions, adult respiratory distress syndrome, sepsis). Sclerotherapy is indicated when variceal ligation is not technically feasible.
• **Transjugular intrahepatic portosystemic shunt (TIPS)** is a radiologic procedure wherein an expandable metal stent is deployed between the hepatic veins and the portal vein to decompress the portal system and reduce portal venous pressure. Indications include refractory variceal bleeding unresponsive to variceal ligation or sclerotherapy, and bleeding from gastric varices in the setting of portal hypertension (*Hepatology 2007;46:922–938*). Encephalopathy may occur in up to 25% of patients but is usually controlled with medical therapy (see Chapter 16, Liver Diseases). Shunt stenosis is another complication that may respond to balloon dilation. Screening for shunt stenosis with duplex Doppler ultrasound is recommended if the patient redevelops variceal bleeding or has recurrence of esophageal or gastric varices on endoscopy.

Surgical Management

• **Emergent total colectomy** may rarely be required as a lifesaving maneuver for massive, unlocalized, colonic bleeding; this should be preceded by emergent EGD to rule out a rapidly bleeding upper source whenever possible. Certain lesions (e.g., neoplasia, Meckel's diverticulum) require surgical resection for a cure.
• **Total or partial colectomy** may be required for diverticular bleeding. Ongoing bleeding with transfusion requirements exceeding 4 to 6 units over 24 hours or 10 units overall, or more than two to three recurrent bleeding episodes from the same source have been considered indications for surgery.
• **Splenectomy** is curative in bleeding gastric varices from splenic vein thrombosis.
• **Shunt surgery** (portacaval or distal splenorenal shunt) should be considered in patients with good hepatic reserve if the patient (a) fails endoscopic or pharmacologic therapy, (b) is unable to return for follow-up visits, (c) is at high risk of death from recurrent bleeding because of cardiac disease or difficulty in obtaining blood products, or (d) lives far from medical care. Although bleeding may be controlled

in 95% of cases, hospital death rates are high, and there is a significant incidence of postoperative encephalopathy, especially among patients with higher grades of Child's classification (see Chapter 16 (Liver)).

Dysphagia and Odynophagia

GENERAL PRINCIPLES

Definition

- **Oropharyngeal dysphagia** consists of difficulty in transferring food from the mouth to the esophagus, often associated with symptoms of nasopharyngeal regurgitation and pulmonary aspiration.
- **Esophageal dysphagia** is the sensation of impairment in passage of food down the esophagus.
- **Odynophagia** is pain on swallowing food and fluids, and may indicate the presence of esophagitis, particularly infectious esophagitis and pill esophagitis.

Etiology

- **Oropharyngeal dysphagia** is typically caused by neuromuscular or structural disorders involving the pharynx and proximal esophagus (*Gastroenterology 1999;116:452*).
- **Esophageal dysphagia** can occur from an obstructive process in the esophagus (*Gastroenterology 1999;117:233*). Progressive dysphagia may be seen with neoplasia, while intermittent symptoms can result from webs or rings. Acute onset of dysphagia in temporal relationship to a meal may suggest food impaction. In the absence of a structural obstructive process, an esophageal motility disorder may be responsible for symptoms (achalasia, diffuse esophageal spasm, incomplete LES relaxation).

DIAGNOSIS

Oropharyngeal dysphagia

- Assessment is initiated with a detailed neurologic exam.
- Barium videofluoroscopy (modified barium swallow) evaluates the oropharyngeal swallow mechanism and may identify laryngeal penetration.
- Ear, nose, and throat exam including flexible nasal endoscopy may identify structural etiologies. Imaging studies (CT scans) also evaluate for a structural process.
- Laboratory tests for polymyositis, myasthenia gravis, and other neuromuscular disorders can be considered in the absence of neurologic and structural etiologies.

Esophageal dysphagia

- Endoscopy is typically used for initial investigation of esophageal dysphagia. Endoscopy provides information on mucosal abnormalities, allows tissue sampling, and offers the option of dilation if a narrowing is seen (*Gastroenterology 1999;117:233*).
- Barium swallow is also a suitable initial test for esophageal dysphagia, although biopsies and esophageal dilation require endoscopy. Subtle rings and webs may not be visualized unless a barium swallow is performed using a solid bolus or a barium pill.
- Esophageal manometry can characterize esophageal motor disorders when other studies are normal or suggest a motility disorder.
- Acute esophageal obstruction is best investigated with endoscopy.

TREATMENT

- Modification of diet and swallowing maneuvers may benefit patients with dysphagia, especially oropharyngeal dysphagia.
- Enteral feeding through a gastrostomy tube may be indicated in patients with frank tracheal aspiration on attempted swallowing.
- Endoscopic retrieval of an obstructing food bolus can result in dramatic resolution of acute dysphagia from food impaction.
- Nutrition needs to be addressed in patients with prolonged dysphagia causing weight loss; patients with dysphagia are typically advised to chew their food well and eat foods of soft consistencies.

Medications

- Mucosal inflammation from reflux disease can be treated with acid suppression.
- Odynophagia generally responds to specific therapy of the condition causing esophagitis (e.g., PPIs for reflux disease, antimicrobial agents for infectious esophagitis). Viscous lidocaine swish-and-swallow solutions may afford symptomatic relief.
- Patients with oropharyngeal dysphagia and drooling of saliva can be treated with anticholinergic medication (e.g., transdermal scopolamine).
- **Glucagon** (2 to 4 mg IV bolus) can be attempted in acute dysphagia from food impaction. Sublingual **nitroglycerin** can also be given, but meat tenderizer should not be administered.

Other Nonoperative Therapies

Endoscopic therapy

- Esophageal dilation is performed for anatomic narrowing visualized during endoscopy. Empiric dilation is sometimes performed even when a defined narrowing is not identified and may result in symptomatic benefit.
- Aggressive pneumatic dilation of the LES is sometimes performed for achalasia (see Esophageal Motor Disorders), but laparoscopic myotomy is gaining popularity over pneumatic dilation. Botulinum toxin injections to the LES may result in temporary symptom relief in achalasia and in errors of LES relaxation.
- Esophageal stent placement can alleviate dysphagia in inoperable neoplasia.

Nausea and Vomiting

GENERAL PRINCIPLES

Etiology

- Nausea and vomiting may result from side effects of medications, systemic illnesses, central nervous system (CNS) disorders, and primary GI disorders.
- Vomiting that occurs during or immediately after a meal can result from acute pyloric stenosis (e.g., pyloric channel ulcer) or from functional disorders.
- Vomiting within 30 to 60 minutes after a meal may suggest gastric or duodenal pathology.
- Delayed vomiting after a meal with undigested food from a previous meal can suggest gastric outlet obstruction or gastroparesis.
- Symptoms lasting longer than 1 month in duration are considered chronic (*Gastroenterology 2001;120:261*).

DIAGNOSIS

Clinical Presentation

History

- **Bowel obstruction and pregnancy should be ruled out.**
- Medication lists should be scrutinized, and systemic illnesses (acute and chronic) should be evaluated as etiologies or contributing factors.

TREATMENT

- Correction of fluid and electrolyte imbalances is an important supportive measure.
- Oral intake should be withheld or limited to clear liquids. Many patients with self-limited illnesses require no further therapy.
- NG decompression may be required for patients with bowel obstruction or protracted nausea and vomiting of any etiology.
- Patients with protracted nausea and vomiting may sometimes require enteral feeding through jejunal tubes, or rarely even total parenteral nutrition.

Medications

Empiric pharmacotherapy is often initiated while investigation is in progress, or when the etiology is thought to be self-limited.

- **Phenothiazines and related agents.** Prochlorperazine (Compazine), 5 to 10 mg PO tid–qid, 10 mg IM or IV q6h, or 25 mg PR bid; promethazine (Phenergan), 12.5 to 25.0 mg PO, IM, or PR q4–6h; and trimethobenzamide (Tigan), 250 mg PO tid–qid, 200 mg IM tid–qid, or 200 mg PR tid–qid are effective. Drowsiness is a common side effect, and acute dystonic reactions or other extrapyramidal effects may occur.
- **Dopamine antagonists** include metoclopramide (10 mg PO 30 minutes before meals and at bedtime, or 10 mg IV prn), a prokinetic agent that also has central antiemetic effects. Drowsiness and extrapyramidal reactions may occur, and a warning has been issued by the FDA regarding the risk of tardive dyskinesia with high dose or long-term use; tachyphylaxis may limit long-term efficacy. Domperidone is an alternate agent that does not cross the blood–brain barrier and therefore has no CNS side effects; however, it is not uniformly available.
- **Antihistaminic agents** are most useful for nausea and vomiting related to motion sickness, but may also be useful for other causes. Agents used include diphenhydramine (Benadryl, 25 to 50 mg PO q6–8h, or 10 to 50 mg IV q2–4h), dimenhydrinate (Dramamine, 50 to 100 mg PO or IV q4–6h), and meclizine (Antivert, 12.5 to 25 mg 1 hour before travel).
- **Serotonin 5-HT$_3$ receptor antagonists. Ondansetron** (Zofran, 0.15 mg/kg IV q4h for three doses or 32 mg IV infused over 15 minutes beginning 30 minutes before chemotherapy) is effective in chemotherapy-associated emesis. It can also be used in emesis that is refractory to other medications (4 to 8 mg PO or IV up to q8h), especially the sublingual formulation. **Granisetron** (Kytril, 10 mcg/kg IV for one to three doses 10 minutes apart, or 1 mg PO bid) is also effective.
- **Neurokinin-1 (NK-1) receptor antagonist. Aprepitant** (Emend, 125 mg PO day 1, 80 mg PO days 2 and 3) is an alternative agent currently indicated **only for chemotherapy-induced nausea and vomiting.**

Diarrhea

GENERAL PRINCIPLES

Definition

- **Acute diarrhea** consists of abrupt onset of increased frequency and/or fluidity of bowel movements. Infectious agents, toxins, and drugs are the major causes of acute diarrhea. In hospitalized patients, pseudomembranous colitis, antibiotic or drug associated diarrhea, and fecal impaction should be considered (*Gastroenterology 2004;127:287*).
- **Chronic diarrhea** consists of passage of loose stools with or without increased stool frequency for more than 4 weeks.

DIAGNOSIS

- Most acute infectious diarrheal illnesses last less than 24 hours and could be viral in etiology; therefore, stool studies are unnecessary in short-lived episodes without fever, dehydration, or presence of blood or pus in the stool (*NEJM 2004;350:38*).
- Stool cultures, *Clostridium difficile* toxin assay, ova and parasite examinations, and flexible sigmoidoscopy may be warranted in patients with severe, prolonged, or atypical symptoms.
- The fecal osmotic gap can be calculated in patients with chronic diarrhea and voluminous watery stools as follows: $290 - 2(\text{stool } [Na^+] + \text{stool } [K^+])$.
  - **Secretory diarrhea:** Stool osmotic gap is <50 mOsm/kg.
  - **Osmotic diarrhea:** Stool osmotic gap is >125 mOsm/kg.
- A positive fecal occult blood test or fecal leukocyte test suggests inflammatory diarrhea.
- Steatorrhea is traditionally diagnosed by demonstration of fat excretion in stool of >7 g/d in a 72-hour stool collection while the patient is on a 100-g/d fat diet. Sudan staining of a stool specimen is an alternate test; >100 fat globules per high-power field is suggestive of steatorrhea.
- Laxative screening should be considered in any patient with chronic diarrhea that remains undiagnosed.

Clinical Presentation

- **Acute diarrhea**
  - **Bacterial and viral infections.** Viral enteritis and bacterial infections with *Escherichia coli, Shigella, Salmonella, Campylobacter,* and *Yersinia* species constitute the most common causes of acute diarrhea.
  - **Pseudomembranous colitis** is usually seen in the setting of antimicrobial therapy and is caused by toxins produced by *C. difficile.*
  - **Giardiasis** is confirmed by identification of *Giardia lamblia* trophozoites in the stool, in duodenal aspirate, or in small-bowel biopsy specimens. A stool immunofluorescence assay is also available for rapid diagnosis.
  - **Amebiasis** may cause acute diarrhea, especially in travelers to areas with poor sanitation and in homosexual men. Demonstration of trophozoites or cysts of *Entamoeba histolytica* in the stool, or a serum antibody test, confirms the diagnosis.
  - **Diarrhea related to medication use.** Common offending agents include laxatives, antacids, cardiac medications (e.g., digitalis, quinidine), colchicine, and

antimicrobial agents. Symptoms usually respond to discontinuation of the offending agent.

- **Graft-versus-host disease** needs to be considered in patients who develop diarrhea after organ transplantation, especially bone marrow transplantation.
- **Chronic diarrhea.** After a careful history, thorough physical examination, and routine laboratory tests, chronic diarrhea can typically be classified into one of the following categories: watery diarrhea (secretory or osmotic), inflammatory diarrhea, or fatty diarrhea (steatorrhea) (*Gastroenterology 2004;127:287–293*).

TREATMENT

- Adequate hydration is an essential initial step in the therapy of diarrheal disease. IV hydration is required in severe cases. Long-term IV fluids or parenteral nutrition is sometimes necessary in refractory diarrhea.
- Symptomatic therapy is recommended in simple self-limiting GI infections where diarrhea is frequent or troublesome, while diagnostic workup is in progress, when specific management fails to improve symptoms, or when a specific etiology is not identified.
  - **Loperamide,** 2 to 4 mg up to four times a day, **opiates** (tincture of opium; belladonna; and opium capsules), and **anticholinergic agents** (diphenoxylate and atropine [Lomotil], 15 to 20 mg/d of diphenoxylate in divided doses) are the most effective nonspecific antidiarrheal agents.
  - **Pectin** and **kaolin** preparations (bind toxins) and **bismuth subsalicylate** (antibacterial properties) are also useful in symptomatic therapy of acute diarrhea.
  - **Bile acid–binding resins** (e.g., cholestyramine, 1 g up to qid) are beneficial in bile acid–induced diarrhea.
  - **Octreotide** (100 to 200 μg bid–qid PRN) is useful in hormone-mediated secretory diarrhea, but can be of benefit in refractory diarrhea.

Medications

- **Empiric antibiotic therapy** is only recommended in patients with moderate to severe disease and associated systemic symptoms, while awaiting stool cultures. Antibiotics can increase the possibility of hemolytic–uremic syndrome associated with shiga toxin producing *E. coli* infections (*E. coli* O157:H7) (*NEJM 2000;342: 1930–1936*).
  - **Fluoroquinolones** (ciprofloxacin, 500 mg PO bid for 3 days, or norfloxacin, 400 mg PO bid for 3 days)
  - **Trimethoprim–sulfamethoxazole** (160 mg/800 mg PO bid for 5 days)
- Oral **metronidazole** is the treatment of choice for pseudomembranous colitis. Oral **vancomycin** is reserved for resistant cases or intolerance to metronidazole (for further details, see Chapter 11, Treatment of Infectious Diseases).
- Treatment of symptomatic amebiasis is with **metronidazole,** 750 mg PO tid or 500 mg IV q8h for 5 to 10 days. This should be followed by **paromomycin,** 500 mg PO tid for 7 days, or **iodoquinol,** 650 mg PO tid for 20 days, to eliminate cysts.
- Therapy for giardiasis consists of metronidazole, 250 mg PO tid for 5 to 7 days, or tinidazole, 2-g single dose. Quinacrine, 100 mg PO tid for 7 days, is an alternative agent. More prolonged therapy may be necessary in the immunocompromised patient.

SPECIAL CONSIDERATIONS

Diarrhea in HIV disease

- Opportunistic agents, including *Cryptosporidium, Microsporidium,* cytomegalovirus (CMV), *Mycobacterium avium* complex, and *Mycobacterium tuberculosis,* may cause diarrhea in patients with advanced HIV (CD4 counts < 50 cells/μL) and should be looked for specifically with stool studies and endoscopic biopsies from the colon and small bowel. However, opportunistic infections have fallen in frequency since HAART became popular, and *C. difficile* is fast becoming the most commonly identified bacterial pathogen (*Gut 2008;57:861*).
- Venereal infections (syphilis, gonorrhea, chlamydiosis, herpes simplex virus [HSV] infection) as well as other nonvenereal infections (amebiasis, giardiasis, salmonellosis, shigellosis) may also cause diarrhea.
- Other causes of diarrhea in this population include intestinal lymphoma and Kaposi sarcoma. Stool studies (ova and parasites, culture), endoscopic biopsies, and serologic testing may assist diagnosis.
- The most likely cause of undiagnosed diarrhea is missed pathogens; however, drugs, antibiotics, HIV acting as a pathogen, autonomic disturbance, and abnormal intestinal motility may also contribute to diarrhea. Management consists of specific therapy if pathogens are identified; symptomatic measures may be of benefit in idiopathic cases.

Constipation

GENERAL PRINCIPLES

Definition

Constipation consists of infrequent (and frequently incomplete) bowel movements, sometimes associated with straining and passage of pellet-like stools.

Etiology

- A recent change in bowel habits may indicate an organic cause, whereas constipation of several years' duration is more likely due to a functional disorder.
- Medication (e.g., calcium blockers, opiates, anticholinergics, iron supplements, barium sulfate) and systemic disease (e.g., diabetes mellitus, hypothyroidism, systemic sclerosis, myotonic dystrophy) may contribute.
- Other predisposing factors include lack of exercise, disorders that cause pain on defecation (e.g., anal fissures, thrombosed external hemorrhoids), and prolonged immobilization.

DIAGNOSIS

Diagnostic Testing

- Colonoscopy and barium studies help rule out structural disease and may be particularly important in individuals >50 years without prior colorectal cancer screening, or with other alarm situations such as anemia, blood in the stool, and new onset symptoms (*Gastroenterology 2000;119:1761*).
- Colonic transit studies, anorectal manometry, and defecography are reserved for resistant cases without a structural explanation after initial workup.

TREATMENT

- Regular exercise and adequate fluid intake are nonspecific measures.
- **Fiber supplementation.** An increase in dietary fiber intake to 20 to 30 g/d may be beneficial in many adults with constipation. Fecal impactions should be resolved before fiber supplementation is initiated. A fiber supplement such as wheat bran or psyllium with water two to four times a day can be initiated; fluid intake should be increased with these preparations. Transient bloating often occurs.

Medications

- **Laxatives**
  - **Emollient laxatives** consist of docusate salts and mineral oil. Docusate sodium, 50 to 200 mg PO daily, and docusate calcium, 240 mg PO daily, allow water and fat to penetrate the fecal mass. Mineral oil (15 to 45 mL PO q6–8h) can be given orally or by enema. Tracheobronchial aspiration of mineral oil can result in lipoid pneumonia.
  - **Stimulant cathartics** such as castor oil, 15 mL PO, stimulate intestinal secretion and increase intestinal motility. Anthraquinones (cascara, 5 mL PO daily; senna, one tablet PO daily to qid) stimulate the colon by increasing fluid and water accumulation in the proximal colon. Chronic use can result in benign staining of the colonic mucosa (melanosis coli) and colonic atony from smooth muscle atrophy and damage to the myenteric plexus. Bisacodyl (10 to 15 mg PO at bedtime, 10-mg rectal suppositories) is structurally similar to phenolphthalein and stimulates colonic peristalsis. Lubiprostone (8 to 24 mcg PO bid) is a selective intestinal chloride channel activator, causing movement of fluid into the bowel lumen and stimulating peristalsis.
  - **Osmotic cathartics** include nonabsorbable salts or carbohydrates that cause water retention in the lumen of the colon. Magnesium salts include milk of magnesia (15 to 30 mL q8–12h) and magnesium citrate (200 mL PO); they should be avoided in renal failure. Lactulose (15 to 30 mL PO bid–qid) can cause bloating as a side effect.
- **Enemas.** Sodium biphosphate (Fleet) enemas (one to two rectally PRN) can be used for mild to moderate constipation and for bowel cleansing before sigmoidoscopy. However, these should be avoided in patients with renal failure because of the risk of developing hyperphosphatemia and subsequent hypocalcemia. Tap water enemas (1 L) are also useful for bowel cleansing. Oil-based enemas (cottonseed colace, hypaque) are reserved for refractory constipation.
- **Other agents.** Polyethylene glycol in powder form (MiraLax, 17 g PO daily to bid) can be used regularly or intermittently for the treatment of constipation. Lubiprostone (Amitiza, 24 mcg bid) is a synthetic bicyclic fatty acid that increases frequency of bowel movements.
- **Bowel-cleansing agents.** Patients should be placed on a clear liquid diet the previous day and kept NPO for 6 to 8 hours or overnight prior to the bowel examination (colonoscopy or barium enema). Care should be taken to avoid dehydration. Patients may experience mild abdominal discomfort, nausea, and vomiting with the bowel preparation (*Am J Health-Syst Pharm 2009;66:27*).
  - An iso-osmotic **polyethylene glycol solution** (GoLYTELY or NuLYTELY, 1 gallon, administered at a rate of 8 oz every 10 minutes) is commonly used as a bowel-cleansing agent before colonoscopy. The large volume required for adequate cleansing is the biggest hindrance to its tolerability. Smaller volume preparations

(half gallon) have been designed, administered in conjunction with a laxative. When the preparation is inadequate, more of the iso-osmotic solution can be administered until the stool is clear.

- **Nonabsorbable phosphate** (Fleet phosphosoda, 20 to 45 mL with 10 to 24 oz liquid, taken the day before and morning of the procedure), a hyperosmotic solution, draws fluid into the gut lumen and produces bowel movements in 0.5 to 6 hours. The dose can be taken with 4 oz of liquid and followed with at least 8 oz more of liquid, or 15 mL each can be mixed with three 8-oz glasses of liquid and taken within 30 minutes. It is also available in pill form (Visicol or Osmoprep, 32 to 40 tablets, taken at the rate of 3 to 4 tablets every 15 min with 8 oz fluid).
  - ○ Phosphosoda can result in severe dehydration, hyperphosphatemia, hypocalcemia, hypokalemia, hypernatremia, and acidosis. A dreaded rare complication is acute phosphate nephropathy, where calcium phosphate deposits cause irreversible dysfunction of renal tubules resulting in renal failure. Risk factors for **acute phosphate nephropathy** include age > 55 years, hypovolemia or dehydration, abnormal kidney function, bowel obstruction, active colitis, and medications that affect kidney perfusion (diuretics, angiotensin-converting enzyme inhibitors, angiotensin receptor blockers, and NSAIDs).
- **Split preparations.** Proximity of bowel preparation to procedure time improves effectiveness of cleansing and visualization during the procedure. Therefore, preparations can be administered in two doses, one dose administered the evening prior, and the second dose the morning of the procedure (*Endoscopy 2007;39: 616*). This approach may be particularly useful for colonoscopy scheduled in the afternoon hours.
- **Two-day bowel preparation** is sometimes indicated in elderly or debilitated individuals when conventional bowel preparation is contraindicated, not tolerated, or ineffective. This consists of magnesium citrate (120 to 300 mL PO) administered on 2 consecutive days while the patient remains on a clear liquid diet; bisacodyl (30 mg PO or 10-mg suppository) can also be administered on both days.
- **Tap water enemas** (1-L volume, repeated one to two times) can cleanse the distal colon when colonoscopy is indicated in patients with proximal bowel obstruction.

LUMINAL GASTROINTESTINAL DISORDERS

Gastroesophageal Reflux Disease

GENERAL PRINCIPLES

Definition

Gastroesophageal reflux disease (GERD) is defined as symptoms and/or complications resulting from reflux of gastric contents into the esophagus and more proximal structures.

DIAGNOSIS

Clinical Presentation

- Typical **esophageal symptoms** of GERD include heartburn and regurgitation.

- GERD can also present as **atypical chest pain,** where an important priority is to exclude a cardiac source before considering GERD (*AJG 2006;101:1900*).
- **Extraesophageal manifestations** include cough, laryngitis, asthma, and dental erosions. A GERD association has been proposed for sinusitis, pulmonary fibrosis, pharyngitis, and recurrent otitis media under certain circumstances (*AJG 2006;101: 1900*).
- Symptom response to a therapeutic trial of PPIs can be diagnostic, but a negative response does not exclude GERD (*Gastroenterology 2008;135:1392*).

Differential Diagnosis

Other disorders that can result in esophagitis include:

- **Eosinophilic esophagitis** is characterized by eosinophilic infiltration of esophageal mucosa, which can cause symptoms similar to GERD. Atopy (allergic rhinitis, eczema, asthma) is common, and food allergens may trigger the process. This condition is most common in young males, and should also be considered if GERD symptoms do not improve with maximal antisecretory therapy. The most common symptoms include food impaction requiring emergency endoscopy, dysphagia, heartburn, chest and abdominal pain. Common endoscopic findings include furrows, luminal narrowing, corrugations (with a trachea-like appearance), and whitish plaques in the esophageal mucosa. Histopathology demonstrates eosinophilic infiltration with >15 eosinophils/HPF; multiple biopsy specimens from multiple levels increase sensitivity. Food allergen testing can be considered, but the yield is typically low. Treatment options include topical (swallowed fluticasone, 880 to 1,760 μg/d in two to four divided doses) and less commonly systemic corticosteroids, elimination of dietary allergens when identified, mast cell stabilizers, and anti-IL5 antibodies, but there is no consensus on optimal therapy at present. Cautious dilation of tight strictures can be considered if steroid therapy is unsuccessful (*Gastroenterology 2007; 133:1342*).
- **Infectious esophagitis** is seen most often in immunocompromised states (AIDS, organ transplant recipients), esophageal stasis (abnormal motility [e.g., achalasia, scleroderma]; mechanical obstruction [e.g., strictures]), malignancy, diabetes mellitus, and antibiotic use. However, HSV and varicella esophagitis can rarely occur in the normal healthy host. The presence of typical oral lesions (thrush, herpetic vesicles) may suggest an etiologic agent. The usual presenting symptoms are dysphagia and odynophagia.
  - ***Candida* esophagitis** is the most common esophageal infection, and typically occurs in the setting of esophageal stasis, impaired cell-mediated immunity from immunosuppressive therapy (e.g., with steroids or cytotoxic agents), malignancies, or AIDS. When concurrent oropharyngeal thrush is present, empiric therapy is recommended, reserving endoscopy for refractory symptoms. Visualization of typical whitish plaques at endoscopy has near 100% sensitivity for diagnosis. **Fluconazole** 100 to 200 mg/d or **itraconazole** 200 mg/d for 14 to 21 days is recommended as initial therapy for *Candida* esophagitis. For infections refractory to azoles, a short course of parenteral **amphotericin B** (0.3 to 0.5 mg/kg/d) can be considered (*Best Pract Res Clin Gastroenterol 2008;22:639*).
  - **HSV esophagitis** is characterized by small vesicles and well-circumscribed ulcers on endoscopy, and typical giant cells on histopathology. Viral antigen or DNA can be identified by immunofluorescent antibodies. Treatment consists of **acyclovir** 400 to 800 mg PO five times a day for 14 to 21 days or 5 mg/kg IV q8h for 7

to 14 days. **Famciclovir** and **valacyclovir** are alternate agents. The condition is usually self-limited in immunocompetent hosts even without treatment (*Curr Opin Gastroenterol 2008;24:496*).

- **CMV esophagitis,** which occurs exclusively in immunocompromised hosts, can cause erosions or frank ulcerations. IV therapy with **ganciclovir, foscarnet,** or **cidofovir** is effective for a variety of GI **CMV** infections. **Ganciclovir** 5 mg/kg IV q12h or **foscarnet** 90 mg/kg IV q12h for 3 to 6 weeks can be used as initial therapy. Oral **valganciclovir** may also be effective.
- Symptomatic relief can be achieved with 2% viscous **lidocaine** swish and swallow (15 mL PO q3–4h PRN) or **sucralfate** slurry (1 g PO qid). Concomitant acid suppression should also be administered.
- **Chemical esophagitis**
  - Ingestion of caustic agents (alkalis, acids) or medications such as oral potassium, doxycycline, quinidine, iron, NSAIDs, aspirin, and bisphosphonates can result in mucosal irritation and damage.
  - Cautious early endoscopy is recommended to evaluate the extent and degree of mucosal damage. With caustic ingestions, the optimal time to perform endoscopy is 24 to 72 hours from ingestion.
  - The offending medication should be discontinued if possible. Mucosal coating agents (sucralfate) and acid suppressive agents may help. A second caustic agent to neutralize the first is contraindicated.
- **Nonspecific ulceration** can be seen with medications, malignancy, or AIDS (idiopathic ulcer).
  - Multiple biopsies, brushings, and culture specimens should be obtained at endoscopy.
  - Idiopathic ulcer of AIDS may respond to oral steroid or thalidomide therapy.
  - Concomitant acid suppression should always be administered.

Diagnostic Testing

- **Endoscopy** is primarily indicated for avoiding misdiagnosis of alternate causes of esophageal symptoms (e.g., eosinophilic esophagitis), identification of complications, and evaluation of treatment failures. Patients with symptoms refractory to empiric acid suppression may also benefit from endoscopy, although yield for diagnosis of esophagitis is low in this setting. **Warning symptoms** of dysphagia, odynophagia, early satiety, weight loss, or bleeding should prompt endoscopy (*NEJM 2008; 359:1700*).
- **Ambulatory pH or pH-impedance monitoring** is used to quantify esophageal acid exposure and reflux events, and for symptom–reflux correlation in patients with ongoing symptoms despite acid suppression (especially if endoscopy is negative) or those with atypical symptoms. It is also used to determine adequacy of acid suppression in patients with established GERD and ongoing symptoms.
- **Esophageal manometry,** particularly high-resolution manometry, may identify motor processes contributing to refractory symptoms, but this test is not routinely needed.

TREATMENT

Medications

- Over-the-counter **antacids, histamine-2 receptor antagonists (H_2RAs),** and **PPIs** are effective in patients with mild or intermittent symptoms, and can be used intermittently or prophylactically.

- **PPIs** are more effective than standard-dose H_2RA and placebo in symptom relief and endoscopic healing of GERD. Efficacy is similar for currently available PPIs. Modest gain is achieved by doubling the PPI dose in severe esophagitis or persistent symptoms. Continuous long-term PPI therapy is effective in maintaining remission of GERD symptoms, but the dose should be decreased after 8 to 12 weeks to the lowest dose that achieves symptom relief (*NEJM 2008;359:1700*). Long term PPI use has been associated with bone demineralization, enteric infections, community acquired pneumonia, and reduced circulating levels of vitamin B12 in observational studies, but benefits continue to outweigh risks. An exception is when co-administered with clopidogrel (Plavix), where PPIs may competitively inhibit the cytochrome P-450 enzyme that activates clopidogrel. Substitution with an H_2RA, or administration 12 hours apart from clopidogrel are alternative approaches when appropriate.
- Standard doses of **H_2RAs** (Table 2) can result in symptomatic benefit and endoscopic healing in up to half of the patients (*NEJM 2008;359:1700*). Dosage adjustments are required in renal insufficiency.

Surgical Management

Indications for **fundoplication** include the need for continuous or increasing doses of medication in patients who are good surgical candidates. Patients who require aggressive long-term medical therapy can be offered the surgical option. Other indications

Table 2	Dosage of Acid-Suppressive Agents		
Medication Therapy	**Peptic Ulcer Disease**	**GERD**	**Parenteral**
Cimetidine[a]	300 mg qid 400 mg bid 800 mg at bedtime	400 mg qid 800 mg bid	300 mg q6h
Ranitidine[a]	150 mg bid 300 mg at bedtime	150–300 mg bid–qid	50 mg q8h
Famotidine[a]	20 mg bid 40 mg at bedtime	20–40 mg bid	20 mg q12h
Nizatidine[a]	150 mg bid 300 mg at bedtime	150 mg bid	
Omeprazole	20 mg daily	20–40 mg daily–bid	
Esomeprazole	40 mg daily	20–40 mg daily–bid	20–40 mg q24h
Lansoprazole Dexlansoprazole	15–30 mg daily	15–30 mg daily–bid 30–60 mg daily	30 mg q12–24h
Pantoprazole	20 mg daily	20–40 mg daily–bid	40 mg q12–24h or 80 mg IV, then 8 mg/hr infusion

GERD, gastroesophageal reflux disease.
[a]Dosage adjustment required in renal insufficiency.

include noncompliance or intolerance to medical therapy, and ongoing nonacid reflux despite adequate medical therapy and patient preference for surgery.

- Elevated esophageal acid exposure and correlation of symptoms to reflux events on ambulatory pH monitoring predict a higher likelihood of a successful outcome.
- Patients with medical treatment failures need careful evaluation to determine whether symptoms are indeed related to acid reflux before surgical options are considered; these patients often have other diagnoses including eosinophilic esophagitis, esophageal motor disorders, visceral hypersensitivity, and functional heartburn.
- Potential complications of surgery include dysphagia, inability to belch and gasbloat syndrome, and bowel symptoms including flatulence, diarrhea, and abdominal pain.

Lifestyle/Risk Modification

- Patients with nocturnal GERD symptoms may benefit from elevating the head of the bed by 6 to 8 in. and avoiding eating within 2 to 3 hours before bedtime.
- Weight loss may benefit certain overweight patients with GERD.
- Avoiding foods that trigger reflux (fatty foods, chocolate, coffee, cola) or foods that result in heartburn (spicy foods, tomato, citrus, carbonated drinks) may be prudent in the appropriate setting. Smoking cessation is also thought to be beneficial.
- Lifestyle modifications alone are unlikely to resolve symptoms in the majority of GERD patients, and should be recommended in conjunction with medications.

COMPLICATIONS

- Esophageal erosion and ulceration (esophagitis) can rarely lead to overt bleeding and iron-deficiency anemia.
- Strictures can form when esophagitis heals, leading to dysphagia. Endoscopic dilation and maintenance PPI therapy typically resolve dysphagia from strictures.
- Barrett's esophagus is a reflux-triggered change from normal squamous esophageal epithelium to specialized intestinal metaplastic epithelium, and carries a 0.5% per year risk of progression to esophageal adenocarcinoma. Endoscopic screening for Barrett's esophagus is performed in patients ≥ 50 years or with a symptom history that exceeds 5 to 10 years (*Gastroenterology 2008;135:1392*).

Esophageal Motor Disorders

GENERAL PRINCIPLES

Definition

- **Achalasia** is the most easily recognized motor disorder of the esophagus, characterized by failure of the lower esophageal sphincter (LES) to relax completely with swallowing and aperistalsis of the esophageal body (*AJG 1999;94:3406*).
- **Diffuse esophageal spasm** is a spastic disorder characterized by simultaneous, nonperistaltic contractions in the esophageal body. Concomitant incomplete LES relaxation may be present. Nonspecific spastic disorders have limited spastic features from esophageal inhibitory dysfunction (*Gastroenterologist 1997;5:112*).
- **Esophageal hypomotility disorders** are characterized by feeble or absent esophageal peristalsis, sometimes with LES hypomotility, leading to reflux symptoms.

DIAGNOSIS

Clinical Presentation

- Presenting symptoms in achalasia can include dysphagia, regurgitation, chest pain, weight loss, and aspiration pneumonia.
- Diffuse esophageal spasm and other spastic disorders may have obstructive symptoms (dysphagia, regurgitation), but also perceptive symptoms (chest pain) from heightened visceral sensitivity.
- Hypomotility disorders typically present with reflux symptoms. LES hypomotility diminishes barrier function and esophageal body hypomotility affects esophageal clearance of refluxed material, which can lead to prolonged reflux exposure and reflux complications.

Diagnostic Testing

- **Esophageal manometry** is the gold standard for diagnosis. High-resolution manometry has better sensitivity than conventional manometry in identification of atypical achalasia and spastic syndromes (*Gastroenterology 2008;135:756*). Characteristic findings in achalasia consist of nonrelaxing LES and aperistalsis of the esophageal body. Multiple (typically >30%) simultaneous contractions are seen in diffuse esophageal spasm. Hypomotility disorders demonstrate varying degrees of failed and fragmented peristalsis, low-amplitude contractions and low LES basal pressures.
- **Barium radiographs** may demonstrate a typical achalasia appearance of a dilated intrathoracic esophagus with impaired emptying, an air–fluid level, absence of gastric air bubble, and tapering of the distal esophagus with the appearance of a bird's beak. A beaded or corkscrew appearance may be seen with diffuse esophageal spasm, sometimes with epiphrenic diverticula. A dilated esophagus with an open LES and free gastroesophageal reflux may be seen with severe esophageal hypomotility.
- **Endoscopy** may help exclude a stricture or neoplasia of the distal esophagus in achalasia and spastic disorders; the esophageal body may be dilated and contain food debris, whereas the LES, although pinpoint, typically allows passage of the endoscope into the stomach with minimal resistance. Hypomotility disorders may also manifest a dilated esophagus, but with a gaping gastroesophageal junction and evidence of reflux disease.

TREATMENT

Medications

- **Smooth muscle relaxants** such as nitrates or calcium channel blockers administered immediately before meals may afford short-lived symptom relief in spastic disorders and achalasia. Overall, smooth muscle relaxants are not very effective in achalasia symptom relief.
- **Botulinum toxin** injection at endoscopy can improve dysphagia symptoms for several weeks to months in achalasia and spastic disorders with incomplete LES relaxation. This approach may be useful in elderly and frail patients who are poor surgical risks or as a bridge to more definitive therapy (*Ann Surg 2009;249:45*).
- **Neuromodulators** (e.g., low-dose tricyclic antidepressants) may improve perceptive symptoms (such as chest pain) associated with spastic motor disorders and achalasia.
- **Antisecretory therapy** with a PPI is recommended for reflux associated with esophageal hypomotility disorders.

- No specific promotility therapy exists. Antireflux surgery should be approached with caution in advanced hypomotility disorders.

Surgical Management

Disruption of the circular muscle of the LES using **pneumatic dilation** or surgical incision **(Heller myotomy)** can result in durable symptom relief in achalasia (*Ann Surg 2009;249:45*). Gastroesophageal reflux can result, treated with lifelong acid suppression or concurrent partial fundoplication at myotomy. Esophageal perforation occurs in 3% to 5% with pneumatic dilation, requiring prompt surgical repair. Surgical myotomy is rarely indicated for diffuse esophageal spasm when incomplete LES relaxation is thought to contribute significantly to dysphagia symptoms.

COMPLICATIONS

- Complications of achalasia include aspiration pneumonia and weight loss.
- Achalasia is associated with a 0.15% risk of squamous cell cancer of the distal esophagus, a 33-fold higher risk relative to the nonachalasic population.

Peptic Ulcer Disease

GENERAL PRINCIPLES

Definition

Peptic ulcer disease (PUD) consists of mucosal breaks in the stomach and duodenum when corrosive effects of acid and pepsin overwhelm mucosal defense mechanisms. Peptic ulcers can also occur in the esophagus, in the small bowel adjacent to gastroenteric anastomoses, and within a Meckel's diverticulum.

Etiology

- *Helicobacter pylori,* a spiral, gram-negative urease-producing bacillus, is thought to be responsible for at least half of all PUD, and the majority of ulcers that are not due to NSAIDs. Overall, 10% to 15% of patients with *H. pylori* infection develop PUD (*JCG 1997;24:2*).
- PUD can develop in 15% to 25% of chronic NSAID and aspirin users. Past history of PUD, age > 60 years, concomitant corticosteroid or anticoagulant therapy, high-dose or multiple NSAID therapy, and presence of serious comorbid medical illnesses increase risk for PUD from NSAID or aspirin use (*JCG 1997;24:2*).
- A gastrin-secreting tumor or **gastrinoma** accounts for <1% of all peptic ulcers from uncontrolled acid production.
- Gastric cancer or lymphoma may manifest as a gastric ulcer.
- When none of the above etiologies are evident, PUD is designated idiopathic. Most idiopathic PUD could be due to undiagnosed *H. pylori* or undetected NSAID use.
- Cigarette smoking doubles the risk for peptic ulcers.

DIAGNOSIS

Clinical Presentation

- Epigastric pain or dyspepsia may be presenting symptoms; however, symptoms are not always predictive of the presence of ulcers. Epigastric tenderness may be elicited on abdominal palpation.
- Ten percent may present with a complication (see below).

- In the presence of alarm symptoms (weight loss, early satiety, bleeding, anemia, persistent vomiting, epigastric mass, and lack of appropriate response to acid suppression), endoscopy is indicated to evaluate for a complication or an alternate diagnosis (*BMJ 2008;337:a1400.doi:1136/bmj.a1400*).

Diagnostic Testing

- **Endoscopy** is the gold standard for diagnosis of peptic ulcers.
- **Barium studies** also have good sensitivity for diagnosis of ulcers, but smaller ulcers and erosions may be missed, and tissue sampling for *H. pylori* or cancer cannot be performed.
- **Serum *H. pylori* antibody testing** is the cheapest noninvasive test with a sensitivity of 85% and a specificity of 79% for the diagnosis of *H. pylori* infection. The antibody remains detectable as long as 18 months after successful eradication, and therefore, this test cannot be used to document successful eradication of the organism (*BMJ 2008;337:a1400.doi:1136/bmj.a1400*).
- **Stool *H. pylori* antigen testing** has 91% sensitivity and 93% specificity for the diagnosis of *H. pylori* infection. This test can be used to confirm eradication of *H. pylori* after triple therapy.
- **Rapid urease assay** (e.g. *Campylobacter*-like organism [CLO] test) and histopathologic examination of endoscopic biopsy specimens are commonly used for diagnosis in patients undergoing endoscopy; these tests may be falsely negative in patients on PPI therapy.
- **Carbon-labeled urea breath testing** is the most accurate noninvasive test for diagnosis, with sensitivity and specificity of 95%; often used to document successful eradication after therapy of *H. pylori* infection (*BMJ 2008;337:a1400.doi: 1136/bmj.a1400*).

TREATMENT

Medications

- Regardless of etiology, **acid suppression** forms the mainstay of therapy of PUD. Gastric ulcers are typically treated for 12 weeks, and duodenal ulcers for 8 weeks.
- Oral PPI or H_2RA therapy will suffice in most instances; parenteral administration of PPIs is necessary in the presence of GI bleeding or when oral administration is not tolerated or not possible (see Table 2). Abdominal pain and diarrhea are common side effects of PPI therapy, see segment on GERD for long term side effects. Headache and mental status abnormalities (lethargy, confusion, depression, hallucinations) can result from H_2RA therapy while hepatotoxicity, thrombocytopenia, and leukopenia are rare. Dosage intervals should be prolonged for H_2RAs in the presence of renal insufficiency. Cimetidine can impair metabolism of many drugs, including warfarin anticoagulants, theophylline, and phenytoin.
- **Triple therapy.** Two antibiotics and a PPI form a standard eradication regimen for *H. pylori*. Eradication promotes healing and markedly reduces recurrence of gastric and duodenal ulcers. Several antimicrobial and antisecretory agent regimens are available (Table 3). Patients previously exposed to a macrolide antibiotic should be treated with a regimen that does not include clarithromycin. Clarithromycin resistance and poor compliance with therapy affect eradication rates, metronidazole resistance does not (*Gastroenterology 2007;133:985*).
- NSAIDs and aspirin should be avoided if possible. If these agents need to be continued, maintenance PPI therapy or a mucosal protective agent (misoprostol, 400 to 800 µg/d) are recommended.

Table 3	Examples of Regimens Used for Eradication of *Helicobacter pylori*

Medications	Dose	Comments
Clarithromycin	500 mg bid	First line
Amoxicillin	1 g bid	
PPI[a]	bid	
Metronidazole	500 mg bid	First line with history of exposure to clarithromycin
Amoxicillin	1 g bid	
PPI	bid	
Pepto-Bismol	524 mg qid	First line in penicillin-allergic patients
Metronidazole	250 mg qid	Salvage regimen if three-drug regimen fails
Tetracycline	500 mg qid	
PPI[a] or H$_2$RA[b]	bid	
Clarithromycin	500 mg bid	Alternate regimen if four-drug therapy is not tolerated
Metronidazole	500 mg bid	
PPI[a]	bid	
Levofloxacin	250 mg bid	Alternate salvage regimen
Amoxicillin	1 g bid	
PPI[a]	bid	
Rifabutin	300 mg daily	Alternate salvage regimen
Amoxicillin	1 g bid	
PPI	Bid	
Furazolidine	200–400 mg daily	Alternate salvage regimen
Amoxicillin	1 g bid	
PPI[a]	bid	

PPI, proton pump inhibitor.
Duration of therapy: 10 to 14 days. When using salvage regimens after initial treatment failure, choose drugs that have not been used before.
[a]Standard doses for PPI: omeprazole 20 mg, lansoprazole 30 mg, pantoprazole 40 mg, rabeprazole 20 mg, all twice a day. Esomeprazole is used as a single 40-mg dose once a day.
[b]Standard doses for H$_2$RA: ranitidine 150 mg, famotidine 20 mg, nizatidine 150 mg, cimetidine 400 mg, all twice a day.

- **Sucralfate** acts by coating the mucosal surface without blocking acid secretion and can be as effective as H$_2$RAs in healing duodenal ulcers. This agent is used in stress ulcer prophylaxis. Side effects include constipation and reduction of bioavailability of certain drugs (e.g., cimetidine, digoxin, fluoroquinolones, phenytoin, and tetracycline) when administered concomitantly.
- **Antacids** are rarely used as primary therapy for PUD but can be useful as supplemental therapy for pain relief.
- **Nonpharmacologic measures.** Cigarette smoking doubles the risk of peptic ulcer development, delays healing, and promotes recurrence; therefore, cessation of cigarette smoking should be encouraged. Alcohol in high concentrations can damage the gastric mucosal barrier, but no evidence exists to link alcohol with ulcer recurrence.

Surgical Management

Surgery is still occasionally required for intractable symptoms, GI bleeding, Zollinger–Ellison syndrome, and other complications of PUD. Surgical options vary depending on the location of the ulcer and the presence of associated complications.

SPECIAL CONSIDERATIONS

Zollinger–Ellison syndrome

- This syndrome is caused by a gastrin-secreting, non–β islet cell tumor of the pancreas or duodenum. Multiple endocrine neoplasia type I can be associated with this syndrome in 25% of patients. The resultant hypersecretion of gastric acid can cause multiple peptic ulcers in unusual locations, ulcers that fail to respond to standard medical therapy, or recurrent ulceration after surgical therapy. Diarrhea and gastroesophageal reflux symptoms are common.
- Gastric acid output is typically >15 mEq/L, and gastric pH is <1.0. A fasting serum gastrin level while off acid suppression for at least 5 days serves as a screening test in patients who make gastric acid; a value >1,000 pg/mL is seen in 90% of patients with Zollinger–Ellison syndrome. When serum gastrin is elevated but <1,000 pg/mL, a secretin stimulation test may demonstrate a paradoxical 200-pg increment in serum gastrin level after IV secretin in patients with gastrinomas (*APT 2009;29:1055*). PPIs are generally required in higher doses than those used for PUD. Specialized nuclear medicine scans (octreotide scans) can be useful in localizing the neoplastic lesion for curative resection (*Expert Opin Pharmacother 2009;10:1145*).

COMPLICATIONS

- **GI bleeding** (see Gastrointestinal Bleeding)
- **Gastric outlet obstruction** is more likely to occur with ulcers that are close to the pyloric channel. Nausea and vomiting, sometimes several hours after meals, may occur. Plain abdominal radiographs often show a dilated stomach with an air–fluid level. NG suction should be maintained for 2 to 3 days to decompress the stomach while repleting fluids and electrolytes intravenously.
  - Although medical management may be temporarily effective, recurrence is common, and endoscopic balloon dilation or surgery is often necessary for definitive correction.
- **Perforation** occurs in a small number of PUD patients and usually necessitates emergency surgery. Perforation may occur in the absence of previous symptoms of PUD and may be asymptomatic in patients who are receiving glucocorticoids. A plain upright radiograph of the abdomen may demonstrate free air under the diaphragm.
- **Pancreatitis** can result from penetration into the pancreas, most commonly seen with ulcers in the posterior wall of the duodenal bulb. The pain becomes severe and continuous, radiates to the back, and is no longer relieved by antisecretory therapy. Serum amylase may be elevated. Computed tomography (CT) scanning may be diagnostic. These patients frequently require surgery.

MONITORING/FOLLOW-UP

- EGD or upper GI series should be performed 8 to 12 weeks after initial diagnosis of all gastric ulcers to document healing; repeat endoscopic biopsy should be considered for nonhealing ulcers to exclude the possibility of a malignant ulcer.
- Duodenal ulcers are almost never malignant, and therefore, documentation of healing is unnecessary in the absence of symptoms.

Inflammatory Bowel Disease

GENERAL PRINCIPLES

Definition

- **Ulcerative colitis (UC)** is an idiopathic chronic inflammatory disease of the colon and rectum, characterized by mucosal inflammation and typically presenting with bloody diarrhea. Rectal involvement is almost universal.
- **Crohn's disease (CD)** is characterized by transmural inflammation of the gut wall and can affect any part of the tubular GI tract.

DIAGNOSIS

Clinical Presentation

- Both disorders can present with diarrhea, weight loss, and abdominal pain. UC typically presents with bloody diarrhea. CD can also present with fistula formation, strictures, abscesses, or bowel obstruction.
- Extracolonic manifestations of inflammatory bowel disease (IBD) include arthritis, primary sclerosing cholangitis, ocular and skin lesions.

Diagnostic Testing

- **Endoscopy** remains the preferred method for diagnosis, especially for UC where contiguous inflammation is seen starting at the rectum and extending varying distances into the colon. Endoscopy may demonstrate colonic involvement in CD (erosions or ulcers with a patchy distribution and skip lesions); ileoscopy during colonoscopy may demonstrate terminal ileal involvement. **Histopathology** demonstrates chronic mucosal inflammation with crypt abscesses and cryptitis in UC, and may demonstrate multinucleated giant cells and noncaseating granulomas in CD.
- Cross-sectional **imaging studies** (CT and MRI scans) have value in the evaluation of CD, especially when luminal narrowing (stricture) or extraluminal complications (abscess, fistula) are suspected. MR and CT enterography can evaluate for small-bowel mural inflammation and/or strictures. Contrast radiography (small bowel follow through series, barium enema) may also be useful, particularly in CD.
- **Serologic markers** play a limited role as adjuncts for diagnosis. Anti-*Saccharomyces cerevisiae* antibodies are typically seen in CD, and perinuclear antineutrophil cytoplasmic antibodies (pANCA) in UC; the finding of one in the absence of the other antibody may help differentiate indeterminate colitis (*Gastroenterology 2002;122: 1242*). C-reactive protein and erythrocyte sedimentation rate (ESR) are sometimes useful as correlates for disease activity.
- The incidence of *C. difficile* colitis is higher in IBD patients compared to non-IBD population; therefore, **stool studies** are warranted to look for this organism with disease flares (*CGH 2007;5:339*). CMV superinfection can occur in patients on immunosuppressive agents and can be diagnosed by histopathology during endoscopy (*AJG 2006;101:2857*).

TREATMENT

Medications

Treatment is based on the severity of disease, the location, and associated complications. Management aims are to resolve the acute presentation and reduce future recurrences.

Both UC and CD can be categorized into three categories of severity for management purposes:

- **Mild to moderate disease** applies to patients with little to no weight loss, good functional capacity, and ability to maintain adequate oral intake. UC patients have less than four bowel movements with no rectal bleeding or anemia, normal vital signs and normal ESR, while Crohn's patients have little or no abdominal pain. Treatment typically begins with aminosalicylates, but can include antibiotics and glucocorticoids, depending on location of disease.
  - **5-Aminosalicylates (5-ASA).** The mechanism of action remains unknown but involves decreasing the production of arachidonic acid metabolites, particularly leukotrienes. Various formulations are available, each targeting different parts of the tubular gut, and useful for both inducing and maintaining remission in mild to moderate disease. Infrequent hypersensitivity reactions include pneumonitis, pancreatitis, hepatitis, and nephritis.
    - ○ **Sulfasalazine** reaches the colon intact, where it is metabolized to 5-ASA and a sulfapyridine moiety. Benefit is therefore limited to UC or CD limited to the colon, either as initial therapy (0.5 g PO bid, increased as tolerated to 0.5 to 1.5 g PO qid) or to maintain remission (1 g PO bid–qid). The sulfapyridine moiety is responsible for side effects of headache, nausea, vomiting, and abdominal pain, which may respond to dose reduction. Rare hypersensitivity reactions include skin rash, fever, agranulocytosis, hepatotoxicity, and paradoxical exacerbation of colitis. Reversible reduction in sperm counts can be seen in males. Folic acid supplementation is recommended as sulfasalazine can impair folate absorption.
    - ○ **Mesalamine.** Newer 5-ASA preparations lack the sulfa moiety of sulfasalazine and are associated with fewer side effects. They can be more expensive.
      - - **Asacol** is an oral formulation of 5-ASA released at a pH of 7 in the distal ileum. It is useful in UC and ileocecal/colonic CD at doses of 800 to 1,600 mg PO tid.
      - - **Pentasa** has a time- and pH-dependent release mechanism that allows drug availability throughout the small bowel and colon. It is useful in diffuse small bowel involvement with CD, but can also be used in UC in doses of 0.5 to 1.0 g PO qid.
      - - **Apriso** also has a pH dependent release mechanism, and distributes mesalamine throughout the colon when administered in doses of 1.5 g PO once daily.
      - - **Balsalazide (Colazal)** is cleaved by colonic bacteria to mesalamine and an inert molecule. It is therefore only useful for colonic disease, at doses of 2.25 g PO tid for active disease and 1.5 g PO bid for maintenance.
      - - **Multimatrix delivery system mesalamine (Lialda)** uses a novel drug delivery system that allows sustained 5-ASA release throughout the colon while decreasing frequency of administration, and is therefore useful in colonic disease at doses of 1.2 to 2.4 g PO qd–bid.
    - ○ **Olsalazine (Dipentum)** is a 5-ASA dimer cleaved by colonic bacteria, and therefore useful in colonic disease. It can be associated with significant diarrhea that limits its use.
  - **Antibiotics** are commonly used clinically in mild to moderate CD as well as perianal disease, but not UC where the role of bacteria has not been established. Despite frequent usage, controlled studies have failed to consistently show efficacy for luminal inflammation. Their role should be limited to colonic or ileocolonic CD, perianal disease, fistulas, and abscesses. Typical antibiotics used are **metronidazole** (250 to 500 mg PO tid) and **ciprofloxacin** (500 mg PO bid), usually concurrently, for 2 to 6 weeks.

- **Budesonide** (6 to 9 mg PO qd) is a synthetic corticosteroid with first pass liver metabolism that limits systemic toxicity while retaining local efficacy from high affinity to the glucocorticoid receptor, similar to oral corticosteroids. It is effective and safe for short-term use in mild to moderate ileocolonic CD and can replace mesalamine in inducing remission (*AJG 2009;104:465*). Efficacy has not been reported in UC.
- **Topical therapy** is useful in IBD limited to distal left colon. Ulcerative proctitis or UC limited to the rectosigmoid colon can be treated effectively with 5-ASA and/or glucocorticoid enemas or suppositories administered once to twice a day; concurrent systemic therapy is administered in severe cases (*AJG 2004;99:1371*). Sitz baths, analgesics, hydrocortisone creams, and local heat may provide symptomatic benefit in perianal CD, in conjunction with conventional systemic therapy.
- **Moderate to severe disease** refers to CD patients who fail to respond to treatment for mild to moderate disease, or those with significant weight loss, anemia, fever, abdominal pain or tenderness, and intermittent nausea and vomiting without bowel obstruction (*AJG 2009;104:465*), or UC patients with more than six bloody bowel movements a day, fever, mild anemia, and elevated ESR. The goal of therapy is to induce remission rapidly with corticosteroids, and to maintain remission with immunosuppressive agents and/or biologic agents as appropriate. Treatment is typically continued until the patient fails to respond to a particular agent, or the agent is no longer tolerated.
  - **Glucocorticoids** are effective in inducing remission in moderate to severe disease, especially with flare-ups of disease activity. Extracolonic manifestations of inflammatory bowel disease (ocular lesions, skin disease, and peripheral arthritis) also respond to glucocorticoids.
    - **Prednisone** is started orally (40 to 60 mg PO qd) and continued until symptom improvement. The dose can then be reduced by 5 to 10 mg weekly until the dose of 20 mg, following which taper can be continued by 2.5 to 5 mg weekly. Glucocorticoids are not recommended for maintenance therapy, and alternatives should be sought for the patient who appears dependent on these medications.
    - **Oral or parenteral glucocorticoids should not be prescribed before ruling out an infectious process and should not be initiated for the first time over the telephone.**
    - Patients treated with at least 5 mg prednisone for >2 months need to be continually monitored for osteoporosis (*JAMA 2001;285:785*). Other risk factors for osteoporosis include smoking, low body mass, sedentary lifestyle, family history of osteoporosis, and nutritional deficiencies (*Gastroenterology 2003;124:791*).
  - **Immunosuppressive agents**
    - **6-Mercaptopurine** (1.0 to 1.5 mg/kg/d PO), a purine analog, and **azathioprine** (1.5 to 2.5 mg/kg/d PO), its S-imidazole precursor, cause preferential suppression of T-cell activation and antigen recognition and are useful in maintaining a glucocorticoid-induced remission in both UC and CD. Both agents have more favorable side effect profiles than do glucocorticoids and are used as steroid-sparing agents in severe or refractory inflammatory bowel disease. Response may be delayed for up to 1 to 2 months, with optimal response occurring about 4 months after treatment initiation. Side effects include reversible bone marrow suppression, pancreatitis, and allergic reactions.
      - Determination of **thiopurine methyltransferase (TPMT)** enzyme activity prior to initiation of therapy will identify genetic polymorphisms that may predispose to toxicity with the use of these agents (*Gastroenterology 2006;130:935*).

- Routine blood cell counts should be performed, initially every 1 to 2 weeks to monitor for acute or delayed bone marrow suppression. On stable doses, testing can be performed every 3 months.
  ○ **Methotrexate** (15 to 25 mg IM or PO weekly) is effective as a steroid-sparing agent in CD but not UC. Side effects include hepatic fibrosis, bone marrow suppression, alopecia, pneumonitis, allergic reactions, and teratogenicity.
    - Baseline CXR should be performed at initiation of therapy, and monitoring of CBC and liver functions tests should be performed routinely.
    - Patients with abnormal transaminases may require a liver biopsy to assess for hepatic fibrosis prior to treatment, and subsequent biopsies are performed for significant elevations thereafter.
- **Antitumor necrosis factor alpha (anti-TNF-α) monoclonal antibodies** modify immune system function and are beneficial in moderate to severe CD refractory to other approaches including immunosuppressives, both for induction and maintenance of remission. Benefit has also been demonstrated in moderate to severe UC (*Gastroenterology 2009;136:1182*). **Infliximab** (5 mg/kg IV infusions at weeks 0, 2, and 6, followed by maintenance infusions every 8 weeks), **adalimumab** (160 mg SQ at week 0, then 80 mg SQ at week 2, followed by 40 mg SQ every 2 weeks), and **certolizumab pegol** (400 mg SQ at weeks 0, 2, and 4, followed by maintenance doses every 4 weeks) are the available anti-TNF agents.
  ○ Anti-TNF-α therapy has been associated with reactivation of latent tuberculosis, hence placement of a PPD and chest x-ray are essential prior to initiation of therapy. Opportunistic infections as well as infectious complications can develop, and congestive heart failure may worsen during therapy.
  ○ Acute and delayed hypersensitivity reactions, antibodies to infliximab and anti-double-stranded DNA antibodies can develop with infliximab infusions. Local injection site reactions have been reported with adalimumab and certolizumab pegol therapy.
- **Natalizumab** (300-mg infusions at weeks 0, 4, and 8, followed by monthly infusions thereafter) is a humanized monoclonal antibody to alpha-4 integrin, a cellular adhesion molecule, used for moderate to severe CD refractory to all other approaches including anti-TNF-α antibodies. This agent may induce reactivation of human JC polyoma virus causing progressive multifocal leukoencephalopathy (PML). Risk for PML can be minimized by avoiding concomitant immunosuppressive agents and close monitoring (*AJG 2009;104:465*). Infusion can also result in other infectious complications and acute hypersensitivity reactions.
- **Severe or fulminant disease** describes patients typically hospitalized due to the severity of their symptoms. Fulminant CD patients have persistent symptoms despite conventional glucocorticoids or anti-TNF-α therapy, or have high fevers, persistent vomiting, intestinal obstruction, intra-abdominal abscess, peritoneal signs, or cachexia (*AJG 2009;104:465*). Fulminant colitis (both CD and UC) can present with profuse bloody bowel movements, significant anemia, systemic signs of toxicity (fever, sepsis, electrolyte disturbances, dehydration), and elevated laboratory markers of inflammation (*Arch Surg 2005;140:300*). **Toxic megacolon** occurs in 1% to 2% of UC patients, wherein the colon becomes atonic and modestly dilated, with significant systemic toxicity.
- Supportive therapy consists of NPO status with NG suction if there is evidence of small-bowel ileus. Dehydration and electrolyte disturbances are treated vigorously, and blood transfusions administered for severe anemia. Anticholinergic and opioid medication should be discontinued in toxic megacolon.

- Initial investigation includes cross-sectional imaging (CT, MRI) to evaluate for intra-abdominal abscess. A cautious flexible sigmoidoscopy may be appropriate to determine severity of colonic inflammation in fulminant colitis and for biopsies to exclude CMV colitis. Blood cultures and stool studies to exclude superimposed *C. difficile* colitis are performed.
- Intensive medical therapy with IV **corticosteroids** (methylprednisolone 1 mg/kg body weight or equivalent to 40 to 60 mg of prednisone) and broad-spectrum antimicrobials should be initiated.
- If no response is noted, patients can be started on **cyclosporine** infusion (2 to 4 mg/kg/d, to achieve blood levels of 200 to 400 ng/mL). Data are most consistent with this approach in fulminant UC colitis. Tacrolimus infusions are also an option. Once improved, the patient can gradually be transitioned to an equivalent oral regimen, supplemented with immunosuppressive agents (*Arch Surg 2005;140:300*).
- Nutritional support is administered as appropriate after 5 to 7 days; total parenteral nutrition is often indicated if enteral nutrition is not tolerated.
- Clinical deterioration/lack of improvement despite 7 to 10 days of intensive medical management, evidence of bowel perforation, or peritoneal signs are indications for urgent total colectomy.
- Surgical evaluation should be pursued in those with concern for abscess formation or GI obstruction. If the patient is refractory to medical management, surgical excision of affected area should be considered. Strictureplasty is an accepted procedure for focal tight strictures; biopsies should be obtained to rule out cancer at stricture sites.

Surgical Management

- Surgery is generally reserved for patients with fistulas, obstruction, abscess, perforation, or bleeding, and rarely for medically refractory disease and neoplastic transformation.
- In CD, recurrence close to the resected margins is common after bowel resection. Efforts should be made to avoid multiple resections in CD because of the risk of short-bowel syndrome. Immunosuppressive agents should be discontinued before surgery and reinstituted if necessary during the postoperative period.
- In UC, total colectomy is curative, and for some patients is preferred over long-term immunosuppressive or biologic therapy.

Lifestyle/Risk Modification

Diet

- A low-roughage diet often provides symptomatic relief in patients with mild to moderate disease or in patients with strictures. Elemental diets have been used in acute phases of the diseases, especially CD, but are unpalatable and disliked by patients.
- Patients with Crohn's ileitis or ileocolonic resection may need vitamin B_{12} supplementation. Specific oral replacement of calcium, magnesium, folate, iron, vitamins A and D, and other micronutrients may be necessary in patients with small-bowel CD.
- Patients with intermittent obstructive symptoms should avoid highly indigestible foods such as nuts, pits, hulls, skins, seeds, and pulps that may precipitate obstruction.
- **Total parenteral nutrition** can be administered in patients with food intolerance for greater than 4 or 5 days. Bowel rest has not been shown to reduce time to remission,

but can be used for nutritional maintenance and symptom relief while waiting for the effects of medical treatment, or as a bridge to surgery.

SPECIAL CONSIDERATIONS

- **Colon cancer surveillance.** In patients with colitis lasting longer than 8 to 10 years (both UC and Crohn's colitis), annual colonoscopic surveillance for neoplasia with four-quadrant mucosal biopsies every 5 to 10 cm is recommended. Histopathologic evidence of any grade of dysplasia is an indication for total colectomy.
- **Smoking cessation** is generally warranted for all patients with IBD. There is epidemiological evidence of a protective effect on a limited number of patients with UC. However, nicotine has been shown to increase metabolism of many medications routinely used to treat IBD, decreasing their efficacy.
- **Symptom control** is important as adjunct to therapy but must be used cautiously.
  - **Antidiarrheal agents** may be useful as an adjunctive therapy in selected patients with mild exacerbations or post resection diarrhea. They are contraindicated in severe exacerbations and toxic megacolon.
  - **Narcotics** should be used sparingly for pain control, as the chronicity of symptoms can lead to potential for dependence.

Functional Gastrointestinal Disorders

GENERAL PRINCIPLES

Definition

- Functional GI disorders are characterized by the presence of abdominal symptoms in the absence of a demonstrable organic disease process. Symptoms can arise from any part of the luminal gut.
- **Irritable bowel syndrome (IBS),** primarily characterized by abdominal pain linked to altered bowel habits of at least 3 months duration, is the best-recognized functional bowel disease (*Gastroenterology 2006;130:1480*).

DIAGNOSIS

- Clinical evaluation and investigation should be directed toward prudently excluding organic processes in the involved area of the gut while initiating therapeutic trials when functional symptoms are suspected.
- In the absence of alarm features (anemia, weight loss, family history of colorectal cancer, IBD, or celiac sprue), symptom-based diagnosis of IBS is generally accurate (*AJG 2009;104(Suppl 1):S1*).
- **Serologic tests for celiac sprue** are recommended in IBS patients with a component of diarrhea. The prevalence of celiac sprue in this subset of IBS patients is estimated at 3.6%, compared to 0.7% of the general population (*AJG 2009;104(Suppl 1):S1*).
- Patients >50 years with new-onset bowel symptoms, patients with alarm symptoms (GI bleeding, anemia, weight loss, early satiety), and patients with symptoms not responding to empiric treatment need further workup with endoscopy. Routine cross-sectional imaging is not recommended in patients without alarm features with typical functional symptoms.

- In young individuals with short-lived symptoms and no other explanation for dyspepsia, noninvasive testing for *H. pylori* (serology or urea breath test) can be considered (*BMJ 2008;337:a1400.doi:10.1136/bmj.a1400*).

TREATMENT

Patient education, reassurance, and help with diet and lifestyle modification are key to an effective physician–patient relationship. The psychosocial contribution to symptom exacerbation should be determined, and its management may be sufficient for many patients.

Medications
- **Symptomatic management**
  - **Antiemetic agents** are useful in functional nausea and vomiting syndromes, in addition to neuromodulators.
  - When pain and bloating are the predominant symptoms, **antispasmodic** or **anticholinergic** medications (hyoscyamine, 0.125 to 0.25 mg PO/sublingual up to qid; dicyclomine, 10 to 20 mg PO qid) may provide short-term relief.
  - Constipation-predominant IBS may report increased stool frequency from increased dietary fiber (25 g/d) supplemented with laxatives PRN, but abdominal pain may not improve.
  - **Loperamide** (2 to 4 mg, up to qid/PRN) can reduce stool frequency, urgency, and fecal incontinence.
  - Short-term treatment with a nonabsorbable **antibiotic** may improve bloating and diarrhea-predominant symptoms; long-term treatment has not been adequately studied. Certain **probiotics** (e.g., bifidobacteria) may also be beneficial in certain patients (*AJG 2009;104(Suppl 1):S1*).
  - **Lubiprostone** (8 μg bid), a selective chloride channel activator, may improve constipation-predominant IBS symptoms in women.
  - **Alosetron** (Lotronex, 1 mg daily to bid), a 5-HT$_3$ antagonist, is useful in women with diarrhea-predominant IBS; its use is restricted to women with symptoms refractory to other measures because of the potential for ischemic colitis in a small proportion of patients.
- **Neuromodulators**
  - Low-dose **TCAs** (e.g., amitriptyline, nortriptyline, imipramine, doxepin: 25 to 100 mg at bedtime) have neuromodulatory and analgesic properties that are independent of their psychotropic effects and can be beneficial, especially in pain-predominant functional GI disorders.
  - **Selective serotonin reuptake inhibitors** (e.g., fluoxetine, 20 mg; paroxetine, 20 mg; sertraline, 50 mg; duloxetine 20 to 60 mg) may also have efficacy, sometimes with better side effect profiles.
  - Patients with **cyclic vomiting syndrome** (stereotypic episodes of vigorous vomiting with asymptomatic intervals between episodes) benefit from treatment with low-dose TCAs or antiepileptic medications (Zonegran, Keppra) as maintenance options (*CGH 2007;5:44*). Anecdotal evidence suggests that these patients may also benefit from sumatriptan (25 to 50 mg PO, 5 to 10 mg transnasally, or 6 mg SC at the beginning of an episode), especially if administered during a prodrome or early in the episode.

Acute Intestinal Pseudo-Obstruction (Ileus)

GENERAL PRINCIPLES

Definition

- **Acute intestinal pseudo-obstruction or ileus** consists of impaired transit of intestinal contents and obstructive symptoms (nausea, vomiting, abdominal distension, lack of bowel movements) from diminished gut peristalsis without a mechanical explanation (*MCNA 2008;92:649*).
- **Acute colonic pseudo-obstruction** or **Ogilvie syndrome** on the other hand describes massive colonic dilation without mechanical obstruction in the presence of a competent ileocecal valve, resulting from impaired colonic peristalsis (*Br J Surg 2009;96:229*).

Etiology

Ileus is frequently seen in the postoperative period. Narcotic analgesics administered for postoperative pain control may contribute, as can other medications that slow intestinal peristalsis (calcium channel blockers, anticholinergic medications, tricyclic antidepressants, antihistamines). Other predisposing causes include virtually any medical insult, particularly life-threatening systemic diseases, infection, vascular insufficiency, and electrolyte abnormalities. Etiology is similar for acute colonic pseudo-obstruction, but this condition is much less common and will not be focused on in this section.

DIAGNOSIS

- A careful history and physical exam is essential in the initial evaluation of these patients.
- Conventional laboratory studies (blood cell count, complete metabolic profile, amylase, lipase) help in assessing for a primary intra-abdominal inflammatory process.
- **Obstructive series** (supine and upright abdominal radiograph with a chest radiograph) determines the distribution of intestinal gas and assesses for the presence of free intraperitoneal air.
- **Additional imaging studies** may be required to assess for mechanical obstruction and inflammatory processes and include **CT scanning, contrast enema, and small-bowel series.**

TREATMENT

- Basic supportive measures consist of nothing by mouth (NPO), fluid replacement, and correction of electrolyte imbalances. Prompt antimicrobial therapy is indicated if an infectious process is suspected. Medications that slow GI motility (adrenergic agonists, TCAs, sedatives, narcotic analgesics) should be withdrawn or doses reduced. The ambulatory patient is encouraged to remain active and to undertake short walks.
- **Intermittent NG suction** prevents swallowed air from passing distally. In protracted cases, gastric decompression, either using an NG tube or a percutaneous endoscopic gastrotomy tube, eliminates upper GI secretions and decreases vomiting and gastric distension.
- **Rectal tubes** help decompress the distal colon; more proximal colonic distension may necessitate **colonoscopic decompression,** especially when the cecal diameter

approaches 9 to 10 cm. A flexible decompression tube can be left in the proximal colon during colonoscopy. Turning the patient from side to side may potentiate the benefit of colonoscopic decompression.

- Temporary total parenteral nutrition may be required in protracted cases.

Medications

- **Neostigmine** (2 mg IV administered slowly over 3 to 5 minutes) is beneficial in selected patients with acute colonic distension. The drug can induce rapid reestablishment of colonic tone and is contraindicated if mechanical obstruction remains in the differential diagnosis. Side effects include abdominal pain, excessive salivation, symptomatic bradycardia, and syncope. A trial of neostigmine may be warranted before colonoscopic decompression in patients without contraindications (*NEJM 1999;341:137*).
- **Erythromycin** (200 mg IV) acts as a motilin agonist and stimulates upper gut motility; it has been used with some success in refractory postoperative ileus.

Surgical Management

- **Surgical consultation** is required when the clinical picture is suggestive of mechanical obstruction or if peritoneal signs are present.
- **Cecostomy** is rarely required when colonoscopic decompression fails in acute colonic distension.
- Surgical exploration is reserved for acute cases with peritoneal signs, ischemic bowel, or other evidence for perforation.

PANCREATOBILIARY DISORDERS

Acute Pancreatitis

GENERAL PRINCIPLES

Definition

Acute pancreatitis consists of inflammation of the pancreas and peripancreatic tissue from activation of potent pancreatic enzymes within the pancreas, particularly trypsin.

Etiology

The most common causes are alcohol and gallstone disease, accounting for 75% to 80% of all cases. Less common causes include abdominal trauma, hypercalcemia, hypertriglyceridemia, and a variety of drugs. Post endoscopic retrograde cholangiopancreatography (ERCP) pancreatitis occurs in 5% to 10% of patients undergoing ERCP.

DIAGNOSIS

Clinical Presentation

Typical symptoms consist of acute onset epigastric abdominal pain, nausea, and vomiting often exacerbated by food intake. Systemic manifestations can include fever, shortness of breath, altered mental status, anemia, and electrolyte imbalances, especially with severe episodes.

Diagnostic Testing

Laboratories

- Serum **lipase** is more specific and sensitive than serum **amylase,** though both are usually elevated to two to three times the upper limits of normal. These values do not correlate with severity or resolution of symptoms. Patients with renal insufficiency may have elevated enzymes at baseline from impaired clearance.
- A complete blood cell count may demonstrate elevated hemoglobin levels from hemoconcentration; blood urea nitrogen and serum creatinine levels may be elevated.
- Hepatic function testing may identify biliary obstruction as a possible etiology, and a lipid panel may suggest hypertriglyceridemia as the cause of acute pancreatitis.

Imaging

- **Dual-phase (pancreatic protocol) CT scanning** is useful in the initial evaluation of severe acute pancreatitis and is considered the gold standard for diagnosis by some. It should be reserved for patients with severe or prolonged symptoms or if the diagnosis is still unclear (*MCNA 2008;92:889*).
- **MRI with gadolinium** can also be used with at least similar efficacy. It may not be appropriate for patients who are hemodynamically unstable, and should be reserved for patients with contraindications to CT. MRCP is useful to detect a biliary source for pancreatitis before ERCP is performed (*MCNA 2008;92:889*).

TREATMENT

- Aggressive volume repletion with IV fluids must be undertaken, with careful monitoring of fluid balance and awareness of the potential for significant fluid sequestration within the abdomen. Serum electrolytes, calcium, and glucose levels should be monitored and supplemented as necessary. Patients with severe pancreatitis with hemodynamic instability often require admission to the ICU.
- Urine output, hemodynamics, and laboratory parameters help assess adequacy of volume repletion.
- Patients should receive **nothing by mouth** until they are free of pain and nausea. NG suction is reserved for patients with ileus or protracted emesis. TPN may be necessary when inflammation is slow to resolve (around 7 days) or if an ileus is present. Enteral nutrition through a tube placed distal to the ligament of Treitz is usually tolerated, and is safer and more cost-effective than TPN (*SCNA 2007;87: 1403*).
- **Acid suppression** may be necessary in severely ill patients with risk factors for stress ulcer bleeding (see Gastrointestinal Bleeding), though has not been shown to decrease symptom duration or severity (*Gastroenterology 2007;132:2022*).
- Ranson criteria (Table 4) may provide prognostic information.

Medications

- **Narcotic analgesics** are usually necessary for pain relief.
  - **Dilaudid** is often used initially, but other narcotic analgesics (e.g., **meperidine**) are alternatives. **Patient-controlled analgesia** is frequently necessary for adequate relief of pain.
- Prophylactic antibiotics are not indicated in the absence of any signs or symptoms of systemic infection.

Table 4	Ranson Criteria for Severity Assessment in Acute Pancreatitis[a]	
	Alcoholic Pancreatitis	**Nonalcoholic Pancreatitis**
On admission		
Age	>55 yr	>70 yr
WBC count	>16,000/mcL	>18,000/mcL
Blood glucose	>200 mg/dL	>220 mg/dL
LDH	>350 International Units/L	>400 International Units/L
AST	>250 units/L	>440 units/L
During the first 48 hr of admission		
Fall in hematocrit	>10%	>10%
Serum calcium	<8 mg/dL	<8 mg/dL
Base deficit	>4.0 mEq/L	>5.0 mEq/L
Increase in blood urea	>5 mg/dL	>2 mg/dL
Fluid sequestration	>6 L	>6 L
Arterial PO$_2$	<60 mm Hg	<60 mm Hg

AST, aspartate aminotransferase; LDH, lactic dehydrogenase; PO$_2$, oxygen tension; WBC, white blood cell.
[a]The presence of three or more criteria indicates severe pancreatitis.

Other Nonoperative Therapies

Endoscopic therapy. Urgent **ERCP and biliary sphincterotomy** within 72 hours of presentation can improve the outcome of severe gallstone pancreatitis in the presence of elevated liver numbers and/or a dilated common bile duct. This is thought to result from reduced biliary sepsis rather than true improvement of pancreatic inflammation.

COMPLICATIONS

- **Necrotizing pancreatitis** represents a severe form of acute pancreatitis, usually identified on dynamic dual-phase CT scanning with IV contrast. The presence of radiologically identified pancreatic necrosis increases the morbidity and mortality of acute pancreatitis. Increasing abdominal pain, fever, marked leukocytosis, and bacteremia suggest infected pancreatic necrosis that requires broad-spectrum antibiotics and often surgical debridement. **Carbapenems** or a combination of a **fluoroquinolone** and **metronidazole** have good penetration into necrotic tissue. CT-guided percutaneous aspiration for Gram stain and culture can confirm the diagnosis of infected necrosis. Surgical debridement is required in severe cases.
- The presence of **pseudocysts** is suggested by persistent pain or high amylase levels. Complications include infection, hemorrhage, rupture (pancreatic ascites), and obstruction of adjacent structures. Generally, asymptomatic nonenlarging pseudocysts can be followed clinically with serial imaging studies, and tend to resolve within a few weeks. Decompression of symptomatic or infected pseudocysts can be performed by percutaneous, endoscopic, or surgical techniques (*Gastrointest Endosc Clin N Am 2007;17:559*).

- **Infection.** Potential sources of fever include pancreatic necrosis, abscess, infected pseudocyst, cholangitis, and aspiration pneumonia. Cultures should be obtained, and broad-spectrum antimicrobials appropriate for bowel flora should be administered. In the absence of fever or other clinical evidence for infection, prophylactic antimicrobial therapy has no clear role in acute pancreatitis.
- **Pulmonary complications.** Atelectasis, pleural effusion, pneumonia, and acute respiratory distress syndrome can develop in severely ill patients (see Chapter 7, Pulmonary Diseases).
- **Renal failure.** Severe intravascular volume depletion or acute tubular necrosis can cause renal failure.
- **Other complications.** Metabolic complications include hypocalcemia, hypomagnesemia, and hyperglycemia. GI bleeding can result from stress gastritis, pseudoaneurysm rupture, or gastric varices from splenic vein thrombosis.

Chronic Pancreatitis

GENERAL PRINCIPLES

Definition

- Chronic pancreatitis represents inflammation, fibrosis, and atrophy of acinar cells resulting from recurrent acute or chronic inflammation of the pancreas.
- Most commonly seen with chronic alcohol abuse, it can also result from dyslipidemia, hypercalcemia, autoimmune disease, and exposure to various toxins. An inherited form is rarely seen (*Gastroenterology 2007;132:1557*).

DIAGNOSIS

Clinical Presentation

Chronic abdominal pain, exocrine insufficiency from acinar cell injury and fibrosis (manifesting as weight loss, and steatorrhea), and **endocrine insufficiency** from destruction of islet cells (manifesting as brittle diabetes) are the main clinical manifestations.

Diagnostic Testing

Laboratories
- **Lipase** and **amylase** may be elevated but are frequently normal and are nonspecific. **Bilirubin, alkaline phosphatase,** and **transaminases** may be elevated if there is concomitant biliary obstruction. A **lipid panel** and **serum calcium** should also be assessed.
- Pancreatic function testing (such as secretin stimulation, fecal fat, and fecal elastase) can be obtained but are not widely available and difficult to perform. In the presence of steatorrhea, a serum trypsinogen level of <20 ng/mL is diagnostic of chronic pancreatitis with exocrine insufficiency (*Am Fam Physician 2007;76:1679*).

Imaging
- Calcification of the pancreas can be seen on plain films and ultrasound. Contrast-enhanced CT has a sensitivity of 75% to 90% and a specificity of 85% for the

diagnosis of chronic pancreatitis, while MRCP is equivalent and a suitable alternative (*Gastroenterology 2007;132:1557*). ERCP is comparatively sensitive and specific but is rarely used because of invasiveness and associated complications.

- **Endoscopic ultrasound** has higher sensitivity (97%) at the cost of lower specificity (60%) for the diagnosis of chronic pancreatitis. It is useful for evaluating lesions concerning for neoplasia in the setting of chronic pancreatitis.

TREATMENT

Medications

- **Narcotic analgesics** are frequently required for control of pain, and narcotic dependence is common. **Neuromodulators** (TCAs, SSRIs) may improve symptoms and decrease reliance on narcotics. In patients with mild to moderate exocrine insufficiency, the addition of oral pancreatic enzyme supplements may be beneficial for pain control.
- **Pancreatic enzyme supplements** are the mainstay of management of pancreatic exocrine insufficiency, in conjunction with a low-fat diet (<50 g fat/d). Enteric-coated preparations (Pancrease or Creon, one to two capsules with meals) are stable at acid pH and should not be given with concomitant acid suppression.
- **Fat-soluble vitamin** supplementation may be necessary, while use of antioxidants may improve symptoms.
- **Insulin** therapy is generally required for endocrine insufficiency, as the resultant diabetes mellitus is characteristically brittle and thus unresponsive to oral agents.
- When identified, treatment of the underlying disorder (e.g., hyperparathyroidism, dyslipidemia) is indicated. Alcohol cessation should be advised.

Other Nonoperative Therapies

- Patients with pancreatic duct obstruction from stones, strictures, or papillary stenosis may benefit from **ERCP and sphincterotomy.**
- Intractable pain may necessitate **celiac ganglion block** or even surgery, such as a **Whipple's procedure.**

Gallstone Disease

GENERAL PRINCIPLES

Definition

- **Asymptomatic gallstones (cholelithiasis)** is a common incidental finding for which no specific therapy is generally necessary. Cholesterol stones are the most common type, but pigmented stones can be seen with hemolysis or infection. Risk factors include obesity, female gender, and family history.
- **Symptomatic cholelithiasis,** when upper abdominal symptoms are thought to be related to the presence of gallstones, is typically treated surgically with cholecystectomy.
- **Acute cholecystitis** is caused most often by obstruction of the cystic duct by gallstones, but acalculous cholecystitis can occur in severely ill or hospitalized patients.

DIAGNOSIS

Clinical Presentation

- Cholelithiasis may present as **biliary colic,** a constant pain lasting for hours, located in the right upper quadrant, radiating to the back or right shoulder, and sometimes associated with nausea or vomiting.
- Other presentations of gallstone disease include acute cholecystitis, acute pancreatitis, and cholangitis. Gallstone disease may rarely be associated with gallbladder cancer.
- Patients with **acute ascending cholangitis** present with right upper quadrant pain, fever with chills, and jaundice (Charcot's triad), usually in the setting of biliary obstruction (choledocholithiasis, neoplasia, sclerosing cholangitis, biliary stent occlusion). Elderly patients may lack abdominal symptoms.

Diagnostic Testing

Imaging

- **Ultrasound scans** have a high degree of accuracy in diagnosis (sensitivity and specificity >95%) and form the preferred initial test.
- Hydroxy iminodiacetic acid **(HIDA)** scan can demonstrate nonfilling of the gallbladder in patients with acute cholecystitis.

TREATMENT

Other Nonoperative Therapies

- **Supportive measures** include IV fluid resuscitation and broad-spectrum antimicrobial agents, especially in the event of complications such as acute cholecystitis with sepsis, perforation, peritonitis, abscess, or empyema formation.
- Percutaneous cholecystotomy and decompression of the gallbladder can be performed under fluoroscopy in severely ill patients with acute cholecystitis who are not surgical candidates.
- **Ursodeoxycholic acid** (8 to 10 mg/kg/d PO in two to three divided doses for prolonged periods) might be prudent in a small select group of patients with small cholesterol stones in normally functioning gallbladders who are at high risk for complications from surgical therapy. Side effects include diarrhea and reversible elevation in serum transaminase levels.

Surgical Management

Cholecystectomy is the therapy of choice for symptomatic gallstone disease and acute cholecystitis. Laparoscopic cholecystectomy compares favorably with the open procedure, with lower morbidity, lower cost, shorter hospital stay, and better cosmetic results (*Lancet 2006;368:230–239*).

COMPLICATIONS

- **Acute pancreatitis.** See section on acute pancreatitis above.
- **Choledocholithiasis.** In patients who have undergone cholecystectomy, retained common bile duct stones can complicate the postoperative course. Common bile duct obstruction, jaundice, biliary colic, cholangitis, or pancreatitis can result. The diagnosis can be made on ultrasonography, CT scanning, or magnetic resonance cholangiography. ERCP with sphincterotomy and stone extraction is curative.

- **Acute ascending cholangitis** represents a medical emergency with high morbidity and mortality if biliary decompression is not performed urgently. The condition should be stabilized with IV fluids and broad-spectrum antibiotics. Drainage of the biliary tree can be performed through the endoscopic (ERCP with sphincterotomy) or percutaneous approach under fluoroscopic guidance.

OTHER GASTROINTESTINAL DISORDERS

Anorectal Disorders

GENERAL PRINCIPLES

- **Thrombosed external hemorrhoids** present as acutely painful, tense, bluish lumps covered with skin in the anal area. The thrombosed hemorrhoid can be surgically excised under local anesthesia for relief of severe pain. In less severe cases, oral analgesics, sitz baths (sitting in a tub of warm water), stool softeners, and topical ointments may provide symptomatic relief (*BMJ 2008;336:380*).
- **Internal hemorrhoids** commonly present with either bleeding or a prolapsing mass with straining. Bulk-forming agents such as fiber supplements are useful in preventing straining at defecation. Sitz baths and Tucks pads (cotton soaked in witch hazel) may provide symptomatic relief. Ointments and suppositories that contain topical analgesics, emollients, astringents, and hydrocortisone (e.g., Anusol-HC Suppositories, one per rectum bid for 7 to 10 days) may decrease edema, but do not reduce bleeding. Hemorrhoidectomy or band ligation can be curative and is indicated in patients with recurrent or constant bleeding (*BMJ 2008;336:380*).
- **Anal fissures** present with acute onset of pain during defecation and are often caused by passage of hard stool. Anoscopy reveals an elliptical tear in the skin of the anus, usually in the posterior midline. Acute fissures generally heal in 2 to 3 weeks with the use of stool softeners, oral or topical analgesics, and sitz baths. Topical nitroglycerin ointment, 0.2%, applied three times a day may be beneficial. Chronic fissures often require surgical therapy.
- **Perirectal abscess** commonly presents as a painful induration in the perianal area. Patients with IBD and immunocompromised states are particularly susceptible. Prompt drainage is essential to avoid the serious morbidity associated with delayed treatment. Antimicrobials directed against bowel flora (metronidazole, 500 mg PO tid, and ciprofloxacin, 500 mg PO bid) should be administered in patients with significant inflammation, systemic toxicity, or immunocompromised states.

Celiac Sprue

GENERAL PRINCIPLES

Definition

- Celiac sprue is a sensitivity to gluten, the protein found in wheat, barley, and rye. The resulting chronic inflammation in the small-bowel mucosa causes malabsorption of dietary nutrients.
- Clinical presentation can vary greatly from asymptomatic iron-deficiency anemia to significant diarrhea and weight loss. Other presenting features can include

osteoporosis, dermatitis herpetiformis, abnormal liver enzymes, and abdominal pain; incidental recognition at endoscopy can also occur (*NEJM 2007;357:1731*).

DIAGNOSIS

Diagnostic Testing

Laboratories
- Noninvasive serologic tests are highly sensitive and specific. Both IgA antiendomysial antibodies and antitissue transglutaminase antibodies have accuracies close to 100% (*NEJM 2007;357:1731*). Quantitative IgA levels should be checked; IgG antibodies against tissue transglutaminase are checked if the patient is IgA deficient.
- Endoscopic biopsy confirmation of the diagnosis is recommended. Classic biopsy findings include blunting or complete absence of villi and a prominent intraepithelial lymphocytosis.
- Almost all patients with celiac sprue carry HLA DQ2 and HLA DQ8 molecules, so absence of these alleles has high negative predictive value when the diagnosis is in question (*Gastroenterology 2006;131:1981*).

TREATMENT

- A gluten-free diet results in prompt improvement in symptoms. Dietary nonadherence is the most frequent cause for persistent symptoms.
- If symptoms persist despite strict gluten-free diet, radiologic and endoscopic evaluation of the small bowel should be performed to rule out complications including collagenous colitis and **small-bowel lymphoma.**

Medications

- Patients may require iron, folate, calcium, and vitamin supplements.
- **Corticosteroids** (prednisone, 10 to 20 mg/d) may be required in refractory cases; immunosuppressive drugs and infliximab have also been used (*NEJM 2007;357: 1731*).

Diverticulosis and Diverticulitis

GENERAL PRINCIPLES

Definition

- **Diverticula** consist of outpouchings in the bowel, most commonly in the colon, but also rarely seen elsewhere in the gut.
- **Diverticular bleeding** can rarely occur from an artery at the mouth of the diverticulum. See segment on Gastrointestinal Bleeding for further details.
- **Diverticulitis** results from microperforation of a diverticulum and resultant extracolonic or intramural inflammation.

DIAGNOSIS

Clinical Presentation

- Diverticulosis is most frequently asymptomatic. Though diverticulosis may be found in patients being investigated for symptoms of abdominal pain and altered bowel habits, a causal link is difficult to establish.

- Typical symptoms of diverticulitis include left lower quadrant abdominal pain, fevers and chills, and alteration of bowel habits. Localized left lower quadrant abdominal tenderness may be elicited on physical examination.

Diagnostic Testing

Laboratories

Diverticulitis may be associated with an elevated white blood cell (WBC) count with a left shift.

Imaging
- Diverticula are frequently seen on screening colonoscopy.
- Imaging studies, most commonly CT scans, are useful in the diagnosis of diverticulitis.
- Colonoscopy is contraindicated for 4 to 6 weeks after an episode of acute diverticulitis but should be performed after that interval to exclude a perforated neoplasm.

TREATMENT

- Increased dietary fiber is generally recommended in patients with diverticulosis, although no hard data exist to support its benefit. No data exist to support exclusion of nuts and popcorn from the diet to prevent acute diverticulitis.
- A low-residue diet is recommended for mild diverticulitis. Oral feedings are withheld in complicated diverticulitis, and parenteral nutrition may be necessary if protracted.

Medications
- Oral **antibiotics** (e.g., ciprofloxacin, 500 mg PO bid, and metronidazole, 500 mg PO tid for 10 to 14 days) may suffice for mild diverticulitis.
- Hospital admission, bowel rest, IV fluids, and broad-spectrum IV antimicrobial agents are typically required in moderate to severe cases.

Surgical Management
- Surgical consultation should be obtained early in moderate to severe diverticulitis, as operative intervention may be necessary should complications arise.
- Surgical resection may also be necessary in recurrent diverticulitis, typically after ≥3 recurrences at the same location.

Gastroparesis

GENERAL PRINCIPLES

Definition

Gastroparesis consists of abnormally delayed emptying of stomach contents into the small bowel in the absence of mechanical obstruction, usually as a result of damage to the nerves or smooth muscle involved in gastric emptying (*AJG 2006;127:287*).

Etiology

- Gastroparesis can result from chronic disorders (diabetes mellitus, scleroderma, intestinal pseudo-obstruction, previous gastric surgery) or, less frequently, from acute metabolic derangements (hypokalemia, hypercalcemia, hypocalcemia, hyperglycemia) or medications (narcotic analgesics, anticholinergic agents, chemotherapy agents);

it is designated idiopathic when a predisposing cause is not identified (*Gastroenterology 2004;127:1589*).
- Mechanical obstruction should always be excluded.

DIAGNOSIS

Clinical Presentation

Symptoms include nausea, bloating, and vomiting, usually hours after a meal.

Diagnostic Testing

Imaging
- A gastric-emptying study consisting of gamma camera scanning after a radiolabeled meal can help with the diagnosis.
- Endoscopic evidence of retained food debris in the stomach after an overnight fast may be an indirect indicator of delayed gastric emptying.

TREATMENT

- Underlying metabolic derangements should be corrected. In particular, precise glucose control using short-acting insulin preparations may improve emptying in early stages of diabetic gastroparesis (*CGH 2005;3:642*).
- High-fat and insoluble fiber in meals can further delay gastric emptying, and should be avoided.
- High-calorie liquid iso-osmotic meals may be beneficial in refractory situations.

Medications

- **Prokinetic agents** have been used with varying degrees of success.
- **Metoclopramide** (10 mg PO qid half an hour before meals) has variable efficacy, and side effects (drowsiness, tardive dyskinesia, parkinsonism) may be limiting.
- **Domperidone** (20 mg PO qid before meals and at bedtime) does not cross the blood–brain barrier, but hyperprolactinemia can result. This medication is not universally available.
- **Erythromycin** (125 to 250 mg PO tid or 200 mg IV) is a motilin receptor agonist and stimulates gastric motility, but tachyphylaxis, abdominal pain, and nausea limit long-term therapy.

Surgical Management

- **Enteral feeding** through a jejunostomy feeding tube may be required for supplemental nutrition and is favored over total parental nutrition.
- **Gastric electrical stimulation** using a surgically implanted stimulator may reduce symptoms of nausea and vomiting in half of medically refractory patients, but gastric emptying is typically not enhanced by this approach (*Gastroenterology 2008;134:665*).

Ischemic Instestinal Injury

GENERAL PRINCIPLES

- Acute mesenteric ischemia results from arterial (or rarely venous) compromise to the superior mesenteric circulation.

- Emboli and thrombus formation are the most common causes of acute mesenteric ischemia, although **nonocclusive mesenteric ischemia** from vasoconstriction can also give rise to the disorder.
- Ischemic colitis results from mucosal ischemia in the inferior mesenteric circulation during a low-flow state (hypotension, arrhythmias, sepsis, aortic vascular surgery) in patients with atherosclerotic disease (*Gastroenterology 2000;118:951*).
- Vasculitis, sickle cell disease, vasospasm, and marathon running can also predispose to ischemic colitis.

DIAGNOSIS

Clinical Presentation

- Patients with acute mesenteric ischemia may present with abdominal pain, but physical examination and imaging studies can be unremarkable until infarction has occurred. As a result, diagnosis is late and mortality is high.
- Ischemic colitis may manifest as transient bleeding or diarrhea; severe insults can lead to stricture formation, gangrene, and perforation.

Diagnostic Testing

Imaging

- Urgent angiography is indicated if the suspicion for acute mesenteric ischemia is high.
- In patients with ischemic colitis, characteristic "thumbprinting" of the involved colon may be seen on plain radiographs of the abdomen.
- Colonoscopy may reveal mucosal erythema, edema, and ulceration, sometimes in a linear configuration; evidence of gangrene or necrosis is an indication for surgical intervention.

TREATMENT

- Treatment of acute mesenteric ischemia is essentially surgical.
- In patients with ischemic colitis, in the absence of peritoneal signs or evidence of gangrene or perforation, expectant management with fluid and electrolyte repletion, broad-spectrum antimicrobials, and maintenance of adequate hemodynamics usually suffices.
- Evidence of gangrene or necrosis in the setting of ischemic colitis is an indication for surgery (*Gastroenterology 2000;118:951*).

Liver Diseases

Anil B. Seetharam and Mauricio Lisker-Melman

Evaluation of Liver Disease

GENERAL PRINCIPLES

- Liver disease can present as a spectrum of clinical conditions that ranges from asymptomatic disease to end-stage liver disease (ESLD).
- A comprehensive investigation combining thorough history and physical examination combined with diagnostic tests, liver histology, and imaging, can often establish a precise diagnosis.

DIAGNOSIS

Clinical Presentation

History

History taking should be focused on the following:

- History of present illnesses
- Medicine usage and toxin exposure (including alcohol)
- Associated symptoms—development of swelling, screening for encephalopathy, gastrointestinal (GI) bleeding
- Family history of liver disease
- Dietary habits
- Risk factors for infection: that is, intravenous/intranasal drug use, body piercings, tattooing, sexual history, travel to foreign countries, occupation

Physical Examination
- Detailed physical exam is necessary. Physical stigmata of acute and chronic liver disease may be subtle or absent.
  - Assess for icterus
  - Ascites—shifting dullness; peripheral edema
  - Hepatomegaly and splenomegaly
  - Gynecomastia, testicular hypotrophy
  - Muscle wasting
  - Telangiectasias, palmar erythema, pubic hair changes
- Specific liver disorders may be associated with distinctive physical abnormalities: that is, arthritis, acne, skin color changes, Kayser–Fleischer rings, clubbing, S3 gallop.

Diagnostic Testing

Laboratories
- **Serum enzymes.** Hepatic disorders associated predominantly with elevation in **aminotransferases** are referred to as **hepatocellular**; hepatic disorders with predominant elevation in **alkaline phosphatase (ALP)** are referred to as **cholestatic**.
  - Elevation of **serum aspartate and alanine aminotransferases (AST and ALT, respectively)** indicates hepatocellular injury and necrosis. Markedly elevated levels

(>1,000 U/L) typically occur with acute hepatocellular injury (e.g., viral, drug induced, or ischemic), whereas mild to moderate elevations may be seen in a variety of conditions (e.g., acute or chronic hepatocellular injury, infiltrative diseases, biliary obstruction). The ratio of serum AST to ALT is typically >2 in alcoholic liver disease. In viral hepatitis, this ratio is characteristically <1.

- **ALP** is an enzyme that is present in a variety of tissues (bone, intestine, kidney, leukocytes, liver, and placenta). The concomitant elevation of other hepatic enzymes (e.g., **γ-glutamyl transpeptidase [GGT] or 5′-nucleotidase**) assists in establishing the hepatic origin of ALP. Serum ALP level is often elevated in biliary obstruction, space-occupying lesions or infiltrative disorders of the liver, and conditions that cause intrahepatic cholestasis (primary biliary cirrhosis [PBC], primary sclerosing cholangitis [PSC], drug-induced cholestasis). The degree of elevation of ALP does not differentiate the site or cause of cholestasis.

- **GGT** is an enzyme that is present in a variety of tissues. Increases in GGT and ALP tend to occur in similar hepatic diseases. GGT may be elevated in individuals who ingest barbiturates, phenytoin, or alcohol even when other liver enzyme and bilirubin levels are normal.

- **5′-Nucleotidase** is comparable to ALP in sensitivity in detecting biliary obstruction, cholestasis, and infiltrative hepatobiliary diseases.

- **Synthetic products**
  - **Serum albumin** concentration is frequently decreased in chronic liver disease. However, chronic inflammation, expanded plasma volume, and GI or renal losses can also lead to hypoalbuminemia. Because the half-life of albumin is relatively long (20 days), serum levels may be normal in acute liver disease.
  - Several important proteins involved in **hemostasis** and **fibrinolysis** (coagulation factors: α_2-antiplasmin, antithrombin, heparin cofactor II, high-molecular-weight kininogen, prekallikrein, protein C and S) are synthesized by the liver. The synthesis of factors II, VII, IX, and X and proteins C and S depends on the presence of vitamin K. The adequacy of hepatic synthetic function can be estimated by the **prothrombin time (PT)** and the **international normalized ratio (INR)**. PT/INR prolongation may result from impaired coagulation factor synthesis or vitamin K deficiency. Normalization of PT/INR after administration of vitamin K indicates vitamin K deficiency.
  - **Cholesterol** is synthesized in the liver. Patients with advanced liver disease may have very low cholesterol levels. However, in PBC, levels of serum cholesterol may be markedly elevated.
  - Other synthetic products whose levels can be measured in specific liver diseases are α_1-**antitrypsin and ceruloplasmin.**

- **Excretory products**
  - **Bilirubin** is a degradation product of hemoglobin and nonerythroid hemoproteins (e.g., cytochromes, catalases). Total serum bilirubin is composed of **conjugated (direct)** and **unconjugated (indirect)** fractions. Unconjugated hyperbilirubinemia occurs as a result of **excessive bilirubin production** (neonatal or physiologic jaundice, hemolysis and hemolytic anemias, ineffective erythropoiesis, and resorption of hematomas), **reduced hepatic bilirubin uptake** (Gilbert's syndrome and drugs such as rifampin and probenecid), or **impaired bilirubin conjugation** (Gilbert's or Crigler–Najjar syndrome). Elevation of conjugated and unconjugated fractions occurs in Dubin–Johnson's and Rotor's syndromes and in conditions associated with **intrahepatic** (from hepatocellular, canalicular, or ductular damage) and **extrahepatic** (from mechanical obstruction) **cholestasis.**

- **Bile acids** are produced in the liver and are secreted into the intestine, where they are required for lipid digestion and absorption. Elevated levels of serum bile acids are specific but not sensitive markers of hepatobiliary disease. Levels of individual bile acids are not useful in the differential diagnosis of liver disorders. Bile acid determination is uncommon in the regular workup of patients with liver disease.
- **α-Fetoprotein (AFP)** is normally produced by fetal liver cells. Its production falls to normal adult levels of <10 ng/mL within 1 year of life. AFP is an insensitive marker for hepatocellular carcinoma (HCC). One-third of HCCs have no increase in AFP level and only 30% have an AFP level > 50 ng/mL (*Aliment Pharmacol Ther 2007;26:1187*). Levels of >400 ng/mL or a rapid doubling time are suggestive of HCC; mild to moderate elevations can also be seen in acute and chronic liver inflammation.

Imaging

- **Ultrasonography** is used to screen for dilation of the biliary tree and to detect gallstones and cholecystitis in patients with right-sided abdominal pain associated with abnormal liver blood tests. It can reveal and characterize liver masses, abscesses, and cysts. Color flow Doppler ultrasonography can assess patency and direction of blood flow in the portal and hepatic veins. Ultrasonography is a frequently used modality for screening of HCC; however, this modality is less sensitive (tumors with diameters < 2 cm) for the detection of HCC compared with CT or MRI.
- **Helical computed tomography (CT)** scan with IV contrast is useful in the evaluation of parenchymal liver disease. It has the added feature of contrast enhancement to define space-occupying lesions (e.g., abscess and tumor) and allows calculation of liver volume. Triple-phase CT (noncontrast, arterial phase, and venous phase) is indicated for liver mass evaluation. A delayed phase is useful when cholangiocarcinoma is suspected.
- **Magnetic resonance imaging (MRI)** offers information similar to that provided by CT scan with the additional advantage of better characterization of liver lesions, fatty infiltration, and iron deposition. It is the modality of choice in patients with an allergy to iodinated contrast.
- **Magnetic resonance cholangiopancreatography (MRCP)** is a specialized version of MRI that provides an alternative noninvasive diagnostic modality for visualizing the intra- and extrahepatic bile ducts.
- **Positron emission tomography (PET)** is a modality that uses differences in metabolism among normal, inflammatory, and malignant tissues. PET scans are helpful in assessing the presence of hepatic metastasis in colorectal cancer. PET scans may also be helpful in diagnosing cholangiocarcinoma.

Diagnostic Procedures

- **Percutaneous transhepatic cholangiography (PTC) and endoscopic retrograde cholangiopancreatography (ERCP)** involve the instillation of contrast into the biliary tree. They are most useful after the preliminary determination of abnormalities detected by ultrasonography, CT, or MRI/MRCP. These procedures allow for diagnostic and therapeutic maneuvers including biopsy, brushings, stenting, and placement of drains.
- **Percutaneous liver biopsy** is an invasive procedure that can be performed with or without radiographic (ultrasound or CT) guidance. In the presence of coagulopathy, thrombocytopenia, and/or ascites, a biopsy can be obtained by the transjugular route. Suspicious liver lesions are usually biopsied with ultrasonographic or CT guidance.

Laparoscopy is an alternative method for obtaining liver tissue. Percutaneous liver biopsy is generally safe and is usually performed as an outpatient procedure. Bleeding, pain, infection, injury to neighboring organs, and (rarely) death are potential complications.

- Noninvasive testing to assess fibrosis/cirrhosis: for example, aspartate aminotransferase to platelet ratio index (APRI), FibroTest, transient elastography, and MR spectroscopy are under investigation and at this point they should be viewed as complementary to liver biopsy.

VIRAL HEPATITIS

The hepatotropic viruses include hepatitis A virus (HAV), hepatitis B virus (HBV), hepatitis C virus (HCV), hepatitis D virus (HDV), and hepatitis E virus (HEV) (Tables 1 and 2). Nonhepatotropic viruses (viruses that indirectly affect the liver) include Epstein–Barr virus, cytomegalovirus, herpes virus, measles, Ebola, and others.

Acute viral hepatitis is defined by the sudden onset of significant aminotransferase elevation as a consequence of diffuse necroinflammatory liver injury. Symptoms may be variable. This condition may resolve or progress to fulminant hepatic failure (FHF) or chronic hepatitis.

Chronic viral hepatitis is defined as the presence of persistent (at least 6 months) necroinflammatory and fibrotic injury. Histopathologic classification of chronic viral hepatitis is based on etiology, grade, and stage. Grading and staging are measures of the severity of the necroinflammatory process and fibrosis, respectively. Chronic viral hepatitis may lead to cirrhosis and HCC.

Hepatitis A Virus

GENERAL PRINCIPLES

Classification

HAV is an **RNA virus** that belongs to the **picornavirus family.**

Etiology

- HAV is the most common cause of viral hepatitis worldwide.
- Approximately 30% of acute viral hepatitis in the United States is caused by HAV.

Pathophysiology

- HAV infection is usually transmitted via **the fecal–oral route.**
- Large-scale outbreaks due to contamination of food and drinking water can occur.
- The period of greatest infectivity is 2 weeks before the onset of clinical illness; fecal shedding continues for 2 to 3 weeks after the onset of symptoms.
- Although the period of viremia is brief, sexual transmission and parenteral transmission may occur.

Risk Factors

High-risk groups include people living in or traveling to developing countries (food and water contamination), men having sex with men, users of injection and noninjection drugs, patients with clotting factor disorders, persons working with nonhuman

Table 1	Clinical and Epidemiologic Features of Hepatotropic Viruses				
Organism	**Hepatitis A**	**Hepatitis B**	**Hepatitis C**	**Hepatitis D**	**Hepatitis E**
Incubation	15–45 d	30–180 d	15–150 d	30–150 d	30–60 d
Transmission	Fecal–oral	Blood	Blood	Blood	Fecal–oral
		Sexual	Sexual (rare)	Sexual (rare)	
		Perinatal	Perinatal (rare)		
Risk groups	Residents of and travelers to endemic regions	Injection drug users	Injection drug users	Any person with hepatitis B virus	Residents of and travelers to endemic regions
	Children and caregivers in daycare centers	Multiple sexual partners	Transfusion recipients	Injection drug users	
		Men having sex with men			
		Infants born to infected mothers			
		Health care workers			
		Transfusion recipients			
Fatality rate	1.0%	1.0%	<0.1%	2–10%	1%
Carrier state	No	Yes	Yes	Yes	No
Chronic hepatitis	None	2–10% in adults; 90% in children <5 yr	70–85%	Variable	None
Cirrhosis	No	Yes	Yes	Yes	No

Table 2	Viral Hepatitis Serologies			
Hepatitis	**Acute**	**Chronic**	**Recovered/Latent**	**Vaccinated**
HAV	IgM anti-HAV+	NA	IgG anti-HAV+	IgG anti-HAV+
HBV	IgM anti-HBc+ HBeAg+ HBsAg+ HBV DNA+	IgG anti-HBc+ HBeAg ± Anti-HBe ± [a] HBsAg+ HBV DNA ± [a]	IgG anti-HBc+ HBeAg– Anti-HBe ± [a] HBsAg– Anti-HBs Ab+ HBV DNA-	Anti-HBs+ only
HCV	All tests possibly negative HCV RNA+ Anti-HCV Ab+ in 8–10 wk	Anti-HCV Ab+ HCV RNA+	Anti-HCV Ab+ HCV RNA–[b]	NA
HDV	IgM anti-HDV+[c] HDV Ag+[c]	IgG anti-HDV+[c]	IgG anti-HDV+[c]	NA[d]
HEV	Available from CDC and research specialty laboratories	NA	Available from CDC and research specialty laboratories	NA

Ab, antibody; CDC, Centers for Disease Control and Prevention; HAV, hepatitis A virus; HBc, hepatitis B core antigen; HBeAg, hepatitis B e antigen; HBsAg, hepatitis B surface antigen; HBV, hepatitis B virus; HCV, hepatitis C virus; HDV, hepatitis D virus; HEV, hepatitis E virus; NA, not applicable.
[a]HBeAg is present during periods of high replication along with HBV DNA. Anti-HBe is present during periods of low replication when HBeAg and HBV DNA may be undetectable.
[b]Negative HCV RNA results should be interpreted with caution. Differences are found in thresholds for detection among assays and among laboratories.
[c]Markers of HBV infection are also present, because HDV cannot replicate in the absence of HBV.
[d]Although no vaccine is available for HDV, immunity to HBV protects against HDV infection.

primates, staff and attendees at daycare centers, and patients with chronic liver disease (increased risk for fulminant hepatitis A).

Prevention

Immunization programs are available (see Treatment section).

DIAGNOSIS

- The diagnosis of acute HAV is made by the detection of **IgM anti-HAV antibody.**
- Aminotransferase elevations range from 10 to 100 times the upper limit of the reference range.
- The **recovery phase** and **immunity phase** are characterized by **IgG anti-HAV antibody.**
- Liver biopsy is rarely needed.

Clinical Presentation

- HAV can be silent (subclinical), especially in children and young adults. Symptoms vary from mild illness to FHF.
- Malaise, fatigue, pruritus, headache, abdominal pain, myalgias, arthralgias, nausea, vomiting, anorexia, and fever are common but nonspecific symptoms.

History

History should include a review of symptoms, temporal course of illness, and assessment for any potential exposures from traveling to developing countries or food and water ingestion.

Physical Examination

Physical examination may reveal jaundice, hepatomegaly, and in rare cases lymphadenopathy, splenomegaly, or a vascular rash.

TREATMENT

- No specific treatment is available.
- Supportive symptomatic treatment is recommended.
- Liver transplantation may be an option for FHF.

Medications
- **Preexposure prophylaxis**
  - **HAV vaccine.** Inactivated HAV vaccines (containing the single HAV antigen) and combination vaccines (containing both HAV and hepatitis B antigens) are available. Vaccinations should be administered intramuscularly into the deltoid muscle in a two-dose regimen (single-antigen HAV vaccine; first dose at time 0 and second dose at 6 to 18 months) or in a three-dose regimen (combination vaccine; first dose at time 0, second dose at 1 month, and third dose at 6 months).
  - Protective antibody levels are present in 94% to 100% of those immunized 1 month after the first dose (*MMWR Recomm Rep 2006 May 19;55(RR-7):1*).
- **Postexposure prophylaxis**
  - Immune globulin (Ig) is a sterile preparation of concentrated antibody made from pooled human plasma that allows for passive transfer of antibodies.
  - No transmission of hepatitis B, hepatitis C, or HIV has been identified with intramuscular injection of Ig.
  - Ig (0.02 mL/kg IM) should be given as soon as possible after known exposure to HAV. Efficacy beyond 2 weeks after exposure has not been established.
  - Hepatitis A vaccine is not licensed for use as postexposure prophylaxis; however, patients who have been administered one dose of vaccine at more than 1 month prior to exposure do not need Ig.
- If HAV vaccine and Ig are recommended, they may be administered simultaneously at separate injection sites.

OUTCOME/PROGNOSIS

- Almost all cases of acute HAV hepatitis will resolve in 4 to 8 weeks.
- Prolonged cholestatic disease, characterized by persistent jaundice, is more frequently seen in adults.

- **Fulminant liver failure** is relatively rare, but risk increases with age: 0.1% in patients younger than 15 years old to >1% in patients older than 40 years old.
- HAV does not induce chronic hepatitis or cirrhosis.

Hepatitis B Virus

GENERAL PRINCIPLES

Classification

- **HBV** is a **DNA virus** that belongs to the **hepadnavirus family.**
- Eight genotypes of HBV have been identified and labeled A through H.

Epidemiology

- Two billion people worldwide have serological evidence of past or present infection and approximately 400 million people are chronic carriers.
- HBV is unevenly distributed throughout the world. In endemic areas such as Asia and sub-Saharan Africa, infection is usually acquired in childhood, while in Western countries where HBV is relatively rare, the infection is acquired in adulthood.
- The prevalence of HBV genotypes varies depending on the geographical location. All known HBV genotypes have been found in the United States, with genotypes A, B, and C being the most prevalent (*Hepatology 2007;45:507*).
- HBV causes 60% to 80% of HCC worldwide.
- While HBV-related mortality is not known, it is estimated that between 500,000 and 1,000,000 deaths occur worldwide per year.
- HBV is the indication for 5% to 10% of cases of liver transplantation.

Pathophysiology

- The liver damage that ensues after HBV infection is immune mediated.
- Modes of transmission include:
  - Parenteral or percutaneous routes (e.g., needlestick injury, injection drug use, hemodialysis, transfusions)
  - Sexual contact (e.g., men who have sex with men, sexual promiscuity, or intercourse with HBV-infected partners)
- Vertical or perinatal transmission (from mother to infant).

Risk Factors

High-risk groups include individuals with a history of multiple blood transfusions, patients on hemodialysis, injection drug users, sexual promiscuity, men having sex with men, household and heterosexual contacts of hepatitis B carriers, residents and employees of residential care facilities, travelers to endemic regions, and individuals born in areas of high or intermediate prevalence (e.g., Alaska, southern Asia, Africa, south Pacific Islands, the Amazon delta in South America).

Prevention

Immunization programs are available. (See section on treatment.)

Associated Conditions

Extrahepatic manifestations include polyarteritis nodosa, glomerulonephritis, cryoglobulinemia, serum sickness–like illness, papular acrodermatitis (predominantly in children), and aplastic anemia.

DIAGNOSIS

Clinical Presentation

- Incubation period after HBV infection ranges from 30 to 160 days.
- According to the natural history of infection, different **clinical phases** have been defined:
  - **Acute hepatitis B:** Can be silent (subclinical), especially in children and young adults. Symptoms vary from mild illness to FHF. Malaise, fatigue, pruritus, headache, abdominal pain, myalgias, arthralgias, nausea, vomiting, anorexia, and fever are common but nonspecific symptoms. Progression to chronicity depends on age of acquisition. Most acute HBV infections are self-limited in adults.
  - **Chronic hepatitis B** runs an indolent course, sometimes for decades. Fatigue is a common symptom. The disease may only become clinically apparent late in the natural course, with symptoms typically associated with ESLD. Chronic HBV infection is a dynamic process that occurs in different phases:
    - **Immune tolerant:** Characterized by high rates of viral replication, yet normal liver enzymes and low levels of inflammation and fibrosis. This phase is frequently seen in children or those infected early in life. It may last for decades.
    - **Immune active:** Characterized by elevation of liver enzymes as a consequence of a vigorous immune response. During this phase, there is active replication with high levels of HBV DNA and hepatitis B e antigen (HBeAg). Histologic activity is manifested by inflammation and fibrosis. This phase is frequently seen in adults and may last for years.
    - **Carrier state with low replication:** Characterized by low or undetectable HBV DNA levels. Usually, these patients have normal liver enzymes and reduced liver inflammation. These individuals do not have progressive disease and have low risk for progression to the development of HCC. *Serologically, this can be identified by seroconversion from HBeAg to HBeAb.* Reactivation with conversion to immune-active or e-antigen negative phases is possible.
    - **Chronic HBeAg negative:** These patients harbor HBV variants with mutations (pre- or basal-core promoter regions) that prevent the production of or have low expression of HBeAg. Despite the absence of HBeAg, HBV DNA levels are high, liver enzymes are elevated, and there is active histologic activity. This is a late phase in the natural history of chronic HBV. This phase is often seen in older patients with more advanced disease and is usually triggered by frequent periods of reactivation.
- **Resolution:** In this phase, eradication of the virus is evidenced by viral clearance (negative HBV DNA). Antigen to antibody seroconversion is the hallmark of this phase. Seroconversion may occur spontaneously (0.5% clear HBsAg yearly). Patients with resolved HBV have normal liver enzymes and a reduced risk to progress to cirrhosis, cirrhosis with decompensation, or HCC.

History

History should include a thorough investigation of risk factors and review of systems.

Diagnostic Testing

The diagnosis of HBV often requires the combination of data obtained from liver chemistries, serology, molecular biology, and histology.

Laboratories

- Liver chemistries usually abnormal in acute hepatitis include AST, ALT, ALP, and total bilirubin. In chronic HBV, the biochemical changes are variable and aminotransferases may fluctuate ranging from normal to increased levels. Recent studies have recommended newer upper limits of normality for ALT in men and women (30 and 19 U/mL, respectively) (*Liver Int 2006;26:445*).

- Tests that measure cholestasis (ALP, GGT, and total bilirubin) or liver synthetic function (albumin and PT/INR) may be abnormal according to the disease stage.
- HBV contains several genes (S, core, and X) that produce proteins (antigens) that elicit a corresponding antibody response.
  - HBV antigens detected in serum and used for diagnostic purposes in clinical practice include **hepatitis B surface antigen (HBsAg) and hepatitis B e antigen (HBeAg).**
  - HBV antigens detected in liver biopsy by immunoperoxidase staining include HBsAg stained in the hepatocyte cytoplasm and **hepatitis B core antigen (HBcAg)** stained in hepatocyte nuclei.
- HBV antibodies are specific to their corresponding antigen and include:
  - Antibody against HBsAg (anti-HBs), antibody against HBeAg (anti-HBe), and IgM and IgG antibodies against HBcAg (IgM and IgG anti-HBc).
- **HBV viral DNA (HBV DNA)** is the most accurate marker of viral replication. It is detected by polymerase chain reaction (PCR) and reported as copies per milliliter or more commonly as International Units per milliliter. Large long-term population-based studies have demonstrated a close correlation between HBV DNA levels and disease progression to cirrhosis and development of HCC (*Gastroenterology 2006;130:678*; *JAMA 2006;295:65*).
- For use of HBV markers in clinical practice, see Table 3.
- Genotypic determination is growing in clinical significance as data are emerging with respect to response to antivirals, disease progression, and risk of HCC.
  - Genotypes A and B have been associated with higher rates of response to interferon therapy (*Am J Gastroenterol 2006;101:297*).
- Genotype B, most commonly seen in Asia, has been associated with earlier HBeAg seroconversion, less severe liver disease, and lower rates of progression to HCC (*Hepatology 2002;35:1274*).

Diagnostic Procedures

Liver biopsy is useful to score the degree of inflammation (grade) and fibrosis (stage) in patients with chronic hepatitis. At times liver histology is a very important adjuvant diagnostic test in guiding treatment decisions.

TREATMENT

- Preventing the progression to ESLD, HCC, and death with improvement in quality of life are the goals of treatment. End points of treatment include:
  - Clearance of HBV DNA
  - HBeAg and HBsAg seroconversion (i.e., antigen loss and antibody appearance)
  - Normalization of liver enzymes
  - Normalization of histology

Medications

- Seven agents are currently available for the treatment of chronic HBV. They are divided into three main groups: interferon-based therapy (interferon-α [IFN-α] and pegylated interferon-α [pIFN-α]), nucleoside analogs (lamivudine, entecavir, and telbivudine), and nucleotide analogs (adefovir and tenofovir).

Table 3	Use of HBV Markers in Clinical Practice					
	Acute	Resolved Acute	High-Replication	Low-Replication	HBV Precore	Vaccination
Test	Hepatitis B	Hepatitis B	Chronic HBV	Chronic HBV	Mutant	
HBsAg	+	–	+	+	+	–
HBeAg	+	–	+	+	–	–
Anti-HBs	–	+	–	–	–	+
Anti-HBe	–	+	–	+	+	–
IgM anti-HBc	+	–	+	–	–	–
IgG anti-HBc	–	+	+	–	+	–
HBV DNA	$>10^5$ copies/mL	Negative	$>10^5$ copies/mL	10^2–10^4 copies/mL	$>10^4$ copies/mL	Negative
ALT/AST	++	Normal	+++	Normal	+/++	Normal

ALT, alanine transaminase; AST, aspartate transaminase; HBc, hepatitis B core antigen; HBeAg, hepatitis B e antigen; HBsAg, hepatitis B surface antigen; HBV, hepatitis B virus.

- Current indications for treatment include chronic hepatitis B (e-antigen positive and e-antigen negative) with HBV DNA > 2,000 IU/mL (about 10,000 copies/mL) and/or elevated ALT and severe necroinflammation/fibrosis on liver biopsy. Patients with compensated or decompensated cirrhosis should be treated even with normal ALT levels or HBV DNA levels < 2,000 IU/mL (*J Hepatol 2009;50:227*).
- The optimal treatment duration has not yet been defined. When pIFN and ribavirin are used, treatment is typically limited to 1 year. In patients with hepatitis B (e antigen positive), treatment is prolonged 6 months after HBeAg seroconversion, but reactivation is a possibility and has to be monitored. In hepatitis B (e antigen negative), treatment should be continued indefinitely or until HBsAg loss is achieved.
- Immune-tolerant patients and those with slight elevations of ALT and mild histology do not require treatment, but follow-up is obligatory. Therapy is not recommended for carriers with low replication.
- Antiviral resistance is a phenomenon observed with the use of nucleoside and nucleotide analogs. Resistance can be detected by commercially available assays and should be suspected initially after an HBV DNA level rebound ($>1 \log_{10}$) from the lowest level of suppression achieved. Nucleoside and nucleotide analogs with high genetic barrier (lowest susceptibility for resistance) are preferred therapeutic agents.

First Line

Entecavir and tenofovir are the analogs (nucleoside and nucleotide, respectively) with the highest genetic barrier to resistance and therefore are the preferred oral medications for the treatment of chronic HBV.

- **Entecavir (ETV)** is a potent anti-HBV **oral nucleoside (guanosine) analog** and is well tolerated. Dose: 0.5 and 1 mg in naïve and lamivudine-resistant patients. In patients with renal impairment, dose adjustment is needed. Long-term observations in HBeAg-positive patients have demonstrated a cumulative rate of HBV DNA clearance of more than 90% with a very low rate of resistance in treatment-naïve patients after 4 years (*J Hepatol 2007;46(Suppl 1):S294*). Patients resistant to lamivudine are prone to develop rapid antiviral resistance to ETV. Pregnancy category C.
- **Tenofovir (TDF)** is a potent anti-HBV oral nucleotide (acyclic) analogue and is well tolerated. Dose: 300 mg daily. Rarely reported to induce renal failure and Fanconi syndrome. Recent 96-week data in HbeAg-positive and HbeAg-negative patients demonstrated undetectable HBV DNA in 79% and 91%, respectively. No clinical resistance identified at 2 years of treatment (*Hepatology 2008;48:158*; *Hepatology 2008;48:146*). Pregnancy category B.
- **IFN-α** and **pIFN-α** are antiviral, immunomodulatory, and antiproliferative glycoproteins that have been used in the treatment of chronic HBV for several years. Dose: subcutaneous 5 million units (mu) daily or 10 mu three times per week for IFN and 180 mcg for pIFN-α 2a weekly. Interferons are parenteral agents, associated with poor tolerability profile, in particular in patients with advanced liver disease. Long-term studies have shown a durable benefit in responders. Neither IFN or pIFN-α induce antiviral resistance. Pregnancy category C.
  - **pIFN-α** has replaced conventional IFN because of its more convenient once-weekly administration facilitated by longer half-life and bioavailability, given its attachment to a polyethylene glycol molecule. Research trials have combined **pIFN** with oral agents to improve the HBV treatment efficacy. Although results are still preliminary, HBsAg loss occurred at a higher rate when compared with oral nucleoside monotherapy. pIFN is associated with higher HBeAg seroconversion and HBeAg loss in patients with genotypes A and B.

Second Line

- **Telbivudine (LdT)** is an oral nucleoside (thymidine) analog and is well tolerated. Dose: 600mg daily. In patients with renal impairment, dose adjustment is needed. It has potent antiviral activity when compared with lamivudine and adefovir. Its resistance profile is better than lamivudine but worse than the first-line agents. Not useful in patients with antiviral resistance to other nucleoside analogs. Pregnancy category B.
- **Adefovir (ADV)** is an oral nucleotide (adenosine) analogue and is well tolerated. Dose: 10 mg daily. In patients with renal impairment, dose adjustment is needed. Despite its improved resistance profile over lamivudine, this agent does not confer a greater degree of viral suppression. Resistance is up to 29% at 5 years in HBeAg-negative patients (*Gastroenterology 2006;131:1743*). Pregnancy category C.
- **Lamivudine (LAM)** is an oral nucleoside (dideoxy-3′-thiacytidine) analog and is well tolerated. Dose: 100 mg daily. In patients with renal impairment, dose adjustment is needed. First oral drug approved for the treatment of chronic HBV. Treatment success is proportional to treatment duration. Its use has diminished given its high rates of resistant mutations (70% at 5 years of treatment). Not useful in patients with antiviral resistance to other nucleoside analogs. Pregnancy category B.

Other Nonoperative Therapies

- **Preexposure prophylaxis**
  - **HBV vaccine** should be considered for everyone, but particularly in individuals who belong to high-risk groups (see Risk Factors section). HBV vaccines have been demonstrated to be safe.
    - HBsAg is used to prepare the HBV vaccine (single-antigen). The HBV vaccine is also available in combination for the prevention of hepatitis A, *Haemophilus influenza* type B, *Neisseria meningitidis*, diphtheria, tetanus, pertussis, and polio.
  - HBV vaccination schedule includes three intramuscular injections at 0, 1, and 6 months in infants or healthy adults. Protective antibody response is >90% after the third dose. The protective antibody response declines with age. Smoking, obesity, genetics, and immunosuppression can contribute to a decreased protective response from vaccination. Response to vaccination is measured by anti-HBs (≥ 10 mIU/mL).
  - Prevaccination screening for previous exposure or infection is recommended in high-risk groups to avoid vaccinating recovered individuals or those with chronic infection. Postvaccination screening (to evaluate vaccine response) is recommended for individuals who belong to high-risk groups.
  - Additional doses, higher doses, or revaccination can be considered in nonresponders and hypo responders to elicit protective levels of immunity. Booster doses may be needed in immunosuppressed individuals.
- **Postexposure prophylaxis**
  - **Infants born to HBsAg-positive mothers should receive HBV vaccine and hepatitis B immunoglobulin (HBIg), 0.5 mL, within 12 hours of birth.** Immunized infants should be tested at approximately 12 months of age for HBsAg, anti-HBs, and anti-HBc. The presence of HBsAg indicates that the infant is actively infected. The presence of both anti-HBs and anti-HBc suggests that infection occurred but was probably modified by immunoprophylaxis and that immunity is likely to be prolonged. The presence of anti-HBs alone is indicative of vaccine-induced immunity.

- Susceptible sexual partners of individuals with HBV and those with needlestick injury should receive HBIg (0.04 to 0.07 mL/kg) and the first dose of HBV vaccine at different sites as soon as possible (preferably within 48 hours but no more than 7 days after exposure). A second dose of HBIg can be administered 30 days after exposure, and the vaccination schedule should be completed.
- Postexposure prophylaxis with HBIg plus a nucleotide or nucleoside analog should be used after liver transplantation to prevent HBV recurrence.

Surgical Management

Liver transplantation is indicated for patients with advanced liver disease and HCC due to infection with HBV.

OUTCOME/PROGNOSIS

- Depending on the age at infection, people may have spontaneous resolution or progression to chronicity.
  - Children younger than 5 years old: 90% will develop chronic HBV infection.
  - Adults: 5% to 10% will develop chronic HBV.
- Chronic hepatitis B
  - Morbidity and mortality in chronic HBV are linked to persistence of viral replication and evolution to cirrhosis or HCC. Spontaneous clearance of HBsAg occurs in 0.5% of patients annually.
  - Once the diagnosis of chronic HBV is established, the 5-year cumulative incidence of developing cirrhosis ranges from 8% to 20%.
  - 5% to 10% of patients with chronic HBV progress to HCC **with or without preceding cirrhosis**.

Hepatitis C

GENERAL PRINCIPLES

Classification

- HCV is an RNA virus that belongs to the **flavivirus** family.
- There are six HCV genotypes recognized worldwide with >60 subtypes.

Epidemiology

- **HCV** is a global health problem with approximately **200 million carriers worldwide.**
- The incidence of hepatitis C has declined in the last 30 years. The prevalence in the United States is 1.8% of the population, making HCV infection the most common chronic blood-borne infection.
- HCV infection occurs primarily through exposure from infected blood. (See Risk Factors.)
  - Transmission by transfusion of blood products (and their derivatives) and organ transplantation has been reduced to near zero in developed countries due to sensitive screening methods.
- In the United States, 4 million people have been infected with this virus, with 2.7 million estimated to have chronic infection, and it is the leading cause of death from chronic liver disease (*NEJM 1999;341:556; Hepatology 2002;36(Suppl 1):S30*).

* Genotype 1 accounts for 75% and genotypes 2 and 3 account for 20% of HCV infections in the United States.
* In industrialized countries, HCV accounts for 20% of cases of acute hepatitis, 70% of cases of chronic hepatitis, 40% of cases of end-stage cirrhosis, 60% of cases of HCC, and 40% of liver transplants.

Pathophysiology

* The liver damage that ensues after HCV infection is immune mediated.
* Modes of transmission include:
  * **Parenteral** (e.g., transfusion, injection drug use, body piercing, needlestick injury)
  * **Sexually (high-risk sexual practices)** and **from mother to offspring (vertical transmission)**, although at a much lower frequency than HBV

Risk Factors

Risk factors for HCV infection include a history of multiple blood transfusions or clotting factors before the institution of modern screening methodology (1992), hemodialysis, injection drug use, multiple sexual partners, and occupational exposure with blood and blood-derived products. Other risk factors may include tattooing, body piercing, sharing "straws" for intranasal cocaine use, sharing razors, and military service, homelessness, and incarceration (*Gastroenterology 2002;123:2082*).

Prevention

No preexposure prophylaxis or vaccine exists. Prevention of high-risk behavior and lifestyle modifications should be encouraged.

Associated Conditions

Extrahepatic manifestations include mixed cryoglobulinemia (10% to 25% of patients with HCV), glomerulonephritis, porphyria cutanea tarda, cutaneous necrotizing vasculitis, lichen planus, lymphoma, diabetes mellitus, and other autoimmune disorders.

DIAGNOSIS

Clinical Presentation

* The incubation period varies from 15 to 150 days.
* **Acute hepatitis** can be silent (subclinical), especially in children and young adults. Symptoms vary from mild illness to FHF. Malaise, fatigue, pruritus, headache, abdominal pain, myalgias, arthralgias, nausea, vomiting, anorexia, and fever are common but nonspecific symptoms.
* **Chronic hepatitis** runs an indolent course, sometimes for decades. **Fatigue is a common symptom.** The disease may only become clinically apparent late in the natural course, when symptoms are associated with advanced liver disease.

Diagnostic Testing

Laboratories

* **Antibodies against HCV (anti-HCV)** may be undetectable for the first 8 weeks after infection. These antibodies are detected by enzyme immunoassay. **The antibody does not confer immunity.** The test has a sensitivity of 95% to 99% and a lower specificity. A false-positive test (anti-HCV positive with HCV RNA negative) may be

detected in the setting of autoimmune hepatitis (AIH) or hypergammaglobulinemia. A false-negative test (anti-HCV negative with HCV RNA positive) may be seen in immunosuppressed individuals and in patients on hemodialysis.

- **HCV RNA** can be detected by **PCR** in serum as early as **1 to 2 weeks after infection** (qualitative and quantitative assays). It is expressed in International Units per milliliter (IU/mL), with lower limits of detection approaching 10 IU/mL. HCV RNA determination is useful for both diagnosis and treatment purposes.
- **HCV genotypes** can be detected by commercially available serologic and molecular assays. HCV genotype influences the duration, dosage, and response to treatment.
- **Liver biopsy** is useful to score the degree of inflammation (grade) and fibrosis (stage) in the liver of chronically infected patients. It is useful to grade the amount of liver steatosis and guides treatment decisions.

TREATMENT

- Therapeutic **goals for treatment** of HCV:
  - Eradication of the virus
  - Decrease disease progression
  - Histological improvement
  - Decrease HCC frequency
- Treatment outcome in HCV is determined by a number of pre- and on-treatment factors.
  - **Pretreatment factors**
    - Viral genotype, viral load, advanced liver disease (amount of liver fibrosis), metabolic (obesity, steatosis, and insulin resistance), race/ethnicity.
  - **On-treatment factors**
    - Adherence to the prescribed regimen: dose and duration of ribavirin and pIFN.
    - Rapidity of viral response.
  - **Treatment definitions**
    - **Rapid virologic response (RVR):** HCV RNA negative at 4 weeks of treatment.
    - **Early virologic response (EVR):** HCV RNA negative; or >2 $\log_{10}$ drop at 12 weeks of treatment.
      - **Complete EVR (cEVR):** no RVR, but HCV RNA negative at week 12.
      - **Partial EVR (pEVR):** no RVR, detectable HCV RNA but >2 $\log_{10}$ drop at 12 weeks of treatment.
      - **Slow responder:** >2 $\log_{10}$ drop at 12 weeks of treatment and HCV RNA negative at week 24.
      - **Partial responder:** >2 $\log_{10}$ drop at 12 weeks of treatment and HCV RNA positive at week 24.
    - **Relapse:** HCV RNA negative at end of treatment but HCV RNA positive after treatment cessation.
    - **Sustained virologic response (SVR):** absence of HCV RNA 6 months postantiviral treatment.
- Defining the virologic response to treatment at weeks 4 and 12 is useful in predicting an SVR.

Medications

Acute infection. IFN-α (standard or pegylated) for 6 months has been associated with a high rate of sustained HCV RNA clearance (*NEJM 2001;345:1452*). The role of **ribavirin** in addition is under investigation.

First Line
Chronic infection

- A combination of pIFN (peginterferon alfa-2a 180 mcg/wk or peginterferon alfa-2b 1.5 mcg/kg/wk, subcutaneous) and oral ribavirin (genotype 1: <75 kg: 1,000 mg daily, >75 kg: 1,200 mg daily; genotypes 2 and 3: 800 mg daily) is administered for 6 (genotypes 2 and 3) or 12 months (genotype 1).
- Overall SVR is better for genotypes 2 and 3 compared with genotypes 1, 4, 5, and 6. SVR is dependent upon pretreatment factors and rapidity of achieving HCV RNA clearance.
- Overall SVR in HCV patients varies from 54% to 63% (genotype 1: 30% to 40%; genotypes 2 and 3: 80% to 85%). Patients who achieve SVR have a very low rate of recurrence (<1%) and are therefore considered cured of the infection.
- Side effects of interferon-based therapy include flu-like symptoms, neuropsychiatric disorders, endocrine dysfunction, and bone marrow suppression.
- Side effects of ribavirin include teratogenicity, hemolytic anemia, and pulmonary symptoms (dyspnea, cough, and pneumonitis). Contraindications to treatment with ribavirin include pregnancy or unwillingness to practice birth control, chronic renal insufficiency, and the inability to tolerate anemia (15% to 30%).

Second Line
Promising new agents with direct antiviral properties are under investigation in association with standard therapy including pIFN and ribavirin (*NEJM 2009;360:1827*; *NEJM 2009;360:1839*).

MONITORING/FOLLOW-UP

The **progression of fibrosis** determines the ultimate prognosis and thus the need and urgency of therapy.

- Liver biopsy is the gold standard to assess fibrosis.

OUTCOME/PROGNOSIS

- **Acute hepatitis** is frequently **clinically silent**.
- **Up to 40%** of people infected with HCV will have **spontaneous resolution**, while **60%** progress to have chronic infection.
- **Progression to cirrhosis** is slow (two to three decades) and is seen in a quarter of patients with chronic HCV.
- **HCC** develops in approximately **1% to 2% of patients per year**, and rarely occurs in the absence of cirrhosis.

Hepatitis D

GENERAL PRINCIPLES

Classification

HDV is considered a subviral particle resembling plant pathogens, viroids, and virusoids. It has a circular RNA genome and it is the only member of the genus *Delta virus*.

Epidemiology

It is found throughout the world and is endemic to the Mediterranean basin, the Middle East, and portions of South America. Outside these areas, infections occur primarily in individuals who have received transfusions or in injection drug users. **HDV requires the presence of HBV for infection and replication.**

Pathophysiology

HDV infection clinically presents as **a coinfection** (acute hepatitis B and D), as a **superinfection** (chronic hepatitis B with acute hepatitis D), or as a **latent infection** (e.g., in the liver transplant setting).

Risk Factors

High-risk groups are similar to HBV (see HBV Epidemiology).

Prevention

Although there is no vaccine to prevent HDV in carriers of HBV, both infections can be prevented by timely administration of the HBV vaccine.

DIAGNOSIS

Clinical Presentation

In patients with coinfection, the course is transient and self-limited. The rate of progression to chronicity is similar to the one reported for acute HBV. In superinfection, the HBV carriers may present with a severe acute hepatitis exacerbation with frequent progression to chronic HDV.

Diagnostic Testing

Laboratories

Diagnosis is made by finding HDV RNA or HDV antigen in serum or liver and by detecting antibody to the HDV antigen.

TREATMENT

Medications

IFN-α is the **treatment of choice** for chronic hepatitis D.

Hepatitis E

GENERAL PRINCIPLES

Classification

HEV is an **RNA virus** that belongs to the ***Hepeviridae*** family.

Epidemiology

- It has been implicated in epidemics in India, Southeast Asia, Africa, and Mexico. Reported cases in the United States have been in travelers to endemic areas.

- Pets and consumption of organ meats may play a role in transmission.
- Hepatitis E is considered a zoonotic disease and reservoirs include pigs and potentially other species (*Virus Res 2007;127:216*).

Pathophysiology

Transmission closely resembles that of HAV (i.e., **fecal–oral route).**

Prevention

There is no approved pre- or postexposure prophylaxis.

DIAGNOSIS

Clinical Presentation

Acute hepatitis E is clinically indistinguishable from other acute viral hepatitis. HEV infection is associated with a high fatality rate in pregnant women in the second and third trimesters.

TREATMENT

Treatment is supportive.

OUTCOME/PROGNOSIS

Although generally considered an acute illness, chronic HEV infection has been detected in immunosuppressed organ transplant patients (*J Hepatol 2008;48: 494*).

DRUG-INDUCED LIVER TOXICITY

GENERAL PRINCIPLES

- Drug-induced liver toxicity (DILT) is the most common circumstance for a drug to be removed from the market.
- Less commonly DILT can cause chronic liver disease, cirrhosis, and HCC.

Classification

- There are three major classifications of DILT that occur as a result of both intrinsic and idiosyncratic hepatotoxicity:
  - **Hepatocellular injury** refers to injury to the liver cell.
  - **Cholestatic injury** refers to injury to the biliary system.
  - **Mixed hepatocellular and cholestatic** injury refers to injury to both the liver cell and the biliary system.
- Other less common types of DILT include chronic hepatitis, chronic cholestasis, granulomatous hepatitis, fibrosis or cirrhosis, and carcinogenesis.

Epidemiology

DILT causes approximately 50% of the cases of acute liver failure (ALF) in the United States, with **acetaminophen being the most common causative agent**.

Pathophysiology

- **Intrinsic hepatotoxicity** results from the **direct hepatotoxic effects** of the drug or its metabolite. The mechanism is predictable and dose dependent. Examples include carbon tetrachloride, elemental phosphorus, and supratherapeutic doses of acetaminophen.
- **Idiosyncratic hepatotoxicity** can be divided into **hypersensitivity (allergic)** and **metabolic (nonallergic).** These reactions depend on multiple variables and are not predictable.
  - **Hypersensitivity responses** occur as a result of stimulation of the immune system by a metabolite of a drug alone or after haptenization (covalently binding) to a liver protein (e.g., allopurinol, diclofenac). The latency of the reaction is variable. Repeated challenge with the same agent leads to prompt recurrence of the reaction.
- **Metabolic hepatotoxicity** occurs in susceptible patients as a result of altered drug clearance or accelerated production of hepatotoxic metabolites (e.g., isoniazid, ketoconazole). The latency of this reaction is variable.

DIAGNOSIS

Clinical Presentation

- The acute presentation can be clinically silent. When symptoms are present, they are nonspecific and include nausea/vomiting, general malaise, fatigue, and abdominal pain.
- In the acute setting, the majority of patients will recover after cessation of the offending drug.
- Fever and rash may also be seen in association with hypersensitivity reactions.

Diagnostic Criteria

- **Clinical suspicion**
- **Temporal relation** of liver injury to drug usage.
- Resolution of liver injury after the suspected agent has been discontinued.

Diagnostic Testing
Laboratories
Biochemical abnormalities

- Hepatocellular injury: **AST and ALT elevation** more than two times the upper limit of normal.
- Cholestatic injury: **ALP and conjugated bilirubin elevation** more than two times the upper limit of normal.
- Mixed injury includes increases in all of the above biochemical abnormalities to more than two times the upper limit of normal.

Diagnostic Procedures
Liver biopsy is sometimes needed.

TREATMENT

- Treatment includes cessation of offending drug and institution of supportive measures.

- An attempt to remove the agent from the GI tract should be made in most cases of acute toxic ingestion using lavage or cathartics (see Chapter 24, Medical Emergencies).
- Management of acetaminophen overdose is a medical emergency (see Chapter 24, Medical Emergencies).

Surgical Management

Liver transplantation may be an option for patients with FHF.

OUTCOME/PROGNOSIS

- Prognosis of DILT is often unique to the offending medication.
- It is important to be attuned to the development of jaundice because this sign is associated with case-fatality rates in the range of 10% to 50% (*NEJM 2006;354:731*).

ALCOHOLIC LIVER DISEASE

GENERAL PRINCIPLES

Alcohol is a potentially **toxic substance** to the liver.

Classification

- The **spectrum** of alcoholic liver disease is broad, and a single patient may be affected by more than one of the following conditions: **fatty liver, alcoholic hepatitis, or alcoholic cirrhosis.**
- **Fatty liver** is the most commonly observed abnormality, and occurs in up to 90% of alcoholics.
- **Alcoholic cirrhosis** is a common cause of ESLD and HCC.

Epidemiology

- Alcoholism is a significant medical and socioeconomic problem. Although ethyl alcohol exerts a direct toxic effect on the liver, significant liver damage develops in only 10% to 20% of chronic alcoholics.
- Average alcohol consumption can be measured by units per week. **One unit** is equal to 7 g of alcohol, one glass of wine, or a can (240 mL) of 3.5% to 4% beer; approximately 30 to 40 units of alcohol per week can induce cirrhosis in 3% to 8% of individuals over a decade.

Risk Factors

Additional factors (e.g., genetic, nutritional, environmental) may be important in the pathogenesis of alcoholic liver disease.

DIAGNOSIS

Clinical Presentation

- **Fatty liver**
  - Patients are usually asymptomatic.
  - Clinical findings include hepatomegaly and mild liver enzyme abnormalities.

- **Alcoholic hepatitis**
  - Alcoholic hepatitis may be clinically silent or severe enough to lead to rapid development of hepatic failure and death (*Alcohol Alcohol 2008;43:393*).
  - Clinical features include fever, abdominal pain, anorexia, nausea, vomiting, weight loss, and jaundice.
  - In severe cases, patients may have hepatic encephalopathy, ascites, and GI bleeding.
- **Alcoholic cirrhosis.** The presentation is variable, from **clinically silent disease** to decompensated cirrhosis.

History
- Patients frequently give a history of drinking up until the onset of symptoms.
- Alcoholics may underestimate or minimize their reporting of alcohol usage.

Diagnostic Testing
Laboratories
- In alcoholic fatty liver, laboratory tests may be normal or demonstrate mild elevation in serum aminotransferases (**AST higher than ALT**) and ALP.
- In alcoholic hepatitis, laboratory tests typically demonstrate elevation in serum aminotransferases (**AST higher than ALT**) and ALP. **Hyperbilirubinemia (conjugated)** and **prolongation of PT/INR** may also be seen.
  - Laboratory abnormalities associated with a poor prognosis include renal failure, leukocytosis, a markedly elevated total bilirubin, and prolongation of the PT/INR that does not normalize with subcutaneous vitamin K.
  - A number of classification systems have been developed to risk stratify patients with alcoholic hepatitis:
    - **A discriminant function (DF)** = $4.6 \times (PT_{patient} - PT_{control})$ + serum bilirubin. A score < 32 has 93% and >32 has 68% 1-month survival, respectively.
    - **The Glasgow Alcoholic Hepatitis Score (GAHS)** incorporates patient age, white blood cell count, blood urea (mMol/L), PT/INR, and serum bilirubin (Table 4). A score < 9 has 87% and >9 has 46% 1-month survival, respectively (*Gut 2007;56:1743*).
- **In alcoholic cirrhosis**, liver function abnormalities and clinical status vary depending on disease severity.

Diagnostic Procedures
Liver biopsy

- The typical histopathologic findings in alcoholic liver disease include Mallory hyaline bodies, neutrophilic infiltrate, necrosis of hepatocytes, collagen deposition, and fatty changes.

Table 4	The Glasgow Alcoholic Hepatitis Score		
	Points given		
Variable	1	2	3
Age	<50	≥50	X
WBC (10^9/L)	<15	≥15	X
Urea (mmol/L)	<5	≥5	X
INR	<1.5	1.5–2.0	>2.0
Bilirubin (μmol/L)	<125	125–250	>250

- The indication of liver biopsy depends on the clinical assessment of the patient. It may be helpful if alternate diagnoses are being considered.

TREATMENT

The cornerstone of treatment is abstinence from alcohol.

Medications

- **Treatment** of acute alcoholic hepatitis with **corticosteroids is controversial.** However, there is evidence that patients with a **DF > 32 and GAHS > 9** may benefit from steroid therapy. An early fall in bilirubin levels after 1 week of treatment portends a better prognosis.
  - Oral prednisolone 40 mg/d for 4 weeks, followed by a taper has been recommended.
- **Pentoxifylline** is a nonselective phosphodiesterase inhibitor with anti-inflammatory properties and an excellent safety profile that has shown improved survival in severe alcoholic hepatitis at dose of 400 mg PO tid for 4 weeks.
- S-Adenosylmethionine, antioxidants, tumor necrosis factor inhibitors, and glutathione prodrugs are under investigation in alcoholic liver disease but studies thus far are inconclusive.

Surgical Management

Patients with cirrhosis and ESLD can be evaluated for liver transplant but are required to abstain from alcohol for 6 months prior to evaluation and maintain abstinence.

Lifestyle/Risk Modification

Rehabilitation (i.e., Alcoholics Anonymous, private counseling, etc.).

Diet

Emphasis must be given to supplemental enteral nutrition to ensure adequate energy and protein intake in patients with severe alcoholic hepatitis (*Clin Nutr 2006;25:285*).

COMPLICATIONS

Potentially dangerous interactions may occur between alcohol and a variety of medications, including sedative-hypnotics, anticoagulants, and acetaminophen because of shared metabolic pathways.

OUTCOME/PROGNOSIS

- Fatty liver may be reversible with abstinence.
- In alcoholic hepatitis prognosis depends on the severity of presentation and alcohol abstinence. The **in-hospital mortality** for severe cases is approximately **50%.**
- In cirrhosis induced by alcohol, **prognosis is variable** and depends on the degree of liver decompensation. Abstinence from alcohol may promote significant liver chemistry improvement even in advanced liver disease.

IMMUNE-MEDIATED LIVER DISEASE

Autoimmune Hepatitis

GENERAL PRINCIPLES

Definition

Autoimmune Hepatitis (AIH) is **a chronic unresolving inflammation** of the liver of unknown cause, associated with circulating autoantibodies and hypergammaglobulinemia.

Classification

Two types of AIH have been proposed based on differences in their immunologic markers. They do not have distinctive etiologies nor vary in response to corticosteroid therapy.

- **Type I AIH** is the most common form of the disease worldwide, and it is associated with antinuclear antibodies (ANAs) and anti–smooth muscle antibodies (SMAs).
- **Type 2 AIH** is characterized by antibodies to liver/kidney microsome type 1 (anti-LKM1). This type is predominately seen in children and young adults (*NEJM 2006;354:54*).
- A less established form of AIH is characterized by the presence of antibodies to soluble liver antigen/liver pancreas (anti-SLA/LP).

Epidemiology

- AIH occurs worldwide.
- The mean annual incidence of AIH among white Northern Europeans is 1.9 per 100,000, and its point prevalence is 16.9 per 100,000 (*Hepatology 2002;36:479*).
- It accounts for approximately 6% of liver transplantations in the United States.
- Women are affected more than men (gender ratio, 3.6:1).
- In North America, cirrhosis is present at initial presentation more often in African American patients than Caucasian patients.

Associated Conditions

Extrahepatic manifestations may be found in 30% to 50% and include celiac disease, Coombs' positive hemolytic anemia, autoimmune thyroiditis, Graves' disease, rheumatoid arthritis, ulcerative colitis, and other less common presentations.

DIAGNOSIS

Clinical Presentation

In approximately 30% of cases, the presentation is **acute** and similar to viral hepatitis. Patients may present in **FHF** or with **asymptomatic elevation** of serum **ALT**. It **presents** with **cirrhosis** in at least **25%** of patients.

History
- The most common symptoms at presentation include fatigue, jaundice, myalgias, anorexia, diarrhea, acne, and right upper quadrant abdominal discomfort.

- Patients with AIH may **overlap** with findings consistent with other liver diseases (e.g., PBC, PSC, and autoimmune cholangitis).

Physical Examination
AIH is not associated with any specific physical examination findings.

Diagnostic Criteria

Diagnostic criteria have been codified and updated by an international panel (*Hepatology 2002;36(2):479*).

Diagnostic Testing

Diagnostic Procedures
Liver biopsy is **essential** for the diagnosis

- "Piecemeal necrosis" or interface hepatitis with lobular or panacinar inflammation (lymphocytic and plasmacytic infiltration) are the histologic hallmarks of the disease.
- Histologic changes, such as ductopenia or destructive cholangitis, may indicate overlap syndromes combining characteristics of AIH, PSC, PBC, or autoimmune cholangitis.

TREATMENT

- Treatment should be instituted in patients with elevated serum aminotransferase levels and hyperglobulinemia.
- Histologic features of interface hepatitis, bridging, or multiacinar necrosis compel therapy.

Medications

First Line
- **Therapy** is initiated with either **prednisone** alone (40 to 60 mg/d) or a **combination of prednisone** and **azathioprine** (1 to 2 mg/kg/d).
- Prednisone is tapered with biochemical and clinical improvement to an eventual discontinuation of treatment. Some patients require lifelong low-dose therapy.

Second Line
Refractory disease (i.e., remission not achieved with first-line therapy) may require "salvage" therapy with cyclosporine, tacrolimus, or mycophenolate mofetil.

Surgical Management

- **Liver transplantation** should be considered in patients with ESLD.
- After transplantation, **recurrent AIH** is seen in approximately **15% of patients. De novo AIH or immunologically mediated hepatitis**, defined as hepatitis with histologic features similar to AIH in patients transplanted for nonautoimmune diseases, has been described in about **5% of transplant recipients.**

MONITORING/FOLLOW-UP

- Ninety percent of adults have improvements in the serum aminotransferase, bilirubin, and γ-globulin levels within 2 weeks of treatment.
- Histologic improvement lags behind clinical and laboratory improvement by 3 to 6 months.

OUTCOME/PROGNOSIS

- **Remission** (normalization of serum bilirubin, immunoglobulin levels, AST, ALT; disappearance of symptoms; resolution of histologic changes) is achieved in **65%** and **80%** of patients within **1.5** and **3 years**, of treatment, respectively.
- **Relapses** occur in at least **20% to 50%** of patients after cessation of therapy. Relapses require retreatment.

Primary Biliary Cirrhosis

GENERAL PRINCIPLES

Definition

Primary biliary cirrhosis (PBC) is a **cholestatic** hepatic disorder of unknown etiology with autoimmune features.

Epidemiology

- It most often affects **middle-aged women** (90% to 95%).
- Although PBC is seen worldwide, it is more commonly described in North America and Northern Europe.

Pathophysiology

- PBC is caused by granulomatous destruction of the interlobular bile ducts, which leads to progressive ductopenia.
- The consequent cholestasis is generally slowly progressive. Fibrosis, cirrhosis, and eventual liver failure can occur.

Associated Conditions

Extrahepatic manifestations include keratoconjunctivitis sicca (Sjögren's), renal tubular acidosis, gallstones, thyroid disease, scleroderma, Raynaud's phenomenon, CREST syndrome, and celiac disease.

DIAGNOSIS

Clinical Presentation

The **course** is highly **variable.**

History
- **Fatigue, jaundice, and pruritus** are often the most troublesome symptoms.
- Patients may, on occasion, present de novo with manifestations of ESLD.

Physical Examination
While there are no exam findings that are specific for PBC, xanthomata and xanthelasma can be a clue to underlying cholestasis.

Diagnostic Testing

Laboratories
- **Antimitochondrial antibodies** are present in >90% of patients.
- Typical features include elevated levels of **ALP**, bilirubin, cholesterol, IgM, and bile acids.

Diagnostic Procedures

Liver biopsy may be helpful for both diagnosis and staging.

TREATMENT

Medications

No curative therapy is available; treatment aims to slow progression of disease.

First Line

Ursodeoxycholic acid (UDCA) (13 to 15 mg/kg/d PO) improves liver function test abnormalities and appears to delay progression of disease when given for long term (>4 years).

- UDCA increases the rate of transport of intracellular bile acids across the hepatocyte into the canaliculus.
- UDCA treatment also reduces intracellular hydrophobic bile acid levels conferring a cytoprotective effect.

Second Line

Trials investigating the use of azathioprine and cyclosporine have not shown a beneficial effect of therapy on survival.

Other Nonoperative Therapies

Symptom-specific therapy for pruritus, steatorrhea, and malabsorption are outlined below.

Surgical Management

- **Liver transplantation** is an option in advanced disease.
- Recurrent PBC after transplantation has been documented.

OUTCOME/PROGNOSIS

- PBC progresses along a path of increasingly severe histologic damage (florid bile duct lesion, ductular proliferation, fibrosis, and cirrhosis).
- Ultimately, progression to **cirrhosis and liver failure may occur** two decades from diagnosis without treatment.

Primary Sclerosing Cholangitis

GENERAL PRINCIPLES

Definition

Primary sclerosing cholangitis (PSC) is a **cholestatic** liver disorder characterized by inflammation, fibrosis, and eventual obliteration of the extrahepatic and intrahepatic bile ducts.

Classification

- Patients with PSC can be subdivided into those with small duct and large duct involvement. Small duct disease is defined as typical histologic features of PSC with a normal cholangiogram. In large duct PSC, characteristic strictures of the biliary tree can be detected by cholangiography (*Curr Opin Gastroenterol 2008;24(3): 377*).

- Approximately 75% of patients have involvement with both small and large ducts; 15% have only small duct and 10% have only large duct disease (*Curr Gastroenterol Rep 2009;11:37*).
- **Patients with small duct disease have a more favorable prognosis.**

Epidemiology

Most patients are **middle-aged men.**

Associated Conditions

PSC is frequently associated with inflammatory bowel disease (70% with ulcerative colitis). The clinical course of these conditions is not correlated.

DIAGNOSIS

Clinical Presentation

- **Clinical manifestations** include intermittent episodes of jaundice, hepatomegaly, pruritus, weight loss, and fatigue.
- **Cholangitis** is a frequent complication in patients with severe strictures of the biliary ducts.
- Patients may progress to **cirrhosis** and **ESLD.**
- **Cholangiocarcinoma** is the most frequent neoplasm associated with PSC and occurs in 6% to 20% of patients.

Diagnostic Testing

Laboratories

- **PSC** should be considered in individuals with **inflammatory bowel disease** who have increased levels of **ALP** even in the absence of symptoms of hepatobiliary disease.
- ANA is positive in up to 50% of cases, and perinuclear antineutrophil cytoplasmic antibody (p-ANCA) is positive in 80% of cases.

Imaging

MRCP is a noninvasive means of demonstrating abnormalities of the biliary ducts. Liver ultrasound may be useful in establishing the diagnosis if ductal dilation is present.

Diagnostic Procedures

- PSC can be confirmed by demonstration of multiple strictures or irregularities of the intrahepatic or extrahepatic bile ducts by ERCP, which also allows for brushings to be obtained to evaluate for associated malignancy. Intraductal endoscopy provides direct visualization of the biliary ducts with the advantage of obtaining biopsy of tissue.
- Liver biopsy is helpful in the diagnosis of small-duct PSC, in the exclusion of other diseases, and in staging.
  - Characteristic findings include concentric periductal fibrosis ("onion-skinning") that progresses to narrowing and obliteration of small bile ducts.
- Fluorescent *in situ hybridization* (FISH) allows for molecular assessment of malignancy from tissue obtained by brushing or biopsy.

TREATMENT

Medications

- **UDCA** (20 to 30 mg/kg) may be beneficial in improving liver biochemistries; long-term effects on histology and survival are currently being investigated.
- Episodes of cholangitis should be managed with IV antibiotics and endoscopic therapy as outlined below.

Other Nonoperative Therapies

ERCP can be performed to dilate and stent dominant strictures.

Surgical Management

- Colectomy for ulcerative colitis does not affect the course of PSC.
- Patients with cirrhosis or recurrent cholangitis should be referred for liver transplantation.
- While in the past cholangiocarcinoma was a contraindication for liver transplantation, it is now being considered in select circumstances.
- Recurrent PSC after liver transplantation has been documented.

COMPLICATIONS OF CHOLESTASIS

Nutritional Deficiencies

GENERAL PRINCIPLES

Any condition that blocks bile excretion (in the liver cells or biliary ducts) is defined as cholestasis. Laboratory manifestations of cholestasis include elevated levels of ALP and bilirubin.

Etiology

- **Nutritional deficiencies** result from fat malabsorption.
- **Fat-soluble vitamin deficiency** (vitamins A, D, E, and K) is often present in advanced cholestatic disease and is particularly common in patients with steatorrhea.

DIAGNOSIS

Clinical Presentation

History
- Patients may give a history of oily, foul-smelling diarrhea that may stick to the toilet bowl or be difficult to flush.
- Characteristic manifestations of vitamin deficiencies are discussed in Chapter 2, Nutrition Support.

Diagnostic Testing

Laboratories
- Stool can be tested for **fecal fat.** Both spot tests and 24-hour collections can be done.
- **25-Hydroxy vitamin D serum concentrations** reflect the **total body stores** of **vitamin D.** Vitamin D deficiency in the setting of malabsorption and steatorrhea is a good clinical marker for total body concentrations of other fat-soluble vitamins.

TREATMENT

Medications
- Vitamin supplements are available to correct deficiencies.
- Fat-soluble vitamin replacement can be accomplished by water-soluble preparations of **vitamin A,** 10,000 to 50,000 IU PO daily; **vitamin K,** 10 mg subcutaneously; and **vitamin E,** 30 to 100 IU PO daily.
- Vitamin D deficiency can be corrected by **25-hydroxyvitamin D3 (25-cholecalciferol),** 50,000 Units PO 3× weekly.
- **Zinc deficiency** may occur in some patients and is corrected with **zinc sulfate,** 220 mg PO daily (50 mg elemental zinc) for 4 weeks.

Lifestyle/Risk Modification
Activity
In patients with steatorrhea, a **low-fat diet** (40 to 60 g/d) helps to decrease symptoms but may compromise total energy intake.

MONITORING/FOLLOW-UP

Serum levels of **25-hydroxy vitamin D** should be **monitored** to assess the adequacy of replacement therapy and avoid toxicity.

Osteoporosis

GENERAL PRINCIPLES

Definition
Osteoporosis is defined as a decrease in the amount of bone (mainly trabecular bone), leading to a decrease in its structural integrity and consequently an increase in the risk of fractures.

Epidemiology
- Osteoporosis is more commonly seen in clinical cholestasis due to **PBC.**
- The relative risk of osteopenia in cholestatic disease is 4.4 times greater than the general population, matched for age and gender.

Pathophysiology
Both decreased osteoblastic activity and increased osteoclastic activity contribute to the development of osteoporosis.

DIAGNOSIS

Clinical Presentation
Osteoporosis is often insidious and is sometimes diagnosed after development of pathologic fracture.

Diagnostic Testing

Imaging

Bone mineral density through **dual energy x-ray absorptiometry (DEXA)** should be measured in all patients at the time of diagnosis and during follow-up (every 1 to 2 years).

TREATMENT

Medications

Treatment of bone disease includes exercise, oral calcium supplementation (1.0 to 1.5 g/d), bisphosphonate therapy, and vitamin D supplementation.

Pruritus

GENERAL PRINCIPLES

Pathophysiology

The pathophysiology is debated and may be due to the accumulation of bile acid compounds or endogenous opioid agonists.

DIAGNOSIS

Clinical Presentation

Patients with cholestasis may present with itching in the setting of a normal or elevated bilirubin level.

TREATMENT

Medications

First Line

- **Pruritus** is best treated with **cholestyramine,** a basic anion exchange resin. It binds bile acids and other anionic compounds in the intestine and inhibits their absorption. The dose is 4 g mixed with water before and after the morning meal, with additional doses before lunch and dinner. The maximum recommended dose is 16 g/d.
  - Cholestyramine should be administered apart from other vitamins or medications to prevent impaired absorption.
- **Colestipol,** another similar resin, is also available.

Second Line

- **Antihistamines** (diphenhydramine or doxepin, 25 mg PO at bedtime) and petrolatum may provide symptomatic relief.
- **Rifampin** (300 to 600 mg/d) and **naltrexone** (25 to 50 mg/d) are reserved for intractable pruritus.

Other Nonoperative Therapies

Plasmapheresis can be administered when medical therapy has failed.

Surgical Management

Liver transplantation is a last resort option for intractable pruritus.

METABOLIC LIVER DISEASE

Wilson's Disease

GENERAL PRINCIPLES

Definition

Wilson's disease (WD) is an **autosomal recessive disorder** (ATP7B gene on chromosome 13) that results in progressive **copper overload.**

Epidemiology

- Incidence is 1 in 30,000.
- Female to male ratio of 2:1.

Pathophysiology

Absent or reduced function of ATP7B protein leads to decreased hepatocellular excretion of copper into bile. This results in hepatic copper accumulation and injury. Eventually, copper is released into the bloodstream and deposited in other organs, notably the brain, kidneys, and cornea.

Associated Conditions

Other extrahepatic manifestations include Kayser–Fleischer rings on slit-lamp examination (gold to brown rings due to copper deposition in the Descemet's membrane in the periphery of the cornea), Coombs-negative hemolytic anemia, renal tubular acidosis, arthritis, and osteopenia.

DIAGNOSIS

Clinical Presentation

- Liver disease can be highly variable, ranging from asymptomatic with only biochemical abnormalities to ALF.
- The diagnosis of WD should be considered in patients with unexplained liver disease with or without neuropsychiatric symptoms, first-degree relatives with WD, or individuals with FHF (with or without hemolysis).
- The average **age at presentation** of liver dysfunction is **6 to 20 years,** but it can manifest later in life.
- **Neuropsychiatric disorders** usually occur later, most of the time in association with cirrhosis. The manifestations include **asymmetric tremor, dysarthria, ataxia, and psychiatric features.**

Diagnostic Testing

Laboratories

- Low serum ceruloplasmin level (<20 mg/dL), elevated serum free copper level (>25 mcg/dL), and elevated 24-hour urinary copper level (>100 mg).
- Most patients with the ALF presentation of WD have a characteristic pattern of clinical findings including Coombs-negative hemolytic anemia with features of acute intravascular hemolysis, rapid progression to renal failure, modest rise in serum aminotransferases (typically <2,000 IU/L) from the beginning of clinical

illness, normal or markedly subnormal serum ALP (typically <40 IU/L) (*Hepatology 2008;47:2090*).

- Mutation analysis by whole-gene sequencing is possible and should be performed on individuals in whom the diagnosis is difficult to establish by clinical and biochemical testing.
  - Many patients are compound heterozygotes for mutations in ATP7B gene, making identification of mutations difficult.

Imaging

Brain imaging (basal ganglia changes) findings are nonspecific.

Diagnostic Procedures

Liver biopsy

- The **liver histology** (massive necrosis, steatosis, glycogenated nuclei, chronic hepatitis, fibrosis, cirrhosis) findings are **nonspecific** and depend on the presentation and stage of the disease.
- Elevated hepatic copper levels of >250 mcg/g dry weight (normal < 40 mcg/g) on biopsy are highly suggestive of WD.

TREATMENT

Medications

Treatment is with copper-chelating agents.

- **Zinc salts,** 50 mg tid, are indicated in patients with chronic hepatitis and cirrhosis in the absence of hepatic failure. Other than gastric irritation, zinc has an excellent safety profile.
- **Penicillamine** 1 to 2 g/d (in divided doses bid or qid) **plus pyridoxine** 25 mg/d to avoid Vitamin B6 deficiency during treatment. It is indicated in patients with hepatic failure. Use may be limited by side effects (hypersensitivity, bone marrow suppression, proteinuria, systemic lupus erythematosus, Goodpasture syndrome). **Penicillamine should never be given as initial treatment to patients with neurologic symptoms.**
- **Trientine** 1 to 2 g/d (in divided doses bid or qid). This has similar side effects as penicillamine, but at a lower frequency. The risk of neurologic worsening with trientine is less than with penicillamine.

Surgical Management

Liver transplantation is the only therapeutic option in FHF or in progressive dysfunction despite chelation therapy.

Lifestyle/Risk Modification

Diet

Patients should avoid intake of foods and water with high concentrations of copper, especially during the first year of treatment.

MONITORING/FOLLOW-UP

- For routine monitoring, serum copper and ceruloplasmin, liver biochemistries, complete blood cell count and urinalysis (especially for those on chelation therapy), and physical examination should be performed regularly, at least twice annually.

- The 24-hour urinary excretion of copper should be measured annually while on medication. More frequent monitoring may be needed if there is suspicion of non-compliance or if dose adjustment is required. The estimated serum free copper may be elevated or low in situations of nonadherence and overtreatment, respectively.

OUTCOME/PROGNOSIS

In the absence of neurologic symptoms, liver transplantation has a good prognosis and requires no further medical treatment.

Hereditary Hemochromatosis

GENERAL PRINCIPLES

Definition
Hereditary hemochromatosis (HH) is an autosomal recessive disorder of iron overload.

Epidemiology
- This is the most common inherited form of iron overload affecting Caucasian populations.
- One in 200 to 400 Caucasian individuals are homozygous for the HFE gene mutations.
- It rarely manifests clinically before middle age (40 to 60 years).

Etiology
- HH is most frequently caused by a missense mutation (C282Y) in the HFE gene located on chromosome 6. Approximately 90% of patients with HH are homozygote for the C282Y mutation.
- In one study, however, only 58% of homozygotes for the HH mutation had the full phenotype with iron overload (*NEJM 1999;341:718*).
- Less frequent mutations include H63D and S65C and the compound heterozygous C282Y/H63D mutation.

Pathophysiology
This systemic disorder is related to abnormal iron absorption in the duodenum that leads to excessive and damaging iron deposition in the liver, heart, pancreas, skin, and endocrine system.

Associated Conditions
Secondary iron overload states include thalassemia major, sideroblastic anemia, chronic hemolytic anemias, chronic hepatitis B and C, alcohol-induced liver disease, porphyria cutanea tarda, and aceruloplasminemia.

DIAGNOSIS

Clinical Presentation
- Presentation varies from **asymptomatic disease** to **cirrhosis.**
- Clinical findings include slate-colored skin, diabetes, cardiomyopathy, arthritis, hypogonadism, and hepatic dysfunction.

Diagnostic Testing

Diagnosis is based on laboratory testing, imaging, and liver biopsy.

Laboratories

- The diagnosis is suggested by **high fasting transferrin saturation (>45%) (serum iron divided by the total iron binding capacity).**
- Other nonspecific laboratory tests include serum iron and ferritin levels. **Ferritin level >1,000 ng/mL is an accurate predictor for the degree of fibrosis in patients with HH.**
- In asymptomatic, symptomatic, and first-degree relatives of HH, genotype analysis should be performed if transferrin saturation and ferritin is elevated. If homozygosity for an HH mutation (C282Y) is demonstrated, proceed to treatment (see below) even in the presence of normal liver biochemistries. In patients with ferritin levels >1,000 ng/mL or elevated biochemistries proceed to liver biopsy before treatment (see below).
- In patients with elevated transferrin saturation and heterozygosity, exclude other liver or hematologic diseases and consider liver biopsy.

Imaging

MRI is the modality of choice for noninvasive quantification of iron storage in the liver. It allows for repeated measures and minimizes sampling error.

Diagnostic Procedures

In patients with iron overload without typical HFE gene mutations, liver biopsy is still a valuable diagnostic tool. Liver biopsy stages the amount of fibrosis and can be used to quantify the amount of iron deposition. Two measures of iron deposition include the hepatic iron concentration (normal $< 1,800 \ \mu g/g$ dry weight) and hepatic iron index (normal < 1.9).

TREATMENT

Therapy consists of **phlebotomy** every 7 to 15 days (500 mL blood) until iron depletion is confirmed by a ferritin level < 50 ng/mL and a transferrin saturation of $<40\%$. Thereafter, maintenance phlebotomy of one to two units of blood three to four times a year is continued for life.

Medications

Deferoxamine is an iron-chelating agent used in the setting of HH if the patient cannot tolerate phlebotomy. It binds free iron and facilitates urinary excretion.

Surgical Management

Liver transplantation may be considered in cases of HH with cirrhosis.

SPECIAL CONSIDERATIONS

- Once a diagnosis has been made, the **patient's family members** should **undergo screening** for HH by measuring fasting transferrin saturation and ferritin levels.
- Genetic testing may also be performed.

OUTCOME/PROGNOSIS

- The survival rate in appropriately treated noncirrhotic patients is identical to that of the general population.
- Patients with cirrhosis are at increased risk for the development of HCC despite therapy.
- Patients who undergo liver transplantation for hemochromatosis tend to have poorer 1- and 5-year survival rates when compared to other liver transplant recipients (*Hepatology 2001;33:1321*).

α_1-Antitrypsin Deficiency

GENERAL PRINCIPLES

Definition

- **α_1-Antitrypsin (α_1AT) deficiency** is an autosomal recessive disease associated with accumulation of misfolded α_1AT in the endoplasmic reticulum of hepatocytes.
- The gene associated with the disease is located on chromosome 14.
- The most common allele is **protease inhibitor M (PiM—normal variant), followed by PiS and PiZ (deficient variants).** Blacks have lower frequency of these alleles.

Epidemiology

- Severe α_1AT deficiency (PiZZ) is found in approximately 1:3,500 live births. It has been described in all races.
- It is commonly a disease of Caucasians. The most prevalent deficiency alleles Z and S are derived from European ancestry (*Am J Gastroenterol 2008;103:2136*).

Associated Conditions

α_1AT can also be associated with emphysema in early adulthood, as well as other extrahepatic manifestations including panniculitis, pancreatic fibrosis, and membranoproliferative glomerulonephritis.

DIAGNOSIS

Clinical Presentation

- The disease may present as neonatal cholestasis or later in life as chronic hepatitis, cirrhosis, or HCC.
- The presence of significant pulmonary and hepatic disease in the same patient is rare (1% to 2%).

Diagnostic Testing

Laboratories

- Low serum α_1-antitrypsin level (10% to 15% of normal).
- Decreased α_1-globulin level on serum electrophoresis.
- Deficient α_1AT phenotype (PiSS, PiSZ, and PiZZ).

Diagnostic Procedures

Liver biopsy. Characteristic periodic acid Schiff–positive, diastase-resistant globules in the periportal hepatocytes.

TREATMENT

- Currently, there is no specific medical treatment.
- Gene therapy for $\alpha_1 AT$ deficiency is a potential future alternative.

Surgical Management

Liver transplantation is an option for those with cirrhosis.

OUTCOME/PROGNOSIS

- Chronic hepatitis, cirrhosis, or HCC may develop in 10% to 15% of patients with the PiZZ phenotype during the first 20 years of life.
- Controversy exists as to whether liver disease develops in heterozygotes (PiMZ, PiSZ, PiFZ, etc.).
- Transplantation is curative, with survival rates of 90% at 1 year and 80% at 5 years.

MISCELLANEOUS LIVER DISORDERS

Nonalcoholic Fatty Liver Disease

GENERAL PRINCIPLES

Definition

- Nonalcoholic fatty liver disease (NALFD) is a clinicopathologic syndrome that encompasses several clinical entities that range from simple steatosis to steatohepatitis, fibrosis, and ESLD in the absence of significant alcohol consumption (*Gastroenterology 2002;123:1705*).
- Nonalcoholic steatohepatitis (NASH) is part of the spectrum of NAFLD and is defined as steatosis with hepatocellular ballooning plus lobular inflammation.

Epidemiology

- NAFLD is a worldwide phenomenon with an estimated prevalence greater than 30% in the general population. The prevalence of NASH ranges from 3% to 9% with substantial variation among ethnic groups. It affects both children and adults, and the incidence increases with age.
- NAFLD is associated with an increasing prevalence of type II diabetes and obesity in the U.S. population. Metabolic syndrome is also associated with NAFLD.
- Up to 70% of cases of **cryptogenic cirrhosis** have NASH as the underlying etiology. Cirrhosis due to NALFD may also be complicated by HCC (13% of all cases of HCC).

Etiology

Apart from metabolic syndrome, other causes include hepatotoxic drugs (amiodarone, nifedipine, estrogens), surgical procedures (jejuno-ileal bypass, extensive small-bowel resection, biliary and pancreatic diversions), and miscellaneous conditions (total parenteral nutrition, hypobetalipoproteinemia, environmental toxins, etc.).

DIAGNOSIS

Clinical Presentation

The disease may vary from asymptomatic liver fatty infiltration to advanced fibrosis with cirrhosis and HCC.

Diagnostic Testing

- The diagnosis of NAFLD is suspected in patients with abnormal liver chemistries and, in many cases, evidence of the metabolic syndrome.
- The distinction between NASH and simple steatosis cannot be reliably made without liver biopsy.

Laboratories
- Liver enzyme elevations are mild. Up to 80% of patients will have normal liver enzymes.
  - Aminotransferases greater than two times normal are predictive of septal bridging and fibrosis across different populations.
- Biochemical abnormalities may reflect the stage of the disease (e.g., cholestasis, hypoalbuminemia, increased INR).

Imaging
- Imaging studies such as ultrasonography, CT scan, and MRI may detect moderate to severe steatosis.
- Magnetic resonance spectroscopy offers a quantitative measurement of liver fat content, but is not commonly available.

Diagnostic Procedures
- **Liver biopsy remains the gold standard** by which the diagnosis is made. However, the decision to perform a liver biopsy should take into account the specific clinical questions that are relevant to each case.
- Noninvasive predictive models, serum biomarkers, imaging studies, and breath tests are currently under evaluation as surrogate measures of liver fibrosis, inflammation, and steatosis (*Hepatology 2009;49:306*).

TREATMENT

No established specific treatment is available for NAFLD.

Medications

- There are many proposed agents being evaluated currently, each targeting a different step in the pathogenesis of hepatic steatosis or progression to steatohepatitis.
- The proper dosing, duration of treatment, safety, and tolerability for agents such as **metformin** and **thiazolidinedione** are under clinical investigation.
- **Statins** have played a role in decreasing mortality among patients with diabetes mellitus and cardiovascular disease. Their role in NAFLD is under investigation.
- Incretin analogs, glucagon-like protein-1-receptor agonists, have been shown to be a useful adjunct in the treatment of diabetes mellitus and may also be beneficial in the treatment of NASH.

Other Nonoperative Therapies

Therapies to correct or control associated conditions are warranted (weight loss through diet and exercise, tight control of diabetes and insulin resistance, appropriate treatment of hyperlipidemia, and discontinuation of possible offending agents).

- A randomized controlled trial documented that the use of an intensive lifestyle intervention program (ILP) in obese patients with NASH reduced weight and improved overall liver health (*Hepatology 2008;48(4 Suppl 1):802A*).

Surgical Management

Liver transplantation should be considered in patients with cirrhosis. Recurrence of NASH after transplantation can develop.

OUTCOME/PROGNOSIS

- An unknown proportion of those with simple steatosis will progress to NASH.
- Approximately 25% of patients with NASH progress to cirrhosis over a 10- to 15-year period (*Semin Liver Dis 2001;21:17*). Of those with cirrhosis, 30% to 40% decompensate and succumb to liver-related death over a 10-year period.

Ischemic Hepatitis

GENERAL PRINCIPLES

Definition

Ischemic hepatitis results from liver hypoperfusion.

Etiology

Clinical circumstances include severe blood loss, severe burns, cardiac failure, heat stroke, sepsis, and sickle cell crisis.

DIAGNOSIS

Clinical Presentation

History

Ischemic hepatitis presents as acute and transient rise of liver enzymes in the thousands during or following a hypotensive episode.

Diagnostic Testing

Laboratories

- Laboratory studies show a rapid rise and fall in levels of serum AST, ALT (>1,000 mg/dL), and lactate dehydrogenase (LDH) within 1 to 3 days of the insult.
- Total bilirubin, ALP, and INR may initially be normal but subsequently rise as a result of reperfusion injury.

Diagnostic Procedures

Liver biopsy is not usually needed for diagnosis.

- Centrilobular necrosis and sinusoidal distortion with inflammatory infiltrates in zone 3 (central areas) are classic histologic features.

TREATMENT

Correct the underlying condition that caused the circulatory collapse.

OUTCOME/PROGNOSIS

Prognosis is determined by rapid and effective treatment of the underlying cause.

Hepatic Vein Thrombosis

GENERAL PRINCIPLES

Definition

Hepatic vein thrombosis (HVT; also known as Budd–Chiari syndrome) causes hepatic venous outflow obstruction. It has multiple etiologies and a variety of clinical consequences.

Etiology

- Thrombosis is the main factor leading to obstruction of the hepatic venous system, frequently in association with myeloproliferative disorders, antiphospholipid antibody syndrome, paroxysmal nocturnal hemoglobinuria, factor V Leiden, protein C and S deficiency, and contraceptive use (*Gut 2008;57:1469*).
- Membranous obstruction of the inferior vena cava (IVC) is an infrequent condition that presents similarly to HVT.
- HVT can occur during pregnancy and in the postpartum period.
- Less than 20% of cases are idiopathic.

DIAGNOSIS

Clinical Presentation

- Patients may present with acute, subacute, or chronic illness characterized by **ascites, hepatomegaly, and right upper quadrant abdominal pain.**
- Other symptoms may include jaundice, encephalopathy, GI bleeding, and lower extremity edema.

Diagnostic Testing

Laboratories
- Serum-to-ascites albumin gradient is >1.1 g/dL. Serum albumin, bilirubin, AST, ALT, and PT/INR are mildly abnormal.
- Laboratory evaluation to identify a possible hypercoagulable state should be performed (see Chapter 17, Disorders of Hemostasis and Thrombosis).

Imaging
- Doppler ultrasound can be used as a screening test.
- Definitive diagnosis is made with magnetic resonance venography or hepatic venography.

TREATMENT

Medications

Nonsurgical treatment includes anticoagulation, thrombolytics, diuretics, angioplasty, stents, and transjugular intrahepatic portosystemic shunt (TIPS).

Surgical Management

Decompression procedures and liver transplantation are therapeutic options.

Sinusoidal Obstruction Syndrome

GENERAL PRINCIPLES

Definition

Sinusoidal obstruction syndrome (SOS; also known as veno-occlusive disease) refers to alterations in the liver microcirculation that may occur in the absence of vascular occlusion (*World J Gastroenterol 2007;13:1912*).

Etiology

Seen in **bone marrow transplant recipients** after therapy with total body irradiation and high-dose cytoreductive chemotherapy, in **renal transplant recipients** who are immunosuppressed with azathioprine, and in association with ingestion of pyrrolizidine alkaloids (Jamaican bush teas).

DIAGNOSIS

Clinical Presentation

- Diagnosis is based on the triad of **hepatomegaly, weight gain** (2% to 5% of baseline body weight), **and hyperbilirubinemia** (>2 mg/dL), generally occurring within 3 weeks after bone marrow transplantation.
- The severity of SOS varies from mild to moderate to severe disease.
- The clinical presentation depends on the severity of the disease.

Diagnostic Testing

Laboratories

The laboratory findings correlate with the clinical disease, from mild to significant elevations in aminotransferases and bilirubin.

Diagnostic Procedures

- A useful approach to the diagnosis is the transjugular measurement of the hepatic venous pressure. A concomitant liver biopsy can be performed during the same procedure.
- The typical histology shows centrilobular congestion with hepatocellular necrosis and accumulation of hemosiderin-laden macrophages. The terminal hepatic venules exhibit minimal edema without obvious fibrin deposition or thrombosis.

TREATMENT

Treatment is largely supportive.

Medications

Defibrotide, a single-stranded polydeoxyribonucleotide drug, has demonstrated ability to affect inflammatory, thrombotic, and angiogenic pathways involved in veno-occlusive disease. It has been used in the treatment of cardiovascular disorders and has shown promise in endothelial complications of allogeneic stem cell transplantation (*Expert Opin Biol Ther 2009;9(6):763*).

SPECIAL CONSIDERATIONS

Altering the myeloablative therapy and reducing the dose of radiation may decrease the incidence of SOS.

OUTCOME/PROGNOSIS

Prognosis depends on the severity of disease.

Portal Vein Thrombosis

GENERAL PRINCIPLES

Etiology

Portal vein thrombosis (PVT) is seen in a variety of clinical settings, including abdominal trauma, cirrhosis, malignancy, hypercoagulable states, intra-abdominal infections, pancreatitis, and after portocaval shunt surgery and splenectomy (*Am J Gastroenterol 2005;21:275*).

DIAGNOSIS

Clinical Presentation

- PVT can present as an acute or a chronic condition.
- The acute phase may go unrecognized. Symptoms include abdominal pain/distension, nausea, anorexia, weight loss, diarrhea, or features of the underlying disorder.
- Chronic PVT may present with variceal hemorrhage or other manifestations of portal hypertension.

Diagnostic Testing

Laboratories

In patients with no obvious etiology, a hypercoagulable workup should be performed.

Imaging

- **Ultrasonographic Doppler** examination is sensitive and specific for establishing the diagnosis.
- Angiography, CT, or magnetic resonance angiography can also be used.

TREATMENT

Medications

Anticoagulation should be considered in the setting of acute PVT.

Other Nonoperative Therapies

In the chronic setting treatment should focus on the complications of portal hypertension including nonselective β-blockers, endoscopic banding for varices, and diuretics for ascites.

Surgical Management

Portosystemic surgery carries a high morbidity and mortality, especially in patients with PVT associated with cirrhosis.

Pyogenic Abscess

GENERAL PRINCIPLES

Etiology

- **Pyogenic abscess** can result from hematogenous infection, spread from intra-abdominal infection, or ascending infection from the biliary tract.
- Approximately 20% of cases are cryptogenic in origin.

DIAGNOSIS

Clinical Presentation

Clinical features include fever, chills, weight loss, jaundice, and abdominal pain from hepatomegaly.

Diagnostic Testing

Laboratories
- Laboratory studies may demonstrate leukocytosis and elevated ALP.
- Blood cultures are often positive at presentation.

Imaging
Diagnosis is confirmed by CT, MRI, or ultrasonography.

TREATMENT

Medications

Treatment includes a prolonged course of antibiotic therapy.

Other Nonoperative Therapies

In select cases, treatment is by imaging-guided percutaneous drainage or surgery (*Am Surg 2008;74(2):178*).

MONITORING/FOLLOW-UP

Repeated imaging is recommended to document resolution.

Amebic Abscess

GENERAL PRINCIPLES

Amebic abscess is a diagnostic consideration in patients from endemic areas (*Expert Rev Anti Infect Ther2007;5(5):893*).

DIAGNOSIS

Clinical Presentation
- Diagnosis requires a high index of clinical suspicion.
- Clinical features include fever, chills, and tender hepatomegaly. Concurrent diarrhea may be present in small proportion of patients and some patients may give a history of dysentery in the previous few months.

Diagnostic Testing
Laboratories
Specific serologic tests for *Entamoeba histolytica* such as the indirect hemagglutination determination are helpful in establishing the diagnosis in low-prevalence areas.

TREATMENT

Medications
Amebic abscesses are treated with **metronidazole.**

Other Nonoperative Therapies
Imaging-guided drainage is reserved for amebic abscesses at risk for rupture or when pyogenic coinfection is suspected.

Granulomatous Hepatitis

GENERAL PRINCIPLES

Definition
Granulomatous hepatitis is the consequence of a nonspecific reaction to a wide spectrum of diverse etiologic stimuli.

Etiology
Etiologies include infections (e.g., brucellosis, syphilis, mycobacterial, fungal, and rickettsial diseases), sarcoidosis, AIDS, drug-induced injury, lymphoma, and idiopathic causes.

DIAGNOSIS

Clinical Presentation
Patients may present with fever, hepatosplenomegaly, and signs of portal hypertension.

Diagnostic Testing
Laboratories
Laboratory studies show elevated liver enzyme levels and ALP.

Diagnostic Procedures
Liver biopsy is the most accurate and specific way to diagnose granulomatous hepatitis.

TREATMENT

- Specific therapy is directed at the underlying cause.
- If clinical suspicion for tuberculosis is high, an empiric trial of antituberculous therapy may be warranted despite negative mycobacterial cultures.
- Corticosteroids should be considered in patients with idiopathic granulomatous liver disease in whom tuberculosis is not suspected.

ACUTE LIVER FAILURE

GENERAL PRINCIPLES

Definition

- Acute liver disease encompasses a wide range of disorders from asymptomatic aminotransferase elevations to liver failure.
- Acute liver failure (ALF) is a rare condition which includes evidence of coagulation abnormalities (usually an INR > 1.5) and any degree of mental alteration (encephalopathy) in a patient without preexisting cirrhosis and with an illness of <26 weeks duration.

Classification

Terms used signifying length of illness in ALF such as hyperacute (<7days), acute (7 to 21 days), and subacute (>21 days to <26 weeks) are not helpful since they do not have prognostic significance distinct from the cause of illness (*Hepatology 2005;41:1179*).

Epidemiology

Approximately 2,000 cases of ALF occur in the United States each year.

Etiology

- Acetaminophen hepatotoxicity and viral hepatitis are the most common causes of ALF.
- Other causes include AIH, drug and toxin exposure, ischemia, acute fatty liver of pregnancy, WD, and Reye's syndrome.
- In 20% of cases, no clear cause is identified.

Pathophysiology

- Histologic changes to the liver are typically those of acute inflammation with varying degrees of necrosis and collapse of the liver's architectural framework.
- These features are in contrast to the changes of cirrhosis and portal hypertension that dominate chronic liver disease.

DIAGNOSIS

Clinical Presentation

- Patients may present with mild to severe mental status changes in the setting of moderate to severe acute hepatitis and coagulopathy.
- Jaundice may or may not be initially present.
- A history of acetaminophen overdose, toxin ingestion, or risk factors for viral hepatitis may be obtained.

- Patients can develop cardiovascular collapse, acute renal failure, cerebral edema, and sepsis.

Diagnostic Testing

Laboratories
- Aminotransferases are typically elevated, and in many cases are >1,000 IU/L.
- INR is ≥1.5.
- Initial workup to determine the etiology of FHF should include:
  - Acute viral hepatitis panel
  - Serum drug screen, which includes acetaminophen
  - Ceruloplasmin
  - AIH serologies
  - Pregnancy test

Imaging
- Right upper quadrant ultrasound with Doppler may be obtained to evaluate obstruction of hepatic venous inflow or outflow.
- CT of the head may be obtained to evaluate and track progression of cerebral edema; however, the radiologic findings may lag behind its development and do not substitute for bedside assessments of neurologic status.

Diagnostic Procedures
Liver biopsy is seldom used to establish etiology or prognosis. Given the presence of coagulopathy, a transjugular approach to liver biopsy may be attempted if necessary.

TREATMENT

- Supportive therapy in the intensive care unit (ICU) setting of a tertiary center with liver transplant capabilities is essential.
- Precipitating factors should be identified and treated if possible.
- Sedation should be avoided to allow for serial assessments of mental/neurologic status.
- Blood glucose, electrolytes, acid–base, coagulation parameters, and fluid status should be monitored serially.
- Fresh frozen plasma and the use of recombinant activated factor VIIa should be considered in the setting of active bleeding or when invasive procedures are required.
- Cerebral edema and intracranial hypertension are related to severity of encephalopathy. In patients that reach grade III or IV encephalopathy, intracranial pressure monitoring should be considered (intracranial pressure should be maintained below 20 to 25 mm Hg, and cerebral perfusion pressure should be maintained above 50 mm Hg). Therapies to decrease cerebral edema include mannitol (0.5 to 1 g/kg IV), hyperventilation (reduce $PaCO_2$ to 25 to 30 mm Hg), hypothermia (32°C to 34°C), and barbiturates.
- Lactulose is *not* indicated for encephalopathy. Its use may result in increased bowel gas that may interfere with surgical approach for liver transplantation.
- Transplantation should be urgently considered in cases of ALF.

OUTCOME/PROGNOSIS

- Prior to transplantation survival was <15%; in the posttransplant era survival is >65% (*Ann Intern Med 2002;137:947*).

- Death often results from progressive liver failure, GI bleeding, cerebral edema, sepsis, or arrhythmia.
- Poor prognostic indicators in acetaminophen-induced ALF include arterial pH < 7.3, INR > 6.5, creatinine > 2.3 mg/dL, and encephalopathy grade III–IV.

CHRONIC LIVER DISEASE

Cirrhosis

GENERAL PRINCIPLES

- Cirrhosis is a chronic condition characterized by diffuse replacement of liver cells by fibrotic tissue, which creates a nodular-appearing distortion of the normal liver architecture. This fibrosis represents the end result of a variety of etiologies of liver injury.
- Cirrhosis affects nearly 5.5 million Americans and is the tenth leading cause of death in the United States.
- The most common etiologies are alcohol-related liver disease, chronic viral infection, and NASH.

Hepatic Encephalopathy

GENERAL PRINCIPLES

Definition

Hepatic encephalopathy is the syndrome of disordered consciousness and altered neuromuscular activity that is seen in patients with acute or chronic hepatocellular failure or portosystemic shunting.

Classification
- Grade I: sleep reversal pattern, mild confusion, irritability, tremor
- Grade II: lethargy, disorientation, inappropriate behavior, asterixis
- Grade III: somnolence, severe confusion, aggressive behavior, asterixis
- Grade IV: coma

Etiology
- The pathogenesis of hepatic encephalopathy is controversial, and numerous mediators have been implicated.
- **Precipitating factors** include azotemia; ALF; use of a tranquilizer, opioid, or sedative-hypnotic medication; GI hemorrhage; hypokalemia and alkalosis (diuretics and diarrhea); constipation; infection; high-protein diet; progressive hepatocellular dysfunction; and portosystemic shunts (surgical or TIPS).

DIAGNOSIS

- Presentation varies from subtle mental status changes to coma.
- Asterixis (flapping tremor) is present in stage I–III encephalopathy. This motor disturbance is not specific to hepatic encephalopathy.
- The electroencephalogram shows slow, high-amplitude, and triphasic waves.

• Determination of blood ammonia level is not a sensitive or specific test for hepatic encephalopathy.

TREATMENT

Medications

Medications include **nonabsorbable disaccharides** (lactulose, lactitol, and lactose in lactase-deficient patients) and **antibiotics** (neomycin, metronidazole, and rifaximin).

• The initial dose of lactulose is 15 to 45 mL PO bid–qid. Maintenance dose should be adjusted to produce three to five soft stools per day. Oral lactulose should not be given to patients with ileus or possible bowel obstruction.
• **Lactulose enemas** (prepared by the addition of 300 mL lactulose to 700 mL distilled water) can also be administered.
• **Neomycin** can be given by mouth (500 to 1,000 mg q6h) or as a retention enema (1% solution in 100 to 200 mL isotonic saline). Approximately 1% to 3% of the administered dose of neomycin is absorbed, with the attendant risk of ototoxicity and nephrotoxicity. The risk of toxicity is increased in patients with renal insufficiency.
• **Metronidazole** (250 mg PO q8h) is useful for short-term therapy when neomycin is unavailable or poorly tolerated. Long-term metronidazole is not recommended due to its associated toxicities.
• **Rifaximin,** 400 mg PO tid, is used as an alternative to neomycin and metronidazole.
• Combination therapy with lactulose and any of the antibiotics mentioned above should be considered in cases that are refractory to either agent alone.

Diet

The rationale and benefit of dietary protein restriction is controversial. Once the patient is able to eat, a diet containing 30 to 40 g of protein per day is initiated. Special diets (vegetable protein or branched-chain amino acid enriched) may be beneficial in patients with encephalopathy that is refractory to the usual measures.

Portal Hypertension

GENERAL PRINCIPLES

• Portal hypertension is the main complication of cirrhosis and is characterized by increased resistance to portal flow and increased portal venous inflow. Portal hypertension is established by determining the pressure difference between the hepatic vein and the portal vein (normal pressure gradient 3 mm Hg).
• Direct and indirect clinical consequences of portal hypertension (generally with a pressure gradient > 10 mm Hg) include esophageal and gastric varices, portal hypertensive gastropathy, ascites, hepatorenal syndrome (HRS), and spontaneous bacterial peritonitis (SBP) (*Curr Opin Gastroenterol 2005;21:313*).

Associated Conditions

Causes of portal hypertension in patients without cirrhosis include idiopathic portal hypertension, schistosomiasis, congenital hepatic fibrosis, sarcoidosis, cystic fibrosis, arteriovenous fistulas, splenic and portal vein thrombosis, myeloproliferative diseases, nodular regenerative hyperplasia, and focal nodular hyperplasia.

DIAGNOSIS

Clinical Presentation

Portal hypertension frequently complicates cirrhosis and presents with ascites, GI bleeding from esophageal or gastric varices or portal hypertensive gastropathy/colopathy, and splenomegaly.

Imaging
Ultrasonography, CT, and MRI showing cirrhosis, splenomegaly, collateral venous circulation, and ascites are suggestive of portal hypertension.

Diagnostic Procedures
- Upper endoscopy showing varices (esophageal or gastric) or portal hypertensive gastropathy.
- Transjugular portal pressure measurements.

TREATMENT

Treatment of GI bleeding due to portal hypertension is covered in Chapter 15, Gastrointestinal Diseases.

Ascites

GENERAL PRINCIPLES

Definition
Ascites is the abnormal (>25 mL) accumulation of fluid within the peritoneal cavity.

Etiology
Causes of ascites besides cirrhosis include cancer (peritoneal carcinomatosis), heart failure, tuberculosis, pancreatic disease, nephrotic syndrome, surgery or trauma to the lymphatic system or ureters, and serositis (*Hepatology 2004;39:841*).

DIAGNOSIS

Clinical Presentation
Presentation ranges from ascites detected only by imaging methods to a distended, bulging abdomen. Percussion of the abdomen may reveal shifting dullness.

Diagnostic Testing
Laboratories
- A **serum to ascites albumin gradient (SAAG)** that is ≥1.1 g/dL indicates portal hypertension–related ascites (97% specificity).
- A SAAG of <1.1 g/dL is found in nephrotic syndrome, peritoneal carcinomatosis, serositis, tuberculosis, and biliary or pancreatic ascites.

Imaging
Ultrasonography, CT, and MRI are sensitive methods to detect ascites.

Diagnostic Procedures

Paracentesis should be performed for diagnosis (e.g., new-onset ascites, suspicion of malignant ascites, or SBP) or as a therapeutic maneuver when tense ascites causes significant discomfort or respiratory compromise.

- Routine diagnostic testing should include fluid cell and differential counts, albumin, total protein, and culture.
- Amylase and triglyceride measurement, cytology, and mycobacterial smear/culture can be performed to confirm specific diagnoses.
- **Bleeding** and **intestinal perforation** are possible complications.
- Rapid large-volume paracentesis (>5 L) may lead to circulatory collapse, encephalopathy, and renal failure. Concomitant administration of IV albumin (5 to 8 g/L ascites removed) can be used to minimize these complications, especially in the setting of renal insufficiency or the absence of peripheral edema.

TREATMENT

Medications

- **Diuretic therapy** is initiated along with **salt restriction**. The goal of diuretic therapy should be a daily weight loss of no more than 1.0 kg in patients with edema and approximately 0.5 kg in those without edema until ascites is adequately controlled. Diuretics should not be administered to individuals with an increasing serum creatinine level.
- **Spironolactone** (100 mg PO in a single daily dose with food) is the diuretic of choice. The daily dose can be increased by 50 to 100 mg every 7 to 10 days until satisfactory weight loss, a maximum dose of 400 mg, or side effects occur. Hyperkalemia and gynecomastia are common side effects. Amiloride or triamterene (potassium-sparing diuretics) are substitutes that can be used in patients in whom painful gynecomastia develops.
- **Loop diuretics,** such as furosemide (20 to 40 mg, increasing to a maximum dose of 160 mg PO daily) or bumetanide (0.5 to 2.0 mg PO daily), can be added to spironolactone.
- Patients should be observed closely for signs of dehydration, electrolyte disturbances, encephalopathy, muscle cramps, and renal insufficiency. Nonsteroidal antiinflammatory agents may blunt the effect of diuretics and increase the risk of renal dysfunction.

Other Nonoperative Therapies

TIPS has been proven effective in the management of refractory ascites (fluid overload that is nonresponsive to a sodium-restricted diet and high-dose diuretic therapy).

- Complications include shunt occlusion, bleeding, infection, cardiopulmonary compromise, and hepatic encephalopathy.

Lifestyle/Risk Modification

Diet

Dietary salt restriction (2 g salt or 88 mmol Na^+/d) should be initiated and continued thereafter unless the renal ability to excrete sodium spontaneously improves. In selected cases, it may be necessary to restrict sodium intake further.

- The use of potassium-containing salt substitutes can lead to serious hyperkalemia.
- Routine water restriction is not necessary. If dilutional hyponatremia (serum Na$^+$ < 120 mmol/L) occurs, fluid restriction to 1,000 to 1,500 mL/d usually suffices.

Spontaneous Bacterial Peritonitis

GENERAL PRINCIPLES

Definition

Spontaneous bacterial peritonitis (SBP) is an infectious complication of portal hypertension–related ascites.

Risk Factors

Risk factors for SBP include ascitic fluid protein concentration < 1 mg/dL, variceal hemorrhage, and a prior episode of SBP.

DIAGNOSIS

Clinical Presentation

Clinical manifestations include abdominal pain and distention, fever, decreased bowel sounds, and worsening hepatic encephalopathy. It may be present in the absence of specific clinical signs. Cirrhotic patients with ascites and evidence of any clinical deterioration should undergo diagnostic paracentesis to exclude SBP.

Diagnostic Testing

Laboratories

The diagnosis is confirmed when the ascitic fluid contains >250 neutrophils/mL. Gram stain reveals the organism in only 10% to 20% of samples.

- Cultures are more likely to be positive when 10 mL ascitic fluid is inoculated into two blood culture bottles at the bedside.
- The most common organisms are *Escherichia coli*, *Klebsiella*, and *Streptococcus pneumoniae*. Polymicrobial infection is uncommon and should lead to the suspicion of secondary bacterial peritonitis.

TREATMENT

Medications

- Patients with ascitic fluid polymorphonuclear leukocyte (PMN) counts ≥ 250 cells/mm^3 should receive **empiric antibiotic therapy,** for example, an **intravenous third-generation cephalosporin** (ceftriaxone, 1 g IV daily; or cefotaxime, 1 to 2 g IV q6–8h, depending on renal function). Paracentesis should be repeated if no clinical improvement occurs in 48 to 72 hours, especially if the initial ascitic fluid culture was negative (*Hepatology 2009;49:2087*).
  - Oral ofloxacin (400 mg twice per day) can be considered a substitute for intravenous cefotaxime in inpatients without prior exposure to quinolones, vomiting, shock, grade II (or higher) hepatic encephalopathy, or serum creatinine > 3 mg/dL (*Hepatology 2009;49:2087*).

- Patients with ascitic fluid PMN counts < 250 cells/mm³ and signs or symptoms of infection (fever or abdominal pain or tenderness) should also receive **empiric antibiotic therapy** (*Hepatology 2009;49:2087*).
- Concomitant use of **albumin** 1.5 g/kg body weight at diagnosis and 1 g/kg body weight on day 3 improves survival and prevents renal failure in SBP (*N Engl J Med 1999;341:403*).
- **Norfloxacin** (400 mg PO daily) can be used as secondary prophylaxis for reducing the frequency of recurrent episodes of SBP. However, the use of antibiotic prophylaxis has not been clearly shown to improve survival and does select resistant gut flora.

Hepatorenal Syndrome

GENERAL PRINCIPLES

Definition

Hepatorenal syndrome (HRS) is a unique form of functional renal impairment in the setting of acute or, more commonly, chronic liver disease. Common precipitating factors include systemic bacterial infections, SBP, and large-volume paracentesis without volume expansion (*J Gastroenterol 2005;100;460*).

DIAGNOSIS

Major and minor diagnostic criteria are summarized in Table 5.

Table 5	Diagnostic Criteria of Hepatorenal Syndrome

Major criteria

Low glomerular filtration rate, as indicated by serum creatinine > 1.5 mg/dL or 24-hr creatinine clearance < 40 mL/min

Absence of shock, ongoing bacterial infection, fluid losses, and current treatment with nephrotoxic drugs

No sustained improvement in renal function (decrease in serum creatinine to 1.5 mg/dL or increase in creatinine clearance to 40 mL/min) after diuretic withdrawal and expansion of plasma volume with 1.5 L of a plasma expander

Proteinuria < 500 mg/dL and no ultrasonographic evidence of obstructive uropathy or parenchymal renal disease

Additional criteria

Urine volume < 500 mL/d

Urine sodium < 10 mEq/L

Urine osmolality greater than plasma osmolality

Urine red blood cells < 50 per high-power field

Serum sodium concentration < 130 mEq/L

Note: All major criteria must be present for the diagnosis of hepatorenal syndrome. Additional criteria are not necessary for the diagnosis but provide supportive evidence.
Adapted from Arroyo V, Gines P, Gerbes AL, et al. Definition and diagnostic criteria of refractory ascites and hepatorenal syndrome in cirrhosis. International Ascites Club. Hepatology 1996;23:164.

- **Type I** HRS is characterized by the acute onset of rapidly progressive (<2 weeks), oliguric renal failure unresponsive to volume expansion. There is a doubling of the initial serum creatinine to a level > 2.5 mg/dL or a 50% reduction in the creatinine clearance to a level < 20 mL/min.
- **Type II** HRS progresses more slowly but relentlessly and often clinically manifests as diuretic-resistant ascites.

TREATMENT

Medications

No clear or established treatments are available for HRS. Systemic vasoconstrictors including vasopressin analogs (terlipressin), somatostatin analogs (octreotide), and α-adrenergic agonists (midodrine and norepinephrine) with plasma expansion have shown a beneficial role in uncontrolled studies.

Other Nonoperative Therapies

- TIPS is a potential treatment alternative; however, data are limited.
- Hemodialysis may be indicated in patients listed for liver transplantations.

Surgical Management

In suitable candidates, liver transplantation may be curative.

OUTCOME/PROGNOSIS

Without treatment, patients with type I HRS have a short-term prognosis, with death occurring within 2 to 3 months of onset. Patients with type II HRS have a median survival of approximately 6 months.

Hepatocellular Carcinoma

GENERAL PRINCIPLES

Epidemiology

- HCC frequently occurs in patients with cirrhosis, especially when associated with viral hepatitis (HBV or HCV), alcoholic cirrhosis, α_1AT deficiency, and hemochromatosis.
- HCC is the fifth most common cancer in men and the ninth most common cancer in women worldwide. It constitutes 84% of primary liver cancer in the United States (mean age at diagnosis is 65).

DIAGNOSIS

Clinical Presentation

- Clinical presentation is directly proportional to the stage of disease. Early disease is asymptomatic, while patients with late-stage disease may present with right upper quadrant abdominal pain, weight loss, and hepatomegaly.
- Suspect HCC in a well-controlled cirrhotic patient who develops manifestations of liver decompensation.

- Surveillance for HCC (sensitive imaging study every 6 to 12 months) is normally indicated for patients with cirrhosis. In patients with hepatitis B, surveillance should begin after age 40 and in those with family history of HCC even in the absence of cirrhosis.

Diagnostic Testing

Laboratories

- α-Fetoprotein (refer back to section Evaluation of Liver Disease).
- Investigational serum markers for HCC include lens culinaris agglutinin-reactive α-fetoprotein, des-gamma-carboxyprothrombin (DCP), alpha-L-fucosidase, and glypican-3 (GPC3).

Imaging

Liver ultrasound, triple-phase CT, and MRI are adequate and frequently used for detection of HCC.

Diagnostic Procedures

Liver biopsy should be considered for suspicious cases with noncharacteristic imaging features.

TREATMENT

Medications

Sorafenib is a small molecule that inhibits tumor cell proliferation and tumor angiogenesis and increases the rate of apoptosis in a wide range of tumor models.

- In patients with advanced HCC, median survival and radiologic progression were nearly 3 months longer for patients treated with sorafenib than for those given placebo (*N Engl J Med 2008;359:378*).

Other Nonoperative Therapies

- Alternative therapy for unresectable tumors includes percutaneous alcohol or acetic acid injection, arterial chemoembolization, microwave coagulation therapy, or radiofrequency ablation.
- These loco-regional therapies can be used as a bridge to liver transplantation in selected cases.

Surgical Management

- Hepatic resection is the treatment of choice in noncirrhotic patients.
- Liver transplantation is the treatment of choice for select cirrhotic patients (single HCC < 5 cm or up to three nodules < 3 cm).

OUTCOME/PROGNOSIS

Early diagnosis is essential, as surgical resection and liver transplantation can improve long-term survival. Survival with no treatment remains very poor: 36% and 17% at 1 and 3 years, respectively.

LIVER TRANSPLANTATION

GENERAL PRINCIPLES

- Liver transplantation is an effective therapeutic option for both irreversible acute and chronic liver diseases for which available therapies have failed.
- Whole cadaveric livers and partial livers (split-liver, reduced-size, and living-related) are used in the United States as sources for liver transplantation.
- Patients who fulfill criteria for **FHF** are potential candidates for liver transplantation.
- Patients with chronic liver disease should be considered for transplant evaluation when they have a **decline in hepatic synthetic or excretory functions,** ascites, hepatic encephalopathy, or complications such as HRS, HCC, recurrent SBP, or variceal bleeding.
- The prioritization for liver transplantation in chronic liver disease is determined by the **Model for End-Stage Liver Disease (MELD)** score. The MELD score is determined by the use of an equation that takes into account serum bilirubin, serum creatinine, and INR (http://www.unos.org/resources/MeldPeldCalculator.asp?index=98).
- General **contraindications** to liver transplant include:
  - Severe and uncontrolled extrahepatic infection
  - Advanced cardiac or pulmonary disease
  - Extrahepatic malignancy
  - Multiorgan failure
  - Unresolved psychosocial issues
  - Medical noncompliance issues
  - Ongoing substance abuse (e.g., alcohol and illegal drugs)

Epidemiology

- In the United States, over 17,000 patients are awaiting liver transplants, 5,000 transplants are performed and approximately 2,000 patients die each year on the waiting list.
- The disparity between supply and demand of suitable livers for transplantation continues to increase.

TREATMENT

- Candidates for liver transplantation are evaluated by a multidisciplinary team that includes hepatologists, transplant surgeons, transplant nurse coordinators, social workers, psychologists, and financial coordinators.
- Immunosuppressive, infectious, and long-term complications are discussed in Chapter 14, Solid Organ Transplant Medicine.

17 Disorders of Hemostasis and Thrombosis

Roger Yusen, Charles Eby, and Brian F. Gage

Hemostatic Disorders

GENERAL PRINCIPLES

Definition

Normal hemostasis involves a complex sequence of interrelated reactions that lead to platelet aggregation (primary hemostasis) and activation of coagulation factors (secondary hemostasis) to produce a durable vascular seal.

- **Primary hemostasis** is an immediate but temporary response to vessel injury. Platelets and von Willebrand factor (vWF) interact to form a primary plug.
- **Secondary hemostasis (coagulation)** results in formation of a fibrin clot (Fig. 1). Injury initiates coagulation by exposing extravascular tissue factor to blood, which initiates activation of factors VII, X, and prothrombin. The subsequent activation of other factors leads to generation of thrombin, conversion of fibrinogen to fibrin, and formation of a durable clot (*Semin Thromb Hemost 2009; 35:9*).

DIAGNOSIS

Clinical Presentation

History

A detailed history can assess bleeding severity, congenital or acquired status, and primary or secondary hemostatic defects.

- Prolonged bleeding after dental extractions, circumcision, menstruation, labor and delivery, trauma, or surgery may suggest an underlying bleeding disorder.
- Family history may suggest an inherited bleeding disorder.

Physical Examination

- Primary hemostasis defects are suggested by mucosal bleeding and excessive bruising.
  - Petechiae: <2 mm subcutaneous bleeding, do not blanch with pressure, typically present in areas subject to increased hydrostatic force: the lower legs and periorbital area (especially after coughing or vomiting).
  - Ecchymoses: >3 mm black-and-blue (or violaceous) patches due to rupture of small vessels from trauma.

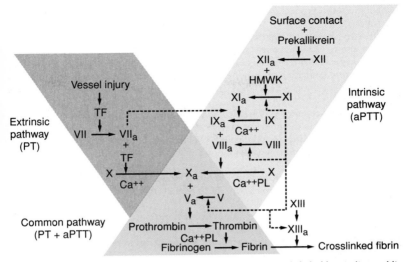

Figure 1. Coagulation cascade. *Solid arrows* indicate activation, and *dashed lines* indicate additional substrates activated by factor VIIa or thrombin. aPTT, activated partial thromboplastin time; HMWK, high-molecular-weight kininogen; PL, phospholipid; PT, prothrombin time; TF, tissue factor.

- Secondary hemostasis defects can produce **hematomas** (localized masses of clotted/unclotted blood), hemarthroses, or delayed bleeding after trauma or surgery.

Diagnostic Testing

Laboratories

The history and physical exam guide test selection. Initial studies should include platelet count, prothrombin time (PT), activated partial thromboplastin time (aPTT), and peripheral blood smear.

- **Primary hemostasis tests**
  - A low **platelet count** requires review of blood smear to rule out platelet clumping artifact (due to the EDTA additive, platelet glycoprotein IIb/IIIa receptor inhibitor drugs), giant platelets.
  - The **bleeding time (BT)** measures time until bleeding cessation from a standardized skin incision, but it does not quantify the peri-operative risk of bleeding (*Arch Pathol Lab Med 1996;120:353*). Many factors can prolong the BT: thrombocytopenia, von Willebrand disease (vWD), abnormal capillary or skin integrity, antiplatelet therapy, uremia, liver failure, anemia, and poor technique.
  - The **PFA-100** (Dade Behring, Deerfield, IL) instrument assesses vWF-dependent platelet activation in flowing citrated whole blood. Most patients with vWD and qualitative platelet disorders have prolonged closure times. Anemia (HCT < 30%)

and thrombocytopenia (platelet count $< 100 \times 10^9$/L) can cause prolonged closure times.

- **In vitro platelet aggregation** studies measure platelet secretion and aggregation in response to platelet agonists (e.g., ADP, collagen, arachidonic acid, epinephrine), and they assist with the diagnosis of qualitative platelet disorders.
- Laboratory evaluation of suspected vWD begins with measurement of von Willebrand factor antigen (**vWF:Ag**) and performance of at least one **vWF activity assay:**
    - **Ristocetin cofactor (vWF:RCo):** measures vWF-mediated agglutination of control platelets in the presence of ristocetin.
    - **Collagen binding assay:** measures vWF affinity for collagen.
    - **"Functional" immunoassay:** monoclonal antibody to vWF domain that binds to platelets.
- **von Willebrand factor multimer analysis** by agarose gel electrophoresis separates vWF multimers by size to classify vWD type 2 subtypes.
- **Secondary hemostasis**
    - **Prothrombin time:** measures time to form a fibrin clot after adding thromboplastin (tissue factor and phospholipid) and calcium to citrated plasma.
        - Sensitive to deficiencies of **extrinsic pathway** (factor VII), **common pathway** (factors X, V, prothrombin), and **fibrinogen.**
        - Reporting a PT ratio as an international normalized ratio (INR) reduces interlaboratory variation (*Thromb Haemost 1983;49:238*).
        - Most PT reagents contain a heparin-neutralizing additive.
        - Point-of-care instruments accurately measure PT/INR from a drop of whole blood.
    - **Activated partial thromboplastin times:** measure the time to form a fibrin clot after activation of citrated plasma by calcium, phospholipid, and negatively charged particles.
    - Besides heparin, deficiencies and inhibitors of coagulation factors of the **intrinsic pathway** (e.g., high-molecular-weight kininogen, prekallikrein, factor XII, factor XI, factor IX, and factor VIII), **common pathway** (e.g., factor V, factor X, prothrombin), and **fibrinogen prolong the** aPTT.
    - **Thrombin time (TT):** measures time to form a fibrin clot after addition of thrombin to citrated plasma. Quantitative and qualitative deficiencies of fibrinogen, fibrin degradation products, heparin, and direct thrombin inhibitor (DTI) drugs prolong the TT.
    - **Fibrinogen:** the addition of thrombin to dilute plasma and the measurement of a clotting time determine the level of fibrinogen. Conditions causing hypofibrinogen and potential for bleeding include decreased hepatic synthesis, massive hemorrhage, and disseminated intravascular coagulation (DIC).
    - **D-dimers** result from plasmin digestion of fibrin. Elevated D-dimer concentrations occur in many disease states that include acute venous thromboembolism (VTE), DIC, trauma, and malignancy.
    - **Mixing studies** determine if a factor deficiency or an inhibitor have prolonged the PT or the aPTT. Mixing patient plasma 1:1 with normal pooled plasma (all factor activities = 100%) restores deficient factors sufficiently to normalize or nearly normalize the PT or the aPTT (Table 1). If mixing partially corrects the prolonged PT or aPTT, a specific factor inhibitor, a nonspecific inhibitor (e.g. lupus anticoagulant), heparin, or a DTI anticoagulant may have caused the prolongation.

Table 1	Factor Deficiencies Cause Prolonged Prothrombin Time and/or Activated Partial Thromboplastin Time That Correct with 50:50 Mix
Abnormal Assay	**Suspected Factor Deficiencies**
aPTT	XII, XI, IX, or VIII
PT	VII
PT and aPTT	II, V, X, or fibrinogen

aPTT, activated partial thromboplastin time; PT, prothrombin time.

PLATELET DISORDERS

Thrombocytopenia

GENERAL PRINCIPLES

Definition

Thrombocytopenia is defined as a platelet count of $<140 \times 10^9$/L at Barnes-Jewish Hospital. In the absence of qualitative platelet defects or vascular damage, spontaneous bleeding does not typically occur with platelet counts $> 30 \times 10^9$/L.

DIAGNOSIS

Differential Diagnosis

Thrombocytopenia occurs from decreased production, increased destruction, or sequestration of platelets (Table 2). Many infectious diseases have an association with thrombocytopenia through complex or poorly understood mechanisms (*Blood 2009;113:6511*).

Immune Thrombocytopenic Purpura

GENERAL PRINCIPLES

Immune thrombocytopenic purpura (ITP), an acquired autoimmune disorder in which antiplatelet antibodies cause shortened platelet survival and suppress megakaryopoiesis, leads to thrombocytopenia and increased bleeding risk. ITP classification consists of idiopathic (primary), associated with coexisting conditions (secondary), and drug induced.

Epidemiology

Adult primary **ITP** has an incidence of 32 cases per 10^6 persons (*Blood 1999;94:909*).

Etiology

- In ITP, autoantibodies bind to platelet surface antigens and cause premature clearance by the reticuloendothelial system, and immune-mediated suppression of platelet

Table 2	Classification of Thrombocytopenia

Decreased platelet production	**Increased platelet clearance**
Marrow failure syndromes	*Immune-mediated mechanisms*
Congenital	Immune thrombocytopenic purpura
Acquired: aplastic anemia, paroxysmal nocturnal hemoglobinuria	Thrombotic thrombocytopenic purpura
Hematologic malignancies	Posttransfusion purpura
Marrow infiltration: cancer, granuloma	Heparin-induced thrombocytopenia
Fibrosis: primary or secondary	*Nonimmune-mediated mechanisms*
Nutritional: vitamin B_{12} and folate deficiencies	DIC
Physical damage: radiation, alcohol, chemotherapy	Local consumption (aortic aneurysm)
	Acute hemorrhage
Increased splenic sequestration	**Infections associated with thrombocytopenia**
Portal hypertension	
Felty's syndrome	HIV, HHV-6, ehrlichiosis, rickettsia, malaria, hepatitis C, CMV, Epstein–Barr, *Helicobacter pylori*, *E. coli* O157
Lysosomal storage disorders	
Infiltrative hematologic malignancies	
Extramedullary hematopoiesis	

production. **Secondary ITP** occurs with systemic lupus erythematosus (SLE), antiphospholipid antibody (APA) syndrome, HIV, hepatitis C virus, *Helicobacter pylori*, and lymphoproliferative disorders (*Blood 2009;113:6511*).

- **Drug-dependent immune thrombocytopenia** results from drug–platelet interactions prompting antibody binding (*NEJM 2007;357:580*). Medications linked to thrombocytopenia include quinidine and quinine; platelet inhibitors abciximab, eptifibatide, tirofiban, and ticlopidine; antibiotics linezolid, rifampin, sulfonamides, and vancomycin; the anticonvulsants phenytoin, valproic acid, and carbamazepine; the analgesics acetaminophen, naproxen, and diclofenac; cimetidine, and chlorothiazide (*Ann Intern Med 2005;142:474*).

DIAGNOSIS

Clinical Presentation

- **ITP** typically presents as mild mucocutaneous bleeding and petechiae or thrombocytopenia discovered incidentally.
- Primary **ITP** often has the scenario of isolated thrombocytopenia in the absence of a likely underlying causative disease or medication.

Diagnostic Testing

Normalization of platelet counts with discontinuation of suspected drug, and confirmation if thrombocytopenia recurs when rechallenged supports the diagnosis of **drug-induced thrombocytopenia.**

Laboratories

- Laboratory tests do not confirm the presence of primary ITP, though they help to exclude some secondary causes.

- Serologic tests for antiplatelet antibodies generally do not help diagnose **ITP** because of poor sensitivity and low negative predictive value (*Am J Hematol 2005;78:193*).

Diagnostic Procedures
Diagnosis of ITP does not typically require bone marrow biopsy and aspirate studies, though these tests help to exclude other causes in select patients such as those with age greater than 60 years and those who do not respond to immune suppression therapy (*Blood 1996;88:3*).

TREATMENT

- The decision to treat **primary ITP** depends upon the severity of thrombocytopenia and concerns about bleeding. Management of **secondary ITP** may include treatment of the underlying disease and the primary ITP therapy. Initial therapy, when indicated, consists of glucocorticoids (typically prednisone 1 mg/kg/d). Nonresponders or patients with active bleeding typically also receive IVIg (1 g/kg × 2 days) or anti-D immunoglobulin (WinRho) if Rh-positive (ineffective postsplenectomy). Most primary ITP patients initially respond to therapy with resolution of thrombocytopenia within 1 to 3 weeks. Nonresponders and 30% to 40% of patients who relapse during a steroid taper have refractory ITP, for whom the therapeutic goal consists of a safe platelet count (30×10^9 to 50×10^9/L) and minimization of treatment-related toxicities.
- Two-thirds of patients with refractory ITP will obtain a durable complete response following splenectomy. Administer pneumococcal, meningococcal, and *Haemophilus influenzae* type B vaccines at least 2 weeks before splenectomy.
- Options for patients who do not undergo splenectomy, or those who fail splenectomy, include single or combined therapies with prednisone, IVIg, androgen therapy with danazol, other immunosuppressive agents, or anti-CD20 monoclonal antibodies (rituximab) (*Blood 1996;88:3; Blood 2001;98:952*).
- In 2008, the FDA approved two small-molecule thrombopoietin receptor (TPO-R) agonists for treatment of refractory primary ITP patients with increased bleeding risk. Romiplostim (Nplate), dosed SQ weekly, and eltrombopag (Promacta), taken orally once a day, produce durable platelet count improvements in a majority of refractory ITP patients beginning 5 to 7 days after initiation. Potential complications include thromboembolic events and bone marrow fibrosis (*Lancet 2009;373:1562*).
  - For **drug-induced thrombocytopenia,** platelet transfusions for severe thrombocytopenia may decrease the risk of bleeding. IVIg, steroids, and plasmapheresis have uncertain benefit.

Thrombotic Thrombocytopenic Purpura and Hemolytic Uremic Syndrome

GENERAL PRINCIPLES

Definition
Thrombotic thrombocytopenic purpura (TTP) and **hemolytic uremic syndrome (HUS),** thrombotic microangiopathies (TMAs) caused by platelet–vWF aggregates and platelet–fibrin aggregates, respectively, result in thrombocytopenia, microangiopathic hemolytic anemia (MAHA), and organ ischemia. Typically, clinical and

laboratory features permit differentiation of TTP from HUS. TMA has an association with DIC, HIV infection, malignant hypertension, vasculitis, organ and stem cell transplant–related toxicity, adverse drug reactions, and, during pregnancy, preeclampsia/eclampsia and HELLP syndrome.

Epidemiology

Sporadic **TTP** has an incidence of approximately 11.3 cases per 10^6 persons and occurs more frequently in women and African Americans (*J Thromb Haemost 2005;3:1432*). HUS usually occurs in outbreaks affecting children. However, adults may present with both typical and atypical variants of HUS.

Etiology

- Autoantibody-mediated removal of plasma vWF-cleaving protease (ADAMTS13), leading to elevated levels of abnormally large vWF multimers, typically causes **sporadic TTP** (*New Engl J Med 1998;339:1578*). The abnormal vWF multimers spontaneously adhere to platelets and may produce occlusive vWF–platelet aggregates in the microcirculation and subsequent microangiopathy. Second-hit events may involve endothelial dysfunction or injury.
- Severe ADAMTS13 deficiency does not cause HUS and other types of TMA, with the exception of some cases associated with HIV and pregnancy.
- **Typical HUS** has an association with *Escherichia coli* (O157:H7) production of Shiga-like toxins. **Atypical HUS** has an association with transplantation, endothelial damaging drugs, and pregnancy (*Kidney Int Suppl 2009;112:S8*). Inherited defects in regulation of the alternative pathway of complement activation cause **familial HUS** (*J Exp Med 2007;204:1245*).

DIAGNOSIS

Clinical Presentation

- The complete clinical pentad of **TTP,** present in <30% of cases, includes consumptive thrombocytopenia, MAHA, fever, renal dysfunction, and fluctuating neurologic deficits.
- The findings of thrombocytopenia and MAHA should raise suspicion for TTP in the absence of other identifiable causes.
- TTP may occur during pregnancy and postpartum, and in association with HIV infection.
- Patients with autosomal recessive inherited ADAMTS13 deficiencies have relapsing TTP (Upshaw–Schulman syndrome).
- Diarrhea, often bloody, and abdominal pain often proceed typical HUS, and more pronounced renal dysfunction occurs.

Diagnostic Testing

Laboratories
- TMAs produce schistocytes and thrombocytopenia on blood smears. The findings of anemia, elevated reticulocyte count, low or undetectable haptoglobin, and elevated lactate dehydrogenase support the presence of hemolysis.
- Sporadic TTP has TMA findings, normal PT and aPTT, mild to moderate azotemia, very low or undetectable ADAMTS13 enzyme activity, and sometimes an ADAMTS13 inhibitory antibody.

- HUS has TMA and acute renal failure. In typical HUS, *E. coli* O157 stool culture has a higher sensitivity than do Shiga toxin assays. However, stool samples obtained after diarrhea has resolved reduce the sensitivity of both tests (*Kid Int 2009;75:S29–S32*). Testing for **sporadic or familial HUS** should include molecular analysis of complement regulator factor H and I genes through reference laboratories.

TREATMENT

- TTP: **The mainstay of therapy consists of rapid treatment with plasma exchange (PEX)** of 1.0 to 1.5 plasma volumes daily. PEX is usually continued for at least 5 or 2 days after normalization of platelet count and lactate dehydrogenase.
  - If PEX is not available or will be delayed, infuse **fresh frozen plasma (FFP)** immediately to replace ADAMTS13.
  - Common practice includes the administration of **glucocorticoids:** prednisone, 1 mg/kg PO or methylprednisolone, 1g IV daily.
  - Transfuse red cells based on signs and symptoms of anemia.
  - Platelet transfusion in the absence of severe bleeding is relatively contraindicated due to potential risk of additional microvascular occlusions.
  - ~ 90% of treated patients have a remission. Relapses may occur within days to years later after remission.
  - Therapy with **rituximab,** an anti-CD20 monoclonal antibody, achieves durable remissions following TTP relapses (*Ann Intern Med 2003;138:105;Thromb Haemost 2009;101:233*).
  - **Immunosuppression** with cyclophosphamide, azathioprine, or vincristine and splenectomy may have success in the treatment of refractory or relapsing TTP (*Ann Hematol 2002;81:7; Blood 2000;96:1223*).
- Treatment of typical HUS remains supportive. Familial HUS often leads to chronic renal failure.
  - HUS does not usually improve with PEX.
  - Antibiotic therapy does not hasten recovery or minimize toxicity for HUS associated with infection.
  - Atypical HUS associated with calcineurin inhibitors (cyclosporine, tacrolimus) usually responds to drug dose reduction or discontinuation.

Heparin-Induced Thrombocytopenia

GENERAL PRINCIPLES

Definition

Heparin-induced thrombocytopenia (HIT) is an acquired hypercoagulable disorder caused by antibodies targeting heparin and platelet factor 4 (PF4) complexes. HIT typically presents with a decreased platelet count by at least 50% from preexposure baseline, though HIT-associated thrombosis can occur prior to the platelet count drop. Exposure to unfractionated heparin (UFH), and less likely with low-molecular-weight heparin (LMWH), and fondaparinux causes HIT. HIT complications include venous and arterial thromboses, skin necrosis at injection sites, and acute systemic reactions after IV bolus administration.

Epidemiology

The incidence of **HIT** varies with clinical setting, anticoagulant formulation, dose, duration of exposure, and previous exposure, and it ranges from 0.1% to 1% in medical and obstetric patients receiving prophylactic and therapeutic UFH to >1% to 5% in patients receiving prophylactic UFH after total hip or knee replacements or cardiothoracic surgery (*Chest 2008;133:340S*). Patients exposed only to LMWH have a low incidence of HIT (*Thromb Res 2009;124:189*). HIT rarely occurs in association with the synthetic pentasaccharide fondaparinux (*NEJM 2007;356: 2653*).

Etiology

Immune-responsive patients produce autoantibodies that bind to PF4/heparin complex, which can activate platelets, cause thrombocytopenia, and lead to clot formation through increased thrombin generation (*Blood 2003;101:31*).

DIAGNOSIS

Clinical Presentation

- Suspect HIT when thrombocytopenia occurs during heparin exposure by any route in the absence of other causes of thrombocytopenia, and when platelet counts recover after cessation of heparin.
- **HIT** usually develops between 5 and 14 days of heparin exposure (**typical-onset HIT).** Exceptions include **delayed-onset HIT,** which occurs after stopping heparin, and **early-onset HIT,** which starts within the first 24 hours of heparin administration in patients with recent exposure to heparin (*Chest 2008;133:340S*). HIT rarely causes severe thrombocytopenia and bleeding.
- Thromboembolic complications, venous more than arterial, occur in 30% to 75% of HIT patients. Thrombosis can precede, be concurrent with, or follow recognition of thrombocytopenia.
- HIT causing venous thrombi at heparin injection sites produces full-thickness skin infarctions sometimes in the absence of thrombocytopenia.
- HIT can cause systemic allergic responses following an IV bolus of heparin characterized by fever, hypotension, dyspnea, and cardiac arrest.

Diagnostic Testing

Laboratories

For suspected HIT, laboratory tests for PF4 antibodies improve diagnostic accuracy. Laboratories use two types of HIT assays: **functional** assays (platelet aggregometry or serotonin release assay to detect activation of control platelets in the presence of patient serum and heparin) and **serologic** enzyme immunoassays (**PF4 EIA**) to detect PF4 antibodies.

- In comparison, functional assays have higher specificity, while serologic tests have higher sensitivity.
- For a low pretest probability of HIT, a functional test should confirm a positive PF4 EIA result.
- For a high clinical suspicion for HIT, despite an initial negative PF4 EIA, the patient should undergo repeat testing (*Am J Hematol 2008;83:212*).

TREATMENT

- Since PF4 antibody test results rarely become immediately available, clinical assessment determines initial management. A scoring system based on 4Ts improves diagnostic accuracy: *t*hrombocytopenia, *t*iming, *t*hrombosis, and o*t*her explanation for thrombocytopenia (*J Thromb Haemost 2006;4:759*).
- When HIT is strongly suspected, begin treatment by eliminating all heparin exposure. Patients with and those at high risk for thrombosis require alternative anticoagulation with a parenteral DTI, either hirudin (**lepirudin**) or **argatroban** (see Anticoagulants).
- Do not substitute LMWH for UFH due to high rates of cross-reactivity with HIT antibodies.
- The safety and efficacy of prophylactic or therapeutic fondaparinux therapy in HIT patients is controversial. (*Thromb Haemost 2008;99:2*).
- Perform lower extremity venous compression ultrasound since it often detects DVT in asymptomatic "isolated" HIT patients and the presence of thrombosis mandates longer duration anticoagulation (*Blood 2003;101:31*).
- Start warfarin only after the platelet count normalizes, at an initial low dose, overlapping with a DTI for 5 days, to reduce the risk of limb gangrene due to ongoing hypercoagulable conditions and depletion of proteins C and S.
- DTIs prolong the INR and require careful monitoring when transitioning from DTI to warfarin (see Anticoagulants section for argatroban and lepirudin dosing guidelines).
  - The recommended duration of anticoagulation therapy for HIT depends on the clinical scenario: typically until the platelet count recovers for **isolated HIT** (without thrombosis) and typical thromboembolism duration for **HIT-associated thrombosis** (see treatment duration in "Approach to Venous Thromboembolism" section).

Posttransfusion Purpura

GENERAL PRINCIPLES

Definition

Posttransfusion purpura (**PTP**), a rare syndrome characterized by the formation of alloantibodies against platelet surface antigens, most commonly HPA-1a, follows blood component transfusion and causes severe thrombocytopenia.

Epidemiology

PTP has an incidence of 1 in 50,000 to 100,000 blood transfusions, although ~2% of the population has a potential risk for PTP based on the frequency of HPA-1b/1b.

Etiology

Platelet glycoprotein IIIa has a polymorphic epitope called HPA-1a/b. **PTP** typically occurs in HPA-1b/1b multiparous women or previously transfused patients when reexposed to HPA-1a by transfusion. An amnestic response produces alloantibodies to the HPA-1a epitope, which appear to recognize the patient's HPA-1a–negative platelets and cause thrombocytopenia. In some cases, alloantibodies recognize different platelet-specific epitopes (HPA-3a/b, HPA-5a/b).

DIAGNOSIS

- In **PTP,** severe thrombocytopenia ($<15 \times 10^9$/L) occurs within approximately 7 to 10 days of transfusion.
- Confirmation of suspected **PTP** requires detection of platelet alloantibodies.

TREATMENT

Although spontaneous platelet recovery eventually occurs, bleeding may require treatment. Effective therapies include IVIg and plasmapheresis. Transfusion with platelets from a donor who lacks the causative epitope (typically HPA-1a) does not clearly have higher efficacy than random platelet transfusion, and most hospitals do not have HPA-1a–negative platelets readily available. Reserve transfusion with platelets of unknown HPA-1 status for patients with PTP and severe bleeding (*Am J Hematol 2004;76:258*).

Gestational Thrombocytopenia

GENERAL PRINCIPLES

Definition
Gestational thrombocytopenia (platelet counts no lower than 70 $\times$ 10^9/L) is a benign, mild thrombocytopenia associated with pregnancy.

Epidemiology
Gestational thrombocytopenia spontaneously occurs in approximately 5% to 7% of otherwise uncomplicated pregnancies.

Etiology
The mechanism of **gestational thrombocytopenia** remains unknown.

DIAGNOSIS

Clinical Presentation
Gestational thrombocytopenia occurs in the third trimester of pregnancy. The mother has no symptoms and the fetus remains unaffected.

Differential Diagnosis
Other causes of thrombocytopenia during pregnancy include **ITP, preeclampsia, eclampsia, HELLP** syndrome, **TTP,** and **DIC.**

Diagnostic Testing
Diagnostic testing for gestational thrombocytopenia includes a thorough evaluation for evidence of hemolysis, infection, hypertension, and liver dysfunction to distinguish between these syndromes.

TREATMENT

Platelet transfusion

- **Platelet products.** Platelets can be separated from units of donated whole blood (random-donor platelets) or collected by apheresis (single-donor platelets). In patients with thrombocytopenia resulting from a platelet production defect, transfusion of either one single-donor apheresis unit or six random-donor units typically produces an immediate increment of approximately $30 \times 10^9/L$.

- **Transfusion threshold.** Prophylactic platelet transfusion seems appropriate for asymptomatic outpatients with platelet counts $< 20 \times 10^9/L$ and asymptomatic inpatients with platelet counts $< 10 \times 10^9/L$. Patients undergoing a major invasive procedure typically have a platelet transfusion threshold below $50 \times 10^9/L$. High-risk surgery may warrant prophylactic transfusion to maintain the platelet count $> 100 \times 10^9/L$.
- Bleeding leads to use of higher platelet transfusion thresholds.
- Shortened platelet survival occurs with sepsis, fever, active bleeding, splenic sequestration, certain drugs, or alloantibody (HLA more likely than platelet specific) development in multiply-transfused patients.
- To assess antibody-mediated refractoriness to platelet transfusions, measure the platelet count before and 60 minutes after transfusion. An increment of $<5 \times 10^9/L$ suggests that antibody-mediated refractoriness rather than shortened survival due to another mechanism has occurred.
- ABO-compatible platelets, HLA-matched single-donor platelets, or platelets from donors lacking alloantibodies produced by the patients may improve platelet increments (*Br J Haematol 2008;142:348*).

COMPLICATIONS

Reaction to platelets

- Removing WBC from random-donor units by filtration and by apheresis for single-donor units can reduce the risk of febrile reactions, alloimmunization, and refractoriness to platelet transfusion in patients who will require chronic platelet support.
- Platelets are stored at room temperature, which facilitates bacterial replication. Mandated screening for bacterial contamination before release of stored platelets has reduced severe and fatal platelet transfusion reactions.
- Not using multiparous platelet donors or screening out those with HLA antibodies reduces the risk of transfusion-related acute lung injury (TRALI) due to donor HLA antibodies that target the recipient leukocytes.

OUTCOME/PROGNOSIS

Gestational thrombocytopenia and thrombocytopenia associated with preeclampsia and eclampsia usually resolve promptly after delivery.

Thrombocytosis

GENERAL PRINCIPLES

Classification

- **Reactive thrombocytosis** may occur in response to recovery from thrombocytopenia, postsplenectomy, iron deficiency, chronic infectious or inflammatory states, and malignancies. Patients with reactive thrombocytosis do not have an increased risk of bleeding or thrombosis. Platelets normalize after improvement of the underlying disorder.

- **Essential thrombocythemia (ET)** is a chronic myeloproliferative disorder. Eventual progression to myelofibrosis, acute myeloid leukemia, or myelodysplastic syndrome occurs in a small minority of ET patients (*Br J Haematol 2005;130:153*).

DIAGNOSIS

Clinical Presentation

ET may present as an incidental discovery or present with thrombotic or hemorrhagic symptoms. The risk of thrombosis increases with age, prior thrombosis, duration of disease, and other comorbidities (*Blood 1999;93:417*). Erythromelalgia, due to microvascular occlusive platelet thrombi, presents as intense burning or throbbing of the extremities, typically involving the feet. Cold exposure usually relieves symptoms. Hemorrhage typically occurs with platelet counts > 1,000 × 10⁹/L, and acquired deficiencies of large vWF multimers often accompany hemorrhage patients with ET (*Blood 1993;82:1749*).

Physical Examination
Approximately 50% of ET patients develop mild splenomegaly. Typical signs of erythromelalgia include erythema and warmth of affected digits.

Diagnostic Criteria

2008 World Health Organization revised criteria for ET require the following:

- Sustained platelet count > 450 × 10⁹/L.
- Bone marrow biopsy showing increased mature megakaryocytes and no increase in erythropoiesis or granulopoiesis.
- CML, polycythemia vera, and primary myelofibrosis not present according to WHO criteria.
- Presence of JAK2V617F mutation or other clonal marker (*Lancet 2005;365:1054*).
- No evidence for reactive thrombocytosis if clonal marker not present (*Leukemia 2008;22:14*).

TREATMENT

Patients requiring platelet reduction therapy include those with age > 60, a prior thrombosis or hemorrhage, hypertension, diabetes, smoking, or hyperlipidemia.

- The majority of thrombotic complications occur at modest platelet count elevations. Treatment typically aims for a platelet count of ≤400 × 10⁹/L. Platelet-lowering drugs include **hydroxyurea** and **anagrelide,** or **interferon-α** in pregnant patients or females in their childbearing years (*Blood 2001;97:863*).
  - Limited evidence suggests that long-term hydroxyurea therapy has a very low leukemogenic potential.
  - Anagrelide side effects include palpitations, atrial fibrillation, fluid retention, and headache.
  - Hydroxyurea and anagrelide provide equivalent platelet count control but anagrelide causes more complications (*NEJM 2005;353:33*).
  - Platelet pheresis rapidly lowers platelet counts to manage acute arterial thrombosis.

Qualitative Platelet Disorders

GENERAL PRINCIPLES

Qualitative platelet disorders present with mucocutaneous bleeding and excessive bruising in the setting of an adequate platelet count, PT and aPTT, and normal screening tests for vWD. Most platelet defects produce prolonged BTs and/or PFA-100 closure times. However, a high clinical suspicion of a disorder in a patient with normal test results should lead to in vitro platelet aggregation studies.

Classification

- **Inherited disorders** of platelet function include receptor, signal transduction, cyclooxygenase, secretory (e.g., storage pool disease), adhesion, or aggregation defects. In vitro platelet aggregation studies can identify patterns of agonist responses consistent with a particular defect such as the rare autosomal recessive disorders of Bernard–Soulier syndrome (lack of platelet glycoprotein [GP] IbIX [vWF receptor]) and Glanzmann thrombasthenia (lack of GP IIb/IIIa [fibrinogen receptor]).
- **Acquired** platelet defects occur more commonly than hereditary platelet qualitative disorders.
  - Conditions associated with acquired qualitative defects include myeloproliferative diseases, myelodysplasia, acute leukemia, monoclonal gammopathy, metabolic disorders (uremia, liver failure), and cardiopulmonary bypass platelet trauma.
  - **Drug-induced** platelet dysfunction occurs as a side effect of many drugs that include high-dose penicillin, aspirin, and other NSAIDs, and ethanol. Other drug classes, such as β-lactam antibiotics, β-blockers, calcium channel blockers, nitrates, antihistamines, psychotropic drugs, tricyclic antidepressants, and selective serotonin reuptake inhibitors, cause platelet dysfunction in vitro but rarely cause bleeding.
  - Certain **foods and herbal products** may affect platelet function including omega-3 fatty acids, garlic and onion extracts, ginger, gingko, ginseng, and black tree fungus. Patients should stop using herbal medications and dietary supplements at least 2 weeks before major surgery (*Thromb Res 2005;117:49*; *Anaesthesia 2002;57: 889*).

TREATMENT

- Conservative management of patients with inherited platelet defects reserves transfusions for major bleeding episodes. Anecdotal reports have described successful control of bleeding with recombinant factor VIIa (rFVIIa).
- Treatment of **uremic** platelet dysfunction includes the following:
  - Dialysis, to improve uremia.
  - Increase of hematocrit to $\geq 30\%$, by transfusion or erythropoietin.
  - Desmopressin (diamino-8-D-arginine vasopressin [DDAVP], **0.3 mcg/kg IV**), to stimulate release of vWF from endothelial cells.
  - Conjugated estrogens (0.6 mg/kg IV daily for 5 days), which may improve platelet function for up to 2 weeks.
  - Platelets transfusions in actively bleeding patients, though transfused platelets rapidly acquire the uremic defect.

- **Reversal of drug-induced platelet dysfunction**
  - Some drugs have irreversible or reversible effects on platelet function:
    - **Aspirin** irreversibly inhibits cyclooxygenase-1 and cyclooxygenase-2. Its effects gradually diminish over 7 to 10 days due to new platelets production.
    - Since other **NSAIDs** reversibly inhibit cyclooxygenase-1 and cyclooxygenase-2, their effect only lasts several days. **Cyclooxygenase-2 inhibitors** have antiplatelet activity in large doses, but they have a minimal effect on platelets at therapeutic doses.
    - **Thienopyridines** (ticlopidine, clopidogrel and prasugrel) inhibit platelet aggregation by irreversibly blocking platelet ADP receptor P2Y12.
    - **Dipyridamole,** alone or in combination with aspirin (Aggrenox), inhibits platelet function by increasing intracellular cyclic adenosine monophosphate (cAMP).
    - **Abciximab, eptifibatide, and tirofiban** block platelet IIb/IIIa–dependent aggregation (see Chapter 3, **Preventative Cardiology and** Ischemic Heart Disease).
    - Platelet transfusion compensates for drug-induced platelet dysfunction, except immediately following tirofiban and eptifibatide therapy.
  - Withhold antiplatelet agents for 7 to 10 days before elective invasive procedures.

INHERITED BLEEDING DISORDERS

Hemophilia A

GENERAL PRINCIPLES

Definition

Hemophilia A is an X-linked recessive coagulation disorder due to mutations in the gene encoding factor VIII.

Epidemiology

Hemophilia A affects ~1 in 5,000 live male births. Approximately 40% of cases occur in families with no prior history of hemophilia, reflecting the high rate of spontaneous germ line mutations in the factor VIII gene (*NEJM 2001;344:1773*).

DIAGNOSIS

Clinical Presentation

- Patients with severe hemophilia experience frequent spontaneous hemarthroses and hematomas, hematuria, and delayed posttraumatic and postoperative bleeding. Repeated bleeding into a "target" joint causes chronic synovitis and hemophilic arthropathy.
- Moderate hemophiliacs have fewer spontaneous bleeding episodes, and mild hemophiliacs may only bleed excessively after trauma or surgery.

Diagnostic Testing

Laboratories

Factor VIII activity determines bleeding risk: severe (<1%), moderate (1% to 5%), and mild (>5% to 40%).

TREATMENT

Medications

First Line

- The severity of factor VIII deficiency and the type of hemorrhage determines the type of therapy. In patients with mild to moderate hemophilia A and a minor bleeding episode, **DDAVP** (0.3 mcg/kg IV in 50 to 100 mL normal saline infused over 30 minutes, or 300 mcg intranasally [Stimate, 1.5 mg/mL] dosed every 12 hour) typically increases factor VIII activity three- to fivefold and has a half-life of 8 to 12 hours. Tachyphylaxis may occur after several doses (*Blood 1997;90:2515*).
- Patients with mild to moderate hemophilia A and major bleeding episodes or those with severe hemophilia A with any hemorrhage require **factor VIII replacement.**
  - Many hemophiliacs infuse **lyophilized factor VIII concentrates** at home. To safeguard from transmission of infectious agents in plasma-derived factor VIII concentrates, donors undergo screening, plasma undergoes nucleic acid testing for pathogens, and the final product undergoes viral inactivation. **Recombinant factor VIII concentrates** have increasingly become available.
  - One to three doses of factor VIII concentrates targeting peak plasma activities of 30% to 50% typically stop mild hemorrhages. Major traumas and surgery require maintenance of factor VIII levels > 80% for extended periods.
  - Plasma factor VIII activity increases approximately 2% for every 1 IU/kg (International Units per kilogram) factor VIII concentrate infused. A 50-IU/kg IV bolus would be expected to raise factor VIII activity to approximately 100% over baseline, and extended treatment then consists of a 25-IU/kg IV bolus q12h.
  - Continuous infusion of factor VIII provides a feasible and efficient alternative to intermittent infusion (*Hematol Oncol Clin North Am 1998;12:1315*).
  - Dose adjustments based on peak and trough factor VIII levels ensure adequate hemostasis.

Second Line

Second-line replacement therapies include **cryoprecipitate** and **FFP.**

Hemophilia B

GENERAL PRINCIPLES

Definition

Hemophilia B is an X-linked recessive coagulation disorder secondary to mutations in the gene encoding factor IX. Hemophilia B affects ~1 in 30,000 male births.

TREATMENT

Hemophilia B remains clinically indistinguishable from hemophilia A, but the distinction is important, as the therapy consists of factor IX replacement with either plasma-derived FIX or recombinant factor IX (BeneFIX).

- **DDAVP** does not increase factor IX levels.
- Postinfusion peak targets, duration of replacement, and laboratory monitoring for treatment of hemophilia B–related bleeding episodes have guidelines similar to those provided for hemophilia A.

- One International Unit of factor IX replacement per kilogram of body weight typically raises plasma factor IX activity by 1%, and factor IX has a half-life of 18 to 24 hours.

COMPLICATIONS

Inhibitors

- Alloantibodies to factors VIII and IX in response to replacement therapy develop in approximately 20% and 12% of severe hemophilia A and B patients, respectively. These alloantibodies neutralize infused factor VIII or factor IX and prevent correction of the coagulopathy.
- Determining the titer of a factor VIII or factor IX inhibitor, using a laboratory assay that reports inhibitor strength in Bethesda units (BUs) predicts inhibitor behavior and guides therapy.
- Treatment options for hemophiliacs with factor VIII or factor IX inhibitors are as follows:
  - rFVIIa (NovoSeven), dosed at 90 mcg/kg every 2 hours until achievement of hemostasis (*Semin Hematol 2001;38(4 Suppl 12):43*).
  - Activated prothrombin complex concentrate (FEIBA VH) contains partially activated vitamin K–dependent coagulation factors XI, X, and VII, and thrombin. The increased risk of thrombotic complications should limit its use.
  - Large doses of factor VIII or factor IX concentrates sometimes decrease bleeding in hemophiliacs with weak inhibitors (BU < 5).

von Willebrand Disease

GENERAL PRINCIPLES

Classification

Classification recognizes three main types of vWD (*J Thromb Haemost 2006;4:2103*) (see Table 4). **Type 1 vWD,** a partial quantitative deficiency of vWF:Ag and activity, accounts for 70% to 80% of cases. **Type 2 vWD includes four subtypes:** 2A: selective loss of large multimers and decreased platelet adhesion; 2B: loss of large and medium multimers due to increased affinity for platelet GPIb; 2M: decreased platelet adhesion without loss of large multimers; 2N: decreased binding affinity for factor VIII. **Type 3 vWD** has a virtual complete deficiency of vWF (*Blood 2001;97:1915*).

Epidemiology

vWD, the most common inherited bleeding disorder, affects an estimated 0.1% of the population.

Etiology

von Willebrand disease (vWD) results from an inherited quantitative or qualitative defect of vWF. Most forms of **vWD** have an autosomal dominant inheritance with variable penetrance, although autosomal recessive forms (types 2N and 3) exist (Table 3). vWF circulates as multimers of variable size, and these facilitate adherence of platelets to injured vessel walls and stabilize factor VIII in plasma.

Table 3   Hemostasis Test Patterns in von Willebrand Disease

	Type I	Type 2A	Type 2B	Type 2M	Type 2N	Type 3
PFA-100 closure time	↑/nl	↑/nl	↑	↑	nl	↑
aPTT	↑/nl	↑/nl	nl/↑	nl/↑	↑/nl	↑
VWF antigen	↓	↓/nl	↓/nl	↓/nl	Normal	Absent
VWF activity	↓	↓↓	↓↓	↓↓	Normal	Absent
Factor VIII:C	↓/nl	↓/nl	↓/nl	↓/nl	↓↓	↓↓
RIPA[a]	Reduced	Reduced	Enhanced	Reduced	Normal	Absent
Multimetric pattern	Normal	Missing large multimers	Missing large multimers	Normal	Normal	None detected
Inheritance	Dominant	Dominant	Dominant	Dominant	Recessive	Recessive

[a]Ristocetin-induced platelet aggregation.

DIAGNOSIS

Clinical Presentation

- The characteristic clinical findings consist of mucocutaneous bleeding (epistaxis, menorrhagia, GI bleeding) and easy bruising.
- Trauma, surgery, or dental extractions may result in life-threatening bleeding in severely affected individuals.
- Patients with mild vWD phenotype may remain undiagnosed into adulthood (*Blood 2001;97:1915*).

Diagnostic Testing

Laboratories

If personal and family bleeding histories support a reasonable pretest likelihood of an inherited primary hemostasis or bleeding disorder, screening for vWD should begin with measurements of vWF antigen and activity and FVIII activity (Table 3).

- vWF:Ag tests measure circulating vWF protein by immunoassay. A deficiency of vWF:Ag detects type 1 and 3 vWD, and low or normal levels may occur with type 2 forms.
- vWF:RCo measures vWF-mediated agglutination of control platelets in the presence of ristocetin. A deficiency of vWF (types 1 and 3), vWF mutations that cause a selective loss of large multimers (types 2A and 2B), or defective platelet binding despite a normal multimer pattern (type 2M) cause decreased platelet agglutination.
- Suspect a quantitative vWF defect (type 1) with low vWF and Ag/RCo activity and a vWF:Ag/RCo ratio of ≥ 0.7.
- A quantitative deficiency of vWF (types 1 and 3) or vWF mutations that reduce FVIII binding to vWF (type 2N) may reduce factor VIII activity.
- Enzyme immunoassays measuring vWF binding affinity for factor VIII can confirm type 2N diagnosis.
- Suspect type 2 vWD when vWF:Ag/RCo activity has a ratio of ≤ 0.7. vWF multimer analysis by gel electrophoresis assesses for the presence (type 2M) or absence (type 2A and 2B) of large vWF multimers, and a ristocetin-induced platelet aggregation test (patient's plasma and platelets plus ristocetin) distinguishes types 2A and 2M (attenuated) from type 2B (exaggerated) platelet aggregation responses.

TREATMENT

- Management of **vWD** consists of raising vWF:RCo and factor VIII activities to ensure adequate hemostasis. **Minor bleeding** in **type 1 vWD** usually responds to **DDAVP** (see Hemophilia A section for dosing guidelines). Test dose administration should confirm clinically acceptable vWF:RCo and FVIII increments. vWF:RCo activities > 50% control most hemorrhages. Recommendations for **minor invasive procedures** include a DDAVP infusion 1 hour before surgery, followed by infusions q12–24h for 2 to 3 days postoperatively, with or without the oral antifibrinolytic drug aminocaproic acid (Amicar).
- DDAVP does not effectively treat some type 2A, 2M, and 2N vWD and all type 3vWD patients. Because of the risk of postinfusion thrombocytopenia, patients with type 2B vWD should not receive DDAVP.
- **Severe bleeding** and **major surgery** in vWD patients require infusion of vWF multimers, available in two brands of FVIII concentrates (Alphanate or Humate-P),

or cryoprecipitate q12–24h to raise vWF:RCo activity to ~100% and maintain it between 50% and 100% until sufficient wound repair occurs (typically 5 to 10 days).

ACQUIRED COAGULATION DISORDERS

Vitamin K Deficiency

GENERAL PRINCIPLES

Etiology

Vitamin K deficiency is usually caused by malabsorption states or poor dietary intake combined with antibiotic-associated loss of intestinal bacterial colonization. Hepatocytes require vitamin K to complete the synthesis (γ-carboxylation) of clotting factors (X, IX, VII, prothrombin) and the natural anticoagulant proteins C, S, and Z.

DIAGNOSIS

Diagnostic Testing

Laboratories

Vitamin K deficiency is suspected when an at-risk patient has a prolonged PT that corrects after a 1:1 mix with normal pooled plasma.

TREATMENT

- **Vitamin K replacement** should be given orally or intravenously. Vitamin K has variable absorption when administered subcutaneously, especially in edematous patients, and intravenous vitamin K carries the risk of anaphylaxis. With adequate replacement therapy, the PT should begin to normalize within 12 hours and should normalize completely in 24 to 48 hours (*Ann Intern Med 2002;137:251*).
- **FFP** rapidly but temporarily (4 to 6 hours) corrects acquired coagulopathies secondary to vitamin K deficiency. Patients with coagulopathy who have been actively bleeding or who require immediate invasive procedures should receive FFP or prothrombin complex concentrate.
  - The usual starting dose of FFP is two to three units (400 to 600 mL), with measurement of the PT and aPTT after the infusion to determine the need for additional therapy. Up to 10 to 15 mL/kg may be needed for severe bleeding with significant PT prolongation.
  - Because factor VII has a half-life of only 6 hours, the PT may again become prolonged and require additional FFP, until adequate production of coagulation factors occurs.
  - Vitamin K replacement should be initiated concomitantly with FFP.

Liver Disease

GENERAL PRINCIPLES

Liver disease can seriously impair hemostasis because the liver produces coagulation factors, with the exception of vWF. Hemostatic abnormalities associated with liver disease typically remain stable unless liver synthetic function rapidly worsens or the patient is not eating normally. Other hemostatic complications of liver disease are hyperfibrinolysis, thrombocytopenia due to splenic sequestration, DIC, spontaneous bacterial peritonitis, gastrointestinal hemorrhage, and cholestasis (which impairs vitamin K absorption).

TREATMENT

- **Vitamin K** replacement may help shorten the PT in liver dysfunction.
- **FFP** is indicated for patients who are bleeding or require an invasive procedure and have abnormal coagulation parameters (PT or aPTT > 1.5 times control).
- **Cryoprecipitate,** a concentrated source of fibrinogen, given at a dose of 1.5 units/10 kg body weight, corrects severe hypofibrinogenemia (<100 mg/dL) in the setting of bleeding or invasive procedures. Periodic measurement of the fibrinogen level determines the need for dosing.
- Reserve **platelet transfusions** for active bleeding or prior to invasive procedures such as liver biopsies in patients with thrombocytopenia.

Disseminated Intravascular Coagulation

GENERAL PRINCIPLES

Etiology

Disseminated intravascular coagulation (DIC) occurs in a variety of systemic illnesses, including sepsis, trauma, burns, shock, obstetric complications, and malignancies (notably, acute promyelocytic leukemia).

Pathophysiology

In DIC, exposure of tissue factor to the circulation generates excess thrombin and its consequences: consumption of coagulation factors (including fibrinogen) and regulators (protein C, protein S, antithrombin), platelet activation, fibrin generation, generalized microthrombi, and reactive fibrinolysis.

DIAGNOSIS

Clinical Presentation

Consequences of **DIC** include bleeding, organ dysfunction secondary to microvascular thrombi and ischemia, and, less often, large arterial and venous thrombosis (*NEJM 1999;341:586*).

Diagnostic Testing

Laboratories

Although no one test confirms a diagnosis of DIC, affected patients commonly have prolonged PT and aPTT, thrombocytopenia, low fibrinogen levels, elevated fibrin degradation products, and a positive d-dimer.

TREATMENT

DIC treatment consists of supportive care, correction of the underlying disorder if possible, and administration of **FFP, cryoprecipitate,** and **platelets** as needed for hypofibrinogen and thrombocytopenia. Though controversy exists regarding the use of heparin to prevent thrombosis in DIC, large-vessel thrombosis in DIC should be treated with adjusted-dose **heparin** (see Anticoagulants). Recombinant activated protein C (drotrecogin alfa) can reduce mortality in patients with severe sepsis and DIC (see Chapter 6, Critical Care), but can also cause major hemorrhage (*J Thromb Haemost 2004;2:1924*).

Acquired Inhibitors of Coagulation Factors

GENERAL PRINCIPLES

Etiology

Acquired inhibitors of coagulation factors may arise de novo (autoantibodies) or may develop in hemophiliacs (alloantibodies) following FVIII or IX infusions. The most common acquired specific inhibitor is directed against factor VIII.

DIAGNOSIS

Clinical Presentation

Patients with coagulation factor inhibitors present with an abrupt onset of bleeding, prolonged aPTT that does not correct after 1:1 mixing, markedly decreased FVIII activity, and a normal PT.

TREATMENT

Bleeding complications in patients with factor VIII inhibitors (autoantibodies) are managed in the same manner as for hemophiliacs with alloantibodies to factor VIII (see Inherited Bleeding Disorders). Long-term therapy consists of immunosuppression with cyclophosphamide, prednisone, rituximab, or vincristine to reduce production of the autoantibody (*Blood 2002;100:3426*).

VENOUS THROMBOEMBOLIC DISORDERS

Approach to Venous Thromboembolism

GENERAL PRINCIPLES

Definition

- **Venous thromboembolism (VTE)** refers to the presence of **deep vein thrombosis (DVT)** or **pulmonary embolism (PE).**
- **Superficial thrombophlebitis** may occur in any superficial veins.
- **APA syndrome** diagnosis requires the presence of at least one clinical and one laboratory criterion (*J Thromb Haemost 2006;4:295*).
  - **Clinical criteria** consist of (a) the occurrence of arterial or venous thrombosis in any tissue or organ and (b) pregnancy morbidities (unexplained late fetal death; premature birth complicated by eclampsia, preeclampsia, or placental insufficiency; at least three unexplained consecutive spontaneous abortions).
  - **Laboratory criteria** consist of persistent (at least 12 weeks apart) detection of autoantibodies (lupus anticoagulant, anticardiolipin antibody, and β_2-glycoprotein-1 antibodies) that react with negatively charged phospholipids.

- The APA syndrome may include other features, such as thrombocytopenia, valvular heart disease, livedo reticularis, neurologic manifestations, and nephropathy.

Classification

The anatomic location of DVT PE, clot burden, and sequelae may affect prognosis and treatment recommendations.

- Thromboses can be classified as **deep** or **superficial** and as **proximal** or **distal.**
  - To avoid confusion about its deep vein location, the term **femoral vein** has replaced the term **superficial femoral vein.**
  - **Proximal** lower extremity DVTs occur in or superior to the popliteal vein (or the confluence of tibial and peroneal veins), whereas **distal** DVTs occur more inferiorly.
- Location in the pulmonary arterial system characterizes **PE**s as **central** (main pulmonary artery, lobar, or segmental) or **distal.**

Epidemiology

- Symptomatic DVTs most commonly develop in the lower limbs.
- Untreated calf vein DVTs may propagate proximally.
- Without treatment, approximately 50% of patients with proximal lower extremity DVT develop PE.
- DVTs in the proximal lower extremities and pelvis produce most PEs.
- DVTs that occur in upper extremities, often secondary to an indwelling catheter, may also cause PE.
- DVT may occur concomitantly with superficial thrombophlebitis.

Etiology

- Venous thromboemboli arise under conditions of **stasis, hypercoagulability,** or venous **endothelial injury.**
- Acute illnesses that lead to prolonged **immobilization** (trauma, surgery, and other major medical illnesses) predispose to development of VTE.
- Hypercoagulable states may have an inherited or acquired etiology.
  - **Acquired hypercoagulable states may arise secondary to malignancy, nephrotic syndrome, estrogen use, and pregnancy.**
  - **Both HIT and the APA syndrome can cause arterial or venous thrombi.**
- **Superficial thrombophlebitis** occurs in association with varicose veins, trauma, infection, and hypercoagulable disorders.
- Other causes of pulmonary arterial occlusion include in situ thrombi (e.g., sickle cell disease), marrow fat embolism, amniotic fluid embolism, pulmonary artery sarcoma, and fibrosing mediastinitis.

Risk Factors

- **Inherited thrombophilic disorders** are suggested by a history of spontaneous VTE at a young age (<50 years), recurrent VTE, VTE in first-degree relatives, thrombosis in unusual anatomic locations, and recurrent fetal loss.
- The most common inherited risk factors for VTE include two gene polymorphisms **(factor V Leiden and prothrombin gene G20210A),** deficiencies of the natural anticoagulants **protein C, protein S,** and **antithrombin, dysfibrinogenemia,** and **hyperhomocysteinemia.**
- **Homocystinuria** caused by deficiency of cystathionine-β-synthase causes extremely high plasma homocysteine and arterial and venous thromboembolic events

beginning in childhood. More commonly, milder homocysteine elevations arise from an interaction between genetic mutations that affect enzymes involved in homocysteine metabolism and acquired factors such as inadequate folate consumption (*NEJM 2001;344:1222*).

- Unusual spontaneous venous thromboses, such as cavernous sinus thrombosis, mesenteric vein thrombosis, or portal vein thrombosis, may be the initial presentation of paroxysmal nocturnal hemoglobinuria **(PNH)** or myeloproliferative disorders.
- **Spontaneous (idiopathic) thrombosis,** despite the absence of an inherited thrombophilia and detectable autoantibodies, predisposes patients to future thromboses (*NEJM 2001;344:1222*).
- **Autoantibodies** associated with HIT and the APA syndrome can cause arterial or venous thrombi. (See Heparin-Induced Thrombocytopenia.)
- At least 10% of patients with SLE have evidence of LAs; however, most patients with LAs do not have SLE.

Prevention

Prevention, by identifying patients at high risk of thromboembolism and instituting prophylactic measures, remains the ideal strategy for dealing with the problem of VTE (DVT or PE) (see Chapter 1, Patient Care in Internal Medicine).

DIAGNOSIS

Clinical Presentation

- **DVT** has neither sensitive nor specific symptoms and signs. However, pretest assessment of the probability of a DVT provides useful information when combined with the results of compression ultrasound or a D-dimer test, or both, in determining whether to exclude or accept the diagnosis of DVT or perform additional imaging studies (*Lancet 1997;350:1795*).
  - DVT may produce pain and edema in the affected extremity.
  - **Superficial thrombophlebitis** presents as a tender, warm, erythematous, and often palpable thrombosed vein. Accompanying DVT may produce additional symptoms and signs.
- **PE** has neither sensitive nor specific symptoms and signs. However, PE may produce shortness of breath, chest pain (pleuritic), hypoxemia, hemoptysis, pleural rub, new right-sided heart failure, and tachycardia (*Ann Intern Med 1998;129:997*).
  - Validated clinical risk factors for a PE in outpatients who present to an emergency department include signs and symptoms of DVT, high suspicion of PE by the clinician, tachycardia, immobility in the past 4 weeks, history of VTE, active cancer, and hemoptysis (*Ann Intern Med 2001;135:98*).
- Clinical **suspicion of DVT or PE should lead to objective testing.**

Differential Diagnosis

- The differential diagnosis for **unilateral lower extremity** symptoms and signs of **DVT,** such as swelling and pain, includes Baker cyst, hematoma, venous insufficiency, postphlebitic syndrome, lymphedema, sarcoma, arterial aneurysm, myositis, cellulitis, rupture of the medial head of the gastrocnemius, and abscess.
  - **Symmetric, bilateral lower extremity edema** suggests the presence of heart, renal, or liver failure rather than a DVT.
  - Additional diseases to consider in association with **lower extremity pain** include musculoskeletal and arteriovascular disorders.

- The **differential diagnosis** of symptoms and signs of **PE** includes dissecting aortic aneurysm, pneumonia, acute bronchitis, broncho carcinoma, pericardial or pleural disease, heart failure, costochondritis, and myocardial ischemia.

Diagnostic Testing

Laboratories

- **D-dimers,** cross-linked fibrin degradation products, may increase during acute illness or VTE.
- Assays used to measure D-dimers differ in accuracy.
- D-dimer testing for DVT or PE has a low positive predictive value and specificity; **patients with a positive test require further evaluation.**
- The negative predictive value of a sensitive quantitative D-dimer assay is high enough to exclude a **DVT** when the objectively defined clinical probability is low and/or a noninvasive test is negative (*Ann Intern Med 2004;140:589; JAMA 2006;295:199*).
- A negative D-dimer in combination with low pretest probability can exclude almost all PEs (*Ann Intern Med 1998;129:1006*).
- In the setting of a moderate to high clinical pretest probability (e.g., patients with cancer), a negative D-dimer does not have sufficient negative predictive value for excluding the presence of DVT or PE (*Ann Intern Med 1999;131:417; Arch Intern Med 2001;161:567*).
- Hypercoagulability testing (Table 4).
- Signs and symptoms of the APA syndrome should lead to laboratory evaluation.
  - Serologic tests (IgG and IgM β_2-glycoprotein-1 antibodies, and IgG and IgM cardiolipin antibodies) or clotting assays (LA) detect APAs.
  - Performing both serologic and clotting assays improves sensitivity.
  - LAs may prolong the aPTT or PT/INR, though they do not predispose to bleeding.
  - To assess for **PNH** in the setting of unusual spontaneous venous thromboses, perform flow cytometry to detect missing antigens on red cells or leukocytes.

Table 4	Laboratory Evaluation of Thrombophilic States
Inherited Thrombophilia	**Laboratory Assessment**
Prothrombin gene mutation G20210A	G20210A mutation
Partial protein C deficiency	Protein C activity
Partial protein S deficiency	Free protein S antigen, protein S activity
Partial antithrombin deficiency	Antithrombin heparin cofactor activity
Factor V Leiden	Activated protein C resistance, if positive; confirm with factor V Leiden PCR
Hyperhomocysteinemia	Fasting plasma homocysteine level
Acquired thrombophilias	**Laboratory assessment**
Antiphospholipid antibody syndrome	Anticardiolipin antibody, β_2-glycoprotein- 1, lupus anticoagulant
Paroxysmal nocturnal hemoglobinuria	RBC or WBC flow cytometry for loss of CD55, CD59
Myeloproliferative disorder	JAK-2 mutation

PCR, polymerase chain reaction; RBC, red blood cell; WBC, white blood cell.

Imaging
- **DVT-Specific Testing**
  - Initial diagnostic testing for symptomatic acute DVT should utilize a **noninvasive test,** typically **compression ultrasound** (called *duplex examination* when performed with Doppler testing) (*Am J Respir Crit Care Med 1999;160:1043*).
    - In addition to assessing for DVT, compression ultrasound, MR venography, and CT venography may detect other pathology (see Differential Diagnosis).
    - Compression ultrasound has low sensitivity for detecting **calf** DVT and may fail to visualize parts of the deep femoral vein, parts of the upper extremity venous system, and the pelvic veins.
    - The presence of an **old DVT** may make noninvasive testing difficult to interpret.
  - **Lower extremity venous compression ultrasonography** provides useful information in a patient with a suspected PE who has a nondiagnostic ventilation/perfusion (V/Q) scan and in a patient with a nondiagnostic or negative chest CT scan with high suspicion of disease, because proximal DVT can serve as a surrogate for PE; ultrasonography also serves as a useful surrogate for PE, if positive, in patients who have contraindications to or difficulty completing imaging for PE (see PE-specific testing).
  - Noninvasive testing has a low sensitivity in **asymptomatic** patients.
  - **Serial testing** can improve the diagnostic yield. If a patient with a clinically suspected lower extremity DVT has a negative initial noninvasive test result, one can withhold anticoagulant therapy and repeat testing at least once 3 to 14 days later.
  - **Simplified compression ultrasound** limited only to the common femoral vein in the groin and the popliteal vein (down to the trifurcation of the calf veins) has lower sensitivity than a **complete** proximal lower extremity venous examination.
    - Repeating simplified noninvasive tests within 10 days improves sensitivity.
    - Concerns about unreliable noninvasive test results or patient follow-up should lead to complete noninvasive testing or venography.
  - **Venography,** the gold-standard technique for diagnosing DVT, requires placement of an IV catheter, administration of iodinated contrast, and exposure to radiation.
    - Patients with suspected DVT should first undergo noninvasive testing.
    - Contraindications to venography include renal dysfunction and dye allergy.
  - **Magnetic resonance imaging (MRI)** has shown good sensitivity for acute, symptomatic proximal DVT in small studies.
  - **CT venography** testing for DVT may be performed in conjunction with a contrast-enhanced spiral CT testing for PE (*NEJM 2006;354:2317; Ann Intern Med 2000; 132:227*).
    - CT venography allows for visualization of the veins in the abdomen, pelvis, and proximal lower extremities.
    - Spiral CT for evaluation of patients with suspected DVT has lower accuracy than CT used for suspected PE (*NEJM 2006;354:2317; Ann Intern Med 2000; 132:227*).
- **PE-specific testing**
  - **Nondefinitive tests** such as electrocardiography (e.g., right-sided strain pattern, with characteristic S wave in lead I, and Q wave in lead III, and T wave inversion in lead III), troponin and brain natriuretic peptide (BNP) levels, blood gases, and chest radiography may help determine the pretest probability, focus the differential diagnosis, and assess the cardiopulmonary reserve, but they do not rule in or rule out PE with acceptable certainty.

- Unless an objectively low clinical probability of PE combined with a negative D-dimer test occurs, the suspicion of PE usually requires further evaluation.
- **Contrast-enhanced spiral (helical) chest CT**
  - PE protocol chest CT requires IV administration of iodinated contrast and exposure to radiation.
  - Contraindications to spiral CT include renal dysfunction and dye allergy.
  - **Multidetector CT** has better sensitivity than single-detector CT for evaluating patients with suspected PE.
- Used according to standardized protocols in conjunction with expert interpretation, spiral CT has good accuracy for detection of large (proximal) PEs, but it has lower sensitivity for detecting small (distal) emboli (*NEJM 2006;354: 2317*).
  - The sensitivity of CT for VTE improves by combining the CT pulmonary angiography results with (a) objective grading of clinical suspicion and (b) proximal lower extremity CT venography that assesses for DVT.
  - Lower extremity compression ultrasonography may provide additional useful information, though negative D-dimer and multidetector chest CT tests exclude most PE (*Lancet 2008;371:1343*).
- **Clinical suspicion discordant with the objective test finding** (e.g., high suspicion with a negative CT scan, or low suspicion with a positive CT scan) **should lead to further testing.**
- Advantages of CT scan over V/Q scan include more diagnostic results (positive or negative), with fewer indeterminate or inadequate studies, and the detection of alternative diagnoses, such as dissecting aortic aneurysm, pneumonia, and malignancy.
- **V/Q scanning**
  - V/Q scanning requires administration of radioactive material (via both inhaled and IV routes).
  - V/Q scans may be classified as normal, nondiagnostic (i.e., very low probability, low probability, intermediate probability), or high probability for PE.
  - V/Q scanning remains most useful in a patient with a normal chest radiograph, because nondiagnostic V/Q scans commonly occur in the setting of an abnormal chest radiograph.
  - Use of clinical suspicion improves the accuracy of V/Q scanning. In patients with normal or high-probability V/Q scans and matching pretest clinical suspicion, the testing has a positive predictive value of 96% (*JAMA 1990;263:2753*).
- **Magnetic resonance angiography (MRA)**
  - MRI requires IV administration of a nonionic contrast agent (e.g., gadolinium).
  - MRI appears to be sensitive for diagnosing acute PE, though large studies have not been performed, and the PIOPED III study aims to better define the accuracy of MRI.
- **Pulmonary angiography (PA)**
  - Angiography requires placement of a pulmonary artery catheter, infusion of IV contrast, and exposure to radiation.
  - Similar to venography and PE-protocol CT scanning, contraindications to angiography include renal dysfunction and dye allergy.
  - Less invasive tests have mostly replaced PA over the past decade.
- **Echocardiography** to assess cardiopulmonary reserve and evidence of end-organ damage (right ventricular dysfunction) in patients with PE has a role in decision making regarding the use of thrombolytic therapy (see Thrombolytic therapy).

TREATMENT

- **VTE therapy** should aim to prevent recurrent VTE, consequences of VTE (i.e., post-phlebitic syndrome [i.e., pain, edema, and ulceration], pulmonary arterial hypertension, and death), and complications of therapy (e.g., bleeding and HIT).
- Clinicians should perform standard laboratory tests (i.e., CBC, PT, and aPTT) before starting anticoagulants.
- Unless contraindications exist, **initial treatment of VTE should consist of parenteral anticoagulation,** either with IV or SC UFH, SC LMWH, or SC pentasaccharide (fondaparinux).

Medications

- **Anticoagulants** (Fig. 1)
  - **Warfarin** is an oral anticoagulant that inhibits reduction of vitamin K to its active form and leads to depletion of the vitamin K–dependent clotting factors II, VII, IX, and X and proteins C, S, and Z.
    - Though warfarin has good oral absorption, it requires 4 to 5 days to achieve the full anticoagulant effect.
      - The initial INR rise primarily reflects warfarin-related depletion of factor VII; the depletion of factor II takes several days due to its relatively long half-life.
      - Because of the rapid depletion of the anticoagulant protein C and slower onset of anticoagulant effect, patients might develop increased hypercoagulability during the first few days of warfarin therapy if warfarin is not combined with a parenteral anticoagulant (*Thromb Haemost 1997;78:785*).
    - The typical **starting dose** of warfarin is 5 mg PO daily, but depends upon age and habitus (e.g., ~3 mg in older, petite patients, ~7 mg in younger, robust patients). Patients with polymorphisms in genes for cytochrome P-450 2C9 or vitamin K epoxide reductase may benefit from cautious warfarin initiation (see www.WarfarinDosing.org). The INR is used to adjust dosing (Table 5).
    - **Treatment of DVT/PE with warfarin requires overlap therapy with a parenteral anticoagulant**; in combination with warfarin, patients should receive a parenteral anticoagulant (UFH, LMWH, or pentasaccharide) for at least 4.5 days and until they achieve INRs of at least 2.0 for 2 consecutive days.
      - For most indications, warfarin has a **target INR** of 2.5 and a therapeutic range of 2 to 3.
      - Patients with most **mechanical heart valves** require a higher level of anticoagulation (INR target range, 2.5 to 3.5) (Table 6).
- **Warfarin nomogram dosing** has more success than nonstandardized dosing (Table 5).
  - **INR monitoring should occur frequently during the first month of therapy (e.g., twice weekly for 1 to 2 weeks, then weekly for 2 weeks, then less frequently).**
    - Patients receiving a stable warfarin dose should have INR monitoring performed monthly, though patients with labile INRs should have more frequent monitoring (e.g., weekly).
    - The addition or discontinuation of medications, especially and antifungal drugs should trigger more frequent INR monitoring.
    - **Long-term anticoagulation with SC LMWH or fondaparinux** provides a treatment option for compliant patients who have unacceptable INR lability, or those with LA and difficulty monitoring due to an elevated baseline INR.

Table 5	Warfarin Nomogram	
Day	INR	Dosage (mg)
2	<1.5	5
	1.5–1.9	2.5
	2.0–2.5	1.0–2.5
	>2.5	0
3	<1.5	5–10
	1.5–1.9	2.5–5.0
	2–3	0–2.5
	>3	0
4	<1.5	10
	1.5–1.9	5
	2–3	0–3
	>3	0
5	<1.5	10
	1.5–1.9	7.5–10.0
	2–3	0–5
	>3	0

Starting dose 5 mg PO daily on day 1.
INR, international normalized ratio.
Adapted from *Ann Intern Med* 1997;127:333.

- Unfractionated heparin **(UFH)** comes from porcine intestinal mucosa.
  - UFH catalyzes the inactivation of thrombin and factor Xa by antithrombin.
  - At usual doses, UFH prolongs the TT and aPTT, and it has a minimal effect on the PT/INR.
  - Because the anticoagulant effects of UFH normalize within hours of discontinuation and **protamine sulfate** reverses it even faster, UFH is the anticoagulant of choice for patients with increased risk of bleeding.
  - Abnormal renal function does not typically affect UFH dosing.
  - For **DVT prophylaxis,** the typical dosage is 5,000 units SC q8–12h, and aPTT monitoring is not necessary.
  - For **therapeutic anticoagulation,** UFH is usually administered IV with a bolus followed by continuous infusion (Table 7).

Table 6	Anticoagulation with Artificial Heart Valves	
Material	Type/Location	INR
Tissue	Any	2.5 for 3 mo, then ASA 325 mg lifelong
Mechanical[a]	St. Jude aortic	2.5
	St. Jude mitral	3.0
	Caged-ball/caged-disk	3.0, add ASA 81 mg

ASA, acetylsalicylic acid.
[a]Add ASA for any caged valve, coronary artery disease, history of stroke or peripheral embolism

Table 7	Weight-Based Heparin Dosing for Venous Thromboembolism[a]
Initial therapy[a]	
Bolus[b]	80 units/kg
Infusion[b]	18 units/kg/hr
Adjustments[c]	
aPTT < 40	80 units/kg bolus; increase infusion by 3 units/kg/hr
aPTT 40–50	40 units/kg bolus; increase infusion by 2 units/kg/hr
aPTT 51–59	Increase infusion by 1 unit/kg/hr
aPTT 60–94	No change
aPTT 95–104	Decrease infusion by 1 unit/kg/hr
aPTT 105–114	Hold for 0.5 hr; decrease infusion by 2 units/kg/hr
aPTT > 115	Hold for 1 hr; decrease infusion by 3 units/kg/hr

Note: Target activated partial thromboplastin time (aPTT) can vary among hospitals depending on reagents and instruments used.
[a]For patients with ST-segment elevation myocardial infarction, typical bolus dose is 60 units/kg (maximum 5,000 units), and typical initial infusion dose is 12 units/kg/hr (maximum 1,000 units/hr).
[b]Round all doses to nearest 100 units.
[c]Draw aPTT 6 hours after any bolus or change in infusion rate.
Adapted from *Ann Intern Med* 1993;119:874).

- **Nomogram**-driven weight-based dosing provides a more rapid and reliable prolongation of the aPTT into the therapeutic range than non-nomogram dosing (Table 7).
  - Bleeding risks lead to use of different-intensity nomograms for different types of patients; patients with VTE often receive larger boluses and higher initial drip rates than patients with unstable angina who receive antiplatelet therapy.
  - **UFH may be administered subcutaneously:** initial dose of 333 U/kg SC, followed by a fixed dose of 250 U/kg every 12 hours (*JAMA 2006;296:935*).
- **LMWHs** are produced by chemical or enzymatic cleavage of UFH.
  ○ Since LMWH inactivates factor Xa to a greater extent than it does thrombin (IIa), LWMH minimally prolongs the aPTT.
  ○ Extensive clinical trials have confirmed the efficacy and safety of weight-based SC LMWH for the treatment of VTE.
  ○ Given a linear dose response, factor Xa monitoring is not normally recommended.
    - In patients experiencing renal dysfunction, obesity, or pregnancy, factor Xa level monitoring may be prudent.
    - For therapeutic anticoagulation, peak factor Xa levels, measured 4 hours after an SC dose, should be 0.6 to 1.0 IU/mL for q12h dosing and 1 to 2 IU/mL for q24h dosing (*Blood 2002;99:3102*).
  ○ Different LMWH preparations have different dosing recommendations (Table 8).
  ○ Given the renal clearance of LMWHs, they are generally contraindicated in patients with CrCl < 10 mL/min, and patients with a CrCl < 30 mL/min require dose adjustments (e.g., enoxaparin 1 mg/kg once daily instead of twice daily). Dose adjustments may also be required in patients with cachexia or obesity, or in women who are pregnant.

Table 8	Low-Molecular-Weight Heparin and Pentasaccharide Dosages for Treatment of Venous Thromboembolism
Drug	**Dosage**
Enoxaparin	Outpatient: 1 mg/kg SC q12h Inpatient: 1 mg/kg SC q12h *or* 1.5 mg/kg SC q24h
Tinzaparin	175 IU/kg SC daily[a]
Dalteparin	200 IU/kg SC daily[b]
Fondaparinux	5 mg SC daily for weight < 50 kg, 7.5 mg SC daily for weight 50–100 kg, and 10 mg SC daily for weight > 100 kg

Caution with use of fondaparinux, tinzaparin, dalteparin, or enoxaparin for pregnancy, morbid obesity, or severe renal dysfunction (CrCl < 30 mL/min); anti-Xa level monitoring is recommended in these settings.
IU, anti-Xa units; for enoxaparin, 1 mg = 100 anti-Xa units.
[a]U.S. Food and Drug Administration (FDA) approved for treatment of PE without DVT.
[b]Not an FDA-approved indication. 200 IU/kg SC daily for month 1, followed by 150 IU/kg SC daily during months 2 to 6 for patients with cancer undergoing prolonged LMWH therapy.

- Though initial SC LMWH overlap therapy with PO warfarin is typically converted to sole PO warfarin long-term therapy, patients with cancer may have reduced recurrent VTE when treated long term solely with LMWH (*NEJM 2003;349:146*) at a slightly reduced dose.
- Protamine only partially reverses LMWH.
- **Because of the SC dosing route, LMWH** facilitates outpatient VTE therapy.
  - Patients selected for outpatient DVT therapy should have no other indications for hospitalization (i.e., complications of VTE or concomitant disease), low risk for VTE recurrence and bleeding, adequate cardiopulmonary reserve, adequate instruction and understanding of the warning signs of bleeding and VTE recurrence, access to a telephone and transportation, ability to inject the drug or a responsible caretaker, and adequate outpatient follow-up with a health care provider who can manage frequent lab testing, complications, etc. (*Chest 1999;115:972*).
- **Long-term anticoagulation with SC LMWH** is the first choice in **pregnant** women (without artificial heart valves) with thrombosis, and it is an alternative for patients with **cancer** and patients who have clearly **failed oral anticoagulation** (objectively confirmed new DVT/PE despite consistently therapeutic INRs) (*NEJM 2003;349:146*).
- **Fondaparinux** is a synthetic pentasaccharide that is structurally similar to the region of the heparin molecule that binds antithrombin and functions as a selective inhibitor of factor Xa.
  - Because fondaparinux inhibits factor Xa and does not inhibit thrombin, it does not significantly prolong the aPTT.
  - Large clinical trials have confirmed the efficacy and safety of weight-based subcutaneously dosed fondaparinux for the treatment of VTE (*Ann Intern Med 2004;140:867*; *NEJM 2003;349:1695*).
  - Similar to the LMWHs, factor Xa monitoring is not normally recommended, but may be necessary for patients with renal dysfunction.
  - Fondaparinux may be used for outpatient VTE therapy.
  - The recommended dose for VTE therapy consists of 5.0, 7.5 or 10 mg SC daily, and the dose used depends on weight (Table 8).

Table 9	Initial Lepirudin Infusion Rates in Renal Impairment[a]	
Creatinine Clearance (mL/min)	Serum Creatinine (mg/dL)	Adjusted Infusion Rate (mg/kg/hr)
45–60	1.6–2.0	0.075
30–44	2.1–3.0	0.045
15–29	3.1–6.0	0.0225
<15	>6	Avoid or stop infusion

[a]Dose adjustment is required for patients on hemodialysis.

- **Lepirudin (Refludan, recombinant hirudin)** is a DTI that is used for the treatment of **HIT.**
  - Lepirudin has a half-life of 1.5 hours.
  - Because of its renal clearance, lepirudin **requires cautious use and dose adjustments in patients with renal insufficiency** (Table 9).
  - Lepirudin dosing for HIT uses a bolus of 0.2 to 0.4 mg/kg (up to 110 kg body weight, maximum dose 44 mg) and then a continuous IV infusion rate of 0.10 to 0.15 mg/kg/hr (up to 110 kg body weight, maximum dose 16.5 mg) (Fig. 2); some experts advise against using the bolus to reduce drug accumulation in patients with renal dysfunction and to reduce the risk of anaphylaxis (*Chest 2008;133(6 Suppl):340S*).

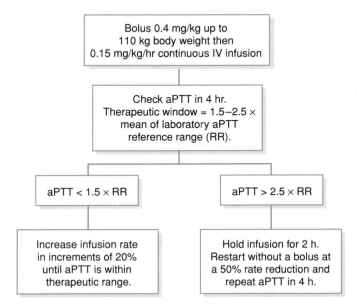

Figure 2. Lepirudin dosing algorithm. aPTT, activated partial thromboplastin time; CIVI, continuous intravenous infusion. (Adapted from Alving BM. How I treat heparin-induced thrombocytopenia and thrombosis. *Blood* 2003;101:31.)

- o aPTT monitoring should occur 4 hours after a dose change, and the dose should undergo adjustment to obtain a target range of 1.5 to 2.5 times the patient's baseline or the mean of the laboratory normal aPTT. A lower target aPTT range (1.5 to 2.0 times baseline) may have similar efficacy and less bleeding risk (*Chest 2008;133(6 Suppl):340S*).
  - o The interpretation of the INRs in patients receiving warfarin must take into account the increased PT/INR caused by lepirudin (*Chest 2008;133 (6 Suppl):340S*).
- **Argatroban** is a synthetic DTI that is used for **HIT** therapy.
  - o Argatroban has a half-life of <1 hour, and a reversal agent is not available.
  - o Argatroban treatment of HIT uses an IV infusion (without a bolus) rate of 2 mcg/kg/min. For patients recovering from cardiac surgery, and those with heart failure, multiple organ failure, or severe anasarca, guidelines recommend a lower initial infusion rate between 0.5 and 1.2 mcg/kg/min (*Chest 2008;133 (6 Suppl):340S*).
  - o aPTT monitoring should occur 2 hours after beginning the infusion, and the infusion rate should undergo adjustment (rate not to exceed 10 mcg/kg/min) to achieve a steady-state therapeutic aPTT (1.5 to 3.0 times the patient's baseline aPTT, not to exceed 100 seconds).
  - o Because of its hepatic clearance, argatroban **requires dose adjustment** (e.g., use an IV infusion rate of 0.5 to 1.0 mcg/kg/min) **in patients with hepatic dysfunction.**
  - o During warfarin coadministration, argatroban should be discontinued when the INR becomes >4, and the INR should undergo remeasurement within 4 to 6 hours (Fig. 2).
    - While off argatroban ≤2 mcg/kg/min for 4 to 6 hours, a subtherapeutic INR (<2) should lead to the resumption of argatroban, and the warfarin dose should undergo daily adjustment until a therapeutic INR (e.g. 2 to 3) occurs during similar testing.
    - For monitoring an argatroban dose > 2 mcg/kg/min, reduce the argatroban infusion to 2 mcg/kg/min before holding the warfarin for 4 to 6 hours later (*Chest 2008;133(6 Suppl):340S*).
- **Thrombolytic therapy**
  - **Thrombolytic therapy** (e.g. alteplase or recombinant tissue plasminogen activator as a 100 mg IV infusion over 2 hours) is appropriate for rare patients with VTE for whom the benefits outweigh the risks of bleeding.
    - o The indications for thrombolytic therapy of **PE** consist of refractory systemic hypotension and PE associated with objectively demonstrated (e.g. echocardiogram, spiral CT) acute, severe right ventricular strain.
      - Though many experts believe that thrombolytic therapy for PE saves lives, clinical trials have failed to demonstrate a survival benefit (*N Engl J Med 2003; 349:631*).
    - o Thrombolytic therapy is uncommonly used for **DVT.** The main indication is DVT leading to venous congestion that compromises the arterial supply to the limb, which is most often seen with massive iliofemoral DVT.
- **Duration of anticoagulation**
  - **Duration of anticoagulation** decisions require individualization based on patient preferences and assessment of the patient's added risk of recurrent VTE off anticoagulant therapy versus the added risk of bleeding complications from continued anticoagulation (*N Engl J Med 2003;349:631*).

- Patients with a **first episode of VTE due to reversible risk factors** (surgery, major trauma) have a low risk of recurrence (<6%/yr), and anticoagulation is recommended for 3 months (*Chest 2008;133:454S*).
- Guidelines recommend a minimum of 3 months of anticoagulant therapy for patients with a **first episode of idiopathic VTE** associated with less compelling and transient risk factors, such as prolonged travel, oral contraceptive pills/hormone replacement therapy, or minor injury (*Chest 2008;133:454S*).
- For patients with unprovoked proximal lower extremity DVT or PE, consider long-term anticoagulation in willing patients with no major risk factors for bleeding and good anticoagulant control. For patients with a strong preference for less frequent INR monitoring, guidelines recommend low-intensity coumarin therapy (INR range 1.5 to 2.0) with less frequent monitoring rather than discontinuation of therapy (*Chest 2008;133:454S*).
- Patients with **cancer and VTE** should undergo anticoagulation until cancer resolution or development of a contraindication. In patients with cancer, VTE recurrence rates are lower with LMWH (e.g., dalteparin 200 IU/kg once daily for 1 month, followed by 150 IU/kg for 5 months) than with standard coumarin therapy (INR of 2 to 3; *NEJM 2003;349:146*).
- For patients with a **first VTE and one inherited hypercoagulable risk factor,** consider an anticoagulation duration of longer than 6 months, depending on the type of thrombophilia.
  - Heterozygous factor V Leiden or heterozygous prothrombin 20210A modestly increases the odds of recurrence (RR 1.6 and 1.4, respectively). Deficiency of protein S, protein C, or AT III carries a greater risk of recurrence than that of heterozygous factor V Leiden or heterozygous prothrombin 20210A (*JAMA 2009;301:2472*).
  - Patients with a **first VTE and APAs or two inherited risk factors** should receive a longer course of anticoagulation (e.g., 12 months) and indefinite therapy should be considered.
- Guidelines recommend that patients with **isolated calf vein DVT** or **upper extremity DVT** often undergo short-duration (e.g., 3 months) anticoagulation.
- Patients with **recurrent idiopathic VTE** should receive anticoagulation indefinitely, unless a contraindication develops, or patient preferences dictate otherwise.
- Patients with a history of VTE, especially those with ongoing risk factors, should possibly receive temporary prophylactic anticoagulation (e.g. low-dose LMWH SQ) during **periods of increased VTE risk,** including surgery, trauma, immobilization, prolonged air travel, hospitalization for medical illnesses, and postpartum.

Other Nonoperative Therapies

- **Leg elevation** is useful for the treatment of edema associated with DVT, though it is not an adequate sole therapy.
- **Ambulation** is encouraged for patients with DVT, especially after improvement of pain and edema, though strenuous lower extremity activity should initially be avoided.
- **Fitted graduated compression stockings** reduce the high incidence of postphlebitic syndrome in patients with lower extremity DVT.
- In patients with **congenital antithrombin (AT) deficiency,** infusion of **AT concentrate** can be used for an acute thrombosis (*Br J Haematol 1982;50:531*).

- **IVC filters** are mainly indicated for acute DVT situations in which there are **absolute contraindications to anticoagulation** (e.g., active bleeding, severe thrombocytopenia, urgent surgery) or **recurrent thromboemboli despite therapeutic anticoagulation.**
- Prophylactic IVC filters in patients with acute DVT/PE reduce the risk of recurrent PE; however, a reduction in overall mortality has not been demonstrated, and they do increase DVT recurrence rates (*Circulation 2005;112:416*).
  - Relative indications for IVC filters include primary or metastatic CNS cancer or limited cardiopulmonary reserve.
  - In patients who had **IVC filters** placed due to **temporary contraindications to anticoagulation,** anticoagulation therapy should be added when safe, to reduce the risk of filter-related thromboses.
  - Several types of removable **IVC filters** exist and can provide a temporary physical barrier against emboli from the lower extremities, but they increase the risk of DVT recurrence. Filter removal requires a second procedure.
- **Catheter embolectomy, often combined with local thrombolytic therapy,** can treat large, acute PE and DVT. The ATTRACT trial is testing whether this dual approach reduces the risk of DVT recurrence or postphlebitic syndrome.

Surgical Management

Surgical embolectomy should be considered in patients with life-threatening massive PE that have contraindications to thrombolytic therapy. Predictors of life-threatening massive PE include elevated plasma BNP, tachycardia, hypotension, right ventricular strain on echocardiogram, and right ventricular enlargement on chest CT (*Circulation 2004;110:3276*).

SPECIAL CONSIDERATIONS

- **Superficial thrombophlebitis** associated with IV infusion therapy does not require systemic anticoagulation, and treatment of discomfort may consist of oral NSAIDs. For patients with spontaneous superficial thrombophlebitis, nonextensive disease does not clearly require systemic anticoagulation. Extensive superficial thrombophlebitis should undergo systemic anticoagulation for at least 4 weeks (*Chest 2008;133:454S*). Treatment with low-dose LMWH (e.g., enoxaparin 40 mg SQ daily) for 8 to 12 days (*Arch Intern Med 2003;163:1657*) may lower the short-term incidence of additional thrombosis. Recurrent superficial thrombophlebitis may be treated with anticoagulation or vein stripping (*Br J Haematol 1982;50:531*).
  - **Perioperative management of anticoagulation** requires close coordination with the surgical service (see Perioperative Medicine in Chapter 1, Patient Care in Internal Medicine) to address timing of interventions and therapeutic changes with the aim of thromboembolism prevention and avoidance of bleeding.
- **Invasive procedures** require discontinuation of warfarin.
  - To achieve a preoperative INR ≤ 1.5, stop warfarin therapy 4 to 5 days before an invasive procedure.
  - In situations where a clinician aims to minimize the patient's time off therapeutic anticoagulation, parenteral anticoagulation should be initiated when the INR becomes subtherapeutic, approximately 3 days after the last warfarin dose but it should be stopped 6 to 24 hours prior to the procedure, depending on the half-life of the parenteral drug.

- o In some instances, intravenous UFH is the preferred choice of therapy (e.g., pregnant woman with a mechanical heart valve undergoing a procedure).
  - o If an INR around 1.7 is acceptable for the procedure, the warfarin dose can be halved for 4 days preoperatively (*Clin Lab Haematol 2003;25:127*).
- After the procedure, resume warfarin (at the previous dose) and/or parenteral anticoagulation as soon as hemostasis and bleeding risk reach an acceptable level, typically within 24 hours.

COMPLICATIONS

- **Bleeding** is the major complication of anticoagulation.
  - Up to 2% of patients who receive short-term UFH, LMWH, or pentasaccharide for VTE therapy experience major bleeding.
  - For patients receiving chronic oral coumarin therapy (INR 2 to 3), the annual incidence of major bleeding is approximately 1% to 3%.
  - Concomitant use of **antiplatelet agents** increases the risk of bleeding.
- **Major bleeding in a patient with an acute VTE should lead to the discontinuation of anticoagulation and consideration of IVC filter placement. Reinitiation of standard-duration anticoagulation should occur after the bleeding concerns have resolved.**
- **INR elevation** on warfarin:
  - Asymptomatic minor INR elevations < 5 should be managed by holding or reducing warfarin dose until the INR returns to the appropriate range and then resuming warfarin at a lower dose (Table 10).

Table 10		Treatment of Elevated INR > 5 (Besides Stopping All Antithrombotic Therapy)
Bleeding	**INR**	**Action**
None	5–9	Evaluate for food and drug interactions and for dosing or laboratory errors
		Repeat INR in 1–4 d
		If INR rising or at high risk for bleeding, give vitamin K 1–2.5 mg PO
	>9	Evaluate for food and drug interactions and for dosing or laboratory errors
		Repeat INR in 12–24 hr and in 48 hr
		Vitamin K 2–10 mg PO; Repeat vitamin K as needed
Minor	Any	Vitamin K 1–5 mg PO or IVPB
		INR q8–24h; repeat vitamin K as needed
		If bleeding not controlled in 24 hr, treat as major bleeding
Major	Any	Vitamin K 10 mg IV over 10–20 min
		FFP (2–3 units), prothrombin complex concentrate (25–50 U/kg)
		Repeat INR in 6–12 hr and continue vitamin K and FFP until INR remains normal AND bleeding has stopped
		Surgical intervention for hemostasis

FFP, fresh frozen plasma; INR, international normalized ratio; PO, by mouth; IVPB, IV Piggyback.

Table 11	HEMORR$_2$HAGES Score
Risk Factor[a]	Definition
Hepatic or renal disease	Albumin < 3.6 g/dL, CrCl < 30 mL/min
ETOH (alcohol) abuse	
Malignancy	
Older age	>75 years
Reduced platelets/platelet function	Plt < 75 × 109/L, on ASA or clopidogrel
Rebleeding	2 points for prior major bleed, 1 point for prior minor bleed
Hypertension	SBP > 160 mm Hg
Anemia	HCT < 30%
Genetic factors	Presence of VKORC1 or CYP2C9 SNPs
Excessive fall risk	
Stroke	Prior ischemic stroke
HEMORR$_2$HAGES Score	**Bleeding Rate Per 100 Patient Years Warfarin (95% CI)**
0	1.9 (0.6–4.4)
1	2.5 (1.3–4.3)
2	5.3 (3.4–8.1)
3	8.4 (4.9–13.6)
4	10.4 (5.1–18.9)
>5	12.3 (5.8–23.1)

ASA, acetylsalicylic acid; CI, confidence interval; CrCl, creatinine clearance; HCT, hematocrit; Plt, platelet; SBP, systolic blood pressure; SNP, single nucleotide polymorphism.
[a]One point for each bleeding risk factor, except a prior major bleed (2 points). Modified from Gage BF, Yan Y, Milligan PE, et al. Clinical classification schemes for predicting hemorrhage: results from the National Registry of Atrial Fibrillation (NRAF). *Am Heart J* 2006;151:713–719.

- Moderate (INR ≥ 5 but < 9) elevation of the INR in asymptomatic patients should be treated by holding one or more warfarin doses. Treatment with oral vitamin K$_1$ 1 to 5 mg probably does not reduce the risk of hemorrhage in this setting as compared to warfarin cessation alone (*Ann Intern Med 2009;150:293*).
- Severe (INR ≥ 9) should be treated with vitamin K (e.g., oral vitamin K$_1$ 2 to 10 mg) (*Thromb Res 2004;113:205*) unless the INR is likely to be spurious.
- **Bleeding with warfarin** (Table 11)
  - Serious hemorrhages should be treated with vitamin K (10 mg) by slow IV infusion and FFP. Because of the long half-life of warfarin (~36 hours, depending on genotype), vitamin K should be repeated every 8 or 12 hours to prevent INR rebound.
  - Though expensive and potentially thrombogenic, **rFVIIa** may stop life-threatening bleeding (*Br J Haematol 2002;116:178*).
- For patients receiving **parenteral anticoagulants:**
  - Discontinuation usually sufficiently restores normal hemostasis.
  - With moderate to severe bleeding, give **FFP.**
  - For patients receiving **UFH** who develop major bleeding, heparin can be completely reversed by infusion of **protamine sulfate** in situations where the potential benefits outweigh the risks (e.g., intracranial bleed, epidural hematoma, retinal bleed).

- ○ Heparin serum concentrations decline rapidly due to a short half-life after IV administration, and the amount of protamine required decreases over time.
- ○ Approximately 1 mg protamine sulfate IV neutralizes 100 units of heparin, up to a maximum dose of 250 mg. The dose can be given as a loading dose of 25 to 50 mg by slow intravenous injection over 10 minutes, with the rest of the calculated dose over 8 to 16 hours by intravenous infusion.
- ○ If 30 minutes to 1 hour has elapsed since a heparin dose, the protamine dose should be reduced to approximately 0.5 mg/100 units heparin.
- ○ If more than 2 hours has elapsed since a heparin dose, 0.25 mg protamine/100 units heparin should be administered.
- ○ If heparin was administered subcutaneously, the same reductions in the protamine dose are adequate.
- For major bleeding associated with **LWMH,** protamine sulfate has less efficacy compared to its effect on UFH since it neutralizes only approximately 60% of LMWH (*Reg Anesth Pain Med 2003;28:172*). Protamine does not reverse **pentasaccharide (e.g., fondaparinux).**
  - ○ For patients with very serious bleeding receiving fondaparinux, concentrated factor VIIa may be used.
- **Occult GI or genitourinary bleeding** is a relative and not absolute contraindication to anticoagulation, though its presence prior to or during anticoagulation warrants an investigation for underlying disease.
- **Warfarin-induced skin necrosis, associated with** rapid depletion of protein C, occurs during initiation of warfarin therapy.
  - ○ Necrosis occurs most often in areas with a high percentage of adipose tissue, such as breast tissue, and it can be life threatening.
  - ○ Therapeutic anticoagulation with an immediate-acting anticoagulant (UFH, LMWH, etc.) and/or avoidance "loading doses" of warfarin prevents warfarin-induced skin necrosis.
- **Warfarin is absolutely contraindicated in early** (i.e., first trimester) **pregnancy** because of the **risk of teratogenicity,** and it is often avoided during the entire **pregnancy** because of the **risk of fetal bleeding,** though it is safe for infants of nursing mothers.
- **Osteoporosis** may occur with long-term heparin or warfarin use (*Arch Intern Med 2006;166:241*).

MONITORING/FOLLOW-UP

- For a suspicious clinical presentation, **testing for intrinsic hypercoagulable risk factors** ideally should wait until the patient is in stable health and off anticoagulation therapy for at least 2 weeks **to avoid false-positive results** for nongenetic testing.
  - However, if reasons exist to screen for hypercoagulable risk factors, collect blood for **activated protein C resistance/factor V Leiden and LA.** Blood collection for **protein C, protein S, and antithrombin** testing should occur before initiating anticoagulation. Although normal protein C, protein S, and antithrombin tests rule out congenital deficiencies, abnormally low results require confirmation through repeat testing or screening first-degree relatives to rule out a temporary deficiency related to the acute thrombosis.
- For patients with suspected lower extremity DVT, an initial negative compression ultrasound, and no satisfactory alternative explanation, **serial compression ultrasonography** within 2 weeks can improve the diagnostic yield.

- If patient preferences or contraindications lead to the withholding of anticoagulant therapy for **calf DVT,** we recommend further evaluation with **a repeat compression ultrasonography** during the next 10 days to assess for proximal extension, which would mandate therapy.
- Though testing for PE in patients with DVT and testing for DVT in patients with PE will produce many positive findings, such testing rarely affects therapy. However, baseline results may provide useful comparison data for patients who return with symptoms of VTE, though studies have not determined the cost-effectiveness of this practice.
- Prolongation of anticoagulation duration in patients with residual thrombosis on **compression ultrasonography at the end of standard duration anticoagulation** for proximal DVT reduces VTE recurrence (but can cause hemorrhage) (*Ann Intern Med 2009;150:577*).

Anemia and Transfusion Therapy

Reshma Rangwala and Morey Blinder

Anemia

GENERAL PRINCIPLES

Definition

Anemia is defined as a decrease in circulating red blood cell (RBC) mass; the usual criteria being hemoglobin (Hb) < 12 g/dL or hematocrit (Hct) < 36% for women and Hb < 14 g/dL or Hct < 41% in men.

Classification

Anemia can be broadly classified into three etiologic groups: **blood loss (acute or chronic), decreased RBC production, and increased RBC destruction (hemolysis).**

DIAGNOSIS

A systematic approach to anemia is best at narrowing down the diagnosis and guiding the subsequent diagnostic workup.

Clinical Presentation

- The clinical presentation of anemia can be accompanied by a variety of signs and symptoms depending on the severity of the anemia, its chronicity, and its pace of development.
- As with any other medical condition, the history and physical exam play key roles in approaching anemia.
- Based on symptoms, one can often discern timeline (acute, subacute, or chronic), severity, and possibly the underlying etiology.
- Patients may be asymptomatic, but patients with an Hb level of <7 g/dL will usually have symptoms.
- Adaptive compensatory mechanisms can mask many signs or symptoms of anemia that have an insidious onset and/or are present over a prolonged period of time.
- In contrast to chronic anemia, patients with abrupt onset of anemia tolerate diminished red cell mass poorly. The anemia may be relatively mild (i.e., Hct > 30%), but the patient may have symptoms of fatigue, malaise, dizziness, syncope, or angina. Acute blood loss most commonly occurs in the gastrointestinal (GI) tract (gastritis due to alcohol or nonsteroidal anti-inflammatory drugs (NSAIDs), diverticulosis, or peptic or gastric ulcer disease) and may be accompanied by epigastric symptoms, nausea and vomiting, or diarrhea.

Physical Examination

Common signs of anemia include pallor, tachycardia, hypotension, dizziness, tinnitus, headaches, loss of concentration, fatigue, weakness occasionally occur. Atrophic glossitis, angular cheilosis, koilonychias (spoon nails), and brittle nails are more common in severe anemia. Reduced exercise tolerance, dyspnea on exertion, and heart failure are seen in more severe anemia. High-output heart failure and shock may be seen in the most severe forms.

Diagnostic Testing

Laboratories
- The complete blood cell (CBC) count measures white blood cells (WBCs), Hb, Hct, platelets, as well as measures of the red cell indices.
- The Hb level is a measure of the concentration of Hb in blood as expressed in g/dL, whereas the Hct level is the percentage of space that the RBC occupies in the blood. Remember that Hb and Hct are unreliable indicators of red cell mass in the setting of rapid shifts of intravascular volume (i.e., an acute bleed).
- The most useful red cell indices include the **mean cellular volume (MCV), red cell distribution width (RDW), and mean cellular Hb (MCH).**
- MCV is the mean volume of the red cells and the normal range is 80 to 96 fL. RBCs can be classified as **microcytic if the MCV is <80 fL, macrocytic when the MCV > 96 fL, and normocytic between 80 and 96 fL.**
- RDW is a reflection of the variability in the size of the red cells and is proportional to the standard deviation of the MCV. **An elevated RDW indicates an increased variability in RBC size.**
- MCH describes the concentration of Hb in each cell and an elevated level is often indicative of spherocytes or a hemoglobinopathy.
- **The reticulocyte count** measures the percentage of immature red cells in the blood and reflects the bone marrow's (BM) response to anemia (i.e., a normal BM response is to increase the production of red cells in anemia so that the observed reticulocyte count increases).
  - A nascent RBC circulates for about 120 days, and the BM is constantly replenishing the bloodstream with new RBCs, with the normal reticulocyte count being ~1%.
  - In the setting of anemia or blood loss, the BM should increase its production of RBC in proportion to loss of RBC and thus a 1% reticulocyte count in the setting of anemia is inappropriate.
  - **The reticulocyte index** (RI) is calculated as % reticulocytes × actual Hct/normal Hct and is important in determining if a patient's BM is responding appropriately to the level of anemia.
  - In normal individuals, RI 1.0 to 2.0 is expected; however, **RI < 2 with anemia indicates decreased production of RBCs (hypoproliferative anemia). RI > 2 with anemia may indicate hemolysis or loss of RBCs** leading to increased compensatory production of reticulocytes (hyperproliferative anemia).
- The **peripheral smear** is a necessary part of the initial hematologic evaluation. RBC shape, size, the presence of inclusions, and orientation of cells in relation to each other are important factors to look for in a smear. RBCs can appear in many abnormal forms, such as acanthocytes, schistocytes, spherocytes, or teardrop cells, and abnormal orientation such as Rouleaux formation.

Diagnostic Procedures
A **BM biopsy** may be indicated in cases of normocytic anemias with a low reticulocyte without an identifiable cause or anemia associated with other cytopenias. The biopsy may confirm myelophthisic process (i.e., presence of teardrop or fragmented

cells, normoblasts, or immature WBCs on peripheral blood smear) in the setting of pancytopenia.

ANEMIAS ASSOCIATED WITH DECREASED RED BLOOD CELL PRODUCTION

Microcytic Anemia

GENERAL PRINCIPLES

Etiology
- **Iron deficiency** is the most common cause of anemia in the ambulatory setting.
- Menstrual blood loss or pregnancy is the most common etiology.
- In the absence of menstrual bleeding, GI blood loss is the presumed etiology in most patients, and the appropriate radiographic and endoscopic procedures should be pursued to identify a source and exclude occult malignancy.
- Diseases of the stomach and proximal small intestine (e.g., *Helicobacter pylori* infection, achlorhydria, celiac disease, and bariatric surgery) often lead to impaired iron absorption.
- Other causes of microcytic anemia include sideroblastic anemia, lead poisoning, thalassemia, and anemia of chronic disease (ACD), which more typically presents as a normocytic anemia.

DIAGNOSIS

Clinical Presentation
Patients may present with fatigue or malaise, which is related to the importance of iron in cellular metabolism and its role in oxygen delivery, as well as pica (consumption of substances such as ice, starch, or clay). Iron deficiency has also been increasingly associated with restless leg syndrome.

History
A careful history relating to menstrual frequency and duration as well as GI blood loss (melena, hematochezia, hematemesis) is essential.

Physical Examination
Splenomegaly, koilonychia ("spoon nail"), and the Plummer-Vinson's syndrome (glossitis, dysphagia, and esophageal webs) are rare findings. The presence of telangiectasias or heme-positive stool may help identify the source of blood loss.

Diagnostic Testing
Laboratories
- The laboratory evaluation depends in part on patient demographics.
- With adequate follow-up, a microcytic anemia in a menstruating female needs only a baseline Hb/Hct value that is repeated 2 to 4 months after the initiation of oral iron therapy.
- Postmenopausal women and men require more detailed evaluation, including evaluation of potential RBC losses, commonly via the GI tract (e.g., peptic ulcer disease,

colon carcinoma) or, rarely, the urinary tract (e.g., paroxysmal nocturnal hemoglobin-uria).

- Because evaluating these patients may require considerable expense and effort, laboratory studies are necessary to document iron deficiency before further evaluation.
- **Ferritin** is the primary storage form for iron in the liver and bone marrow and is the best surrogate marker of iron stores.
  - A ferritin level of <10 ng/mL in women or 20 ng/mL in men is a specific marker of low iron stores.
  - Ferritin is an acute-phase reactant, so normal levels may be seen in inflammatory states despite low iron stores. **A serum ferritin level of >200 ng/mL generally excludes an iron deficiency;** however, in renal dialysis patients, a functional iron deficiency may be seen with a ferritin up to 500 ng/mL.
- **Iron, transferrin, and transferrin saturation** are often used to diagnose iron deficiency anemia but are not as reliable as ferritin for the diagnosis.
  - In this setting, serum iron declines to <50 mg/dL once iron stores are exhausted.
  - Transferrin increases linearly to approximately 400 m/dL once patients are in negative iron balance so that transferrin saturation falls below 16% only when iron stores are exhausted.

Diagnostic Procedures

A **BM biopsy** that shows absent staining for iron is the definitive test for establishing iron deficiency and is helpful when the serum tests fail to confirm the diagnosis.

TREATMENT

- **Oral iron therapy.** In stable patients with mild symptoms, this consists of ferrous sulfate, 325 mg (65 mg elemental iron) PO one to three times per day.
  - Iron is best absorbed on an empty stomach, and between 3 and 10 mg of elemental iron can be absorbed daily.
  - Oral iron ingestion may induce a number of GI side effects, including epigastric distress, bloating, and constipation, as a result noncompliance is a common problem. These side effects can be decreased by initially administering the drug with meals or once per day and increasing the dose as tolerated. Concomitant treatment with a stool softener can also alleviate these symptoms.
  - Ferrous gluconate and fumarate at a similar dose may be better-tolerated alternative therapies.
  - Iron polysaccharide complex (Niferex) contains 150 mg of elemental iron, given twice daily, is as effective as other preparations at a similar cost and seems to have fewer GI side effects.
  - Administration of vitamin C along with the iron improves absorption by maintaining the iron in the reduced state.
- **Parenteral iron therapy.** Parenteral iron therapy may be useful in patients with:
  - Poor absorption (e.g., inflammatory bowel disease, malabsorption).
  - Very high iron requirements that cannot be met with oral supplementation (e.g., ongoing bleeding).
  - Intolerance to oral preparations.
  - The total amount of iron necessary to replete the deficiency can be estimated by a formula using the starting Hb level; however, in practice, parenteral iron is often infused to a dose of 1 to 1.2 g.

- **Iron dextran.** IV iron dextran therapy (INFeD, Dexferrum) can be complicated by serious side effects including **anaphylaxis;** therefore, an **IV test dose** of 25 mg in 50 mL of normal saline (NS) should be administered over 5 to 10 minutes. Methylprednisolone, diphenhydramine, and 1:1,000 epinephrine 1-mg ampule (for subcutaneous administration) should be immediately available at all times during the infusion. For an online dose calculator, go to www.globalrph.com/irondextran.htm.
  - Delayed reactions to IV iron, such as arthralgia, myalgia, fever, pruritus, and lymphadenopathy may be seen within 3 days of therapy and usually resolve spontaneously or with NSAIDs.
- Alternatives to iron dextran include sodium ferric gluconate (Ferrlecit) and iron sucrose (Venofer).
  - The side effect profile for these preparations appears to be better than that of iron dextran, with less hypersensitivity infusion reactions.
  - **However, they cannot be used to replenish the entire iron deficit with a single infusion.**
  - The recommended dosage of sodium ferric gluconate is 125 mg diluted in 100 mL of NS infused IV over 1 hour or as a **slow** IV push over 10 minutes (12.5 mg/min). This can be repeated weekly until circulating iron (to a normal Hct) and storage iron (1 to 3 g) are replenished.
  - Iron sucrose is administered as a 100 to 200 mg IV push or up to 400 mg over a 2.5-hour IV infusion.

Thalassemia

GENERAL PRINCIPLES

Definition

The **thalassemia syndromes** are inherited disorders characterized by reduced Hb synthesis associated with mutations in either the α- or β-chain of the molecule (Table 1).

Epidemiology

Affected individuals are of Mediterranean, Middle Eastern, Indian, African, or Asian descent.

Etiology

- **Beta thalassemia** results in a decreased production of β-globin and a resultant excess of α-globin, forming insoluble α-tetramers and leading to ineffective erythropoiesis.
  - **Thalassemia minor (trait)** occurs with one gene abnormality with variable amounts of β-chain underproduction. Patients are asymptomatic and present with microcytic, hypochromic RBCs, and Hb levels >10 g/dL.
  - **Thalassemia intermedia** occurs with dysfunction in both β-globin genes so that the anemia is more severe (Hb 7 to 10 g/dL).
  - **Thalassemia major** (Cooley anemia) is caused by severe abnormalities of both genes and requires lifelong transfusion support.
- **Alpha thalassemia** occurs with a deletion of one or more of the four α-globin genes leading to a β-globin gene excess.

Table 1	Thalassemias			
	Number of Affected Genes	Hemoglobin (g/dL)	Mean Cellular Volume (fL)	Transfusion Dependent
Alpha thalassemia				
Alpha-thal-2 trait	1	Normal	None	No
Alpha-thal-1 trait	2	>10	<80	No
Hemoglobin H	3	7–10	<70	+/–
Hydrops fetalis	4	Incompatible with life		
Beta thalassemia				
Beta-thal minor (trait)	1	>10	<80	No
Beta-thal intermedia[a]	2	7–10	65–75	+/–
Beta-thal major	2	<7	<70	Yes

[a]Beta thalassemia intermedia has two mutated β-globin genes with impaired but not absent synthesis.

- Mild microcytosis and mild hypochromic anemia (Hb > 10 g/dL) is seen with the loss of one or two genes, whereas Hb H disease (deletion of three α-globin genes) results in splenomegaly and hemolytic anemia.
- Treatment of Hb H disease rarely requires transfusion or splenectomy, but oxidant drugs similar to those that exacerbate glucose-6-phosphate dehydrogenase deficiency should be avoided because increased hemolysis may occur (Table 2).
- Hydrops fetalis occurs with the loss of all four α-globin genes and is incompatible with life.

DIAGNOSIS

Clinical Presentation
- A family history of microcytic anemia or microcytosis is helpful.
- Splenomegaly may be the only physical manifestation.

Diagnostic Testing
Laboratories
- Microcytic hypochromic RBCs are seen, along with poikilocytosis and nucleated RBCs.
- In thalassemia trait, iron studies are normal, as is the red cell distribution width (RDW), which help to differentiate the condition from the microcytosis of iron-deficiency anemia.
- Hb electrophoresis is diagnostic for beta thalassemia showing an increased percentage of Hb A2 and Hb F.
- **Silent carries with a single α-chain loss have an essentially normal electrophoresis.** Those with Hb H disease (loss of three loci) have increased Hb H (β-tetramers). The diagnosis is made by α-globin gene analysis.

Table 2 — Drugs That Can Induce Red Blood Cell Disorders

Sideroblastic Anemia	Aplastic Anemia[a]	Hemolytic Episode in G6PD Deficiency	Immune Hemolytic Anemia		
			Autoantibody	Hapten	Immune Complex[b]
Chloramphenicol	Acetazolamide	Dapsone	α-Methyldopa	Ak-Fluor 25%	Amphotericin B
Cycloserine	Antineoplastic drugs	Furazolidone	Cephalosporins	Cephalosporins	Antazoline
Ethanol	Carbamazepine	Methylene blue	Diclofenac	Penicillins	Cephalosporins
Isoniazid	Chloramphenicol	Nalidixic acid	Ibuprofen	Tetracycline	Chlorpropamide
Pyrazinamide	Gold salts	Nitrofurantoin	Interferon alpha	Tolbutamide	Diclofenac
	Hydantoins	Phenazopyridine	ʟ-Dopa		Diethylstilbestrol
	Penicillamine	Primaquine	Mefenamic acid		Doxepin
	Phenylbutazone	Sulfacetamide	Procainamide		Hydrochlorothiazide
	Quinacrine	Sulfamethoxazole	Teniposide		Isoniazid
		Sulfanilamide	Thioridazine		p-Aminosalicylic acid
		Sulfapyridine	Tolmetin		Probenecid
					Quinidine
					Quinine
					Rifampin
					Sulfonamides
					Thiopental
					Tolmetin

Note: Data compiled from multiple sources. Agents listed are available in the United States.

G6PD, glucose-6-phosphate dehydrogenase.

[a]Drugs with >30 cases reported; many other drugs rarely are associated with aplastic anemia and are considered low risk.

[b]Some sources list mechanisms for many of these drugs as unknown.

Adapted from Cooper DH, Krainik AJ, Lubner SJ, et al., eds. The Washington Manual of Medical Therapeutics. 32nd Ed. Philadelphia: Lippincott Williams & Wilkins, 2007.

TREATMENT

- Those with thalassemia trait require no specific treatment.
- In patients with more severe forms of the disease, RBC transfusions to maintain an Hb level of 9 to 10 g/dL are needed to prevent the skeletal deformities that result from accelerated erythropoiesis.
- In severe forms of thalassemia, the transfusions result in tissue iron overload, which may cause congestive heart failure (CHF), hepatic dysfunction, glucose intolerance, and secondary hypogonadism. **Iron chelation therapy** delays or prevents these complications. Once clinical organ deterioration has begun, it may not be reversible.
- **Chelation therapy** is indicated for transfusion-associated iron overload from any cause. It is indicated in patients with iron infusion burden of >20 units of packed RBCs and ferritin consistently >1,000 ng/mL. Deferoxamine, 40 mg/kg subcutaneously (SC) or intravenously (IV) over 8 to 12 hours continuous infusion (*Am J Hematol 1992;41(1):61–63*). Deferasirox 20 to 30 mg/kg PO Q day is can also be given (*Oncologist 2009;14(5):489*). Side effects of deferasirox include mild to moderate GI disturbances and skin rash. Efficacy is similar to that of deferoxamine. Chelation therapy should be continued until ferritin levels of <1,000 mg/L is maintained.
- Hydroxyurea 15 to 35 mg/kg/d may benefit some patients with beta thalassemia.
- Stem marrow transplant should be considered in young patients with thalassemia major who have human leukocyte antigen (HLA)–identical donors.

Surgical Management

Splenectomy should be considered in patients with accelerated (>2 units/mo) transfusion requirements.

- To decrease the risk of postsplenectomy sepsis, immunization against *Pneumococcus*, *Haemophilus influenzae*, and *Neisseria meningitidis* should be administered at least 2 weeks before surgery if not previously vaccinated (see Appendix A, Immunizations and Postexposure Therapies).
- Not recommended if the patient is younger than 5 to 6 years because of the risk of sepsis.

Myelodysplastic Syndrome

GENERAL PRINCIPLES

Definition

Myelodysplastic syndrome (MDS) is a clonal stem cell disorder characterized by ineffective hematopoiesis resulting in peripheral cytopenias. Some patients progress to develop acute leukemia.

Classification

World Health Organization Classification (Blood *2009 Jul 30;114(5):937–951*)

- Refractory anemia: Erythroid dysplasia, <5% myeloblasts in bone marrow
  - With ring sideroblasts, >15% of nucleated marrow cells
  - Without ring sideroblasts
- Refractory cytopenia with multilineage dysplasia: Evidence of dysplasia in nonerythroid cell lines and <5% myeloblasts in bone marrow.

- Refractory anemia with excess blasts: 5% to 20% myeloblasts in bone marrow.
- 5q-syndrome: Favorable prognosis; may have thrombocytosis.
- MDS; unclassifiable.

Etiology
- **Idiopathic** (70% of patients).
- **Secondary** (30% of patients) to prior radiation, chemotherapy, or toxin exposure.

DIAGNOSIS

Diagnostic Testing
Laboratories
- Complete blood cell count:
  - Cytopenias; anemia is most common, but any combination of low blood counts is possible.
  - Macrocytosis may be present.
- Peripheral smear:
  - Dysplasia: hypogranular or hypolobulated neutrophils (pseudo-Pelger–Hüet anomaly), basophilic stippling, and megaloblastic changes in red cells.
  - Circulating blasts.

Diagnostic Procedures
Bone marrow examination with chromosomal analysis is necessary for diagnosis and classification.

- Iron stain to evaluate for ring sideroblasts.
- Vitamin B_{12} and folate levels to exclude megaloblastic anemia.

TREATMENT

Therapy is based in part upon prognosis at diagnosis. Low-risk MDS is treated primarily with supportive therapies including blood transfusion that may result in clinically significant iron overload (see the Thalassemia section). Patients with intermediate and high risk for MDS can be treated with azacitidine and decitabine. Referral to a hematologist-oncologist is recommended.

Medications
- 5-Azacitidine (Vidaza), 75 mg/m^2 SC × 7 days of a 28-day cycle (*J Clin Oncol 2002;20(10):2429–2440*).
  - Response rate of 15.7% (complete remission + partial remission).
- Slows progression to acute myeloid leukemia and improves survival versus best supportive care (*J Clin Oncol 2002;20(10):2429–2440*).
  - Indicated for patients with high risk for MDS (class INT-2 and high) and for patients who are transfusion dependent.
  - Most common side effects are neutropenia, anemia, and thrombocytopenia.
- Decitabine has also been shown to increase overall improvement rates when compared to supportive therapy (*Cancer 2006;106:1794–1803*).
- Immunosuppressive therapy with antithymocyte globulin, cyclosporine, and glucocorticoids are most effective in patients with a hypocellular (referring to bone marrow cellularity) MDS.

Table 3	**International Prognostic Scoring System**		
Score	Bone Marrow Blasts (%)	Karyotype[a]	Cytopenias
0	<5	Good	0–1
0.5	5–10	Poor	2–3
1			
1.5	11–20		
2	21–30		
Risk group	**Total score[b]**	**Median survival (yr)**	
Low	0	5.7	
INT-1	0.5–1	3.5	
INT-2	1.5–2	1.2	
High	>2.5	0.4	

INT, intermediate.
[a]Good: normal, −Y, 5q, 20q; pcor: complex (>3 abnormalities), chromosome 7 abnormalities.
[b]Score—Total score of bone marrow blasts, karyotype, and cytopenia.

- Iron chelation therapy should be considered in patients with a low or INT-1 risk after 50 to 100 units of RBCs have been transfused.
- Lenalidomide (10 mg PO daily for 21 days of a 28-day cycle) is effective in patients with MDS and 5q-syndrome.

SPECIAL CONSIDERATIONS

- Bone marrow blast count of >20% is diagnostic for acute leukemia.
- Supportive care including RBC transfusions as needed.
- Erythropoietin (Epo) (40,000 units SC every week) or darbepoetin (200 to 300 mg SC every 2 to 3 weeks) may provide some improvement in erythropoiesis.
- Pyridoxine 50 to 200 PO daily, with response rate 20% in patients with ring sideroblasts.
- Stem cell transplant should be considered in patients younger than 50 years who have an HLA-identical sibling.

OUTCOME/PROGNOSIS

- Prognosis is based on WHO classification.
- See Table 3 for the international prognostic scoring system in MDS based on three laboratory features (*Blood 1997;89(6):2079–2088*).

Sideroblastic Anemias

GENERAL PRINCIPLES

Definition

Sideroblastic anemias are hereditary or acquired RBC disorders characterized by abnormal iron metabolism occasionally associated with the presence of ring sideroblasts in the bone marrow aspirate and normal cytogenetics.

Etiology

- Drugs (see Table 2)
- Lead toxicity
- Chronic ethanol use
- Copper deficiency

DIAGNOSIS

Diagnostic Testing

Diagnostic Procedures

A bone marrow examination including cytogenetics may be necessary to evaluate for the presence of ring sideroblasts or other abnormal marrow forms.

TREATMENT

- Remove any possible offending agent.
- Pyridoxine 50 to 200 mg PO daily to treat any underlying nutritional deficiency.

Macrocytic/Megaloblastic Anemia

GENERAL PRINCIPLES

Definition

Megaloblastic anemia is a term used to describe disorders of impaired DNA synthesis in hematopoietic cells but affects all proliferating cells.

Etiology

- Almost all cases are due to folic acid or vitamin B_{12} deficiency.
- **Folate deficiency** arises from a negative folate balance arising from malnutrition, malabsorption, or increased requirement (pregnancy, hemolytic anemia).
  - Patients on slimming diets, alcoholics, the elderly, and psychiatric patients are particularly at risk for nutritional folate deficiency.
  - **Pregnancy and lactation** require higher (three- to fourfold) daily folate needs and are commonly associated with megaloblastic changes in maternal hematopoietic cells, leading to a dimorphic (combined folate and iron deficiency) anemia.
  - Folate malabsorption can also be seen in celiac disease.
  - **Drugs** that can interfere with folate absorption include ethanol, trimethoprim, pyrimethamine, diphenylhydantoin, barbiturates, and sulfasalazine.
  - Patients who are undergoing dialysis require enhanced folate intake because of folate losses.
  - Patients with hemolytic anemia, such as sickle cell anemia, require increased folate for accelerated erythropoiesis and can present with aplastic crisis (rapidly falling RBC counts) with folate deficiency.
- **Vitamin B_{12} deficiency** occurs insidiously over 3 or more years, because daily vitamin B_{12} requirements are low (1 to 3 mg/d), whereas total body stores are 1 to 3 mg.
  - Because multivitamins now contain folic acid, the hematologic manifestations of vitamin B_{12} deficiency may be obscured, leading solely to neurologic presentations.
  - Causes of vitamin B_{12} deficiency include partial (up to 20% of patients within 8 years of surgery) or total gastrectomy and pernicious anemia (PA). Older patients

with gastric atrophy may develop a food-bound vitamin B_{12} deficiency in which vitamin B_{12} absorption is impaired.
- PA occurs in individuals who are older than 40 years (mean onset, age 60 years). Up to 30% of patients have a positive family history. PA is associated with other autoimmune disorders (Graves' disease 30%, Hashimoto's thyroiditis 11%, and Addison's disease 5% to 10%). Of patients with PA, 90% have antiparietal cell IgG antibodies and 60% have anti-intrinsic factor antibodies.
- Other etiologies include pancreatic insufficiency, bacterial overgrowth, and intestinal parasites (*Diphyllobothrium latum*).

DIAGNOSIS

Clinical Presentation
- Folate-deficient patients present with sleep deprivation, fatigue, and manifestations of depression, irritability, or forgetfulness.
- By the time the anemia due to vitamin B_{12} is clinically manifest, neurologic manifestations including peripheral neuropathy, paresthesias, lethargy, hypotonia, and seizures.

Physical Examination
Physical examination may indicate poor nutrition, pigmentation of skin creases and nail beds, or glossitis. Jaundice or splenomegaly may indicate ineffective and extramedullary hematopoiesis. Vitamin B_{12} deficiency may cause decreased vibratory and positional sense, ataxia, paresthesias, confusion, and dementia. Neurologic complications may occur even in the absence of anemia and may not fully resolve despite adequate treatment. **Folic acid deficiency does not result in neurologic disease.**

Diagnostic Testing
Laboratories
- A macrocytic anemia is usually present, and leukopenia and thrombocytopenia may occur.
- The peripheral smear may show anisocytosis, poikilocytosis, and macro-ovalocytes; hypersegmented neutrophils (containing five or more nuclear lobes) are common.
- Lactic dehydrogenase (LDH) and indirect bilirubin are typically elevated, reflecting ineffective erythropoiesis and premature destruction of RBCs.
- **Serum vitamin B_{12} and RBC folate levels** should be measured.
- RBC folate is a more accurate indicator of body folate stores than serum folate, particularly if measured after folate therapy or improved nutrition has been initiated.
- **Serum methylmalonic acid (MMA) and homocysteine (HC)** may be useful when the vitamin B_{12} or folate level is equivocal. MMA and HC are elevated in vitamin B_{12} deficiency; only HC is elevated in folate deficiency.
- A **Schilling test** may be useful in the diagnosis of PA due to vitamin B_{12} deficiency but rarely affects the therapeutic approach. Therefore, it is rarely done anymore.
- Detecting **antibodies to intrinsic factor** is specific for the diagnosis of PA.

Diagnostic Procedures
Bone marrow biopsy may be necessary to rule out MDS or acute leukemia since these disorders may present with findings similar to those of megaloblastic anemia.

TREATMENT

- Treatment is directed toward replacing the deficient factor.
- Potassium supplementation may be necessary when treatment is initiated to avoid potentially serious arrhythmias due to hypokalemia induced by enhanced hematopoiesis.
- Reticulocytosis should begin within 1 week of therapy, followed by a rising Hb over 6 to 8 weeks.
- Coexisting iron deficiency is present in one-third of patients and is a common cause for an incomplete response to therapy.
- Folic acid, 1 mg PO qd, is given until the deficiency is corrected. High doses of folic acid (5 mg PO qday) may be needed in patients with malabsorption syndromes.
- Vitamin B_{12} deficiency is corrected by administering cyanocobalamin. Unless the patient is severely ill (decompensated CHF due to anemia, advanced neurologic dysfunction), treatment with full doses of cyanocobalamin (1 mg/d IM) should await the laboratory diagnosis.
- After 1 week of daily therapy, 1 mg/wk should be given for 4 weeks and then 1 mg/mo for life.
- Patients who decline or cannot take parenteral therapy can be prescribed oral tablets or syrup at 50 mg/d for life.

Anemia of Chronic Renal Insufficiency

GENERAL PRINCIPLES

Anemia of chronic renal insufficiency is attributed primarily to decreased endogenous Epo production and may occur as the creatinine clearance declines below 50 mL/min. Other causes including iron deficiency may contribute to the etiology (see the previous description).

DIAGNOSIS

- Laboratory evaluation reveals a normal MCV in 85% of the cases.
- The Hct level is usually 20% to 30%.
- Peripheral smear: The RBCs are often hypochromic, with the occasional presence of echinocytes (burr cells).
- If the patient's creatinine level is >1.8 mg/dL, the primary cause of the anemia can be assumed to be Epo deficiency and/or iron deficiency, and an Epo level is unnecessary.
- Iron deficiency should be evaluated in patients who are undergoing dialysis due to chronic blood loss via ferritin and transferrin saturation. Oral iron supplementation is not effective in chronic kidney disease (CKD) so that parenteral iron to maintain a ferritin level of >500 ng/mL is recommended. (*Kid Int 2005;68: 2846*)

TREATMENT

- Treatment has been revolutionized by erythropoiesis-stimulating agents (ESAs) including epoetin alfa and darbepoetin alfa (Table 4).
- Therapy is initiated in predialysis patients who are symptomatic.

Table 4	Erythropoietin Dosing	
	Agent and Initial Dose (SC or IV)	
Indication	Erythropoietin[a]	Darbepoetin[b]
Chemotherapy-induced anemia from nonmyeloid malignancy, multiple myeloma, lymphoma; anemia secondary to malignancy, or myelodysplastic syndrome	40,000 units/wk or 150 units/kg three times a week	2.25 µg/kg/wk or 100 µg/wk or 200 µg/2 wk or 500 µg/3 wk
Anemia associated with renal failure	50–150 units/kg three times a week	0.45 µg/kg/wk
Anemia associated with HIV infection	100–200 units/kg three times a week	Not approved
Anemia of chronic disease	150–300 units/kg three times a week	Not approved
Anemia in patients unwilling or unable to receive red blood cells; anemic patients undergoing major surgery	600 units/kg/wk × 3 300 units/kg/d × 1–2 wk	Not recommended

[a]Dose increase after 48 wk up to 900 units/kg/wk or 60,000 units/wk; discontinue if hematocrit (Hct) is >40%; resume when Hct is <36% at 75% of previous dose.
[b]Dose increase after 6 wk up to 4.5 mg/kg/wk or 150 mg/wk or 300 mg/2 wk; hold dose if Hct is >36%; then resume when Hct is <36% at 75% of previous dose.

- Objective benefits of reversing the anemia include enhanced exercise capacity, improved cognitive function, elimination of RBC transfusions, and reduction of iron overload. Subjective benefits include increased energy, enhanced appetite, better sleep patterns, and improved sexual activity.
- Administration of ESAs can be IV (hemodialysis patients) or SC (predialysis or peritoneal dialysis patients). In dialysis and predialysis patients with CKD, **the target hemoglobin should be between 11 and 12 g/dL and should not exceed 13 g/dL.** A hemoglobin and hematocrit should be measured at least monthly while receiving an ESA. Dose adjustments should be made to maintain the target hemoglobin.
- Adverse reactions to ESAs: Targeting higher hemoglobin levels and/or exposure to high doses of ESAs is associated with a greater risk of cardiovascular complications and mortality. In addition, a higher Hct level from ESAs increase the risk of stroke, heart failure, and deep vein thrombosis. (*N Engl J Med 2006;355:2085*)
- **Suboptimal responses to ESA therapy** are a common phenomenon due to iron deficiency, inflammation, bleeding, infection, malignancy, malnutrition, and aluminum toxicity.
  - Because anemia is a powerful determinant of life expectancy in patients on chronic dialysis, IV iron administration has become standard therapy in many individuals who receive ESA therapy and has also been shown to reduce the ESA dosage that is required to correct anemia.
  - A ferritin and transferrin saturation should be tested at least monthly during the initiation of ESA therapy with a goal ferritin level of >200 ng/mL and a transferrin

saturation of >20% in dialysis-dependent patients and a ferritin level of >100 ng/mL and a transferrin saturation of >20% in predialysis or peritoneal dialysis patients.
- Iron therapy is of unlikely benefit if the ferritin level is >500 ng/mL.
- Secondary hyperparathyroidism that causes bone marrow fibrosis and relative ESA resistance may also occur.

Anemia of Chronic Disease

GENERAL PRINCIPLES

ACD often develops in patients with long-standing inflammatory diseases, malignancy, autoimmune disorders, and chronic infection.

Etiology
- The etiology seems to be multifactorial with defective iron mobilization during erythropoiesis, inflammatory cytokine-mediated suppression of erythropoiesis, and impaired Epo response to anemia all play a role.
- ACD is also a common complication of therapy for the underlying disease (e.g., chemotherapy for malignancy, zidovudine for HIV infection).

DIAGNOSIS

Diagnostic Testing
Laboratories
- **At present no laboratory test is diagnostic** for the anemia of chronic disease.
- A normocytic, normochromic anemia is typical.
- Iron studies may be similar to patients with iron deficiency and are difficult to interpret.
- **Serum transferrin receptor** may help distinguish iron-deficiency anemia from anemia of chronic disease (elevated in iron deficiency, normal in anemia of chronic disease).
- Clinical responses to iron therapy can be seen in patients with ferritin levels of up to 100 ng/mL.

Diagnostic Procedures
A BM evaluation for storage iron may be necessary to rule out an absolute iron deficiency accompanying an ACD.

TREATMENT

- Therapy for ACD is directed at the underlying disease and at eliminating exacerbating factors such as nutritional deficiencies and marrow-suppressive drugs.
- ESA therapy should be considered if the patient is transfusion dependent or has symptomatic anemia.
  - Effective doses of Epo are higher than those reported in anemia from renal insufficiency.
  - If no response has been observed at 900 units/kg/wk, further dose escalation is unlikely to be effective.

- The risks of ESA therapy include cardiovascular and arterial and venous thromboembolic events and hypertension.
- Transfusion should be considered for patients with Hct levels of <24% or if symptomatic.

Anemia in Cancer Patients

GENERAL PRINCIPLES

The role of ESAs in patients receiving chemotherapy has come under question. Recent studies indicate that ESA may potentiate cancer growth and decrease disease-free survival. In addition, ESAs have not shown to significantly reduce the need for RBC transfusions in patients not receiving chemotherapy, nor did they increase quality of life. ESA therapy should be considered in transfusion-dependent patients with a target hemoglobin level of 11 to 12 g/dL. (*Lancet 2003;362:1255*, *J Clin Oncol 2005;23:5960*, *J Clin Oncol 2007;25:1027*, *J Clin Oncol 2005;22:9377*, *Lancet Oncol 2003;4:459*)

Anemia Associated with HIV Infection

GENERAL PRINCIPLES

Epidemiology
Anemia is the most common cytopenia in persons with HIV; the prevalence increases as the disease progresses and the CD4 count drops. (*Am J Med 2004;116(Suppl 7A):27S–43S*)

Etiology
Similar mechanism as anemia of chronic disease in which inflammatory mediators cause decreased erythropoiesis.

DIAGNOSIS

Diagnostic Testing
Laboratories
- CBC count: Normochromic, normocytic anemia, although zidovudine and stavudine induce a macrocytic anemia.
- Decreased reticulocyte count.
- Bone marrow exam rarely needed. (See Special Considerations)
- Dysplasia similar to MDS is common.

TREATMENT

Medications
Epo (Table 4) improves the Hct level in patients with an endogenous Epo level of ≤500 mU/mL.

SPECIAL CONSIDERATIONS

- *Mycobacterium avium* complex infections are frequently associated with severe anemia. Diagnosis is established on bone marrow (BM) examination or culture. Treatment of *M. avium* complex is described in Chapter 13, Human Immunodeficiency Virus and Acquired Immunodeficiency Syndrome.
- Parvovirus B19 should be considered in HIV-infected patients with transfusion-dependent anemia and a low reticulocyte count.
  - Laboratory studies: Parvovirus by polymerase chain reaction from blood (serum) or BM.
- Treatment with IV immunoglobulin ([IVIG] 0.4 g/kg IV daily for 5 to 10 days) results in erythropoietic recovery. Relapses have occurred between 2 and 6 months and can be successfully managed with intermittent IVIG at an empiric maintenance dose of 0.4 g/kg IV for 1 day given every 4 weeks (*Ann Intern Med 1990;113(12):926–933*). Further treatment of *M. avium* complex is described in Chapter 13, Human Immunodeficiency Virus and Acquired Immunodeficiency Syndrome.

Aplastic Anemia

GENERAL PRINCIPLES

Aplastic anemia is an acquired abnormality of hematopoietic stem cells that usually presents with pancytopenia.

Etiology

- Most cases are idiopathic
- Approximately 20% of cases are associated with drug or chemical exposure
- Ten percent of cases are associated with viral illnesses (e.g., viral hepatitis, Epstein–Barr virus, cytomegalovirus [CMV]).
- There is a growing body of evidence suggesting that bone marrow failure in aplastic anemia results from immunologic destruction of hematopoietic stem and progenitor cells (*Curr Opin Hematol 2008 May;15(3):162–168*)

DIAGNOSIS

Clinical Presentation

- Usually presents with pancytopenia.
- Presenting symptoms are usually due to anemia (fatigue, malaise, dyspnea) or thrombocytopenia (mucosal bleeding, bruising), although some patients present with fever and leukopenia.

Diagnostic Criteria

- Severe aplastic anemia (*Lancet 1987;2(8565):955–957*)
- Bone marrow cellularity of <30% with normal cytogenetics
- Two of three peripheral blood criteria:
  - Absolute neutrophil count < 500/mm^3
  - Platelet count < 20,000/mm^3
  - Reticulocyte count < 40,000/mm^3
- No other hematologic disease

- Considered moderate aplastic anemia if patients have pancytopenia but do not fulfill criteria.

Diagnostic Testing
Diagnostic Procedures
Bone marrow biopsy is required for diagnosis.

- Morphology of bone marrow biopsy may be difficult to distinguish from hypocellular MDS and paroxysmal nocturnal hemoglobinuria.

TREATMENT

- Suspected offending drugs should be discontinued and exacerbating factors corrected.
- Once the diagnosis is established, care should be provided in a center experienced with aplastic anemia.
- Immunosuppressive treatment with cyclosporine, glucocorticoids, and antithymocyte globulin should be considered in patients who do not undergo an SCT (*Ann Intern Med 2002;136(7):534–546*).
- **Stem cell transplant.** Early referral to a center that is experienced in managing aplastic anemia is recommended. When feasible, SCT from an HLA-identical sibling is generally recommended and has achieved a long-term survival rate of 60% to 70%.
- **Transfusions in aplastic anemia.** Transfusions with RBCs should be kept to a minimum. Prophylactic platelet transfusions are generally recommended if the platelet count is below 10,000/mm^3. Transfusion with blood products from family members should be avoided while SCT is being considered.

ANEMIAS ASSOCIATED WITH INCREASED RED BLOOD CELL DESTRUCTION

Anemias Associated with Increased Erythropoiesis

GENERAL PRINCIPLES

Definition
Anemias associated with increased erythropoiesis (i.e., an elevated reticulocyte count) are caused by bleeding or destruction of RBCs (hemolysis) and may exceed the capacity of normal bone marrow to correct the Hb. Bleeding is much more common than is hemolysis.

Etiology
- Blood loss
- Sites of blood loss are usually readily clinically evident.
  - Suspect occult loss into GI tract, retroperitoneum, thorax, and deep compartments of thigh depending on history (recent instrumentation, trauma, hip fracture, coagulopathy).
- Hemolytic anemias are characterized by the predominant site of hemolysis.
  - Intravascular hemolysis may present with fever, chills, tachycardia, and backache.

- ABO-incompatible RBC transfusion
  - Microangiopathic hemolytic anemia (MAHA)
  - Thrombotic thrombocytopenic purpura (TTP)
    - Disseminated intravascular coagulation (DIC)
    - Mechanical heart valve
    - Malignant hypertension
    - Vasculitis
  - Cold autoimmune hemolytic anemia (cold agglutinin disease)
  - RBC infection (malaria, babesiosis)
- Extravascular hemolysis is characterized by RBC destruction in the reticuloendothelial system, primarily the spleen.
  - Warm autoimmune hemolytic anemia
  - Hereditary spherocytosis

DIAGNOSIS

Diagnostic Testing

Laboratories
- If the presentation is within 5 days of an acute onset, the only abnormal laboratory value may be decreased Hb and Hct levels.
- An elevated reticulocyte response occurs in 3 to 5 days, which is indicative of an appropriate erythropoietic response.
- LDH and bilirubin are increased in most patients reflecting an increase in RBC turnover.
- Serum haptoglobin is decreased with hemolysis due to clearance of intravascular Hb.
- With severe hemolysis, free Hb can be measured in the plasma, and hemosiderin can also be detected in the urine with more chronic hemolysis.
- Examination of the peripheral smear is an important clue to detect hemolysis and may help define the cause. Intravascular hemolysis may reveal red cell fragmentation (schistocytes, helmet cells), whereas spherocytes indicate extravascular, immune-mediated hemolysis.
- Polychromasia and nucleated RBCs can be seen with intense hemolysis and increased erythropoiesis.
- Evaluation for hemolysis includes the direct Coombs test (direct antibody testing [DAT]) for the presence of antibody attached to red cells; the indirect Coombs test indicates the presence of free antibody in the plasma.

Sickle Cell Disease

GENERAL PRINCIPLES

- The sickle cell diseases are a group of hereditary Hb disorders in which the Hb undergoes sickle shape transformation under conditions of deoxygenation.
- The most common are homozygous sickle cell anemia (Hb SS) or other heterozygous conditions (Hb SC, Hb S–beta thalassemia).
- Newborn screening programs for hemoglobinopathies now identify most patients in infancy.

Epidemiology

Sickle cell trait is present in 2.5 million people in the United States, occurring in 8% of African Americans.

Prevention

- **Dehydration and hypoxia** should be avoided because they may precipitate or exacerbate irreversible sickling.
- **Folic acid,** 1 mg PO daily is generally administered to all patients with sickle cell disease because of chronic hemolysis.
- **Antimicrobial prophylaxis** with penicillin VK 125 mg PO bid up to age 3 years and then 250 mg PO bid until 5 years, is effective in reducing the risk of infection. Patients who are allergic to penicillin should receive erythromycin 10 mg/kg PO bid. In most patients, antimicrobial prophylaxis should be discontinued after 5 years of age to decrease the risk of resistant organisms (*J Pediatr 1995;127:685*).
- **Immunizations** against the usual childhood illnesses should be given to children with sickle cell disease, including hepatitis B vaccine. After 2 years of age, a polyvalent pneumococcal vaccine should be administered. Yearly influenza vaccine is recommended.
- **Ophthalmologic examinations** are recommended yearly in adults because of the high incidence of proliferative retinopathy, which leads to vitreous hemorrhage and retinal detachment.
- **Surgery and anesthesia.** Local and regional anesthesia can be used without special precautions. With general anesthesia, measures to avoid volume depletion, hypoxia, and hypernatremia are crucial. For major surgery, RBC transfusions to increase the Hb concentration to 10 g/dL seem to be as effective as more aggressive regimens in most circumstances (*N Engl J Med 1995;333:206*).

Associated Conditions

No hematologic findings are associated with sickle cell trait, which is a benign hereditary condition. Nevertheless, some risks have been reported in patients with sickle cell trait, including high-altitude hypoxia leading to splenic infarction, cerebrovascular complications, and basic training of military recruits associated with increased incidence of sudden death related to extreme exertion and dehydration.

DIAGNOSIS

Clinical Presentation

- Clinical manifestations are variable but generally relate to complications from chronic hemolysis and/or vascular occlusion. Vaso-occlusive complications include pain crises, avascular necrosis, priapism, and acute chest syndrome. Hemolytic complications include pulmonary hypertension, cholelithiasis, and leg ulcers. Strokes and renal medullary infarctions are complications of both.
- Delayed growth and development occur in the pediatric years.
- **Acute intermittent complications** account for much of the care provided to these patients and include the following:
  - **Acute painful episodes ("sickle cell crisis")**
    - Vaso-occlusive pain crises are the most common manifestation of sickle cell disease. Pain is typically in the long bones, back, chest, and abdomen. These crises are precipitated by stress, including vasoreactivity of the microvascular

system along with dehydration or infection or both, and generally last for 2 to 6 days.

- o Although each individual tends to have a consistent pattern of presentation, wide variability is found among patients. Patient-specific factors related to the ability to cope with stress and chronic illness may also contribute to the clinical variability.
- o Some patients have mild disease with rare painful episodes and may be characterized by a higher Hb F levels. Nevertheless, these patients are still at risk of all of the complications of the disease.
- **Acute chest syndrome** occurs when hypoxia (<90% oxygen saturation) leads to increased intravascular sickling and irreversible occlusion of the microvasculature (predominantly pulmonary) circulation. Patients with lung pathology, such as pneumonia, are particularly at risk.
- **Aplastic "crisis"** presents with a sudden decrease in Hb level. The RI is inappropriately low, reflecting suppression of erythropoiesis. The most common etiology in pediatric patients is infection with parvovirus B19; folate deficiency should also be suspected because of the chronic increased requirements for erythropoiesis.
- **Priapism**: Often presents in adolescence and may persist into adulthood.
- **Cerebrovascular events**: Stroke may occur at any age but is most common in children younger than 10 years and is usually caused by cerebral infarction.
- **Infections** in adults typically occur in tissues that are susceptible to vaso-occlusive infarcts (bone, kidney, lung). *Staphylococcus* spp., *Salmonella* spp., and enteric organisms are the most common. Pneumonia is most likely to be caused by *Mycoplasma pneumoniae*, *Staphylococcus aureus*, or *H. influenzae* and must be distinguished from acute chest syndrome.
- **Renal medullary infarction** results in chronic polyuria due to impaired urinary concentration, leading to a chronic risk of dehydration.
- **Renal tubular defects** caused by sickling in the anoxic hyperosmolar environment of the renal medulla may lead to isosthenuria (inability to concentrate urine) and hematuria in both sickle cell trait and disease. These conditions predispose patients to dehydration, which increases the risk of vaso-occlusive events.
- **Cholelithiasis** is present in more than 80% of patients, primarily due to bilirubin stones.
- **Osteonecrosis** of the femoral heads occurs in up to 50% of patients and is a cause of severe pain in adults.
- **Leg ulceration** occurring at the ankle is often chronic and recurring.
- **Pregnancy** in a patient with sickle cell anemia should be considered high risk and is associated with increased spontaneous abortions or premature delivery, along with increased vaso-occlusive crises.

Diagnostic Testing

Laboratories

- Hb electrophoresis or high-pressure liquid chromatography is used to diagnose hemoglobinopathies and distinguishes homozygous sickle cell disease (Hb SS) from other abnormal hemoglobin types.
- The mean Hb in Hb SS disease is about 8 g/dL (range 5 to 10 g/dL). The MCV may be slightly elevated due to reticulocytosis but is low in Hb S–beta thalassemia.
- Leukocytosis (10,000 to 20,000/mm^3) and thrombocytosis (>450,000/mm^3) are common, due to enhanced stimulation of the marrow compartment and to autosplenectomy.

- Peripheral smear shows sickle-shaped RBCs, target cells (particularly in Hb SC and Hb S–beta thalassemia), and Howell–Jolly bodies, indicative of functional asplenism.
- The degree of anemia and reticulocytosis is generally milder in Hb SC disease.

TREATMENT

Acute vaso-occlusive complications

- The full NIH guidelines for pain management are available at http://www.nhlbi. nih.gov/health/prof/blood/sickle/sc_mngt.pdf.
- Management of **acute painful episodes** consists of rehydration (oral fluids, 3 to 4 L/d), evaluation for and management of infections, analgesia, and, if needed, antipyretic and empiric antibiotic therapy.
  - **Opioids** (see Chapter 1, Patient Care in Internal Medicine, the Opioids section) are typically used and are effectively administered by a **patient-controlled analgesia pump,** allowing for the patient to self-administer medication within a set limit of infusions (lockout interval) and basal rate.
    - Morphine (2 mg/hr basal rate with boluses of 2 to 10 mg every 6 to 10 minutes) is the drug of choice for moderate or severe pain. If patient-controlled analgesia is not used, morphine (0.1 to 0.2 mg/kg IV q2–3h) or hydromorphone (0.02 to 0.04 mg/kg IV q2–3h) is recommended.
- Transfusion therapy has no role in the treatment of uncomplicated vaso-occlusive crises.
- Supplemental oxygen does not benefit acute pain crisis unless hypoxia is present.
- **Hydroxyurea** therapy (15 to 35 mg/kg PO daily) has been shown to increase levels of Hb F and significantly decreases the frequency of vaso-occlusive crises and acute chest syndrome in adults with sickle cell disease (*N Engl J Med 1995;332(20):1317–1322*).
- Individuals with suspected **acute chest syndrome** require aggressive transfusion therapy, including red cell exchange. The presentation of acute chest syndrome is clinically indistinguishable from pneumonia; thus, empiric broad-spectrum antibiotics should be administered.
- **Iron chelation therapy** can be used as dictated by transfusion frequency.
- **Priapism** is initially treated with hydration and analgesia. Persistent erections for more than 24 hours may require transfusion therapy or surgical drainage.

SPECIAL CONSIDERATIONS

- Patients with suspected **aplastic crisis** require hospitalization. Therapy includes folic acid, 5 mg/d, as well as RBC transfusions.
- **Cholelithiasis** may lead to acute cholecystitis or biliary colic. Acute cholecystitis should be treated medically with antibiotics and cholecystectomy should be performed when the attack subsides. Elective cholecystectomy for asymptomatic gallstones is controversial.
- Treatment of osteonecrosis consists of local heat, analgesics, and avoidance of weight bearing. Hip and shoulder arthroplasty may be effective in decreasing symptoms and improving function.

- In those with a history of stroke, long-term transfusions to maintain the Hb S concentration to <50% for at least 5 years significantly reduce the incidence of recurrence.
- **Leg ulcers** should be treated with rest, leg elevation, and intensive local care. Wet to dry dressings should be applied three to four times per day. A zinc oxide–impregnated bandage (Unna boot), changed weekly for 3 to 4 weeks, can be used for nonhealing or more extensive ulcers.

G6PD Deficiency

GENERAL PRINCIPLES

This enzymatic deficiency of glucose-6-phosphate dehydrogenase results in RBCs that are more susceptible to oxidant stress than normal RBCs, leading to chronic or episodic hemolysis.

Classification
- A mild form of the deficiency occurs in approximately 10% of men of African heritage and is characterized by hemolytic episodes that are triggered by infections or drug exposure (Table 2).
- A more severe enzyme deficiency, such as the Mediterranean variety, results in hemolysis when susceptible individuals are exposed to fava beans.
- The most severe type causes a chronic, hereditary, nonspherocytic hemolytic anemia in the absence of an inciting cause.

Epidemiology
- This is the most common of the hereditary RBC enzyme deficiencies.
- It is a sex-linked disorder that typically affects men.
- More than 500 different mutations have been identified with variable severity.

DIAGNOSIS

Diagnostic Testing
Laboratories
- The peripheral smear shows "bite cells," and special stains can show **Heinz bodies** (representing denatured Hb) within RBCs.
- Diagnosis is made by demonstrating reduced levels of the enzyme. Because older senescent cells with lower enzyme levels hemolyze first during an acute hemolytic episode, a younger population of RBCs may result in a falsely elevated (normal) enzyme level so that the diagnosis may have to await recovery from the hemolytic episode.

TREATMENT

- Acute hemolytic episodes are largely intravascular and self-limited. Therapy, including hydration and transfusion, is therefore supportive.
- Identification and removal of oxidant stresses such as drugs are paramount.

Autoimmune Hemolytic Anemia

GENERAL PRINCIPLES

Definition

In autoimmune hemolytic anemia (AIHA) autoantibody is targeted to antigens on the patient's own red cells resulting in extravascular hemolysis.

Classification

- Warm AIHA antibodies interact best with RBCs at 37°C.
- Cold AIHA antibodies are most active at temperatures below 37°C.

Etiology

- Warm antibody AIHA is usually caused by an IgG autoantibody.
  - It may be idiopathic or associated with an underlying malignancy (lymphoma, chronic lymphocytic leukemia), collagen vascular disorder, or drug (Table 2).
- Cold antibody AIHA is typically IgM (in cold agglutinin disease).
  - The acute form often secondary to an infection (*Mycoplasma*, Epstein-Barr virus), which is usually transient.
  - The chronic form is due to a paraprotein (lymphoma, chronic lymphocytic leukemia [CLL], Waldenström macroglobulinemia) in approximately one-half of cases and is usually idiopathic in the others.

DIAGNOSIS

Clinical Presentation

- Mild cases of warm antibody AIHA may present with a stable anemia and reticulocytosis. In fulminant cases with an RBC life span of <5 days, the anemia can be severe and the compensatory erythropoiesis inadequate, with a presentation of a rapidly declining Hb, fever, chest pain, and dyspnea. Jaundice, icterus, and dark urine reflect elevated indirect bilirubin from Hb degradation.
- In cold antibody AIHA, severe acute hemolysis may be triggered by exposure to cold ambient temperatures in some patients so that avoiding the cold is of the utmost importance. The disease is otherwise generally characterized by mild anemia with intermittent exacerbations.

Diagnostic Testing

Laboratories

- Decrease in haptoglobin
- Increase in LDH and bilirubin, which may not be dramatic due to extravascular hemolysis.
- Positive direct antiglobulin test DAT:
  - Warm AIHA: IgG+, C3+ or IgG+, C3−
  - Cold AIHA: IgG−, C3−
- Cold agglutinin titers
- Flow cytometry to rule out paroxysmal nocturnal hemoglobinuria.
- Peripheral smear shows spherocytes, polychromasia.
- Consider workup for underlying malignancy.

TREATMENT

- Both warm and cold AIHA therapy should be directed at identifying and treating any underlying cause.
  - Warm AIHA
  - Glucocorticoids, such as prednisone 1 mg/kg. If patients are sensitive to glucocorticoids, response is typically seen in 7 to 10 days. When hemolysis has abated, glucocorticoids can be tapered over 2 to 3 months. Rapid steroid tapers can result in relapse.
  - IVIG is less effective than in ITP, with a response rate of about 40% (*Am J Hematol 1993;44(4):237–242*).
  - Splenectomy should be considered for steroid-resistant AIHA.
  - Rituximab, 375 mg/m² IV weekly for four doses, has shown efficacy in small case series (*Br J Haematol 2001;114(1):244–245*).
- **Idiopathic cold AIHA**
  - Glucocorticoids and splenectomy are not efficacious.
  - Rituximab has been demonstrated to be effective in a case reports (*Blood 2004;103(8):2925–2928*).
  - In severe cases, plasma exchange may be used to remove offending IgM antibody (which is 80% intravascular) to control the disease while other therapies are administered.
  - Warm RBC transfusions to 37°C; keep the patient and room warm to prevent exacerbation of hemolysis.
- **RBC Transfusion in AIHA**
  - **RBC transfusions** may not be as effective in increasing RBC mass due to hemolysis of transfused cells.
    - Transfuse RBCs only when patient is symptomatic or there is decreased oxygen-carrying capacity (e.g., Hb < 6 g/dL).
  - Autoantibodies may confound plasma antibody screens and conventional cross-matches and therefore alloantibodies may go undetected.

Drug-Induced Hemolytic Anemia

GENERAL PRINCIPLES

Drug-induced hemolytic anemia is caused by one of three different mechanisms. Treatment consists of discontinuing the offending agent. Medications that are known to cause these effects are listed in Table 2.

Pathophysiology

- **Drug-induced autoantibodies** present similarly to warm AIHA. The DAT is positive for IgG. α-Methyldopa is the prototype.
- **Haptens** form when a drug (usually an antimicrobial) coats RBC membranes, forming a new antigenic determinant. If antibodies against the drug are present and the patient receives the drug (particularly at high doses), a DAT-positive hemolytic anemia may result.
- **Immune complexes** occur in most cases of drug-induced hemolysis. IgM (occasionally IgG) antibodies may develop against a drug and form a drug–antibody complex that adheres to the RBCs. Because the antibody is usually IgM, the DAT is positive only for C3.

Microangiopathic Hemolytic Anemia

GENERAL PRINCIPLES

Definition

This is a syndrome of traumatic (microangiopathic) intravascular hemolysis.

DIAGNOSIS

MAHA is a morphologic classification in which fragmented RBCs (schistocytes) are seen on peripheral blood smear. It is not a specific diagnosis but suggests a limited differential diagnosis.

Differential Diagnosis

- **Mechanical heart valves can cause direct RBC shear stress, especially if the valve is dysfunctional; this may be difficult to diagnose.**
- Other processes that cause RBC fragmentation and hemolysis include DIC, TTP, hemolytic uremic syndrome, malignant hypertension, the preeclampsia/eclampsia syndromes, vasculitis, adenocarcinoma, and improper use of blood warmers.

Diagnostic Testing

Laboratories
- CBC count: normocytic anemia with thrombocytopenia
- Elevated LDH, reticulocyte count, bilirubin
- Decreased haptoglobin
- Peripheral smear shows schistocytes, polychromasia

TREATMENT

The treatment depends on the underlying etiology of microangiopathy. (For specific recommendations for TTP/hemolytic uremic syndrome, see Disorders of Hemostasis.)

TRANSFUSION MEDICINE

Approach to Transfusion Therapy

GENERAL PRINCIPLES

The benefits and risks of transfusion therapy must be carefully weighed in each situation because blood products are a limited resource with potentially life-threatening side effects.

- **Indications/contraindications**
  - RBC transfusion is indicated to increase the oxygen-carrying capacity of blood in anemic patients. Transfusion threshold (in general):
    - Hemoglobin 7 to 8 g/dL with no cardiac risk.
    - Hemoglobin 10 g/dL with a history of coronary artery disease or risk of ischemia.
  - One unit of RBCs increases the Hb level by 1 g/dL in the average adult.

- If the cause of anemia is easily treatable (e.g., iron or folic acid deficiency) and no cerebrovascular or cardiopulmonary compromise is present, it is preferable to avoid transfusions.
- **Pretransfusion**
  - The type and screen procedure tests the recipient's RBCs for the A, B, and D (Rh) antigens and also screens the recipient's serum for antibodies against other RBC antigens.
  - Cross-matching tests the patient's serum for antibodies against antigens on the donor's RBCs and is performed before a specific unit of blood is dispensed for a patient.
- **Manipulation of blood products**
  - Leukoreduced blood products are recommended in the following circumstances:
    - If the patient has a history of one or more nonhemolytic febrile transfusion reactions that were not responsive to acetaminophen. Blood products are often leukoreduced at the time of collection or preparation. If they are not leukoreduced, bedside filters can leukoreduce the unit as it is being transfused; however, this is not effective in the prevention of nonhemolytic febrile transfusion reactions, which are due to cytokines released from WBCs.
    - To prevent CMV infection in patients who require CMV-negative blood products that are not available.
    - To prevent the formation of platelet alloantibodies.
  - Irradiation of blood products eliminates immunologically competent lymphocytes and is recommended for immunocompromised bone marrow or organ transplant recipients or for any patient who is receiving directed donations from HLA-matched donors or first-degree relatives.
  - Washed RBCs are rarely indicated but should be considered in patients in whom plasma proteins may cause a serious reaction (e.g., IgA-deficient recipients or other anaphylactic reactions).
  - CMV-negative blood products are indicated in immunocompromised bone marrow or organ transplant recipients who are CMV antibody negative. If only CMV-positive products are available, the risk of CMV transmission can be minimized with prestorage leukoreduced units issued with a leukoreduction filter.
- **Procedures**
  - Patient and blood product identification procedures must be carefully followed to avoid mishandling errors.
  - The IV catheter should be at least 18 gauge to allow adequate flow.
  - All blood products should be administered through a 170- to 260-μm "standard" filter to prevent infusion of macroaggregates, fibrin, and debris.
  - Patients should be observed for 5 to 10 minutes of each transfusion for adverse effects and at regular intervals thereafter.
  - Each unit of packed RBCs should be completed within 4 hours of delivery to the bedside.
  - Infusion is typically administered over 2 hours.

SPECIAL CONSIDERATIONS

- Long-term RBC transfusion therapy.
  - If the patient has received >20 units of RBCs, iron chelation therapy should be considered (see the Anemias Associated With Decreased Red Blood Cell Production section).

- Consideration should also be given to performing an expanded RBC antigen panel to determine RBC phenotypic matches and decrease the risk of RBC alloimmunization and delayed hemolytic transfusion reactions.
- Emergency RBC transfusions should be used only in situations in which massive blood loss has resulted in cardiovascular compromise.
  - Volume expansion with normal saline should be attempted initially.
  - Blood typing can be performed in 10 minutes and cross-matching within 30 minutes in emergency situations.
  - If unmatched blood must be used, it should be group O/Rh-negative type that has been previously screened for reactive antibodies.
  - At the first sign of a transfusion reaction, the infusion should be stopped.
- Approach to patients who are unwilling or unable to receive RBC transfusions (e.g., Jehovah's Witness):
  - Management includes reducing blood loss by phlebotomy and obtaining necessary testing in pediatric tubes.
  - Epo is often of benefit (Table 4).
  - In most cases, concurrent use of oral or parenteral iron is also recommended (see the Anemias Associated with Decreased Red Blood Cell Production section). An increase in Hb of 1 to 2 g/dL over approximately a week is generally observed.

COMPLICATIONS

- **Transfusion-transmitted infections**
  - Transfusion-transmitted infections include HIV-1/2, human T-lymphotropic virus type 1/2, hepatitis B virus, hepatitis C virus, syphilis, and West Nile virus.
  - Risk of infectious transmission:
    - Risk of HIV-1, HIV-2, human T-lymphotropic virus type 1, and hepatitis C is estimated to be 1 in 2,000,000 to 3,000,000.
    - Risk of hepatitis B virus transmission is approximately 1 in 50,000.
  - Viral infections occur when donors are in the window period (undetectable to testing).
  - CMV transmission from RBC and platelet transfusion is an important risk in immunocompromised patients.
  - Bacterial transmission may occur from either a donor infection or a contaminant at the time of collection.
    - Platelet transfusions are more likely than RBCs to have bacterial contamination because they are stored at room temperature.
    - Most common organism identified in RBCs is *Yersinia enterocolitica* and in platelets is *Staphylococcus aureus*.
- **Noninfectious hazards of transfusion**
  - **Hemolytic transfusion reactions**
    - **Acute hemolytic reactions** are usually caused by **preformed antibodies** in the recipient and are characterized by intravascular hemolysis of the transfused RBCs soon after the administration of ABO-incompatible blood.
      - **Fever, chills, back pain, chest pain, nausea, vomiting,** and symptoms related to hypotension may develop. Acute renal failure with hemoglobinuria may occur. In the unconscious patient, hypotension or hemoglobinuria may be the only manifestation.
      - If a hemolytic transfusion reaction is suspected, **the transfusion should be stopped immediately and all IV tubing should be replaced.** Clotted and EDTA-treated samples of the patient's blood should be delivered to the blood

bank along with the remainder of the suspected unit for repeat of the cross-match. The direct and indirect Coombs tests are performed, and the plasma and freshly voided urine should be examined for free Hb.

- Management includes preservation of intravascular volume and protection of renal function. Urine output should be maintained at ≥100 mL/hr with the use of IV fluids and diuretics or mannitol, if necessary. The excretion of free Hb can be aided by alkalinization of the urine. Sodium bicarbonate can be added to IV fluids to increase the urinary pH to ≥7.5 (see Renal Diseases).

○ **Delayed hemolytic** transfusion reactions typically occur 3 to 10 days after transfusion and are caused by either a primary or an amnestic antibody response to specific RBC antigens on donor RBCs.
- Hb and Hct levels may fall.
- DAT is positive, resulting in confusion with AIHA.
- Delayed hemolytic transfusion reaction may at times be severe; these cases should be treated similarly to acute hemolytic reactions.

○ **Nonhemolytic** febrile transfusion reactions are characterized by fevers and chills.
- Decreased incidence with leukoreduced products
- White cells or cytokines released from white cells are thought to be the cause.
- The symptoms may be treated with acetaminophen.
- Prophylaxis with acetaminophen and prestorage leukoreduced blood products may prevent future febrile reactions.

○ Allergic reactions are characterized by urticaria and, in severe cases, bronchospasm and hypotension.
- The reactions are due to plasma proteins that elicit an IgE-mediated response. The reaction may be specific to the plasma proteins of a particular donor and therefore the reaction may occur infrequently to blood products or never again.
- If the symptoms are mild, pretreatment with diphenhydramine may prevent future reactions.
- Anaphylactic reactions necessitate the addition of pretreatment glucocorticoids and washed RBCs or volume-reduced platelets.
- If anaphylaxis occurs, check serum immunoglobulins because patients with IgA deficiency who receive IgA-containing blood products may experience anaphylaxis with small exposure to donor plasma.

○ **Transfusion-associated circulatory overload** is a relatively common yet under-recognized complication of blood transfusion. Volume overload with signs of CHF may be seen when patients with cardiovascular compromise are transfused with RBCs. The clinical and radiographic features may be indistinguishable from that of transfusion-related acute lung injury (TRALI) (see the following text). In critically ill patients, more invasive techniques may be required for a definitive diagnosis (*Crit Care Med 2006 May;34(5 Suppl):S109–S113*). Slowing the rate of transfusion and judicious use of diuretics help prevent this complication.

○ **TRALI** is indistinguishable from acute respiratory distress syndrome and occurs within 4 hours of a transfusion.
- Symptoms include dyspnea, hypotension, fever, chills, and hypoxemia.
- Ventilatory assistance may be required.
- Anti-human leukocyte antigen (HLA) or antigranulocyte antibodies in the donor's serum directed to the recipient's WBCs cause the disorder.
- Despite clinical or radiographic findings that suggest edema, data indicate that diuretics have no role and may be detrimental (*Blood 2005;105(6):2266–2273*).

- Hypoxemia resolves rapidly, typically in about 24 hours.
- On recognition, transfusions must be stopped and the blood bank notified so that other products from the donor(s) in question may be quarantined.

○ **Transfusion-associated graft-versus-host** disease is usually seen in immuno-compromised patients and is thought to result from the infusion of immuno-competent T lymphocytes.
- Symptoms include rash, elevated liver function tests, and severe pancytopenia.
- Mortality is >80%.
- This has been reported in immunocompetent patients who share an HLA haplotype with HLA-homozygous blood donors (usually a relative or members of inbred populations).
- **Irradiation** of blood products prevents this disease. Because the chances of shared HLA haplotypes with a random blood donor are extremely low, irradi-ation of nonrelated blood products is not indicated for the immunocompetent patient.

○ **Post-transfusion purpura** is a rare syndrome of severe thrombocytopenia and purpura or bleeding that starts 7 to 10 days after exposure to blood products that contain platelets. The disorder is described in Chapter 17, Disorders of Hemostasis and Thrombosis, the Platelet Disorders section.

- **Adverse effects due to massive transfusion**
  - Administration of blood products greater than the normal blood volume of the patient in a 24-hour period (massive transfusion) may be associated with several additional complications.
  - Hypothermia caused by rapid infusion of chilled blood may cause cardiac dys-rhythmias. A blood-warming device can prevent this problem.
  - Citrate intoxication occurs in patients with hepatic dysfunction.
    ○ This results in **hypocalcemia,** causing paresthesias, tetany, hypotension, and decreased cardiac output. On rare occasions, the patient may require calcium gluconate, 10 mL of a 10% solution IV. Calcium should never be added directly to the transfusion product because it may cause the blood to clot.
  - **Hyperkalemia**
    ○ Hyperkalemia is not usually significant unless the patient was hyperkalemic before transfusion (e.g., because of renal failure or muscle injury).
    ○ Twenty-four hours after massive transfusion, hypokalemia may occur as RBCs become more metabolically active, and take up potassium from the plasma.
  - **Bleeding complications** from dilution of platelets and plasma coagulation factors may be seen during massive transfusion. Correction of platelet and coagulation factor deficiencies should be based on clinical findings and laboratory monitoring rather than an empiric formula.

WHITE BLOOD CELL DISORDERS

Leukocytosis

GENERAL PRINCIPLES

Definition

Leukocytosis is an elevation in the absolute WBC count (>10,000/mm^3).

Etiology

- An elevated WBC count typically reflects the normal response of bone marrow to an infectious or inflammatory process, steroid, β-agonist or lithium therapy, splenectomy, and stress, and usually causes an **absolute neutrophilia.**
- Occasionally, leukocytosis is due to a primary bone marrow abnormality in WBC production, maturation, or death (apoptosis) related to a leukemia or myeloproliferative disorder and can affect any cell in the leukocyte lineage.
- Medications implicated in leukocytosis such as corticosteroids should be considered as an etiology.
- An excessive WBC response (i.e., >50,000/mm^3) associated with a cause outside the bone marrow is termed a "**leukemoid reaction,**" which can be either reactive or malignant in origin.
- Lymphocytosis is less commonly encountered and is associated with a viral infection, medication effect or leukemia.

DIAGNOSIS

Clinical Presentation

- Patients with leukocytosis can present with a wide variety of nonspecific symptoms including fevers, chills, fatigue, and malaise.
- In addition, patients with circulating immature WBCs including blasts or those with extreme leukocytosis may present with signs and symptoms of stasis such as central nervous system (CNS) and visual disturbances.
- Weight loss is a concerning finding for an underlying malignancy.

History

A careful history, including the temporal nature of the symptoms, specific infectious symptomology, and a detailed medication history should be elicited.

Physical Examination

- The physical exam should be directed toward the identification of an infectious process.
- Lymphocytosis secondary to CLL, however, will often present with splenomegaly and lymphadenopathy.
- Patients with chronic myelogenous leukemia (CML) present with leukocytosis and splenomegaly; they will rarely present with lymphadenopathy.
- Clinical findings associated with thrombocytopenia or anemia may also occur.

Diagnostic Testing

Laboratories

- A CBC count with peripheral smear is necessary for the evaluation of WBC disorders.
- The presence of blasts on a peripheral smear is concerning for an acute leukemia and warrants emergent evaluation.
- Unexplained neutrophilia should be assessed with a BCR-abl molecular study for the diagnosis of CML.
- Acute leukemia may also have an associated elevation in LDH and uric acid from the high cell turnover.

Diagnostic Procedures

If a malignant etiology is suspected, a bone marrow biopsy, cytogenetics, and flow cytometry often establish the diagnosis.

TREATMENT

- A number of patients with a neutrophilia will have an infectious or inflammatory etiology and treatment should be directed at the underlying cause.
- See Chapter 19, Medical Management of Malignant Disease, for the treatment of acute and chronic leukemia.

Leukopenia

GENERAL PRINCIPLES

Definition

Leukopenia is a reduction in the WBC count ($<3,500$ cells/mm^3).

Etiology

- It can occur in response to infection, inflammation, malignancy, drugs, environmental exposure to heavy metals or radiation, and vitamin deficiencies, with a majority due to medications such as chemotherapeutic or immunosuppressive drugs; the latter are usually dose-dependent effects.
- Idiosyncratic leukopenia can occur secondary to numerous medications and should be suspected when developing shortly after starting a new agent.

Associated Conditions

- A severe neutropenia with an absolute neutrophil count ([ANC] < 500/mm^3) increases the risk of a life-threatening bacterial infection. If patients develop a neutropenic fever, immediate treatment with broad-spectrum antibiotics should be instituted.
- Growth factor support should be considered in patients with chronic neutropenia and ongoing infections until the neutropenia resolves (see Oncologic Emergencies in Chapter 19, Medical Management of Malignant Disease).

MONOCLONAL GAMMOPATHIES

Monoclonal Gammopathy of Unknown Significance

GENERAL PRINCIPLES

Definition

Monoclonal gammopathy of unknown significance (MGUS) refers to the presence of a monoclonal protein ("M protein") in the absence of related organ failure and a known related disease, such as multiple myeloma (MM) or amyloidosis.

Classification

Most patients identified with a monoclonal gammopathy are classified as having MGUS, while the others are diagnosed with a malignant lymphoproliferative disorder, including MM, amyloidosis, Waldenström macroglobulinemia, lymphoma, or chronic lymphocytic leukemia.

Epidemiology

The incidence of MGUS increases with age; 3% of older than 70 years persons have an MGUS.

DIAGNOSIS

Monoclonal gammopathies are commonly found on serum protein electrophoresis; most of the gammopathies are identified as IgG, but gammopathies in all immunoglobulin classes have been identified.

Diagnostic Criteria

Characteristics of MGUS include a monoclonal gammopathy level of <3 g/dL, no evidence of organ damage (e.g., anemia, hypercalcemia, renal insufficiency, or plasmacytoma). A bone marrow examination must show <10% plasma cells in patients with MGUS. The presence of any of these abnormalities or significant amounts of monoclonal immunoglobulin in the urine suggests a more serious lymphoproliferative disorder.

OUTCOME/PROGNOSIS

MGUS **evolves into a more serious lymphoproliferative malignancy** at a rate of about 1% per year and the risk continues for long term. Most of these malignancies are MM. Therefore, it is recommended that patients with MGUS should be followed indefinitely.

- Three risk factors for progression have been identified: Patients with non-IgG gammopathy (IgM or IgA), abnormal, serum-free, light-chain ratio ($\kappa{:}\lambda$ ratio), and initial gammopathy concentration of >1.5 g/dL each of these factors increases the risk of progressing and the presence of all three confers the highest risk of 58% at 20 years.

Multiple Myeloma

GENERAL PRINCIPLES

Definition

MM is a lymphoproliferative disorder associated with a monoclonal gammopathy that can present with an unexpected skeletal fracture (long bone or vertebral body), renal failure (due to Bence Jones proteinuria), hematologic abnormalities (anemia, neutropenia, thrombocytopenia), hypercalcemia, or a combination of these.

DIAGNOSIS

The diagnosis is usually established by a bone marrow exam with the presence of plasma cells >30% in the marrow.

Diagnostic Criteria

- Clonal bone marrow plasma cells ≥10% (*Leukemia 2009 Jan;23(1):3–9*)
- Presence of serum and/or urinary monoclonal protein
- Evidence of end-organ damage
  - Hypercalcemia: serum calcium ≥ 11.5mg/100mL
  - Renal insufficiency: serum creatinine >1.73mmol/L)
  - Anemia: hemoglobin value <10g/100mL
  - Bone lesions

TREATMENT

Treatment with pulse corticosteroids in combination with other chemotherapy (melphalan, thalidomide, lenalidomide, or bortezomib) is usually successful in achieving a response.

Waldenström Macroglobulinemia

GENERAL PRINCIPLES

Waldenström macroglobulinemia is an uncommon IgM monoclonal disorder also known as lymphoplasmacytic lymphoma, characterized by mild hematologic abnormalities, and accompanied by tissue infiltration including lymphadenopathy, splenomegaly, or hepatomegaly. Because of its high molecular weight and concentration, IgM gammopathy can lead to hyperviscosity (CNS, visual, cardiac) manifestations.

TREATMENT

- Treatment with chemotherapy is usually successful in achieving a response (*Clin Lymphoma Myeloma 2008 Aug;8(4):219–229*).
- Patients with complications of viscosity often benefit from treatment with plasmapheresis to decrease the IgM concentration.

Amyloidosis

GENERAL PRINCIPLES

Primary (AL) amyloidosis is an infiltrative disorder due to monoclonal, light-chain deposition in various tissues. Most often involving the kidney (renal failure, nephrotic syndrome), heart (nonischemic cardiomyopathy), peripheral nervous system (neuropathy), and GI tract/liver (macroglossia, diarrhea, nausea, vomiting). Unexplained findings in any of these organ systems should prompt evaluation for amyloidosis.

DIAGNOSIS

- An M protein in urine or serum is found in >90% of patients and helps establish the diagnosis. Biopsy of an affected organ or bone marrow is often done; diagnosis is made by identification of amyloid protein in the biopsy tissue.

- Several effective chemotherapy regimens have been developed during the last decade (*Haematologica 2009 Aug;94(8):1044–1048*). However, treatment of amyloidosis is difficult and progressive organ failure is frequent.

OUTCOME/PROGNOSIS

Cardiac involvement with amyloidosis has a particularly poor prognosis with a median survival of <1 year.

19 Medical Management of Malignant Disease

Boone Goodgame, Daniel Morgensztern, and Ramaswamy Govindan

Medical Management of Malignant Disease

Cancer is the leading cause of mortality in the developed world and increasingly becoming so in the developing world. Cancer therapy has evolved significantly over the past six decades. The pace of research in oncology has accelerated rather dramatically over the past 10 years thanks to advances in genomics, drug development, and supportive care. There is now significant interest in discerning the critical interacting molecular pathways operative in cancer cells and targeting them effectively to produce meaningful clinical benefit. The successes with trastuzumab in breast cancer, imatinib in gastrointestinal stromal tumors and chronic myeloid leukemia, and gefitinib and erlotinib in patients with non–small-cell lung cancer (NSCLC) that have activating mutations in the epidermal growth factor receptor (EGFR) tyrosine kinase illustrate the promise of this approach. This chapter provides a quick overview of cancer therapy.

Approach to the Cancer Patient

GENERAL PRINCIPLES

Principles of targeted therapy

- Newer "molecular" or "targeted" therapies have lead to marked advances in some malignancies. These agents inhibit the function of specific proteins and have specific toxicities that can be significant.
- The most common classes of drugs are as follows: (1) monoclonal antibodies, given intravenously, and designed to bind to cell surface molecules (cetuximab, panitumumab, bevacizumab, trastuzumab, etc.) and (2) oral receptor tyrosine kinase inhibitors ([TKIs]; e.g., erlotinib, gefitinib, imatinib, lapatinib, sunitinib, sorafenib) (Table 1).
- Most antibodies are used in combination with chemotherapy or radiation, whereas most TKIs are used as single agents.
- The majority of targeted agents have a moderate effect and prolong the time to disease progression, while others have striking benefit, including the following:
  - Imatinib in chronic myeloid leukemia (CML) inhibits the bcr-abl tyrosine kinase and leads to prolonged remissions.
  - Imatinib in gastrointestinal (GI) stromal tumors inhibits C-Kit and leads to marked disease regression.
  - Gefitinib and erlotinib in lung cancer inhibit EGFR, leading to marked benefits in patients with mutations in EGFR (approximately 10% of lung cancer patients).
  - Trastuzumab in resected breast cancer, when used in the adjuvant setting, reduces relapse by 50%.

Table 1	Most Common Cancer Diagnoses and Rates of Death in the United States for 2008					
Sites	New Cases			Deaths		
	Both Sexes	**Male**	**Female**	**Both Sexes**	**Male**	**Female**
Lung	215,020	114,690	100,330	161,840	90,810	71,030
Prostate	186,320	186,320	X	28,660	28,660	X
Breast	184,540	1,990	182,460	40,930	450	40,480
Colon	108,070	53,760	54,310	49,960	24,260	25,700
Non-Hodgkin's lymphoma	66,120	35,450	30,670	19,160	9,790	9,370

- Toxicities of targeted therapies are unique to each agent (summarized in Table 1), but some helpful generalizations can be made.
  - Inhibitors of EGFR frequently cause an acne-like rash on the face and upper chest, which can be severe. Treatment is typically with topical corticosteroids or oral minocycline.
  - Inhibitors of HER2 are associated with a reversible decline in cardiac systolic function and ejection fraction should be monitored.
  - Inhibitors of angiogenesis are associated with endothelial toxicity leading to hypertension, proteinuria, delayed wound healing, mild cardiac toxicity, increased risk of bleeding, thromboembolism, and GI perforation/fistula. All antiangiogenics should be held in the perioperative period.

Epidemiology

- Cancer is the fourth most common cause of death in the United States, causing >500,000 deaths per year and 7 million deaths worldwide. Tables 2 and 3 show rates of the most common malignancies in the United States and worldwide.
- Cancer is associated with aging and has increased as life expectancy has increased. Median age at diagnosis for all cancers in the United States is 67 years (*CA Cancer J Clin 2008;58:71*).

Table 2	Most Common Cancer Diagnoses in Incidence and Mortality Worldwide for 2007		
New Cases		Deaths	
Male	**Female**	**Male**	**Female**
Lung (1,108,731)	Breast (1,301,867)	Lung (974,624)	Breast (464,854)
Prostate (782,647)	Cervical (555,094)	Stomach (511,549)	Lung (376,410)
Stomach (691,432)	Colorectal (536,662)	Liver (474,215)	Cervical (309,808)
Colorectal (630,358)	Lung (440,390)	Colorectal (318,798)	Stomach (288,681)
Liver (502,271)	Stomach (375,111)	Esophagus (300,034)	Colorectal (284,169)

Table 3	ECOG Score
Grade	**ECOG**
0	Fully active, able to carry on all predisease performance without restriction
1	Restricted in physically strenuous activity but ambulatory and able to carry out work of a light or sedentary nature, e.g., light housework, office work
2	Ambulatory and capable of all self-care but unable to carry out any work activities. Up and about >50% of waking hours
3	Capable of only limited self-care, confined to bed or chair >50% of waking hours
4	Completely disabled. Cannot carry on any self-care. Totally confined to bed or chair
5	Dead

Am J Clin Oncol 1982;5:649.

- Tobacco is the most common cause of cancer death and is associated with lung, head and neck, esophageal, gastric, pancreatic, kidney, and bladder cancers.
- Diet, obesity, and inactivity likely contribute to many malignancies.

DIAGNOSIS

- A tissue diagnosis is required prior to any medical or radiation therapy.
- **Cytology** specimens may contain only a few malignant cells and are often the least invasive to obtain. Examples include cervical brushings (Pap smears), endoscopic brushings, and samples of sputum, urine, and pleural, pericardial, or peritoneal fluid. Cytology is not the preferred approach specifically to diagnose and characterize subtypes of lymphoma. Even in other malignancies, the current approach is to get core biopsy with material adequate not just for morphology but also for additional molecular studies. Increasingly, cytology is used mainly either to confirm recurrence of cancer or to confirm the presence of malignancy in an additional site (e.g., cytological analysis of pleural fluid in a patient with biopsy confirmed lung cancer). **Fine needle aspiration (FNA)** provides a cytology specimen. Usually validated by a cytopathologist at the bedside and performed with multiple passes of a small-bore needle into a solid lesion. Tissue architecture cannot be observed.
- **Histology** rather than cytology is preferred for most malignancies and is essential for suspected lymphoma. This can be obtained by a large-core needle biopsy, excisional biopsy, or surgical resection.

TREATMENT

- **Staging and treatment planning**
  - Cancer stage is an assessment of the extent of tumor spread and treatment is based on staging.
  - Most malignancies are staged by the tumor, lymph node, and metastasis (TNM) system from stages I to IV. The T classification is based on the size and extent of local invasion. The N classification describes the extent of lymph node involvement, and the M classification is based on the presence or absence of distant metastasis.

- Appropriate radiologic staging must be performed before therapy, usually including computed tomographic (CT) imaging. Fluorodeoxyglucose-positron emission tomography (FDG-PET) adds to CT in select malignancies. Brain imaging with magnetic resonance imaging ([MRI] preferable) or CT with intravenous contrast should be considered in advanced melanoma and lung and kidney cancer. See tumor type discussion for further details.
- Complete surgical staging provides more accurate extent of the disease than clinical staging and is possible only in patients with resectable disease when surgery is performed with an intent to cure.
- Tumor grade is an assessment by the pathologist of the tumor's similarity to the cell of origin and the proliferation rate, usually low, moderate, or high grade. Tumor grade is rarely used in treatment decisions, except in certain malignancies (i.e., sarcoma).
- Once the staging workup is completed, treatment decisions are made often using a multidisciplinary approach. This process is facilitated by weekly "tumor board" conferences that enable surgeons, radiation oncologists, medical oncologists, radiologists, pathologists, and other support staff collectively plan the treatment approach. Cancer care is truly a team effort.
- Presence or absence of comorbidities and performance status guide extent of therapy. The commonly used scale for assessing performance status is the one developed by the Eastern Cooperative Oncology Group (ECOG) (Table 4).
- **Principles of radiation**
  - Collaboration with a radiation oncologist is critical for the management of most patients. Radiation planning is designed to deliver a precise dose of ionizing radiation to a tumor while sparing surrounding tissues.
  - External beam radiation is the most common modality, but brachytherapy (radioactive implants) is effective in certain settings.
  - **Curative** intent radiotherapy is used in several settings.
    - **Neoadjuvant:** Preoperative therapy intended to reduce both the extent of surgery and the risk of local relapse.
    - **Adjuvant:** Postoperative intended to reduce the risk of local relapse.
    - **Definitive:** High dose with curative intent, usually not followed by surgery.
    - **Concurrent chemoradiation:** Chemotherapy with definitive radiation significantly increases toxicity but increases efficacy in some settings.
  - **Palliative** radiotherapy is used in lower dosing to reduce symptoms, including bony pain, obstruction (esophageal, bronchial), bleeding (GI, gynecologic, bronchial, cutaneous), and neurologic symptoms (brain metastasis)
- **Principles of chemotherapy**
  - Traditional, cytotoxic chemotherapy targets all dividing cells and has broad toxicities.
  - Chemotherapy is typically given in 2-, 3-, or 4-week "cycles." In most regimens, intravenous treatment is given on the first day of the cycle, with no further treatment until the next cycle. In other regimens, treatments are weekly for 2 or 3 weeks, with 1 week off prior to the next cycle.
  - **Curative** intent chemotherapy includes neoadjuvant, adjuvant, and chemoradiation protocols in solid tumors. Chemotherapy alone is curative in many lymphomas, leukemias, and germ cell tumors (GST).
  - **Palliative** chemotherapy is used in advanced solid tumors and hematologic malignancies, with a focus on prolonging survival without overly affecting quality of life. Should only be used in patients with a good performance status.

Table 4 — Most Frequently Used Chemotherapies for Common Malignancies

Legend: ■ Most frequent ▦ Common ☐ Rare

	Gliomas	Head and neck	Lung	Breast	Esophageal/gastric	Pancreas/biliary	Colon/rectal	Kidney	Bladder	Prostate	Germ cell	Gynecologic	Sarcoma	Lymphoma	Leukemia
Platinum agents															
Cisplatin		■	■		■	▦			■		■	■	■	■	▦
Carboplatin		■	■	▦	▦				▦		▦	■		▦	
Oxaliplatin					▦		■								
Antimetabolites															
5-FU		■			■		■		■						
Capecitabine				▦	▦	▦	■								
Gemcitabine				■		■			■				▦		
Methotrexate									▦					▦	
Pemetrexed			■												
Cytarabine															■
Fludarabine															■
Alkylators															
Cyclophosphamide				■										■	▦
Ifosfamide											▦		■	▦	
Temozolamide	■														
Dacarbazine													▦	▦	
Anthracyclines															
Doxorubicin				■					▦	■		▦	■	■	
Epirubicin				▦	■									▦	
Idarubicin															■
Mitoxantrone										▦					
Microtubule agents															
Vincristine											▦			■	▦
Vinorelbine			■	▦											
Paclitaxel		■	■	■	▦							■			
Docetaxel		■	■	■	■					■		▦	▦		
Other															
Etoposide			■								■		■	▦	▦
Irinotecan					▦		■								
Topotecan			▦									■			
Bleomycin											■			■	

752

- Specific chemotherapy protocols are beyond the scope of this text. Table 5 lists the most common malignancies and the chemotherapy agents that are most frequently used in each protocol but is not all-inclusive.
- Chemotherapy toxicities are widely variable and potentially life threatening. Table 6 lists the most clinically significant toxicities for common chemotherapy agents but should not be considered all-inclusive. Toxicities are also entirely dependent on the dose and route of administration. Toxicity management is discussed at the end of this chapter.
- Most agents have a very narrow therapeutic index and dosing is based on body surface area (mg/m^2).

Surgical Management

- Goals of therapy, cure versus palliation, must guide any surgical intervention.
- Surgical resection is often performed only when there is a possibility of cure, though palliative surgery is performed to relieve discomfort (mastectomy for local control in a patient with metastatic disease) in some malignancies.
- Complete lymph node staging provides useful information for postoperative treatment planning (adjuvant therapy).
- Surgical resection of isolated metastatic sites in select patients can improve survival. Examples include solitary brain metastases, pulmonary metastases from colorectal cancer or sarcomas, and liver metastases from colorectal cancer.

OUTCOME/PROGNOSIS

- The goal of therapy (cure vs. palliation) must be clear to the patient. High-risk or highly toxic therapies are not appropriate in a noncurative setting.
- Patients diagnosed with cancer often expect to hear an estimate of life expectancy, and physicians often feel obligated to provide such estimates. However, such temporal estimates are often incorrect and unhelpful, given the variability in disease and response to treatment.
- It is more accurate and easier to describe the likelihood of surviving to a defined time point (i.e., 1-year or 5-year survival rate) rather than giving an individual a specific time frame (i.e., median survival). It is important to underscore the enormous variability in the outcomes even within a seemingly homogenous group (e.g., stage I NSCLC] due to molecular heterogeneity of cancer. It is critical to emphasize the difference between accurately describing a group statistic ("1-year survival of patients with metastatic NSCLC is around 40%") and erroneously attributing the median survival as a true measure of one's individual's life expectancy ("you have 9 months to live").

Lung Cancer

GENERAL PRINCIPLES

Epidemiology

Most common cause of cancer death in the United States (160,000 per year) and worldwide. More than 90% of cases are tobacco related. Risk remains greater even

Table 5 Most Frequent Toxicities for Common Chemotherapy Agents

Legend: ■ = Frequent/Severe ▨ = Less common/Mild (blank) = Uncommon

	Cytopenias	Nausea	Mucositis	Diarrhea	Nephrotoxicity	Cardiac	Neuropathy	Fatigue	Vesicant	Late leukemia	Hair loss	Unique toxicity
Platinum agents												
Cisplatin	▨	■			■	▨	■	■				Hearing loss, low Mg/K
Carboplatin	■	▨			▨			▨				Low Mg/K
Oxaliplatin	▨	▨					■	▨				Cold sensitivity
Antimetabolites												
5-FU	▨		▨	■		▨		▨				Hand-foot syndrome
Capecitabine				▨				▨				Hand-foot syndrome
Gemcitabine	▨							▨				TTP/HUS
Methotrexate	■	▨	■		■			▨			▨	Accumulates in effusions
Pemetrexed	▨											
Alkylators												
Cyclophosphamide	■	■	▨		▨	▨		▨			■	Hemorrhagic cystitis
Ifosfamide	■	▨	▨				■	▨			■	Encephalopathy, cystitis
Temozolamide	▨	▨						▨			▨	
Anthracyclines												
Doxorubicin	■	■				■		▨	■	▨	■	
Epirubicin	■	■				▨		▨	▨	▨	■	
Mitoxantrone	▨	▨				▨		▨	▨	▨	▨	
Microtubule agents												
Vincristine	▨	▨					■	▨	▨		■	Constipation
Vinorelbine	▨	▨					▨	▨	▨			Constipation
Paclitaxel	■	▨		▨			■	▨				
Docetaxel	■	▨	▨				■	■			▨	Nail loss, fluid retention
Other												
Etoposide	■	▨		▨				■		▨	■	
Irinotecan	■	▨		■				▨			▨	Acute hypercholinergic reaction
Topotecan	■	▨						▨			▨	
Bleomycin				▨				▨	■		▨	Pulmonary fibrosis

■ Frequent/Severe   ▨ Less common/Mild   ☐ Uncommon

Table 6	Most Frequently Used Targeted Therapies for Common Malignancies and Typical Side Effects

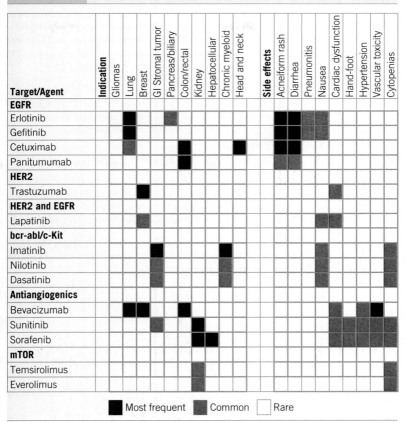

Most frequent ■ Common ▓ Rare ☐

20 to 30 years after quitting smoking. Asbestos exposure is strongly linked to mesothelioma (cancer of the pleura) and other lung cancers, particularly in smokers. High radon exposure is also risk factor.

Pathology

More than 85% of cases are of NSCLC. Most common histologic subtypes are adenocarcinoma and squamous cell carcinoma, with large cell, bronchoalveolar, and other subtypes being less common. Distinction between squamous cell and other forms of NSCLC is important for the selection of medical therapy. Small-cell (formerly "oat-cell") carcinoma is of neuroendocrine origin and is treated in a manner different from that of NSCLC.

DIAGNOSIS

Clinical Presentation

- Most common local symptoms are cough, dyspnea, postobstructive pneumonia, hemoptysis, or chest wall pain. Less common symptoms are Pancoast syndrome from superior sulcus tumors (shoulder pain, brachial plexus symptoms, and Horner's syndrome); superior vena cava compression (SVC syndrome) with face and arm plethora or swelling; or voice hoarseness from recurrent laryngeal nerve involvement. Widespread disease presents with fatigue, cachexia, bone pain, or neurologic symptoms from central nervous system (CNS) metastasis.
- **Paraneoplastic syndromes** include hypercalcemia (usually caused by squamous cell), hyponatremia, syndrome of inappropriate antidiuretic hormone secretion (usually caused by small-cell carcinoma), and hypertrophic pulmonary osteoarthropathy (clubbing, joint pain, swelling).

Diagnostic Testing

- Routine screening is not currently recommended. Any patient with a smoking history and pulmonary symptoms should have a chest CT scan. A normal chest radiograph does not exclude lung cancer. Diagnosis can be made from pleural fluid cytology, bronchoscopy with biopsy, brushings, or washings, or ultrasound/CT-guided needle biopsy. Core needle biopsy is preferable to FNA.
- **Staging evaluation:** In all patients, it should include CT scan of chest and abdomen, bone scan, brain MRI (preferred), or head CT scan. In potentially curable patients, evaluation includes PET scan and mediastinoscopy (Table 7).

TREATMENT

- **NSCLC**
  - **General:**
    - Stage I: Surgery is preferred with no further therapy; 70% chance of cure.
    - Stage II: Surgery followed by adjuvant chemotherapy; 50% chance of cure (*J Clin Oncol 2008;26:3552*).
    - Stage III: Usually concurrent radiation and chemotherapy; surgery in selected patients; <15% chance of cure.
    - Stage IV: Palliative chemotherapy, not curable; 40% of patients have 1-year survival.
  - **Chemotherapy:** In the metastatic setting, improves survival and quality of life. A combination of cisplatin or carboplatin and a second chemotherapy agent is standard for patients with a good performance status (*N Engl J Med 2002;346:92–98*).

Table 7	Simplified TNM Staging System for Lung Cancer		
Tumor	**Lymph Node Involvement**		
	None	**Hilar**	**Mediastinal**
T1–T2: <7 cm, no local invasion	I	II	III
T3: Invasive but resectable	II	III	III
T4: Usually unresectable	III	III	III
Pleural or distant spread	IV	IV	IV

Bevacizumab (an angiogenesis inhibitor) may improve survival in select patients (*N Engl J Med 2006;355:2542*). Erlotinib and gefitinb, oral inhibitors of EGFR TKI, are effective in second-line treatment (*N Engl J Med 2005;353:123*). Lung cancers with activating mutations in the *EGFR* gene are highly sensitive to these inhibitors (*N Engl J Med 2004;350:2129*). These mutations are seen most often in never-smokers.

- **Small-Cell Lung Cancer**
  - "Limited stage" (stages I to III): Concurrent chemotherapy (cisplatin and etoposide) and radiation lead to a 10% to 20% chance of cure.
  - "Extensive stage" (stage IV): Combination chemotherapy (cisplatin with etoposide or irinotecan) has very high response rate, but all patients relapse with treatment-resistant disease. One-year survival is 30% from time of diagnosis (*J Clin Oncol 2006;24:2038*).
  - Prophylactic cranial irradiation is used in select patients to prevent brain metastasis.

Breast Cancer

GENERAL PRINCIPLES

Epidemiology

Most common cause of cancer in women in developed countries. Approximately 180,000 cases per year in the United States and one-fifth as many deaths. One percent of cases are reported in men. Eleven percent of all women in the United States develop breast cancer.

Pathology

- Noninvasive: Ductal carcinoma in situ (DCIS) and lobular carcinoma in situ (LCIS).
- Invasive: Ductal carcinoma is more common than lobular carcinoma.
- Estrogen receptor (ER): Positive in 60% of cases; confers a good prognosis and sensitivity to endocrine therapies.
- Progesterone receptor (PR): Usually correlates with ER.
- HER2, measured by immunohistochemistry (IHC) or fluorescent in situ hybridization (FISH): Positive in 25% of cases; confers not only poor prognosis but also sensitivity to targeted therapies (trastuzumab, lapatinib).

Risk Factors

- Risk factors include a family history, early menarche, late menopause, late first pregnancy, obesity, and hormone replacement therapy (*N Engl J Med 2009;360:573*).
- **Genetics:** BRCA1 and BRCA2 mutations are associated with approximately 50% lifetime risk of breast cancer. BRCA1 is also associated with ovarian cancer.

Prevention

- Prophylactic mastectomy/oophorectomy is recommended for carriers of BRCA1 or BRCA2 mutations.
- Monthly self-exam starting age 20 years. Age 20 to 40 years, clinical breast exam every 3 years. Annual mammogram and clinical breast exam age 40 to 70 years.

DIAGNOSIS

Clinical Presentation

Premenopausal women: A breast mass can be observed 1 month for change.

Diagnostic Testing

Imaging
- Bilateral mammogram and subsequent biopsy for any clinically concerning mass, even with a normal mammogram.
- Chest radiograph in most patients, CT if lymph node–positive disease.

TREATMENT

- **Endocrine therapies.**
  - Tamoxifen, an estrogen antagonist, in breast cancer treatment (agonist in bone/endometrium).
  - Oophorectomy/ovarian suppression with LHRH agonists (goserelin, leuprolide) for premenopausal women.
  - Aromatase inhibitors (AIs) block androgen to estrogen conversion (letrozole, anastrozole, exemestane) in peripheral tissues for postmenopausal women.
  - Fulvestrant, an estrogen receptor antagonist, for postmenopausal women
- **Treatment of DCIS:** Lumpectomy with adjuvant radiation. Repeat resections for positive margins are often necessary. Tamoxifen if ER positive.
- **Treatment of LCIS:** Usually multifocal disease, no role for multiple resections. Prophylactic mastectomy is an option, otherwise tamoxifen is recommended.
- **Adjuvant medical therapy for resectable breast cancer**
  - Neoadjuvant chemotherapy can be used to facilitate surgery in large tumors.
  - Adjuvant endocrine therapy is recommended for ER/PR+ tumors: With tamoxifen (if premenopausal) or an AI (if postmenopausal). Treatment duration is 5 to 10 years.
  - Adjuvant chemotherapy is recommended for lymph node–positive disease, any tumor > 2 cm, tumors > 1 cm if ER/PR negative, and tumors > 0.5 cm if HER2+.
  - The most common adjuvant chemotherapy regimens in the United States are AC + T (adriamycin and cyclophosphamide, followed by paclitaxel) and TC (docetaxel and cyclophosphamide) but many regimens are excellent options.
  - Adjuvant trastuzumab (Herceptin, anti-HER2 antibody) for 1 year improves survival and is used for most HER2+ tumors (*N Eng J Med 2005;353:1673*). Trastuzumab is associated with congestive heart failure (usually reversible), and cardiac function should be monitored.
- **Treatment of metastatic breast cancer**
  - Many patients with ER/PR+ metastatic disease live for >5 years with endocrine therapy alone. The goal of therapy is to prevent symptoms/progressive disease with minimal impact on quality of life.
  - Radiation therapy is preferred for symptomatic bone or brain metastases.
  - Endocrine therapy is recommended in ER/PR+ patients except in the case of symptomatic visceral metastases. Multiple endocrine agents should be tried before chemotherapy.
  - Single agent rather than combination chemotherapy is preferred in most patients.

- Trastuzumab improves outcomes with endocrine or chemotherapy in HER2+.
- Lapatinib is an oral inhibitor of EGFR and HER2 and is used in combination with capecitabine (*N Eng J Med 2006;355:2733*).
- Bevacizumab (Avastin, anti-VEGF antibody) improves progression-free survival in combination with paclitaxel (*N Engl J Med 2008;358:1637*).

Surgical Management

- Lumpectomy (breast conservation therapy) with adjuvant radiation is equivalent to mastectomy (*N Engl J Med 1995;332:907*).
- Sentinel lymph node biopsy at the time of surgery, if the result is negative, can substitute for complete axillary lymph node dissection.

Head and Neck Cancer

GENERAL PRINCIPLES

Epidemiology

Includes squamous cell carcinoma of the lip, oral cavity, pharynx, and larynx. Approximately 35,000 diagnoses per year with 7,000 deaths. Frequently associated with tobacco and alcohol. Human papillomavirus (HPV) infection is also implicated.

DIAGNOSIS

Clinical Presentation

Oral mass/ulcer, dysphagia, voice hoarseness, or neck mass (lymph node involvement).

Diagnostic Testing

- Complete ENT evaluation with biopsy of primary lesion and laryngoscopy.
- **Staging evaluation:** Examination under anesthesia. CT of head, neck, and chest. PET in select patients.

TREATMENT

- **Stage Classification:** Stage I to II disease is resectable with no lymph node involvement. Stage III tumors are larger or have isolated lymph node involvement. Local invasion or significant lymph node involvement is stage IVa/b and distant metastasis is stage IVc.

Treatment by stage:

- Early stage (I to II): Either surgery or definitive radiation can be curative.
- Locally advanced (stage III to IVa/b): Combination of chemotherapy, extensive surgery, and/or chemoradiation.
- Metastatic (IVc): Palliative chemotherapy.
- **Supportive care:** Complete dental extraction prior to radiation therapy is often necessary; feeding tube placement is often needed.

- **Chemotherapy:** Cisplatin is used most commonly in definitive chemoradiation therapy. Taxane combinations are used neoadjuvantly to improve resectability.
- **Targeted therapy:** Cetuximab, an antibody to EGFR, can also be used with definitive radiation (*N Engl J Med 2006;354:567*).
- **Complications** of treatment can be extensive. Surgery may lead to loss of speech (laryngectomy), permanent tracheostomy, and disfigurement. Swallowing can be impaired and lead to aspiration. Radiation can lead to severe xerostomia.

Sarcoma

GENERAL PRINCIPLES

Epidemiology

Sarcomas account for approximately 12,000 diagnoses per year in the United States. These comprise a minority of adult malignancies but 7% of pediatric malignancies. Risk increases with age and is also associated with prior radiation, chemical, and chemotherapy exposures.

Etiology

Genetics: Neurofibromatosis type I is linked to neurofibrosarcoma. Li-Fraumeni syndrome (loss of p53) has a high rate of osteosarcoma and other sarcomas. Patients with Gardner's syndrome and tuberous sclerosis are also at risk. Several sarcomas have been linked to specific, acquired translocations including Ewing's sarcoma: t(11;22), synovial sarcoma: t(X;18), alveolar rhabdomyosarcoma: t(2;13), and myxoid liposarcoma: t(12;16).

Pathology

The most common sarcomas in adults are "soft tissue sarcomas," with the most common locations being in the extremities or retroperitoneum, and are treated similarly. These include malignant fibrous histiocytoma, liposarcoma, and leiomyosarcoma. Gastrointestinal stromal tumor (GIST), osteosarcoma, and Ewing's sarcoma have unique features and are treated differently.

DIAGNOSIS

Clinical Presentation

Varies according to the site of disease.

Diagnostic Testing

Imaging
- MRI for extremities or pelvis.
- CT for abdominal sites.

TREATMENT

- **Soft tissue sarcoma/osteosarcoma:** Resection followed by adjuvant chemotherapy and/or radiation for high-grade tumors. Metastatic sites should be resected if feasible.

- **GIST:** Most common site is stomach, followed by small bowel. Surgery should be performed if feasible. Most GISTs overexpress c-KIT and are highly responsive to imatinib (oral TKI). Adjuvant imatinib can be considered in select patients.
- **Ewing's sarcoma:** Treated similarly to soft tissue sarcoma but more responsive to chemotherapy. Metastatic disease may still be cured with chemotherapy.

GASTROINTESTINAL MALIGNANCIES

Esophageal Cancer

GENERAL PRINCIPLES

Epidemiology

Seventh most common and sixth most lethal malignancy worldwide. Risk factors include tobacco, alcohol, obesity, gastroesophageal reflux disease, Barrett's esophagus, achalasia, and caustic injury.

Pathology

Adenocarcinomas are most common in the lower third of the esophagus and at the gastroesophageal junction and have had a sharp increase in incidence over the past few decades in the United States. Squamous cell carcinomas more common in the upper and middle esophagus.

DIAGNOSIS

Clinical Presentation

Usually progressive dysphagia and weight loss. Other symptoms include odynophagia, cough, and hoarseness.

Diagnostic Testing

- CT of the chest and abdomen. If no metastatic disease, endoscopic ultrasound (EUS) for the definition of tumor depth and lymph node status and FDG-PET to rule out regional and distant metastases.
- Upper endoscopy with biopsy.

TREATMENT

- Early-stage disease: Usually defined as no invasion through the adventitia (T1 to T2) and no nodal or distant metastases. Patients who are medically fit should undergo esophagectomy.
- Locally advanced disease: Patient diagnosed with esophageal cancer with invasion of the adventitia (T3) or lymph node involvement are best considered for potentially curative concurrent chemoradiation, though some prefer to resect these tumors after induction therapy.
- Metastatic disease is usually treated with palliative chemotherapy.

Gastric Cancer

GENERAL PRINCIPLES

Epidemiology

Fourth most common malignancy worldwide with approximately 1 million new cases and second most lethal malignancy with 800,000 deaths estimated in 2007. Highest incidence in Eastern Asia, former Soviet Union, and South America. Risk factors include *Helicobacter pylori* infection, previous partial gastrectomy for benign ulcer, cigarette smoking, and blood group A.

Pathophysiology

More than 90% are adenocarcinomas, subdivided according to Lauren's classification into intestinal or diffuse types. Intestinal type is more common in older patients and has a better prognosis. Diffuse type is more prevalent in younger patients and women, is not associated with dietary patterns, and is the most common subtype in the United States.

DIAGNOSIS

Clinical Presentation

- Most common symptoms are decreased appetite, weight loss, and abdominal discomfort. Dysphagia may occur with gastroesophageal junction tumors and persistent vomiting if there is pyloric obstruction. Physical exam may show metastases to the left supraclavicular node (Virchow's node) or periumbilical node (Sister Mary Joseph's node).
- Diagnosis is established by upper endoscopy. CT of the chest and abdomen in all patients, and CT of the pelvis in women exclude ovarian involvement (Krukenberg tumor). Other tests include *H. pylori* testing, EUS, and PET scan. Staging laparoscopy may be indicated prior to surgery in patients with otherwise resectable tumors.

TREATMENT

Medically fit patients with resectable disease should undergo surgery. Chemotherapy or chemoradiotherapy are commonly used, either before or after the resection, except in patients with very early stage disease. Patients with unresectable disease are treated with palliative chemotherapy.

Colorectal Cancer

GENERAL PRINCIPLES

Epidemiology

Third most common malignancy worldwide, with approximately 1.1 million cases estimated for the year 2007. Incidence is higher in Western industrialized countries, with 110,000 cases per year in the United States. Risk factors include age >50 years, physical inactivity, obesity, diet with increased red meat and decreased fiber, personal history of polyps or colorectal cancer and inflammatory bowel disease, and hereditary syndromes (familial adenomatous polyposis) and hereditary nonpolyposis colorectal cancer [HNPCC]).

DIAGNOSIS

Clinical Presentation

Most common symptoms include bleeding, abdominal pain, change in bowel habits, and obstruction. Any unexplained iron deficiency anemia should be evaluated with upper and lower endoscopy to evaluate for a GI malignancy.

Diagnostic Testing

- Diagnosis is typically made through colonoscopy with biopsy.
- Imaging studies include CT scan of the chest, abdomen, and pelvis. FDG-PET scan is not routinely indicated.
- Additional studies include serum carcinoembryonic antigen (CEA) levels.

TREATMENT

- **Treatment of colon cancer**
  - **Localized disease** should be treated with surgical resection. Adjuvant chemotherapy is indicated in patients with stage III disease and may also be beneficial in selected patients with stage II disease (Table 8).
    - **Surveillance** after successful therapy includes (1) history, physical exam, and CEA levels every 3 to 6 months for 2 years and then every 6 months for 3 years; (2) CT scan for the first 3 years; and (3) colonoscopy within 1 year of resection, at 3 years, and then every 5 years.
  - **Metastatic disease** is treated with combination chemotherapy, usually including 5-FU, leucovorin, oxaliplatin (FOLFOX), or irinotecan (FOLFIRI). The combination of bevacizumab, a vascular endothelial growth factor (VEGF) monoclonal antibody, and chemotherapy improves survival compared with chemotherapy alone (*J Clin Oncol 2007;25:1539*). Cetuximab, an antibody against the EGFR, is also associated with improved outcomes if the *K-ras* gene is not mutated.
  - **Isolated liver metastases** may be treated with surgical resection, preceded or not by neoadjuvant chemotherapy, with curative intention.
- **Treatment of rectal cancer:** Patients without metastatic disease should undergo endorectal ultrasound for the evaluation of T and N status. Adjuvant or neoadjuvant therapy is indicated for patients with stage II or III disease. Concurrent neoadjuvant chemoradiation is commonly used to decrease the risk of local recurrence and

Table 8	Simplified TNM Staging System for Colorectal Cancer	
T Status	**Lymph Node Involvement**	
	None	**Present**
T1–T2: No serosal invasion	I	III
T3–T4: Local invasion	II	III
Distant metastases	IV	IV

downsize the tumor, facilitating sphincter preserving surgery (Table 8). Patients with metastatic disease should be treated similarly to those with colon cancer.

Pancreatic Cancer

GENERAL PRINCIPLES

Epidemiology

Pancreatic adenocarcinoma is the fourth most common cause of cancer death for men in the United States. Incidence increases with age, with median age at diagnosis between 60 and 80 years. Risk factors include cigarette smoking, diabetes mellitus, and inherited syndromes (*BRCA2* mutation, HNPCC).

DIAGNOSIS

Clinical Presentation

Common symptoms include jaundice, anorexia, weightloss, and abdominal pain. Pancreatic cancer should be suspected when diabetes mellitus develops suddenly in patients older than 50 years, particularly if associated with abdominal pain, anorexia, or weight loss.

Diagnostic Testing
Imaging

Diagnosis is usually suspected by the presence of a pancreatic mass or dilated biliary duct on CT scan or ultrasound. Pancreas protocol CT with thin slices is recommended to evaluate for resectability defined as absence of distant metastases, patent superior mesenteric and portal veins, and absence of celiac and superior mesenteric artery involvement.

Diagnostic Procedures
- In case of metastatic disease, biopsy of the metastatic lesion is preferred.
- Those with resectable disease may have a tissue diagnosis by ERCP or EUS-guided FNA.

TREATMENT

- **Treatment of localized disease:** Surgical resection is the only potentially curative therapy. Approximately 20% of patients are candidates for surgery, which is typically a pancreaticoduodenectomy (Whipple procedure). Patients who have adequately recovered from surgery may benefit from adjuvant chemotherapy or chemoradiotherapy. More than 80% of patients suffer relapse even with optimal therapy.
- **Treatment of unresectable disease:** Locally invasive disease may be treated with chemotherapy or chemoradiotherapy, whereas those with metastatic disease are typically treated with chemotherapy. The most frequently used chemotherapy for metastatic pancreatic carcinoma is gemcitabine, either alone or in combination with erlotinib (*J Clin Oncol 2007;25:1960*).

Hepatocellular Carcinoma

GENERAL PRINCIPLES

Epidemiology

Hepatocellular carcinoma (HCC) is the sixth most common cancer and third most common cause of cancer death. Estimated 710,000 new cases and 680,000 annually worldwide. Incidence is increasing in the United States. Risk factors include chronic viral hepatitis B or C, alcohol abuse, autoimmune hepatitis, and hemochromatosis. Approximately 80% to 90% of the patients with HCC have cirrhosis.

DIAGNOSIS

Clinical Presentation

Common symptoms include abdominal pain, anorexia with weight loss, jaundice, and vomiting. Invasion of the hepatic veins may cause Budd–Chiari syndrome, characterized by tender hepatomegaly and tense ascites. HCC should be suspected in patients with stable cirrhosis and rapid decompensation, including ascites, encephalopathy, and variceal bleeding. Most common paraneoplastic syndromes include hypoglycemia, hypercalcemia, and erythrocytosis. α-Fetoprotein (AFP) levels are increased in approximately 50% of patients in the United States.

Diagnostic Testing

- The classic feature of HCC in CT or MRI is rapid enhancement during the arterial phase of contrast administration, followed by "washout" during the later venous phases. Patients with liver lesions >2 cm, AFP level >200 ng/mL, and radiologic features suggestive of HCC on two imaging modalities may be diagnosed without biopsy. Lesions <1 cm have low probability of being HCC and should be followed with repeated imaging to detect growth suspicious of malignancy (*Hepatology 2005;42:1208*). PET scan may identify extrahepatic metastases.
- Those with lesions between 1 and 2 cm should undergo percutaneous biopsy.

TREATMENT

Other Nonoperative Therapies

- **Local therapy:** For nonsurgical candidates, local therapy, including percutaneous ethanol injection, radiofrequency ablation, cryoablation, transarterial chemoembolization, and liver radiation, may be used for palliation or to control tumor growth while waiting for transplant.
- **Chemotherapy** has minimal efficacy in HCC, with doxorubicin being the most common agent used. The small molecule TKI sorafenib is well tolerated and improves survival modestly compared to best supportive care (*N Engl J Med 2008;359:378*).

Surgical Management

The only potentially curative treatment is surgical resection, which can be considered in lesions <5 cm not involving major vessels. Liver transplant is an option for selected patients with cirrhosis since it addresses both the malignancy and the underlying disease. Indications for liver transplant include the following: (1) absence of distant metastases; (2) not a candidate for liver resection; (3) absence of major vessel involvement; (4) single tumor < 5 cm; (5) three or fewer tumors, not larger than 3 cm.

GENITOURINARY MALIGNANCIES

Renal Cancer

GENERAL PRINCIPLES

Epidemiology

Approximately 30,000 cases per year in the United States, with 12,000 deaths. More common in men (1.5:1) and increases with age. Risk factors include smoking, obesity, and hypertension. Medullary renal carcinoma is associated with sickle cell disease.

Etiology

Genetics: Vast majority of cases are sporadic. Von-Hippel Lindau syndrome (VHL) carries a high risk of clear cell renal cell carcinoma (RCC). *VHL* gene mutations increase hypoxia-inducible factor, which increases angiogenesis.

Pathology

RCC is a malignancy of the renal parenchyma. Clear cell RCC is most common (80%), followed by papillary (15%) and chromophobic (5%) RCCs. Cancer of the renal pelvis (transitional cell carcinoma [TCC]) is similar to bladder cancer.

DIAGNOSIS

Clinical Presentation

Known as "the internist's tumor" because of its multiple manifestations. Most diagnoses in the United States are incidental findings on CT scan. Most common symptoms are anemia, hematuria, cachexia, and fever. The classic triad of flank pain, hematuria, and a palpable mass is uncommon. Erythrocytosis from erythropoietin production can also be seen but is uncommon.

Diagnostic Testing
Imaging
- Cystic renal lesions (by ultrasound) require no further evaluation. CT is highly sensitive and specific for RCC.
- **Staging evaluation:** Preoperative CT for the evaluation of lymph nodes, metastatic disease, and tumor thrombus is typically sufficient. PET does not have a role.

Diagnostic Procedures
Most lesions can be resected without a biopsy.

TREATMENT

Medical treatment of RCC has changed more in the past 5 years than the treatment of any solid tumor. Cytotoxic chemotherapy is ineffective.

- **Adjuvant therapy** is not currently indicated.
- **Molecularly targeted therapy** is standard. Sunitinib and sorafenib are oral inhibitors of VEGF and other tyrosine kinases and are effective and tolerable. Metastatic disease can be controlled for >1 year and median survival is >2 years (*N Engl J Med 2007;356:115*). Bevacizumab is effective when used in combination with interferon (*Lancet 2007;22:2103*). The mTOR inhibitors temsirolimus and everolimus are also approved for RCC and are typically used in high-risk patients or after the progression of VEGF-targeted therapy (*N Engl J Med 2007;356:2271, Lancet 2008;372: 449*).
- **Immunotherapy** was standard for eligible patients prior to targeted therapies. High dose IL-2 has significant toxicities but has reported complete response rates of 5%. Interferon given subcutaneously can also lead to a response and disease control in some patients.

Surgical Management

Surgical treatment is of primary importance.

- Early disease (stage I/II, no local invasion, no lymph nodes) is treated with radical nephrectomy, or partial nephrectomy in select patients. Laparoscopic nephrectomies are increasing.
- Locally invasive tumors should be resected if possible, sometimes requiring partial liver resection or partial resection of the SVC.
- In metastatic disease, resection of the primary tumor should be considered if the overall burden of disease is low.
- Resection of isolated metastases (brain, lung, adrenal) improves survival in select patients.

Bladder Cancer

GENERAL PRINCIPLES

Epidemiology

Very common (almost 70,000 cases per year in the United States) but less frequently fatal (one-fifth as many deaths). Most are TCC, which is strongly associated with tobacco as well as benzene and other industrial chemicals. Schistosome infection is linked to squamous cell bladder cancer.

DIAGNOSIS

Clinical Presentation

Ninety percent of patients present with hematuria, often with frequency, urgency, and dysuria.

Diagnostic Testing

- Gross hematuria should be evaluated with urine culture and cytology, imaging (IVP or CT), and cystoscopy.
- **Staging:** Based primarily on findings of transurethral resection (TUR), which determines depth of invasion. Lymph node involvement is stage IV.

TREATMENT

Treatment by stage:

- **Superficial tumors** (no muscle invasion, stages 0 to I) are treated cystoscopically with TUR, often needing multiple resections and frequent cystoscopy (q3 months). Intravesical bacillus Calmette-Guérin reduces recurrence. Mitomycin-C and other intravesical chemotherapies may also be used.
- **Muscle invasive disease** (invades bladder muscle or adjacent tissue; stages II to III) is usually treated with radical cystectomy and pelvic lymph node dissection. An ileal conduit is typically created. The ureters are attached to a segment of ileum that is attached to the abdominal wall. Neoadjuvant or adjuvant chemotherapy can be used in stage III disease. Radiation, often with concurrent chemotherapy, is an alternative to surgery if resection cannot be safely performed.
- **Metastatic disease** (includes node-positive or distant disease) is highly responsive to chemotherapy but inevitably relapses if not resected. The most common regimens are gemcitabine + cisplatin, and MVAC (methotrexate, vinblastine, doxorubicin, and cisplatin).

Prostate Cancer

GENERAL PRINCIPLES

Epidemiology

The most common cancer in men in the United States, with 180,000 cases per year but only 28,000 deaths. Risk factors include black race, family history, and a high-fat/low-vegetable diet.

Prevention

Screening with annual prostate-specific antigen (PSA) and digital rectal exam (DRE) has not been definitively shown to improve survival but should be discussed with patients older than 50 years.

DIAGNOSIS

Clinical Presentation

Most common presentation in the United States is asymptomatic elevation in PSA. DRE findings of asymmetric induration or nodules are suggestive. Less common symptoms are obstructive symptoms, new onset erectile dysfunction, hematuria, or hematospermia.

Diagnostic Testing

Specific indications for biopsy are controversial. An abnormal PSA should be repeated for confirmation prior to biopsy. Biopsy should be performed if PSA is >10 ng/mL. For PSA of 4 to 10 ng/mL, biopsy will be positive in approximately 25% and is usually recommended. For PSA > 2.6 ng/mL, biopsy is recommended if PSA is increasing to 0.75 ng/mL/yr (PSA velocity). Suggestive findings on DRE should lead to biopsy.

TREATMENT

- Most important predictors of risk are pretreatment PSA, Gleason score, and clinical stage.
- Gleason score is determined by transrectal biopsy or resection on a scale of 2 to 10, with most scores being 6 to 7.
- T stage is determined by exam and ultrasound with early-stage disease (T1 to T2), defined as no extension beyond the prostate, and locally advanced disease (T3 to T4), defined as local invasion. Nodal involvement is considered stage IV.
- **Early-stage disease:** Outcomes are equivalent with radical prostatectomy, external beam radiation, or brachytherapy. Late toxicities are variable among modalities but rates of incontinence and erectile dysfunction are 10% to 20%. Robotic assisted prostatectomy reduces recovery time but does not improve outcomes. Active surveillance is a suitable option for men with low-risk disease.
- **Locally advanced disease:** Can be treated with a combination of surgical, radiation, and hormonal therapy.
- **Metastatic disease:** Is incurable but can be managed with hormonal therapy for 2 to 10 years. Medical castration with GnRH agonists (leuprolide, goserelin) is the most common first-line therapy. After progression on GnRH agonists, oral androgen receptor blockade ([ARB] bicalutamide or flutamide) is usually effective. Other hormonal treatments include discontinuation of ARB, ketoconazole, and estrogens. Chemotherapy with docetaxel improves survival in hormone refractory disease (*N Engl J Med 2004;351:1502*).

Testicular Cancer and Germ Cell Tumors

GENERAL PRINCIPLES

Epidemiology

Uncommon overall (8,000 per year in the United States), but the most common tumor in men aged 15 and 35 years. Nonseminoma is more common in younger men and seminoma more common after age 30 years. Incidence is higher in Caucasians than in others. Other risk factors are cryptorchidism and Klinefelter's syndrome.

Pathology

Fifty percent of GCT are seminoma and the remainder are nonseminomas or mixed histology. Nonseminomas include embryonal, teratoma, choriocarcinoma, and yolk sac tumor. Pure seminomas have a better prognosis.

DIAGNOSIS

Clinical Presentation

Most commonly, a painless testicular mass but can also present with testicular pain, hydrocele, or gynecomastia.

Diagnostic Testing

Laboratories

Tumor markers (AFP, β-hCG, and lactate dehydrogenase [LDH]) should be obtained. AFP is not elevated, and β-hCG is not usually elevated in pure seminoma. AFP is elevated in 50% of nonseminomas.

Imaging

- Transillumination or ultrasound can distinguish solid from cystic masses.
- Preoperative CT of the abdomen and pelvis and chest radiograph should be performed.

TREATMENT

- **Staging** is based on TNM status and serum markers. In general, disease limited to the scrotum is stage I, lymph node involvement is stage II, visceral metastases are stage III, and there is no stage IV. Risk stratification for patients requiring chemotherapy is based on histology, sites of metastasis, and tumor markers.
- Solid masses should be treated with orchiectomy.
- **Treatment by stage**
  - Stage I: Orchiectomy followed by adjuvant chemotherapy or radiation to retroperitoneal nodes results in cure in almost 100%.
  - Stages II–III: Chemotherapy with BEP (bleomycin, etoposide, and cisplatin) results in high rates of cure, particularly in seminomas. Lymph node dissection is performed for residual tumor (usually in retroperitoneal nodes). Intermediate-risk patients have an 80% cure rate with BEP and poor risk patients have a 45% chance of cure. High-dose chemotherapy with stem cell rescue (autologous stem cell transplant) is appropriate for refractory patients.

GYNECOLOGIC MALIGNANCIES

Cervical Cancer

GENERAL PRINCIPLES

Epidemiology

Second most common malignancy in woman and third most common cause of cancer death worldwide. Most common cause of cancer death in women from developing countries. Decreasing incidence and mortality in developed countries due to effective screening. Most important risk factor is persistent HPV infection, found in more than 95% of cases, usually HPV 16 and 18. Other risk factors include early onset of coitus, large number of sexual partners, history of sexually transmitted disease, and chronic immunosuppression.

Prevention

The prophylactic tetravalent vaccine against HPV 6, 11, 16, 18 (Gardasil) is currently approved for women aged 9 to 26 years. It is more effective if given before the initiation of sexual intercourse. Vaccinated women should continue routine Pap smears because the vaccine is not effective against all HPV subtypes (*N Engl J Med 2007;356: 1915*).

DIAGNOSIS

Clinical Presentation

Patients with early-stage lesions are commonly asymptomatic and diagnosed incidentally on Pap smear. More advanced disease may present with vaginal bleeding.

Diagnostic Testing

Diagnosis obtained through cervical cytology and biopsy. Cone biopsy is recommended if cervical biopsy is inadequate to define the invasiveness of the lesion.

TREATMENT

Patients with small, early-stage lesions may be treated with simple hysterectomy, whereas more advanced stage disease is treated with concurrent chemoradiotherapy or chemotherapy alone.

Endometrial Cancer

GENERAL PRINCIPLES

Epidemiology

Most common gynecologic cancer in the United States and more common in developed countries. Risk factors include obesity, exogenous estrogen (without progestin), low parity, early menarche, and late menopause.

Pathology

Two distinct subtypes are as follows:

- Type I: More common in younger woman. Associated with unopposed estrogen, endometrioid histology, and slow growth.
- Type II: More common in late postmenopause. Not related to estrogen and shows nonendometrioid histologies (serous, clear cell) and aggressive behavior.

DIAGNOSIS

Clinical Presentation

Most common presentation is postmenopausal vaginal bleeding. Any vaginal bleeding in a postmenopausal woman should be evaluated.

Diagnostic Testing

- Occasionally diagnosed by an abnormal Pap smear.
- Definitive diagnosis is made by endometrial biopsy.
- Dilatation and curettage are less commonly used.

TREATMENT

- Patients with cervical extension (stage II) may benefit from adjuvant radiotherapy and those with metastatic disease are treated with chemotherapy.
- Surgery is indicated for staging and treatment.

Ovarian Cancer

GENERAL PRINCIPLES

Epidemiology

Leading cause of gynecologic mortality in the United States. More common in developed countries. The median age for epithelial tumors is 60 years. Risk factors include family history, nulliparity, and familial syndromes (BRCA1 and BRCA2 mutations, HNPCC).

Pathology

More than 85% of the tumors are epithelial. Other types are of germ cell–sex cord-stromal origin.

DIAGNOSIS

Clinical Presentation

Usually vague symptoms including abdominal bloating, dyspepsia, anorexia, and constipation. Most cases are initially treated for gastritis or irritable bowel syndrome. More advanced stages may be associated with adnexal mass or ascites.

Diagnostic Testing

Laboratories

CA-125 is elevated in approximately 80% of patients but is not specific.

Imaging

- Ultrasound may confirm the presence of an adnexal mass.
- CT scan is used to evaluate for metastases.
- Rarely are patients diagnosed by ultrasound-guided biopsy or paracentesis.

TREATMENT

- Surgery is usually performed without prior histologic diagnosis and is necessary for tumor debulking.
- Stage I (without pelvic extension): surgery alone.
- Stage II (extension to uterus, tubes, or other pelvic tissues): surgery and adjuvant chemotherapy.
- Advanced stage (peritoneal/hepatic involvement): debulking/cytoreductive surgery and systemic chemotherapy.
- **Germ cell ovarian cancers** are rare, typically occur in younger women, and are highly curable with chemotherapy.

- **Stromal tumors** usually present in early stage and are commonly cured with resection alone.

Cancer of Unknown Primary

GENERAL PRINCIPLES

Pathology

Cancer of unknown primary may be subdivided by routine microscopy into adenocarcinoma, poorly differentiated carcinoma, squamous cell carcinomas, and undifferentiated tumors. Immunoperoxidase staining, IHC, and cytogenetic studies may help narrow the differential diagnosis.

DIAGNOSIS

Diagnostic Testing

Biopsy-proven malignant tumor whose primary site cannot be identified during pretreatment evaluation.

TREATMENT

Most patients have unfavorable disease and are treated with empiric combination chemotherapy, usually carboplatin and paclitaxel.

OUTCOME/PROGNOSIS

Favorable subsets include women with isolated axillary adenopathy, papillary serous adenocarcinoma of the peritoneal cavity, squamous cell carcinoma of the cervical or inguinal lymph nodes, and single metastatic site.

HEMATOLOGIC MALIGNANCIES

Acute Myeloid Leukemia

GENERAL PRINCIPLES

Epidemiology

Most common type of acute leukemia in adults. Median age at presentation is 65 years. Risk factors include prior exposure to chemotherapy, radiotherapy, antecedent hematologic disorder such as myelodysplastic syndrome (MDS) or myeloproliferative disorder (MPD), and congenital disorders (Down's syndrome, Fanconi's anemia).

Pathology

Current World Health Organization (WHO) classification includes the following: (1) acute myeloid leukemia (AML) with recurrent genetic abnormalities; (2) AML with multilineage dysplasia (prior MDS); (3) AML therapy related; (4) AML not otherwise categorized, which includes the FAB subtypes M0 (AML minimally differentiated),

M1 (AML without maturation), M2 (AML with maturation), M4 (acute myelomonocytic leukemia), M5 (acute monocytic leukemia), M6 (acute erythroleukemia), and M7 (acute megakaryoblastic leukemia). M3 (acute promyelocytic anemia) is usually classified as AML with recurrent genetic abnormalities due to the presence of t(15;17).

DIAGNOSIS

Clinical Presentation

Symptoms usually related to bone marrow failure, including fatigue, fever, bruising, or bleeding. Most patients present with pancytopenia and circulating blast forms. Patients with white blood cell count above 100,000/µL are at risk for leukostasis, manifested by dyspnea, chest pain, headaches, confusion, and cranial nerve palsies.

Diagnostic Testing

- Bone marrow specimens should be evaluated for cytochemistry, flow cytometry, and cytogenetics. Markers for AML include positive myeloperoxidase staining, CD33, CD13, CD41, and glycophorin A. AML is classified by cytogenetic findings into three prognostic groups: favorable, intermediate, and unfavorable.
- Diagnosis is confirmed by the presence at least 20% myeloblasts in the bone marrow aspirate.

TREATMENT

- **Remission induction:** Usually with cytarabine for 7 days and an anthracycline for 3 days (7 + 3 regimen).
- **Consolidation:** Therapy with high-dose cytarabine in patients younger than 60 years who achieved complete remission.
- **Stem cell transplant:** High-dose chemotherapy followed by donor stem cell transplant may be considered in young patients with poor cytogenetic features or antecedent hematological disorders.
- Acute promyelocytic leukemia (AML-M3) is characterized by the translocation t(15;17), disseminated intravascular coagulopathy, and increased cure rates with the use of all-trans retinoic acid.

Acute Lymphoblastic Leukemia

GENERAL PRINCIPLES

Epidemiology

Most common childhood leukemia. Median age at presentation is 35 years. Bimodal distribution with one peak at 4 to 5 years and a second gradual increase after the age of 50 years.

Pathology

Subdivided into three groups: precursor B cell, mature B cell (Burkitt's lymphoma), and T cell.

DIAGNOSIS

Clinical Presentation

Symptoms include fatigue, fever, and bleeding. Extremity joint pain may be the only manifestation in children. Leukostasis is uncommon, even with high white blood cell counts. Lymphadenopathy and splenomegaly are present in approximately 20% of cases.

Diagnostic Testing

Bone marrow aspiration with cytochemical analysis, flow cytometry, and cytogenetics.

TREATMENT

Complex and may be subdivided into induction (initial chemotherapy to achieve a complete remission), consolidation (postremission therapy to destroy clinically occult disease), and maintenance (prolonged low-dose chemotherapy to prevent relapse, given usually for 2 to 3 years). Because of the high risk of CNS, relapse prophylactic intrathecal therapy is administered during the induction and consolidation phases. Allogeneic stem cell transplant may be used at relapse or in patients with high-risk disease.

Chronic Myeloid Leukemia

GENERAL PRINCIPLES

Epidemiology

Accounts for 14% of leukemias in the United States. Median age at diagnosis is 65 years.

Pathophysiology

Characterized by the presence of the Philadelphia chromosome (Ph) or t(9;22), which results from the translocation of the *abl* gene from chromosome 9 to the *bcr* gene on chromosome 22, forming the chimeric *bcr-abl* gene.

DIAGNOSIS

Clinical Presentation

May present in any of three phases: chronic, accelerated, and blastic. Approximately 90% present in chronic phase, usually diagnosed incidentally by an abnormal blood cell count. Symptoms are usually related to splenomegaly (pain, left abdominal mass, early satiety) or anemia. Peripheral blood counts show increased white blood cell cells with all levels of granulocytic differentiation, from myeloblasts to segmented neutrophils. Transformation from chronic phase may be insidious through accelerated phase or abrupt-to-blastic phase.

Diagnostic Testing

- Made by bone marrow aspirate with cytogenetics and FISH for the bcr-abl rearrangement.
- The Philadelphia chromosome is not pathognomonic for CML, as it may also be detected in acute lymphoblastic leukemia (ALL; 15% to 30% adults) and AML (2%).

TREATMENT

Most patients are initially treated with oral imatinib, a potent inhibitor of the bcr-abl tyrosine kinase. Young patients with HLA-identical siblings or imatinib failures may benefit from stem cell transplant.

Chronic Lymphocytic Leukemia

GENERAL PRINCIPLES

Epidemiology
Most common form of leukemia in Western countries. Median age at presentation is 65 years.

DIAGNOSIS

Staging (Rai system): low-risk (lymphocytosis and adenopathy), intermediate-risk (hepatomegaly or splenomegaly), and high-risk (anemia or thrombocytopenia).

Clinical Presentation
Usually asymptomatic and diagnosed incidentally by routine blood cell counts. Symptoms may include night sweats, weight loss, lymphadenopathy, and splenomegaly. Peripheral blood typically shows absolute lymphocyte count above 5,000/μL and "smudge cells" caused by damage of the fragile lymphocytes during smear preparation. Anemia and thrombocytopenia may also be present.

Diagnostic Testing
Diagnosis is confirmed by flow cytometry showing CD5+, CD23+ cells. Identical disease to small lymphocytic lymphoma (SLL).

TREATMENT

Many patients do not require treatment. Indications for treatment include bulky disease, cytopenias, recurrent infections, rapid progression, and transformation to large cell lymphoma (Richter syndrome). Treatment options include oral alkylating agents (chlorambucil, cyclophosphamide), purine analogues (fludarabine, cladribine), and monoclonal antibodies such as rituximab (anti-CD20) and alemtuzumab (anti-CD52), either as single agents or in combination.

Hairy Cell Leukemia

GENERAL PRINCIPLES

Epidemiology
Rare disorder, most common in elderly men.

DIAGNOSIS

Characteristic "hairy" appearing leukocytes on peripheral smear. Flow cytometry is positive for CD20, CD11c, CD103, and tartrate-resistant acid phosphatase.

Clinical Presentation

Usually present with fatigue or infections related to cytopenias and splenomegaly.

TREATMENT

The standard therapy is one cycle of cladribine.

Hodgkin's Lymphoma

GENERAL PRINCIPLES

Epidemiology

Bimodal distribution with the first peak at age 25 years and second peak after the age of 50 years.

Pathology

Hodgkin's lymphoma (HL) is subdivided into nodular lymphocyte-predominant and classical HL (nodular sclerosis, lymphocyte-rich, mixed cellularity, lymphocyte depleted).

DIAGNOSIS

Clinical Presentation

Most patients present with painless lymphadenopathy in the cervical or supraclavicular region. Systemic or "B" symptoms (drenching night sweats, fever, and weight loss) are more common in advanced stages.

Diagnostic Testing

- Made with excisional biopsy showing Reed-Sternberg cells within a background of reactive inflammatory cells. FNA is insufficient. Workup includes history and physical, complete blood cell (CBC) count, chemistry, LDH, erythrocyte sedimentation rate, CT, PET, and bone marrow exam.
- **Staging:** The Ann Arbor staging system subdivides the lymphomas into four stages (Table 9).

Table 9	Ann Arbor Staging[a]
Stage	**Description**
I	Involvement of a single lymph node region (I) or single extralymphatic organ (IE)
II	Involvement of ≥2 lymph node regions in the same side of the diaphragm
III	Involvement of lymph node regions in both sides of the diaphragm
IV	Diffuse or disseminated involvement of one or more extralymphatic organs

[a]**Modifying features:** A, absence of B features; B, presence of B features; E, involvement of a single extranodal site contiguous or proximal to the involved nodal site; S, spleen involvement; X, bulky disease defined as lymph node ≥ 10 cm than one-third of mediastinum.

TREATMENT

Includes chemotherapy with ABVD (Adriamycin, bleomycin, vinblastine, dacarbazine). Radiation may be added in the early-stage or bulky disease. Relapsed disease should be treated with salvage chemotherapy. Stem cell transplant should be considered in patients younger than 70 years.

Non-Hodgkin's Lymphoma

GENERAL PRINCIPLES

Epidemiology

Fifth most common malignancy in the United States. Risk factors include immunodeficiency, autoimmune disorders, bacterial infections (*H. pylori*), viral infections (human immunodeficiency virus [HIV], Epstein-Barr virus, human herpesvirus 8, human T-cell leukemia virus-1), and previous transplant, either solid organ or stem cell.

Pathology

Broadly divided into indolent (follicular, marginal, small lymphocytic), aggressive (diffuse large cell, mantle cell, peripheral T cell, anaplastic T cell), and very aggressive (Burkitt's lymphoma, lymphoblastic) tumors.

DIAGNOSIS

- Clinical manifestations, staging, and therapy depend on the histological subtype. Essential workup includes history, physical exam, CBC count, chemistry, CT scans, and bone marrow exam. The cerebrospinal fluid (CSF) evaluation is indicated in patients with high-grade lymphomas, those with HIV-related lymphomas, and those with involvement of the epidural space, nasopharynx, and paranasal sinuses.
- **Staging:** Patients are staged by the Ann Arbor classification. Patient with aggressive lymphoma are usually stratified according to the International Prognostic Index, which uses five adverse prognostic factors: age < 60 years; Ann Arbor stage III or IV; abnormal serum LDH; two or more extranondal sites involved; and performance status ECOG 2 or higher. Five-year survival rates for patients with 0–1, 2, 3, or 4–5 risk factors are 73%, 51%, 43%, and 26%, respectively (*N Engl J Med 1993;329: 987*).

TREATMENT

- **Follicular lymphoma:**
  - Second most common NHL and most common indolent lymphoma. Patients are usually older adults with asymptomatic adenopathy and generalized involvement. Bone marrow involvement is common.
  - The cytogenetic hallmark is the t(14;18), which causes overexpression of bcl-2 and protection from apoptosis. Subdivided into three grades according to the microscopic pattern. Grades 1 (0–5 large, noncleaved cells/high-power field [hpf]) and 2 (6–15 large, noncleaved cells/hpf) usually follow an indolent course, whereas

grade 3 (>15 large, noncleaved cells/hpf) behaves as an aggressive tumor and is treated like diffuse large cell lymphoma.

- Prognosis system most commonly used is the Follicular Lymphoma International Prognostic Index, which uses five independent poor prognostic factors including age > 60 years, Ann Arbor stage III or IV, hemoglobin < 12 g/dL, less than four involved nodal areas, and abnormal serum LDH. Five-year survival for patients with 0–1, 2, or 3–5 risk factors are 90%, 77%, and 52%, respectively (*Blood 2004;104:1258*). Patients with stage I and II lesion are usually treated with radiation therapy and patients with stage III or IV lesion may be observed or treated with chemotherapy.

- **Small Lymphocytic Lymphoma (SLL)** is a different manifestation of chronic lymphocytic leukemia, diagnosed in the absence of lymphocytosis. Treatment of the two disorders is the same.

- **Marginal zone lymphoma** may be subdivided into extranodal marginal zone B-cell lymphoma of the mucosa-associated lymphoid tissue, nodal marginal zone, and splenic marginal zone. Extranodal marginal zone is the most common subtype and most commonly involves the stomach. *H. pylori* is commonly found in these patients and antibiotic therapy for early-stage results in higher rates of cure, particularly in the absence of t(11;18). Advanced stage patients are usually treated similarly to other indolent lymphomas.

- **Diffuse, large B-cell lymphoma** is the most common subtype of NHL. Stage I and II lymphomas are treated with rituximab and CHOP (cyclophosphamide, doxorubicin, vincristine, and prednisone) with or without involved field radiotherapy. Stage III and IV lymphomas are treated with chemotherapy alone. Relapsed tumors should be treated with salvage chemotherapy, followed by autologous stem cell transplant if feasible.

- **Peripheral T-cell lymphomas and anaplastic large cell lymphomas** are treated similarly to diffuse large B-cell lymphoma, with the exception that there is no role for rituximab.

- **Mantle cell lymphoma** usually presents as advanced disease in elderly patients. GI tract is frequently involved and the characteristic abnormality is t(11;14), leading to overexpression of cyclin D1. Standard chemotherapy with CHOP is suboptimal, and fit patients are commonly treated with more aggressive regimens.

- **Burkitt's lymphoma** may be subdivided into endemic (young patients, common involvement of the jaw), sporadic, and HIV-associated. The typical histological pattern of benign, clear macrophages in a background of darker malignant cells reveals the "starry sky" appearance. The characteristic feature is t(8;14) translocation, leading to overexpression of *c*-myc. Treated with very aggressive, complex chemotherapy regimens, similar to ALL.

- **Lymphoblastic lymphomas** may be of B-cell or T-cell origin, usually present with widespread disease, and are treated with complex regimens. Treated similarly to ALL.

Multiple Myeloma

GENERAL PRINCIPLES

Epidemiology

Second most frequent hematological malignancy after NHL. Median age at diagnosis is 68 years.

DIAGNOSIS

- Initial evaluation includes history, physical exam, CBC count, chemistry, β_2-microglobulin, serum protein electrophoresis, urine protein electrophoresis, bone survey, and bone marrow exam. The diagnosis is confirmed by the presence of 10% of more plasma cells in the bone marrow and monoclonal protein in the serum or urine.
- **Staging:** The International Stage System for multiple myeloma (MM) uses β_2-microglobulin (B2M) and albumin to stratify patients into three stages: stage I (B2M < 3.5 mg/dL and albumin > 3.5 g/dL), stage II (albumin < 3.5 g/dL or B2M 3.5–5.5 mg/dL), and stage III (B2M > 5.5 mg/dL). Median survival in months for stages I, II, and III are 62, 44, and 29, respectively.

Clinical Presentation

Most common presentation is bone pain. Anemia, renal failure, and hypercalcemia are also common.

TREATMENT

Treatment is usually reserved for symptomatic myeloma, including bone lesions, hypercalcemia, renal insufficiency, and anemia. Nontransplant candidates, usually elderly patients or those with significant comorbidities, are treated with melphalan and prednisone (MP). Recent studies have shown improved survival with the addition of thalidomide (MPT) or Velcade (MPV). Transplant candidates are usually treated with a combination of dexamethasone and thalidomide, or other induction regimens, followed by autologous stem cell transplant.

Principles of Stem Cell Transplant

GENERAL PRINCIPLES

- **Background:** Hematopoietic stem cell transplant (HSCT) involves the infusion of autologous (patient) or allogenic (donor) stem cells after a "conditioning" regimen of chemotherapy and/or radiation. This allows for an intensification of chemotherapy with the hope of eradicating malignancy (auto- and allotransplant), and a graft versus tumor effect (allo only). More than 40,000 HSCTs are performed each year worldwide.
- **Indications:** Transplant can be considered for patients who have progressive or residual disease that is thought to be chemoresponsive (auto) or susceptible to graft versus tumor effect (allo). MM and lymphoma are the most common indications for autotransplant, and myelodysplastic syndrome (MDS) and leukemia are the most common indications for allotransplant. Autotransplant is also used for refractory germ cell tumors.
- **Donor selection:** Appropriate allogenic donors are selected on the basis of the following:
  - HLA typing: Major histocompatibility class I and II alleles trigger immune activation. Six to 10 alleles are tested for compatibility and at least a 5 of 6 match is required.

- Blood group: ABO-incompatible transplants are feasible but complex.
- Cytomegalovirus (CMV)-negative donors are preferred for CMV-negative patients.
- **Source of stem cells:**
  - Bone marrow was historically used and is obtained under anesthesia from repeated aspirations from the iliac crest but is becoming less common.
  - Peripheral blood stem cells have become the most common product. Stem cells routinely circulate in low numbers but can be "mobilized" by granulocyte colony-stimulating factor (G-CSF) and then collected by leukopheresis. Stem cells are limited when patients have received multiple cytotoxic agents, and plerixafor (a subcutaneous CXCR4 antagonist) was recently approved to increase stem cell collection in such patients.
  - Umbilical cord blood can be used but is limited by the low volume of cord blood in each cord.

COMPLICATIONS

- **Hematopoietic:** Stem cells may fail to engraft leading to prolonged cytopenias or failure after engraftment. Prolonged requirements for platelet and red blood cell transfusion are not uncommon. ABO incompatibility may lead to acute or delayed hemolysis.
- **Graft versus host disease (GVHD):** Occurs when the donor T cells react with recipient tissues leading to acute and chronic inflammation. Most common tissues affected include skin, cornea, gut, and lungs. Acute, mild GVHD is common but acute, severe GVHD is almost uniformly fatal. Chronic GVHD leads to diarrhea, nausea, sclerodermatous type skin changes, and corneal irritation. Prophylaxis and treatment of GVHD rely on corticosteroids and a myriad of immunosuppressants.
- **Infectious:** During the immediate transplant period, patients are susceptible to infections associated with neutropenia, including overwhelming gram-negative sepsis, gram-positive infections of indwelling catheters, *Candida* infections, and herpes simplex virus (HSV) reactivation. The postengraftment period is complicated by impaired cell–mediated immunity, with susceptibility to CMV, *Pneumocystis carinii* pneumonia, and *Aspergillus* infections.

ONCOLOGIC EMERGENCIES

Febrile Neutropenia

GENERAL PRINCIPLES

Definition

Febrile neutropenia (FN) is defined as an absolute neutrophil count (ANC) of $<500/\text{mm}^3$, with a single core temperature of $>38.3°C$ or a persistent temperature (>1 hour) of $>38.0°C$.

Risk Factors

Risk of FN is proportional to the duration of neutropenia. Most solid tumor chemotherapy regimens have, if any, a brief (<5 day) duration of neutropenia. The highest risk for FN is with leukemia and transplant regimens, in which neutropenia may persist for weeks. Risk is also increased with regimens that cause mucositis (inflammation and ulceration of the oral and GI mucosa).

DIAGNOSIS

- Evaluation should include a complete physical exam, including an assessment for mucositis, of catheter sites, and of the perianal region. DRE should not be performed because of the potential risk of bacterial translocation.
- Cultures of blood and urine in all patients and stool studies and sputum cultures of symptomatic patients should be obtained.
- Chest x-ray should be performed in all patients.

TREATMENT

- Should be treated as an emergency case with immediate intravenous antibiotics to prevent life-threatening, gram-negative sepsis.
- **Antimicrobial treatment:**
  - Immediate, empiric intravenous antibiotics with coverage of gram-positive cocci and gram-negative bacilli (including *Pseudomonas aeruginosa*) must be included.
  - Empiric coverage of methicillin-resistant *Staphylococcus aureus* (MRSA) (i.e., with vancomycin) is not recommended unless patients are unstable, have active, oral mucositis, have evidence of a catheter-related infection, or had a recent infection with MRSA.
  - Antimicrobials should be modified according to the source of infection if one is identified (i.e., *Clostridium difficile*, MRSA, anaerobes, *P. carinii*).
  - Persistent fever does not warrant an empiric change in antibacterial therapy.
  - Empiric antifungal therapy should be considered if fever persists for >72 hours.
  - Gram-negative coverage should continue until ANC is $>500/mm^3$.
  - Low-risk patients (afebrile for 24 hours after antibiotics, negative culture results, and expected duration of myelosuppression for <1 week) can be treated as outpatients with oral, broad-spectrum antibiotics such as fluoroquinolone, amoxicillin/clavulanic acid, or trimethoprim-sulfamethoxazole.

SPECIAL CONSIDERATIONS

- Patients should be kept in reverse isolation.
- Consuming raw fruits and vegetables had been discouraged in the past but more recently has been found not to lead to excessive risk.
- **White cell growth factors (G-CSF, GM-CSF)**
  - These may reduce the duration of hospitalization for FN but do not improve survival. G-CSF is the most commonly used agent, given subcutaneously in doses of 5 mg/kg/d.
  - CSFs should not be given <24 hours after chemotherapy or during radiation because of the potential for increased myelosuppression.
  - Prophylactic G-CSF is used in the curative setting to (1) prevent FN when the risk is $>15\%$ and (2) reduce the duration of neutropenia to prevent chemotherapy delays.

- Use of G-CSF for FN prophylaxis in the palliative setting is controversial since chemotherapy regimens with high rates of FN are usually not appropriate.

Tumor Lysis Syndrome

GENERAL PRINCIPLES

- Group of metabolic disturbances resulting from significant tumor breakdown with release of intracellular products into the circulation.
- Tumor lysis syndrome (TLS) occurs only in tumors that are rapidly growing and sensitive to chemotherapy. Highest incidence in acute leukemias and high-grade lymphomas.
- Risk is increased in cases of bulky tumors, high leukocyte counts, elevated pretreatment levels of LDH or uric acid, and compromised renal function.

DIAGNOSIS

Manifestations can be divided into laboratory and clinical (Table 10) (*Br J Hematology 2004;127:3*).

TREATMENT

- The most important intervention to prevent TLS is aggressive hydration, using, whenever possible, 3 L/m^2/d to maintain the urine output of at least 100 mL/m^2/hr. The addition of bicarbonate to intravenous fluids for urine alkalinization remains controversial.
- Hyperuricemia is usually treated with the xanthine oxidase inhibitor allopurinol. Rasburicase is a recombinant urate oxidase enzyme that degrades uric acid. Rasburicase is indicated in patients with elevated uric acid prior to treatment and those at high risk for developing hyperuricemia such as elevated white blood cell levels, acute leukemias, high-grade lymphomas, and high LDH levels.
- Hyperkalemia is the main immediate threat and should be treated aggressively. Calcium administration should be restricted in patients with symptomatic hypocalcemia or in the treatment of symptomatic hyperkalemia, since it may cause metastatic calcifications in patients with hyperphosphatemia. Hyperphosphatemia should be treated with phosphate binders such as aluminum hydroxide.

Table 10	Classification of Tumor Lysis Syndrome
Manifestation	Features
Laboratory	1. Uric acid ≥ 8 mg/dL or 25% increase from baseline
	2. Potassium ≥ 6 mEq/dL or 25% increase from baseline
	3. Phosphorus ≥ 6.5 mg/dL or 25% increase from baseline
	4. Calcium ≤ 7 mg/dL or 25% decrease from baseline
Clinical	1. Creatinine ≥ 1.5 upper normal limit
	2. Cardiac arrhythmia or sudden death
	3. Seizure

Malignant Hypercalcemia

GENERAL PRINCIPLES

- Most common paraneoplastic syndrome, occurring in 10% to 20% of patients with cancer.
- Usually caused by squamous cell lung cancer, breast cancer, MM, and lymphoma.
- The three main mechanisms include focal bone destruction, humoral hypercalcemia due to the production of PTH-related protein (PTH-rP), and tumor production of vitamin D analogues.

DIAGNOSIS

Classic symptoms usually develop with total calcium levels above 12 mg/dL and include polyuria, polydipsia, anorexia, constipation, nausea, vomiting, and confusion. Patients usually have severe hypovolemia due to excessive fluid losses and limited intake.

TREATMENT

The most important treatment consists of aggressive fluid replacement with normal saline. Diuretics should not be used unless volume overload is present. Intravenous bisphosphonates, which inhibit bone resorption by osteoclasts, may also be used. The two agents of choice are pamidronate 90 mg and zoledronic acid 4 mg. Refractory cases may be treated with calcitonin. Hypercalcemia caused by tumor production of vitamin D analogues may respond to corticosteroids.

Malignant Spinal Cord Compression

GENERAL PRINCIPLES

- Common problem affecting approximately 5% to 10% of patients with cancer.
- Most common primary tumors are those of lung, breast, prostate, and lymphoma. When malignant spinal cord compression (MSCC) occurs in patients without a history of previous malignancy, the most common causes are lung cancer, lymphoma, and myeloma.

DIAGNOSIS

The study of choice for MSCC is MRI of the entire spine. Plain radiography may also be helpful when there are delays in obtaining the MRI, since approximately 80% of the patients with MSCC have abnormal radiographic findings.

Clinical Presentation

The majority of patients present with back pain and tenderness to palpation in the involved vertebral body. The pain is usually worsened by recumbent position, sneezing, coughing, and Valsalva maneuver. Other symptoms include motor weakness, sensory loss, and dysfunction of the bladder and bowel.

TREATMENT

- Patients with suspicion for MSCC should be treated immediately with glucocorticoids. If there is a delay in obtaining imaging, treatment should begin even before the diagnostic test. The most commonly used corticosteroid regimen is dexamethasone in a 10- to 16-mg loading dose, followed by 4 mg every 4 hours. Higher doses, up to 100 mg, may be associated with slightly better pain control but are associated with increased toxicity and unclear effect on neurologic recovery.
- External-beam radiation therapy is the mainstay of treatment and should begin as soon as the diagnosis is made. The role for surgery remains controversial, but it may be useful for selected patients with bone compression, previous radiation therapy, radioresistant tumors, neurologic progression during or shortly after the radiation, and single site of compression (*J Clin Oncol 2005;23:2028*). Patients with very chemosensitive tumors may be treated with systemic chemotherapy alone.

Brain Metastases with Increased Intracranial Pressure

GENERAL PRINCIPLES

- Brain metastases are common in patients with malignancies, with yearly incidence estimated between 90,000 and 170,000 cases. Many patients are asymptomatic and remain undiagnosed until the autopsy.
- Most common causes are lung cancer, breast cancer, and melanoma.
- Most lesions are supratentorial and located at gray–white matter junction, where the change in blood vessel size acts as a trap for emboli.

DIAGNOSIS

Clinical Presentation

Most patients have known cancer, and approximately one-third remain asymptomatic despite the brain metastases. The most common symptoms include headaches, confusion, and focal weakness.

Diagnostic Testing

Brain metastasis should be suspected in patients with cancer who develop neurologic symptoms and is confirmed by brain imaging with either CT scan with intravenous contrast or MRI.

TREATMENT

- Untreated patients usually die because of increasing peritumoral edema causing increased intracranial pressure and cerebral herniation.
- Symptomatic treatment with dexamethasone at the initial dose of 16 mg, followed by 4 mg every 6 hours, usually relieves symptoms.
- Whole-brain radiation is the treatment of choice for patients with multiple lesions. Chemotherapy may have a role in sensitive tumors, particularly in previously radiated patients.
- Anticonvulsants are indicated only in patients with seizures, with no benefit as prophylaxis.

- Selected patients with a solitary lesion in an accessible site and a controlled primary tumor may undergo surgery with curative intent. Stereotactic radiosurgery may also be used in similar patients.

Superior Vena Cava Syndrome

DIAGNOSIS

Typically diagnosed by history and physical with careful evaluation for airway compression. Venous thrombosis should be ruled out, using CT with intravenous contrast.

Clinical Presentation

It is most commonly associated with primary lung tumors and less commonly with lymphoma, germ cell tumors, or other mediastinal masses. Presents as facial and upper extremity erythema, swelling, and venous engorgement. Severe cases are associated with headache and confusion. Most commonly a subacute rather than emergent presentation.

TREATMENT

Empiric corticosteroids can reduce swelling and temporarily reduce symptoms. Urgent initiation of radiotherapy is usually indicated for most solid tumors. Chemotherapy is preferable for lymphomas, germ cell tumors, or small cell lung cancer.

MANAGEMENT OF TREATMENT TOXICITIES

Nausea

GENERAL PRINCIPLES

- Historically, nausea was one of the most debilitating side effects of chemotherapy, but with improved antiemetics and newer chemotherapy agents, nausea is less burdensome for patients.
- Incidence of chemotherapy-induced nausea and vomiting (CINV) is widely variable among chemotherapy agents and is dosed dependent. (See Table 6 for a general summary.) With aggressive antiemetics, vomiting is very uncommon for the great majority of chemotherapy regimens.
- CINV is divided into acute (<24 hours) and delayed (>24 hours). Acute CINV is the most important predictor of delayed CINV.

Prevention

Prevention is by far more effective than treatment when it occurs.

- Dexamethasone is an active antiemetic and is frequently given intravenously prior to chemotherapy and often continued orally for 2 to 3 days.
- 5HT3 receptor antagonists (ondansetron, granisetron, dolasetron, palonosetron, etc.) are widely used chemotherapy premedications as CINV prophylaxis and are highly effective.
- Aprepitant is a newer agent that is indicated only with regimens with high rates of CINV.

TREATMENT

- Posttreatment nausea should not be immediately assumed to be secondary to chemotherapy, particularly since many agents lead to little or no nausea (Table 6). Secondary causes, including bowel obstruction, brain metastasis with cerebral edema, constipation, narcotics, and gastroenteritis, should all be considered.
- Initial treatment with prochlorperazine is often effective. Lorazepam or other anxiolytics have antiemetic properties. 5HT3 antagonists are less effective in treatment than in prevention but are frequently used. Olanzapine has also been studied and found to be active.

Diarrhea

GENERAL PRINCIPLES

Diarrhea is a common side effect of many chemotherapies (irinotecan, 5-FU, capecitabine) and targeted agents (erlotinib, cetuximab, sunitinib).

TREATMENT

- Empiric and aggressive treatment with loperamide is essential for avoiding volume depletion, particularly with irinotecan.
- When loperamide is ineffective, diphenoxylate, atropine ("Lomotil"), or other agents can be used.

Cytopenias

GENERAL PRINCIPLES

- **Neutropenia** management and prevention are discussed in the previous text with febrile neutropenia.
- **Anemia** is common with many chemotherapy regimens.
  - Evaluation for iron deficiency (ferritin, serum Fe, and total iron-binding capacity) should take place in all patients. Hemolysis or blood loss should be considered if anemia is acute.
  - Red blood cell transfusion should be avoided unless hemoglobin is <8 g/dL or <10 g/dL with cardiac disease or symptoms.
  - Erythropoietin analogues (erythropoietin, darbepoetin) reduce the rate of blood transfusions but should not be used in the absence of significant anemia (<10 mg/dL) and are best reserved for use in patients with incurable malignancies, as there are some concerns that these agents are associated with increased mortality from disease progression and/or thromboembolism.
  - Intravenous iron supplementation may further reduce the need for transfusion and can be considered in patients with a serum ferritin level of <100 ng/mL.
- **Thrombocytopenia** is common with many regimens but no preventative agents are currently available. Chemotherapy may need to be held or dose reduced for platelet counts <50,000. Patients with hematologic malignancies, particularly after stem cell transplant, may have prolonged thrombocytopenia and require platelet transfusions to keep platelet counts >5,000 or to treat bleeding.

Mucositis

GENERAL PRINCIPLES

Mucositis (inflammation and ulceration of the oral and GI mucosa) is common with many chemotherapy regimens and is worst with chemoradiation and stem cell transplant regimens.

Prevention

Oral saline or bicarbonate rinses are minimally effective.

DIAGNOSIS

- Presents as oral pain/ulcers, odynophagia/dysphagia, abdominal pain, or diarrhea.
- HSV stomatitis should be ruled out in immunocompromised patients.

TREATMENT

Viscous lidocaine for oral or esophageal pain, with oral or intravenous narcotics for refractory pain. Acid suppression may improve abdominal pain, and antimotility agents should be used aggressively for diarrhea.

Pneumonitis

GENERAL PRINCIPLES

Definition

Pneumonitis is an uncommon but potentially life-threatening complication of thoracic radiation, EGFR-targeted therapies, and bleomycin.

DIAGNOSIS

New cough, shortness of breath, or hypoxia in susceptible patients should be evaluated with a chest radiograph and CT if there is any suspicion for pneumonitis.

TREATMENT

Treatment with corticosteroids (prednisone 50 mg/d) usually improves symptoms but chronic fibrosis may develop.

SUPPORTIVE CARE: COMPLICATIONS OF CANCER

Cancer Pain

GENERAL PRINCIPLES

- Pain is one of the most common manifestations in cancer, with an estimated incidence of 25% at diagnosis and at least 75% in advanced stages.

- The two main mechanisms for pain are nociceptive (somatic or visceral) and neuropathic. Nociceptive pain is caused by stimulation of pain receptors and neuropathic pain by direct injury to the peripheral or central nervous system. Somatic pain typically occurs in bone metastases, musculoskeletal inflammation, or after surgery and is characterized by a well-localized, dull or aching pain. Visceral pain results from tumor infiltration and compression or distention of viscera and is described as diffuse, deep, squeezing, and pressure-like sensation. Neuropathic pain occurs due to tumor infiltration of peripheral nerves, plexi, roots, or spinal cord, as well as chemical injury caused by chemotherapy, radiotherapy, or surgery. This pain is described as sharp or burning sensation. These three types of pain may occur alone or in combination in the same patient.
- Cancer pain in adults may be classified into three levels on the basis of a 0 to 10 numerical scale: mild pain (1 to 3), moderate pain (4 to 6), and severe pain (7 to 10).

TREATMENT

- The treatment is usually based on the WHO ladder, with a stepwise approach according to the level of pain. Patients with mild pain and not taking opioids may be treated with nonopioid analgesics including nonsteroidal anti-inflammatory drugs (NSAIDs) or acetaminophen (step 1). Patients with no response to nonopioids or moderate pain are treated with weak opioids such as codeine, hydrocodone, and oxycodone, alone or in combination with acetaminophen (step 2). Severe pain is treated with morphine, hydromorphone, methadone, or transdermal fentanyl (step 3). Tramadol, which has weak affinity to μ-opioid receptors and is considered a nonopioid medicine, may be used in patients with mild to moderate pain not responding to NSAIDs and who wish to defer opioid treatment. The oral route is usually the most appropriate route because of easier administration and lower costs.
- Patients with mild pain may be reevaluated at the next appointment, whereas those with moderate or severe pain should be reevaluated within 24 to 48 hours. Dose titration should be done aggressively to expedite symptom relief.
- Coanalgesics should be considered in specific cases. Systemic corticosteroids may be useful in pain caused by bone metastases, increased cranial pressure, spinal cord compression, and nerve compression or infiltration. Tricyclic antidepressants, such as nortriptyline, and anticonvulsants, such as gabapentin, are commonly indicated in neuropathic pain, which is usually less responsive to opioids. Bisphosphonates (zoledronic acid and pamidronate) and radiolabeled agents (strontium-89 and samarium-153) may help treat pain resulting from bone metastases.
- Common side effects of opioid therapy include constipation, nausea, respiratory depression, and sedation.
  - Constipation should be prevented with the prophylactic use of combined stimulant laxative and stool softener (senna + docusate). If symptoms persists, patients may benefit from the addition of a third agent, including lactulose, magnesium citrate, or polyethylene glycol, or enema.
  - Nausea may develop during the treatment and should be aggressively treated. Respiratory depression may occur with short-acting agents, but patients usually develop tolerance to repeated administration.
  - Sedation and drowsiness may be treated by decreasing the individual dose or by increasing the frequency of administration or changing to an agent with shorter half-life.

- Patients who experience inadequate pain control despite aggressive opioid therapy or who cannot tolerate opioid titration due to side effects may benefit from interventional therapies including regional infusion of analgesics and neuroablative or neurostimulatory procedures.

Bone Metastasis

GENERAL PRINCIPLES

Most common in prostate, breast, lung, kidney, and bladder cancers and MM.

DIAGNOSIS

Bone scan (nuclear imaging with technetium-99m) is sensitive for blastic lesions and but will not detect lytic lesions (i.e., MM). Concerning lesions on bone scan should be evaluated with plain x-ray films or CT to identify lesions at risk for pathologic fracture.

TREATMENT

- Pain should be managed aggressively with opioids. NSAIDS may give additional relief.
- Lesions at risk for fracture should be treated with radiation therapy. Bisphosphonates may reduce the risk for fracture and reduce pain.

Pleural Effusion

GENERAL PRINCIPLES

Pleural effusions are common in primary lung cancer and mesothelioma, as well as in advanced breast cancer and lymphoma. Effusions may be malignant (positive fluid cytology or pleural biopsy) or paramalignant (caused by indirect tumor effects). This distinction is critical in lung cancer since patients with malignant effusions are not considered for potentially curative therapies (classified as stage IV disease).

DIAGNOSIS

Discussed in detail in Chapter 7, Pulmonary Diseases, but, briefly, routine thoracentesis with cytologic evaluation is typically adequate. However, effusions with negative cytology should be further evaluated with thoracoscopy or open pleural biopsy.

TREATMENT

- Prompt and complete drainage by therapeutic thoracentesis is necessary to avoid chronic fibrosis and trapped lung. Observation for rate of reaccumulation after initial drainage is appropriate for most patients. Rapidly reaccumulating effusions (<1 month) should be treated aggressively.
- Pleurodesis (obliteration of the pleural space by fibrosis) by complete drainage and instillation of a sclerosant (usually talc) will prevent recurrence of most malignant

effusions. Requires hospitalization and chest tube placement and causes significant temporary pain.

- Placement of an indwelling pleural catheter for intermittent outpatient drainage is an alternative. Pleural fibrosis and resolution of the effusion occurs over several weeks in most patients.
- Medical therapy may be sufficient in breast cancer or lymphoma but is otherwise ineffective.
- Radiation of the pleural space is not feasible, but treatment of central masses will often alleviate paramalignant effusions.

Venous Thromboembolism

GENERAL PRINCIPLES

Any malignancy is a hypercoagulable state, which manifests as a spectrum of diseases from migratory superficial thrombophlebitis (Trousseau's syndrome) to life-threatening venous thromboembolism (VTE). VTE is most frequent in hematologic malignancies and adenocarcinomas of the lung and GI tract.

Prevention

Empiric prevention with warfarin, unfractionated heparin, or low-molecular-weight heparins (LMWH) is not recommended in patients without known VTE.

TREATMENT

- Anticoagulant treatment in patients with cancer is associated with more recurrent VTE and bleeding complications than in patients without cancer.
- Treatment with LMWH is superior to warfarin in patients with cancer (recurrent VTE in 8% vs. 16%) with no difference in bleeding, but cost and daily injections are prohibitive for many patients. Dalteparin is approved for this indication in the United States (*N Engl J Med 2003;349:146*).
- Treatment with warfarin is complicated by more frequent treatment failures, as well as varying oral intake due to anorexia and chemotherapy, and requires vigilant INR monitoring.
- Treatment should continue indefinitely or until the malignancy resolves.

Fatigue

GENERAL PRINCIPLES

- Common symptom in cancer, occurring in an estimated 80% of patients with advanced disease.
- Underlying depression should be managed appropriately, including antidepressants when indicated.

TREATMENT

First step in the treatment is the identification of treatable contributing factors such as pain, poor nutrition, emotional distress, sleep disturbance, activity level, and comorbidities (anemia, infection, organ dysfunction). Pain management, nutrition support, sleep therapy, exercise, and optimization therapy for comorbidities may improve the fatigue symptoms.

Medications

- Erythropoietin may be helpful in patients with anemia.
- Methylphenidate may provide rapid improvement and dose escalations may be required over time to maintain benefit.
- Modanafil improves fatigue in multiple sclerosis and may be useful in cancer patients.

Anorexia and Cachexia

GENERAL PRINCIPLES

- Anorexia is defined as loss of appetite in cancer patients with associated weight loss.
- Cachexia is a metabolic syndrome characterized by profound involuntary weight loss.

TREATMENT

- In addition to caloric supplementation, patients may benefit from pharmacologic therapy.
- Megestrol acetate is active, with symptomatic improvement in <1 week. Despite the quick increase in the appetite, it may take several weeks to achieve weight gain. Megestrol is also associated with an increased risk of thromboembolism.
- Dexamethasone provides a short-lived improvement, usually without significant weight gain.
- Dronabinol has limited benefits in anorexia and is associated with sedation.

20 Diabetes Mellitus and Related Disorders

Janet B. McGill

Diabetes Mellitus

GENERAL PRINCIPLES

- **Diabetes mellitus (DM)** is a group of metabolic diseases characterized by hyperglycemia resulting from defects in insulin secretion, insulin action, or both.
- DM is present in 10.7% of the U.S. adult population older than 20 years, but 17% of affected persons are not diagnosed. The prevalence increases to 23.1% of persons older than 60 years. Type 2 diabetes (T2DM) represents 90% to 95% of all cases of diabetes, with type 1 diabetes (T1DM) and other causes representing the remaining 5% to 10% (see http://www.cdc.gov/diabetes/pubs).
- Persons with diabetes are at risk for microvascular complications, including retinopathy, nephropathy, and neuropathy, and are at increased risk for macrovascular disease.
- T2DM is accompanied by hypertension in about 75% and hyperlipidemia in more than half of adult patients and is considered a "cardiac risk equivalent" because of the excess risk for macrovascular disease, cardiovascular disease (CV) events, and mortality (*Diabetes Care 2010;33(Suppl 1):S11–S61*).

Classification

DM is classified into four clinical classes (*Diabetes Care 2010;33(Suppl 1):S62–S67*).

- T1DM accounts for <10% of all cases of DM and results from a cellular-mediated autoimmune destruction of the beta (β) cells of the pancreas.
  - The rate of destruction of β cells is rapid in infants and children and slower in adults. Thus, the presentation in young people is often ketoacidosis, whereas older persons may have a longer symptomatic prodrome and may be diagnosed on the basis of hyperglycemia and positive autoantibodies.
  - T1DM is characterized by severe insulin deficiency. Exogenous insulin is required to control blood glucose (BG) level, prevent diabetic ketoacidosis (DKA), and preserve life. When insulin is withheld from a person with T1DM, ketosis will develop in 8 to 16 hours and ketoacidosis in 12 to 24 hours.
  - Early in the course of T1DM, some insulin secretory capacity remains and the insulin requirement may be lower than expected (0.3 to 0.4 units/kg). Tight control of BG level from the onset has been shown to preserve the residual β-cell function and prevent or delay later complications.
  - Latent autoimmune diabetes in adults (LADA) is characterized by mild to moderate hyperglycemia at presentation that often responds to noninsulin therapies but progresses over months to years to insulin dependency. Adults with LADA will have one or more autoantibodies and tend to require insulin therapy sooner than patients with T2DM.

- T2DM accounts for >90% of all cases of diabetes. T2DM is characterized by insulin resistance followed by reduced insulin secretion from β cells that are unable to compensate for the increased insulin requirements.
  - T2DM is usually a disease of adults, with both incidence and prevalence increasing at older ages. T2DM is no longer uncommon in children and adolescents, accounting for up to one-third of new cases of diabetes diagnosed over the age of 5 years.
  - T2DM is associated with obesity, family history of diabetes, history of gestational diabetes or prediabetes, hypertension, physical inactivity, and race/ethnicity. African Americans, Latinos, Asian Indians, Native Americans, Pacific Islanders, and some groups of Asians have a greater risk of developing T2DM than do Caucasians.
  - T2DM may be asymptomatic and therefore remain undiagnosed in a large number of affected individuals.
  - Insulin secretion is usually sufficient to prevent ketosis, but DKA or hyperosmolar nonketotic coma can develop during severe stress. Some persons with T2DM can present with or later develop DKA but have adequate insulin reserves to be treated with noninsulin therapies after resolution of the acute event.
- **Other specific types of DM** include those that result from genetic defects in insulin secretion or action, pancreatic surgery or disease, endocrinopathies (e.g., Cushing syndrome, acromegaly), drugs, and diabetes associated with other syndromes.
- **Gestational DM** (GDM) is defined as any degree of glucose intolerance, with onset or diagnosis during pregnancy. About 60% of affected women will develop T2DM in the ensuing 5 to 10 years and all remain at an increased risk for the development of T2DM later in life.
  - All patients with GDM should undergo diagnostic testing 6 to 12 weeks postpartum to determine whether abnormal carbohydrate metabolism has persisted and annually thereafter.
  - Weight loss and resumption of exercise are encouraged to decrease the risk of persistent prediabetes or T2DM after delivery.

DIAGNOSIS

- **The diagnosis of DM** can be established using any of the following criteria:
  - **A_{1C} ≥6.5%** using a NGSP certified method
  - **Plasma glucose ≥126 mg/dL** (7.0 mmol/L) after an overnight fast. A positive value should be confirmed with a repeat test.
  - **Symptoms of diabetes** (polyuria, polydipsia fatigue, weight loss) and a random plasma glucose level of ≥200 mg/dL (11.1 mmol/L).
  - **Oral glucose tolerance test** (OGTT) that shows a plasma glucose level of ≥200 mg/dL (11.1 mmol/L) at 2 hours after ingestion of 75 g of glucose.
- **Categories of increased risk for diabetes. Impaired fasting glucose (IFG) and impaired glucose tolerance (IGT)** refer to intermediate states between normal glucose tolerance and T2DM. IFG and IGT are risk factors for T2DM and micro- and macrovascular complications.
  - **IFG** is defined by fasting plasma glucose between 100 and 125 mg/dL.
  - **IGT** is defined by a 2-hour glucose value of 140 to 199 mg/dL after ingesting 75 g of glucose during an OGTT.
  - Progression from IFG or IGT to T2DM occurs at the rate of 2% to 22% (average, about 12%) per year depending on the population studied.
  - Lifestyle modification, including a balanced hypocaloric diet and regular exercise, is recommended for persons with IFG or IGT to prevent progression to T2DM

(*Diabetes Care 2010;33(Suppl 1):S11–S61*). Metformin, thiazolidinediones (TZDs), acarbose, and orlistat have been shown to delay progression to T2DM; however, FDA approval for the use of drugs to prevent diabetes is lacking. Metformin is recommended for persons at highest risk for progression, defined as those with other risk factors for CV disease and/or both IFG and IGT.

TREATMENT

Principles of Management of DM

- **Goals of therapy** are alleviation of symptoms, achievement of glycemic, blood pressure, and lipid targets, and prevention of acute and chronic complications of diabetes.
  - Glycemic control recommendations are the same for type 1 and type 2 diabetes: Fasting and preprandial capillary BG values of 70 to 130 mg/dL (3.9 to 7.2 mmol/L), postprandial capillary BG values of <180 mg/dL (<10 mmol/L), and A_{1C} of <7% or as close to normal as possible while avoiding significant hypoglycemia (*Diabetes Care 2009;32(Suppl 1):S1–S98*). This degree of glycemic control has been associated with the lowest risk for microvascular complications in patients with T1DM (*N Engl J Med 1993;329:978–986*) as well as T2DM (*Lancet 1998; 352:837–853*).
  - The blood pressure target for patients with diabetes is <130/80 mm Hg; and the use of either an angiotensin-converting enzyme (ACE) inhibitor or an angiotensin receptor blocker (ARB) is recommended as first-line therapy. For those patients not at goal, a thiazide diuretic should be added if the glomerular filtration rate (GFR) is >30 mL/min/1.73 m^2 and a loop diuretic if the GFR is <30 mL/min/1.73 m^2.
  - The lipid targets are as follows: low-density lipoprotein (LDL) < 100 mg/dL, total cholesterol < 150 mg/dL, and high-density lipoprotein (HDL) > 40 mg/dL in men and >50 mg/dL in women. In patients with known CV disease or two risk factors in addition to DM, the LDL should be <70 mg/dL, preferably using high-dose statin therapy.
  - Aspirin therapy should be advised in patients with diabetes and older than 40 years or who have other risk factors. Low doses (75–162 mg) are appropriate for primary prevention.
- **Assessment of glycemic control** consists of the following:
  - **Self-monitoring of blood glucose (SMBG)** is recommended for all patients who take insulin and provides useful information for those on noninsulin therapies. Patients using multiple daily injections or insulin pumps should test three or more times daily. Less frequent testing may be appropriate for those on noninsulin therapies. While most SMBG is done before meals and at bedtime, periodic testing 1 to 2 hours after eating may be necessary to achieve postprandial glucose targets.
  - **Continuous glucose monitoring (CGM)** has been shown to reduce A_{1C} in adults older than 25 years on intensive insulin therapy. CGM measures interstitial glucose, which provides a close approximation of BG values. Hypoglycemia and hyperglycemia alarms may help patients with widely fluctuating BG levels or hypoglycemia unawareness.
  - **A_{1C}** (also known as A_{1C}, hemoglobin A_{1C} or A_{1C}) provides an integrated measure of BG values over the preceding 2 to 3 months. A_{1C} should be obtained every 3 months in patients not at goal or when either diabetes therapy or clinical condition changes. It can be tested twice yearly in well-controlled patients. A_{1C} should confirm

results of SMBG, and discordant values should be investigated. An A_{1C} level that is higher than expected should be evaluated by a diabetes educator to ensure meter accuracy, appropriate technique, and frequency of testing. When the A_{1C} is lower than expected, blood loss, transfusion, hemolysis, and hemoglobin variants should be considered. The correlation between A_{1C} and mean plasma glucose is sufficiently strong that laboratory reports may include both the A_{1C} result and the estimated average glucose.

- **Ketones** can be detected in a fingerstick blood sample by measuring β-hydroxybutyrate with the handheld glucose/ketone meter, Precision Xtra. Urine ketones can be qualitatively identified, using Ketostix or Acetest tablets. Patients with T1DM should test for ketones, using one of these methods during febrile illness or persistent elevated glucose (>300 mg/dL) or if signs of impending DKA (e.g., nausea, vomiting, abdominal pain) develop. Testing for β-hydroxybutyrate is useful in emergency departments to determine whether a patient with hyperglycemia has ketonemia (*Acad Emerg Med 2006;13(6):683–685*). Hospital laboratories measure serum ketones including acetone, acetoacetate, and β-hydroxybutyrate.

Medications

Medications for diabetes are more effective when instituted as part of a comprehensive management approach that includes instruction in management principles, diet, and exercise.

Diet

- **Medical nutrition therapy** includes dietary recommendations for a healthy, balanced diet to achieve adequate nutrition and maintain an ideal body weight.
- Caloric restriction is recommended for overweight individuals, with individualized targets that may be as low as 1,000 to 1,500 kcal/d for women and 1,200 to 1,800 kcal/d for men depending on activity level and starting body weight.
- Caloric intake is usually distributed as follows: 45% to 65% of total calories as carbohydrates, 10% to 30% as protein, and $<30\%$ as total fat ($<7\%$ saturated fat) with <300 mg/d of cholesterol.
- In patients with LDL cholesterol >100 mg/dL, total fat should be restricted to $<25\%$ of total calories, saturated fat to $<7\%$, and <200 mg/d of cholesterol.
- Patients with progressive kidney disease may benefit from restriction of protein intake to 0.8 g/kg/d. Patients with severe chronic kidney disease (CKD) will need additional restrictions of potassium- and phosphorus-containing foods.
- "Carbohydrate counting" is useful skill for patients on intensified insulin therapy who adjust insulin doses based on carbohydrate intake at each meal and snack. Of note, 1 carbohydrate "exchange" is 15 g and 60 kcal.

Activity

Exercise improves insulin sensitivity, reduces fasting and postprandial BG levels, and offers numerous metabolic, cardiovascular, and psychological benefits in diabetic patients. Patients may need individualized guidance regarding exercise, and they are more likely to exercise when counseled by their physician to do so.

PATIENT EDUCATION

Patient education is integral to the successful management of diabetes. Diabetes education is necessary to teach basic skills of SMBG and insulin administration and more advanced skills necessary to achieve tight glucose control with complex regimens (*Diabetes Care 2010;33(Suppl 1):S89–S96*).

Diabetes Mellitus in Hospitalized Patients

GENERAL PRINCIPLES

Indications for hospitalization in diabetic patients

- **DKA** is characterized by a plasma glucose level of >250 mg/dL in association with an arterial pH < 7.30 or serum bicarbonate level of <15 mEq/L and moderate ketonemia or ketonuria.
- **Hyperosmolar nonketotic** state includes marked hyperglycemia (≥400 mg/dL) and elevated serum osmolality (>315 mOsm/kg), often accompanied by impaired mental status.
- **Hypoglycemia** is an indication for hospitalization if induced by a sulfonylurea (SFU) medication, is due to a deliberate drug overdose, or results in coma, seizure, injury, or persistent neurologic change.
- **Newly diagnosed T1DM** or newly recognized GDM can be indications for hospitalization, even in the absence of ketoacidosis (see Type 1 Diabetes and Diabetic Ketoacidosis).
- **Patients with T2DM** are rarely admitted to the hospital for initiation or change in insulin therapy unless hyperglycemia is severe and associated with mental status change or other organ dysfunction.

TREATMENT

Management of diabetes in hospitalized patients

- Hyperglycemia is a common finding in hospitalized patients and may be due to previously diagnosed diabetes, undiagnosed diabetes, or stress-induced hyperglycemia. Up to 40% of general medical and surgical patients exhibit hyperglycemia and approximately 80% of intensive care unit (ICU) patients will demonstrate transient or persistent hyperglycemia.
  - A_{1C} can help identify previously undiagnosed diabetes in hospitalized patients and may assist with the evaluation of prior glucose control. A_{1C} is not accurate in patients who are severely anemic, bleeding, or hemolyzing or who have been transfused.
  - Observational studies have shown a strong, nearly linear relationship between the level of BG and adverse outcomes in hospitalized patients. Accumulating evidence suggests that tight glycemic control improves mortality and morbidity in patients after coronary artery bypass graft, stroke, and cardiac surgery; however, discrepancies have emerged as the number of randomized clinical trials has increased.
    - Intensive glucose control (achieved BG 110 mg/dL compared to conventional therapy with achieved BG 153 mg/dL) in surgical ICU patients significantly decreased in-hospital sepsis, acute renal failure requiring dialysis or hemofiltration, transfusion requirements, polyneuropathy, and days on mechanical ventilation.
    - However, in medical ICU patients, intensive insulin therapy significantly reduced morbidity but not the overall mortality. Mortality was only significantly decreased in medical ICU patients with intensive insulin therapy who stayed for ≥3 days,

and hypoglycemia was identified as an independent risk factor for death in medical ICU patients.

- The NICE-SUGAR study in 6,104 ICU patients showed increased mortality at 90 days (odds ratio, 1.14; confidence interval, 1.02–1.28) in patients undergoing tight glycemic control with achieved BG level of 118 mg/dL compared to conventional therapy with achieved BG level of 144 mg/dL. Both regimens used intravenous (IV) insulin as needed to reach the target glucose values (*N Engl J Med 2009;360:1283–1297*).
- Hypoglycemia was increased in the intensive treatment arms of several ICU studies and was associated with adverse outcomes. Avoidance of hypoglycemia should be a priority for both ICU and non-ICU inpatients.
- **Glucose targets in hospitalized patients.** Optimal target BG values may depend on the severity of illness, comorbid conditions, and other factors. Glucose levels should be kept close to 140 mg/dL in the ICU. In the noncritical care units, preprandial glucose should be 90 to 130 mg/dL and maximal glucose <180 mg/dL (*Ann Intern Med 1999;131:281–303*).
- **Patients hospitalized for reasons other than diabetes and are eating normally** may continue the outpatient diabetes treatment, unless specifically contraindicated.
  - The common practice of giving the entire insulin allotment as "sliding scale" has been shown to provide suboptimal glycemic control when compared to a basal/bolus regimen. Any patient with a BG level of >150 mg/dL should be considered for basal/bolus therapy, leaving "sliding scale" only to patients with intermittent minor elevations in BG levels.
  - For patients naive to insulin, a starting dose of basal insulin should equal 0.2 units/kg or 0.1 units/lb. If the presenting BG level is >200 mg/dL, adding premeal insulin is appropriate. The dose should be 0.2 units/kg divided by three meals.
    - Example: Your patient weighs 80 kg and has a BG level of 250 mg/dL. The starting insulin dose should be 16 units of long-acting insulin plus 5 units of rapid-acting insulin before each meal. A correction dose of 1 to 2 units per 50 mg/dL of BG, beginning at 150 mg/dL, can be added to the premeal doses.
  - Insulin doses should be given in relation to meals and should be adjusted according to glucose levels (*Arch Intern Med 1997;157:545–552*). BG levels should be monitored four times per day, especially in patients treated with insulin.
  - Adjustments in the next-day basal or premeal insulin doses are indicated if correction doses of insulin are frequently required. Extreme values (>300 or <60 mg/dL) from bedside capillary BG meters should be confirmed using laboratory measurements and may warrant immediate action.
  - If significant or persistent hyperglycemia is observed in hospitalized patients, ketoacidosis should be ruled out with an assessment of acid–base status and plasma ketone measurement. Insufficient insulin replacement or missed doses can have serious consequences in insulin-deficient patients.
- **Oral medications** for diabetes should be reviewed with regard to potential toxicities, risk of hypoglycemia, and other problems before ordering for hospitalized patients. It may be appropriate to restart home medications in stable patients after most of the diagnostic testing has been completed and the patient is on a stable treatment regimen.
  - **SFUs** and other insulin secretagogues may put hospitalized patients at risk for hypoglycemia and in general should not be used unless patients are eating regularly and are otherwise stable.

- **Metformin** should be withheld 1 day before any diagnostic evaluation that involves the use of iodinated radiocontrast dyes. It can be restarted 48 hours after radiocontrast exposure and documentation of normal renal function. Metformin is contraindicated in the presence of sepsis, congestive heart failure (CHF), renal dysfunction, or other conditions that predispose to lactic acidosis.
- **TZDs** should not be administered to patients with edema, CHF, or hepatic dysfunction as indicated by elevated serum transaminase levels.
- **Glucosidase inhibitors** may be continued if the patient is eating usual meals and not having gastrointestinal (GI) problems.
- **Dipeptidyl peptidase 4** (DPP-IV) inhibitors may be continued in patients eating normally, but dose adjustment will be required if renal function declines.
- **Glucagon-like peptide (GLP) 1** mimetics and agonists may be continued in stable patients if the doses can be appropriately timed with meals. These agents cause nausea, diarrhea, and other GI problems in a significant number of patients, so therapy with these agents should not be initiated in the hospital.
- **Colesevelam** is not absorbed and does not cause hypoglycemia, so it can be continued in hospitalized patients. Care must be taken so that it does not interfere with absorption of other medications, especially those with a narrow therapeutic index such as warfarin sodium, digoxin, and levothyroxine.
- **Patients hospitalized for reasons other than diabetes and who are required to fast** should discontinue oral antidiabetic medications.
  - In patients requiring insulin, IV insulin infusion is recommended for critical illness or major surgery (see Diabetes Mellitus in Surgical Patients, Chapter 1, Patient Care in Internal Medicine). Alternative treatment is to continue basal insulin with a modest dose reduction and to supplement with sliding scale.
  - An IV infusion of 5% dextrose in water (D5W) at 25 to 100 mL/hr should be provided to prevent ketosis and to maintain plasma glucose between 90 and 150 mg/dL. Alternatively, 10% dextrose in water (D10W) can be infused at a rate of 10 to 50 mL/hr to provide a steady, consistent source of calories.
  - It is recommended that transition from insulin drip to SC insulin occur before a meal, preferably before breakfast. The insulin drip should be discontinued 30 minutes to 1 hour after patients have received SC regular insulin and intermediate-acting insulin; however, if a rapid-acting insulin is used, the insulin drip can be discontinued shortly after SC insulin has been administered.
  - For patients requiring basal insulin, half of the anticipated basal insulin dose can be given as NPH (neutral protamine Hagedorn) or detemir at breakfast in addition to the usual short-acting insulin and the usual dose of glargine or detemir resumed in the evening. If the insulin drip is discontinued at another time point during the day, a prorated basal insulin should be provided until the usual dose schedule can be resumed.
- **Diabetic patients with emergency surgery**
  - Exclude DKA and neuropathy complications mimicking surgical emergencies.
  - Assess glycemic, acid–base, electrolyte (potassium, magnesium, and phosphate), and fluid status.
  - Restore circulating volume and correct acidosis and potassium abnormalities if surgery can be delayed.
  - Administer IV insulin, supplemented with glucose, and potassium as needed to achieve target BG levels (see "Glucose targets in hospitalized patients"). Hourly glucose measurements are mandatory to adjust insulin and glucose infusions.

Potassium should be monitored at least every 2 hours and replaced aggressively as required.

- **Enteral nutrition (*Mayo Clin Proc 1996;71:587–594*).** Intermittent tube feeds should be matched by either short-acting insulin or intermediate-acting insulin. Patients with baseline hyperglycemia may need a basal insulin dose in addition to the doses given to cover tube feeds. For example, nighttime enteral feeding lasting 6 to 8 hours should be managed with NPH, with or without a basal insulin dose. NPH can be given three to four times daily for continuous tube feeds, allowing a change in insulin dose if the feeding is interrupted.
- Total parenteral nutrition (TPN). Individuals with T2DM who require TPN are likely to require large amounts of insulin. See Chapter 2, Nutrition Support, for insulin management of patients on TPN.

TYPE 1 DIABETES AND DIABETIC KETOACIDOSIS

Type 1 Diabetes

GENERAL PRINCIPLES

A comprehensive approach is necessary for successful management of T1DM. A team approach that includes the expertise of physicians, diabetes educators, dietitians, and other members of the diabetes care team offers the best chance of success.

TREATMENT

Treatment of T1DM requires lifelong insulin replacement.

- **Insulin preparations.** After SC injection, there is individual variability in the duration and peak activity of insulin preparations and day-to-day variability in the same subject (Table 1).
  - **Rapid-acting insulins** include regular insulin, insulin lispro, insulin aspart, and insulin glulisine. Regular insulin can be administered intravenously, intramuscularly, or subcutaneously. An IV bolus of regular insulin exerts maximum effect in 10 to 30 minutes and lasts up to 1 hour.
  - **Intermediate-acting insulin,** NPH (isophane), is the only available insulin in this class. NPH is released slowly from SC sites and peaks in 6 to 12 hours, followed by gradual decline.
  - **Long-acting insulins** are absorbed more slowly than the intermediate-acting preparations. Long-acting insulins provide a steady "basal" supply of circulating insulin when administered once or twice a day. Glargine and detemir are "peakless" bioengineered human insulin analogues with an extended duration of activity. These insulins are generally administered once daily as a SC injection at bedtime, in a regimen that includes premeal rapid-acting insulin. Some patients with T1DM have improved control when the basal insulin is given twice a day rather than every day.
  - **Concentration.** The standard insulin concentration is 100 units/mL (U-100), with vials containing 1,000 units in 10 mL. A highly concentrated form of regular insulin containing 500 units/mL (Humulin U-500) is available for the rare patient

Table 1	Approximate Kinetics of Human Insulin Preparations After Subcutaneous Injection		
Insulin Type	Onset of Action (hr)	Peak Effect (hr)	Duration of Activity (hr)
Rapid acting			
Lispro, aspart, glulisine	0.25–0.50	0.50–1.50	3–5
Regular	0.50–1.00	2–4	6–8
Intermediate acting			
NPH	1–2	6–12	18–24
Long acting			
Glargine	4–6	None[a]	18–24
Detemir	3–4		18–24

[a]Insulin dosage and individual variability in absorption and clearance rates affect pharmacokinetic data. Duration of insulin activity is prolonged in renal failure. After a lag time of approximately 5 hours, insulin glargine has a flat peakless effect over a 24-hour period.

with severe insulin resistance (usually T2DM). The vial size for U-500 insulin is 20 mL.

- **Mixed insulin therapy.** Short- and rapid-acting insulins (regular, lispro, aspart, and glulisine) can be mixed with NPH insulin in the same syringe for convenience. The rapid-acting insulin should be drawn first, cross contamination should be avoided, and the mixed insulin should be injected immediately. Commercial premixed insulin preparations do not allow dose adjustment of individual components but are convenient for patients who are unable or unwilling to do the mixing themselves.

- **SC insulin administration.** The abdomen, thighs, buttocks, and upper arms are the preferred sites for SC insulin injection. Absorption is fastest from the abdomen, followed by the arm, buttocks, and thigh, probably as a result of differences in blood flow. Injection sites should be rotated within the regions, rather than randomly across separate regions, to minimize erratic absorption. Exercise or massage over the injection site may accelerate insulin absorption.

- **Insulin requirement** for optimal glycemic control is approximately 0.5 to 0.8 units/kg/d for the average nonobese patient. A conservative total daily dose (TDD) of 0.4 units/kg/d is given initially to a newly diagnosed patient; the dose is then adjusted, using SMBG values.

- A regimen of **multiple daily insulin injections** that include basal, premeal, and correction doses is preferred to obtain optimal control in both hospitalized patients and outpatients. This regimen implies that capillary glucose monitoring will occur four times daily, 10 to 30 minutes before meals and at bedtime.

  - Basal insulin can be provided by NPH given twice daily, insulin detemir given once or twice daily, or insulin glargine generally dosed once daily. A reasonable starting dose is 0.2 units/kg or 0.1 units/lb for the day, either divided into two parts or given once. Basal insulin should provide 40% to 50% of the TDD of insulin and should be adjusted by 5% to 10% daily until the fasting glucose is consistently <130 mg/dL. In general, basal insulin is given regardless of NPO or dietary status and should not be held without a direct order.

○ Premeal insulin is strongly recommended for patients consuming full liquids or regular food. The total premeal complement should roughly equal the total basal dose, with one-third given before or after each meal. Rapid-acting insulin (lispro, aspart, or glulisine) are preferred, but regular human insulin can be used. Orders should be written to hold premeal insulin doses if the patient is NPO, off the medical floor, or not able to eat at least half of the meal provided.

○ The third component of a comprehensive insulin regimen is "correction factor" insulin, which is similar to sliding scale, adjusted according to the premeal fingerstick glucose testing and the patients estimated insulin sensitivity. In general, thinner patients should use a lower scale than heavier or more insulin-resistant patients. Correction factor and premeal doses should utilize the same insulin and be given together in the same syringe.

• **Continuous SC insulin infusion** using an insulin pump is a tool for intensive diabetes control in selected patients.

○ A typical regimen provides 50% of total daily insulin as basal insulin and the remainder as multiple preprandial boluses of insulin, using a programmable insulin pump.

○ Patients who utilize an insulin pump at home may be allowed to continue this therapy if mental status is not compromised and the regimen can be ordered and supervised by a knowledgeable physician. Specific order sets may be needed for these patients.

• **Sliding scale** only regimens are contraindicated in patients with T1DM and should be reserved for patients with minor elevations in BG levels during hospitalization. Regimens that include intermediate- or long-acting insulin give superior results in patients with previously diagnosed diabetes (*Arch Intern Med 1997;157:545–552*).

MONITORING/FOLLOW-UP

BG levels should be monitored at least four times a day (preprandially and at bedtime) in hospitalized patients with either T1DM or T2DM. The A_{1C} should be obtained if a recent result is unavailable. Blood or urine should be tested for ketones whenever hyperglycemia (>300 mg/dL) persists on more than one measurement.

Diabetic Ketoacidosis

GENERAL PRINCIPLES

Epidemiology

DKA, a potentially fatal complication, occurs in up to 5% of patients with T1DM annually; it is seen much less frequently in T2DM.

Pathophysiology

DKA results from severe insulin deficiency, often in association with stress and activation of counterregulatory hormones (e.g., catecholamines, glucagon).

Risk Factors

Precipitating factors for DKA include inadvertent or deliberate interruption of insulin therapy, sepsis, trauma, myocardial infarction (MI), and pregnancy. DKA may be the first presentation of T1DM and, rarely, T2DM.

Prevention

Every episode of DKA suggests a breakdown in clinical communication. Diabetes education should therefore be reinforced at every opportunity, with special emphasis on (a) self-management skills during sick days; (b) the body's need for more, rather than less, insulin during such illnesses; (c) testing of blood or urine for ketones; and (d) procedures for obtaining timely and preventive medical advice.

DIAGNOSIS

A high index of suspicion is warranted because clinical presentation may be nonspecific.

Clinical Presentation

History

Patients may describe a variety of symptoms including polyuria, polydipsia, weight loss, nausea, vomiting, and vaguely localized abdominal pain.

Physical Examination

- Tachycardia; decrease of capillary filling; rapid, deep, and labored breathing (Kussmaul respiration); and fruity breath odor are common physical findings.
- Prominent GI symptoms and abdominal tenderness on exam may give rise to suspicion for intra-abdominal pathology.
- Dehydration is invariable and respiratory distress, shock, and coma can occur.

Diagnostic Testing

Laboratories

- Labs will show an anion gap metabolic acidosis and positive serum β-hydroxybutyrate or ketones (a semiquantitative measurement of acetone, acetoacetate, and β-hydroxybutyrate).
- Plasma glucose level usually is elevated, but the degree of hyperglycemia may be moderate (≤ 300 mg/dL) in 10% to 15% of patients with DKA. Pregnancy and alcohol ingestion are associated with "euglycemic DKA."
- Urine ketones are generally present in DKA.
- Hyponatremia, hyperkalemia, azotemia, and hyperosmolality are other findings.
- Serum amylase, transaminase, and/or triglyceride levels may be elevated.
- A focused search for a precipitating infection is recommended if clinically indicated.
- An electrocardiogram (ECG) should be obtained to evaluate electrolyte abnormalities and for unsuspected myocardial ischemia.

TREATMENT

Management of DKA should preferably be conducted in an ICU. **If treatment is conducted in a non-ICU setting, close monitoring is mandatory until ketoacidosis resolves and the patient's condition is stabilized.** The therapeutic priorities are fluid replacement, adequate insulin administration, and potassium repletion. Administration of bicarbonate, phosphate, magnesium, or other therapies may be advantageous in selected patients.

- **IV access and supportive measures** should be instituted without delay.
- **Fluid** deficits of several liters are common in DKA patients and can be estimated by subtracting the current weight from a recently known dry weight. The

average degree of dehydration for most patients is approximately 7% to 9% of body weight. Hypotension indicates a loss of > 10% of body fluids (*Diabetes Care 2004;27: S94–S102*).

- **Restoration of circulating volume** using isotonic (0.9%) saline should be the initial therapeutic intervention. The first liter should be infused rapidly (if cardiac function is normal) and should be followed by additional fluids at a rate of 0.5 to 1 L/hr until vital signs have stabilized and urine output has been established, usually in 2 to 3 hours. The remaining volume deficit can be corrected more slowly. Hypotonic saline (0.45%) can be used in patients with severe hypernatremia (>150 mEq/L) and after stabilization of blood pressure.
- The next goal is to **replenish total body water deficits;** this can be accomplished using a 0.45% saline infusion at 150 to 500 mL/hr if the corrected serum sodium level is normal or elevated; 0.9% NaCl at a similar rate is appropriate if the corrected serum sodium level is low. The rate of the fluid replacement depends on the degree of dehydration and cardiac and renal status. Do not exceed a change in osmolality >3 mOsm/kg/hr. The success of the fluid replacement is judged by improvement in blood pressure, urine output, and clinical examination.
- **Maintenance fluid replacement** is continued until the fluid intake/output records indicate an overall positive balance similar to the estimated fluid deficit. Complete fluid replacement in a typical DKA patient may require 12 to 24 hours to accomplish.
- **Insulin therapy**. Sufficient insulin must be administered to turn off ketogenesis and correct hyperglycemia.
  - **An IV bolus of regular insulin,** 10 to 15 units (0.15 units/kg), should be administered immediately. This should be followed by a continuous infusion of regular insulin at an initial rate of 5 to 10 units/hr (or 0.1 units/kg/hr). A solution of regular insulin, 100 units in 100 mL of 0.9% saline, infused at a rate of 10 mL/hr delivers 10 units/hr of insulin.
  - **A decrease in BG levels of 50 to 75 mg/dL/hr** is an appropriate response; lesser decrements suggest insulin resistance, inadequate volume repletion, or inadequate insulin dose or delivery. If insulin resistance is suspected, the hourly dose of regular insulin should be increased progressively by 50% to 100% until an appropriate glycemic response is observed.
  - **Excessively rapid correction of hyperglycemia** at rates > 100 mg/dL/hr should be avoided to reduce the risk of osmotic encephalopathy.
  - **Maintenance insulin infusion rates of 1 to 2 units/hr** can be continued (indefinitely) until the patient is clinically improved, the serum bicarbonate level rises to ≥15 mEq/L, and the anion gap has closed. Once oral intake resumes, insulin can be administered SC and the parenteral route can be discontinued. It is prudent to give the first SC injection of insulin 30 to 60 minutes before stopping the IV insulin infusion. Both basal and premeal doses of insulin will need to be restarted, so stopping at a logical time, for example, before breakfast or in the evening, makes sense.
- **Dextrose (5%)** in 0.45% saline should be infused once plasma glucose level decreases to 250 mg/dL and the insulin infusion rate should be decreased to 0.05 units/kg/hr to prevent dangerous hypoglycemia. Consider starting a separate dextrose-containing infusion of 50 to 100 mL/hr and adjusting the fluid replacement accordingly. Rapid rates of dextrose infusion with reduced insulin doses may result in rebound hyperglycemia.
- **Potassium deficit** should always be assumed or anticipated regardless of plasma levels on admission. Insulin administration results in a rapid shift of potassium into the intracellular compartment.

- The goal is to maintain plasma potassium level in the normal range and thereby prevent the potentially fatal cardiac effects of hypokalemia. Potassium status should be documented from the outset; this includes ECG to rule out rare life-threatening hyperkalemia.
- Potassium should be added routinely to the IV fluids (consider starting with the second or third liter of fluid replacement) at a rate of 10 to 20 mEq/hr except in patients with hyperkalemia (>6.0 mmol/L and/or ECG evidence), renal failure, or oliguria confirmed by bladder catheterization.
- Patients who present with hypokalemia should receive higher doses of potassium, ≥40 mEq/hr, depending on severity.
- Potassium chloride is an appropriate initial choice, but this can later be changed to potassium phosphate to reduce chloride load in patients without severe renal impairment.
- **Monitoring of therapy**
  - BG levels should be monitored hourly, serum electrolyte levels every 1 to 2 hours, and arterial blood gas values as often as necessary for a severely acidotic or hypoxic patient.
  - Serum sodium tends to rise as hyperglycemia is corrected; failure to observe this trend suggests that the patient is being overhydrated with free water.
  - Serial serum ketone assays are not necessary because ketonemia lags behind clinical recovery and because the most commonly used assays measure all ketones. Repeating a β-hydroxybutyrate measurement if available may be more accurate. Restoration of renal buffering capacity by normalization of the serum bicarbonate level and closure of the anion gap are more reliable indices of metabolic recovery.
  - Use of a flowchart is an efficient method of tracking clinical data (e.g., weight, fluid balance, mental status) and laboratory results during the management of DKA.
  - Continuous ECG monitoring may be required for proper management of potassium in patients with oliguria or renal failure.
- **Bicarbonate therapy** is not routinely necessary and may be deleterious in certain situations.
  - Bicarbonate therapy may be considered for DKA patients who develop (a) shock or coma, (b) severe acidosis (pH < 7.1), (c) severe depletion of buffering reserve (plasma bicarbonate <5 mEq/L), (d) acidosis-induced cardiac or respiratory dysfunction, or (e) severe hyperkalemia.
  - Sodium bicarbonate, 50 to 100 mEq in 1 L of 0.45% saline infused over 30 to 60 minutes, can be given in these situations. Bicarbonate treatment should be guided by arterial pH measurement and continued until the indications are no longer present.
  - Care should be taken to avoid hypokalemia; an additional dose of potassium, 10 mEq, should be included with each infusion of bicarbonate unless hyperkalemia is present.
- **Phosphate and magnesium** stores are reduced in DKA patients, and plasma levels (particularly phosphate) decline further during insulin therapy. The clinical significance of these changes is unclear, and routine replacement of phosphate or magnesium is not necessary, especially if the patient is able to resume usual caloric intake.
  - In hypophosphatemic patients with compromised oral intake, the use of potassium phosphate in maintenance IV fluids can be considered (see Chapter 9, Fluid and Electrolyte Management).
  - Magnesium therapy is indicated in patients with ventricular arrhythmia and can be administered as magnesium sulfate (50%) in doses of 2.5 to 5.0 mL (10 to 20 mEq of magnesium) IV.

- **IV antimicrobial therapy** should be started promptly for documented bacterial, fungal, and other treatable infections. Empiric broad-spectrum antibiotics can be started in septic patients, pending results of blood cultures (see Chapter 13, Human Immunodeficiency Virus Infection and Acquired Immunodeficiency Syndrome). Note that DKA is not typically accompanied by fever, so infection must be considered in a febrile patient.

COMPLICATIONS

Complicationsof DKA includes life-threatening conditions that must be recognized and treated promptly.

- **Lactic acidosis** may result from prolonged dehydration, shock, infection, and tissue hypoxia in DKA patients. Lactic acidosis should be suspected in patients with refractory metabolic acidosis and a persistent anion gap despite optimal therapy for DKA. Adequate volume replacement, control of sepsis, and judicious use of bicarbonate constitute the approach to management.
- **Arterial thrombosis** manifesting as stroke, MI, or an ischemic limb occurs with increased frequency in DKA. However, routine anticoagulation is not indicated except as part of the specific therapy for a thrombotic event.
- **Cerebral edema,** a dire complication of DKA, is observed more frequently in children than in adults.
- Symptoms of increased intracranial pressure (e.g., headache, altered mental status, papilledema) or a sudden deterioration in mental status after initial improvement in a patient with DKA should raise suspicion for cerebral edema.
  - Overhydration with free water and excessively rapid correction of hyperglycemia are known risk factors.
  - A fall in serum sodium level or failure to rise during therapy for DKA is a clue to imminent or established overhydration with free water. Neuroimaging with a computed tomographic (CT) scan can establish the diagnosis. Prompt recognition and treatment with IV mannitol is essential and may prevent neurologic sequelae in patients who survive cerebral edema.
- **Rebound ketoacidosis** can occur due to premature cessation of IV insulin infusion or inadequate doses of SC insulin after the insulin infusion has been discontinued. All patients T1DM and patients with T2DM who develop DKA (indicating severe insulin deficiency) require both basal and premeal insulin in adequate doses to avoid recurrence of metabolic decompensation.

TYPE 2 DIABETES AND NONKETOTIC HYPEROSMOLAR SYNDROME

Type 2 Diabetes

GENERAL PRINCIPLES

Pathophysiology

- T2DM results from defective insulin secretion followed by loss of β-cell mass in response to increased demand as a result of insulin resistance.
- The loss of pancreatic β cells is progressive; however, insulin secretion is usually sufficient to prevent ketosis under basal conditions. T2DM patients can develop

DKA when hyperglycemia is severe or prolonged or when exposed to severe stress.
- The mechanisms underlying the β-cell loss in T2DM are unknown, but programmed cell death in response to genetic and environmental factors has been demonstrated in animal models.

TREATMENT

Medications

- Recommended glycemic goals for patients with T2DM are the same as in T1DM, $A_{1C} < 7\%$ or as low as can be achieved safely. Near normalization of glucose values may be safely achievable in many patients with T2DM.
- The achievement of these goals requires individualized therapy and a comprehensive approach that incorporates lifestyle and pharmacologic interventions. Several considerations should be taken into account before choosing oral agents (Table 2) in patients with T2DM:
  - Oral therapy should be initiated early in conjunction with diet and exercise.
  - Monotherapy with maximum doses of insulin secretagogues, metformin, or TZDs yields comparable glucose-lowering effects.
  - The glucose-lowering effects of metformin, insulin secretagogues, and DPP-IV inhibitors and GLP mimetics are observed within days to weeks, while the maximum effects of TZDs may not be observed for several weeks to months.
  - Combination therapy with two or more oral agents may be needed to achieve the A_{1C} and glucose targets in patients presenting with significant hyperglycemia and may be needed as β-cell function deteriorates over time in most patients.
  - Glycemic control with monotherapy is less likely to occur in patients with very high glucose readings (>200 mg/dL) at the time of diagnosis (*Ann Intern Med 1999;131:281–303*). Combination therapy or insulin should be considered as first-line therapy for these patients.
  - Because pancreatic β-cell function is required for the glucose-lowering effects of all noninsulin therapies, many patients with advanced T2DM do not respond satisfactorily to these agents and insulin therapy may become necessary.
  - Moreover, the toxicity profile of some oral agents may preclude their use in patients with preexisting illnesses.
- **Insulin secretagogues**
  - **SFUs** increase insulin secretion by binding to specific receptors in β cells. All SFUs are equally effective in controlling hyperglycemia at equivalent doses but have variable pharmacokinetics.
    - These agents should be taken 30 to 60 minutes before food and should never be administered to fasting patients.
    - Glyburide has an active metabolite with significant renal excretion and **should be avoided in the setting of impaired renal function and used with caution in elderly patients.**
    - Glipizide has a short duration of action and should be administered two to three times per day or once daily in a modified long-acting formulation. Glimepiride has the longest duration of action and can be administered once per day.
    - Therapy should be initiated with the lowest effective dose and increased gradually over several days or weeks to the optimal dose.
    - Good responders to SFU include newly diagnosed type 2 diabetics with mild to moderate fasting hyperglycemia.

Table 2   Noninsulin Medications for Diabetes

	Daily Dosage Range	Doses Per Day	Duration of Action (hours)	Main Adverse Effects
Oral antidiabetic medications for type 2 diabetes				
Insulin secretagogues				
SFUs (second generation)				
Glyburide (glibenclamide)	1.25–20 mg	qd or bid	12–24	Hypoglycemia, weight gain
Glipizide	2.5–40 mg	qd or bid	12–24	
Glimepiride	1–8 mg	qd or bid	24	
Gliclazide (not available in the United States)	40–320 mg	bid	12	
Non-SFU secretagogues				
Nateglinide	180–320 mg	tid before meals	4	Hypoglycemia, weight gain; not as severe as SFUs
Repaglinide	1.5–16 mg	tid before meals	4 to 6	
Biguanide				
Metformin (available in liquid and long-acting formulations)	500 mg–2.5 g	bid or tid	12 to 18	Diarrhea, nausea, abdominal pain or cramping, lactic acidosis
α-Glucosidase inhibitors				
Acarbose	75–300 mg	tid before meals	2 to 3	Gas, bloating, diarrhea, abdominal pain
Miglitol	75–300 mg	tid before meals	2 to 3	
Thiazolidinediones				
Rosiglitazone (rosiglitazone has been associated with increased risk of myocardial infarction)	2–8 mg	qd or bid	24+	Weight gain, edema, congestive heart failure, anemia, increased fractures in women
Pioglitazone	15, 30, 45	qd	24+	
Dipeptidyl peptidase-4 inhibitors				
Sitagliptin (dose adjustment for CKD: use 50 mg if CrCl ≤ 50 mL/min; use 25 mg if CrCl ≤ 25 mL/min)	25, 50, 100	qd	24	Angioedema, Stevens-Johnson syndrome, URI

Saxagliptin (dose adjustment for CKD, use 2.5 mg if CrCl ≤ 50 mL/min)	2.5 or 5 mg	qd		Urticaria, facial edema, URI
Vildagliptin (not available in the United States and not indicated in severe renal or hepatic impairment, LFT ≥ 3× upper limit of normal)	50–100 mg	qd- or bid	24	Blistering skin lesions in animals, increased LFTs,
Bile acid sequestrant				
Colesevelam hydrochloride (contraindicated in bowel obstruction or GI motility disorders)	3.8 g (each tablet is 625 mg)	3 tablets bid	12	Constipation, reduced absorption of some medications
Dopamine receptor agonist				
Bromocriptine mesylate (do not use with other dopamine agonists or antagonists)	0.8–4.8 mg	1–6 tablets qd	24	Nausea, asthenia, dizziness, headache, constipation, diarrhea
Injectable medications for type 2 diabetes				
GLP agonists				
Exenatide	5–10 μg	bid	9	Nausea, vomiting, GI distress, reported cases of pancreatitis
Liraglutide (not approved in the United States at the time of this writing)	0.6–1.8 mg	qd	24	Nausea, vomiting, GI distress; increased calcitonin and goiter
Injectable medications for type 1 or type 2 diabetes				
Amylin analogue				
Pramlintide acetate (given as a separate injection with meals, insulin dose reduction is required when starting)	15–120 μg	tid before meals	2	Nausea, vomiting, diarrhea, headache, hypoglycemia

CKD, chronic kidney disease; CrCl, creatinine clearance; GI, gastrointestinal; GLP, glucagon-like peptide; LFT, liver function test; SFU, sulfonylurea; URI, upper respiratory infection.

- ○ Hypoglycemia is seen with all SFUs but is the most common with glyburide.
- ○ Weight gain is also a notable adverse effect.
- **Repaglinide** is a meglitinide analog that augments food-stimulated insulin secretion with a similar glucose-lowering effect as SFUs. Unlike SFUs, however, the meglitinides have a very short onset of action and a short half-life.
  - ○ Repaglinide can be used as a single agent or in a combination with metformin in patients with T2DM.
  - ○ The dose range is 0.5 to 4.0 mg PO with two to four meals daily; the drug should be taken within 30 minutes before meals and skipped if no meal is planned.
  - ○ Adverse effects include hypoglycemia and weight gain.
- **Nateglinide,** a d-phenylalanine derivative chemically distinct from other insulin secretagogues, acts directly on the pancreatic β cells to stimulate early insulin secretion (*Diabetes Care 2000;23:202–207*).
  - ○ It is taken 10 minutes before breakfast, lunch, and dinner and leads to significant insulin secretion within 15 minutes, with a return to baseline in 3 to 4 hours, effectively controlling postprandial hyperglycemia. The maximum effective dosage is 120 mg three times daily.
  - ○ Nateglinide is metabolized by the cytochrome P-450 system, so it has potential for drug interactions.
  - ○ The drug is well tolerated and the risk of hypoglycemia appears minimal.
- **Metformin,** the only biguanide in current clinical use, inhibits hepatic glucose output and stimulates glucose uptake by peripheral tissues. It is the preferred initial agent for most patients with T2DM and particularly those in whom weight gain is not desirable.
  - ○ Metformin should be taken with food and beginning with a single 500- or 850-mg tablet, the dose is increased every few days to weeks until optimal glycemic effect is achieved or 2,000 mg/d is reached.
  - ○ GI symptoms occur in 20% to 30% of patients and can be managed by dose titration or adjustment; however, about 10% of patients do not tolerate any dose.
  - ○ Lactic acidosis, the most serious adverse effect, has an incidence of approximately 3 per 100,000 patient-years and a significant mortality rate. Risk factors for lactic acidosis include renal dysfunction, hypovolemia, tissue hypoxia, infection, alcoholism, and cardiopulmonary disease.
  - ○ A serum creatinine level of >1.5 mg/dL in men (>1.4 mg/dL in women) or a GFR of <70 mL/min are contraindications to metformin use.
  - ○ Metformin should be discontinued at the time of the radiographic contrast procedure and not restarted for 48 hours.
  - ○ Other situations in which metformin therapy should be avoided include cardiogenic or septic shock, CHF requiring pharmacologic therapy, severe liver disease, pulmonary insufficiency with hypoxemia, and severe tissue hypoperfusion (*N Engl J Med 1996;334:574–579*).
- **α-Glucosidase inhibitors** block polysaccharide and disaccharide breakdown and decrease postprandial hyperglycemia when administered with food. Two members of this class, acarbose and miglitol, exert maximal effects at a dosage of approximately 300 mg/d. Voglibose is a similar drug used in Japan.
  - ○ Each drug should be initiated at low doses (25 mg PO daily–tid, with food) and increased slowly in weekly steps of 25 mg to minimize GI intolerance.
  - ○ Monotherapy with these agents provides A_{1C} lowering of 0.4% to 0.7%, which is modest but without risk of hypoglycemia.

- ○ Dose-related adverse effects are diarrhea, bloating, abdominal cramping, and flatulence in 25% to 50% of individuals.
- ○ Acarbose has been associated with elevation in liver enzymes and therefore periodic monitoring of transaminases is recommended.
- ○ Hypoglycemia in patients who are receiving regimens that include α-glucosidase inhibitors should be treated with glucose, not sucrose.
- **TZDs** increase insulin sensitivity in muscle, adipose tissue, and liver. Therefore, patients with considerable endogenous insulin secretion respond better to these agents. The two TZDs currently available, rosiglitazone and pioglitazone, appear to have similar efficacy on glycemia.
  - ○ Edema is the most common adverse effect and may range from none to mild peripheral edema to precipitation of CHF. Therapy with these agents is not recommended in patients with compromised cardiac function (New York Heart Association class 3 and 4 cardiac status). Before starting TZDs, the physician should determine the existence of cardiac disease, concomitant use of medications associated with fluid retention, edema, and shortness of breath. The risk of CHF is increased in patients with history of heart failure, coronary artery disease (CAD), hypertension, long-standing diabetes, left ventricular hypertrophy, preexisting edema, edema after TZD therapy, insulin therapy, advanced age, renal failure, and aortic and mitral valve disease (*Diabetes Care 2004;27:256–263*).
  - ○ The risk of drug-induced hepatotoxicity with pioglitazone and rosiglitazone is considered rare; however, periodic monitoring of liver function is recommended.
  - ○ TZDs have been associated with mild decrements in hemoglobin and/or pancytopenia. This has been attributed to increased plasma volume, but there may also be subclinical bone marrow suppression.
  - ○ TZDs may increase the risk of fracture in women, particularly smaller bones. The presumed mechanism is inhibition of osteoblast activity.
  - ○ Resumption of ovulation may occur during TZD therapy in some premenopausal women with anovulatory cycles. Therefore, contraceptive practice should be reviewed to prevent unintended pregnancy.
  - ○ **Rosiglitazone** can be used in combination with metformin or an SFU.
    - - The usual starting dosage is 4 mg PO daily (or 2 mg PO bid) taken with or without food. This can be advanced to 8 mg PO daily (or 4 mg PO bid) after 12 weeks if glycemic response is inadequate.
    - - Although data from clinical trials suggest a low propensity for hepatotoxicity, regular monitoring of hepatic transaminases is required in patients treated with rosiglitazone.
    - - Potential drug interaction with phenobarbital, rifampin, amiodarone, and fluconazole can occur.
    - - Rosiglitazone may increase LDL levels.
    - - Recent analyses of clinical trial data have suggested an increase in MI with rosiglitazone; however, this effect has not been observed in trials designed to interrogate CV effects.
  - ○ **Pioglitazone** can be used as a single agent (as an adjunct to diet and exercise) or in combination with SFU, metformin, sitagliptin, exenatide, or insulin.
    - - The initial dosage is 15 or 30 mg PO daily, taken with or without food; this can be increased after several weeks to 45 mg PO daily for optimal effect.
    - - Regular monitoring of hepatic transaminases is required during pioglitazone therapy.

- Pioglitazone alters the levels of medications metabolized by cytochrome P-450 isoform CYP 3A4 (carbamazepine, cyclosporine, felodipine, and some oral contraceptives, among others). The risk of edema and CHF increases when pioglitazone is used with insulin.
- **DPP-IV inhibitors** are orally administered inhibitors of DPP-IV, the enzyme that breaks down endogenous GLP, which is an incretin secreted from the intestinal L cells. Increased levels of GLP reduce BG concentration by inhibiting glucagon secretion from the pancreatic α cells and by stimulating insulin secretion. Pancreatitis has been reported in rare cases in conjunction with DPP-IV inhibitor therapy, and allergic reactions may include angioedema and Steven-Johnson syndrome.
  - ○ **Sitagliptin** is given once daily at a usual dose of 100 mg. It has been studied for use as monotherapy or in conjunction with metformin, SFUs, TZDs, and insulin. It is well tolerated and without significant adverse effects. Its elimination pathway is predominantly renal, so dose reduction is recommended in patients with reduced renal function (give 50 mg if estimated glomerular filtration rate [eGFR] is <50 mL/min/1.73 m^2, 25 mg daily if eGFR is <25 m/min/1.73 m^2).
  - ○ **Vildagliptin** is approved for use in Europe at doses of 50 or 100 mg administered once daily. It has been studied for use as monotherapy and in conjunction with metformin, SFU, TZD, and insulin. It is not indicated in patients with impaired renal function.
  - ○ **Saxagliptin** is also administered once daily in doses of 2.5 or 5 mg. The lower dose should be used in patients with creatinine clearance < 50 mL/min. The main side effects are urticaria and facial edema.
- **Colesevelam hydrochloride** is a bile acid sequestrant that has been shown to have glucose-lowering properties. When given at full dose of three (625 mg) tablets bid, it lowers A$_{1C}$ by 0.4% to 0.8% when used as monotherapy or in conjunction with metformin or SFUs. It is also indicated for LDL lowering. The major side effect is constipation, and caution is advised for patients with preexisting GI problems or disease. It should not be used in patients with significant hypertriglyceridemia, as it may raise triglycerides. Colesevelam hydrochloride should be taken on an empty stomach, and before or after other medications so as not to interfere with their absorption. Colesevelam hydrochloride has a pregnancy category B rating and can be used in patients with renal insufficiency and hepatic insufficiency because it is not absorbed.
- **GLP agonists/mimetics.** These peptides are structurally similar to endogenous GLP1 but resist breakdown by DPP enzymes. Thus, they have a longer half-life than native GLP1 and reach higher blood and tissue levels. GLP1 agonists and mimetics are given by injection and in addition to glucose-lowering properties may improve satiety and assist with weight loss.
  - ○ Exenatide was the first GLP1 mimetic available. It is given in doses of 5 or 10 μg twice daily before meals. Expected A$_{1C}$ lowering is 0.6% to 1.2%, which is accompanied by an average weight loss of 4 kg. Postmarketing cases of pancreatitis have been reported.
  - ○ Liraglutide is approved for use in Europe. The dose is 0.6 to 1.8 mg once daily by subcutaneous injection. The main side effects are nausea, vomiting, dizziness, and headache. Increased calcitonin levels and goiters have been described.
- **Insulin therapy** in T2DM is indicated in the following:
  - ○ Patients in whom oral agents failed to sustain glycemic control
  - ○ DKA
  - ○ Nonketotic hyperosmolar crisis

- ○ Newly diagnosed patients with severe hyperglycemia
- ○ Pregnancy and other situations in which oral agents are contraindicated
- **The success of insulin therapy** depends on the use of sufficient doses of insulin (0.6 to >1.0 units/kg of body weight per day) to achieve target glucose and A_{1C} values rather than any specific pattern of insulin administration.
  - ○ A once-daily injection of intermediate- or long-acting insulin at bedtime or before breakfast can be added to an oral agent regimen to achieve the target A_{1C} goal.
  - ○ Premeal insulin may be required if basal insulin plus oral agents is not adequate. Short- or rapid-acting insulin administered before meals can be added to a basal insulin, or a premixed insulin can be given twice daily before breakfast and dinner. In general, the secretagogues are discontinued when premeal insulin is added, but sensitizing and other agents are continued on the basis of the individual patient needs.
  - ○ The dose(s) of insulin required vary widely in patients with T2DM based on body mass index, the continuation of oral agents, and the presence of comorbid conditions. Large doses of insulin (>100 units/d) may be required for optimal glycemic control. Weight gain with insulin use is a concern.
  - ○ The risk of insulin-induced hypoglycemia, the most dangerous side effect, may increase cardiovascular event rates and death. Avoidance of hypoglycemia while achieving an A_{1C} as low as can safely be achieved requires close collaboration between physician, patient, and diabetes educators. The frequency of hypoglycemia increases as patients approach normal A_{1C} levels or when deterioration of kidney function occurs.
- **Combination therapy.** About 60% of patients on monotherapy may have worsening of metabolic control during the first 5 years of therapy, and concurrent use of two or more medications with different mechanisms of action may be necessary (United Kingdom Prospective Diabetes Study [UKPDS]).
  - ○ Dose increase and addition of agents should be performed in a short period of time until glucose control is achieved.
  - ○ Combination therapy using a secretagogue and an insulin sensitizer should be considered as a first-line therapy in patients with A_{1C} levels of ≥9%. Widely used regimens include an SFU plus metformin (most common), a TZD plus SFU or metformin plus a DPP IV inhibitor.
  - ○ The combination of a TZD plus insulin is less accepted because of a higher incidence of CHF exacerbations.
  - ○ Several combinations of two antidiabetic medications are available in one tablet.

Nonketotic Hyperosmolar Syndrome

GENERAL PRINCIPLES

Nonketotic hyperosmolar syndrome (NKHS) is one of the most serious life-threatening complications of T2DM.

Epidemiology

- Hyperosmolar hyperglycemic state (HHS) occurs primarily in patients with T2DM and in 30% to 40% of cases; NKHS is the initial presentation of a patient's diabetes (*Emerg Med Clin North Am 2005;23:629–648*).

- NKHS is significantly less common than DKA with an incidence of <1 case per 1,000 person-years.

Pathophysiology

- Ketoacidosis is absent because the ambient insulin level may effectively prevent lipolysis and subsequent ketogenesis yet is inadequate to facilitate peripheral glucose uptake and to prevent hepatic residual gluconeogenesis and glucose output.
- Precipitating factors include dehydration, stress, infection, stroke, noncompliance with medications, dietary indiscretion, and alcohol and cocaine abuse. Impaired glucose excretion is a contributory factor in patients with renal insufficiency or prerenal azotemia.

DIAGNOSIS

Clinical Presentation

In contrast to DKA, the onset of NKHS is usually insidious. Several days of deteriorating glycemic control are followed by increasing lethargy. Clinical evidence of severe dehydration is the rule. Some alterations in consciousness and focal neurologic deficits may be found at presentation or may develop during therapy. Therefore, repeated neurologic assessment is recommended.

Differential Diagnosis

The differential diagnosis of NKHS includes any cause of altered level of consciousness, including hypoglycemia, hyponatremia, severe dehydration, uremia, hyperammonemia, drug overdose, and sepsis. Seizures and acute stroke-like syndromes are common presentations.

Diagnostic Testing

Laboratories

Clinical findings include (a) hyperglycemia, often >600 mg/dL; (b) plasma osmolality >320 mOsm/L; (c) absence of ketonemia; and (d) pH > 7.3 and serum bicarbonate level of >20 mEq/L. Prerenal azotemia and lactic acidosis can develop. Although some patients will have detectable urine ketones, most patients do not have a metabolic acidosis. Lactic acidosis may develop from an underlying ischemia, infection, or other cause.

TREATMENT

- **The goals of therapy are as follows:**
  - Restoration of hemodynamic stability and intravascular volume by fluid replacement.
  - Correction of electrolyte abnormalities.
  - Gradual correction of hyperglycemia and hyperosmolarity with fluid replacement and insulin therapy.
  - Detection and treatment of underlying disease states and precipitating causes. However, such efforts should not delay fluid replacement and insulin therapy.
- **Initial treatment** can make a difference in the frequency of complications and outcome. Therapy must be individualized on the basis of the degree of dehydration and underlying cause (sepsis and renal and cardiac function). Rapid vein access and urinary catheterization are essential.

- **Restoring hemodynamic stability** is the first aim. Restoration of intravascular volume should be followed by correction of total body water deficit. Compared to DKA, patients with NKHS may require as much as 10 to 12 L of positive fluid balance over 24 to 72 hours to restore total deficits.
- **Electrolyte management**
  - Although the potassium level may be initially normal or even high, all patients with NKHS are potassium depleted. Rehydration and insulin therapy usually result in hypokalemia, and this should be corrected.
  - If the initial potassium levels are low, replacement should begin immediately after urine output is ensured. Lactic acidosis requiring bicarbonate therapy may develop as a complication of NKHS or metformin therapy.
- **Insulin therapy.** Insulin plays a secondary role in the initial management of NKHS, and fluid therapy always should precede insulin administration.
  - In patients with marked hyperglycemia (>600 mg/dL), regular insulin, 5 to 10 units IV, should be given immediately, followed by continuous infusion of 0.1 to 0.15 units/kg/hr. Lower doses of a regular insulin bolus can be used for less severe hyperglycemia.
  - Once plasma glucose decreases to 250 to 300 mg/dL, insulin infusion can be decreased to 1 to 2 units/hr and 5% dextrose should be added to the IV fluids. After full rehydration and clinical recovery, regular insulin can be given SC and patients can thereafter resume their usual diabetes therapy.
- **Underlying illness.** Detection and treatment of any underlying predisposing illness are critical in the treatment of NKHS. Antibiotics should be administered early, after appropriate cultures, in patients in whom infection is known or suspected as a precipitant to a HHS. A high index of suspicion should be maintained for underlying pancreatitis, GI bleeding, renal failure, and thromboembolic events, especially acute MI.

COMPLICATIONS

Complications of NKHS include thromboembolic events (cerebral and MI, mesenteric thrombosis, pulmonary embolism, and disseminated intravascular coagulation), cerebral edema, adult respiratory distress syndrome, and rhabdomyolysis.

MONITORING/FOLLOW-UP

- **Monitoring of therapy.** Use of a flowchart is helpful for tracking clinical data and laboratory results.
- Initially, BG levels should be monitored every 30 to 60 minutes and serum electrolyte levels every 1 to 2 hours; frequency of monitoring can be decreased during recovery.
- Neurologic status must be reassessed frequently; persistent lethargy or altered mentation indicates inadequate therapy. On the other hand, relapse after initial improvement in mental status suggests too-rapid correction of serum osmolarity.

CHRONIC COMPLICATIONS OF DIABETES MELLITUS

Prevention of long-term complications is one of the main goals of diabetes management. Appropriate treatment of established complications may delay their progression and improve quality of life.

Microvascular complications include diabetic retinopathy, nephropathy, and neuropathy. These complications are directly related to hyperglycemia. Tight glycemic control has been shown to reduce the development and progression of these complications.

Diabetic Retinopathy

GENERAL PRINCIPLES

Classification

- Diabetic retinopathy (DR) is classified as background retinopathy (microaneurysms, retinal infarcts or hemorrhage) with or without *macular edema* and proliferative retinopathy. Background retinopathy is also known as pre-proliferative retinopathy.
- Other ocular abnormalities associated with diabetes include cataract formation, dyskinetic pupils, glaucoma, optic neuropathy, extraocular muscle paresis, floaters, and fluctuating visual acuity. The latter may be related to changes in BG levels.
- The presence of floaters may be indicative of preretinal or vitreous hemorrhage; immediate referral for ophthalmologic evaluation is warranted.

Epidemiology

DR is diagnosed in 80% and 90% of patients with T1DM after 10 and 15 years of diagnosis, respectively. DR is less frequent in T2DM, but maculopathy may be more severe. DR is the leading cause of vision loss in adults younger than 65 years.

DIAGNOSIS

Annual examination by an ophthalmologist is recommended at the time of diagnosis of all T2DM patients and at the beginning at puberty or 3 to 5 years after diagnosis for patients with T1DM. Dilated eye examination should be repeated annually by an optometrist or ophthalmologist since progressive DR can be completely asymptomatic until sudden loss of vision occurs. Early detection of DR is critical as therapy is more effective before severe maculopathy or proliferation develops. In general, any diabetic with visual symptoms or abnormalities should be referred for ophthalmologic evaluation.

TREATMENT

Background retinopathy usually is not associated with loss of vision and may remain stable for years. However, the development of macular edema or proliferative retinopathy (particularly new vessels near the optic disk) requires elective laser photocoagulation therapy to preserve vision. Vitrectomy is indicated for patients with vitreous hemorrhage or retinal detachment.

Diabetic Nephropathy

GENERAL PRINCIPLES

Epidemiology

Approximately 25% to 45% of patients with T1DM develop clinically evident diabetic nephropathy during their lifetime, and this is the leading cause of end-stage renal disease (ESRD) (*Med Clin North Am 2004;88:1001–1036*). The risk of nephropathy seems to be equivalent in the two types of diabetes (*Diabetes 1995;44:739–743*).

Risk Factors

Microalbuminuria precedes overt proteinuria (>300 mg of albumin/d) by several years in T1DM and T2DM. The mean duration from diagnosis of type 1 diabetes to the development of overt proteinuria is 17 years and the time from the occurrence of proteinuria to ESRD averages 5 years. In T2DM, microalbuminuria can be present at the time of diagnosis.

Prevention

Screening for microalbuminuria is mandatory because patients with nephropathy are often asymptomatic and because a number of effective intervention strategies can slow disease progression. Annual screening should be performed in type 1 diabetic patients who have had diabetes for >5 years and all type 2 diabetic patients starting at diagnosis.

Associated Conditions

- Patients with proteinuria (albumin/creatinine > 300 mg/g) are at higher risk for anemia due to loss of transferrin and poor production of erythropoietin and should be screened at any stage of CKD and treated.
- **Patients with CKD are at higher risk for CV disease and mortality**, so management of other CV risk factors is particularly important in this group of patients.

DIAGNOSIS

Diagnostic Testing

Laboratories
- Measurement of the microalbumin-to-creatinine ratio (normal, <30 mg of albumin/g of creatinine) in a random urine sample is recommended for screening. At least two to three measurements within a 6-month period should be performed to establish the diagnosis (*Diabetes Care 2003;26:S94–S98*).
- Measurement of serum creatinine and serum urea nitrogen should be performed annually, along with calculation of the eGFR. Patients with diabetes may have reduced kidney function without manifesting albumin in their urine. Testing and treatment of associated disorders such as anemia, secondary hyperparathyroidism, hyperkalemia, and acid–base disturbances should begin when the eGFR is <60 mL/min/1.73 m^2, or stage 3 CKD (see Chapter 10, Renal Diseases).

TREATMENT

Intensive control of both diabetes and hypertension is important to reduce the rate of progression of CKD due to diabetes. Achieving the blood pressure target of <130/80 mm Hg is recommended for all patients with diabetes, especially those with evidence of CKD.

Medications

First Line
- Antihypertensive treatment with ACE inhibitor or ARB drugs is recommended as first-line therapy for all patients with diabetes and hypertension. These agents have

been shown to reduce progression of both retinopathy and nephropathy and may be considered in patients with normal blood pressure or prehypertension.

- In type 2 diabetic patients with hypertension, creatinine > 1.5 mg/dL, and macroal-buminuria, angiotensin II receptor blockers (ARBs) delay progression of nephropathy.

Second Line
Diuretics are considered second line, followed by calcium channel blockers, β-blockers, or centrally acting agents (*Diabetes Care 2004;27:S79–S83*).

Lifestyle/Risk Modification

- Dietary protein restriction may be beneficial in some patients to slow progression.
- Avoidance of renal toxins is important for preservation of kidney function.

Diabetic Neuropathy

GENERAL PRINCIPLES

Classification

Diabetic neuropathy can be classified in (a) subclinical neuropathy, determined by abnormalities in electrodiagnostic and quantitative sensory testing; (b) diffuse clinical neuropathy with distal symmetric sensorimotor and autonomic syndromes; and (c) focal syndromes.

Epidemiology

Peripheral diabetic neuropathy (PDN) is the most common neuropathy in developed countries and accounts for more hospitalizations than all the other diabetic complications combined. Sensorimotor diabetic peripheral polyneuropathy is a major risk factor for foot trauma, ulceration, and Charcot arthropathy and is responsible for 50% to 75% of nontraumatic amputations (*Med Clin N Am 2004;88:947–999*).

Prevention

- Sensation in the lower extremities should be documented at least annually, using a combination of modalities such as a light-touch monofilament, tuning fork (frequency of 128 Hz), pinprick, or temperature.
- Foot examination should be conducted at least annually to evaluate the presence of musculoskeletal deformities, skin changes, and pulses, in addition to the sensory examination.

TREATMENT

- **Painful peripheral neuropathy** responds variably to treatment with tricyclic antidepressants (e.g., amitriptyline, 10 to 150 mg PO at bedtime), topical capsaicin (0.075% cream), or anticonvulsants (e.g., carbamazepine 100 to 400 mg PO bid, gabapentin 900 to 3600 mg/d, or pregabalin 50 to 300 mg should be 150 to 300 mg/d). Patients should be warned about adverse effects, including sedation and anticholinergic symptoms (tricyclics), burning sensation (capsaicin), and blood dyscrasias (carbamazepine). α-Lipoic acid (600 mg bid) and high-dose thiamine (50 to 100 mg tid) have been tested in early PDN.

- **Orthostatic hypotension** is a manifestation of autonomic neuropathy, but common etiologies (e.g., dehydration, anemia, medications) should be excluded. Treatment is symptomatic: Postural maneuvers, use of compressive garments (e.g., Jobst stockings), and intravascular expansion using sodium chloride 1 to 4 g PO qid and fludrocortisone 0.1 to 0.3 mg PO daily. Hypokalemia, supine hypertension, and CHF are some adverse effects of fludrocortisone.
- **Intractable nausea and vomiting** in diabetes are manifestations of impaired GI motility from autonomic neuropathy. **Surveillance for DKA** is warranted in insulin-treated patients with nausea and vomiting because interruption of insulin therapy is widespread among such patients. Other causes of nausea and vomiting should be excluded.
  - **Management of diabetic gastroenteropathy** can be challenging. Frequent, small meals (six to eight per day) of soft consistency that are low in fat and fiber provide relief for some patients. Parenteral nutrition may become necessary in some individuals. Improvement in glycemic control also is beneficial because hyperglycemia delays gastric emptying.
  - **Pharmacologic therapy** includes the prokinetic agent metoclopramide, 10 to 20 mg PO (or as a suppository) before meals and at bedtime, and erythromycin, 125 to 500 mg PO qid. Extrapyramidal side effects (tremor and tardive dyskinesia) from the antidopaminergic actions of metoclopramide may limit therapy.
  - **Cyclical vomiting** that is unrelated to a GI motility disorder or other clear etiology may also occur in diabetic patients and appears to respond to amitriptyline 25 to 50 mg PO at bedtime.
- **Diabetic cystopathy,** or bladder dysfunction, results from impaired autonomic control of detrusor muscle and sphincteric function. Manifestations include urgency, dribbling, incomplete emptying, overflow incontinence, and urinary retention. Recurrent urinary tract infections are common in patients with residual urine. Treatment with bethanechol 10 mg tid or intermittent self-catheterization may be required to relieve retention.
- **Chronic, persistent diarrhea** in patients with diabetes is probably multifactorial. Celiac disease and inflammatory bowel diseases should be ruled out, particularly in patients with T1DM. Pancreatic mass is reduced with longstanding diabetes, so the possibility of exocrine pancreatic dysfunction should be considered. Bacterial overgrowth has been considered as an etiology but is difficult to diagnose. Empiric treatment with broad-spectrum antibiotics (e.g., azithromycin, tetracycline, cephalosporins) along with metronidazole may be beneficial. Antifungal agents and probiotic replacement can be tried. If diarrhea persists, loperamide or octreotide 50 to 75 mg SC bid can be effective in patients with intractable diarrhea.

MACROVASCULAR COMPLICATIONS OF DM

Coronary Heart Disease

GENERAL PRINCIPLES

- Coronary heart disease (CHD), stroke, and peripheral vascular disease (PVD) are responsible for 80% of deaths in persons with diabetes (*Lancet 1997;350 (Suppl 1):SI23–SI28*). (see Chapter 3, Preventative Cardiology and Ischemic Heart Disease)

- **CAD** occurs at a younger age and may have atypical clinical presentations in patients with diabetes (*Lancet 1997;350(Suppl 1):S123–S128*).
  - MI carries a worse prognosis, and angioplasty gives less satisfactory results in diabetic patients.
  - Persons with diabetes have an increased risk of ischemic and nonischemic heart failure and sudden death.

Risk Factors

Risk factors for macrovascular disease that are common in persons with diabetes include insulin resistance, hyperglycemia, microalbuminuria, hypertension, hyperlipidemia, cigarette smoking, and obesity.

Prevention

- Cardiovascular risk factors should be assessed at least annually and treated aggressively (see treatment goals in the following text). ECG should be obtained yearly, and there should be a low threshold for ordering stress tests.
- Screening with cardiac stress test has not been shown to reduce mortality or events in asymptomatic patients with T2DM. It has been recommended in patients with a history of peripheral or carotid occlusive disease, sedentary lifestyle, age > 35 years, and who plan to begin a vigorous exercise program, or in patients with two or more of the following CHD risk factors: dyslipidemia, hypertension, smoking, a positive family history of premature coronary disease, and the presence of micro- or macroalbuminuria (*Diabetes Care* 1994;17:1514–1522).
- Aspirin 81 to 325 mg/d is of proven benefit in secondary prevention of MI or stroke in diabetic patients.

TREATMENT

- Aggressive risk factor reduction lowers the risk of both micro- and macrovascular complications in patients with diabetes.
  - Glycemic control should be optimized to A_{1C} < 7% and as close to normal as possible in the first few years after diagnosis. Patients with long-standing T2DM may have increased risk of mortality with very tight glycemic control (A_{1C} < 6.5%), particularly if multiple agents are required and the risk of hypoglycemia increases.
  - Hypertension should be controlled to a target blood pressure of <130/80 mm Hg (or < 125/75 mm Hg in patients with proteinuria).
  - Hyperlipidemia should be treated appropriately, with a target LDL cholesterol level of <100 mg/dL, or < 70 mg/dL in patients with known CHD. HDL cholesterol levels of >50 mg/dL and triglyceride levels of <150 mg/dL should be achieved.
  - Cigarette smoking should be actively discouraged, and weight loss should be promoted in obese patients.
- **Management of diabetes after acute MI**
  - Hyperglycemia (glucose > 110 mg/dL), with or without a history of diabetes, is an independent predictor of in-hospital mortality and CHF in patients admitted for acute MI (*Lancet 2000;355:773–778*). However, the results of the studies that investigated tight glucose control with insulin in the setting of acute MI in type 2 diabetic patients are inconclusive (*BMJ 1997;314:1512–1515, J Am Coll Cardiol*

1995;26:57–65, Eur Heart J 2005;26:650–661). Nevertheless, given the consistent epidemiologic association, it is reasonable to expect that glucose-lowering effects in acute conditions could lead to clinical benefit.

Peripheral Vascular Disease

GENERAL PRINCIPLES

Risk Factors

Diabetes and smoking are the strongest risk factors for PVD. In diabetic patients, the risk of PVD is increased by age, duration of diabetes, and presence of peripheral neuropathy. PVD is a marker for systemic vascular disease involving coronary, cerebral, and renal vessels. Diabetic patients with PVD have increased risk for subsequent MI or stroke regardless of the PVD symptoms.

DIAGNOSIS

Clinical Presentation

Symptoms of PVD include intermittent claudication, rest pain, tissue loss, and gangrene, but most of the patients are asymptomatic due to concomitant neuropathy.

Physical Examination

Physical examination findings including diminished pulses, dependent rubor, pallor on elevation, absence of hair growth, dystrophic toenails, and cool, dry, fissured skin are signs of vascular insufficiency.

Diagnostic Testing

- The ankle-to-brachial index (ABI) defined as the ratio of the systolic blood pressure in the ankle divided by the systolic blood pressure at the arm is the best initial diagnostic test. An ABI < 0.9 by a handheld, 5- to 10-MHz Doppler probe has a 95% sensitivity for detecting angiogram-positive PVD (*Int J Epidemiol 1988;17:248–254*).
- Screening ABI should be performed in (a) diabetic patients older than 50 years, (b) diabetic patients younger than 50 years who have other PVD risk factors (e.g., smoking, hypertension, hyperlipidemia, or duration of diabetes 10 years) (*Diabetes Care 2003;26:3333–3341*), and (c) patients with symptoms of PVD.

TREATMENT

- Risk factors should be controlled, with similar goals described for CAD (see in the previous text).
- Antiplatelets agents such clopidogrel (75 mg/d) have additional benefits when compared with aspirin in diabetic patients with PVD (*Diabetes Care 2003;26:3333–3341*).
- Therapy for intermittent claudication could also benefit from exercise rehabilitation and cilostazol (100 mg bid). This medication is contraindicated in patients with CHF.

MISCELLANEOUS COMPLICATIONS

Erectile Dysfunction

GENERAL PRINCIPLES

Epidemiology

It is estimated that 40% to 60% of men with diabetes have erectile dysfunction (ED), and the prevalence varies depending on the age of the patient and duration of diabetes. In addition to increasing age, ED is associated with smoking, poor glycemic control, low HDL, neuropathy, and retinopathy.

Etiology

ED in diabetic patients is multifactorial. It can result from nerve damage, impaired blood flow (vascular insufficiency), adverse drug effects, low testosterone, psychological factors, or a combination of these etiologies.

DIAGNOSIS

Diagnostic Testing

Laboratories

Evaluation should include a measurement of total or bioavailable testosterone. If the total testosterone is <300 mg/dL, the test should be repeated in the morning (does not have to be fasting, but a blood draw before 9:00 AM is appropriate) along with a prolactin and prostate-specific antigen (PSA).

TREATMENT

- If testosterone is low, and both PSA and prostate examination are normal, then testosterone replacement can be tried with either testosterone enanthate, 200 mg every 2 to 3 weeks, or a topical gel (AndroGel or Testim).
- A trial of phosphodiesterase type 5 inhibitors (sildenafil, tadalafil, vardenafil) is often warranted in addition to hormonal correction (if indicated). Typical doses include sildenafil 50 to 100 mg or vardenafil 10 mg 1 hour prior to sexual activity and tadalafil 10 mg/d prior to sexual activity. Referral to urology specialist should be considered if the problem persists. Cardiovascular status should be considered before starting these agents. **This drug class should not be used concurrently with nitrates** to prevent severe and potentially fatal hypotensive reactions. Macular edema should also be ruled out before starting these agents.

Diabetic Foot Ulcers

GENERAL PRINCIPLES

Epidemiology

The prevalence of foot ulcers is 4% to 10% and the lifetime incidence is as high as 25% (*JAMA 2005;293:217–228*).

Etiology

Causative factors include peripheral sensory neuropathy, excessive plantar pressure, and repetitive trauma. Vascular insufficiency, poor healing, and polymicrobial infection are major contributors to ulcer formation. Poor footwear can add to the risk of ulceration.

Prevention

- **Screening to identify patients at risk for ulcers** includes detection of loss of protective sensation by monofilament (see discussion on peripheral neuropathy) and PVD.
- Patients with prior foot ulcers are at high risk for recurrence and may need ongoing specialized care and footwear.

TREATMENT

- Poorly managed foot ulcers may result in limb loss from amputation. Patient education should emphasize the following prevention: daily foot examination, application of moisturizing lotion, use of proper footwear, and early treatment of tinea and other minor foot infections. Patients should use caution with self-pedicure and seek assistance with nail care if body habitus, limited vision, or thick toenails precludes self-care.
- The exposed feet should be inspected and palpated at every patient encounter; significant findings, such as calluses, hammertoes or other deformities, infections, and soft tissue lesions, should be evaluated.
- Diabetic foot infections should be treated aggressively. Proper management includes a multidisciplinary approach that includes orthopedic surgeons, specialized nursing care, and close monitoring. Evaluation of PVD and referral to a vascular specialist should be considered as an integral part of the management of food ulcers. The presence of deep infection with abscess, cellulitis, gangrene, or osteomyelitis is an indication for hospitalization and prompt surgical drainage. Acute treatment of foot infections is dependent on severity, as outlined in the following text.
- **Mild to moderate cellulitis.** Rest, elevation of the affected foot and relief of pressure are essential components of treatment and should be initiated at first presentation. In localized cellulitis and new ulcers, *Staphylococcus aureus* and streptococci are the most frequent pathogens. Therapy with oral dicloxacillin, first-generation cephalosporin, amoxicillin/clavulanate, or clindamycin is recommended. IV antibiotics may be necessary due if the cellulitis does not respond immediately to oral antibiotics.
- **Moderate to severe cellulitis.** This type of involvement requires IV therapy and admission to the hospital. Consultation for debridement and aerobic and anaerobic cultures are necessary when necrotic tissue is present. IV oxacillin/nafcillin, a first-generation IV cephalosporin, ampicillin/sulbactam, clindamycin, and vancomycin are options for therapy. Antibiotic coverage should subsequently be tailored according to the clinical response of the patient, culture results, and sensitivity testing.
- **Moderate to severe cellulitis with ischemia or significant local necrosis.** It is important to determine the presence of bone involvement and PVD since failure to diagnose osteomyelitis and ischemia often results in failure of wound healing.
  - Bone involvement is present if bone is seen at the base of the ulcer or is easily detected by gentle probing with a blunt sterile probe. Radiographs are not very sensitive for diagnosis and leukocyte scanning or magnetic resonance imaging offers better specificity.

- Presence of PVD is suspected by the absence of pedal pulses or decreased capillary filling.
- IV antibiotics, bed rest, surgical debridement, culture obtained from the base of the ulcer, and bone culture help direct antibiotic therapy.
- Ampicillin/sulbactam and ticarcillin/clavulanate are first-line agents; piperacillin/tazobactam, clindamycin plus ciprofloxacin, ceftazidime, cefepime, cefotaxime, or ceftriaxone plus metronidazole are good alternatives for initial therapy.
- In the presence of osteomyelitis, 6 to 12 weeks of IV antibiotic therapy is recommended. Ulcers with localized or generalized gangrene require surgical amputation, often limited to a toe or metarsal head.

Hypoglycemia

GENERAL PRINCIPLES

Classification

Hypoglycemia is uncommon in patients not treated for diabetes. Iatrogenic factors usually account for hypoglycemia in the setting of diabetes, whereas hypoglycemia in the nondiabetic population could be classified as fasting or postprandial hypoglycemia.

- **Iatrogenic hypoglycemia** complicates therapy with insulin or SFUs and is a limiting factor to achieve glycemic control during intensive therapy in patients with DM (*Diabetes Care 2003;26:1902–1912*).

Risk Factors

Hypoglycemia resulting from too intensive diabetes therapies may increase the risk of mortality in older patients with a long duration of diabetes and should be avoided.

- Risk factors for iatrogenic hypoglycemia include skipped or insufficient meals, unaccustomed physical exertion, misguided therapy, alcohol ingestion, and drug overdose.
- Recurrent episodes of hypoglycemia impair recognition of hypoglycemic symptoms, thereby increasing the risk for severe hypoglycemia (hypoglycemia unawareness).
- Hypoglycemia unawareness results from defective glucose counterregulation with blunting of autonomic symptoms and counterregulatory hormone secretion during hypoglycemia. Seizures or coma may develop in such patients without the usual warning symptoms of hypoglycemia.
- Hypoglycemia unrelated to diabetes therapy is an infrequent problem in general medical practice.

DIAGNOSIS

Clinical Presentation

- Hypoglycemia is a clinical syndrome in which low serum (or plasma) glucose levels lead to symptoms of sympathetic–adrenal activation (sweating, anxiety, tremor, nausea, palpitations, and tachycardia) from increased secretion of counterregulatory hormones (e.g., epinephrine).
- Neuroglycopenia occurs as the glucose levels decrease further (fatigue, dizziness, headache, visual disturbances, drowsiness, difficulty speaking, inability to concentrate, abnormal behavior, confusion, and ultimately loss of consciousness or seizures).

Differential Diagnosis

Plasma or capillary BG values should be obtained, whenever feasible, to confirm hypoglycemia.

- Any patient with a serum glucose concentration of <60 mg/dL should be suspected of having a hypoglycemic disorder, and further evaluation is required if the value is <50 mg/dL.
- Absence of symptoms with these levels of glucose suggests the possibility of artifactual hypoglycemia. These levels are usually accompanied by symptoms of hypoglycemia. Detailed evaluation is usually required in a healthy-appearing patient, whereas hypoglycemia may be readily recognized as part of the underlying illness in a sick patient (*N Engl J Med 1986;315:1245–1250*). Major categories include fasting and postprandial hypoglycemia.
- **Fasting hypoglycemia** can be caused by inappropriate insulin secretion (e.g., insulinoma), alcohol abuse, severe hepatic or renal insufficiency, hypopituitarism, glucocorticoid deficiency, or surreptitious injection of insulin or ingestion of an SFU.
  - These patients present with neuroglycopenic symptoms but episodic autonomic symptoms may be present. Occasionally, patients with recurrent seizures, dementia, and bizarre behavior are referred for neuropsychiatric evaluation, which may delay timely diagnosis of hypoglycemia.
  - **Definitive diagnosis** of fasting hypoglycemia requires hourly BG monitoring during a supervised fast lasting up to 72 hours and measurement of plasma insulin, C-peptide, and SFU metabolites if hypoglycemia (<50 mg/dL) is documented. Patients who develop hypoglycemia and have measurable plasma insulin and C-peptide levels without SFU metabolites require further evaluation for an insulinoma.
- **Postprandial hypoglycemia** often is suspected, but seldom proven, in patients with vague symptoms that occur 1 or more hours after meals.
  - **Alimentary hypoglycemia** should be considered in patients with a history of partial gastrectomy or intestinal resection in whom recurrent symptoms develop 1 to 2 hours after eating. The mechanism is thought to be related to too-rapid glucose absorption, resulting in a robust insulin response. These symptoms should be distinguished from dumping syndrome, which is not associated with hypoglycemia and occurs in the first hour after food intake. Thus, frequent small meals with reduced carbohydrate content may ameliorate symptoms.
  - **Functional hypoglycemia.** Symptoms that are possibly suggestive of hypoglycemia, which may or may not be confirmed by plasma glucose measurement, occur in some patients who have not undergone GI surgery. This condition is referred to as "functional hypoglycemia." The symptoms tend to develop 3 to 5 hours after meals. Current evaluation and management of functional hypoglycemia are imprecise; some patients show evidence of IGT and may respond to dietary therapy.

TREATMENT

Isolated episodes of mild hypoglycemia may not require specific intervention. Recurrent episodes require a review of lifestyle factors; adjustments may be indicated in the content, timing, and distribution of meals, as well as medication dosage and timing. Severe hypoglycemia is an indication for supervised treatment.

- **Readily absorbable carbohydrates** (e.g., glucose and sugar-containing beverages) can be administered orally to conscious patients for rapid effect. Alternatively, milk, candy bars, fruit, cheese, and crackers may be used in some patients with mild hypoglycemia. Hypoglycemia associated with acarbose or miglitol therapy should preferentially be treated with glucose. Glucose tablets and carbohydrate supplies should be readily available to patients with DM at all times.

- **IV dextrose** is indicated for severe hypoglycemia, in patients with altered consciousness, and during restriction of oral intake. An initial bolus, 20 to 50 mL of 50% dextrose, should be given immediately, followed by infusion of D5W (or D10W) to maintain BG level above 100 mg/dL. Prolonged IV dextrose infusion and close observation is warranted in SFU overdose, in the elderly, and in patients with defective counterregulation.

- **Glucagon**, 1 mg IM (or SC), is an effective initial therapy for severe hypoglycemia in patients unable to receive oral intake or in whom an IV access cannot be secured immediately. Vomiting is a frequent side effect and therefore care should be taken to prevent the risk of aspiration. A glucagon kit should be available to patients with a history of severe hypoglycemia; family members and roommates should be instructed in its proper use.

PATIENT EDUCATION

- **Education** regarding etiologies of hypoglycemia, preventive measures, and appropriate adjustments to medication, diet, and exercise regimens are essential tasks to be addressed during hospitalization for severe hypoglycemia.

- **Hypoglycemia unawareness** can develop in patients who are undergoing intensive diabetes therapy. These patients should be encouraged to monitor their BG levels frequently and take timely measures to correct low values (<60 mg/dL). In patients with very tightly controlled diabetes, slight relaxation in glycemic control and scrupulous avoidance of hypoglycemia may restore the lost warning symptoms.

DISORDERS OF THE THYROID GLAND

Evaluation of Thyroid Function

GENERAL PRINCIPLES

The major hormone secreted by the thyroid is **thyroxine (T_4),** which is converted by deiodinases in many tissues to the more potent **triiodothyronine (T_3)**. Both are bound reversibly to plasma proteins, primarily **thyroxine-binding globulin (TBG).** Only the free (unbound) fraction enters cells and produces biological effects. T_4 secretion is stimulated **by thyroid-stimulating hormone (TSH).** In turn, TSH secretion is inhibited by T_4, forming a negative feedback loop that keeps free T_4 levels within a narrow normal range. Diagnosis of thyroid disease is based on clinical findings, palpation of the thyroid, and measurement of plasma TSH and thyroid hormones (*Endocrinol Metab Clin North Am 2007;36:579*).

DIAGNOSIS

Clinical Presentation
Physical Examination
Thyroid palpation determines the size and consistency of the thyroid and the presence of nodules, tenderness, or a thrill.

Diagnostic Testing
Laboratories
- **Plasma TSH is the initial test of choice in most patients with suspected thyroid disease,** except when thyroid function is not in a steady state. TSH levels are elevated in very mild primary hypothyroidism and are suppressed to <0.1 microunits/mL in very mild hyperthyroidism. Thus, **a normal plasma TSH level excludes hyperthyroidism and primary hypothyroidism.** Because even slight changes in thyroid hormone levels affect TSH secretion, **abnormal TSH levels are not specific for clinically important thyroid disease.** Changes in plasma TSH lag behind changes in plasma T_4, and TSH levels may be misleading when plasma T_4 levels are changing rapidly, as during treatment of hyperthyroidism.
  - **Plasma TSH is mildly elevated** (up to 20 microunits/mL) in some euthyroid patients with **nonthyroidal illnesses** and in mild (or subclinical) hypothyroidism.
  - **TSH levels may be suppressed to <0.1 microunits/mL** in severe **nonthyroidal illness,** in mild (or subclinical) hyperthyroidism, and during treatment with dopamine or high doses of glucocorticoids. Also, TSH levels remain <0.1 microunits/mL for some time after hyperthyroidism is corrected.
  - **TSH levels are usually within the reference range in secondary hypothyroidism** and are not useful for detection of this rare form of hypothyroidism.

Table 1	Effects of Drugs on Thyroid Function Tests
Effect	**Drug**
Decreased free and total T$_4$	
True hypothyroidism (TSH elevated)	Iodine (amiodarone, radiographic contrast)
	Lithium
Inhibition of TSH secretion	Glucocorticoids
	Dopamine
Multiple mechanisms (TSH normal)	Phenytoin
Decreased total T$_4$ only	
Decreased TBG (TSH normal)	Androgens
Inhibition of T$_4$ binding to TBG (TSH normal)	Furosemide (high doses)
	Salicylates
Increased free and total T$_4$	
True hyperthyroidism (TSH < 0.1 microunits/mL)	Iodine (amiodarone, radiographic contrast)
Inhibited T$_4$ to T$_3$ conversion (TSH normal)	Amiodarone
Increased free T$_4$ only	
Displacement of T$_4$ from TBG in vitro (TSH normal)	Heparin, low-molecular-weight heparin
Increased total T$_4$ only	
Increased TBG (TSH normal)	Estrogens, tamoxifen

T$_3$, triiodothyronine; T$_4$, thyroxine; TBG, thyroxine-binding globulin; TSH, thyroid-stimulating hormone.

- **Plasma free T$_4$** confirms the diagnosis and assesses the severity of hyperthyroidism when plasma TSH is <0.1 microunits/mL. It is also used to diagnose secondary hypothyroidism and adjust thyroxine therapy in patients with pituitary disease. Most laboratories measure free T$_4$ by analog immunoassays. Total T$_4$ assays are less reliable and should not be used, except when free T$_4$ is artifactually elevated by heparin treatment (Table 1).
  - **Free T$_4$ measured by equilibrium dialysis** is the most reliable measure of clinical thyroid status, but results seldom are rapidly available. It is needed only in rare cases in which the diagnosis is not clear from measurement of plasma TSH and free T$_4$ by analog immunoassay.
- **Effect of nonthyroidal illness on thyroid function tests** (*Endocrinol Metab Clin North Am 2007;36:657*). Many illnesses alter thyroid tests without causing true thyroid dysfunction (the nonthyroidal illness or euthyroid sick syndrome). These changes must be recognized to avoid mistaken diagnosis and therapy.
  - **The low T$_3$ syndrome** occurs in many illnesses, during starvation, and after trauma or surgery. Conversion of T$_4$ to T$_3$ is decreased, and plasma T$_3$ levels are low. Plasma free T$_4$ and TSH levels are normal. This may be an adaptive response to illness, and thyroid hormone therapy is not beneficial.
  - **The low T$_4$ syndrome** occurs in severe illness. Plasma total T$_4$ levels fall due to decreased levels of TBG and perhaps due to inhibition of T$_4$ binding to TBG. **Plasma free T$_4$ measured by equilibrium dialysis usually remains normal.**

However, when measured by commonly available analog immunoassays, free T_4 may be low. **TSH levels decrease early in severe illness,** sometimes to <0.1 microunits/mL. **During recovery, they rise, sometimes to levels higher than the normal range** (although rarely >20 microunits/mL).

- Some drugs affect thyroid function tests (Table 1). Iodine-containing drugs (**amiodarone** and radiographic contrast media) may cause hyperthyroidism or hypothyroidism in susceptible patients. Other drugs alter thyroid function tests, especially plasma total T_4, without causing true thyroid dysfunction. In general, plasma TSH levels are a reliable guide to determine whether true hyperthyroidism or hypothyroidism is present.

Hypothyroidism

GENERAL PRINCIPLES

Etiology

- **Primary hypothyroidism** (due to disease of the thyroid itself) accounts for >90% of cases.
- **Chronic lymphocytic thyroiditis (Hashimoto's disease)** is the most common cause and may be associated with Addison's disease and other endocrine deficits. Its prevalence is greater in women and increases with age.
- **Iatrogenic hypothyroidism** due to thyroidectomy or radioactive iodine (RAI, ^{131}I) therapy is also common.
- Transient hypothyroidism occurs in postpartum thyroiditis and subacute thyroiditis, usually after a period of hyperthyroidism.
- **Drugs that may cause hypothyroidism** include iodine-containing drugs, lithium, interferon-a, interleukin-2, and thalidomide.
- Secondary hypothyroidism due to TSH deficiency is uncommon but may occur in any disorder of the pituitary or hypothalamus. However, it rarely occurs without other evidence of pituitary disease.

DIAGNOSIS

Clinical Presentation

Most symptoms of hypothyroidism are nonspecific and develop gradually. They include cold intolerance, fatigue, somnolence, poor memory, constipation, menorrhagia, myalgias, and hoarseness.

History

Hypothyroidism is readily treatable and should be suspected in any patient with compatible symptoms, especially in the presence of a diffuse goiter or a history of RAI therapy or thyroid surgery.

Physical Examination

Signs include slow tendon reflex relaxation, bradycardia, facial and periorbital edema, dry skin, and nonpitting edema (myxedema). Mild weight gain may occur, but hypothyroidism does not cause marked obesity. Rare manifestations include hypoventilation, pericardial or pleural effusions, deafness, and carpal tunnel syndrome.

Diagnostic Testing

Laboratories

- Laboratory findings may include hyponatremia and elevated plasma levels of cholesterol, triglycerides, and creatine kinase.
- In suspected primary hypothyroidism, plasma TSH is the best initial test.
  - A normal value excludes primary hypothyroidism, and a markedly elevated value (>20 microunits/mL) confirms the diagnosis.
  - Mild elevation of plasma TSH (<20 microunits/mL) may be due to nonthyroidal illness, but usually indicates **mild (or subclinical) primary hypothyroidism,** in which thyroid function is impaired but increased secretion of TSH maintains plasma free T_4 levels within the reference range. These patients may have nonspecific symptoms that are compatible with hypothyroidism and a mild increase in serum cholesterol and low-density lipoprotein cholesterol. They develop clinical hypothyroidism at a rate of 2.5% per year.
- If secondary hypothyroidism is suspected because of evidence of pituitary disease, plasma free T_4 should be measured.
  - Plasma TSH levels are usually within the reference range in secondary hypothyroidism and cannot be used alone to make this diagnosis. Patients with secondary hypothyroidism should be evaluated for other pituitary hormone deficits and for a mass lesion of the pituitary or hypothalamus (see Disorders of Anterior Pituitary Gland Dysfunction).
- **In severe nonthyroidal illness,** the diagnosis of hypothyroidism may be difficult. Plasma total T_4 and free T_4 measured by routine assays may be low.
  - **Plasma TSH is the best initial diagnostic test.** A normal TSH value is strong evidence that the patient is euthyroid, except when there is evidence of pituitary or hypothalamic disease or in patients treated with dopamine or high doses of glucocorticoids. Marked elevation of plasma TSH (>20 microunits/mL) establishes the diagnosis of primary hypothyroidism.
  - Moderate elevations of plasma TSH (<20 microunits/mL) may occur in euthyroid patients with nonthyroidal illness and are not specific for hypothyroidism. Plasma free T_4 should be measured if TSH is moderately elevated, or if secondary hypothyroidism is suspected, and patients should be treated for hypothyroidism if plasma free T_4 is low. Thyroid function in these patients should be reevaluated after recovery from illness.

Electrocardiography

The electrocardiogram (ECG) may show low voltage and T-wave abnormalities.

TREATMENT

Medications

Thyroxine is the drug of choice. The average replacement dose is 1.6 mcg/kg PO daily, and most patients require doses between 75 and 150 mcg/d. In elderly patients, the average replacement dose is lower. The need for lifelong treatment should be emphasized. Thyroxine should be taken 30 minutes before a meal, since some foods interfere with its absorption, and should not be taken with medications that affect its absorption (see below).

- **Initiation of therapy.** Young and middle-aged adults should be started on 100 mcg/ daily. This regimen gradually corrects hypothyroidism, as several weeks are required to reach steady-state plasma levels of T_4. Symptoms begin to improve within a few weeks. In otherwise healthy elderly patients, the initial dose should be 50 mcg/daily. Patients with cardiac disease should be started on 25 to 50 mcg/daily and monitored carefully for exacerbation of cardiac symptoms.

- **Dose adjustment and follow-up.**
  - **In primary hypothyroidism, the goal of therapy is to maintain plasma TSH within the normal range.** Plasma TSH should be measured 6 to 8 weeks after initiation of therapy. The dose of thyroxine should then be adjusted in 12- to 25-mcg increments at intervals of 6 to 8 weeks until plasma TSH is normal. Thereafter, annual TSH measurement is adequate to monitor therapy. TSH should also be measured in the first trimester of pregnancy, since the thyroxine dose requirement increases at this time (see below). Overtreatment, indicated by a subnormal TSH, should be avoided since it increases the risk of osteoporosis and atrial fibrillation.
  - **In secondary hypothyroidism, plasma TSH cannot be used to adjust therapy.** The goal of therapy is to maintain the **plasma free T_4** near the middle of the reference range. The dose of thyroxine should be adjusted at 6- to 8-week intervals until this goal is achieved. Thereafter, annual measurement of plasma free T_4 is adequate to monitor therapy.
  - **Coronary artery disease** may be exacerbated by the treatment of hypothyroidism. The dose of thyroxine should be increased slowly in patients with coronary artery disease, with careful attention to worsening angina, heart failure, or arrhythmias.

COMPLICATIONS

- **Situations in which thyroxine dose requirements change.** Difficulty in controlling hypothyroidism is most often due to **poor compliance** with therapy. Observed therapy may be necessary in some cases. Other causes of increasing thyroxine requirement include the following:
  - Malabsorption due to intestinal disease or drugs that interfere with thyroxine absorption (e.g., calcium carbonate, ferrous sulfate, cholestyramine, sucralfate, aluminum hydroxide)
  - Drug interactions that increase thyroxine clearance (e.g., estrogen, rifampin, carbamazepine, phenytoin) or block conversion of T_4 to T_3 (amiodarone)
  - Pregnancy, in which thyroxine requirements often increase in the first trimester (see below)
  - Gradual failure of remaining endogenous thyroid function after RAI treatment of hyperthyroidism
- **Pregnancy. Thyroxine dose increases by an average of 50% in the first half of pregnancy** (*J Clin Endocrinol Metab 2007;92:S1*). In women with primary hypothyroidism, plasma TSH should be measured as soon as pregnancy is confirmed and monthly thereafter through the second trimester. The thyroxine dose should be increased as needed to maintain plasma TSH within the normal range.
- **Subclinical hypothyroidism** should be treated with thyroxine if any of the following are present: (a) **symptoms compatible with hypothyroidism,** (b) a **goiter,** (c) **hypercholesterolemia** that warrants treatment, or (d) the **plasma TSH is >10 microunits/mL** (*Endocr Rev 2008;29:76*). Untreated patients should be monitored annually, and thyroxine should be started if symptoms develop or serum TSH increases to >10 microunits/mL.
- **Urgent therapy** for hypothyroidism is rarely necessary. Most patients with hypothyroidism and concomitant illness can be treated in the usual manner. However,

hypothyroidism may impair survival in critical illness by contributing to hypoventilation, hypotension, hypothermia, bradycardia, or hyponatremia.

- Hypoventilation and hypotension should be treated intensively, along with any concomitant diseases. Confirmatory tests (plasma TSH and free T_4) should be obtained before thyroid hormone therapy is started.
- **Thyroxine, 50 to 100 mcg IV, can be given q6–8h for 24 hours,** followed by 75 to 100 mcg IV daily until oral intake is possible. Replacement therapy should be continued in the usual manner if the diagnosis of hypothyroidism is confirmed. No clinical trials have determined the optimum method of thyroid hormone replacement, but this method rapidly alleviates thyroxine deficiency while minimizing the risk of exacerbating underlying coronary disease or heart failure. **Such rapid correction is warranted only in extremely ill patients. Vital signs and cardiac rhythm should be monitored carefully to detect early signs of exacerbation of heart disease. Hydrocortisone,** 50 mg IV q8h, is usually recommended during rapid replacement of thyroid hormone, because such therapy may precipitate adrenal crisis in patients with adrenal failure.

Hyperthyroidism

GENERAL PRINCIPLES

Etiology

- **Graves' disease** (*NEJM 2008;358:2594*) causes most cases of hyperthyroidism, especially in young patients. This autoimmune disorder may also cause **proptosis** (exophthalmos) and pretibial myxedema, neither of which is found in other causes of hyperthyroidism.
- **Toxic multinodular goiter (MNG)** is a common cause of hyperthyroidism in older patients.
- Unusual causes include **iodine-induced hyperthyroidism** (usually precipitated by drugs such as **amiodarone** or radiographic contrast media), thyroid adenomas, subacute thyroiditis (painful tender goiter with transient hyperthyroidism), painless thyroiditis (nontender goiter with transient hyperthyroidism, most often seen in the postpartum period), and surreptitious ingestion of thyroid hormone. TSH-induced hyperthyroidism is extremely rare.

DIAGNOSIS

Clinical Presentation

- Symptoms include heat intolerance, weight loss, weakness, palpitations, oligomenorrhea, and anxiety.
- **In the elderly,** hyperthyroidism may present with only atrial fibrillation, heart failure, weakness, or weight loss, and a high index of suspicion is needed to make the diagnosis.

History

Hyperthyroidism should be suspected in any patient with compatible symptoms, as it is a readily treatable disorder that may become very debilitating.

Physical Examination

- Signs include brisk tendon reflexes, fine tremor, proximal weakness, stare, and eyelid lag. Cardiac abnormalities may be prominent, including sinus tachycardia, atrial fibrillation, and exacerbation of coronary artery disease or heart failure.

Table 2	Differential Diagnosis of Hyperthyroidism
Type of Goiter	**Diagnosis**
Diffuse, nontender goiter	Graves' disease or painless thyroiditis
Multiple thyroid nodules	Toxic multinodular goiter
Single thyroid nodule	Thyroid adenoma
Tender painful goiter	Subacute thyroiditis
Normal thyroid gland	Graves' disease, painless thyroiditis, or factitious hyperthyroidism

- Key differentiating physical exam findings include (Table 2) the following:
  - The presence of proptosis or pretibial myxedema, seen only in Graves' disease (although many patients with Graves' disease lack these signs)
  - A diffuse nontender goiter, consistent with Graves' disease or painless thyroiditis
  - Recent pregnancy, neck pain, or recent iodine administration, suggesting causes other than Graves' disease

Diagnostic Testing

In rare cases, **24-hour RAI uptake (RAIU)** is needed to distinguish Graves' disease or toxic MNG (in which RAIU is elevated) from postpartum thyroiditis, iodine-induced hyperthyroidism, or factitious hyperthyroidism (in which RAIU is very low).

Laboratories

In suspected hyperthyroidism, plasma TSH is the best initial diagnostic test.

- A TSH level > 0.1 microunits/mL excludes clinical hyperthyroidism. If plasma TSH is <0.1 microunits/mL, **plasma free T_4** should be measured to determine the severity of hyperthyroidism and as a baseline for therapy. If plasma free T_4 is elevated, the diagnosis of clinical hyperthyroidism is established.
- **If plasma TSH is <0.1 microunits/mL but free T_4 is normal,** the patient may have clinical hyperthyroidism due to elevation of plasma T_3 alone; and plasma T_3 should be measured in this case.
- Very **mild (or subclinical) hyperthyroidism** may suppress TSH to <0.1 microunits/mL, and thus suppression of TSH alone does not confirm that symptoms are due to hyperthyroidism.
- TSH may also be suppressed by **severe nonthyroidal illness** (see Evaluation of Thyroid Function).

TREATMENT

- Some forms of hyperthyroidism (subacute or postpartum thyroiditis) are transient and require only **symptomatic therapy.**
  - A **β-adrenergic antagonist** (such as **atenolol** 25 to 100 mg daily) is used to relieve symptoms of hyperthyroidism, such as palpitations, tremor, and anxiety, until hyperthyroidism is controlled by definitive therapy, or until transient forms of hyperthyroidism subside. The dose is adjusted to alleviate symptoms and tachycardia, then reduced gradually as hyperthyroidism is controlled.
  - Verapamil at an initial dose of 40 to 80 mg PO tid can be used to control tachycardia in patients with contraindications to β-adrenergic antagonists.

- Three methods are available for definitive therapy (none of which controls hyperthyroidism rapidly): RAI, thionamides, and subtotal thyroidectomy.
  - **During treatment, patients are followed by clinical evaluation and measurement of plasma free T$_4$.** Plasma TSH is useless in assessing the initial response to therapy, as it remains suppressed until after the patient becomes euthyroid.
  - Regardless of the therapy used, all patients with Graves' disease require lifelong follow-up for recurrent hyperthyroidism or development of hypothyroidism.
- **Choice of definitive therapy**
  - **In Graves' disease, RAI therapy is the treatment of choice for almost all patients.** It is simple and highly effective, but **cannot be used in pregnancy. Propylthiouracil (PTU) should be used to treat hyperthyroidism in pregnancy.** Thionamides achieve long-term control in fewer than half of patients with Graves' disease and they carry a small risk of life-threatening side effects. Thyroidectomy should be used in patients who refuse RAI therapy and who relapse or develop side effects with thionamide therapy.
  - **Other causes of hyperthyroidism.** Toxic MNG and toxic adenoma should be treated with RAI (except in pregnancy). Transient forms of hyperthyroidism due to thyroiditis should be treated symptomatically with atenolol. Iodine-induced hyperthyroidism is treated with thionamides and atenolol until the patient is euthyroid. Although treatment of some patients with amiodarone-induced hyperthyroidism with glucocorticoids has been advocated, **nearly all patients with amiodarone-induced hyperthyroidism respond well to thionamide therapy** (*Circulation 2002;105:1275*).
- **RAI therapy**
  - A single dose permanently controls hyperthyroidism in 90% of patients, and further doses can be given if necessary.
  - A **pregnancy test** is done immediately before therapy in potentially fertile women.
  - A 24-hour RAIU is usually measured and used to calculate the dose.
  - Thionamides interfere with RAI therapy and should be stopped at least 3 days before treatment. If iodine treatment has been given, it should be stopped at least 2 weeks before RAI therapy.
  - Most patients with Graves' disease are treated with 8 to 10 mCi, although treatment of toxic MNG requires higher doses.
  - **Follow-up.** Usually, several months are needed to restore euthyroidism. Patients are evaluated at 4- to 6-week intervals, with assessment of clinical findings and plasma free T$_4$.
    - **If thyroid function stabilizes within the normal range,** the interval between follow-up visits is gradually increased to annual intervals.
    - If symptomatic hypothyroidism develops, thyroxine therapy is started (see Hypothyroidism).
    - **If symptomatic hyperthyroidism persists after 6 months, RAI treatment is repeated.**
  - **Side effects**
    - **Hypothyroidism** occurs in most patients within the first year and continues to develop at a rate of approximately 3% per year thereafter.
    - Because of the release of stored hormone, a slight rise in plasma T$_4$ may occur in the first 2 weeks after therapy. This development is important only in **patients with severe cardiac disease,** which may worsen as a result. Such patients should be treated with thionamides to restore euthyroidism and to deplete stored hormone before treatment with RAI.

- There is no convincing evidence that RAI has a clinically important effect on the course of Graves' eye disease.
- It does not increase the risk of malignancy or cause congenital abnormalities in the offspring of women who conceive after RAI therapy.
- **Thionamides** (*NEJM 2005;352:905*). Methimazole and PTU inhibit thyroid hormone synthesis. PTU also inhibits extrathyroidal deiodination of T_4 to T_3. Once thyroid hormone stores are depleted (after several weeks to months), T_4 levels decrease. These drugs have no permanent effect on thyroid function. **In the majority of patients with Graves' disease, hyperthyroidism recurs within 6 months after therapy is stopped.** Spontaneous remission of Graves' disease occurs in approximately one-third of patients during thionamide therapy and, in this minority, no other treatment may be needed. Remission is more likely in mild, recent-onset hyperthyroidism and if the goiter is small.
  - **Initiation of therapy.** Before starting therapy, patients must be warned of side effects and precautions. Usual starting doses are PTU, 100 to 200 mg PO tid, or methimazole, 10 to 40 mg PO daily; higher initial doses can be used in severe hyperthyroidism.
  - **Follow-up.** Restoration of euthyroidism takes up to several months.
    - Patients are evaluated at 4-week intervals with assessment of clinical findings and plasma free T_4. If plasma free T_4 levels do not fall after 4 to 8 weeks, the dose should be increased. Doses as high as PTU, 300 mg PO qid, or methimazole, 60 mg PO daily, may be required.
    - Once the plasma free T_4 level falls to normal, the dose is adjusted to maintain plasma free T_4 within the normal range.
    - No consensus exists on the optimal duration of therapy, but periods of 6 months to 2 years are used most commonly. Patients must be monitored carefully for recurrence of hyperthyroidism after the drug is stopped.
  - **Side effects** are most likely to occur within the first few months of therapy.
    - Minor side effects include rash, urticaria, fever, arthralgias, and transient leukopenia.
    - **Agranulocytosis** occurs in 0.3% of patients treated with thionamides. Other life-threatening side effects include **hepatitis,** vasculitis, and drug-induced lupus erythematosus. These complications usually resolve if the drug is stopped promptly.
    - **Patients must be warned to stop the drug immediately if jaundice or symptoms suggestive of agranulocytosis develop (e.g., fever, chills, sore throat)** and to contact their physician promptly for evaluation. Routine monitoring of the white blood cell (WBC) is not useful for detecting agranulocytosis, which develops suddenly.
- **Subtotal thyroidectomy.** This procedure provides long-term control of hyperthyroidism in most patients.
  - Surgery may trigger a perioperative exacerbation of hyperthyroidism, and patients should be prepared for surgery by one of the two methods.
    - **A thionamide** is given until the patient is nearly euthyroid. **Supersaturated potassium iodide (SSKI),** 40 to 80 mg (one to two drops) PO bid, is then added 1 to 2 weeks before surgery. Both drugs are stopped postoperatively.
    - **Atenolol** (50 to 100 mg daily) is started 1 to 2 weeks before surgery. The dose of atenolol is increased, if necessary, to reduce the resting heart rate below 90 beats/min and is continued for 5 to 7 days postoperatively. SSKI is given as above.
  - **Follow-up.** Clinical findings and plasma free T_4 and TSH should be assessed 4 to 6 weeks after surgery.

- ○ If thyroid function is normal, the patient is seen at 3 and 6 months, then annually.
- ○ If symptomatic hypothyroidism develops, thyroxine therapy is started (see Hypothyroidism).
- ○ Mild hypothyroidism after subtotal thyroidectomy may be transient, and asymptomatic patients can be observed for further 4 to 6 weeks to determine whether hypothyroidism will resolve spontaneously.
- ○ Hyperthyroidism persists or recurs in 3% to 7% of patients.
- **Complications** of thyroidectomy include **hypothyroidism** in 30% to 50% of patients and **hypoparathyroidism** in 3%. Rare complications include permanent vocal cord paralysis, due to recurrent laryngeal nerve injury, and perioperative death. The complication rate appears to depend on the experience of the surgeon.

SPECIAL CONSIDERATIONS

- **Subclinical hyperthyroidism** is present when the plasma TSH is suppressed to <0.1 microunits/mL but the patient has no symptoms that are definitely caused by hyperthyroidism, and plasma levels of free T_4 and T_3 are normal (*J Clin Endocrinol Metab 2007;92:3*).
  - Subclinical hyperthyroidism increases the risk of **atrial fibrillation** in patients older than 60 years and those with heart disease, and predisposes to **osteoporosis** in postmenopausal women; it should be treated in these patients.
  - Asymptomatic young patients with mild Graves' disease can be observed for spontaneous resolution of hyperthyroidism, or the development of symptoms or increasing free T_4 levels that warrant treatment.
- **Urgent therapy** is warranted when hyperthyroidism exacerbates heart failure or acute coronary syndromes, and in rare patients with severe hyperthyroidism complicated by fever and delirium. Concomitant diseases should be treated intensively, and confirmatory tests (serum TSH and free T_4) should be obtained before therapy is started.
- **PTU, 300 mg PO q6h,** should be started immediately.
- **Iodide (SSKI,** two drops PO q12h) should be started 1 hour after the first dose of PTU to inhibit thyroid hormone secretion rapidly.
- **Propranolol,** 40 mg PO q6h (or an equivalent dose IV), should be given to patients with angina or myocardial infarction, and the dose should be adjusted to prevent tachycardia. Propranolol may benefit some patients with heart failure and marked tachycardia but can further impair left ventricular systolic function. In patients with clinical heart failure, it should be given only with careful monitoring of left ventricular function.
- Plasma free T_4 is measured every 4 to 6 days. When free T_4 approaches the normal range, the doses of PTU and iodine are gradually decreased. RAI therapy should be scheduled 2 weeks after iodine is stopped.
- **Hyperthyroidism in pregnancy.** If hyperthyroidism is suspected, plasma TSH should be measured. Plasma TSH declines in early pregnancy, but rarely to <0.1 microunits/mL (*Endocrinol Metab Clin North Am 2006;35:117*).
  - If TSH is <0.1 microunits/mL, the diagnosis should be confirmed by measurement of plasma free T_4.
  - RAI is contraindicated in pregnancy, and therefore, patients should be treated with PTU. The dose should be adjusted at 4-week intervals to maintain the plasma free T_4 near the upper limit of the normal range to avoid fetal hypothyroidism. The dose required often decreases in the later stages of pregnancy.

- Atenolol, 25 to 50 mg PO daily, can be used to relieve symptoms while awaiting the effects of PTU.
- The fetus and neonate should be monitored carefully for hyperthyroidism.

Euthyroid Goiter and Thyroid Nodules

GENERAL PRINCIPLES

- The diagnosis of euthyroid goiter is based on palpation of the thyroid and evaluation of thyroid function. If the thyroid is enlarged, the examiner should determine whether the enlargement is **diffuse or multinodular, or whether a single palpable nodule is present.** All three forms of euthyroid goiter are common, especially in women.
- Thyroid scans or ultrasonography provide no useful additional information about goiters that are diffuse or multinodular by palpation and should not be performed in these patients.
- Between 30% and 50% of people have nonpalpable thyroid nodules that are detectable by ultrasound. These nodules rarely have any clinical importance, but their incidental discovery may lead to unnecessary diagnostic testing and treatment (*Clin Endocrinol 2004;60:18–20*).

Classification
- **Diffuse goiter**
  - Almost all euthyroid diffuse goiters in the United States are due to **chronic lymphocytic thyroiditis (Hashimoto's thyroiditis).** Since Hashimoto's thyroiditis may also cause hypothyroidism, plasma TSH should be measured even in patients who are clinically euthyroid.
  - Diffuse goiters are usually asymptomatic, and therapy is seldom required. Patients should be monitored regularly for the development of hypothyroidism.
- **Multinodular goiter**
  - MNG is common in older patients, especially women. Most patients are asymptomatic and require no treatment.
  - In a few patients, **hyperthyroidism** (toxic MNG) develops (see Hyperthyroidism).
  - In rare patients, the gland compresses the trachea or esophagus, causing dyspnea or dysphagia, and treatment is required. Thyroxine treatment has little, if any, effect on the size of MNGs. RAI therapy reduces gland size and relieves symptoms in most patients (*Clin Endocrinol 2007;66:757–764*). Subtotal thyroidectomy can also be used to relieve compressive symptoms.
  - The risk of malignancy in MNG is low, comparable to the frequency of incidental thyroid carcinoma in clinically normal glands. Evaluation for thyroid carcinoma with needle biopsy is warranted if one nodule is disproportionately enlarged.
- **Single thyroid nodules**
  - **Single palpable thyroid nodules** are usually benign, but about 5% are thyroid carcinomas (*Thyroid 2006;16:1–33*).
  - Clinical findings that increase the likelihood of carcinoma include the presence of cervical lymphadenopathy, a history of radiation to the head or neck in childhood, and a family history of medullary thyroid carcinoma or multiple endocrine neoplasia syndromes types 2A or 2B. A hard, fixed nodule, recent nodule growth, or hoarseness due to vocal cord paralysis also suggests malignancy.
  - Most patients with thyroid carcinomas have none of these risk factors, and all **palpable single thyroid nodules should be evaluated with needle aspiration**

biopsy. Patients with thyroid carcinoma should be managed in consultation with an endocrinologist.

- Nodules with benign cytology should be reevaluated periodically by palpation. Thyroxine therapy has little or no effect on the size of single thyroid nodules and is not indicated.
- Imaging studies cannot distinguish benign from malignant nodules and are not needed for the evaluation of a palpable thyroid nodule. The management of non-palpable thyroid nodules discovered incidentally by ultrasound is controversial (*Clin Endocrinol 2004;60:18*).

DISORDERS OF ADRENAL FUNCTION

Adrenal Failure

GENERAL PRINCIPLES

Etiology

- Adrenal failure may be due to disease of the adrenal glands (**primary adrenal failure, Addison's disease**), with deficiency of both cortisol and aldosterone and elevated plasma adrenocorticotropic hormone (ACTH), or due to ACTH deficiency caused by disorders of the pituitary or hypothalamus (**secondary adrenal failure**), with deficiency of cortisol alone.
  - **Primary adrenal failure** is most often due to **autoimmune adrenalitis,** which may be associated with other endocrine deficits (e.g., hypothyroidism).
  - Infections of the adrenal gland such as **tuberculosis** and **histoplasmosis** may also cause adrenal failure.
  - **Hemorrhagic adrenal infarction** may occur in the postoperative period, in coagulation disorders and hypercoagulable states, and in sepsis. Adrenal hemorrhage often causes abdominal or flank pain and fever; computed tomography (CT) scan of the abdomen reveals high-density bilateral adrenal masses.
  - Adrenal failure may develop in patients with AIDS, caused by disseminated cytomegalovirus, mycobacterial or fungal infection, or adrenal lymphoma.
  - Less common etiologies include adrenoleukodystrophy that causes adrenal failure in young males, and drugs such as ketoconazole and etomidate that inhibit steroid hormone synthesis.
- **Secondary adrenal failure** is most often due to **glucocorticoid therapy;** ACTH suppression may persist for a year after therapy is stopped. Any disorder of the pituitary or hypothalamus can cause ACTH deficiency, but other evidence of these disorders is usually obvious.

DIAGNOSIS

Clinical Presentation

- Adrenal failure should be suspected in patients with hypotension, weight loss, persistent nausea, hyponatremia, or hyperkalemia.
- **Clinical findings** in adrenal failure are nonspecific, and without a high index of suspicion, the diagnosis of this potentially lethal but readily treatable disease is easily missed.

- Symptoms include **anorexia, nausea, vomiting, weight loss, weakness, and fatigue. Orthostatic hypotension** and **hyponatremia** are common.
- Symptoms are usually chronic, but **shock** may develop suddenly, and is fatal unless promptly treated. Often, this adrenal crisis is triggered by illness, injury, or surgery. All these symptoms are due to cortisol deficiency and occur in both primary and secondary adrenal failure.
- **Hyperpigmentation** (due to marked ACTH excess) and **hyperkalemia** and **volume depletion** (due to aldosterone deficiency) occur only in primary adrenal failure.

Diagnostic Testing

Laboratories

- **The cosyntropin (Cortrosyn) stimulation test** is used for diagnosis (*Ann Intern Med 2003;139:194*). Recent literature suggests that the use of cosyntropin 1 mcg may detect adrenal failure in patients who would not have been diagnosed using 250 mcg (*Endocr Pract 2008;14(2):233–238*). However, given the ease of administration, 250-mcg dosing is still used in clinical practice. Cosyntropin, 250 mcg, is given IV or IM, and **plasma cortisol is measured 30 minutes later.** The normal response is a stimulated plasma cortisol > 20 mcg/dL. This test detects primary and secondary adrenal failure, except within a few weeks of onset of pituitary dysfunction (e.g., shortly after pituitary surgery; see Disorders of Anterior Pituitary Gland Dysfunction).
- **The distinction between primary and secondary adrenal failure** is usually clear.
  - Hyperkalemia, hyperpigmentation, or other autoimmune endocrine deficits indicate primary adrenal failure, whereas deficits of other pituitary hormones, symptoms of a pituitary mass (e.g., headache, visual field loss), or known pituitary or hypothalamic disease indicate secondary adrenal failure.
  - If the cause is unclear, the **plasma ACTH** level distinguishes primary adrenal failure (in which it is markedly elevated) from secondary adrenal failure.
  - Most cases of primary adrenal failure are due to autoimmune adrenalitis, but other causes should be considered. Radiographic evidence of adrenal enlargement or calcification indicates that the cause is infection or hemorrhage.
  - Patients with secondary adrenal failure should be tested for other pituitary hormone deficiencies and should be evaluated for a pituitary or hypothalamic tumor (see Disorders of Anterior Pituitary Gland Dysfunction).

TREATMENT

- **Adrenal crisis** with hypotension must be treated immediately. Patients should be evaluated for an underlying illness that precipitated the crisis.
- **If the diagnosis of adrenal failure is known, hydrocortisone, 100 mg IV q8h,** should be given, and **0.9% saline with 5% dextrose** should be infused rapidly until hypotension is corrected. The dose of hydrocortisone is decreased gradually over several days as symptoms and any precipitating illness resolve, then changed to oral maintenance therapy. Mineralocorticoid replacement is not needed until the dose of hydrocortisone is <100 mg/d.
- **If the diagnosis of adrenal failure has not been established,** a single dose of **dexamethasone,** 10 mg IV, should be given, and a rapid infusion of 0.9% saline with 5% dextrose should be started. A **Cortrosyn stimulation test** should be performed. Dexamethasone is used because it does not interfere with measurement of plasma

cortisol. After the 30-minute plasma cortisol measurement, hydrocortisone, 100 mg IV q8h, should be given until the test result is known.

- **Maintenance therapy** in all patients requires cortisol replacement with prednisone. Most patients with primary adrenal failure also require replacement of aldosterone with fludrocortisone.
  - **Prednisone,** 5 mg PO every morning, should be started. The dose is then adjusted with the goal being the lowest dose that relieves the patient's symptoms, to prevent osteoporosis and other signs of Cushing's syndrome. Most patients require doses as high as 7.5 mg PO daily. Concomitant therapy with rifampin, phenytoin, or phenobarbital accelerates glucocorticoid metabolism and increases the dose requirement.
  - **During illness, injury, or the perioperative period, the dose of prednisone must be increased.**
    - For minor illnesses, the patient should double the dose for 3 days. If the illness resolves, the maintenance dose is resumed.
    - **Vomiting requires immediate medical attention,** with IV glucocorticoid therapy and IV fluid. Patients can be given a 4-mg vial of dexamethasone to be self-administered IM for vomiting or severe illness if medical care is not immediately available.
    - **For severe illness or injury,** hydrocortisone, 50 mg IV q8h, should be given, with the dose tapered as severity of illness wanes. The same regimen is used in **patients undergoing surgery,** with the first dose of hydrocortisone given preoperatively. The dose can be tapered to maintenance therapy by 2 to 3 days after uncomplicated surgery.
- **In primary adrenal failure, fludrocortisone, 0.1 mg PO daily,** should be given. The dose is adjusted to maintain blood pressure (supine and standing) and serum potassium within the normal range; the usual dosage is 0.05 to 0.2 mg PO daily.
- **Patients should be educated in management of their disease,** including adjustment of prednisone dose during illness. They should wear a medical identification tag or bracelet.

Cushing's Syndrome

GENERAL PRINCIPLES

Etiology

- Cushing's syndrome (*Lancet 2006;367:1605*) is most often **iatrogenic,** due to therapy with glucocorticoid drugs.
- **ACTH-secreting pituitary microadenomas (Cushing's disease)** account for 80% of cases of endogenous Cushing's syndrome.
  - Adrenal tumors and ectopic ACTH secretion account for the remainder.

DIAGNOSIS

Clinical Presentation

Physical Examination

- Findings include truncal obesity, rounded face, fat deposits in the supraclavicular fossae and over the posterior neck, hypertension, hirsutism, amenorrhea, and depression. More specific findings include thin skin, easy bruising, reddish striae, proximal muscle weakness, and osteoporosis.

- Hyperpigmentation or hypokalemic alkalosis suggests Cushing's syndrome due to ectopic ACTH secretion.
- Diabetes mellitus develops in some patients.

Diagnostic Testing

Laboratories
- **Diagnosis** is based on increased cortisol excretion and lack of normal feedback inhibition of ACTH and cortisol secretion.
- The best initial test is the **24-hour urine cortisol** measurement test. Alternatively, an **overnight dexamethasone suppression test** (1 mg dexamethasone given PO at 11:00 p.m.; plasma cortisol measured at 8:00 a.m. the next day; normal range: plasma cortisol < 2 mcg/dL) may be performed. Both tests are very sensitive, and a normal value virtually excludes the diagnosis. If the overnight dexamethasone suppression test is abnormal, 24-hour urine cortisol should be measured.
  - If the 24-hour urine cortisol excretion is more than four times the upper limit of the reference range in a patient with compatible clinical findings, the diagnosis of Cushing's syndrome is established.
  - In patients with milder elevations of urine cortisol, a **low-dose dexamethasone suppression test** should be performed. Dexamethasone, 0.5 mg PO q6h, is given for 48 hours, starting at 8:00 a.m. Urine cortisol is measured during the last 24 hours, and plasma cortisol is measured 6 hours after the last dose of dexamethasone. Failure to suppress plasma cortisol to <2 mcg/dL and urine cortisol to less than the normal reference range is diagnostic of Cushing's syndrome.
  - Testing should not be done during severe illness or depression, which may cause false-positive results. Phenytoin therapy also causes a false-positive test by accelerating metabolism of dexamethasone.
- Random plasma cortisol levels are not useful for diagnosis, because the wide range of normal values overlaps those of Cushing's syndrome. After the diagnosis of Cushing's syndrome is made, tests to determine the cause are best done in consultation with an endocrinologist.

Incidental Adrenal Nodules

GENERAL PRINCIPLES

- Adrenal nodules are a common incidental finding on abdominal imaging studies.
- Most incidentally discovered nodules are benign adrenocortical tumors that do not secrete excess hormone.

DIAGNOSIS

In patients without a known malignancy elsewhere, the **diagnostic issues are whether a syndrome of hormone excess or an adrenocortical carcinoma is present.**

Clinical Presentation

Physical Examination

Patients should be evaluated for hypertension, symptoms suggestive of pheochromocytoma (episodic headache, palpitations, and sweating) and signs of Cushing's syndrome (see Cushing's Syndrome).

Differential Diagnosis

- The differential diagnosis includes adrenal adenomas causing Cushing's syndrome or primary hyperaldosteronism, pheochromocytoma, adrenocortical carcinoma, and metastatic cancer (*NEJM 2007;356:601*).
- The imaging characteristics of the nodule may suggest a diagnosis but are not specific enough to obviate further evaluation.

Diagnostic Testing

Laboratories

- **Plasma potassium, metanephrines, and dehydroepiandrosterone sulfate** should be measured, and an **overnight dexamethasone suppression** test should be performed.
- **Patients who have potentially resectable cancer elsewhere** and in whom an adrenal metastasis must be excluded may require positron emission tomography.
- Patients with hypertension and hypokalemia should be evaluated for primary hyperaldosteronism by measuring the ratio of plasma aldosterone (in ng/dl) to plasma renin activity (in ng/mL/hr). If the ratio is less than 20, the diagnosis of primary hyperaldosteronism is excluded, while a ratio greater than 50 makes the diagnosis very likely. Patients with an intermediate ratio should be further evaluated in consultation with an endocrinologist.
- An abnormal overnight dexamethasone suppression test should be evaluated further (see Cushing's Syndrome).
- Elevation of plasma dehydroepiandrosterone sulfate or a large nodule suggests adrenocortical carcinoma.

TREATMENT

- Most incidental nodules are <4 cm in diameter, do not produce excess hormone, and do not require therapy. At least one **repeat imaging procedure** 3 to 6 months later is recommended to ensure that the nodule is not enlarging rapidly (which would suggest an adrenal carcinoma).
- A policy of resecting all nodules > 4 cm in diameter appropriately treats the great majority of adrenal carcinomas while minimizing the number of benign nodules that are removed unnecessarily.
- If clinical or biochemical evidence of a pheochromocytoma is found, the nodule should be resected after appropriate α-adrenergic blockade with phenoxybenzamine.

DISORDERS OF ANTERIOR PITUITARY FUNCTION

Anterior Pituitary Gland Dysfunction

GENERAL PRINCIPLES

- The anterior pituitary gland secretes **prolactin, growth hormone,** and four **trophic hormones,** including corticotropin (ACTH), thyrotropin (TSH), and the gonadotropins, luteinizing hormone and follicle-stimulating hormone. Each trophic hormone stimulates a specific target gland.

- Anterior pituitary function is regulated by hypothalamic hormones that reach the pituitary via portal veins in the pituitary stalk. **The predominant effect of hypothalamic regulation is to stimulate secretion of pituitary hormones, except for prolactin,** which is inhibited by hypothalamic dopamine secretion.
- **Secretion of trophic hormones is also regulated by negative feedback** by their target gland hormone, and the normal pituitary response to target hormone deficiency is increased secretion of the appropriate trophic hormone.
- **Anterior pituitary dysfunction** can be caused by disorders of either the pituitary or hypothalamus.

Etiology

- **Pituitary adenomas** are the most common pituitary disorder. They are classified by size and function.
  - **Microadenomas** are <10 mm in diameter and cause clinical manifestations only if they produce excess hormone. They are too small to produce hypopituitarism or mass effects.
  - **Macroadenomas** are >10 mm in diameter and may produce any combination of pituitary hormone excess, hypopituitarism, and mass effects (headache, visual field loss).
  - **Secretory adenomas** produce prolactin, growth hormone, or ACTH.
  - **Nonsecretory macroadenomas** may cause hypopituitarism or mass effects.
  - **Nonsecretory microadenomas** are common incidental radiographic findings, seen in approximately 10% of the normal population, and do not require therapy.
- **Other pituitary or hypothalamic disorders,** such as head trauma, pituitary surgery or radiation, and postpartum pituitary infarction (Sheehan's syndrome) may cause hypopituitarism. Other tumors of the pituitary or hypothalamus (e.g., craniopharyngioma, metastases), inflammatory disorders (e.g., sarcoidosis, histiocytosis X), and infections (e.g., tuberculosis) may cause hypopituitarism or mass effects.

DIAGNOSIS

Clinical Presentation

- Pituitary and hypothalamic disorders may present in several ways.
- In **hypopituitarism** (deficiency of one or more pituitary hormones), gonadotropin deficiency is most common, causing amenorrhea in women and androgen deficiency in men. Secondary hypothyroidism or adrenal failure rarely occurs alone. Secondary adrenal failure causes deficiency of cortisol but not of aldosterone; hyperkalemia and hyperpigmentation do not occur, although life-threatening adrenal crisis may develop.
- **Hormone excess** most commonly results in **hyperprolactinemia,** which can be due to a secretory adenoma or due to nonsecretory lesions that damage the hypothalamus or pituitary stalk. Growth hormone excess **(acromegaly)** and ACTH and cortisol excess **(Cushing's disease)** are caused by secretory adenomas.
- **Mass effects** due to pressure on adjacent structures, such as the optic chiasm, include **headaches** and **loss of visual fields or acuity.** Hyperprolactinemia may also be due to mass effect. **Pituitary apoplexy** is sudden enlargement of a pituitary tumor due to hemorrhagic necrosis.

Diagnostic Testing

Imaging

- **Asymptomatic pituitary adenomas**
- **If a microadenoma is found** on imaging done for another purpose, the patient should be evaluated for clinical evidence of hyperprolactinemia, Cushing's disease, or acromegaly.
- Plasma prolactin should be measured, and tests for acromegaly and Cushing's syndrome should be performed if symptoms or signs of these disorders are evident.
- If no pituitary hormone excess exists, therapy is not required. Whether such patients need repeat imaging is not established, but the risk of enlargement is clearly small.
- **Incidental discovery of a macroadenoma** is unusual. Patients should be evaluated for hormone excess and hypopituitarism. Most macroadenomas should be treated since they are likely to grow further.

Hypopituitarism

DIAGNOSIS

Clinical Presentation

Hypopituitarism may be suspected in the presence of clinical signs of target hormone deficiency (e.g., hypothyroidism) or pituitary mass effects.

Diagnostic Testing

Laboratories

- **Laboratory evaluation** for hypopituitarism begins with evaluation of **target hormone function,** including **plasma free T_4** and a **Cortrosyn stimulation test** (see Adrenal Failure).
  - If recent onset of secondary adrenal failure is suspected (within a few weeks of evaluation), the patient should be treated empirically with glucocorticoids and should be tested 4 to 8 weeks later, since the Cortrosyn stimulation test cannot detect secondary adrenal failure of recent onset.
  - In men, **plasma testosterone** should be measured. The best evaluation of gonadal function in women is the **menstrual history.**
- **If a target hormone is deficient,** its trophic hormone is measured to determine whether target gland dysfunction is secondary to hypopituitarism. An elevated trophic hormone level indicates primary target gland dysfunction. In hypopituitarism, trophic hormone levels are not elevated and are usually within (not below) the reference range. Thus, **pituitary trophic hormone levels can be interpreted only with knowledge of target hormone levels,** and **measurement of trophic hormone levels alone is useless in the diagnosis of hypopituitarism.** If pituitary disease is obvious, target hormone deficiencies may be assumed to be secondary, and trophic hormones need not be measured.

Imaging

Anatomic evaluation of the pituitary gland and hypothalamus is done best by magnetic resonance imaging (MRI). However, hyperprolactinemia and Cushing's disease may be caused by microadenomas too small to be seen with current techniques. The prevalence of incidental microadenomas should be kept in mind when interpreting MRIs. Visual acuity and **visual fields** should be tested when imaging suggests compression of the optic chiasm.

TREATMENT

- Deficient target hormones should be replaced.
- Secondary adrenal failure should be treated immediately, especially if patients are to undergo surgery (see Adrenal Failure).
- Treatment of secondary hypothyroidism should be monitored by measurement of **plasma free T$_4$** (see Hypothyroidism).
- Infertility due to gonadotropin deficiency may be correctable, and patients who wish to conceive should be referred to an endocrinologist.
- Treatment of growth hormone deficiency in adults has been advocated by some, but the benefits, risks, and cost-effectiveness of this therapy are not established (*Ann Intern Med 2002;137:190*).
- Treatment of pituitary macroadenomas generally requires transsphenoidal surgical resection, except for prolactin-secreting tumors.

Hyperprolactinemia

GENERAL PRINCIPLES

- In women, the most common causes of pathologic hyperprolactinemia are prolactin-secreting pituitary **microadenomas** and **idiopathic hyperprolactinemia** (Table 3).
- In men, the most common cause is a prolactin-secreting **macroadenoma.**
- Hypothalamic or pituitary lesions that cause deficiency of other pituitary hormones often cause hyperprolactinemia.
- **Medications** are an important cause in both men and women (*Pituitary 2008; 11:209*).

DIAGNOSIS

Clinical Presentation

- In women, hyperprolactinemia causes **amenorrhea** or irregular menses and **infertility.** Only approximately half of these women have **galactorrhea.** Prolonged estrogen deficiency increases the risk of **osteoporosis.** Plasma **prolactin should be measured**

Table 3	Major Causes of Hyperprolactinemia

Pregnancy and lactation
Prolactin-secreting pituitary adenoma (prolactinoma)
Idiopathic hyperprolactinemia
Drugs (e.g., phenothiazines, metoclopramide, risperidone, verapamil)
Interference with synthesis or transport of hypothalamic dopamine
    Hypothalamic lesions
    Nonsecretory pituitary macroadenomas
Primary hypothyroidism
Chronic renal failure

in women with amenorrhea, whether or not galactorrhea is present. Mild elevations should be confirmed by repeat measurements.
- In men, hyperprolactinemia causes **androgen deficiency** and **infertility** but not gynecomastia; **mass effects and hypopituitarism** are common.

History

The history should include medications and symptoms of pituitary mass effects or hypothyroidism.

Diagnostic Testing

Imaging

Testing for hypopituitarism is needed only in patients with a macroadenoma or hypothalamic lesion. **Pituitary imaging** should be performed in most cases, as large nonfunctional pituitary or hypothalamic tumors may present with hyperprolactinemia.

TREATMENT

- **Microadenomas and idiopathic hyperprolactinemia** (*Endocr Rev 2006;27:485*).
- Most patients are treated because of **infertility** or to prevent **estrogen deficiency and osteoporosis.**
- Some women may be observed without therapy by periodic follow-up of prolactin levels and symptoms. In most patients, hyperprolactinemia does not worsen, and prolactin levels sometimes return to normal. Enlargement of microadenomas is rare.
- **The dopamine agonists bromocriptine** and **cabergoline** suppress plasma prolactin and restore normal menses and fertility in most women.
  - Initial dosages are bromocriptine, 1.25 to 2.5 mg PO at bedtime with a snack, or cabergoline, 0.25 mg twice a week.
  - Plasma prolactin levels are initially obtained at 2- to 4-week intervals, and doses are adjusted until the lowest dose required to maintain prolactin in the normal range is reached. In general, the maximally effective doses are bromocriptine 2.5 mg tid and cabergoline 1.5 mg twice a week.
  - **Side effects** include **nausea** and **orthostatic hypotension,** which can be minimized by increasing the dose gradually, and usually resolve with continued therapy. Side effects are less severe with cabergoline.
  - Initially, patients should use barrier contraception, as fertility may be restored quickly.
    - **Women who want to become pregnant** should be managed in consultation with an endocrinologist.
    - **Women who do not want to become pregnant** should be followed with clinical evaluation and plasma prolactin levels every 6 to 12 months. Every 2 years, plasma prolactin should be measured after bromocriptine has been withdrawn for several weeks, to determine whether the drug is still needed. Follow-up imaging studies are not warranted unless prolactin levels increase substantially.
  - Transsphenoidal resection of prolactin-secreting microadenomas is used only in the rare patient who does not respond to or cannot tolerate dopamine agonists. Prolactin levels usually return to normal, but up to one-half of patients experience relapse.
- **Prolactin-secreting macroadenomas** should be treated with a dopamine agonist, which usually suppresses prolactin levels to normal, reduces tumor size, and improves or corrects abnormal visual fields in 90% of cases.

- If mass effects are present, the dose should be increased to maximally effective levels over a period of several weeks. Visual field tests, if initially abnormal, should be repeated 4 to 6 weeks after therapy is started.
- Pituitary imaging should be repeated 3 to 6 months after initiation of therapy. If tumor shrinkage and correction of visual abnormalities are satisfactory, therapy can be continued indefinitely, with periodic monitoring of plasma prolactin levels.
- The full effect on tumor size may take more than 6 months. Further pituitary imaging is probably not warranted unless prolactin levels rise despite therapy.
- **Transsphenoidal surgery** is indicated to relieve mass effects if the tumor does not shrink or if visual field abnormalities persist during dopamine agonist therapy. However, the likelihood of surgical cure of a prolactin-secreting macroadenoma is low, and most patients require further therapy with a dopamine agonist.
- **Women with prolactin-secreting macroadenomas should not become pregnant** unless the tumor has been resected surgically, as the risk of symptomatic enlargement during pregnancy is 15% to 35%. Barrier contraception is essential during dopamine agonist treatment.

Acromegaly

GENERAL PRINCIPLES

Acromegaly is the syndrome caused by growth hormone excess in adults and is due to a growth hormone–secreting pituitary adenoma in the vast majority of cases (*NEJM 2006;355:2558*).

DIAGNOSIS

Clinical Presentation

Clinical findings include thickened skin and enlargement of hands, feet, jaw, and forehead. Arthritis or carpal tunnel syndrome may develop, and the pituitary adenoma may cause headaches and vision loss. Mortality from cardiovascular disease is increased.

Diagnostic Testing

Laboratories
- **Plasma insulin-like growth factor 1 (IGF-1),** which mediates most effects of growth hormone, is the best diagnostic test. Marked elevations establish the diagnosis.
- If IGF-1 levels are only moderately elevated, the diagnosis can be confirmed by giving 75 mg glucose orally and measuring serum growth hormone q30min for 2 hours. Failure to suppress growth hormone to <1 ng/mL confirms the diagnosis of acromegaly. Once the diagnosis is made, the pituitary should be imaged.

TREATMENT

The treatment of choice is transsphenoidal resection of the pituitary adenoma. Most patients have macroadenomas, and complete tumor resection with cure of acromegaly is often impossible. If IGF-1 levels remain elevated after surgery, radiotherapy is used to prevent regrowth of the tumor and to control acromegaly.

Medications

- The somatostatin analog **octreotide** in depot form can be used to suppress growth hormone secretion while awaiting the effect of radiation. A dose of 10 to 30 mg IM monthly suppresses IGF-1 to normal in most patients. Side effects include cholelithiasis, diarrhea, and mild abdominal discomfort.
- **Pegvisomant** is a growth hormone antagonist that lowers IGF-1 to normal in almost all patients. The dose is 10 to 30 mg SC daily. Few side effects have been reported, but patients should be monitored for pituitary adenoma enlargement and transaminase elevation.

METABOLIC BONE DISEASE

Osteomalacia

GENERAL PRINCIPLES

- Osteomalacia is characterized by defective mineralization of osteoid. Bone biopsy reveals increased thickness of osteoid seams and decreased mineralization rate, assessed by tetracycline labeling.
- Suboptimal vitamin D nutrition, indicated by plasma 25-hydroxy vitamin D (25(OH)D) levels below 30 ng/mL, is very common, and contributes to the development of osteoporosis.

Etiology

- Dietary vitamin D deficiency
- **Malabsorption** of vitamin D and calcium due to intestinal, hepatic, or biliary disease
- Disorders of vitamin D metabolism (e.g., renal disease, vitamin D–dependent rickets)
- Vitamin D resistance
- Chronic hypophosphatemia
- Renal tubular acidosis
- Hypophosphatasia
- Therapy with anticonvulsants, fluoride, etidronate, or aluminum compounds

DIAGNOSIS

Clinical Presentation

Clinical findings include diffuse skeletal pain, proximal muscle weakness, waddling gait, and propensity to fractures.

History

Osteomalacia should be suspected in a patient with osteopenia, elevated serum alkaline phosphatase, and either hypophosphatemia or hypocalcemia.

Diagnostic Testing

Laboratories

- Serum alkaline phosphatase is elevated. Serum phosphorus, calcium, or both may be decreased.
- **Serum 25(OH)D** levels may be low, establishing the diagnosis of vitamin D deficiency or malabsorption.

Imaging
- Radiographic findings include osteopenia and radiolucent bands perpendicular to bone surfaces (pseudofractures or Looser zones).
- Radiography of the chest, pelvis, and hips may reveal characteristic pseudofractures.

TREATMENT

Medications

- **Dietary vitamin D deficiency** can initially be treated with ergocalciferol 50,000 International Units (IU) PO weekly for 8 weeks to replete body stores, followed by long-term therapy with 400 to 1,000 IU/d. Preparations include calcium supplements that contain vitamin D (Os-Cal + D, 125 IU/250- or 500-mg tablet), many multivitamins (400 IU/tablet), and vitamin D drops (200 IU/drop or 8,000 IU/mL).
- **Malabsorption of vitamin D** may require continued therapy with high doses such as 50,000 IU PO per week. The dose should be adjusted to maintain serum 25(OH)D levels within the normal range. Calcitriol, 0.5 to 2.0 mcg PO daily, can also be used. Calcium supplements, 1 g PO daily–tid, may also be required. Serum 25(OH)D, serum calcium, and 24-hour urine calcium should be monitored every 3 to 6 months to avoid hypercalcemia or hypercalciuria. If the underlying disease responds to therapy, the dose of vitamin D must be reduced accordingly.

Paget's Disease

GENERAL PRINCIPLES

Paget's disease of bone is a focal skeletal disorder characterized by rapid, disorganized bone remodeling. It usually occurs after the age of 40 years and most often affects the pelvis, femur, spine, and skull (*NEJM 2006;355:593*).

DIAGNOSIS

Clinical Presentation

- Clinical manifestations include bone pain and deformity, degenerative arthritis, pathologic fractures, neurologic deficits due to nerve root or cranial nerve compression (including deafness), and rarely, high-output heart failure and osteogenic sarcoma.
- Most patients are asymptomatic, with disease discovered incidentally because of elevated serum alkaline phosphatase or a radiograph taken for other reasons.

Diagnostic Testing

Laboratories
Serum alkaline phosphatase is elevated, reflecting the activity and extent of disease. Serum and urine calcium are usually normal but may increase with immobilization, as after a fracture.

Imaging
The radiographic appearance is usually diagnostic. A bone scan will reveal areas of skeletal involvement, which can be confirmed by radiography.

TREATMENT

Indications for therapy include (a) bone pain due to Paget's disease, (b) nerve compression syndromes, (c) pathologic fracture, (d) elective skeletal surgery, (e) progressive skeletal deformity, (f) immobilization hypercalcemia, and (g) asymptomatic involvement of weight-bearing bones or the skull.

Medications

- **Bisphosphonates** inhibit excessive bone resorption, relieve symptoms, and restore serum alkaline phosphatase to normal in most patients. The effectiveness of therapy is monitored by measuring serum alkaline phosphatase every 3 months. Therapy can be repeated when serum alkaline phosphatase rises above normal. Bisphosphonates may cause esophagitis, and are not recommended in patients with renal insufficiency. Typical courses of therapy include the following:
  - **Alendronate,** 40 mg/d for 6 months
  - **Risedronate,** 30 mg/d for 2 months
  - **Pamidronate,** 30 mg IV over 4 hours on 3 consecutive days, or
  - **Zoledronic acid,** 5 mg IV by a single infusion

22 Arthritis and Rheumatologic Diseases

Hector Molina, Christopher Phillips, and Vladimir Despotovic

Basic Approach to the Rheumatic Diseases

GENERAL PRINCIPLES

Definition

Arthritis is any medical process affecting a joint or joints, causing pain, swelling, and stiffness. It has to be distinguished from a periarticular process. The pain from a true articular process is usually present throughout the complete range of motion of a particular joint. The pain from a periarticular process is usually evident at a single point of the range of motion and it is elicited by palpation in a specific area corresponding to a tendon, ligament, or bursa.

Classification

Once it is established that the clinician is dealing with an arthritic process, it can be categorized in an inflammatory versus a noninflammatory process and by the number and type of joints involved (see Fig. 1 and Table 1).

DIAGNOSIS

The history and physical exam are essential. In the history, evidence of an inflammatory process includes the presence of morning stiffness lasting more than an hour and worsening of symptoms with inactivity. The review of systems is instrumental in searching for the presence of symptoms related to a particular arthropathy or connective tissue disease (skin rashes, uveitis, iritis, mouth ulcers, and serositis among others). There may be associated swelling, warmth, erythema, or constitutional symptoms. Synovial fluid aspiration helps in the diagnosis. Analysis of the synovial fluid should include a cell count, microscopic examination for crystals, Gram stain, and cultures. Ancillary lab test and imaging techniques are helpful in supporting a diagnosis if their use is directed by the specific findings on the history and physical exam (Table 1).

TREATMENT

The etiology of most rheumatologic disorders is unknown. Therapeutic approaches involve either local or systemic administration of analgesic, anti-inflammatory, immunomodulatory, or immunosuppressive drugs. The initial general therapeutic

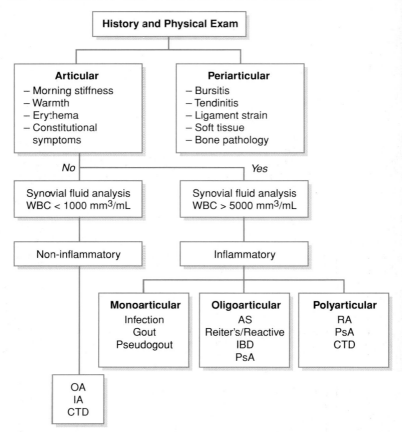

Figure 1. Initial general evaluation of a patient with arthritis. WBC, white blood cells; OA, osteoarthritis; IA, internal dearrangement; CTD, connective tissue disease; AS, ankylosing spondylitis; IBD, inflammatory bowel disease; PsA, psoriatic arthritis; RA, rheumatoid arthritis.

options will be discussed here. Specific immunomodulatory and immunosuppressive therapies will be discussed in association with the disease process for which the therapeutic agent is most commonly used.

Medications

- **Nonsteroidal anti-inflammatory drugs (NSAIDs)** exert their effects by inhibiting the constitutive (COX-1) and inducible (COX-2) isoforms of cyclooxygenase, producing a mild to moderate anti-inflammatory and analgesic effect. Individual responses to these agents are variable. If one drug is not effective during a 2- to 3-week trial, another should be tried.

Table 1   General Features of the Most Common Arthritis

Diagnosis	Type	Additional Features	Laboratory and Imaging
Osteoarthritis	Noninflammatory; monoarticular, oligoarticular, or polyarticular	Bone spurs; knees, hips, PIP, DIP, first MTP, first CMC preferentially affected	Normal ESR/CRP, Osteophytes, bone sclerosis
Gout	Inflammatory; monoarticular, oligoarticular, or polyarticular	Tophi; acute attacks followed by spontaneous resolution	Elevated uric acid; positive uric acid crystals in joint fluid; elevated ESR/CRP; erosions with overhanging borders
Pseudogout	Inflammatory; monoarticular or polyarticular	Acute attacks or chronic	Elevated ESR/CRP; positive CPPD crystals in joint fluid; chondrocalcinosis
Septic joint	Inflammatory; monoarticular, rarely polyarticular (immunosuppression)	Sepsis, fever	Positive cultures; elevated ESR/CRP; leucocytosis
Rheumatoid arthritis	Inflammatory; polyarticular	Extra-articular manifestations; DIP not affected	Positive RF, CCP; elevated ESR/CRP; erosions; periarticular osteoporosis
Psoriatic arthritis	Inflammatory; oligoarticular; polyarticular	Psoriatic skin rash; asymmetric sacroiliac joint involvement; spondylitis; syndesmophytes	Erosions; Ankylosis
Ankylosing spondylitis	Inflammatory	Spondylitis (bamboo spine); syndesmophytes, symmetric sacroiliac involvement	Ankylosis

PIP, proximal interphalangeal joint; DIP, distal interphalangeal joint; MTP, metatarsophalangeal joint; CMC, carpometacarpal joint; ESR, erythrocyte sedimentation rate; CRP, C-reactive protein; CPPD, calcium pyrophosphate dehydrate; RF, rheumatoid factor; CCP, citrullinated peptide.

- **Side effects**
  - **Gastrointestinal (GI) toxicity** manifests clinically as dyspepsia, nausea, vomiting, or GI bleeding. Nausea and dyspepsia often respond to the addition of a histamine-2 (H_2)-blocking agent or proton pump inhibitor or to a change NSAIDs. Direct GI irritation can be minimized by administration after food, by the use of enteric-coated preparations, and by use of the lowest effective dose. All NSAIDs, however, have a systemic effect on the GI mucosa, resulting in increased permeability to gastric acid. Most serious GI bleeds during NSAID use occur without prior GI symptoms. **Risk factors for GI bleed** include a history of duodenal–gastric ulceration, age, smoking, ethanol use, and concomitant use of corticosteroids. **Misoprostol,** a synthetic prostaglandin E analog, decreases the risk of NSAID-induced gastric or duodenal ulceration but may cause diarrhea and is an abortifacient. An alternative is high-dose **famotidine,** 40 mg PO bid, or **omeprazole,** 20 mg daily.
  - **Acute renal failure** is the most common form of renal toxicity, and nephrotic syndrome and acute interstitial nephritis may also occur. **Risk factors** for acute renal failure include pre-existing renal dysfunction, congestive heart failure (CHF), cirrhosis with ascites, **and concomitant angiotensin-converting enzyme (ACE) inhibitor or angiotensin-receptor blockers.** Periodic monitoring of renal function is recommended, particularly in elderly patients.
  - **Platelet dysfunction** can be caused by all NSAIDs, particularly aspirin which is a covalent inhibitor of cyclooxygenase. NSAIDs should be used cautiously or avoided in patients with a bleeding diathesis and those taking warfarin. NSAIDs should be discontinued 5 to 7 days before surgical procedures.
  - **Hypersensitivity reactions** are often seen in patients with a history of asthma, nasal polyps, or atopy. NSAIDs may cause a variety of type I hypersensitivity-like reactions, including urticaria, asthma, and anaphylactoid shock, presumably by increasing leukotriene synthesis. Patients with a hypersensitivity reaction to one NSAID should avoid all NSAIDs and selective COX-2 inhibitors.
  - **Other side effects. Central nervous system** (CNS) toxicity (headaches, dizziness, dysphoria, confusion, aseptic meningitis) is uncommon. Tinnitus and deafness can complicate NSAID use, particularly with high-dose salicylates. **Blood dyscrasias** including aplastic anemia have been observed as isolated case reports with ibuprofen, piroxicam, indomethacin, and phenylbutazone. **Dermatologic reactions** and **elevations in transaminases** have also been described. **Acid-base imbalance** is seen with high doses of salicylates. Nonacetylated salicylates have been reported to have less toxicity but also may be less effective. The use of NSAIDs in general may be associated with an increased risk for **cardiovascular thrombotic events.**
- **Selective COX-2 inhibitors** exhibit selective inhibition of COX-2, thereby inhibiting inflammation while preserving the homeostatic functions of constitutive COX-1–derived prostaglandins. Their anti-inflammatory and analgesic efficacy are similar to that of traditional NSAIDs. Celecoxib is the only selective COX-2 inhibitor approved in the United States.
- **Side effects**
  - Some data demonstrate that **GI symptoms** and **GI ulcerations** are reduced with these agents in comparison to NSAIDs. The potential gastroduodenal-sparing effect of selective COX-2 inhibitors may be eliminated by concurrent low-dose aspirin therapy for primary or secondary prevention of cardiovascular or cerebrovascular disease (*JAMA 2000; 284:1247–1255*).

- ○ **Platelet function** is not impaired, making selective COX-2 inhibitors a good anti-inflammatory option for patients with thrombocytopenia, hemostatic defects, or chronic anticoagulation. In patients who are taking warfarin, however, the international normalized ratio (INR) should be monitored after the addition of a COX-2 inhibitor (as with any medication change). In addition, there has been controversy as to whether the inhibition of prostacyclin but not thromboxane by these agents may promote clotting slightly.
  - ○ Patients with hypersensitivity reactions to NSAIDs should not use a COX-2 inhibitor. It has been suggested that individuals with a sulfonamide allergy should not use celecoxib although some recent studies have found no untoward effect of this medication in patients allergic to sulfonamide. However, further investigations are required to confirm this concern.
  - ○ An increase in blood pressure has also been associated with the use of celecoxib. A dose-related increased in cardiovascular events has been associated with the use of this medication.
- **Glucocorticoids** exert a pluripotent anti-inflammatory effect via the inhibition of inflammatory mediator gene transcription.
  - **Preparations, dosages, and routes of administration.** The goal of glucocorticoid therapy is to suppress disease activity with the minimum effective dosage. Prednisone (PO) and methylprednisolone (IV) are generally the preferred drugs because of cost and half-life considerations. IM absorption is variable and therefore is not advised. The dose, route, and frequency of administration are determined by the type of disease and the severity of the disease manifestations. The following are **relative anti-inflammatory potencies** of common glucocorticoid preparations: cortisone, 0.8; hydrocortisone, 1; prednisone, 4; methylprednisolone, 5; dexamethasone, 25.
  - **Side effects.** Adverse effects are related to dosage and duration of administration and, except for cataracts and osteoporosis, can be minimized by alternate-day administration once the disease is controlled (twice the daily dose given every other day).
    - ○ **Adrenal suppression.** Glucocorticoids suppress the hypothalamic–pituitary–adrenal axis. Assume functional suppression in patients receiving more than 20 mg of prednisone (or the equivalent) daily for more than three weeks or in patients with Cushingoid appearance. Adrenal suppression is unlikely if the patient has received any dose of steroids for less than 3 weeks or if using alternate-day therapy. The degree of adrenal suppression is uncertain in patients receiving 10 to 20 mg of prednisone for more than 3 weeks. Adrenal suppression is minimized by dosing in the morning and using a single daily low dose of a short-acting preparation, such as prednisone, for a short period. In patients who are receiving chronic glucocorticoid therapy, hypoadrenalism (anorexia, weight loss, lethargy, fever, and postural hypotension) may occur at times of severe stress (e.g., infection, major surgery) and should be treated with stress doses of glucocorticoids. Mineralocorticoid activity, however, is preserved. These patients should wear a medical-alert bracelet or carry identification.
    - ○ **Immunosuppression.** Glucocorticoid therapy reduces resistance to infections. **Bacterial infections** in particular are related to the dosage of glucocorticoids and are a major cause of morbidity and mortality. Thus, minor infections may become systemic, quiescent infections may be activated, and organisms that usually are nonpathogenic may cause disease. Local and systemic signs of infection may be partially masked, although fever associated with infection generally is

not suppressed completely by glucocorticoids. When possible, a skin test for tuberculosis should be placed before glucocorticoid therapy is instituted, and, if it is positive, appropriate prophylaxis is indicated.

o **Endocrine abnormalities.** Possible endocrine abnormalities include a cushingoid habitus and hirsutism. Hyperglycemia may be induced or aggravated by glucocorticoids but usually is not a contraindication to therapy. Insulin therapy may be required, although ketoacidosis is rare. Fluid and electrolyte abnormalities include hypokalemia and sodium retention, which may induce or aggravate hypertension.

o **Osteoporosis** with vertebral compression fractures is common among patients who are receiving long-term glucocorticoid therapy. Supplemental calcium, 1.0 to 1.5 g/d PO, should be given along with vitamin D, **400–800 units daily PO,** as soon as steroid therapy is begun. A bisphosphonate may be indicated in postmenopausal women or in men or premenopausal women who are at high risk for osteoporosis, and calcitonin can be considered for those who cannot tolerate a bisphosphonate. Teriparatide (recombinant human parathyroid hormone [1–34]) is another alternative (*N Engl J Med 2007;357:2028–2039*). Determination of baseline bone density is appropriate in these patients. A judicious exercise program may be beneficial in stimulating bone formation.

o **Steroid myopathy** generally involves the hip and shoulder girdle musculature. Muscles are weak but not tender and, in contrast to inflammatory myositis, serum creatine kinase, aldolase, and electromyography are normal. The myopathy usually resolves slowly with a reduction in glucocorticoid dosage and an aggressive exercise program.

o **Ischemic bone necrosis** (aseptic necrosis, avascular necrosis) caused by glucocorticoid use often is multifocal, most commonly affecting the femoral head, humeral head, and tibial plateau. Early changes can be demonstrated by bone scan or magnetic resonance imaging (MRI).

o **Other adverse effects.** Changes in **mental status** ranging from mild nervousness, euphoria, and insomnia to severe depression or psychosis may occur. **Ocular effects** include increased intraocular pressure (sometimes precipitating glaucoma) and the formation of posterior subcapsular cataracts. **Hyperlipidemia, menstrual irregularities,** increased perspiration with **night sweats,** and **pseudotumor cerebri** also may occur.

• **Immunomodulatory and immunosuppressive drugs** include a number of pharmacologically diverse agents that exert anti-inflammatory or immunosuppressive effects. Often such agents are referred to as *disease-modifying antirheumatic drugs.* They are characterized by a delayed onset of action and the potential for serious toxicity. Consequently, they should be prescribed with the guidance of a rheumatologist or other physician who is experienced in their use and given only to well-informed, cooperative patients who are willing to comply with meticulous follow-up. The specific agents will be discussed in relation to the diseases for which they are indicated (see below).

• **Complications**
  • Postinjection synovitis may develop rarely as a result of phagocytosis of glucocorticoid ester crystals. Such reactions usually resolve within 48 to 72 hours. More persistent symptoms suggest the possibility of iatrogenic infection, which occurs very rarely (in <0.1% of patients).
  • Localized skin depigmentation and atrophy may result after glucocorticoid injection. Accelerated deterioration of bone and cartilage also may occur when frequent

injections are administered over an extended period. Therefore, any single joint should be injected no more frequently than every 3 to 6 months.

Other Nonoperative Therapies

Joint aspiration should be performed (a) when an effusion is present in a single joint and its etiology is unclear, (b) for symptomatic relief in a patient with a known arthritis diagnosis, and (c) to monitor the response to therapy in patients with infectious arthritis. Intra-articular glucocorticoid therapy can be used to suppress inflammation when only one or a few peripheral joints are inflamed and infection has been excluded. The joint should be aspirated to remove as much fluid as possible before glucocorticoid injection. Glucocorticoid preparations include methylprednisolone acetate, triamcinolone acetonide, and triamcinolone hexacetonide. The dose used is arbitrary, but the following guidelines based on volume are useful: large joints (knee, ankle, shoulder), 1 to 2 mL; medium joints (wrists, elbows), 0.5 to 1.0 mL; and small joints of the hands and feet, 0.25 to 0.5 mL. Lidocaine (or its equivalent), up to 1 mL of a 1% solution, can be mixed in a single syringe with the glucocorticoid to promote immediate relief but is not generally used in the digits.

- **Technique.** The site of aspiration should be cleansed with povidone–iodine solution. Topical ethyl chloride spray can be used as a local anesthetic. The site can also be infiltrated with local anesthetic in preparation for the procedure, particularly if there is little or no joint effusion or if there is notable joint space narrowing.
- **Contraindications.** Infection overlying the site to be injected is an absolute contraindication. Significant hemostatic defects and bacteremia are relative contraindications to joint aspiration and injection.

Infectious Arthritis and Bursitis

GENERAL PRINCIPLES

Classification

Infectious arthritis is generally categorized into gonococcal and nongonococcal disease.

Etiology

- **Nongonococcal infectious arthritis** in adults tends to occur in patients with previous joint damage or compromised host defenses. It is caused most often by *Staphylococcus aureus* (60%) and *Streptococcus* species. Gram-negative organisms are less common and typically seen with IV drug abuse, neutropenia, concomitant urinary tract infection, or postoperative status.
- In contrast **gonococcal arthritis** causes one-half of all septic arthritis in otherwise healthy, sexually active young adults.

DIAGNOSIS

Clinical Presentation

- **Nongonococcal infectious arthritis** usually presents with fever and an acute monarticular arthritis, although multiple joints may be affected by hematogenous spread of pathogens.

- The clinical spectrum of **gonococcal arthritis** often includes migratory or additive polyarthralgias, followed by tenosynovitis or arthritis of the wrist, ankle, or knee and vesiculopustular skin lesions on the extremities or trunk.

Diagnostic Testing

- **Joint fluid examination,** including Gram stain of a centrifuged pellet, a joint fluid leukocyte count, and cultures are mandatory to make a diagnosis and to guide management. Synovial fluid Gram stain may be positive in 50% to 70% of non-gonococcal infectious arthritis (*Infect Dis Clin North Am 2005;19:799–817*). Cultures of blood and other possible extra-articular sites of infection also should be obtained.
- In contrast to nongonococcal infectious arthritis, Gram staining of synovial fluid and cultures of blood or synovial fluid often are negative in cases of gonococcal arthritis.
  - Bacteriologic assessment of the throat, cervix, urethra, and rectum may aid in establishing the diagnosis.

TREATMENT

- **Initial antimicrobial therapy** is based on the clinical situation.
  - With a positive Gram stain, antibiotic coverage can be focused accordingly.
  - With a nondiagnostic Gram stain, antibiotics should be chosen to cover *S. aureus, Streptococcus* species, and *Neisseria gonorrhoeae* in otherwise healthy patients, whereas broad-spectrum antibiotics are appropriate in immunosuppressed patients.
  - IV antimicrobials usually are given for at least 2 weeks, followed by 1 to 2 weeks of oral antimicrobials, with the course of therapy tailored to the patient's response.
  - Treatment of gonococcal arthritis is with an IV antibiotic for the first 1 to 3 days, generally ceftriaxone, 1 to 2 g IV daily. After clinical improvement is noted, therapy is continued with an oral antibiotic to complete 7 to 14 days of treatment. Fluoroquinolones are no longer recommended for treatment of gonococcal infections (*MMWR 2007;56:332*). Cefixime 400 mg PO bid or amoxicillin/clavulanate, 500 to 350 mg PO bid may be used. Treatment of coexisting *Chlamydia* infection should also be considered.
  - Oral or intra-articular antimicrobials are not appropriate as initial therapy.
- **An NSAID** is often useful to reduce pain and increase joint mobility but should not be used until response to antimicrobial therapy has been demonstrated by symptomatic and laboratory improvement.
- **Surgical drainage** or arthroscopic lavage and drainage are indicated for (a) a septic hip; (b) joints in which either the anatomy, large amounts of tissue debris, or loculation of pus prevent adequate needle drainage (most commonly the shoulder); (c) septic arthritis with coexistent osteomyelitis; (d) joints that do not respond in 3 to 5 days to appropriate therapy and repeated arthrocenteses; and (e) prosthetic joint infection.
- **General supportive** measures include splinting of the joint, which may help to relieve pain. However, prolonged immobilization can result in joint stiffness.
- **Hospitalization** is indicated to ensure drug compliance and careful monitoring of the clinical response.
- **Repeated arthrocentesis** should be performed daily or as often as necessary to prevent reaccumulation of fluid. Arthrocentesis is indicated to (a) remove destructive inflammatory mediators, (b) reduce intra-articular pressure and promote

antimicrobial penetration into the joint, and (c) monitor response to therapy by documenting sterility of synovial fluid cultures and steadily decreasing leukocyte counts.

SPECIAL CONSIDERATIONS

Nonbacterial infectious arthritis is common with many viral infections, especially hepatitis B, rubella, mumps, infectious mononucleosis, parvovirus, enterovirus, and adenovirus.

- It is generally self-limiting, lasting for <6 weeks, and responds well to a conservative regimen of rest and NSAIDs.
- Arthralgias (often severe) or a reactive arthritis can also be a manifestation of HIV infection.
- A variety of fungi and mycobacteria can cause septic arthritis and should be considered in patients with chronic monoarticular arthritis.

Septic Bursitis

DIAGNOSIS

- Usually involving the olecranon or prepatellar bursa, it can be differentiated from septic arthritis by localized, fluctuant superficial swelling and by relatively painless joint motion (particularly extension).
- Most patients have a history of previous trauma to the area or an occupational predisposition (e.g., "housemaid's knee," "writer's elbow").
- *S. aureus* is the most common pathogen of septic bursitis.

TREATMENT

- Septic bursitis should be treated with aspiration, which can be repeated if fluid reaccumulates. Oral antibiotics (guided by Gram stain and culture of bursa fluid) and outpatient management are usually appropriate, and surgical drainage is indicated only if adequate needle drainage is not possible.
- Preventive measures (e.g., knee pads) should be used in patients with occupational predispositions to septic bursitis.

Lyme Disease

GENERAL PRINCIPLES

Etiology

Lyme disease is caused by the tick-borne spirochete *Borrelia burgdorferi*.

DIAGNOSIS

- Typical manifestations begin with an erythematous annular rash (erythema migrans) and flulike symptoms.
- Arthralgias, myalgias, meningitis, neuropathy, and cardiac conduction defects may follow in weeks to a few months. Months later, an intermittent or chronic arthritis in

one or a few joints, characteristically including the knee, may develop in untreated patients.
- The diagnosis is based on the clinical picture and exposure in an endemic area, and supported by serology.

Diagnostic Testing

A two-tiered serologic assay with ELISA and IgG western blot for *B. burgdorferi* is uniformly positive by the time frank arthritis develops. False positives occur, however, and may signify prior infection. *B. burgdorferi* DNA can be detected by PCR in synovial fluid in 85% of cases.

TREATMENT

- Antibiotic therapy is required, generally with doxycycline 100 mg PO bid or amoxicillin 500 mg PO tid for 28 days (*Infect Dis Clin North Am* 2008;22:289–300).
- NSAIDs are a useful adjunct for arthritis.

Crystal-Induced Synovitis

GENERAL PRINCIPLES

Definition

Deposition of microcrystals in joints and periarticular tissues results in **gout, pseudogout,** and **apatite disease.**

Classification

- The clinical phases of gout can be divided into (a) asymptomatic hyperuricemia, (b) acute gouty arthritis, and (c) chronic arthritis.
- **Asymptomatic hyperuricemia** (uric acid levels > 7 mg/dL in men and > 6 mg/dL in women).

Epidemiology

Men are much more commonly affected by gouty arthritis than women; most premenopausal women with gout have a family history of the disease.

Etiology

- **Primary gouty arthritis** is characterized by hyperuricemia that is usually because of underexcretion of uric acid (90% of cases) rather than its overproduction. Urate crystals may be deposited in the joints, subcutaneous tissues (tophi), and kidneys.
- **Secondary gout,** like primary gout, can be caused by either defective renal excretion or overproduction of uric acid. Intrinsic renal disease, diuretic therapy, low-dose aspirin, cyclosporine, and ethanol all interfere with renal excretion of uric acid. Starvation, lactic acidosis, dehydration, preeclampsia, and diabetic ketoacidosis also can induce hyperuricemia.
- **Pseudogout** results when calcium pyrophosphate dihydrate crystals deposited in bone and cartilage are released into synovial fluid and induce acute inflammation. **Risk factors** include older age, advanced osteoarthritis (OA), neuropathic joint, gout, hyperparathyroidism, hemochromatosis, diabetes mellitus, hypothyroidism, and hypomagnesemia.

DIAGNOSIS

Clinical Presentation

- **Acute gouty arthritis** presents as an excruciating attack of pain, usually in a single joint of the foot or ankle. Occasionally, a polyarticular onset can mimic rheumatoid arthritis (RA).
- **Chronic gouty arthritis.** With time, acute gouty attacks occur more frequently, asymptomatic periods are shorter, and chronic joint deformity may appear. Overproduction of uric acid occurs in myeloproliferative and lymphoproliferative disorders, hemolytic anemia, polycythemia, and cyanotic congenital heart disease.
- **Pseudogout** may present as an **acute monarthritis or oligoarthritis** mimicking gout or as a **chronic polyarthritis** resembling RA or OA. Usually the knee or wrist is affected, although any synovial joint can be involved.
- **Apatite disease** may present with periarthritis or tendonitis, particularly in patients with chronic renal failure. An episodic oligoarthritis also may occur.

History

Acute gouty arthritis attacks can be precipitated by surgery, dehydration, fasting, binge eating, or heavy ingestion of alcohol. Although the acute gouty attack will subside spontaneously over several days, prompt treatment can abort the attack within hours.

Diagnostic Testing

Laboratories

- A definitive diagnosis of gout or pseudogout is made by finding intracellular crystals in joint fluid examined with a compensated polarized light microscope. Urate crystals, which are diagnostic of gout, are needle shaped and strongly negatively birefringent. The calcium pyrophosphate dihydrate crystals seen in pseudogout are pleomorphic and weakly positively birefringent. Hydroxyapatite complexes, diagnostic of apatite disease, and basic calcium phosphate complexes can be identified only by electron microscopy and mass spectroscopy. In most cases, the arthritides associated with these compounds are suspected clinically but never confirmed.
- **Acute gouty arthritis.** The serum uric acid level is normal in 30% of patients with acute gout and, if elevated, should not be manipulated until an attack has resolved.
- Apatite disease should be suspected when no crystals are present in the synovial fluid.

Imaging

- Erosive arthritis may be seen.
- If pseudogout is suspected, films of the wrists, knees, and pubic symphysis may be ordered. These are the most common sites for chondrocalcinosis, a finding that is supportive of (but not diagnostic for) pseudogout.

TREATMENT

- **Asymptomatic hyperuricemia** is not routinely treated because of expense and the potential drug toxicity.
- **Management of secondary gout** includes treatment of the underlying disorder and urate-lowering therapy.
- The treatment of **apatite disease** is similar to that for pseudogout.

Medications

- **Acute gout**
  - NSAIDs are the treatment of choice due to ease of administration and low toxicity. Clinical response may require 12 to 24 hours, and initial doses should be high, followed by rapid tapering over 2 to 8 days. One approach is to use indomethacin, 50 mg PO q6h for 2 days, followed by 50 mg PO q8h for 3 days and then 25 mg PO q8h for 2 to 3 days. The long-acting NSAIDs generally are not recommended for acute gout.
  - Glucocorticoids are useful when NSAIDs are contraindicated. An intra-articular injection of glucocorticoids produces rapid dramatic relief. Alternatively, prednisone, 40 to 60 mg PO daily, can be given until a response is obtained and then should be tapered rapidly.
  - **Colchicine is most effective if given in the first 12 to 24 hours** of an acute attack and usually brings relief in 6 to 12 hours. In view of the efficacy and tolerability of a short course of NSAIDs, colchicine is not commonly used to treat gout but is useful when NSAIDs or glucocorticoids are contraindicated or not tolerated.
    - ○ **Oral administration** is often associated with severe GI toxicity. The dosage during an acute attack is 0.6 mg q1–2h for three dosages started at the first sign of the attack. Alternatively, colchicine 0.6 mg tid can be used (*Ann Rheum Dis 2006; 65:1312–1324*). The previous dosage regimen of 0.6 mg q1–2h or 1.0 to 1.2 mg q2h until symptoms abate, GI toxicity develops, or the maximum dose of 6 mg in a 24-hour period is reached is not recommended as primary treatment for most cases due to toxicity. The lower dose regimen has recently been shown to be equally effective with less toxicity.
    - ○ **IV colchicine** is not recommended for general use and its administration in almost all circumstances is questionable.
- **Chronic gouty arthritis**
  - **Colchicine** (0.6 mg PO daily or bid) can be used prophylactically for acute attacks. The dosage needs to be adjusted in patients with renal insufficiency. Colchicine 0.6 mg every other day or every 3 days should be considered in patients with a creatinine clearance between 10 and 34 mL/min. Aspirin (uricoretentive), diuretics, large alcohol intake, and foods high in purines (sweetbreads, anchovies, shellfish, sardines, liver, and kidney) should be avoided. Weight loss should be encouraged. Frequent gout attacks, tophi, joint damage, and urate nephropathy are indications for urate-lowering therapy. **Maintenance colchicine, 0.6 mg PO bid, should be given for a few days before manipulation of the uric acid level to prevent precipitation of an acute attack.** In patients without tophi, prophylactic colchicine can be discontinued 6 months after the target serum urate levels have been obtained and no acute attacks have been documented by the patient. In patients with tophi, duration of prophylaxis is uncertain but consider discontinuation 6 months after resolution of tophi.
  - **Allopurinol,** a xanthine oxidase inhibitor, is effective therapy for hyperuricemia in most patients.
    - ○ **Dosage and administration.** The initial dosage is usually 300 mg PO daily. Daily doses can be increased by 100 mg every 2 to 4 weeks to achieve the minimum maintenance dosage that will keep the uric acid level below 6 mg/dL, which is the below the limit of solubility of monosodium urate in serum. In patients with impaired renal function, the starting daily dose should be reduced by 50 mg for each 20-mL/min decrease in the creatinine clearance. For patients

with a creatinine clearance below 20 mL/min, the starting dosage is 100 mg every other or every third day. The daily dose should be decreased also in patients with hepatic impairment. The concomitant use of a uricosuric agent may hasten the mobilization of tophi. **If an acute attack occurs during treatment with allopurinol, it should be continued at the same dosage while other agents are used to treat the attack.**

○ **Side effects. Hypersensitivity reactions** from a minor skin rash to a diffuse exfoliative dermatitis associated with fever, eosinophilia, and a combination of renal and hepatic injury occur in up to 5% of patients. Patients who have mild renal insufficiency and are receiving diuretics are at greatest risk. Severe cases are potentially fatal and usually require glucocorticoid therapy. Allopurinol may potentiate the effect of oral anticoagulants and blocks metabolism of azathioprine and 6-mercaptopurine, necessitating a 60% to 75% reduction in dosage of these cytotoxic drugs.

- **Febuxostat** is a nonpurine selective inhibitor of the xanthine oxidase that has recently been approved in the United States. Its urate-lowering effect is equal or greater to that of allopurinol, with less risk of hypersensitivity reactions and greater efficacy in patients with chronic kidney disease (*Arthritis Rheum 2008;59:1540–1548*). It is significantly more expensive than Allopurinol. The starting dose is 40 mg/d, with titration to 80 mg/d if needed.

- **Uricase** catabolizes uric acid to the more soluble compound, allantoin. It is available in the United States for the treatment of tumor lysis syndrome in a recombinant form (Rasburicase).

- **Uricosuric drugs** lower serum uric acid levels by blocking renal tubular reabsorption of uric acid. A 24-hour measurement of creatinine clearance and urine uric acid should be obtained before therapy is started, as these drugs are **ineffective with glomerular filtration rates of <50 mL/min.** They are also not recommended for patients who already have high levels of urine uric acid (800 mg/24 hr) because of the risk of urate stone formation. This risk can be minimized by maintaining a high fluid intake and by alkalinizing the urine. If these drugs are being used when an acute gouty attack begins, they should be continued while other drugs are used to treat the acute attack.

○ **Probenecid**
  - Initial dosage is 500 mg PO daily, which can be raised in 500-mg increments every week until serum uric acid levels normalize or urine uric acid levels exceed 800 mg/24 hr. The maximum dose is 3,000 mg/d. Most patients require a total of 1.0 to 1.5 g/d in two to three divided doses.
  - Salicylates and probenecid are antagonistic and should not be used together.
  - Probenecid decreases renal excretion of penicillin, indomethacin, and sulfonylureas.
  - Side effects are minimal.

○ **Sulfinpyrazone** has uricosuric efficacy similar to that of probenecid; however, it also inhibits platelet function. The initial dosage of 50 mg PO bid can be increased in 100-mg increments weekly until serum uric acid levels normalize, to a maximum dose of 800 mg/d. Most patients require 300 to 400 mg/d in three to four divided doses.

- **Pseudogout**
  - As in gout, the therapy of choice for most patients is a brief high-dose course of an NSAID

- **Oral corticosteroids** can be used and **colchicine** also may relieve symptoms promptly, but toxicity limits its use. Dosage and administration are similar to the ones used in the treatment of gout.
- Maintenance daily PO colchicine may diminish the number of recurrent attacks. Allopurinol or uricosuric agents have no role in treating pseudogout.
- Aspiration of the inflammatory joint fluid often results in prompt improvement and intra-articular injection of glucocorticoids may hasten the response.

Rheumatoid Arthritis

GENERAL PRINCIPLES

Definition

RA is a systemic disease of unknown etiology that is characterized by symmetric inflammatory polyarthritis, extra-articular manifestations (rheumatoid nodules, pulmonary fibrosis, serositis, vasculitis), and serum rheumatoid factor in up to 80% of patients.

DIAGNOSIS

Clinical Presentation

- Most patients describe the insidious onset of pain, swelling, and morning stiffness in the hands and/or wrists.
- Synovitis may be evident upon exam of the metacarpophalangeal, proximal interphalangeal, wrists, or other joints. Rheumatoid nodules may be palpated most commonly on extensor surfaces.
- The course of RA is variable but tends to be chronic and progressive.
- Clinical criteria for the diagnosis of RA is available (Table 2).

Diagnostic Testing

Rheumatoid factor may be positive in 80% of patients, and anti-CCP (cyclic citrullinated peptide) is positive in 80% to 90% of patients.

- CCP antibodies are more specific (90%) for RA than is the RF, which can also be elevated in the setting of Hepatitis C and other chronic infections.

Table 2	The American College of Rheumatology 1987 Classification Criteria[a]

Morning stiffness (>60 min)
Arthritis of three or more joint areas
Arthritis of hand joints
Symmetric arthritis
Rheumatoid nodules
Serum rheumatoid factor
X-ray changes (erosions or decalcification)

[a]Four of the seven criteria should be met, with criteria 1 to 4 being present for more than 6 weeks

- Hand and wrist x-rays may show early changes of erosions or periarticular osteopenia.
- Musculoskeletal MRI is more sensitive than plain x-ray and may be used in equivocal cases to demonstrate clinically inapparent synovitis or erosions.

TREATMENT

Most patients can benefit from an early aggressive treatment program that combines medical, rehabilitative, and surgical services designed with three distinct goals: (a) early suppression of inflammation in the joints and other tissues, (b) maintenance of joint and muscle function and prevention of deformities, and (c) repair of joint damage to relieve pain or improve function.

Medications

- **DMARDs (disease-modifying antirheumatic drugs)** appear to alter the natural history of RA by retarding the progression of bony erosions and cartilage loss. Because RA may lead to substantial long-term disability (and is associated with increased mortality), the standard of care is to initiate therapy with such agents early in the course of RA. Once a clinical response has been achieved, the chosen drug usually is continued indefinitely at the lowest effective dosage to prevent relapse.
  - **An established diagnosis of RA along with any evidence of disease activity is an indication to initiate disease-modifying therapy.** Initial monotherapy with NSAIDs or steroids is no longer considered appropriate under usual circumstances.
  - **DMARD selection** is tailored to the character of the patient's disease, taking into account the potential toxicity of these agents (see below). **Methotrexate** typically is the initial choice for moderate to severe RA. **Hydroxychloroquine or sulfasalazine** can be used as the initial choice in very mild RA. If response to the initial agent is unsatisfactory after an adequate trial (or if limiting toxicity supervenes), an alternate agent, such as leflunomide, a tumor necrosis factor (TNF) blocker, or abatacept can be added or substituted. Rituximab, a monoclonal antibody directed against the B-cell surface molecule CD20, is approved for patients who have failed TNF therapy. Abatacept is a fusion protein comprising the CTLA4 molecule and the Fc portion of IgG1. It blocks selective costimulation of T cells.
- **Methotrexate,** a purine inhibitor and folic acid antagonist, is useful in treating synovitis, regardless of the underlying disease process. RA is its most common indication. It is also useful for myositis, and may improve the leukopenia of Felty syndrome.
  - **Dosage and administration.** Typically, methotrexate is administered as a single PO dose once a week starting with 7.5 to 10 mg. Clinical response is usually noted in 4 to 8 weeks. The dosage can be increased by 2.5 to 5.0-mg increments every 2 to 4 weeks to a maximum of 25 mg/wk or until improvement is observed. Dosages above 20 mg/wk are generally given by SC injection to promote absorption.
  - **Contraindications and side effects.** Methotrexate is **teratogenic** and should not be used during pregnancy. It should also be avoided in patients with significant hepatic or renal impairment. **Folic acid supplementation** at a dosage of 1 to 2 mg daily may reduce toxicity without attenuating efficacy. Concomitant use of trimethoprim/sulfamethoxazole should be avoided.
    - **Minor side effects** include GI intolerance, stomatitis, rash, headache, and alopecia.
    - **Bone marrow suppression** may occur, particularly at higher doses. Blood and platelet counts should be obtained before initiation, every 2 to 4 weeks during

the first 3 to 4 months or if the dose is changed, and every 8 weeks thereafter. Macrocytosis may herald serious hematologic toxicity and is an indication for folate supplementation, dose reduction, or both.

- ○ **Cirrhosis** may occur rarely with long-term use. Aspartate transaminase (AST), alanine transaminase (ALT), and serum albumin should be obtained every 2 to 4 weeks during the first 3 to 4 months of therapy or if the dose is changed, and then every 8 to 12 weeks. Liver biopsy should be considered if the liver function tests are persistently elevated, if the AST is elevated in five of nine determinations or if the serum albumin level falls below the normal range. Alcohol consumption increases the risk of methotrexate hepatotoxicity.
- ○ **Hypersensitivity pneumonitis** may occur but usually is reversible. Distinction from the ILD associated with RA may be difficult. Patients with pre-existing pulmonary parenchymal disease may be at increased risk. **New or worsening symptoms of dyspnea in a patient on methotrexate should prompt evaluation for pneumonitis.**
- ○ **Rheumatoid nodules** may develop or worsen, paradoxically, in some patients on methotrexate.
- **Sulfasalazine** is useful for treating synovitis in the setting of RA and the seronegative spondyloarthropathies.
  - **Dosage.** The initial dosage is 500 mg PO daily, with increases in 500-mg increments weekly until a total daily dose of 2,000 to 3,000 mg (given in evenly divided doses) is reached. Clinical response usually occurs in 6 to 10 weeks.
  - **Contraindications and side effects. Sulfasalazine should not be used in patients with glucose-6-phosphate dehydrogenase deficiency or sulfa allergy.** Nausea is the principal adverse effect and can be minimized by the use of the enteric-coated preparation of the drug. Hematologic toxicity including a reduction in any cell line and aplastic anemia rarely occurs. Periodic monitoring of blood and platelet counts is, however, recommended.
- **Hydroxychloroquine** is an antimalarial agent that is used to treat dermatitis, alopecia, and synovitis in systemic lupus erythematosus (SLE) and mild synovitis in RA.
  - **Dosage.** Hydroxychloroquine typically is given at a dosage of 4 to 6 mg/kg PO daily (200 to 400 mg) after meals to minimize dyspepsia and nausea.
  - **Contraindications and side effects. Hydroxychloroquine should not be used in patients with porphyria, glucose-6-phosphate dehydrogenase deficiency, or significant hepatic or renal impairment.** It is probably safe during pregnancy. The most common side effects are allergic skin eruptions and nausea. Serious ocular toxicity occurs but is rare with currently recommended dosages. Ophthalmologic evaluation should be performed on an annual basis.
- **Leflunomide** is a pyrimidine inhibitor that has been approved for the treatment of RA.
  - **Dosage and administration.** Treatment is begun with 10 or 20 mg PO daily. Clinical response is generally seen within 4 to 8 weeks.
  - **Contraindications and side effects.** Leflunomide is **teratogenic** and has a very long half-life. Women who plan to become pregnant must discontinue the drug and complete a course of elimination therapy with cholestyramine, 8 g PO tid for 11 days. Plasma levels should then be verified to be <0.02 mg/L on two separate tests at least 14 days apart before pregnancy is considered. Leflunomide is **contraindicated** in patients with significant hepatic dysfunction or in those who are receiving rifampin. **GI side effects** are the most common. **Diarrhea** occurs in up to 20% of patients and may require discontinuation of the drug. Dosage

reduction to 10 mg/d may provide relief while maintaining efficacy, and loperamide can be used for symptomatic relief. **Elevations in serum transaminase levels** may occur, and transaminase levels should be measured at baseline and then monitored monthly. The dosage should be reduced for confirmed twofold elevations, and greater elevations should be treated with cholestyramine and discontinuation of leflunomide. **Rash** and **alopecia** may occur during therapy.

- **Anticytokine therapies** directed at specific cytokines have been developed. These agents may all be considered **biologic DMARDs.**
  - **TNF inhibitors** have been approved for treatment of RA and seronegative spondyloarthropathies, and have also been useful in some forms of vasculitis. In general, these agents are used in patients with moderate to severe RA who have failed a trial of one or more disease-modifying antirheumatic drugs as listed above. The effect of these agents on RA synovitis can be dramatic, with responsive patients reporting the onset of symptomatic benefits within 1 to 2 weeks. In addition to their symptomatic benefits, these agents appear to retard joint damage significantly. Three preparations are currently available, with similar efficacy and toxicity profiles.
    - **Etanercept** is a fusion protein that consists of the ligand-binding portion of the human TNF receptor linked to the Fc portion of human immunoglobulin G (IgG). It binds to TNF, blocking its interaction with cell surface receptors, thus inhibiting the inflammatory and immunoregulatory properties of TNF. This preparation is given in a dosage of 25 mg SC twice a week or 50 mg SC weekly.
    - **Infliximab** is a chimeric monoclonal antibody that binds specifically to human TNF-α, blocking its proinflammatory and immunomodulatory effects. It is given by IV infusion in conjunction with methotrexate to reduce production of neutralizing antibodies against infliximab. The recommended treatment regimen includes infliximab infusions of 3 mg/kg at initiation, at 2 and 6 weeks, and every 8 weeks thereafter, along with methotrexate at a dose of at least 7.5 mg/wk.
    - **Adalimumab** is a recombinant human IgG-1 monoclonal antibody that is specific to human TNF-α. It can be given in a dosage of 40 mg SC every other week.
- **Contraindications and side effects**
  - **Serious infections and sepsis,** including fatalities, have been reported during the use of TNF-blocking agents. These drugs are contraindicated in patients with acute or chronic infections, and if serious infection or sepsis occurs, the drug should be stopped. Those with a history of recurrent infections and those with underlying conditions that may predispose to infection should be treated with caution and counseled to be vigilant for signs and symptoms of infection. Upper respiratory and sinus infections are most common. Tuberculosis has also been noted, and a tuberculin skin test and chest radiograph should be obtained before beginning therapy. These agents are also contraindicated in patients with CHF. Patients who are undergoing elective surgical procedures can omit the last dose of the drug that is scheduled to be given before surgery, as well as the next dose scheduled to follow the surgery.
  - **Local injection site reactions** are common with etanercept and adalimumab, particularly during the first month of therapy. These reactions are generally self-limited and do not require discontinuation of therapy. Serious systemic allergic reactions are rare but may occur with infliximab infusions.
  - **Other adverse effects** may include induction of antinuclear antibodies and, rarely, a lupus-like illness. A demyelinating disorder has been described as well as

exacerbations of pre-existing multiple sclerosis. It is unclear whether the frequency of occurrence of lymphoma may be increased in patients who receive these agents.

- **Interleukin inhibitors.** While only one interleukin inhibitor is currently available for patients with rheumatic diseases, several are in development.
  - **Anakinra** is a recombinant IL-1– receptor antagonist that is approved for use in RA. It blocks binding of IL-1 to its receptor, thus inhibiting the proinflammatory and immunomodulatory actions of IL-1.
    - It is given in a **dosage** of 100 mg SC daily. Like the TNF blockers, it should not be prescribed to patients with ongoing or recurrent infections.
    - **Adverse effects** include an increased frequency of bacterial infections and injection site reactions.
  - **Tocilizumab** is an antagonist of soluble and membrane bound IL-6 receptors. It is approved for RA in Japan and is awaiting approval in the United States. It is given as an IV infusion. Side effects include increased infections, neutropenia, and elevations in cholesterol.
- **B-cell–directed therapy.** One biologic agent targeting B cells, rituximab, is currently available. Several more are in development.
  - **Rituximab** is a monoclonal antibody directed against CD20, a cell surface receptor found on B cells. CD20-positive B cells in peripheral blood are rapidly depleted after 2 infusions of 1 g of rituximab 2 weeks apart. Methotrexate is generally used as background therapy. It is redosed in 6 to 12 month intervals, based on patient symptoms. It is FDA-approved for patients having failed anti-TNF therapy.
    - **Contraindications and side effects.** Rituximab has rarely been reported to cause reactivation of JC virus, leading to the clinical syndrome of progressive multifocal leukoencephalopathy, which is uniformly fatal.
    - **Infusion reactions** are more common with the first dose, and have rarely been fatal. Antihistamines, IV steroids, and acetaminophen are routinely given prior to infusion.
    - **Infectious complications** are a concern as with all biologics, but appear to be less frequent than in TNF-treated patients.
- **Abatacept** is a fusion protein comprising the CTLA4 molecule and the Fc portion of IgG1. It blocks selective costimulation of T cells. It is given as an IV infusion of 500 to 1000 mg every 4 weeks. It is approved in patients with an inadequate response to biologic or nonbiologic DMARDs.
  - **Infections** occur slightly more often than in placebo-treated patients. Opportunistic infections have not been observed. **Infusion reactions** are much less common than with rituximab.
  - **COPD exacerbations and respiratory infections** are more common in patients with obstructive lung disease when treated with abatacept.
- **Combinations of DMARDs** can be used if the patient has a partial response to the initial agent.
  - Common combination therapies include methotrexate with either hydroxychloroquine, sulfasalazine, or both. Methotrexate is commonly combined with TNF antagonists as there is evidence for additive efficacy and for a decrease in the formation of HACAs (human antichimeric antibodies) against the TNF blocker. Methotrexate is often used in combination with rituximab or abatacept. Methotrexate and leflunomide may have additive hepatotoxicity, and this combination should be used cautiously.
- **Combination therapy including two biologic agents is contraindicated because of increased infectious complications.**

- **NSAIDs or selective COX-2 inhibitors** may be used as an adjunct to DMARD therapy. A longer-acting NSAID may facilitate patient compliance.
- **Glucocorticoids** are not curative and probably do not alter the natural history of RA; however, they are among the most potent anti-inflammatory drugs available (see General Principles under Basic Approach to the Rheumatic Diseases).
  - **Indications** for glucocorticoids include (a) symptomatic relief while waiting for a response to a slow-acting immunosuppressive or immunomodulatory agent, (b) persistent synovitis despite adequate trials of DMARDs and NSAIDs, and (c) severe constitutional symptoms (e.g., fever and weight loss) or extra-articular disease (vasculitis, episcleritis, or pleurisy).
  - **Oral administration** of prednisone 5 to 20 mg daily usually is sufficient for the treatment of synovitis, whereas severe constitutional symptoms or extra-articular disease may require up to 1 mg/kg PO daily. Although alternate-day glucocorticoid therapy reduces the incidence of undesirable side effects, some patients do not tolerate the increase in symptoms that may occur on the off day.
  - **Intra-articular administration** may provide temporary symptomatic relief when only a few joints are inflamed. The beneficial effects of intra-articular steroids may persist for days to months and may delay or negate the need for systemic glucocorticoid therapy.

Other Nonoperative Therapies

- **Acute care** of inflammatory arthritides involves joint protection and pain relief. Proper joint positioning and splints are important elements in joint protection. Heat is a useful analgesic.
- **Subacute disease** therapy should include a gradual increase in passive and active joint movement.
- **Chronic care** encompasses instruction in joint protection, work simplification, and performance of activities of daily living. Adaptive equipment, splints, orthotics, and mobility aids may be useful. Specific exercises designed to promote normal joint mechanics and to strengthen affected muscle groups are useful. Overall cardiac conditioning also improves functional status.

Surgical Management

- **Corrective surgical procedures** including synovectomy, total joint replacement, and joint fusion, may be indicated in patients with RA to reduce pain and to improve function.
- **Carpal tunnel syndrome** is common, and surgical repair may be curative if local injection therapy is unsuccessful.
- **Synovectomy** may be helpful if major involvement is limited to one or two joints and if a 6-month trial of medical therapy has failed, but usually it is only of temporary benefit.
- **Prophylactic synovectomy and débridement of the ulnar styloid** should be considered for patients with severe wrist disease to prevent rupture of the extensor tendons.
- Other procedures that may be beneficial include **total joint replacement** of the hip and knee joints, resection of metatarsal heads in patients with bunion deformities, and subluxation of the toes. Reconstructive hand surgery may be useful in carefully selected patients.
- **Surgical fusion of joints** usually results in freedom from pain but also in total loss of motion; this is tolerated well in the wrist and thumb.

- Cervical spine fusion of C1 and C2 is indicated for significant cervical subluxation (>5 mm) with associated neurologic deficits.
- Patients with RA undergoing elective surgical procedures should have a lateral cervical spine radiograph in flexion and extensions performed to screen for this subluxation.

COMPLICATIONS

- **Patients with RA and a single joint inflamed out of proportion to the rest of the joints must be evaluated for coexistent septic arthritis.** This complication occurs with increased frequency in RA and carries a 20% to 30% mortality.
- **Sjögren's syndrome,** characterized by failure of exocrine glands, occurs in a subset of patients with RA, producing sicca symptoms (dry eyes and mouth), parotid gland enlargement, dental caries, and recurrent tracheobronchitis.
  - Treatment is symptomatic with artificial tears and saliva, or with Pilocarpine up to 5 mg PO qid. Assiduous dental and ophthalmologic care is recommended, and drugs that suppress lacrimal–salivary secretion further should be avoided.
- **Felty syndrome,** the triad of RA, splenomegaly, and granulocytopenia, also occurs in a small subset of patients, and these patients are at risk for recurrent bacterial infections and non-healing leg ulcers.
- Approximately 70% of patients show irreversible joint damage on radiography within the first 3 years of disease. Work disability is common and life span may be shortened.

REFERRAL

Rehabilitative therapy should be managed by a team of physicians, physical and occupational therapists, nurses, social workers, and psychologists. This approach may benefit patients with any form of arthritis.

PATIENT EDUCATION

Patient education, including pamphlets and support groups, is available in many communities through local chapters of the Arthritis Foundation.

Osteoarthritis

GENERAL PRINCIPLES

Definition

OA, or **degenerative joint disease,** is characterized by deterioration of articular cartilage with subsequent formation of reactive new bone at the articular surface. The joints affected most commonly are the distal and proximal interphalangeal joints of the hands, hips, knees, and cervical and lumbar spine.

Epidemiology

The disease is more common in the elderly but may occur at any age, especially as a sequelae to joint trauma, chronic inflammatory arthritis, or congenital malformation. OA of the spine may lead to spinal stenosis (neurogenic claudication), with aching or pain in the legs or buttocks on standing or walking.

TREATMENT

Medications

- **Acetaminophen** in a dosage of up to 1,000 mg qid is the initial pharmacologic treatment.
- **Low-dose NSAIDs or selective COX-2 inhibitors** are the next step, followed by full-dose treatment (see Treatment under Basic Approach to Rheumatic Disease). Because this patient population is often elderly and may have concomitant renal or cardiopulmonary disease, NSAIDs should be used with caution. NSAID-induced GI bleeding also is increased in the elderly population.
- The data for **glucosamine sulfate,** 1,500 mg PO daily, is contradictory. Some studies suggest it may reduce symptoms as well as the rate of cartilage deterioration, especially with the preparations used in Europe (*Cochrane Database 2005;2:CD002946*). Some studies suggest **chondroitin sulfate** may also be of benefit (*Arth Rheum 2009;60:524–533*). **Intra-articular glucocorticoid injections** often are beneficial but probably should not be given more than every 3 to 6 months (see General Principles under Basic Approach to the Rheumatic Diseases).
- Systemic steroids should be avoided. The μ-opioid agonist **tramadol** may be useful as an alternative analgesic agent. Narcotic agents should be avoided for long term use. Narcotics may be useful for short term pain relief and in patients in which other therapeutic modalities are contraindicated or have failed.
- **Topical NSAIDS or capsaicin** may provide symptomatic relief with minimal toxicity.
- Synthetic and naturally occurring hyaluronic acid derivatives **(Hyalgan, Synvisc)** can be administered intra-articularly. They may reduce pain and improve mobility in select patients.

Other Nonoperative Therapies

- **Nonpharmacologic approaches** may complement drug treatment of arthritis. Activities that involve excessive use of the joint should be identified and avoided. Brief periods of rest for the involved joint can relieve pain. Poor body mechanics should be corrected and malalignments such as pronated feet may be aided by orthotics. An exercise program to prevent or correct muscle atrophy can also provide pain relief. When weight-bearing joints are affected, support in the form of a cane, crutches, or a walker can be helpful. Weight reduction may be of benefit, even for non–weight-bearing joints. Thumb splints may be useful for OA of the first carpometacarpal joint. Consultation with occupational and physical therapists may be helpful.
- **OA of the spine** may cause radicular symptoms from pressure on nerve roots and often produces pain and spasm in the paraspinal soft tissues.
  - Physical supports (cervical collar, lumbar corset), local heat, and exercises to strengthen cervical, paravertebral, and abdominal muscles may provide relief in some patients.
- **Epidural steroid injections** may reduce radicular symptoms.

Surgical Management

- When serious disability results from severe pain or deformity, **surgery** can be considered. Total hip or knee replacement usually relieves pain and increases function in selected patients.

- **Laminectomy and spinal fusion** should be reserved for patients who have severe disease with intractable pain or neurologic complications. Lumbar spinal stenosis may require extensive decompressive laminectomy for relief of symptoms.

Spondyloarthropathies

GENERAL PRINCIPLES

Definition

The **spondyloarthropathies** are an interrelated group of disorders characterized by one or more of the following features: (a) spondylitis, (b) sacroiliitis, (c) enthesopathy (inflammation at sites of tendon insertion), and (d) asymmetric oligoarthritis. Extra-articular features of this group of disorders may include inflammatory eye disease, urethritis, and mucocutaneous lesions. The spondyloarthropathies aggregate in families, where they are associated with HLA-B27.

Ankylosing Spondylitis

DIAGNOSIS

Clinical Presentation

Ankylosing spondylitis (AS) clinically presents as inflammation and ossification of the joints and ligaments of the spine and of the sacroiliac joints.

- Patients classically describe low back pain and stiffness, which improves with exercise.
- Hips and shoulders are the peripheral joints that are most commonly involved. Progressive fusion of the apophyseal joints of the spine occurs in many patients and cannot be predicted or prevented.

TREATMENT

Behavioral

- Physical therapy emphasizing extension exercises and posture is recommended to minimize possible late postural defects and respiratory compromise.
- Patients should be instructed to sleep supine on a firm bed without a pillow and to practice postural and deep-breathing exercises regularly.
- Cigarette smoking should be discouraged strongly.

Medications

- **Non-salicylate NSAIDs,** such as indomethacin, are used to provide symptomatic relief, and **selective COX-2 inhibitors** are also effective (see General Principles under Basic Approach to the Rheumatic Diseases).
- **Methotrexate and sulfasalazine** provide benefit for peripheral disease in some patients (see Treatment under Rheumatoid Arthritis).
- **TNF blockade** has been shown to be of benefit even in some patients with apparent fixed deformities.
- Glucocorticoids and immunosuppressive therapy have been used occasionally in patients who do not respond to other agents.

Surgical Management

Many patients develop osteoporosis in the fused spondylitic spine and are at risk of spinal fracture. Surgical procedures to correct some spine and hip deformities may result in significant rehabilitation in carefully selected patients.

REFERRAL

Acute anterior uveitis occurs in up to 25% of patients with AS and should be managed by an ophthalmologist. Generally, this problem is self-limited, although glaucoma and blindness are unusual secondary complications.

Arthritis of Inflammatory Bowel Disease

GENERAL PRINCIPLES

Arthritis of inflammatory bowel disease occurs in 10% to 20% of patients with Crohn's disease or ulcerative colitis and is similar to that of AS. It may also occur in some patients with intestinal bypass and diverticular disease.

DIAGNOSIS

Clinical Presentation

Clinical features include **spondylitis, sacroiliitis,** and **peripheral arthritis,** particularly in the knee and ankle. Although peripheral joint disease may correlate with the activity of the colitis, spinal disease does not.

TREATMENT

Medications

- As in AS, **NSAIDs** are the initial treatment of choice, and **selective COX-2 inhibitors** are also effective. However, GI intolerance of NSAIDs may be increased among this group of patients, and misoprostol may cause unacceptable diarrhea (see General Principles under Basic Approach to the Rheumatic Diseases).
- **Sulfasalazine** also may be beneficial for this form of arthritis (see Treatment under Rheumatoid Arthritis).
- **TNF antagonists** may benefit both the colitis and arthritis.
- Local **injection of glucocorticoids** and **physical therapy** are useful adjunctive measures.

Reactive Arthritis

GENERAL PRINCIPLES

- Reactive arthritis refers to the inflammatory arthritis, which occasionally follows certain GI or genitourinary infections. The triad of arthritis, conjunctivitis, and urethritis has classically been referred to as Reiter syndrome.
- *Chlamydia trachomatis* is the most commonly implicated genitourinary infection. *Shigella flexneri, Salmonella* species, *Yersinia enterocolitica,* or *Campylobacter jejuni* are the most commonly implicated GI infections.

- 60% to 80% of patients are HLA-B27 positive. Males and females are equally affected after GI infections, though males more commonly develop the classical Reiter syndrome after *Chlamydia* infection.

DIAGNOSIS

Clinical Presentation

The clinical syndrome may include **asymmetric oligoarthritis, urethritis, conjunctivitis,** and characteristic **skin and mucous membrane lesions.** The syndrome is usually transient, lasting from one to several months, but chronic arthritis may develop in 4% to 19% of patients.

Diagnostic Testing

The triggering infection may have been asymptomatic. Testing for stool pathogens is low yield if the diarrheal illness has resolved, but urine testing for *Chlamydia* may be helpful if the clinical syndrome is consistent with reactive arthritis.

TREATMENT

Medications

- Conservative therapy is indicated for control of pain and inflammation in these diseases.
- Spontaneous remissions are common, making evaluation of therapy difficult.
- **NSAIDs** (especially indomethacin) are often useful, and **selective COX-2 inhibitors** also provide relief (see General Principles under Basic Approach to the Rheumatic Diseases).
- **Sulfasalazine** or **methotrexate** may be of benefit for arthritis that does not resolve after several months (see Treatment under Rheumatoid Arthritis).
- In unusually severe cases, **glucocorticoid therapy** may be required to prevent rapid joint destruction (see General Principles under Basic Approach to the Rheumatic Diseases).
- Appropriate treatment for chlamydial infection, if detected, is appropriate. Prolonged empiric antibiotic therapy has not been shown to be beneficial.

REFERRAL

Conjunctivitis is usually transient and benign, but ophthalmologic referral and treatment with topical or systemic glucocorticoids are indicated for **iritis.**

Psoriatic Arthritis

GENERAL PRINCIPLES

Classification

Five major patterns of joint disease occur: (a) asymmetric oligoarticular arthritis, (b) distal interphalangeal joint involvement in association with nail disease, (c) symmetric rheumatoid-like polyarthritis, (d) spondylitis and sacroiliitis, and (e) arthritis mutilans.

Epidemiology

Seven percent of patients with psoriasis have some form of inflammatory arthritis.

TREATMENT

Medications

* **NSAIDs,** particularly indomethacin, are used to treat the arthritic manifestations of psoriasis, in conjunction with appropriate measures for the skin disease.
* **Intra-articular glucocorticoids** may be useful in the oligoarticular form of the disease, but injection through a psoriatic plaque should be avoided. Severe skin and joint diseases generally respond well to **methotrexate** (see TREATMENT under RHEUMATOID ARTHRITIS).
* **Sulfasalazine and leflunomide** may also have disease-modifying effects in polyarthritis (*J Rheum 2006;33:1417–1421*).
* **TNF-α blockers** may produce dramatic improvement in both skin and joint disease.

COMPLICATIONS

When reconstructive joint surgery is performed, colonization of psoriatic skin with *S. aureus* increases the risk of wound infection.

Systemic Lupus Erythematosus .

GENERAL PRINCIPLES

Definition

SLE is a multisystem disease of unknown etiology that primarily affects women of childbearing age. The usual female to male ratio is 9:1. It is most common in the second and third decade of life and more common in African Americans.

Pathophysiology

Pathophysiology is multifactorial and incompletely understood, with interplay of genetic predisposition and environmental factors. The genetic predisposition is complex and likely involves dozens of genes.

DIAGNOSIS

Clinical Presentation

* The course of this disease is highly variable and unpredictable.
* Disease manifestations are protean, ranging in severity from fatigue, malaise, weight loss, arthritis or arthralgias, fever, photosensitivity, rashes, and serositis to potentially life-threatening thrombocytopenia, hemolytic anemia, nephritis, cerebritis, vasculitis, pneumonitis, myositis, and myocarditis.
* Current American College of Rheumatology diagnostic criteria is used primarily in clinical studies and for research purposes but are helpful to review, if suspicion arises. They include the following manifestations. (4 or more of these 11 criteria establish the diagnosis in clinical studies):
  * Malar rash
  * Discoid rash

- Photosensitivity
- Oral and nasopharyngeal ulcers
- Nonerosive arthritis and arthralgias
- Serositis
- Proteinuria and cellular casts
- Seizures and psychosis
- Autoimmune hemolytic anemia, leukopenia or lymphopenia, and thrombocytopenia
- They also include positive serologic tests such as:
  - Anti-nuclear antibodies (ANA) (nonspecific)
  - Anti-double stranded DNA antibodies (highly specific, increased renal disease), anti-SM antibodies (highly specific) and antiphospholipid antibodies
- Commonly associated positive serologies include anti-SSA (Ro) and SSB (La) antibodies in around 30% of patients, and anti-RNP in 40% of patients. Complement reduction (C3 and C4) is nonspecific, but is common in lupus flares, and low levels are more commonly associated with renal disease.
- Patients with lupus have accelerated coronary and peripheral vascular disease, especially with high disease activity and chronic steroid use and their cardiovascular risk factors should be managed aggressively.

TREATMENT

Medications

- **NSAIDs** usually control SLE-associated arthritis, arthralgias, fever, and mild serositis but not fatigue, malaise, or major organ system involvement (see General Principles under Basic Approach to the Rheumatic Diseases). The response to **selective COX-2 inhibitors** is similar. Hepatic and renal toxicities of the NSAIDs appear to be increased in SLE. NSAIDs should be avoided in patients with active nephritis.
- **Hydroxychloroquine** 200 mg bid may be effective in the treatment of rash, photosensitivity, arthralgias, arthritis, alopecia, and malaise associated with SLE and in the treatment of **discoid and subacute cutaneous lupus erythematosus.** Skin lesions may begin to improve within a few days, but joint symptoms may require 6 to 10 weeks to subside. The drug is not effective for treating fever or renal, CNS, and hematologic problems, but long-term usage may decrease incidence of flares and renal and CNS involvement. Complications are rare, but for potential ophthalmologic complications patient needs a yearly eye examination.
- **Glucocorticoid therapy**
  - **Indications** for systemic glucocorticoids include (a) life-threatening manifestations of SLE, such as glomerulonephritis, CNS involvement, thrombocytopenia, and hemolytic anemia; and (b) debilitating manifestations of SLE (fatigue, rash) that are unresponsive to conservative therapy.
  - **Dosage.** Patients with severe or potentially life-threatening complications of SLE should be treated with prednisone, 1 to 2 mg/kg PO daily, which can be given in divided doses. After disease is controlled, prednisone should be tapered slowly, the dosage being reduced by no more than 10% every 7 to 10 days. More rapid reduction may result in relapse. Alternate-day therapy may reduce many of the adverse effects of long-term glucocorticoid therapy. **IV pulse therapy** in the form of methylprednisolone, 500 mg IV q12h for 3 to 5 days, has been used in SLE in such life-threatening situations as rapidly progressive renal failure, active CNS disease, and severe thrombocytopenia. Patients who do not show improvement with this

regimen probably are unresponsive to steroids, and other therapeutic alternatives must be considered. A course of oral prednisone should follow completion of pulse therapy.

- **Immunosuppressive therapy**
  - **Indications** for immunosuppressive therapy in SLE include (a) such life-threatening manifestations of SLE as glomerulonephritis, CNS involvement, thrombocytopenia, and hemolytic anemia; and (b) the inability to reduce corticosteroid dosage or severe corticosteroid side effects.
  - **Choice of an immunosuppressive therapy** is individualized to the clinical situation. Often, **cyclophosphamide** is used for life-threatening manifestations of SLE. High-dose monthly IV pulse cyclophosphamide (0.5 to 1.0 g/m^2) may be less toxic but also less immunosuppressive than is low-dose daily PO cyclophosphamide (1.0 to 1.5 mg/kg/d). **Azathioprine** (1.5 mg/kg/d) and **mycophenolate mofetil** (500 to 1000 mg bid) are also used as steroid-sparing agents for serious lupus manifestations. There is increasing evidence that mycophenolate mofetil may be as effective as cyclophosphamide in certain classes of lupus nephritis with fewer side effects, and mycophenolate is particularly preferred in younger population where fertility maintenance is a concern. Methotrexate (7.5 to 20 mg weekly) is often used for musculoskeletal and skin manifestations. **Rituximab**, a monoclonal antibody directed against the B-cell surface molecule CD20, causes depletion of B cells and has been shown in uncontrolled observational studies to be effective in cases of severe SLE not responding to conventional treatment, however, placebo controlled studies to date have been disappointing.
- **Nonpharmacologic therapies**
  - **Conservative therapy** alone is warranted if the patient's manifestations are mild.
  - **General supportive measures** include adequate sleep and fatigue avoidance, as mild disease exacerbations may subside after a few days of bed rest.
  - For all patients, especially those with photosensitive rashes, sunscreens with SPF 30 or greater, protective clothing, such as a hat and long sleeves and sun avoidance are recommended. Isolated skin lesions may respond to topical steroids.

SPECIAL CONSIDERATIONS

- **Transplantation and chronic hemodialysis** have been used successfully in SLE patients with renal failure. Clinical and serologic evidence of disease activity often disappears when renal failure ensues. The survival rate in these patients is equivalent to that of patients with other forms of chronic renal disease. Recurrence of nephritis in the allograft rarely occurs.
- **Pregnancy in SLE.** An increased incidence of second-trimester spontaneous abortion and stillbirth has been reported in some women with antibodies to cardiolipin or the lupus anticoagulant. Neonatal lupus may occur in offspring of anti-Ro/SSA positive mothers, with skin rash and heart block as the most common manifestations. SLE patients may experience an exacerbation in the activity of their disease in the third trimester or peripartum period. Differentiation between active SLE and preeclampsia is often difficult. Women whose SLE is well controlled when they become pregnant are less likely to have a flare of disease during pregnancy.
- **Drug-induced lupus** is usually of sudden onset with an equal male to female ratio. It is associated with musculoskeletal and rare renal or CNS manifestations. Drug-induced lupus is commonly seen with positive ANA and anti-histone antibodies, negative anti-SM and anti-double stranded DNA antibodies, and normal

complement levels. The disease usually resolves with drug discontinuation, typically in a few weeks. Culprit drugs include procainamide, hydralazine, minocycline, diliazem, penicillamine, INH, quinidine, methyldopa, anti-TNF, and IFN-α.

Systemic Sclerosis

GENERAL PRINCIPLES

Definition

Systemic sclerosis (scleroderma) is a systemic illness of unknown etiology characterized by thickening and hardening of the skin and visceral organs. Most of the manifestations of scleroderma have a vascular basis (Raynaud's phenomenon, telangiectasias, nailfold capillary changes, early edematous skin changes, nephrosclerosis), but frank vasculitis is rarely seen.

Classification

Scleroderma can be subdivided based on anatomic skin distribution into localized scleroderma (morphea and linear scleroderma) and systemic sclerosis (diffuse cutaneous, limited cutaneus and systemic sclerosis sine scleroderma). The limited cutaneous form involves extremities distal to the knees and elbows and the face (limited scleroderma was formerly known as the **CREST syndrome: c**alcinosis, **R**aynaud's phenomenon, **e**sophageal dysmotility, **s**clerodactyly, **t**elangiectasias). Diffuse cutaneus scleroderma in addition involves the skin of the proximal extremities and the trunk. Systemic sclerosis without scleroderma affects the internal organs without skin involvement.

DIAGNOSIS

Clinical Presentation

- Nearly all patients with systemic sclerosis have **Raynaud's phenomenon.**
- **Diffuse scleroderma** is characterized by extensive skin disease, the potential for hypertensive "renal crisis," and shortened survival. Multiple internal organs are affected.
  - **GI involvement.** Decreased motility of bowel segments can occur, leading to bacterial overgrowth, malabsorption, diarrhea, and weight loss. Classic endoscopic findings include colonic wide mouth diverticula, patulous esophagus and gastric antral vascular ectasia (GAVE) also known as watermelon stomach.
  - **Renal involvement.** The appearance of sudden hypertension and renal insufficiency indicate potential scleroderma renal crisis. This phenomenon occurs in approximately 10% of systemic sclerosis patients and is associated with a microangiopathic hemolytic anemia and carries a poor prognosis.
  - **Cardiopulmonary involvement.** Patchy myocardial fibrosis can result in CHF or arrhythmias. Pulmonary involvement includes pleurisy with effusion, inflammatory alveolitis (radiographically seen as ground glass infiltrates) leading to interstitial fibrosis, pulmonary hypertension, and cor pulmonale.
  - **Other organ systems.** Skin: Initially edematous and erythematous with "salt and pepper" pigmentation changes, progressing to skin tightening and thickening. Musculoskeletal manifestations range from arthralgias to frank nonerosive arthritis with joint contractures due to the regional skin involvement.

- **Limited scleroderma** may be associated with primary pulmonary hypertension (in the absence of interstitial lung disease) or biliary cirrhosis and is distinguished by skin thickening that is limited to the face and the distal forearms and hands.
- **Nephrogenic systemic sclerosis** is a recently recognized complication of MRI with gadolinium contrast in the presence of renal failure (acute, chronic and End-Stage Renal Disease). It is associated with skin thickening and internal organ fibrosis resembling scleroderma, without Raynaud's phenomenon or ANA positivity.

Diagnostic Testing

More than 95% of scleroderma patients are ANA positive, 20% to 40% are anti-Scl-70 (associated with diffuse disease) positive. Up to 70% of patients with limited scleroderma have anticentromere antibody, which is not seen in individuals with diffuse scleroderma.

TREATMENT

Medications

No curative therapy for scleroderma exists. Treatment focuses on particular organ involvement in a problem-oriented manner.

- **Skin and periarticular changes.** No therapeutic agent is clearly effective for these cutaneous manifestations, although penicillamine or methotrexate is sometimes used. **Physical therapy** is important to retard and reduce joint contractures.
- **GI involvement**
  - Reflux esophagitis generally responds to standard therapy (e.g., **H_2-receptor antagonists, proton pump inhibitors,** and **promotility agents.**)
  - Treatment with broad-spectrum antimicrobials in a rotating sequence including **metronidazole** often improves the malabsorption. Metoclopramide may reduce bloating and distention.
  - Occasionally, esophageal strictures require mechanical esophageal dilation.
  - Rarely, severe constipation or intestinal pseudo-obstruction may occur.
- **Renal involvement.** Aggressive blood pressure control with **ACE inhibitors** may delay, prevent, or even reverse the onset of uremia in patients with suspected scleroderma renal crisis. Angiotensin-receptor blockade does not appear to be as effective.
- **Cardiopulmonary involvement.** Coronary artery vasospasm can cause angina pectoris and may respond to calcium channel antagonists. Pulmonary involvement includes pleurisy with effusion, interstitial fibrosis, pulmonary hypertension, and cor pulmonale. Standard therapies for these conditions are used. Patients with rapidly progressive pulmonary parenchymal disease may benefit from a course of cyclophosphamide.

Raynaud's Phenomenon

GENERAL PRINCIPLES

Definition

Raynaud's phenomenon is a reversible vasospasm of the digital arteries that can result in ischemia of the digits.

TREATMENT

Medications

Most pharmacologic approaches have had limited success.

- **Calcium channel antagonists** (e.g., nifedipine) are the preferred initial agents, although they may exacerbate gastroesophageal reflux and constipation in these patients.
- Alternative vasodilators such as prazosin are occasionally helpful, but significant side effects including orthostatic hypotension may preclude their use.
- Daily low-dose aspirin therapy is often prescribed for its antiplatelet effects.
- **Sympathetic ganglion blockade** with a long-acting anesthetic agent may be useful when a patient has progressive digital ulceration that fails to improve with conservative therapy.
- Newer vasodilating agents used for pulmonary hypertension such as sildenafil and bosentan are showing promising results in severe ulcerating disease.

Surgical Management

Surgical digital sympathectomy may be beneficial.

PATIENT EDUCATION

Patients must be instructed to avoid exposure of the entire body to cold, protect the hands and feet from cold and trauma, and discontinue cigarette smoking.

Necrotizing Vasculitis

GENERAL PRINCIPLES

Definition

Necrotizing vasculitis is characterized by inflammation and necrosis of blood vessels leading to tissue damage. This diagnosis includes a broad spectrum of disorders that have various causes and involve vessels of different types, sizes, and locations.

Etiology

Although in most cases the inciting antigen has not been identified, vasculitic syndromes have been associated with chronic hepatitis B and C.

Pathophysiology

The immunopathogenic process often involves immune complexes.

DIAGNOSIS

Clinical Presentation

Table 3 summarizes clinical features and diagnostic and treatment approaches to the most common forms of vasculitis. **Clinical features** are diverse and depend in part on the size of the vessel involved. Systemic manifestations including fever and weight loss are also common. The response to therapy and the long-term prognosis of these disorders are highly variable.

Table 3 Clinical Features and Diagnostic and Treatment Approaches to Vasculitis

Vasculitic Syndrome	Clinical Features	Diagnostic Approach	Treatment
Large-vessel involvement			
Giant-cell arteritis	Headache Jaw claudication	Temporal artery biopsy	Prednisone, 60–80 mg/d
Takayasu arteritis	Finger ischemia Arm Claudication	Aortic arch arteriogram	Prednisone, 60–80 mg/d
Medium-vessel involvement			
Polyarteritis nodosa	Skin ulcers Nephritis Mononeuritis Mesenteric ischemia	Skin biopsy Renal biopsy Sural nerve biopsy Mesenteric angiogram Hepatitis B, C testing	Prednisone 60–100 mg/d cyclophospha-mide, 1–2 mg/kg/d can be added
c-ANCA vasculitis	Sinusitis Pulmonary infiltrates Nephritis	Skin biopsy c-ANCA Lung biopsy Renal biopsy	Prednisone, 60–100 mg/d Prednisone, 60–100 mg/d *and* cyclophosphamide, 1–2 mg/kg/d
Microscopic polyangiitis	Pulmonary infiltrates Nephritis	p-ANCA Renal biopsy	Prednisone, 60–100 mg/d cyclophospha-mide, 1–2 mg/kg/d can be added
Vasculitis in SLE or RA	Skin ulcers Polyneuropathy	Skin or sural nerve biopsy	Prednisone, 60–80 mg/d cyclophospha-mide, 1–2 mg/kg/d, can be added
Small-vessel involvement			
Hypersensitivity vasculitis	Palpable purpura	Skin biopsy	Prednisone, 20–60 mg/d Discontinue inciting drug Supportive treatment
Henoch-Schönlein purpura	Palpable purpura Nephritis Mesenteric ischemia	Skin biopsy Renal biopsy	Prednisone, 20–60 mg/d, may be needed

c-ANCA, cytoplasmic antineutrophil cytoplasmic antibodies; p-ANCA, perinuclear antineutrophil cytoplasmic antibodies; RA, rheumatoid arthritis; SLE, systemic lupus erythematosus.

Differential Diagnosis

Vasculitis "mimics" should be considered, including bacterial endocarditis, HIV infection, atrial myxoma, paraneoplastic syndromes, cholesterol emboli, and cocaine and amphetamine use.

TREATMENT

Medications

- **Glucocorticoids** are the usual initial therapy and are beneficial in most vasculitis. Although vasculitis that is limited to the skin may respond to lower doses of corticosteroids, the initial dosage for visceral involvement should be high (prednisone, 1 to 2 mg/kg/d). **If life-threatening manifestations are present** a brief course of high-dose pulse therapy with methylprednisolone, 500 mg IV q12h for 3 to 5 days, should be considered.
- **Immunosuppressives,** in particular oral cyclophosphamide, often are used in the initial management of necrotizing vasculitis, especially when major organ system involvement (e.g., lung, kidney, or nerve) is present. Methotrexate, azathioprine and mycophenolate mofetil are often used for maintenance therapy and as initial therapy in less severe presentations.
- **Trimethoprim/sulfamethoxazole** has been used in variants of Wegener's granulomatosis limited to the upper airway and may also be useful in preventing relapse. This drug is not sufficient treatment for systemic disease.
- The use of **biologic agents** is under study, with limited promising data on rituximab.

REFERRAL

Management should include consultation with a physician experienced in the treatment of these disorders. Treatment should be tailored to the severity of organ system involvement.

Polymyalgia Rheumatica and Temporal Arteritis

DIAGNOSIS

Clinical Presentation

- **Polymyalgia rheumatica (PMR)** presents in elderly patients as proximal limb girdle pain, morning stiffness, and constitutional symptoms.
- **Temporal arteritis (TA)** is a form of vasculitis that presents with headache, scalp tenderness, jaw or tongue claudication, vision disturbances (including blindness), stroke, and, in up to 40% of patients, symptoms of PMR.

Diagnostic Testing

Laboratories
- PMR: elevated erythrocyte sedimentation rate (ESR)
- TA: elevated ESR (often >100)

Diagnostic Procedures

The diagnosis of TA should be confirmed by **temporal artery biopsy,** which is not altered by 3 to 5 days of prednisone therapy.

TREATMENT

Medications

- **Polymyalgia rheumatica**
  - If PMR is present without evidence of TA, prednisone, 10 to 15 mg PO daily, usually produces dramatic clinical improvement within a few days.
  - The ESR should return to normal during initial treatment, but subsequent therapeutic decisions should be based on ESR and clinical status.
  - Glucocorticoid therapy can be tapered gradually to a maintenance dosage of 5 to 10 mg PO daily but should be continued for at least 1 year to minimize the risk of relapse.
  - NSAIDs may facilitate reduction in prednisone dosage.
- **Temporal arteritis**
  - Patients who are suspected of having TA should be treated promptly with **prednisone,** 1 to 2 mg/kg/d PO daily, to prevent irreversible blindness.
  - High-dose steroid therapy should be continued until symptoms have abated and the ESR has returned to normal. The dosage then should be tapered gradually to 10 to 20 mg, with close monitoring of the ESR and clinical status, and should be maintained for 1 to 2 years. Methotrexate is occasionally used as a steroid-sparing agent, however studies to date are controversial about its effectiveness.

Cryoglobulin Syndromes

GENERAL PRINCIPLES

Definition

Cryoglobulins are serum immunoglobulins that reversibly precipitate in the cold.

Classification

Cryoglobulinemia is traditionally categorized as monoclonal (formerly type 1) or polyclonal (mixed; formerly types 2 and 3).

Etiology

- Patients with **monoclonal cryoglobulinemia** usually have an underlying lymphoproliferative disorder such as myeloma, lymphoma or Waldenström's macroglobulinemia.
- The majority of patients with **mixed cryoglobulinemia** have hepatitis C; the remainder of cases are found in association with autoimmune disorders such as SLE or RA, infectious processes (such as bacterial endocarditis, EBV and CMV) or are idiopathic.

DIAGNOSIS

Clinical Presentation

- Symptoms in monoclonal (formerly type 1) cryoglobulinemia are related to hyperviscosity (blurring of vision, digital ischemia, headache, lethargy) and respond to treatment of the underlying disorder, although plasmapheresis can be used in the acute setting.
- Clinical manifestations of mixed cryoglobulinemia are mediated by immune complex deposition (arthralgias, purpura, glomerulonephritis, and neuropathy).

TREATMENT

Therapy for secondary cryoglobulinemic states is directed at the underlying disease.

Medications
- Treatment of hepatitis C with interferon-α and ribavirin effectively reduces cryoglobulins, although they may recur when treatment is stopped.
- Prednisone or immunosuppressive agents can be used to treat cryoglobulinemia due to SLE or RA but may exacerbate hepatitis C.
- Plasmapheresis can be used in addition to immunosuppression in severe disease.

Polymyositis and Dermatomyositis

GENERAL PRINCIPLES

Definition
- **Polymyositis (PM)** is an inflammatory myopathy that presents as weakness and occasionally tenderness of the proximal musculature.
- **Dermatomyositis (DM)** is another inflammatory myopathy associated with a characteristic skin rash.

Classification
PM and DM can occur in three forms: (a) alone, (b) in association with any of the other autoimmune diseases, or (c) with a variety of neoplasms.

Risk Factors
Risk factors for malignancy in the setting of myositis include the presence of DM, cutaneous vasculitis, male sex and advanced age.

DIAGNOSIS

Diagnostic Testing
Laboratories
- Associated with elevated muscle enzyme levels (creatine kinase, aldolase, AST, LDH).
- Certain subsets of disease are associated with myositis-specific antibodies such as Jo-1 (one of the antisynthetase antibodies) and signal recognition particle. These antibodies have therapeutic and prognostic implications, and levels should therefore be measured in all patients.

Imaging
Associated with an abnormal electromyogram. MRI is useful for the localization of inflammation and necrosis.

Diagnostic Procedures
A muscle biopsy is important to establish a diagnosis.

TREATMENT

Medications

- **Prednisone**
  - When PM or DM occurs without associated disease, it usually responds well to **prednisone,** 1 to 2 mg/kg PO daily.
  - Systemic complaints, such as fever and malaise, respond to therapy first, followed by muscle enzymes and, finally, muscle strength.
  - Once serum enzyme levels normalize, the prednisone dosage should be reduced slowly to maintenance levels of 10 to 20 mg PO daily or 20 to 40 mg PO every other day.
  - The appearance of steroid-induced myopathy and hypokalemia may complicate therapeutic assessment.
- IV infusion of **immunoglobulin** may hasten improvement of severe dysphagia.
- PM or DM associated with neoplasia tends to be less responsive to glucocorticoid therapy but may improve after removal of an associated malignant tumor.
- Patients who do not respond or cannot tolerate the side effects of glucocorticoids may respond to methotrexate or azathioprine.
- The use of **biologic agents, particularly rituximab,** is showing promising results, with randomized controlled studies currently in progress.

Other Nonoperative Therapies

Physical therapy is essential in the management of myositis. Bed rest with active assisted range of motion is appropriate during very active disease, with more active exercise prescribed to improve strength once inflammation has been controlled.

SPECIAL CONSIDERATIONS

Screening for common neoplasms, such as colon, lung, breast, and prostate cancer, should be considered in these patients as well as individual risk based assessment.

Neurologic Disorders
Victoria Sharma and Beau Ances

Alterations in Consciousness

GENERAL PRINCIPLES

Definition
- **Coma** is a state of complete behavioral unresponsiveness to external stimulation. Because some causes of coma may lead to irreversible brain damage, expeditious evaluation and treatment should be performed concurrently. The need for neurosurgical intervention must be determined promptly.
- Acute confusional state **(delirium)** results from diffuse or multifocal cerebral dysfunction and is characterized by relatively rapid reduction in the ability to focus, sustain, or shift attention, a change in cognition, fluctuations in consciousness; disorientation and sometimes hallucinations.

Epidemiology
- About 30% of older patients (>60 years old) experience delirium at some time during hospitalization.
- Patients who experience delirium may have prolonged hospitalizations, more rapid functional decline, and are at higher risk for long-term institutionalization.

Etiology
- Coma results from diffuse or multifocal dysfunction within cerebral hemispheres or the reticular activating system in the brainstem.
- Etiologies for delirium are listed in Table 1.
- *Mild systemic illness (i.e., UTI) commonly produces delirium in an elderly or demented patient, especially in combination with new medications, fever, or sleep deprivation.*

Risk Factors
Can be divided into those that increase vulnerability (underlying neurodegenerative disorder or stroke) and precipitating event (trauma or toxin ingestion).

DIAGNOSIS
- Initial assessment should focus on recognizing the development and progression of altered consciousness. Examiner should query for history of trauma, seizures, medication changes, alcohol or drug use, and existing medical conditions as possible etiologies.
- If trauma has or may have occurred, **immobilize the spine immediately** while arranging radiographs to identify or exclude fracture or instability.

Clinical Presentation
Physical Examination
- Search for signs of systemic illness associated with coma (e.g., cirrhosis, hemodialysis shunt, rash of meningococcemia) or signs of head trauma (e.g., lacerations, periorbital or mastoid ecchymosis, hemotympanum).

Table 1	Causes of Altered Mental Status

Metabolic derangements/diffuse etiologies
Hyper/hyponatremia
Hypercalcemia
Hyper/hypoglycemia
Hyper/hypothyroidism
Acute intermittent porphyria
Hypertensive encephalopathy
Hypoxia/hypercapnia
Global cerebral ischemia from hypotension
Infections
Meningitis/encephalitis
Sepsis
Systemic infectious with spread to CNS
Drugs/toxins/poisons
Prescription medications and side effects of medications
Drugs of abuse
Withdrawal situations
Medication side effects
Inhaled toxins
Inborn errors of metabolism
Nutritional deficiency (i.e., thiamine)
Seizures
Subclinical seizures
Postictal state
Head trauma
Structural
Ischemic stroke (only certain stroke locations cause altered mental status)
Hemorrhage
Hydrocephalus
Tumor
Systemic organ failure
Hepatic failure
Renal failure
Psychiatric

- The physical and neurologic examination may reveal systemic illness (e.g., pneumonia) or neurologic signs (meningismus or paralysis) to narrow the differential diagnosis.
- The diagnosis of brain herniation **must be recognized and treated immediately** (serial examinations should be performed to detect and intervene if clinical deterioration occurs).
- Neurologic examination should focus on the ability of the patient to focus, sustain, or shift attention. Repeated neurologic examination may be required due to fluctuations in status.
- **Level of consciousness** can be assessed semiquantitatively and followed by all levels of caregivers with the Glasgow Coma Scale. Scores range from 3 (unresponsive) to 15 (normal).

- **Respiratory rate and pattern**
  - Cheyne–Stokes respirations (rhythmic crescendo–decrescendo hyperpnea alternating with periods of apnea) occur in metabolic coma and supratentorial lesions, as well as in chronic pulmonary disease and congestive heart failure (CHF).
  - Hyperventilation is usually a sign of metabolic acidosis, hypoxemia, pneumonia, or other pulmonary disease but may be caused by upper brainstem injury.
  - Apneustic breathing (long pauses after inspiration), cluster breathing (breathing in short bursts), and ataxic breathing (irregular breaths without pattern) are signs of brainstem injury and warn of impending respiratory arrest.
- **Pupil size and light reactivity**
  - Anisocoria (asymmetric pupils) in a patient with altered mental status requires immediate diagnosis and treatment, or exclusion, of possible herniation. Anisocoria may be physiologic or produced by mydriatics (e.g., scopolamine, atropine).
  - Small but reactive pupils are seen in narcotic overdose, metabolic encephalopathy, and thalamic or pontine lesions.
  - Midposition fixed pupils imply midbrain lesions and occur in transtentorial herniation.
  - Bilaterally fixed and dilated pupils are seen with severe anoxic encephalopathy or intoxication with drugs such as scopolamine, atropine, glutethimide, or methyl alcohol.
- **Eye movements**
  - The oculocephalic (doll's eyes) test is performed (if no cervical injury is present) by quickly turning the head laterally or vertically. In coma with intact brainstem oculomotor function, eyes move conjugately opposite the direction of head movement.
  - The oculovestibular (cold caloric) test is used if cervical trauma is suspected or if eye movements are absent with the oculocephalic test. Verify intact tympanic membrane and patent auditory canal. Elevate the head 30 degrees above horizontal, with the patient supine. Lavage external auditory canal with 10 to 50 mL of ice water. In coma with intact brainstem oculomotor function, eyes move conjugately toward the lavaged ear. Vertical gaze can be assessed with simultaneous lavage of both ears (cold water → eyes depress, warm water → eyes elevate).
  - Absence of all eye movements indicates a bilateral pontine lesion or drug-induced ophthalmoplegia (e.g., barbiturates, phenytoin, paralytics).
  - Disconjugate gaze suggests a brainstem lesion.
  - A gaze preference conjugately to one side suggests a unilateral pontine or frontal lobe lesion. An associated hemiparesis and oculocephalic and oculovestibular tests help localize the lesion. In pontine lesions, gaze preference is toward the paretic side, and eyes may move toward but do not cross midline. In frontal lobe lesions, gaze preference is away from the paresis, and eyes move conjugately across midline to both sides.
  - Impaired vertical eye movement occurs in midbrain lesions and central herniation. Conjugate depression and impaired elevation suggest a tectal lesion (pinealoma) or hydrocephalus.
- **Motor responses** help to assess the level of impaired consciousness. Asymmetric motor responses (spontaneous or stimulus induced) have localizing value.
- **Herniation** occurs when mass lesions or edema cause shifts in brain tissue. Prompt diagnosis and treatment are necessary to prevent irreversible brain damage and death.

- **Nonspecific signs and symptoms of increased intracranial pressure** include headache, nausea, vomiting, hypertension, bradycardia, papilledema, sixth nerve palsy, transient visual obscurations, and alterations in consciousness.
- **Uncal herniation** is caused by unilateral supratentorial lesions and may progress rapidly. The earliest sign is a dilated pupil ipsilateral to the mass, diminished consciousness, and hemiparesis, first contralateral to the mass and later ipsilateral to the mass (Kernohan notch syndrome).
- **Central herniation** is caused by medial or bilateral supratentorial lesions. Signs include progressive alteration of consciousness, Cheyne–Stokes or normal respirations followed later by central hyperventilation, midposition and unreactive pupils, loss of upward gaze, and posturing of the extremities.
- **Tonsillar herniation** occurs when pressure in the posterior fossa forces the cerebellar tonsils through the foramen magnum, compressing the medulla. Signs include altered level of consciousness and respiratory irregularity or apnea.

Diagnostic Testing

Laboratories

Obtain serum electrolytes, creatinine, glucose, calcium, complete blood count, and urinalysis. Drug levels should be ordered if appropriate. Toxic screen of blood and urine should be considered.

Imaging

A head CT should be obtained to evaluate for structural abnormalities.

Diagnostic Procedures

- Lumbar puncture (LP) should be considered in patients with fever and headaches or those at high risk of infection.
- Electroencephalography (EEG) can be considered to rule out seizures, or confirm the diagnosis of certain metabolic or infectious encephalopathies. These include periodic lateralized epileptiform discharges (PLEDs) in encephalitis (e.g., herpes simplex virus [HSV]), triphasic waves in hepatic or uremic encephalopathy, and β activity or voltage suppression in barbiturate or other sedative intoxications.

TREATMENT

- Ensure adequate airway and ventilation, administer oxygen as needed, and maintain normal body temperature.
- Establish secure IV and adequate circulation.
- Arterial, central venous, and intracranial pressures may need to be monitored and treated depending on clinical circumstances.
- Make repeated attempts to reorient the patient and possibly have a sitter present if patient remains confused.
- A quiet, well-lit room with close observation is necessary. Physical restraints should be used only as a last resort and with appropriate documentation in the medical record. If restraints are needed they should be carefully adjusted and checked periodically to prevent excessive constriction.

Medications

- IV thiamine (100 mg), followed by dextrose (50 mL of 50% dextrose in water = 25 g dextrose), should be administered. Thiamine is administered first because dextrose administration in thiamine-deficient patients may precipitate Wernicke's encephalopathy.

- IV naloxone (opiate antagonist), 0.01 mg/kg, should be administered if opiate intoxication is suspected (coma, respiratory depression, small reactive pupils). Naloxone may provoke opiate withdrawal syndrome in addicted patients.

- Flumazenil (benzodiazepine antagonist), 0.2 mg IV, may reverse benzodiazepine intoxication, but its duration of action is short, and additional doses may be needed. Flumazenil can cause seizures.

- In delirious patients, sedatives should be avoided if possible, but if necessary low doses of lorazepam (1 mg) or chlordiazepoxide (25 mg) can be used.

Other Nonoperative Therapies

- If herniation is identified or suspected, treatment consists of measures to lower intracranial pressure while surgically treatable etiologies are identified or excluded. All of the listed measures are only temporizing methods. Consultation with neurosurgery should be performed concurrently.
  - Endotracheal intubation is usually performed to enable hyperventilation to a PCO_2 of 25 to 30 mm Hg, which reduces intracranial pressure within minutes by cerebral vasoconstriction. Bag-mask ventilation can be performed if manipulation of the neck is precluded by possible or established spinal instability. Reduction of PCO_2 below 25 mm Hg is not recommended because it may reduce cerebral blood flow excessively.

- Administration of mannitol IV, 1 to 2 g/kg over 10 to 20 minutes, osmotically reduces free water in the brain via elimination by the kidneys. This effect peaks at 90 minutes.

- Dexamethasone, 10 mg IV, followed by 4 mg IV q6h, reduces the edema surrounding a tumor or an abscess.

- Coagulopathy should be corrected if intracranial hemorrhage is diagnosed and before surgical treatment or invasive procedures (e.g., LP) are performed. Each patient's circumstances should be carefully assessed before therapeutic anticoagulation is reversed.

Surgical Management

Surgical evacuation of epidural, subdural, or intraparenchymal (e.g., cerebellar) hemorrhage, shunting for acute hydrocephalus, may be lifesaving, but clinical circumstances dictate the need for, and urgency of, intervention. Some structural lesions are not amenable to surgical treatment.

SPECIAL CONSIDERATIONS

- **Brain death** occurs from irreversible brain injury sufficient to permanently eliminate all cortical and brainstem functions. Because the vital centers in the brainstem sustain cardiovascular and respiratory functions, brain death is incompatible with survival despite mechanical ventilation and cardiovascular and nutritional supportive measures. Brain death is distinguished from persistent vegetative state, in which the absence of higher cortical function is accompanied by intact brainstem function. Patients in a persistent vegetative state are unable to think, speak, understand, or meaningfully respond to visual, verbal, or auditory stimuli, yet with nutritional and supportive care their cardiovascular and respiratory functions can sustain viability for many years.

- Brain death criteria vary somewhat by institution. Refer to your institution's policy for details.
- **Alcohol withdrawal** typically occurs when illness or hospitalization interrupts alcohol intake.
- Tremulousness, irritability, anorexia, and nausea characterize minor alcohol withdrawal. Symptoms usually appear within a few hours after reduction or cessation of alcohol consumption and resolve within 48 hours. Treatment includes a well-lit room, reassurance, and the presence of family or friends. **Thiamine,** 100 mg IM/IV, followed by 100 mg PO daily; multivitamins containing **folic acid;** and a balanced diet as tolerated should be administered. **Chlordiazepoxide** (25 to 100 mg PO q6h) with dosage adjusted until the patient is calm may reduce the incidence of seizures and delirium tremens. Serial evaluation for signs of major alcohol withdrawal is essential.
- Alcohol withdrawal seizures, typically one or a few brief generalized convulsions, occur 12 to 48 hours after cessation of ethanol intake. **Antiepileptic drugs (AEDs) are not indicated for typical alcohol withdrawal seizures.** Other causes for seizures (see Seizures) must be excluded. If hypoglycemia is present, thiamine should be administered before glucose.
- Severe withdrawal or delirium tremens consists of tremulousness, hallucinations, agitation, confusion, disorientation, and autonomic hyperactivity (fever, tachycardia, diaphoresis), typically occurring 72 to 96 hours after cessation of drinking. Symptoms generally resolve within 3 to 5 days. Delirium tremens complicates 5% to 10% of cases of alcohol withdrawal, with mortality up to 15%. Other causes of delirium must be considered in the differential diagnosis (see Table 1). One should administer supportive management as follows:
  - Chlordiazepoxide is an effective sedative for delirium tremens, 100 mg IV or PO q2–6h as needed (maximum dose, 500 mg in the first 24 hours). One-half the initial 24-hour dose can be administered over the next 24 hours; the dosage can be reduced by 25 to 50 mg/d each day thereafter. Longer-lasting benzodiazepines facilitate smoother tapering, but shorter-acting agents (i.e., lorazepam, 1 to 2 mg PO or IV q6–8h as needed) may be desirable in older patients and those with reduced drug clearance. In patients with severe hepatic failure, oxazepam (15 to 30 mg PO, q6–8h as needed), which is excreted by the kidney, can be used instead of chlordiazepoxide.
  - Maintenance of fluid and electrolyte balance is important. Alcoholic patients are susceptible to hypomagnesemia, hypokalemia, hypoglycemia, and fluid losses, which may be considerable due to fever, diaphoresis, and vomiting.

Alzheimer's Disease

GENERAL PRINCIPLES

- A neurodegenerative disorder of uncertain etiology that usually affects older individuals (>60 years old).
- Typically characterized by memory problems and dementia.

Epidemiology

- Prevalence is <1% before age 65, 5% to 10% at age 65, and up to 40% to 50% by age 85.

- Slightly higher risk in females than males.
- Inherited forms of AD manifest typically before age 65.
- Lifetime risk doubles with a sibling or parent diagnosed with AD.

Pathophysiology

- Senile or neurofibrillary tangles contain an amyloid core.
- Neurofibrillary plaques are composed of abnormal tau microtubules.
- Genetic disorders (~10%) are due to defects in amyloid precursor protein (APP) gene on chromosome 21, presenilin-1 gene on chromosome 14, and presenilin-2 gene on chromosome 1.

DIAGNOSIS

Clinical Presentation

- Memory impairment is required for diagnosis of AD.
- Episodic memory for newly acquired information is impaired while memory for more remote events is not affected.
- Declarative memory for facts and events is affected while procedural memory and motor learning are spared at earlier stages of the disease.
- With progression of disease, language, visuospatial skills, abstract reasoning, and executive function deteriorate. Also apraxia, alexia, and delusions can be present.

Differential Diagnosis

Frontotemporal dementia (changes in personality, behavior, and executive functioning), vascular dementia (stepwise course due to repeated stroke-like events), dementia with Lewy bodies (visual hallucinations, cognitive fluctuations, Parkinsonism, sensitivity to neuroleptics), normal pressure hydrocephalus, vitamin B12 deficiency, thyroid dysfunction, HIV, etc.

Diagnostic Testing

Progression of disease can be assessed by the Mini-Mental State Examination (MMSE) and the Clinical Dementia Rating Scale (CDR).

Laboratories

- Definitive diagnosis of AD requires histopathologic examination.
- Reversible causes of dementia such as B_{12} deficiency, neurosyphilis, and thyroid abnormalities should be ruled out.

Imaging

- Brain magnetic resonance imaging (MRI) can suggest potential alternative diagnoses.
- MRI may show diffuse atrophy with hippocampal atrophy.
- [^{18}F] Fluorodeoxyglucose positron emission tomography (FDG-PET) or perfusion single-photon emission computed tomography (SPECT) will demonstrate distinct hypometabolism and hypoperfusion, respectively, within the precuneus and lateral parietotemporal cortex.
- More recently amyloid PET tracers (i.e., ^{11}C-labeled Pittsburgh compound-B [PIB]) can measure amyloid deposition in the brain.

Diagnostic Procedures

Neuropsychological testing can establish a baseline. This testing can sometimes differentiate dementia from depression.

- Neuropsychological testing can establish a baseline. This testing can sometimes differentiate dementia from depression.
- Cerebral spinal fluid (CSF) measures of reduced AB_{42} and increased tau maybe diagnostic for AD.

TREATMENT

Medications

- Cholinesterase inhibitors including donepezil, rivastigmine, and galantamine can be considered for early AD.
- Memantine—a noncompetitive N-methyl-D-aspartate receptor antagonist (NMDA)—can be considered for moderate to severe dementia.

Seizures

GENERAL PRINCIPLES

Definition

- Seizure: Uncontrolled excessive electrical discharges in the brain which may produce a sudden change in brain function causing physical convulsion, minor physical signs, thought disturbances, or a combination of symptoms.
- Epilepsy is a state of recurrent seizures.
- Status epilepticus: Greater than 30 minutes of continuous seizure activity or recurrent seizures without full recovery between episodes.
  - Practically, a seizure lasting >5 minutes should be treated as status epilepticus.
- Nonconvulsive status epilepticus: Status epilepticus with electrographic seizures with clinically absent or subtle motor activity and impairment or loss of consciousness.
- Aura: Simple partial seizure producing sensory, autonomic, or psychic manifestations.
- Prodrome: Sensation or feeling that a seizure will soon occur.

Classification

- Partial seizures begin focally.
  - **Simple partial:** Consciousness is not impaired. Can be motor (hand jerking), sensory (focal tingling), autonomic (sensation of epigastric rising), and psychic (déjà vu).
  - **Complex partial:** Consciousness is impaired. Include temporal (automatisms such as lip smacking or picking at clothes, staring, behavior arrest), frontal (hypermotor behaviors, bicycling, pelvic thrusting, and automatisms), or occipital (unformed images, visual hallucinations)
- Generalized seizures originate from bilateral hemispheres. Consciousness is lost.
  - May begin as generalized or partial seizures with secondary generalization.
  - Include tonic, clonic, tonic–clonic, atonic, myoclonic, and absence.

Etiology

- Of all patients presenting with seizures, etiology is found in 33% (*Lancet Neurol 2005 Oct;4(10):627*).
- Etiologies for seizures include those listed in Table 2.
  - For patients with a known seizure disorder presenting with an increasing seizure frequency also consider anticonvulsive medication noncompliance, subtherapeutic anticonvulsant levels, or any infection.

Table 2	Causes of Seizures

- CNS infections
- Fever
- Hypoxic brain injury
- Stroke (ischemic or hemorrhagic)
- Tumors
- Head injury
- Eclampsia
- Hyperthyroidism
- Congenital brain malformations
- Genetics (phenylketonuria, Sturge–Weber, tuberous sclerosis, etc.)
- Toxic metabolic (porphyria, uremia, liver failure)
- Drug withdrawal (alcohol, barbiturates, benzodiazepine, AEDS)
- Drug intoxication (TCAs, cocaine, amphetamine)
- Electrolyte abnormalities
  - Hyponatremia
  - Hypocalcemia
  - Hypomagnesemia
  - Hypoglycemia/hyperglycemia

AEDs, antiepileptic drugs; TCAs, tricyclic antidepressants.

Pathophysiology

Persistent seizures produce brain injury, cardiovascular and respiratory insufficiency, and other life-threatening complications.

DIAGNOSIS

Clinical Presentation

History

- Query for family history of epilepsy, developmental delay, trauma, medical historical information including preexisting medical conditions, current and recently discontinued medications, drug allergies, recreational drug use, and possible precipitating events.
- Ask the patient about any prodrome/aura. Obtain witness account of events. Inquire about **incontinence, tongue biting,** and how the patient behaved after the event ended.

Physical Examination

- Convulsive seizures are usually easily identified.
- Carefully observe for subtle signs of nonconvulsive seizures, such as automatisms, facial or extremity twitching, eye deviation, and periods of relatively preserved mental status alternating with periods of impaired consciousness.
- Patients may present during the postictal period, defined as the time between the end of the seizure until the return to baseline mental status. During this time, patients may act confused, obtunded, and have amnesia for events since the seizure. This period can typically last from minutes to hours.
- Postictal paresis (also called Todd's paralysis) is a transient neurologic deficit that lasts for hours or rarely days after an epileptic seizure.

Differential Diagnosis

Alternate diagnoses that may mimic seizures include:

* Syncope, especially convulsive syncope in which seizure-like motor activity is observed (*J Am Coll Cardiol 2000 Jul;36(1):181*)
* Pseudoseizures
* Toxic-metabolic encephalopathy
* Tremors, dyskinesias
* Nonepileptic myoclonus following a hypoxic event
* Rigors

Diagnostic Testing

Laboratories

Initial laboratory studies should include electrolytes, calcium, magnesium, CBC, urinalysis, urine drug screen, and antiepileptic drugs levels if indicated.

Imaging

Neuroimaging is usually indicated to identify structural etiologies.

* Start with a head CT in the acute setting. The administration of contrast can assist in diagnosis of possible tumors.
* Brain MRI with contrast may be indicated, especially in evaluating new-onset seizures.

Diagnostic Procedures

* LP should be done if there is concern for CNS infection. Send for routine CSF studies as well as HSV-PCR.
* EEG is not required for initial diagnosis and management of generalized convulsive status epilepticus. If mental status is not improving as expected after seizures stop, EEG may be necessary to exclude conversion to nonconvulsive status epilepticus.
* Routine EEG is indicated for new-onset seizures.

TREATMENT

* **Starting an antiepileptic drug (AED) is usually not indicated after a single unprovoked seizure** as about two-thirds of patients who had a single seizure will not have seizure recurrence (*N Engl J Med 1998 Feb 12;338(7):429*). Therapy is not required if a first seizure is provoked by factors that resolve.
* A diagnosis of epilepsy is made after two or more unprovoked seizures. AED treatment is generally started after the second seizure as the patient has a substantially increased risk for repeated seizures.
* Treatment of status epilepticus must be prompt as efficacy of treatment decreases with increased seizure duration (*Semin Neurol 2008 Jul;28(3):342*). (See Fig. 1 for treatment of status epilepticus.)

Medications

* The selection of a specific AED for a patient must be individualized according to the drug effectiveness for seizure type(s), potential adverse effects of the drug, interactions with other possible medications, cost, and mechanism of drug action (*Epilepsia 2006;47:1094*).

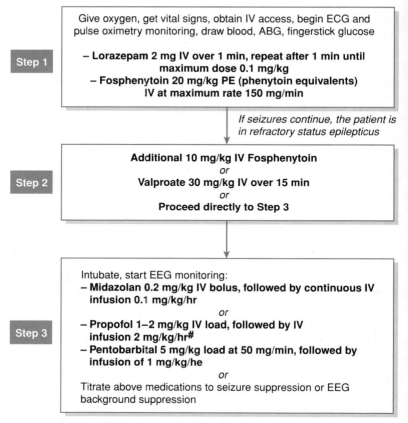

Give oxygen, get vital signs, obtain IV access, begin ECG and pulse oximetry monitoring, draw blood, ABG, fingerstick glucose

Step 1
– **Lorazepam 2 mg IV over 1 min, repeat after 1 min until maximum dose 0.1 mg/kg**
– **Fosphenytoin 20 mg/kg PE (phenytoin equivalents) IV at maximum rate 150 mg/min**

If seizures continue, the patient is in refractory status epilepticus

Step 2
Additional 10 mg/kg IV Fosphenytoin
or
Valproate 30 mg/kg IV over 15 min
or
Proceed directly to Step 3

Step 3
Intubate, start EEG monitoring:
– **Midazolan 0.2 mg/kg IV bolus, followed by continuous IV infusion 0.1 mg/kg/hr**
or
– **Propofol 1–2 mg/kg IV load, followed by IV infusion 2 mg/kg/hr#**
– **Pentobarbital 5 mg/kg load at 50 mg/min, followed by infusion of 1 mg/kg/he**
or
Titrate above medications to seizure suppression or EEG background suppression

Figure 1. Treatment of status epilepticus. (Modified from Arif H, Hirsch LJ. Treatment of status epilepticus. *Semin Neurol* 2008 Jul;28(3):342–354. Epub 2008 Jul 24.)

- About half of all patients with a new diagnosis of epilepsy will become seizure free with the first AED prescribed (*Epilepsia 2001;42:1255*).
- Treatment should be started with a single drug that can be titrated until adequate control or until side effects are experienced.
- **Combination therapy (polytherapy) should be attempted only after at least two adequate sequential trials of single agents have failed.**

Lifestyle/Risk Modification

- Patients should not start other medications (i.e., over-the-counter medications, or herbal remedies) without contacting their physician as there may be drug interactions.
- Patients should keep a seizure calendar to identify possible seizure triggers.
- Patients should maintain adequate sleep regimen.

Diet
- Patients should reduce alcohol intake as heavy consumption (three or more drinks per day) is associated with increased risk of seizures.

REFERRAL

Neurologic consultation may be helpful for managing status epilepticus, and for evaluation and management of new-onset seizures.

PATIENT EDUCATION

Patients with epilepsy do have a small increased risk of sudden death in epilepsy (SUDEP) (*Seizure 1999;8:347*). Patients with epilepsy should not swim unsupervised, bathe in a bathtub of standing water, use motorized tools, or be in position to fall from heights during a seizure. Driver licensing requirements for patients with epilepsy vary from state to state. A complete listing of state laws can be found at: http://www.epilepsyfoundation.org/living/ wellness/transportation/driverlicensing.cfm.

MONITORING/FOLLOW-UP

- Regular follow-up visits should be scheduled to check drug concentrations, blood counts, and hepatic and renal function. Side effects after initiating AED should be followed.
- Correctable causes for seizures (e.g., hyponatremia, drug toxicity) do not require long-term anticonvulsant therapy.

Cerebrovascular Disease

GENERAL PRINCIPLES

- Stroke is a medical emergency that requires rapid diagnosis and treatment.
- The hallmark of stroke is the abrupt interruption of blood flow to a specific brain region resulting in neurologic deficits.
- Fluctuation of functional deficits after stroke onset or a brief deficit known as transient ischemic attack suggests tissue at risk for infarction that may be rescued by reestablishing perfusion.

Epidemiology

More than 500,000 strokes occur per year and it is the third leading cause of death in the United States.

Etiology

- **Ischemic stroke** can be subclassified into atherothrombotic, embolic, or hypoperfusion related.
  - **Atherothrombosis** results from reduced flow within an artery or embolism of thrombus into distal segment of artery.
    - Atherosclerosis is the most common etiology of thrombus formation in large vessels.
    - Less common etiologies include dissection, fibromuscular dysplasia, Moyamoya, giant cell arteritis.
    - Lipohyalinosis, usually due to hypertension, is the most common etiology of small-vessel disease.

- **Cardioembolic** strokes account for about 20% of all ischemic strokes.
  - High-risk cardiac sources include atrial fibrillation, sustained atrial flutter, rheumatic valve disease, atrial or ventricular thrombus, dilated cardiomyopathy, prosthetic valve, bacterial endocarditis, nonbacterial endocarditis (antiphospholipid antibody syndrome, marantic endocarditis, Libman–Sachs endocarditis), sick sinus syndrome, and CABG surgery.
- **Hypoperfusion** occurs due to general circulatory problems and often results in bilateral symptoms. Infarction commonly occurs in border zones between large vessels, resulting in watershed infarcts.
- Hypercoagulable states may predispose to arterial thrombosis. These include sickle cell disease, polycythemia vera, essential thrombocythemia, TTP, antiphospholipid antibody syndrome, etc.
- Factor V Leiden, protein C and S deficiency, and AT-III deficiency typically result in venous, not arterial infarcts.
- **Hemorrhagic stroke** occurs in about 20% of all cases.
  - The location of an **intraparenchymal hemorrhage (IPH)** may suggest its etiology.
    - Hemorrhage in basal ganglia, thalamus, or pons is often due to chronic systemic hypertension.
    - Amyloid angiopathy typically causes lobar hemorrhages and is a common etiology in the elderly.
    - Head trauma, anticoagulants, drugs (cocaine, or amphetamines), arteriovenous malformation, tumor, blood dyscrasia, hemorrhagic conversion of an ischemic stroke, and vasculitis are other etiologies for hemorrhagic stroke.
  - **Subarachnoid hemorrhage (SAH)** is caused by the rupture of an arterial aneurysm resulting in bleeding into the CSF.
    - Hypertension, cigarette smoking, genetic factors, and septic emboli (result in mycotic aneurysms) contribute to aneurysm formation.
- **Cerebral venous sinus thrombosis** is the occlusion of the venous sinuses by thrombus.
  - Occurs in hypercoagulable states such as late pregnancy, postpartum, cancer, and thrombophilias; as well as with trauma and adjacent inflammation.
  - May result in infarcts and/or hemorrhage.

Risk Factors

Risk factors for ischemic stroke include hypertension, TIA, prior stroke, carotid stenosis, DM, hyperlipidemia, cigarette smoking, alcohol consumption, oral contraceptive use, obesity, genetics, and age.

DIAGNOSIS

Clinical Presentation

History

- Time of onset is critical if thrombolytic therapy is to be administered.
- Onset of symptoms is typically sudden. Ask about progression or fluctuation of symptoms and when patient was last normal.
- Prior TIA symptoms (e.g., transient monocular loss of vision, aphasia, dysarthria, paresis, or sensory disturbance) suggest atherosclerotic vascular disease, the most common cause for stroke.

- Inquire about cardiac arrhythmias and atherosclerotic risk factors.
- A history of neck trauma or recent chiropractic maneuvers warrants evaluation for extracerebral arterial dissection.
- SAH may present with only sudden onset of severe "worst headache of my life." Lethargy or coma, fever, vomiting, seizures, and low back pain may also be present.
- IPH presents with neurologic deficits accompanied by headache, vomiting, and possibly lethargy.
- Venous sinus thrombosis often presents with signs and symptoms of elevated intracranial pressure, such as headache, blurred vision, and papilledema.

Physical Examination
- A careful neurologic examination reliably establishes the anatomic location of a stroke.
- In general, carotid artery distribution strokes (anterior circulation) produce combinations of functional deficits (hemiparesis, hemianopsia, cortical sensory loss, often with aphasias or agnosias) contralateral to the affected hemisphere.
- Vertebral-basilar strokes (posterior circulation) produce unilateral or bilateral motor/sensory deficits, usually accompanied by cranial nerve and brainstem signs (vertigo, diplopia, ataxia).
- Horner's syndrome (ptosis, miosis, anhidrosis) contralateral to an acute hemiparesis suggests carotid dissection.
- General physical exam should be focused on possible etiologic factors. Examine for abnormal pulses, arrhythmias, murmurs, carotid bruits, and embolic phenomena.

Differential Diagnosis

Mimics of stroke include postseizure paralysis (Todd's paralysis), migraine with neurologic deficit, and hypoglycemia.

Diagnostic Testing

Laboratories
- Acute laboratory studies should include CBC with platelets, PT/INR, activated PTT, electrolyte panel, blood glucose, and troponin.
- Lipid profile, HgA1C, LFTs (for possible statin therapy), erythrocyte sedimentation rate and blood cultures (if suspect endocarditis), RPR, antinuclear antibody, anticardiolipin antibody, drug toxicology screen, or other specific tests may be required as indicated to establish a specific diagnosis.

Electrocardiography
ECG should be done to look for atrial fibrillation or ischemic changes.

Imaging
- **Noncontrast head CT** scan should be obtained acutely to rapidly differentiate hemorrhagic from ischemic strokes. It can identify acute hemorrhages in most cases. It is insensitive for acute ischemic strokes.
- **MRI** scan is the most sensitive imaging study for stroke diagnosis. Diffusion-weighted images detect stroke earliest. If a diagnosis of stroke is clear from clinical exam, MRI is not always necessary.
- Head CT scan is diagnostic of SAH, demonstrating blood in the sulci and cisternae in 90% of SAH patients in the first 24 hours.

- MR angiography and venograms are useful noninvasive tests to evaluate large arteries and veins, respectively.
- **Carotid Doppler** studies enable noninvasive estimation of carotid stenosis and should be done for anterior circulation strokes.
- **Transthoracic two-dimensional echocardiography** is helpful to demonstrate intracardiac thrombi, valve vegetations, valvular stenosis or insufficiency, and right-to-left shunting (contrast echocardiogram). In some patients, transesophageal echocardiography is necessary to evaluate the left atrium for thrombi.

Diagnostic Procedures
- **Cerebral angiography** is the definitive study for vascular malformations, but may miss small aneurysms.
- It is often necessary prior to carotid endarterectomy (CEA).
- If suspicion for SAH is high and head CT is negative, **lumbar puncture** is necessary to confirm the diagnosis.
  - Tubes 1 and 4 should be sent for cell count. If the number of RBCs decreases dramatically from tube 1 to tube 4, traumatic LP is more likely than SAH.
  - Bloody CSF should be centrifuged and examined for xanthochromia (yellow color). Xanthochromia results from RBC lysis and takes several hours to develop, indicating SAH rather than traumatic LP.

TREATMENT

- Vital signs, including oximetry and continuous telemetry, should be monitored.
- Hypertension management after ischemic stroke:
  - Perfusion pressure in areas of the brain distal to the arterial occlusion may be low.
  - Cerebral perfusion depends in part upon mean systemic arterial pressure.
  - Thus, a degree of hypertension may be necessary to maintain adequate perfusion pressure to injured areas.
  - Aggressive lowering of blood pressure has been associated with neurologic deterioration (*Neurology 2003 Oct 28;61(8):1047*).
  - Patients with acute stroke often present hypertensive. Blood pressure tends to fall on its own over several days following a stroke.
  - While management of hypertension in the setting of acute stroke remains controversial, blood pressure should not be lowered acutely unless necessary for treatment of ACS, CHF, hypertensive crisis with end-organ involvement or systolic BP > 220 or diastolic BP > 120 (*Stroke 2007 May;38(5):1655*).
    - Blood pressure lowering should proceed cautiously, with 15% during the first 24 hours being a reasonable goal.
- Treatment of intracranial hemorrhage consists of supportive care, gradual reduction in BP, and elevation of head of bed by 15 degrees.
- Treatment of SAH depends on etiology. Saccular aneurysms are usually treated surgically.
  - Supportive measures include bed rest, sedation, analgesia, and laxatives to prevent sudden increases in intracranial pressure.
  - Volume expansion, induced hypertension, and balloon dilation can occasionally be used to reverse neurologic deterioration due to vasospasm.

Medications

- Recombinant tissue plasminogen activator (rt-PA) is the only proven therapy for acute ischemic stroke.

- Administration of rt-PA must commence within 4.5 hours of stroke onset (*N Engl J Med 2008 Sep 25;359(13):1317*).
- rt-PA treatment increases risk for symptomatic brain hemorrhage, but with comparable 3- and 12-month mortality versus placebo.
- Exclusion criteria for 0- to 3-hour window include symptoms rapidly improving; recent surgery, head trauma, or gastrointestinal (GI) or urinary hemorrhage; history of intracranial hemorrhage; seizure at stroke onset; platelets < 100,000/mL or anticoagulation with prolonged PT/PTT (patients on anticoagulants with INR ≤ 1.7 can be treated with rt-PA); received heparin in last 48 hours; sustained hypertension (systolic > 185 mm Hg, diastolic > 110 mm Hg), and serum glucose <50 or >400 (*Stroke 2007 May;38(5):1655*).
- There are a few additional exclusion criteria for the 3- to 4.5-hour window (i.e., patients >80 years old, those with an NIH Stroke Scale score > 25, those with a combination of previous stroke and diabetes, and those on anticoagulants regardless of INR).
- Aspirin, heparin, and warfarin should not be given during the first 24 hours post rt-PA.
- Other treatments, including intra-arterial thrombolysis and clot retrieval, are available at some centers.
- Aspirin reduces atherosclerotic stroke morbidity and mortality and is recommended at an initial dose of 325 mg within 24 to 48 hours of stroke onset. The dose may be reduced to 81 mg in the post acute stroke period.
- Other antiplatelet-aggregating drugs (clopidogrel, aspirin/dipyridamole) are available and may be of benefit for certain patients.
- Heparin, low-molecular-weight heparin (LMWH), or warfarin anticoagulation are not recommended for acute ischemic stroke.
- Anticoagulation with warfarin is indicated to prevent recurrent embolic strokes due to atrial fibrillation, target INR 2 to 3 (*Stroke 2007 May;38(5):1655*).
- Nimodipine, a calcium channel blocker, improves outcome in SAH patients and may reduce the incidence of associated cerebral infarction with few side effects.
- Anticoagulation with heparin/LMWH followed by warfarin is indicated for venous sinus thrombosis with and without hemorrhagic infarcts.

Other Nonoperative Therapies

- Physical, occupational, and speech therapy can aid in stroke rehabilitation.
- Patients should be kept NPO until an experienced individual can assess their swallowing abilities.

Surgical Management

- CEA decreases the risk of stroke and death in patients with recent TIAs or nondisabling strokes and ipsilateral high-grade (70% to 99%) carotid stenosis (*N Engl J Med 1991 Aug 15;325(7):445*).
- CEA for asymptomatic high-grade carotid stenosis (≥60%) reduces the 5-year risk of ipsilateral stroke in men, provided that the surgical/angiography complication rate is <3% (*JAMA 1995 May 10;273(18):1421; Stroke 2004 Oct;35(10): 2425*).
- Hemicraniectomy may increase survival in patients with large hemispheric infarcts and severe edema.
- Cerebellar infarction or hematomas may result in brainstem compression or obstructive hydrocephalus, which warrant urgent neurosurgical intervention.

Lifestyle/Risk Modification

- Blood pressure reduction even in normotensive stroke patients is beneficial (*Lancet 2001 Sep 29;358(9287):1033*).
- Oral contraceptives may need to be discontinued in women with stroke.

COMPLICATIONS

- Cerebral edema following ischemic stroke peaks at 48 to 72 hours post stroke and patients need to be watched closely during this time.
- Hemorrhagic conversion of an ischemic stroke is more likely in patients who are receiving anticoagulation or in patients with large strokes.

Headache

GENERAL PRINCIPLES

Classification

- **Primary headache syndromes** include migraines with (classic) or without (common) aura, tension headaches, and cluster headaches.
- **Secondary headaches** have specific etiologies, and symptomatic features vary depending on the underlying pathology (i.e., SAH or tumor or hypertension).
- **Migraine without aura:** Usually five attacks that last 4 to 72 hours. Symptoms usually include unilateral location, pulsating or throbbing, moderate to severe in intensity, and aggravated by activity. Often accompanied by nausea/vomiting, photophobia, and phonophobia.
- **Migraine with aura:** Same as above, except associated aura that lasts from 4 minutes to 1 hour.
- **Cluster headache:** Unilateral orbital or temporal pain with lacrimation, conjunctival injection, nasal congestion, rhinorrhea, facial swelling, miosis, ptosis, and eyelid edema.
- **Rebound headache** occurs after chronic use of analgesics or narcotics.
- **Trigeminal neuralgia** presents as episodic sharp stabbing pain that is unilateral. Rule out multiple sclerosis.
- **Temporal arteritis** presents as dull unilateral headache with thick tortuous artery over temporal region. Seen in older adults with jaw claudication, low-grade fever, and elevated ESR.

Etiology

Secondary headache etiologies include:

- Subdural hematoma, intracerebral hematoma, SAH, arteriovenous malformation, brain abscess, meningitis, encephalitis, vasculitis, obstructive hydrocephalus, and cerebral ischemia or infarction.
- Idiopathic intracranial hypertension (pseudotumor cerebri) presents with headache, papilledema, diplopia, and elevated CSF pressure (>20 cm H_2O in relaxed lateral decubitus position).
- Extracranial causes include giant cell arteritis, sinusitis, glaucoma, optic neuritis, dental disease (including temporomandibular joint syndrome), and disorders of the cervical spine.

- Systemic causes include fever, viremia, hypoxia, carbon monoxide poisoning, hypercapnia, systemic hypertension, allergy, anemia, caffeine withdrawal, and vasoactive or toxic chemicals (nitrites).
- Depression is a common cause of long-standing, treatment-resistant headaches. Specific inquiry about vegetative signs of depression and exclusion of other causes help to support this diagnosis.

Risk Factors

In some patients, triggers may start an attack or worsen a preexisting headache.

DIAGNOSIS

Clinical Presentation

History
- The sudden onset of severe headache (*worst headache of my life*) or a severe persistent headache that reaches maximal intensity within a few seconds or minutes warrants immediate investigation for possible SAH.
- History should focus on:
  - Age at onset
  - Frequency, intensity, and duration of attacks
  - Triggers, associations (menstrual cycle), associated symptoms (photophobia, phonophobia, nausea, vomiting, etc.) and alleviating factors
  - Location and quality of pain (sharp, dull, etc.)
  - Number of headaches per month, including number of disabling headaches
  - Family history of migraines
  - Sleep and diet hygiene (caffeine intake)
  - Use of pain medications, including over-the-counter medications

Physical Examination
- On general examination check blood pressure and pulse, listen for possible bruits, palpate head and neck muscles, and check temporal arteries.
- If neck stiffness and meningismus (resistance to passive neck flexion) observed on exam consider meningitis.
- If papilledema observed on exam consider an intracranial mass, meningitis, or idiopathic intracranial hypertension.

Diagnostic Testing

Imaging
Neuroimaging is generally not indicated for primary headache syndromes, but may be required to exclude secondary etiologies in cases that have not been previously diagnosed, that present with atypical features or abnormal findings.

Diagnostic Procedures
LP is indicated in a patient with severe headache with suspicion of SAH even if the head CT scan is negative.

TREATMENT

- **Acute treatment of migraine,** the most common primary headache syndrome, is directed at aborting the headache. This is easier at onset and often very difficult when the attack is well established. Patients have often used nonprescription analgesics (acetylsalicylic acid [ASA], acetaminophen, NSAIDs) and oral prescription medications (butalbital with aspirin or acetaminophen), which are first-line treatments most effective early in the course of an attack. Emergent treatments include serotonin agonists and other parenteral medications.

- **Triptans** (serotonin receptor $5HT_{1B}$ and $5HT_{1D}$ agonists) are effective abortive medications available in multiple formulations and may be effective even in a protracted attack.
  - Triptans should not be used in patients with coronary artery disease, cerebrovascular disease, uncontrolled hypertension, hemiplegic migraine, or vertebrobasilar migraine.
- **Dihydroergotamine** (DHE) is a potent venoconstrictor with minimal peripheral arterial constriction.
- Cardiac precautions are indicated in those with a history of angina, peripheral vascular disease, or elderly patients.
- **Ergotamine** is a vasoconstrictive agent effective for aborting migraine headaches, particularly if administered during the prodromal phase. Ergotamine should be taken at symptom onset in the maximum dose tolerated by the patient; nausea often limits the dose. Rectal preparations are better absorbed than oral agents.
- Chronic daily headaches should not be treated with narcotic analgesics to prevent addiction, rebound headaches, and tachyphylaxis.
- Treatment of secondary headaches is directed at the primary etiology, such as surgical treatment of cerebral aneurysm causing SAH, evacuation of subdural hematoma, or shunting obstructive hydrocephalus.
- **Prophylactic medications** should be considered if a patient has at least three disabling migraines per month.
  - It is important to review a patient's use of all medications and comorbidities as they may influence choice of medication.
  - Possible prophylaxis included verapamil, β-blockers, topiramate, and antidepressants (amitriptyline, serotonin reuptake inhibitor [SSRI]).

Lifestyle/Risk Modification

Patients should keep a headache calendar to identify possible triggers.

Diet

Patients should reduce alcohol, caffeine, and other triggers that may increase risk of migraines.

REFERRAL

Neurosurgical consultation is indicated for managing SAH.

Head Trauma

GENERAL PRINCIPLES

Definition

- **Traumatic brain injury (TBI)** can occur with head injury due to contact and/or acceleration/deceleration forces.
- **Concussion:** Trauma-induced alteration in mental status with normal radiographic studies that may or may not involve loss of consciousness.

- **Contusion:** Trauma-induced lesion consisting of punctate hemorrhages and surrounding edema.

Classification

- Closed head injuries may produce axonal injury.
- Contusion or hemorrhage can occur at site of initial impact "coup injury" or opposite side of impact, "countercoup injury."
- Penetrating injuries (including depressed skull fracture) or foreign objects cause brain injury directly.
- Secondary increases in intracranial pressure may compromise cerebral perfusion.

DIAGNOSIS

Clinical Presentation

- Patients will often present with confusion and amnesia, including loss of memory for the traumatic event as well as inability to recall events both immediately before and after trauma.
- Patients may complain of nonspecific signs including headache, vertigo, nausea, vomiting, and personality changes.
- Intracerebral hematomas may be present initially or develop after a contusion.
- Epidural hematoma is usually associated with skull fractures across a meningeal artery and may cause precipitous deterioration after a lucid interval.
- Subdural hematoma is most common in aged, debilitated, and alcoholic individuals and in anticoagulated patients. Antecedent trauma may be minimal.

Physical Examination
- Careful examination for penetrating wounds and other injuries.
- Hemotympanum, mastoid ecchymosis (Battle's sign), periorbital ecchymosis ("raccoon eyes"), and CSF otorrhea/rhinorrhea are indicative of a basilar skull fracture.
- Neurologic examination should focus on the level of consciousness, focal deficits, and signs of herniation. Glasgow Comma Scale should be assessed. Serial examinations must be performed and documented to identify neurologic deterioration.

Diagnostic Testing

Imaging
- Head CT should be considered for patients with GCS < 15 two hours after trauma, suspected skull fracture, repeated episodes of vomiting after trauma, >65 years old, dangerous mechanism (pedestrian struck by motor vehicle, occupant ejected from motor vehicle, fall from ≥3 ft or ≥5 stairs), drug or alcohol intoxication, or persistent anterograde amnesia.
- Noncontrast head CT scan in ER can rapidly identify intracranial hemorrhage and contusion.
  - A lenticular-shaped extra-axial hematoma is characteristic of epidural hematoma.
  - Bone window views may locate fractures.
- Cervical radiographs must be performed to exclude fracture or dislocation.
- MRI can assist in evaluation of TBI patients with persistent sequelae as it is more sensitive for demonstrating small areas of contusion or petechial hemorrhage, axonal injury, and small extra-axial hematomas.

TREATMENT

- Hospital admission is recommended for patients at risk for immediate complications from head injury (*Neurosurgery 1990 Apr;26(4):638*; *J Neurosurg 1986 Aug;65(2):203*). These include patients with GCS < 15, abnormal CT scan, intracranial bleeding, cerebral edema, seizures, or abnormal bleeding parameters.
- Awake and alert patients with a concussion can be sent home if a responsible adult is able to watch them for 24 hours, waking the patient up every 2 hours to ascertain continued stability.
- When admitted, continuously monitor vital signs and oximetry. ECG should be performed. Arterial pressure monitoring in conjunction with intracranial monitoring may be needed to optimize cerebral perfusion.
- Immobilize the neck in a hard cervical collar to avoid spinal cord injury from manipulating an unstable or fractured cervical spine.
- Avoid hypotonic fluids to limit cerebral edema.
- Steroids are not indicated for head injury.
- Avoid hypoventilation and systemic hypotension as they may reduce cerebral perfusion.
- Anticipate and conservatively treat increased intracranial pressure:
  - Head midline and elevated 30 degrees.
  - In the mechanically ventilated patient, modest hyperventilation (PCO$_2$ ~35 mm Hg) reduces intracranial pressure by cerebral vasoconstriction; excessive hyperventilation may reduce cerebral perfusion.
- **Brain herniation requires immediate countermeasures** (see Alterations in Consciousness).
- Neurologic deterioration after head injury of any severity requires an immediate repeat head CT scan to differentiate between an expanding hematoma that necessitates surgery from diffuse cerebral edema that requires monitoring and reduction of intracranial pressure.

Surgical Management

- Neurosurgical consultation is indicated for patients with contusion, intracranial hematoma, cervical fracture, skull fractures, penetrating injuries, or focal neurologic deficits.
- In some cases of closed head injury complicated by increased intracranial pressure, intracranial pressure monitoring assists medical management.
- Evacuation of chronic subdural hematoma is determined by the symptoms and degree of mass effect.

Acute Spinal Cord Dysfunction

GENERAL PRINCIPLES

- Spinal cord dysfunction is demonstrated by a level below which motor, sensory, and autonomic functions are interrupted.
- **Traumatic spinal cord injury** (TSCI) may be obvious from history or exam but should also be considered in unconscious, confused, or inebriated patients with trauma.
- **Spinal cord concussion** refers to posttraumatic spinal cord symptoms and signs that resolve rapidly (hours to days).

Etiology

- Etiologies include tumor (primary or metastatic), herniated disk, congenital conditions, epidural abscess or hematoma, trauma leading to fracture of bony elements, ischemia (sometimes after aortic surgery), and vascular malformation.
- Transverse myelitis (inflammation of the spinal cord) occurs with multiple sclerosis, entero viruses, herpes zoster, HIV, tuberculosis or other granulomatous disease, syphilis, and systemic lupus erythematosus.
- Transverse myelopathy (disease of the spinal cord) is caused by infarction (cardiogenic, fibrocartilaginous, or gaseous embolus; hypotension; aortic dissection or surgery) and HIV.

DIAGNOSIS

Clinical Presentation

- **Spinal cord compression** often presents with back pain at the level of compression, progressive walking difficulties, sensory impairment, urinary retention with overflow incontinence, and diminished rectal tone. Rapid deterioration may occur.
- **Transverse myelitis or myelopathy** present with symptoms and signs similar to cord compression.
- **Spinal shock** with hypotonia and areflexia may be present soon after traumatic event.
- Acute presentations suggest traumatic or vascular insults, while a subacute course suggests an enlarging mass lesion or infectious process.
- **Radicular signs** (lancinating pain, paresthesias, and numbness in the dermatomal distribution of a nerve root, with weakness and decreased tone and reflexes in muscles supplied by the root) imply inflammation or compression of the nerve root. Tenderness to spinal percussion over the lesion may be present.
- **Spinal cord syndromes include:**
  - **Complete cord syndrome:** Bilateral flaccid paralysis (quadriplegia or paraplegia) and loss of all sensation (anesthesia) below a dermatomal level, initially with areflexia and sphincter dysfunction (urinary retention/loss of rectal tone). With time hypertonia and hyperreflexia below the lesion, and extensor plantar responses (Babinski signs).
  - **Brown-Séquard's syndrome:** Unilateral cord lesion resulting in contralateral pain and temperature loss, with ipsilateral weakness and proprioceptive loss.
  - **Anterior cord syndrome** often results from anterior spinal artery lesion and produces bilateral pain and temperature loss and weakness below the site of the lesion with preserved proprioception and vibratory sensation.
  - **Cauda equina syndrome** from compression of the lower lumbar and sacral roots produces sensory loss in a saddle distribution, flaccid leg weakness, decreased reflexes, and urinary/bowel incontinence.
  - **Central cord syndrome** is often characterized by motor impairment in upper extremities, more than lower extremities; bladder dysfunction; and variable degree of sensory loss at the site of the lesion.

Diagnostic Testing

Imaging
- The presence and extent of spinal cord injuries should be confirmed with neuroimaging.

- Plain radiographs of the spine may reveal metastatic disease, osteomyelitis, discitis, fractures, or dislocation.
- Emergent MRI scan or CT of the entire cord can confirm exact level and extent of the lesion(s). Myelography is rarely if ever used.

Diagnostic Procedures
- Lumbar puncture: Inflammatory and infectious etiologies often require CSF analysis for pleocytosis, malignant cells, abnormal protein/glucose, and tests for specific pathogens. Imaging should be performed prior to LP with caution used if procedure attempted.

TREATMENT

- Vital signs should be continuously monitored, and adequate oxygenation and perfusion ensured.
- Respiratory insufficiency from high cervical cord injuries requires immediate airway control and ventilatory assistance, without manipulation of the neck.
- Immobilization, especially of the neck, is essential to prevent further injury while the patient's condition is stabilized and radiographic and neurosurgical assessment of the injuries is performed.
- Autonomic dysfunction may occur leading to fluctuating vital signs and BP.

Medications
- Treatable infections require appropriate antibiotics (i.e., acyclovir for herpes zoster).
- **Dexamethasone,** 10 to 20 mg IV bolus followed by 4 mg IV q6h, is often administered for compressive lesions, tumors, or spinal cord infarction, although benefit has not been proven for all etiologies.
- For traumatic spinal cord injury **methylprednisolone,** 30 mg/kg IV bolus, followed by an infusion of 5.4 mg/kg/hr for 24 hours when initiated within 3 hours of injury, and infusion for 48 hours when initiated within 3 to 8 hours of injury, may improve neurologic recovery (*J Neurosurg 1992;76:23*).
- LMWH can be considered to reduce chance of venous thromboembolism and pulmonary embolism.

Surgical Management
Neurosurgical consultation should be obtained because many causes for spinal cord compression can be decompressed and stabilized. Penetrating injury, foreign bodies, comminuted fractures, misalignment, and hematoma may require surgical treatment.

SPECIAL CONSIDERATIONS

Emergent radiation therapy combined with high-dose steroids is usually indicated for cord compression due to malignancy and generally requires a histologic diagnosis.

MONITORING/FOLLOW-UP

- Long-term supportive care is important for patients with spinal cord dysfunction. Pulmonary and urinary infections, skin breakdown, joint contractures, and irregular bowel and bladder elimination are common long-term problems.

- Bladder distension can cause sympathetic overactivity (headache, tachycardia, diaphoresis, and hypertension) as a result of autonomic dysreflexia.

Parkinson's Disease

GENERAL PRINCIPLES

- A chronic, progressive neurodegenerative disease characterized by at least two of three cardinal features: resting tremor, bradykinesia, and rigidity. Often postural instability is seen later in the disease.
- Diagnosis is made by clinical examination.
- Cognitive dysfunction and dementia can be seen with Parkinson's disease (PD) with the prevalence as high as 41% in the community setting.

Epidemiology

Over 1 million people in the United States have been diagnosed with PD. Usually, onset of diagnosis is after 40 years of age.

DIAGNOSIS

Clinical Presentation

- The Parkinsonian tremor is a resting pill rolling tremor (3 to 7 Hz) that is often asymmetrical (*Lancet Neurol 2006 Jan;5(1):75*).
- Bradykinesia is characterized by generalized slowness of movement, especially in finger movement dexterity and gait (often shuffling).
- Cogwheel rigidity is often observed with ratchety pattern of resistance and relaxation as examiner moves limbs.
- Postural instability can be assessed by the "pull" test, where the examiner pulls the patient by the shoulders while standing behind them.
- Other signs that are often associated but not required for diagnosis include masked-like facies, decreased eye blink, increased salivation, hypokinetic dysarthria, micrographia, and sleep disorders (rapid eye movement [REM] sleep behavior disorder).
- Dementia seen with PD is typically subcortical with psychomotor retardation, memory difficulty, and altered personality.

Differential Diagnosis

Essential tremor (action tremor), dementia with Lewy bodies (DLB) (visual hallucinations, fluctuating cognition, sensitivity to neuroleptics), Alzheimer's disease (AD), frontotemporal dementia (FTD) (changes in personality), corticobasal degeneration, Huntington's disease, drug-induced (neuroleptics, other dopamine receptor antagonists), metabolic (Wilson's disease, neurodegeneration with brain iron accumulation), toxic (carbon monoxide, manganese), etc.

Diagnostic Testing

- An acute dopaminergic challenge with levodopa to determine if improvement occurs can help in diagnosis.
- MRI of the brain should be performed to exclude specific structural abnormalities.

TREATMENT

Medications

- **Parkinson's patients should not be given neuroleptics or any dopamine-blocking medications** (Prochlorperazine, Metoclopramide) as this may lead to worsening and prolongation of Parkinson's symptoms (*Expert Opin Drug Saf 2006 Nov;5(6):759*). If a neuroleptic is absolutely necessary, Quetiapine and Clozapine cause the least Parkinsonian symptoms.
- Treatment of PD can be divided into neuroprotective and symptomatic therapy.
- Initiation of symptomatic treatment for a PD patient is determined by the degree to which the patient is functionally impaired.

First Line

- Sinemet is the most effective symptomatic therapy for PD and is often considered when both the patient and physician decide that quality of life of the patient is being affected by PD.
- Dopamine agonists (Pramipexole, Ropinirole) can be used as monotherapy or in combination with other antiparkinsonian drugs. They are ineffective in patients who show no response to levodopa. They may possibly delay initiation of Sinemet-induced dyskinesia and motor fluctuations, but are less efficacious and have increased adverse effects.
- Anticholinergic drugs are used only in younger patients in whom tremor is the predominant symptom.

COMPLICATIONS

- Patients can develop neuroleptic malignant syndrome (NMS) after sudden withdrawal of levodopa or dopamine agonists.
- Serotonin syndrome can occur when monoamine oxidase inhibitors (MAOIs) are combined with tricyclic antidepressants (TCAs) or SSRIs.

NEUROMUSCULAR DISEASE

Guillain–Barré Syndrome

GENERAL PRINCIPLES

Definition

Guillain–Barré syndrome (GBS) is an acute inflammatory polyneuropathy characterized by weakness and areflexia, typically following viral infection, vaccination, or surgery.

Classification

- The **demyelinating type** is most common.
- **Axonal type** is characterized by axonal degeneration, rather than demyelination.
  - Includes acute motor axonal neuropathy (only motor axons affected) and acute motor–sensory axonal neuropathy (both sensory and motor axons affected).
- Miller–Fisher variant consists of ophthalmoparesis, ataxia, and areflexia.
  - Associated with presence of GQ1b antibody in serum.

Pathophysiology

- Infections such as *Campylobacter jejuni*, CMV, EBV, or *Mycoplasma pneumonia* often precede GBS by days to weeks.
- GBS is thought to result from an antibody-mediated attack on these infections. These antibodies cross-react with the myelin or axon components of nerves due to molecular mimicry.

DIAGNOSIS

Clinical Presentation

- GBS typically presents with progressive, symmetric ascending paralysis.
- Reflexes are hypoactive or absent.
- Sensory symptoms, such as paresthesias in the hands and feet, are often present, but objective sensory loss is uncommon.
- Facial and oropharyngeal weakness occurs in about 50% of affected patients.
- Respiratory failure, necessitating intubation, occurs in 25% to 30% of patients (*Lancet Neurol 2008 Oct;7(10):939*).
- Pain in the back, hips, and thighs is common.
- Autonomic instability is common and potentially life threatening.
  - Includes tachy/bradycardia, hypotension alternating with hypertension, and ileus.

Differential Diagnosis

- Differential diagnosis includes sarcoidosis, lyme disease, postdiphtheritic paralysis, tick paralysis, botulism, arsenic neuropathy, acute intermittent porphyria, myelo-radiculopathy, carcinomatous meningitis, and critical illness neuropathy.
- Acute paralysis from poliovirus, HIV, West Nile virus, and polio-type illness from enteroviruses usually has fever and CSF pleocytosis. Paralysis is often asymmetric.

Diagnostic Testing

Imaging

MRI of the spine is occasionally performed to rule out myeloradiculopathy.

Diagnostic Procedures

- **LP should be performed.**
- CSF protein is usually elevated about 1 week after symptoms onset. It may be normal if checked earlier.
- CSF leukocytosis is uncommon and if present an alternative diagnosis should be considered.
- Nerve conduction studies demonstrate demyelination in the demyelinating form and axonal damage in the axonal form. These may be normal early in the course of the disease.

TREATMENT

- Follow **respiratory function closely,** including oximetry, frequent bedside vital capacity (VC), and negative inspiratory force (NIF). Declining VC (<10 to 15 mL/kg) and NIF (<25 cm H_2O) are indications for ventilatory assistance and often occur before hypoxia, dyspnea, and acidosis.

- Paroxysmal hypertension should not usually be treated with antihypertensive medications, but if indicated, titratable short-acting agents are preferred.
- Hypotension is usually caused by decreased venous return and peripheral vasodilation. Mechanically ventilated patients are particularly prone to hypotension. Treatment consists of intravascular volume expansion; occasionally vasopressors may be required (see Chapter 6, Critical Care).
- Continuous ECG monitoring is necessary to monitor for cardiac arrhythmias.
- Prevention of exposure keratitis, venous thrombosis, and vigilance for hyponatremia (including syndrome of inappropriate diuretic hormone [SIADH]) should be priorities.

Medications

- **Plasmapheresis and IV immunoglobulin (IVIG)** are comparably effective in improving outcomes and shortening duration when administered early to patients who cannot walk or have respiratory failure (*Brain 2007 Sep;130(Pt 9):2245*).
  - Fewer complications may occur with IVIG.
- Corticosteroids are not indicated.
- Neuropathic pain medications may be needed.

Other Nonoperative Therapies

Physical therapy to prevent contractures and improve strength and function should be started early.

COMPLICATIONS

Complications from prolonged hospitalization and ventilation may occur. These include aspiration pneumonia, sepsis, pressure ulcers, and pulmonary embolism.

OUTCOME/PROGNOSIS

- Disease typically progresses over 2 to 4 weeks, with almost all patients reaching their nadir by 4 weeks.
- This is followed by a plateau of several weeks duration.
- Recovery takes place over months.
  - Overall, about 80% of patients recover completely or have only minor deficits (*Lancet 2005 Nov 5;366(9497):1653*).
  - 5% to 10% of patients have disabling deficits and 3% remain wheelchair bound.
- 5% of patients die despite optimal medical therapy.

Myasthenia Gravis

GENERAL PRINCIPLES

Definition

Myasthenia gravis (MG) is an autoimmune disorder that involves antibody-mediated disruption of the neuromuscular junction of skeletal muscle resulting in fatigable weakness.

Classification

- Generalized disease is most common and affects a variable combination of ocular, bulbar, respiratory, and skeletal muscles.

- Ocular MG is confined to eyelid and oculomotor function.
  - Accounts for about 20% of all MG cases (*Neurologist 2006 Sep;12(5):231*).

Epidemiology

Bimodal distribution with peak incidence in women in the second and the third decades and in men in the sixth decade.

Pathophysiology

MG is an acquired autoimmune disorder resulting from the production of autoantibodies against the postsynaptic acetylcholine receptor (AChR) or less commonly against a receptor-associated protein, muscle-specific tyrosine kinase (MuSK).

Associated Conditions

- MG is often associated with thymus hyperplasia; 10% may have a malignant thymoma.
- Autoimmune thyroiditis is associated with MG.

DIAGNOSIS

Clinical Presentation

History

- The cardinal feature of MG is fluctuating weakness that is worse after exercise or prolonged activity and improve after rest.
- More than 50% of patients present with ptosis, this may be asymmetric.
- Other common complaints include blurred vision or diplopia, trouble smiling, and chewing.
- Limb weakness (especially proximal) and abnormal or quieter voice are other complaints.
- **Myasthenic crisis** consists of respiratory failure or the need for airway protection and occurs in approximately 10% of MG patients. Patients with bulbar and respiratory muscle weakness are particularly prone to respiratory failure, which may develop rapidly and unexpectedly.
- Respiratory infection, surgery (e.g., thymectomy), medications (e.g., aminoglycosides, quinine, quinolones, β-blockers, lithium, magnesium sulfate), pregnancy, and thyroid dysfunction can precipitate crisis or exacerbate symptoms.

Physical Examination

- Presenting signs include ptosis, diplopia, dysarthria, hypophonia (or nasal quality to speech), dysphagia, extremity weakness, and respiratory difficulty.
- Fatigability on examination is a useful diagnostic feature.
  - Ptosis may worsen after prolonged upward gaze.
- Carefully evaluate the airway, handling of secretions, ventilation, and the work of breathing.
- NIF and forced vital capacity (FVC) are useful at the bedside to assess for respiratory muscle weakness.

Differential Diagnosis

- Lambert–Eaton myasthenic syndrome (LEMS) is an autoimmune disease affecting the neuromuscular junction. It is frequently associated with malignancy (small cell lung cancer). LEMS also presents with fluctuating weakness, but the weakness improves after exercise.

- Amyotrophic lateral sclerosis (ALS) may present with bulbar weakness. However, ALS can be differentiated from MG by presence of upper motor neuron signs in the former.

Diagnostic Testing

Laboratories
- Serum **AChR antibodies** are detected in 80% to 90% of generalized MG patients.
- **MuSK antibodies** are detected in about 50% of AChR (−) MG patients.
- Thyroid function should be checked to evaluate for autoimmune thyroiditis.

Imaging
Chest CT is indicated to identify **thymoma.**

Diagnostic Procedures
Electrodiagnostic studies are an important step in diagnosing MG.

- Repetitive nerve stimulation (at 2 to 5 Hz) typically shows >10% decrement in the amplitude of the compound muscle action potential (CMAP) in MG. In the Lambert–Eaton syndrome, the response is incremental with fast repetitive nerve stimulation (20 to 50 Hz).

TREATMENT

- Treatment of MG is individualized and depends on the severity of the disease, age, comorbidities, and response to therapy.
- **Myasthenic crisis** requires prompt recognition and aggressive support.
  - Consider ICU level care and elective intubation for NIF < 30 cm H_2O or (FVC) < 15 mL/kg.
  - Eliminate precipitating medications; treat infections and metabolic derangements.
  - **Plasmapheresis** is used to treat acute exacerbations of MG. **IVIG** is less commonly used (*Neurotherapeutics 2008 Oct;5(4):535*).
  - As the effects of plasmapheresis or IVIG are rapid, but short lived, corticosteroids are typically started shortly after initiating plasmapheresis or IVIG.
  - Anticholinesterases should be temporarily withdrawn from patients who are receiving ventilation support; this avoids uncertainties about overdosage ("cholinergic crisis") and avoids cholinergic stimulation of pulmonary secretions.
  - Neuromuscular blocking agents should be avoided.

Medications

First Line
Anticholinesterase drugs can produce symptomatic improvement in all forms of MG.

- **Pyridostigmine** should be started at 30 to 60 mg PO tid–qid and titrated for symptom relief.

Second Line
- Immunosuppressive drugs are typically used when additional benefit is needed after cholinesterase inhibitors.
- High doses of **prednisone** can be used to achieve rapid improvement. **However, up to 50% of patients experience a transient worsening of weakness.**
- An alternative is to start low-dose prednisone and then titrate up slowly.

- Azathioprine, mycophenolate mofetil, cyclosporine A, and cyclophosphamide are steroid-sparing immunomodulatory agents used to treat MG.

Surgical Management

- Thymectomy may induce remission or reduce medication dependence (*Neurology 2000 Jul 12;55(1):7*).
- Thymectomy in MG patients is indicated in the presence of thymoma and typically in patients younger than 60 with or without thymoma.

Other Neuromuscular Disorders

GENERAL PRINCIPLES

- **Myopathies:** Rapidly progressive proximal muscle weakness can be caused by ethanol, steroids, cholesterol-lowering drugs, HIV, and hypothyroidism.
  - **Critical illness myopathy** is increasingly recognized in patients with critical illness and is commonly associated with the use of steroids and neuromuscular blocking agents.
  - **Polymyositis and dermatomyositis** should also be considered, particularly if muscle pain is prominent (see Chapter 22, Arthritis and Rheumatologic Diseases).
- **Rhabdomyolysis** may produce rapid muscle weakness leading to hyperkalemia, myoglobinuria, and renal failure (for management, see Chapter 9, Fluid and Electrolyte Management; and Chapter 10, Renal Diseases).
  - Etiologies include muscle compression from crush injury or immobilization, strenuous exercise, hypokalemia or hypophosphatemia, enzyme deficiencies, drugs (statins, cocaine, etc.), convulsive seizures, and metabolic myopathies.
- **Botulism** is a disorder of the **neuromuscular junction** caused by ingestion of an exotoxin produced by *Clostridium botulinum*, acquired through a wound, or via an iatrogenic route.
  - The exotoxin interferes with release of acetylcholine from presynaptic terminals at the neuromuscular junction.
  - In infants it may occur after ingestion of raw honey.
  - Symptoms begin within 12 to 36 hours of ingestion in food-borne botulism and within 10 days in wound botulism.
  - Symptoms include **autonomic dysfunction** (xerostomia, blurred vision, urinary retention, and constipation), followed by **cranial nerve palsies, descending weakness, and possibly respiratory distress.**
  - **Serum assays for botulinum toxin** may be helpful in diagnosis in adults.
  - Management includes removing nonabsorbed toxin with **cathartics;** neutralizing absorbed toxin with **equine trivalent antitoxin,** and supportive care. Penicillin G is often administered but no formal clinical trials have been performed.

Neuromuscular Disorders with Rigidity

GENERAL PRINCIPLES

- **NMS** is associated with the use of neuroleptic drugs, certain antiemetic drugs (e.g., metoclopramide, promethazine), or withdrawal of dopamine agonists (L-dopa in Parkinson's disease).

- Typical features include hyperthermia, altered mental status, muscular rigidity, and dysautonomia.
- Laboratory abnormalities include elevated creatine kinase, myoglobinuria, and leukocytosis.
- Treatment includes discontinuing precipitating drug(s), cooling, monitoring and supporting vital functions (arrhythmias, shock, hyperkalemia, acidosis, renal failure), and administering dantrolene and/or bromocriptine.
- **Serotonin syndrome** results from excessive serotonergic activity, especially following recent dosage changes of SSRIs, monoamine oxidase inhibitors (MAOIs), and TCAs.
  - It presents as a **triad of mental status change, autonomic overactivity, and neuromuscular abnormalities** and may be hard to distinguish from NMS.
  - Hyperthermia, tremor, nausea, vomiting, and clonus are common signs.
  - Treatment includes removal of offending drugs, aggressive supportive care, cyproheptadine, and benzodiazepines (*N Engl J Med 2005 Mar 17;352(11):1112*).
- **Malignant hyperthermia** is the acute development of high fever, obtundation, and muscular rigidity following triggering factors (e.g., halothane anesthesia, succinylcholine).
  - It is a genetic disorder with a mutation in the ryanodine receptor (RyR1), predisposing to abnormal elevation in intracytoplasmic calcium triggered by certain anesthetics.
  - **Serum creatine kinase is markedly elevated.** Renal failure from myoglobinuria and cardiac arrhythmias from electrolyte imbalance can be life threatening.
  - Successful management requires prompt recognition of the syndrome, discontinuation of the offending anesthetic agent, aggressive supportive care that focuses on oxygenation/ventilation, circulation, correction of acid–base and electrolyte derangements, and **dantrolene sodium,** 1 to 10 mg/kg/d, to reduce muscular rigidity.
- **Tetanus** typically presents with generalized muscle spasm (especially trismus) caused by the exotoxin (tetanospasmin) from *Clostridium tetani.*
  - The organism usually enters the body through wounds. Onset typically occurs within 14 days of an injury (*Expert Rev Anti Infect Ther 2008 Jun;6(3):327*).
  - Patients who are **unvaccinated or have reduced immunity** are at risk, underscoring the importance of prevention by tetanus toxoid boosters following wounds. Tetanus may occur in **drug abusers who inject subcutaneously.**
  - Management consists of supportive care, particularly airway control (laryngospasm) and treatment of muscle spasms (benzodiazepines, barbiturates, analgesics, and sometimes neuromuscular blockade). Cardiac arrhythmias and fluctuations in BP can occur.
  - The patient should be kept in quiet isolation, sedated but arousable.
  - Specific measures include wound debridement, **penicillin G or metronidazole, and human tetanus immunoglobulin** (3,000 to 6,000 units IM).
  - **Active immunization** is needed after recovery (total of three doses of tetanus and diphtheria toxoid spaced at least 2 weeks apart).

24 Medical Emergencies

S. Eliza Halcomb, Stephan Brenner, and
Michael E. Mullins

AIRWAY EMERGENCIES

Acute Upper Airway Obstruction

GENERAL PRINCIPLES

Airway obstruction must be recognized and addressed quickly as failure to do so can result in dire consequences.

Etiology

- In awake patients without ventilation, airway obstruction is commonly due to the presence of a foreign body (commonly food) or angioedema.
- In unconscious patients without intact ventilation, airway obstruction can be caused by obstruction by the tongue, foreign body, trauma, infection, or angioedema.

DIAGNOSIS

Clinical Presentation

History

A history is commonly unavailable. In awake patients with adequate ventilation, take a rapid history focused on the causes listed.

Physical Examination

- Manifestations in the **conscious patient** include stridor, impaired phonation, sternal or suprasternal retractions, display of the universal choking sign, and respiratory distress.
- Manifestations in the **unconscious patient** include labored breathing or apnea. Suspect airway obstruction if a nonbreathing patient is difficult to ventilate.
- In all patients, look for urticaria, angioedema, fever, and evidence of trauma.
- Partial obstruction in the awake patient with adequate ventilation:
  - Perform a directed physical examination, looking for airway swelling, trismus, pharyngeal obstruction, respiratory retractions, angioedema, stridor, wheezing, grossly swollen lymph nodes, and neck masses.
  - Observe the patient closely and be prepared to intervene to maintain an airway.
- Airway obstruction in an unconscious patient without intact ventilation:
  - Examine the upper airway visually for evidence of obstruction as part of the resuscitative effort.

Differential Diagnosis

Trauma to the face and neck, foreign body, infection (croup, epiglottitis, Ludwig's angina, retropharyngeal abscess, and diphtheria), tumor, angioedema, laryngospasm, anaphylaxis, retained secretions, or blockage of the upper airway by the tongue (in the unconscious patient).

Diagnostic Testing

Imaging

Partial obstruction in the awake patient with adequate ventilation:

- **Soft tissue radiography** of the neck (posteroanterior and lateral views) is less sensitive and specific than direct examination but may be a valuable adjunct. Such radiography should be performed in the emergency department as a portable study, as the patient should not be left unattended.
- **Rapid computed tomography (CT)** of the airway with constant attendance is an alternative approach where available.

Diagnostic Procedures

Partial obstruction in the awake patient with adequate ventilation:

- If the patient's condition is stable, perform indirect **laryngoscopy** or **fiberoptic nasopharyngolaryngoscopy.** A careful examination is unlikely to cause acute airway obstruction in an adult.

TREATMENT

Therapy is directed at **rapid relief of obstruction** to prevent cardiopulmonary arrest and anoxic brain damage.

- **Airway obstruction in the awake patient without ventilation:**
  - Perform the **Heimlich maneuver** (subdiaphragmatic abdominal thrust) repeatedly until the object is expelled from the airway or patient becomes unconscious. Up to half of patients may require a second technique (i.e., back slaps, chest thrusts) for success (*Circulation 2005;112(Suppl 24):IV19–IV34*).
- **Airway obstruction in an unconscious patient without intact ventilation:**
  - Perform the head tilt–chin lift maneuver if cervical spine trauma is not suspected. Perform a jaw thrust if cervical spine trauma is suspected.
  - If these maneuvers are effective, place an oral or nasal airway. If ineffective, attempt to ventilate the patient with a bag-valve-mask apparatus. If these attempts are also unsuccessful, rapidly examine the oropharynx and hypopharynx. Avoid a blind finger sweep if it is possible to examine the airway directly using a laryngoscope and McGill forceps (if necessary) to remove a foreign body.
  - If laryngoscopy cannot be performed immediately and a foreign body is suspected, perform **the supine Heimlich maneuver** (straddling the supine patient and applying repeated subdiaphragmatic thrusts). Chest thrusts may generate higher airway pressures and may be successful when abdominal thrusts have failed.
  - Substitute chest thrusts if the patient is very obese or is in late pregnancy.

Surgical Management

Airway obstruction in an unconscious patient without intact ventilation:

- Failure of the supine Heimlich maneuver should prompt an attempt at direct laryngoscopy and endotracheal intubation.
- Establish a surgical airway if the patient cannot be intubated.

- If a surgeon is not immediately available, perform needle cricothyrotomy using a 12- to 14-gauge over-the-needle catheter with high-flow oxygen (15 L/min from a 50-psi wall source).
- **Cricothyrotomy** is a preferred alternative.

Pneumothorax

GENERAL PRINCIPLES

- Pneumothorax may occur spontaneously or as a result of trauma.
- **Primary spontaneous pneumothorax** occurs without obvious underlying lung disease.
- **Secondary spontaneous pneumothorax** results from underlying parenchymal lung disease including chronic obstructive pulmonary disease, interstitial lung disease, necrotizing lung infections, *Pneumocystis jiroveci* pneumonia, and cystic fibrosis.
- **Traumatic pneumothoraces** may occur as a result of penetrating or blunt chest wounds.
- **Iatrogenic pneumothorax** occurs after thoracentesis, central line placement, transbronchial biopsy, transthoracic needle biopsy, and barotrauma from mechanical ventilation and resuscitation.
- **Tension pneumothorax** results from continued accumulation of air in the chest that is sufficient to shift mediastinal structures and impede venous return to the heart, resulting in hypotension, abnormal gas exchange, and, ultimately, cardiovascular collapse. It can occur as a result of barotrauma due to mechanical ventilation, a chest wound that allows ingress but not egress of air, or a defect in the visceral pleura that behaves in the same way ("ball-valve" effect).
  - Suspect tension pneumothorax when a patient experiences hypotension and respiratory distress on mechanical ventilation or after any procedure in which the thorax is pierced by a needle.

DIAGNOSIS

Clinical Presentation

History
- Patients commonly complain of ipsilateral chest or shoulder pain. The discomfort is usually of acute onset. A history of recent chest trauma or medical procedure can suggest the diagnosis.
- Dyspnea is usually present.

Physical Examination
- Although examination of the patient with a small pneumothorax may be normal, classic findings include decreased breath sounds, decreased vocal fremitus, and a more resonant percussion note.
- With a larger pneumothorax or with underlying lung disease, there may be tachypnea and respiratory distress. The affected hemithorax may be noticeably larger (due to decreased elastic recoil of the collapsed lung) and relatively immobile during respiration.
- If the pneumothorax is very large, and particularly if it is under tension, the patient may exhibit severe distress, diaphoresis, cyanosis, and hypotension.

- If the pneumothorax is the result of penetrating trauma or pneumomediastinum, subcutaneous emphysema may be felt.

Diagnostic Testing

Electrocardiography

An **electrocardiogram (ECG)** may reveal diminished anterior QRS amplitude and an anterior axis shift. In extreme cases, tension pneumothorax may cause electromechanical dissociation.

Imaging

- A chest **radiograph** will reveal a separation of the pleural shadow from the chest wall. A small pneumothorax is more easily seen on a film taken during expiration. Air travels to the highest point in a body cavity; thus, a pneumothorax in a supine patient may be detected as an unusually deep costophrenic sulcus and excessive lucency over the upper abdomen caused by the anterior thoracic air. This observation is particularly important in the critical care unit, where radiographs of the mechanically ventilated patient are often obtained with the patient supine.
- Although tension pneumothorax is a clinical diagnosis, radiographic correlates include mediastinal and tracheal shift away from the pneumothorax and depression of the ipsilateral diaphragm.

TREATMENT

- Treatment depends on cause, size, and degree of physiologic derangement.
- **Primary pneumothorax**
  - A small, primary, spontaneous pneumothorax without a continued pleural air leak may resolve spontaneously. Air is resorbed from the pleural space at roughly 1.5% daily, and therefore, a small (~15%) pneumothorax is expected to resolve without intervention in approximately 10 days.
  - Confirm that the pneumothorax is **not increasing in size** (repeat the chest radiograph in 6 hours if there is no change in symptoms) and send the patient home if he or she is asymptomatic (apart from mild pleurisy). Obtain follow-up radiographs to confirm resolution of the pneumothorax in 7 to 10 days. Air travel is discouraged during the follow-up period, as a decrease in ambient barometric pressure results in a larger pneumothorax.
  - If the pneumothorax is **small but the patient is mildly symptomatic,** far from home, or unlikely to cooperate with follow-up, admit the patient and administer high-flow oxygen; the resulting nitrogen gradient will speed resorption.
  - If the pneumothorax is **larger than 15% to 20% or is more than mildly symptomatic,** insert a thoracostomy tube.
  - **Pleural sclerosis** to prevent recurrence is recommended by some experts but in most cases is not used after a first episode unless a persistent air leak is present.
- **Secondary pneumothorax**
  - Individuals with a secondary spontaneous pneumothorax are usually symptomatic and require lung reexpansion.
  - Often a bronchopleural fistula persists and a larger thoracostomy tube and suction are required.
  - **Consult a pulmonologist** about pleural sclerosis for persistent air leak and to prevent recurrence.

- **Surgery** may be required for persistent air leak and should be considered for high-risk patients for prevention of recurrence.
- **Iatrogenic pneumothorax**
  - Iatrogenic pneumothorax is generally caused either by introducing air into the pleural space through the parietal pleura (e.g., thoracentesis, central line placement) or by allowing intrapulmonary air to escape through breach of the visceral pleura (e.g., transbronchial biopsy). Often no further air leak occurs after the initial event.
  - If the pneumothorax is small and the patient is minimally symptomatic, he or she can be managed conservatively. If the procedure that caused the pneumothorax required sedation, admit the patient, administer oxygen, and repeat the chest radiograph in 6 hours to ensure the patient's stability. If the patient is completely alert and the chest radiograph shows no change, the patient can be discharged.
  - If the patient is symptomatic or if the pneumothorax is too large for expectant care, a pneumothorax catheter with aspiration or a one-way valve is usually adequate and can often be removed the following day.
  - Iatrogenic pneumothorax due to barotrauma from mechanical ventilation almost always has a persistent air leak and should be managed with a chest tube and suction.
- **Tension pneumothorax**
  - When the clinical situation and physical examination strongly suggest this diagnosis, decompress the affected hemithorax immediately with a 14-gauge needle attached to a fluid-filled syringe. Release of air with clinical improvement confirms the diagnosis. Seal any chest wound with an occlusive dressing and arrange for placement of a thoracostomy tube.

Near-Drowning

GENERAL PRINCIPLES

Definition

- Near-drowning is defined as the survival for at least 24 hours after submersion in a liquid medium.
- Risk factors include youth, inability to swim, alcohol and drug use, barotrauma (in scuba diving), head and neck trauma, and loss of consciousness associated with epilepsy, diabetes, syncope, or dysrhythmias.
- Much has been made of the differences in pathophysiology between fresh- and salt-water drownings. However, the **major insults** (i.e., hypoxemia and tissue hypoxia related to ventilation–perfusion [V/Q] mismatch, acidosis, and hypoxic brain injury with cerebral edema) are common to both.
- Hypothermia, pneumonia, and, rarely, DIC, acute renal failure, and hemolysis may also occur.

DIAGNOSIS

Diagnostic Testing

Laboratories

Obtain serum electrolytes, complete blood cell count (CBC), and arterial blood gases (ABGs). Monitor the cardiac rhythm continuously. Obtain blood alcohol level and drug screen if the mental status is not normal.

Electrocardiography
Obtain ECG.

TREATMENT

Resuscitation

- Begin with resuscitation, focusing on airway management and ventilation with 100% oxygen.
- Establish an IV line with 0.9% saline or lactated Ringer solution.
- The Heimlich maneuver is not indicated unless upper airway obstruction is present (*J Emerg Med 1995;13:397*).
- **Immobilize the cervical spine,** as trauma may be present.
- **Treat hypothermia** vigorously (see Cold-Induced Illness).

Medications

- **Reserve antibiotics for documented infection.** Pneumonia may be due to waterborne organisms such as *Pseudomonas, Aeromonas,* and *Proteus.*
- **Prophylactic glucocorticoids** have no role (*Heart Lung 1987;16:474*).

COMPLICATIONS

- **Cerebral edema**
  - Cerebral edema may occur suddenly within the first 24 hours and is a major cause of death. Treatment of cerebral edema does not appear to increase survival, and intracranial pressure monitoring does not appear to be effective (*Crit Care Med 1986;14:529*). Nevertheless, if cerebral edema occurs, hyperventilate the patient to a PCO_2 not lower than 25 mm Hg (to avoid excessive vasoconstriction) and administer mannitol (1 to 2 g/kg q3–4h) or furosemide (1 mg/kg IV q4–6h).
  - Treat seizures aggressively with phenytoin.
  - The routine administration of glucocorticoids is not recommended.
  - Hypothermia or barbiturate "coma" is not indicated (*Pediatrics 1988;81:630*).
  - It may be necessary to sedate and paralyze the patient to reduce oxygen consumption and facilitate intracranial pressure management.
- **Pulmonary complications**
  - Administer 100% oxygen initially, titrating thereafter by ABGs.
  - Intubate the patient endotracheally and begin mechanical ventilation with positive end-expiratory pressure (PEEP) if the patient is apneic, is in severe respiratory distress, or has oxygen-resistant hypoxemia.
  - Administer bronchodilators if bronchospasm is present.
  - Artificial surfactant has not been shown to be useful (*Acad Emerg Med 1995;2:204*; *Pediatr Emerg Care 1995;11:153*).
- **Metabolic complications:** Manage metabolic acidosis with mechanical ventilation, sodium bicarbonate (if the pH is persistently <7.2), and blood pressure (BP) support.
- **Disposition**
  - Admit patients who have survived severe episodes of near-drowning to an intensive care unit (ICU). Noncardiogenic pulmonary edema may still develop in those individuals with less severe immersions.

- Admit any patient with pulmonary signs or symptoms, including cough, bronchospasm, abnormal ABGs or oxygen saturation as measured by pulse oximetry (SpO_2), or abnormal chest radiograph.
- Observe the asymptomatic patient with a questionable or brief water immersion for 4 to 6 hours and discharge the patient if the chest radiograph and ABGs are normal (*Ann Emerg Med 1986;15:1048*). However, if a documented long submersion, unconsciousness, initial cyanosis or apnea, or even a brief requirement for resuscitation has occurred, the patient must be admitted for at least 24 hours.

HEAT-INDUCED INJURY

Heat Exhaustion

GENERAL PRINCIPLES

Definition

Heat exhaustion occurs in unacclimatized individuals who exercise in the heat and is partly a result of loss of salt and water.

DIAGNOSIS

Clinical Presentation

- The patient notes headache, nausea, vomiting, dizziness, weakness, irritability, and cramps.
- The patient is diaphoretic, demonstrates piloerection, has postural hypotension, and has normal or minimally increased core temperature.

TREATMENT

- **Treatment** consists of resting the patient in a cool environment, accelerating heat loss by fan evaporation, and repleting fluids with salt-containing solutions.
- If the patient is not vomiting and has stable BP, an oral, commercial, balanced salt solution is adequate.
- If the patient is vomiting or hemodynamically unstable, check electrolytes and give 1 to 2 L 0.9% saline IV.

Lifestyle/Risk Modification

Activity

The patient should avoid exercise in a hot environment for 2 to 3 additional days.

Heat Syncope

GENERAL PRINCIPLES

Definition

- Heat syncope affects unacclimatized individuals.
- Exercise in a hot environment results in peripheral vasodilation and pooling of blood, with subsequent loss of consciousness. The affected individual regains consciousness

promptly when supine, and the body temperature is normal. These factors separate this syndrome from heat stroke.

TREATMENT

Treatment consists of rest in a cool environment, fluid repletion, and a more gradual approach to building exercise endurance.

Heat Stroke

GENERAL PRINCIPLES

Heat stroke occurs in two varieties, classic and exertional, both of which have high core temperatures that result in direct thermal tissue injury. Secondary effects include acute renal failure from rhabdomyolysis. Even with rapid therapy, mortality rates can be very high for body temperatures above 41.1°C (106°F).

- **Classic heat stroke** occurs after several days of heat exposure. Patients at risk include those who are chronically ill, dehydrated, elderly, or obese; those who have chronic cardiovascular disease; those who abuse alcohol; and those who use sedatives, hypnotics, α-adrenergic antagonists, diuretics, anticholinergics, or antipsychotics.
  - Abuse of phencyclidine, cocaine, and amphetamines may also contribute.
  - Many patients will have an infection present upon diagnosis.
  - Typically, these patients have **core temperatures higher than 40.5°C (105°F)** and are comatose and anhidrotic.
- **Exertional heat stroke**
  - Exertional heat stroke occurs rapidly in unacclimatized and unfit individuals who exercise in conditions of high ambient temperature and humidity.
  - Those **at risk** include athletes, soldiers, and laborers, particularly if they lack access to water. Some of the risks associated with classic heat stroke may also be present, and certain congenital diseases that impair sweating may contribute. The core temperature may be lower than 40.5°C; 50% of patients are still sweating at presentation.
  - Individuals with exertional heat stroke are more likely than are those with classic heat stroke to have **disseminated intravascular coagulation (DIC), lactic acidosis, and rhabdomyolysis.**

DIAGNOSIS

Diagnosis is based on the history of exposure or exercise, a core temperature usually of 40.6°C (105°F) or higher, and changes in mental status ranging from confusion to delirium and coma.

Differential Diagnosis

- Malignant hyperthermia after exposure to anesthetic agents
- Neuroleptic malignant syndrome (NMS) associated with antipsychotic drugs
  - It is worth noting that NMS and malignant hyperthermia are both accompanied by severe muscle rigidity.
- Anticholinergic poisoning

- Sympathomimetic toxicity (including cocaine)
- Severe hyperthyroidism
- Sepsis
- Meningitis
- Cerebral malaria
- Encephalitis
- Hypothalamic dysfunction due to stroke or hemorrhage
- Brain abscess

Diagnostic Testing

Laboratories
- Laboratory studies should include CBC; partial thromboplastin time; prothrombin time; fibrin degradation products; electrolytes; blood urea nitrogen (BUN); creatinine, glucose, calcium, and creatine kinase levels; liver function tests (LFTs); ABGs; urinalysis; and ECG.
- If an infectious etiology is suspected, obtain appropriate cultures.

Imaging
If a central nervous system (CNS) etiology is considered likely, CT imaging followed by spinal fluid examination is appropriate.

TREATMENT

- **Immediate cooling** is necessary.
  - The best method of cooling is controversial. No study has directly compared ice water application with tepid spray. However, ice water lowers body temperature twice as quickly and is the procedure chosen when exertional heat stroke is anticipated (long-distance races, military training) (*Ann Intern Med 2000;132:678; Int J Sports Med 1998;19(Suppl 2):S150*).
  - Wrap the patient in sheets that are continuously wetted with ice water.
  - If response is insufficiently rapid, submerge the patient in ice water, recognizing that this may interfere with resuscitative efforts (*Am J Emerg Med 1996;14:355*).
  - Most emergency facilities that do not care for large numbers of heat illness cases are not equipped for this treatment. In this case, mist the patient continuously with tepid water (20°C to 25°C). Cool the patient with a large electric fan with maximum body surface exposure.
  - Ice packs should be placed at points of major heat transfer, such as the groin, axillae, and chest, to further speed cooling.
  - If severely elevated core temperature does not respond to these maneuvers, **gastric lavage with ice water** may be helpful, although this treatment is controversial (*Crit Care Med 1987;15:748*).
  - Cold peritoneal lavage is discouraged.
- **Dantrolene sodium** does not appear to be effective for the treatment of heat stroke (*Crit Care Med 1991;19:176*).
- If it is necessary to treat **severe hypertension,** nitroprusside may be preferable, as it theoretically promotes more rapid heat loss via peripheral vasodilation.
- Shivering and vasoconstriction impair cooling and should be prevented by administration of **chlorpromazine,** 10 to 25 mg IM, or **diazepam,** 5 to 10 mg IV.

- Monitor core temperatures continuously by rectal probe as oral and tympanic membrane temperature may be inaccurate.
- Discontinue cooling measures when the core temperature reaches 39°C (102.2°F), which should ideally be achieved within 30 minutes. A temperature rebound may occur in 3 to 6 hours and should be retreated.
- **For hypotension, administer crystalloids;** if refractory, treat with vasopressors and monitor hemodynamics. Avoid pure α-adrenergic agents, as they cause vasoconstriction and impair cooling. Administer crystalloids cautiously to normotensive patients.

COMPLICATIONS

- **Treat rhabdomyolysis** or urine output of <30 mL/hr with adequate volume replacement, mannitol (12.5 to 25 g IV), and bicarbonate (44 to 100 mEq/L in 0.45% normal saline) to promote osmotic diuresis and urine alkalinization. Despite these measures, **renal failure** may still complicate cases of heat stroke.
- **Hypoxemia and acute respiratory distress syndrome (ARDS)** may occur. Treat as described in Chapter 6, Critical Care.
- Treat seizures with diazepam and phenytoin.
- Provide supportive care for hepatic injury, congestive heart failure (CHF), and coagulopathy.

MONITORING/FOLLOW-UP

Patients should be placed on telemetry.

COLD-INDUCED ILLNESS

Exposure to the cold may result in several different forms of injury. Risk factor is accelerated heat loss, which is promoted by exposure to high wind or by immersion. Extended cold exposure may result from alcohol or drug abuse, injury or immobilization, and mental impairment.

Chilblains

GENERAL PRINCIPLES

Definition
- Chilblains are among the mildest form of cold injury and result from exposure of bare skin to a cold, windy environment (33°F to 60°F).
- The ears, fingers, and tip of the nose typically are injured, with itchy, painful erythema on rewarming.

TREATMENT

Treatment involves rapid rewarming (see Frostnip), moisturizing lotions, and analgesics and instructing the patient to avoid reexposure.

Immersion Injury (Trench Foot)

GENERAL PRINCIPLES

Definition

Immersion injury is caused by prolonged immersion (longer than 10 to 12 hours) at a temperature $< 50°F$.

TREATMENT

Treat by rewarming followed by dry dressings. Treat secondary infections with antibiotics.

Frostnip

GENERAL PRINCIPLES

Definition

- Frostnip is the mildest form of frostbite.
- It occurs most frequently on the distal extremities, the nose, or the ear.
- It is marked by tissue blanching and decreased sensitivity.

TREATMENT

Rapid rewarming, in a water bath at $104°F$ to $108°F$ ($40°C$ to $42°C$), is the treatment of choice for all forms of frostbite. The water temperature should never exceed $112°F$.

Superficial Frostbite

DIAGNOSIS

Clinical Presentation

- Superficial frostbite involves the skin and subcutaneous tissues.
- Areas with first-degree involvement are white, waxy, and anesthetic; have poor capillary refill; and are painful on thawing. Second-degree involvement is manifested by clear or milky bullae.

TREATMENT

The **treatment of choice** is rapid rewarming. Immerse the affected body part for 15 to 30 minutes; hexachlorophene or povidone-iodine can be added to the water bath. Narcotic analgesics may be necessary for rewarming pain. Typically, no deep injury ensues and healing occurs in 3 to 4 weeks.

Deep Frostbite

GENERAL PRINCIPLES

Deep frostbite involves death of skin, subcutaneous tissue, and muscle (third degree) or deep tendons and bones (fourth degree).

Risk Factors

Diabetes mellitus, peripheral vascular disease (PVD), an outdoor lifestyle, and high altitude are the additional **risk factors.**

DIAGNOSIS

- The tissue appears frozen and hard.
- On rewarming, there is no capillary filling.
- Hemorrhagic blisters form, followed by eschars. Healing is very slow, and demarcation of tissue with autoamputation may occur.
- The majority of deep frostbite occurs at temperatures < $6.7°C$ ($44°F$) with exposures longer than 7 to 10 hours.

TREATMENT

- The treatment is rapid rewarming as described above. **Rewarming should not be started until there is no chance of refreezing.**
- Administer analgesics (IV opioids) as needed.
- Admit the patient to a surgical service.
- **Elevate** the affected extremity, prevent weight bearing, separate the affected digits with cotton wool, prevent tissue maceration by using a blanket cradle, and prohibit smoking.
- Update tetanus immunization.
- Intra-arterial vasodilators, heparin, dextran, prostaglandin inhibitors, thrombolytics, and sympathectomy are not routinely justified.
- Use antibiotics only for documented infection.
- Amputation is undertaken only after full demarcation has occurred.

Hypothermia

GENERAL PRINCIPLES

Definition

Hypothermia is defined as a core temperature of <$35°C$ ($95°F$).

Classification

Classification of severity by temperature is not universal. One scheme defines hypothermia as mild at $34°C$ to $35°C$, moderate at $30°C$ to $34°C$, and severe at <$30°C$.

Etiology

- The most common cause of hypothermia in the United States is cold exposure due to alcohol intoxication.
- Another common cause is cold water immersion.

DIAGNOSIS

Clinical Presentation

Presentation varies with the temperature of the patient at presentation. All organ systems can be involved.

- **CNS effects**
  - At temperatures **below 32°C,** mental processes are slowed and the affect is flattened.
  - At **32.2°C (90°F),** the ability to shiver is lost, and deep tendon reflexes are diminished.
  - At **28°C,** coma often supervenes.
  - **Below 18°C,** the electroencephalogram (EEG) is flat. On rewarming from severe hypothermia, central pontine myelinolysis may develop.
- **Cardiovascular effects**
  - After an initial increased release of catecholamines, there is a decrease in cardiac output and heart rate with relatively preserved mean arterial pressure. ECG changes, manifest initially as sinus bradycardia with T-wave inversion and QT-interval prolongation, may progress to atrial fibrillation at temperatures of <32°C.
  - Osborne waves (J-point elevation) may be visible, particularly in leads II and V_6.
  - An increased susceptibility to ventricular arrhythmias occurs at temperatures **below 32°C.**
  - At temperatures of **30°C,** the susceptibility to ventricular fibrillation is increased significantly, and unnecessary manipulation or jostling of the patient should be avoided.
  - A decrease in mean arterial pressure may also occur, and, at temperatures of **28°C,** progressive bradycardia supervenes.
- **Respiratory effects**
  - After an initial increase in minute ventilation, respiratory rate and tidal volume decrease progressively with decreasing temperature.
  - ABGs measured with the machine set at 37°C should serve as the basis for therapy without correction of pH and carbon dioxide tension (PCO_2) (*Arch Intern Med 1998;148:1643; Ann Emerg Med 1989;18:72*).
- **Renal manifestations:** Cold-induced diuresis and tubular concentrating defects may be seen.

Differential Diagnosis

- Cerebrovascular accident
- Drug overdose
- Diabetic ketoacidosis
- Hypoglycemia
- Uremia
- Adrenal insufficiency
- Myxedema

Diagnostic Testing

Laboratories

- Basic laboratory studies should include CBC; coagulation studies; LFTs; BUN; electrolytes; creatinine, glucose, creatine kinase, calcium, magnesium, and amylase levels; urinalysis; ABGs; and ECG.
- Obtain toxicology screen if mental status alteration is more profound than expected for temperature decrease.
- Serum potassium is often increased.
- Elevated serum amylase may reflect underlying pancreatitis.
- Hyperglycemia may be noted but should not be treated as rebound hypoglycemia may occur with rewarming.
- DIC may also occur.

Imaging

Obtain chest, abdominal, and cervical spine radiographs to evaluate all patients with a history of trauma or immersion injury.

TREATMENT

Medications

- Administer supplemental oxygen.
- Give **thiamine** to most patients with cold exposure, as exposure due to alcohol intoxication is common.
- Administration of **antibiotics** is a controversial issue; many authorities recommend antibiotic administration for 72 hours, pending cultures. In general, the patients with hypothermia due to exposure and alcohol intoxication are less likely to have a serious underlying infection than those who are elderly or who have an underlying medical illness.

Other Nonoperative Therapies

- **Rewarming:** The patient should be rewarmed with the goal of increasing the temperature by 0.5 to 2.0°C/hr, although the rate of rewarming has not been shown to be related to the outcome.
- **Passive external rewarming**
  - This method depends on the patient's ability to shiver.
  - It is effective only at core temperatures of **32°C or higher.**
  - Remove wet clothing, cover patient with blankets in a warm environment, and monitor.
- **Active external rewarming**
  - Application of heating blankets (40°C to 45°C) or warm bath immersion. This type of therapy has been feared to cause paradoxical core acidosis, hyperkalemia, and decreased core temperature, as cold stagnant blood returns to the central vasculature (*J Royal Naval Med Serv 1991;77:139*), although Danish naval research supports arm and leg rewarming as effective and safe (*Aviat Space Environ Med 1999;70:1081*).
  - Pending further investigation, active rewarming is best reserved for young, previously healthy patients with acute hypothermia and minimal pathophysiologic derangement.
- **Active core rewarming is preferred for treatment of severe hypothermia,** although few data are available on outcomes (*Resuscitation 1998;36:101*).
- **Heated oxygen** is the initial therapy of choice for the patient whose cardiovascular status is stable. This therapeutic maneuver can be expected to raise core temperatures by 0.5 to 1.2°C/hr (*Ann Emerg Med 1980;9:456*). Administration through an endotracheal tube results in more rapid rewarming than delivery via face mask. Administer heated oxygen through a cascade humidifier at a temperature of 45°C or lower.
  - **IV fluids** can be heated in a microwave oven or delivered through a blood warmer; give fluids only through peripheral IV lines.
  - **Heated nasogastric or bladder lavage** is of limited efficacy because of low-exposed surface area and is reserved for the patient with cardiovascular instability.

- **Heated peritoneal lavage** with fluid warmed to 40°C to 45°C is more effective than heated aerosol inhalation, but it should be reserved for patients with cardiovascular instability. Only those who are experienced in its use should perform heated peritoneal lavage, in combination with other modes of rewarming.
- Closed thoracic lavage with heated fluid by thoracostomy tube has been recommended but is unproved (*Ann Emerg Med 1990;19:204*).
- **Hemodialysis** can be used for the severely hypothermic, particularly when due to an overdose that is amenable to treatment in this way.
- **Extracorporeal circulation** (cardiac bypass) is used only in hypothermic individuals who are in cardiac arrest; in these cases, it may be dramatically effective (*N Engl J Med 1997;337:1500*).
  - Extracorporeal circulation may raise the temperature as rapidly as 10 to 12°C/hr but must be performed in an ICU or operating room.
- **Resuscitation**
  - Maintain airway and administer oxygen.
  - If intubation is required, the most experienced operator should perform it (see Airway Management and Tracheal Intubation in Chapter 6, Critical Care).
  - Conduct **cardiopulmonary resuscitation (CPR)** in standard fashion. Perform simultaneous vigorous core rewarming; as long as the core temperature is severely decreased, it should not be assumed that the patient cannot be resuscitated. Reliable defibrillation requires a core temperature of 32°C or higher; prolonged efforts (to a core temperature of 35°C) may be justified because of the neuroprotective effects of hypothermia. **Do not begin CPR if an organized ECG rhythm is present,** as inability to detect peripheral pulses may be due to vasoconstriction, and CPR may precipitate ventricular fibrillation.
  - Do not perform Swan–Ganz catheterization, as it may precipitate ventricular fibrillation.
  - If ventricular fibrillation occurs, begin CPR as per the advanced cardiac life support (ACLS) protocol. Amiodarone may be administered as per the protocol, although there is no evidence to support its use or guide dosage; some experts suggest reducing the maximum cumulative dose by half. Avoid procainamide because it may precipitate ventricular fibrillation and increase the temperature that is necessary to defibrillate the patient. Rewarming is key.
  - Monitor ECG rhythm, urine output, and, possibly, central venous pressure in all patients with an intact circulation.
- **Disposition**
  - Admit patients with an underlying disease, physiologic derangement, or core temperature < 32°C, preferably to an ICU.
  - Discharge individuals with mild hypothermia (32°C to 35°C) and no predisposing medical conditions or complications when they are normothermic and an adequate home environment can be ensured.

MONITORING/FOLLOW-UP

- Monitor core temperature.
- A standard oral thermometer registers only to a lower limit of 35°C. Monitor the patient continuously with a rectal probe with a full range of 20°C to 40°C.
- Equal efficacy of ear thermistor monitoring has **not** been demonstrated.

OVERDOSES

Overdose, General

GENERAL PRINCIPLES

- According to the American Association of Poison Control Centers, there were 2.5 million exposures and 1,597 fatalities related to toxins in 2007 (*Clin Toxicol 46(10):927–1057*). Overdoses are common in the emergency department, and although they are rarely fatal, it is important to follow some general guidelines while caring for the poisoned patient.
- Patients who present to the hospital with an overdose can be challenging for the clinician. This section will begin with a review of the general approach to the poisoned patient, followed by a discussion of specific ingestions.
- When managing the poisoned patient, as with all patients, it is vital to make sure the patient has no airway compromise, intact breathing, and palpable pulses. Beyond the basics of general emergency management, it is important to remember physiologic principles when approaching the poisoned patient. Quite often, patients can be categorized into one of the five toxidromes based on simple clinical examination findings.

Definition

A **toxidrome,** or toxic syndrome, is a constellation of clinical examination findings that assists in the diagnosis and treatment of the patient who presents with an exposure to an unknown agent. The toxicologic physical examination should include documentation of **vital signs, pupillary diameter, skin findings** (dry, flushed, or diaphoretic), as well as the presence or absence of **bowel sounds** and **urinary retention.**

Classification

There are **five general toxidromes** that encompass a variety of xenobiotic exposures. They include the following:

- **Sympathomimetic:** This toxidrome is characterized by widespread activation of the sympathetic nervous system. The vital sign abnormalities include **hypertension** due to α-adrenergic stimulation and **tachycardia** due to increased β-adrenergic tone. Patients may also present with pyrexia. Physical examination will reveal **pupillary dilatation, diaphoresis,** and occasionally altered mental status. Drugs that can cause this type of toxidrome include cocaine and the amphetamines. Likewise, vasopressors and β-adrenergic agonists can cause a partial syndrome depending on which agent is being used.
- **Cholinergic:** This toxidrome is characterized by the widespread activation of the parasympathetic nervous system. Classically, the vital signs associated with a cholinergic toxidrome include **bradycardia** due to increased vagal tone, **respiratory depression** due to paralysis, and **decreased oxygen saturations** on pulse oximetry, due to **bronchoconstriction** and **bronchorrhea.** Excess acetylcholine (ACh) affects muscarinic receptors leading to the development of pinpoint pupils and the SLUDGE syndrome of **salivation, lacrimation, urination, defecation, gastrointestinal (GI) distress, and emesis.** Excess ACh at the neuromuscular junction results in a depolarizing blockade of the muscles, leading to **fasciculations** and **paralysis.** In the

CNS, cholinergic overload is associated with the development of **seizures** and **coma.** Agents linked with the development of this toxidrome all block the function of acetylcholinesterase (AChE), resulting in the accumulation of ACh in the synapse. These agents include organophosphate insecticides and nerve gases, as well as carbamate pesticides. Carbamates are also used therapeutically in anesthesia, myasthenia gravis, and the treatment of anticholinergic toxidromes.

* **Anticholinergic:** This toxidrome should perhaps be more appropriately described as an antimuscarinic syndrome. Its features include **tachycardia** due to vagal blockade and **hyperthermia** (which may be mild to severe). CNS effects include **agitation, delirium,** and in severe cases, seizures. Other peripheral effects include **mydriasis, dry,** flushed skin, **urinary retention,** and **decreased intestinal motility.** Therapeutic agents that cause this toxidrome include atropine, scopolamine, and antihistamines.

* **Opiate:** The opioids produce a classic vital sign combination of **respiratory depression** and oxygen desaturations in conjunction with **miosis, decreased GI motility,** and **coma.** Opioids produce this toxidrome by binding to one of the four G protein receptors on the cell membrane, leading to analgesia. However, respiratory depression, miosis, and physical dependence are secondary, undesirable effects. Other agents that produce a similar toxidrome include the imidazolines, including clonidine, tetrahydrozoline, and oxymetazoline.

* **Sedative hypnotic:** The benzodiazepines bind to GABA receptors in the brain and cause a clinical picture of **sedation or coma** in the setting of **NORMAL** vital signs. A common misconception is that ingested benzodiazepines cause respiratory depression. While this may be true in the setting of intravenously administered benzodiazepines, patients with a **benzodiazepine ingestion generally do not develop respiratory compromise.**

DIAGNOSIS

Diagnostic Testing

If patients do not fall into any of the above categories, suspect a mixed or undifferentiated exposure, and several diagnostic tests should be ordered.

Laboratories

* **Finger stick:** This test should be considered one of the vital signs in the patient with altered mental status.

* **Chemistry:** A basic metabolic profile should be ordered on any patient with a toxic exposure. The two important pieces of information gleaned from the basic metabolic panel (BMP) include the presence or absence of a low bicarbonate and the creatinine. If the patient has a low bicarbonate, a metabolic acidosis is present and the clinician should calculate the **anion gap.** Patients who present with an elevated anion gap acidosis are often subjected to a battery of unnecessary studies because the differential diagnosis is enormous. In order to tailor the diagnosis, the clinician should focus on a mechanistic approach and check serum **ketones** and **lactate.** If these are negative and the **creatinine** is normal, then one should suspect the presence of a toxic alcohol and send the appropriate studies.

* **Blood gas:** In most cases of intoxication, oxygenation is not an issue of great relevance. Instead, the feature of interest is the pH. Therefore, it is reasonable to send **venous blood gases** (VBGs) rather than ABGs in routine cases of poisoning. However, if concerns about adequate oxygenation are a concern (e.g., cyanide, CO poisoning, methemoglobinemia) then an ABG should be sent.

- **Serum drug screen:** In general, the studies included on this panel include acetaminophen, salicylate, and ethanol concentrations. Some laboratories include a tricyclic antidepressant (TCA) screen as well.
  - In practice, the piece of information that is critical on this panel is the serum **acetaminophen** (APAP) since patients with this ingestion are often asymptomatic upon presentation and approximately 1/500 overdoses have been found to have an unsuspected and treatable APAP concentration (*Ann Emerg Med 1985;14:562–567*).
  - Acute **salicylate** ingestions, while very serious, produce a clinical syndrome that is readily identifiable at the bedside. Chronic salicylate toxicity should be suspected in elderly patients taking aspirin who present with altered mental status and tachypnea.
  - **Ethanol** concentrations are NOT predictive of intoxication, despite the forensic definition of 80 mg/dL as the legal limit for driving. Intoxication is a clinical diagnosis. One of the pitfalls of routinely obtaining ethanol levels is that serious medical conditions may coexist in these often fragile patients. These conditions are frequently missed when the patient is thought to be drunk.
  - **TCA** screens are notoriously unreliable and cross-react with many therapeutic agents. In the absence of the characteristic ECG findings and vital sign abnormalities, a positive result is meaningless and is the source of confusion, leading to unnecessary treatment.
- **Urine drug screen:** Rarely contributes to the management of the patient. Many of the assays produce false-positive or false-negative results and may, in fact, cause harm by leading the clinician to attribute a patient's condition to intoxication rather than a medical emergency. Additionally, these tests are expensive to conduct and therefore are of limited value in the management of the poisoned patient. The urine drug screen tends to vary between hospitals but often tests for the following substances:
  - **Amphetamines:** The assay for amphetamines commonly cross-reacts with over-the-counter cold medications.
  - **Opioids:** This assay frequently misses the presence of the synthetic opioids such as fentanyl and meperidine; therefore, it is important to rely on the toxidrome for the diagnosis.
  - **Cocaine:** This assay is not directed at the parent compound, rather it detects the metabolite benzoylecgonine. Since the parent compound is very short lived, this test is very reliable for the identification of recent use, but in no way confirms intoxication.
  - **Cannabinoids:** Like cocaine, detection of the tetrahydrocannabinolic acid (THCA) metabolite is a reliable indicator of use; however, its presence does not have any bearing upon the diagnosis of intoxication.
  - **Benzodiazepines:** The detection of benzodiazepines most commonly relies upon the detection of oxazepam; however, some commonly used benzodiazepines (such as lorazepam) are therefore often missed by this screening (*Clin Chem 2003;49:357–379*). Given that benzodiazepine overdoses tend to be benign, the utility of this component is questionable at best.
  - **Phencyclidine (PCP):** Screening assays may cross-react with dextromethorphan, ketamine, and diphenhydramine to produce a false-positive result. Once again, the clinical picture is more important in the diagnosis of PCP intoxication and the presence of PCP on a drug screen does not alter the management of a patient.
- Specific laboratory testing will be further addressed below.

Electrocardiography
- The ECG is a critical part of the toxicologic evaluation, and certain overdoses produce characteristic ECG changes, that guide diagnosis and treatment plans.
- In general, the important cardiac toxins tend to prolong the PR interval (reflecting nodal blockade), the QRS (reflecting sodium channel blockade), or the QT interval (potassium channel blockade).
- Electrocardiographic changes specific to certain toxins will be further discussed below.

Imaging
- In general, there is a limited role of diagnostic imaging in toxicology. However, there are a few cases when imaging may be helpful in the diagnosis and management of the poisoned patient. The most useful imaging study in overdose is the abdominal radiograph, which may reveal radiodense material in the stomach or gut in the following ingestions (*Goldfrank's Toxicologic Emergencies. 8th Ed. 2006:62*):
  - **C**hloral hydrate
  - **H**eavy metals
  - **I**ron
  - **P**henothiazines
  - **E**nteric-coated preparations
  - **S**ustained-release preparations
- Occasionally, subtle abnormalities on the abdominal film will detect the presence of "rosettes" or elongated packets in the GI tract of body packers. The abdominal film is of limited utility in body stuffers (*Ann Emerg Med 1997;29:596–601*).

TREATMENT

As with any patient, it is crucial to maintain the airway, check for adequacy of breathing and circulation, and check a finger stick blood glucose in the patient with altered mental status or coma.

- **Prevention of absorption:** Traditionally, gastric emptying by either inducing **emesis** or **lavage** has been a mainstay in the treatment of the acutely overdosed patient. However, the literature regarding these methods of decontamination suggests that they are of little benefit (*Med J Aust 1995;163:345–349*). Furthermore, numerous studies have suggested that patients present approximately 3 to 4 hours after ingestion on average, which tends to make it less likely that there will be a large recovery of pills (*Ann Emerg Med 1985;14:562–567*). Therefore, the routine administration of **ipecac** to children and "stomach pumping" has fallen by the wayside except in very specific circumstances.
  - **Activated charcoal (AC)** has largely replaced both of these methods of gastric emptying and has been shown to be effective in the management of acute overdoses (*Ann Emerg Med 2002;39:273–286*). However, the clinical utility of this method of decontamination is limited if the ingestion occurred more than 1 hour prior to presentation (*J Toxicol Clin Toxicol 1997;35:721–741*). Certain ingestions benefit from multidose AC as they either bind to concretions in the stomach (aspirin), or they decrease enterohepatic or enteroenteric reabsorption (phenobarbital, phenytoin, theophylline). AC should be dosed at 1 g/kg body weight.
  - **Whole-bowel irrigation** is appropriate in patients who have ingested sustained-release medications, body packing, or metals that do not bind to AC. The optimal dose of polyethylene glycol is 1 to 2 L/hr until the rectal effluent is clear. This dose

is a large amount of fluid to ingest, so it is often necessary to place a nasogastric tube to achieve this rate of emptying.

- In cases **of life-threatening** ingestions such as colchicine or nondihydropyridine calcium channel blockers (CCBs), it is appropriate to consider **lavage** as well as **AC.**
- **Cathartics** have no role in the management of overdose. They are often present in the premixed AC solutions. If this is the case, only one dose should be administered.
- All of the above interventions are **contraindicated** in the presence of airway compromise, persistent vomiting, and the presence of an ileus, bowel obstruction, or GI perforation.

- **Enhanced elimination**
  - **Forced diuresis** with normal saline and Ringer's lactate enhances the elimination of low-molecular-weight agents such as lithium in dehydrated individuals. This should be carefully monitored and diuretics should be avoided in these patients.
  - **Urinary alkalinization** with intravenous sodium bicarbonate enhances the elimination of weak acids and is useful in the setting of salicylate overdose. Typical doses are 1 to 2 mEq/kg, with a goal of maintaining the urinary pH at approximately 7 to 8. Specific recommendations will be further discussed below.
  - There is no role for **urinary acidification** in the management of overdoses.
  - **Hemodialysis and hemoperfusion** are reserved for life-threatening ingestions of substances that have a low volume of distribution, a molecular weight of less than 500 Da, a low endogenous clearance, are water soluble and have little protein binding. This treatment modality will be further discussed under specific substances.

- **Antidotes** will be discussed under specific toxicities. The regional poison center should be contacted for specific guidelines for treatment.
- **Disposition**
  - Patients who have taken an overdose as a suicidal gesture should all receive a psychiatric evaluation prior to discharge.
  - Most cases of unintentional overdose do not result in significant morbidity, and in cases where the patient is stable and asymptomatic, a brief period of observation may be all that is necessary.
  - In cases where potentially toxic agents have been ingested, patients should be monitored for 4 to 6 hours before discharge.

Acetaminophen

GENERAL PRINCIPLES

N-acetyl-*para*-aminophenol (APAP) is available worldwide as an over-the-counter analgesic and antipyretic and has become the most common pharmacologic agent involved in toxicologic fatalities (*Am J Emerg Med 2005;23(5):589–666*). The recommended maximum dose for adults is 4 g/d.

Classification

- An analgesic. Within the United States, APAP is sold under the trade name Tylenol. The most common trade name for APAP outside the United States is Paracetamol.
- Because of its use as an analgesic and antipyretic, APAP has become a common ingredient in various cold and flu remedies. It is also used in the treatment of fevers, headaches, and acute and chronic pain.

- APAP is often sold in combination preparations together with nonsteroidal anti-inflammatory drugs (NSAIDs), opiate analgesics, or sedatives (e.g., Tylenol #3, Percocet, Darvocet, Vicodin, NyQuil, Tylenol PM).

Epidemiology

APAP is the leading cause of toxicologic fatalities per year in the United States, and APAP-induced hepatotoxicity is the most frequent cause of acute liver failure (*Hepatology 2005;42(6):1364–1372*).

Etiology

- APAP is available as tablets, capsules, liquids, and suppositories. In addition to the more common immediate-release form, there is also an extended-release preparation (e.g., Tylenol Arthritis Pain).
- Unintentional overdosing is much more common than intentional ingestion in suicide attempts, especially in elderly patients on chronic pain regimen with several APAP-containing painkillers (*Hepatol Res 2008;38:3–8*).
- All patients with presumed APAP overdose should be adequately assessed, evaluated, and treated. However, only the minority of poisoned patients require inpatient care (*AEM 1999;6(11):1115–1120*).

Pathophysiology

- **Absorption:** APAP serum levels peak 30 to 60 minutes after oral ingestion; the extended-release preparations peak after 1 to 2 hours. Absorption is often delayed in overdose and peak levels are usually reached after 2 to 8 hours. The overdose kinetics of extended-release APAP are not yet well established.
- **Overdose:** The hepatic conjugation pathways become saturated in overdose. A cascade of biochemical changes occurs in the liver and centrilobular cell necrosis results (*Clin Pharmacol Ther 1974;16(4):676–684*).

Risk Factors

- Decreased glutathione stores (fasting, malnutrition, anorexia nervosa, chronic alcoholism, febrile illness, chronic disease).
- P450 enzyme inducers (ethanol, INH, phenytoin and other anticonvulsants, barbiturates, smoking).

DIAGNOSIS

Clinical Presentation

- **First 24 hours**—asymptomatic stage:
  - Early symptoms are very nonspecific and primarily related to the GI tract (nausea, vomiting, anorexia).
  - High-dose APAP can cause pallor or lethargy in some patients.
  - This initial phase is rare in symptoms and patients appear pretty unremarkable. Therefore, always think of other coingestants if a patient exhibits extreme vital sign abnormalities or other significant symptoms during the first 24 hours.
- **24 to 48 hours**—hepatotoxic stage:
  - RUQ tenderness is the most common symptom.
  - Transaminitis, bilirubinemia, and elevated PT/INR are also common findings during the second phase.

- **2 to 4 days**—fulminant hepatic failure stage: Significant hepatic dysfunction develops (i.e., a peak in hepatic enzyme elevation along with jaundice, coagulopathy with high risk of spontaneous bleeding, hypoglycemia, anuria, and cerebral edema with coma or even death).
- **4 to 14 days**—recovery stage: If stage 3 is survived, the hepatic dysfunction usually resolves over the following days/weeks.

History

- In order to predict the risk of hepatotoxicity after acute overdose, a reliable time of ingestion must be obtained from the patient or family/friends.
- Also obtain information about the amount of APAP that has been ingested, in what form (e.g., combination preparations, extended-release form), and over what period of time.
- Inquire about other coingestants (alcohol, other medications, other drugs).

Physical Examination

Assess airway, breathing, and circulation (ABCs) and mental status. Especially in patients who are nauseated or vomiting, the assessment of mental status is crucial to intervene with airway protection in time.

Diagnostic Criteria

- In general, a dose of 150 mg APAP per kilogram is the potentially toxic limit that requires therapeutic intervention. This limit includes an added 25% safety margin that was added by the FDA to adjust for patients with multiple risk factors for increased liver toxicity (*BMJ 1998;316(7146):1724–1725*).
- If the total amount of ingested APAP is above 150 mg/kg or cannot be obtained from the patient history, it is crucial to predict the risk of toxicity.
- Obtain an APAP serum level at 4 hours or later after ingestion.
- Plot the APAP concentration on the Rumack–Matthew nomogram (APAP serum concentration vs. time after ingestion) to assess the possibility of hepatic toxicity. NOTE: The nomogram should only be used for acute ingestions.
- During treatment of APAP overdose, it is important to assess the risk of progressive liver failure. The King's College Hospital Criteria provide prognostic markers that help to predict the probability of severe liver damage to develop (*Gastroenterology 1989;97(2):439–445*):
  - pH < 7.3 two days post ingestion.
  - All of the following: PT > 100, serum creatinine > 3.3 mmol/L, severe hepatic encephalopathy (grade III or IV).
- Elevated serum phosphate levels > 1.2 mmol/L on days 2 to 4 (additional criterion, not originally part of KCH criteria) (*Hepatology 2002;36(3):659–665*).
- Arterial serum lactate > 3.0 mmol/L after fluid resuscitation (additional criterion, not originally part of KCH criteria) (*Lancet 2002;359(9306):558–563*).

Diagnostic Testing

Laboratories

- **APAP serum level at 4 hours** after ingestion or later (see above).
- **LFT**—AST is a relatively sensitive nonprognostic marker for hepatic injury.
- **PT/INR, serum bicarbonate, blood pH,** serum **lactate, renal function panel,** and serum **phosphate** level are the prognostic markers for hepatic injury.

- APAP may interfere with some blood sugar test kits causing measurements higher or lower than actual; always recheck FSBS over the course of hospitalization (*AJCP 2000;113(1):75–86*).

TREATMENT

Gastric lavage is not useful in APAP overdose; however, it may be indicated in presence of certain other coingestants.

Medications

- **Activated charcoal:** Only indicated in patients with isolated APAP exposure (with no other evidence of mentally altering substances) who present less than 4 hours after ingestion. Give **1 g/kg PO.**
- **N-acetylcysteine (NAC):** NAC is the specific antidote to prevent APAP-related hepatotoxicity (*Toxicol Sci 2004;80(2):343–349*). NAC replenishes depleted GSH glutathione stores. It should be administered early (i.e., within 8 hours after ingestion) to prevent any liver damage. NAC is a nonspecific antioxidant and will still provide some liver protection if given beyond this time window (*JCI 1983;71(4):980–991*).
  - **Oral dosing:** Loading dose of 140 mg/kg PO, then 70 mg/kg PO every 4 hours for a total of 17 doses (i.e., 1,330 mg/kg over 72 hours) (*NEJM 1988;319(24):1557–1562*).
  - **IV dosing:** Prepare the infusion by adding 30 g of a 20% NAC solution (150 mL) to 1 L D_5W. This will result in a final concentration of 30 mg/mL. Load with a dose of 150 mg/kg NAC IV over 1 hour. Thereafter continue to give 14 mg/kg/hr IV for 20 hours (i.e., 430 mg/kg over 21 hours) (According to IV NAC treatment protocol used by Toxicology Service at Barnes-Jewish Hospital. See also *Ann Pharmacother 2008;42(12):1914–1915*).
  - **NAC administration** can be safely stopped prior to the completion of the total regimen as soon as the APAP level returns to 0, INR < 2.0, and AST normalizes (or reaches less than half of the peak level during acute intoxication).
- **NAC indications:** NAC treatment should be started in the following:
  - Any patient after acute poisoning with a toxic APAP level according to the nomogram.
  - Patients who present beyond 8 hours after acute ingestion. Start NAC therapy while awaiting the initial APAP serum level. Continue treatment if the serum concentration is in the toxic range per nomogram.
  - Patients who present more than 24 hours after acute ingestion and still have a detectable serum APAP level or elevated AST.
  - Patients with chronic APAP exposure (i.e., >4 g/d in adults, > 120 mg/kg/d in children) who present with elevated transaminases.
  - Patients with signs of fulminant hepatic failure. NAC treatment should be started immediately and transfer to a transplant center arranged without fail. NAC has been shown to improve survival of patients in fulminant failure (*Lancet 1990;335(8705):1572–1573*; *NEJM 1991;324(26):1852–1857*; *BMJ 1991;303 (6809):1026–1029*).
- **Oral Versus IV NAC:**
  - IV administration of NAC is the preferred route as it is used in all of the studies of patients with fulminant hepatic failure.

- Oral administration may be slightly safer compared to the IV form; however, NAC has a rather bad odor and taste. Rash, flushing, urticaria, nausea/vomiting, angioedema, bronchospasm, tachycardia, and hypotension have been reported as adverse reactions to IV administration (*Br Med J 1984;289(6439):217–219*).
- If oral NAC is given, dilute the NAC with juice, provide a drinking straw, give IV antiemetics (e.g., Reglan, Zofran).
- Consider oral over IV NAC in patients who are prone to anaphylactoid reactions (e.g., severe asthmatics).
- NAC is effective either way when given within 8 hours after ingestion (*NEJM 1988;319(24):1557–1562*).
- AC adsorbs oral NAC. Both, PO and IV NAC regimens provide enough excess of the drug to ensure adequate therapeutic effects. Nevertheless, it is advised to administer AC 2 hours apart from NAC when given PO.

COMPLICATIONS

- Overdose with extended-relief APAP (*Ann Emerg Med 1997;30(1):104–108*):
  - Get APAP serum level 4 hours post ingestion.
  - If toxic per nomogram, treat with full NAC course.
  - If below toxic level per nomogram, get repeat APAP at 8 hours post ingestion.
  - If now toxic, treat with full course. If remains below toxic level, no therapy necessary.
- Patients with progressing liver failure need to be admitted to an ICU bed with close monitoring for hyperglycemia, electrolyte imbalances, GI bleeding, acid–base disturbances, cerebral edema, infections, and renal failure.

REFERRAL

- Involve a clinical toxicologist in all cases where toxic APAP levels are documented. Discuss the initiation of NAC treatment with the toxicology service where possible.
- Inform your regional Poison Control Center (1-800-222-1222).
- Involve the liver or transplant service early in patients presenting with poor prognostic factors for hepatic failure.
- Patients with toxic liver failure should be transferred to a transplant center as early as possible (*BMJ 1991;303(6796):221–223; J R Soc Med 1997;90(7):368–370*).

Colchicine

GENERAL PRINCIPLES

Definition

Colchicine is the active alkaloid extracted from two plants of the Liliacea family: *Colchicum autumnale* (autumn crocus) and *Gloriosa superba* or Glory Lily. It has been used in the therapy of gout for centuries.

Etiology

Colchicine has a very narrow therapeutic index. Severe poisoning and death can result from the ingestion of as little as 0.8 mg/kg of body weight (*Nouv Presse Med 1977;6:1625–1629*).

Pathophysiology

Colchicine is an effective inhibitor of intracellular microtubule formation, leading to impaired leukocyte chemotaxis and phagocytosis resulting in a decrease in the inflammatory cascade (*JAMA 2003;289:2857–2860*). In overdose, colchicine causes mitotic arrest, leading to cellular dysfunction and death (*J Emerg Med 1994;12:171–177*).

Prevention

Patients who are started on colchicine for gout symptoms should be explicitly directed to stop taking the medication as soon as symptoms of diarrhea occur. They should also be told that increasing the dose in an acute flare can result in significant toxicity; therefore, if they are unable to control the symptoms at home, they should seek expert care early.

DIAGNOSIS

Clinical Presentation

Patients who present with a colchicine overdose tend to develop a syndrome that progresses through three phases. The initial phase usually begins several hours after the overdose and is characterized by nausea, vomiting, and diarrhea. Over the next 1 to 7 days, patients may develop multiorgan failure requiring intensive support; death is common at this stage. In the final phase, patients develop alopecia and myoneuropathies.

History

Patients with inadvertent overdoses will present with a recent history of an acute gouty flare, followed by the development of nausea, vomiting, and diarrhea within a few hours after the overdose. Intentional overdoses may present late and should be suspected in patients with a GI syndrome followed by multiorgan failure.

Physical Examination

The exam tends to be somewhat unremarkable in these patients. They may exhibit signs of dehydration with tachycardia and dry mucous membranes. They may also have decreased urine output. As the toxicity progresses, patients may develop signs of worsening distress and confusion requiring aggressive resuscitation measures. As the disease evolves, fatal cardiac arrhythmias and refractory cardiovascular collapse may occur, usually within a week of overdose (*J Forensic Sci 1994;39:280–286*). Reversible alopecia has been reported in survivors (*J Emerg Med 1994;12:171–177*).

Differential Diagnosis

As with any ingestion, the differential diagnosis is large. However, GI symptoms are common in patients with overdoses of methylxanthines, podophyllin, digoxin and other cardioactive steroids, chemotherapeutic agents, heavy metals, and salicylates.

Diagnostic Testing

There is a very interesting sequence of laboratory findings that should lead one to consider colchicine poisoning in patients.

Laboratories

CBC: In the initial phase of poisoning that lasts for approximately 12 to 24 hours, patients develop a leukocytosis. In the next 48 to 72 hours, signs of bone marrow suppression evolve starting with a profound decline in the leukocyte count and subsequent pancytopenia.

- **BMP:** Colchicine poisoning has also been associated with renal failure and adrenal hemorrhage (*J Anal Toxicol 1991;15:151–154*); therefore, electrolytes should be monitored.
- **HFP:** Colchicine overdoses have been reported to cause hepatotoxicity; therefore, LFTs should be monitored.
- **Coagulation studies:** DIC occasionally occurs; therefore, a full panel, including fibrinogen and fibrin split products should be obtained.
- **Colchicine concentrations:** Colchicine has a narrow therapeutic index, and plasma concentrations > 3 ng/mL may produce significant toxicity. However, this laboratory test is not readily available, so toxicity should be suspected, given the constellation of clinical symptoms and laboratory studies. This test should be thought of as a confirmatory study.
- **Other studies:** CK, troponin, lipase, and other electrolytes should be obtained depending on the clinical scenario.

Electrocardiography

An ECG should be obtained at presentation, given the patient's predilection for developing cardiac arrhythmias, and the patient should be admitted with continuous cardiac monitoring.

Imaging

Colchicine toxicity has been associated with the development of ARDS. Therefore, a chest x-ray should be obtained.

TREATMENT

Colchicine overdoses are often fatal and require aggressive supportive measures. As always, airway protection is of paramount importance followed by adequacy of breathing and support of circulation.

Medications

In cases of severe neutropenia, consider **G-CSF** administration.

Other Nonoperative Therapies

- If the patient is **not** vomiting, consider **gastric lavage** and **AC**. If the patient is altered and vomiting, consider early **endotracheal intubation. Fluids** and direct acting **vasopressors** should be used in cases of hypotension. **Hemodialysis** is not useful for clearing colchicine, given its large volume of distribution; however, it should be used in the setting of colchicine-induced renal failure.
- All symptomatic patients should be admitted to the ICU. Patients without symptoms should be monitored for 8 to 12 hours prior to discharge.

SPECIAL CONSIDERATIONS

Given its narrow therapeutic window and pharmacokinetics, colchicine should be used cautiously in patients with underlying renal or liver dysfunction. Likewise, colchicine is a P450 drug and is subject to many drug–drug interactions (*Biochem Pharmacol 1997;10:111–116*). A thorough review of the patient's medication list should be conducted before starting the patient on this agent as toxic concentrations can accumulate rapidly. In this setting, consider using alternative therapies for the management of acute gouty flares.

Nonsteroidal Anti-Inflammatory Drugs

GENERAL PRINCIPLES

NSAIDS are widely prescribed as analgesics for the management of inflammatory diseases. There are many different classes available; however, the discussion below relates to over-the-counter preparations available in the USA and includes ibuprofen, ketoprofen, and naproxen as well as the selective COX-2 inhibitors.

Pathophysiology

NSAIDS exert their therapeutic effects by inhibiting cyclooxygenase and thereby preventing the formation of prostaglandins. This mechanism accounts for both their therapeutic and toxic side effects, which include ulceration of the GI mucosa and renal dysfunction. In the vast majority of cases, overdose is benign.

DIAGNOSIS

Clinical Presentation

Overdose histories are often unreliable. Consider NSAID overdose in patients who present with **GI distress.**

- **Massive overdose** with ibuprofen occasionally presents with **coma and seizures.**

Diagnostic Testing

Laboratories

Obtain a **BMP** to evaluate renal function and hydration status. An **APAP** concentration should be obtained as many patients confuse over-the-counter analgesics.

TREATMENT

Usually supportive care is all that is necessary for the management of this overdose. IV fluids are beneficial for maintaining hydration in vomiting patients.

Medications

- Consider **AC** 1 g/kg for GI decontamination.
- **Antiemetics and antacids** are beneficial in patients with significant distress.
- **Benzodiazepines** should be used for the management of seizures associated with massive ibuprofen overdose.

Opioids

DIAGNOSIS

Clinical Presentation

Symptoms of opioid overdose are respiratory depression, a depressed level of consciousness, and **miosis.** However, the pupils may be dilated with acidosis or hypoxia or after overdoses with meperidine or diphenoxylate plus atropine. Overdose with fentanyl or derivatives such as α-methylfentanyl ("China white") may result in negative urine toxicology screens.

Diagnostic Testing

Laboratories

Drug concentrations and other standard laboratory tests are of little use. Pulse oximetry and **ABG**s are useful for monitoring respiratory status. Although less widely available, capnography measuring end-tidal CO_2 is more sensitive in detecting impending respiratory arrest as hypercapnia precedes hypoxemia.

Electrocardiography

- **Methadone** has been reported to cause a **prolonged QT_c.** Obtain an ECG in suspected overdose.
- **Propoxyphene** exhibits type IA antidysrhythmic effects due to sodium channel blockade and may present with a **wide complex QRS** on ECG (*Acta Pharmacol Toxicol 1978;42:171–178*).

Imaging

A chest radiograph should be obtained if pulmonary symptoms are present.

TREATMENT

- Treatment includes airway maintenance, ventilatory support, and judicious use of opioid antagonist.
- Avoid gastric lavage.
- Limit use of whole-bowel irrigation to body packers. Body packers rarely require surgery, except in cases of intestinal obstruction.
- Endoscopic removal should not be attempted due to the danger of rupture.

Medications

- **Naloxone hydrochloride** specifically reverses opioid-induced respiratory and CNS depression and hypotension.
- The lowest effective dose should be used. The goal of treatment is adequate spontaneous respiration and not necessarily alertness. The initial dose is 0.04 to 2 mg IV, although the lowest effective dose should be used.
- Larger doses (up to 10 mg IV) may be required to reverse the effects of propoxyphene, diphenoxylate, buprenorphine, or pentazocine.
- In the absence of an IV line, naloxone can be administered sublingually (*Ann Emerg Med 1987;16:572*), via endotracheal tube, or intranasally (*Emerg Med J 2006;23:221*). Isolated opioid overdose is unlikely if there is no response to a total of 10 mg naloxone. Repetitive doses may be required (duration of action is 45 minutes), and this should prompt hospitalization despite the patient's return to an alert status.

- Methadone overdose may require therapy for 24 to 48 hours, whereas levo-α-acetylmethadol may require therapy for 72 hours. A continuous IV drip that provides two-thirds of the initial dose of naloxone hourly, diluted in D_5W, may be necessary to maintain an alert state (*Ann Emerg Med 1986;15:566*).
- Ventilatory support should be provided for the patient who is unresponsive to naloxone and for pulmonary edema.
- **Disposition**
  - If the patient is alert and asymptomatic for 4 to 6 hours after a single dose of naloxone, or for 4 hours after a single treatment for an IV overdose, he or she can be discharged safely.
  - Body packers should be admitted to an ICU for close monitoring of the respiratory rate and level of consciousness and remain so until all packets have passed, as documented by CT.

SPECIAL CONSIDERATIONS

- Heroin may be adulterated with scopolamine, cocaine, clenbuterol, or caffeine, complicating the clinical picture. Less common complications include hypotension, bradycardia, and pulmonary edema.
- Be aware of body packers who smuggle heroin in their intestinal tracts. Deterioration of latex or plastic containers may result in drug release and death (*Am J Forensic Med Pathol 1997;18:312*).

Salicylates

GENERAL PRINCIPLES

Definition

- Salicylate toxicity may result from **acute or chronic** ingestion of acetylsalicylic acid (aspirin is a generic name in the United States, but a brand name in the rest of the world). Toxicity is usually mild after acute ingestions of <150 mg/kg, moderate after ingestions of 150 to 300 mg/kg, and generally severe with overdoses of 300 to 500 mg/kg.
- Toxicity from chronic ingestion is typically due to intake of >100 mg/kg/d over a period of several days and usually occurs in elderly patients with chronic underlying illness. Diagnosis is often delayed in this group of patients, and mortality is approximately 25%. Significant toxicity due to chronic ingestion may occur with blood concentrations lower than those associated with acute ingestions.
- Topical preparations containing methylsalicylate or oil of wintergreen can cause toxicity with excessive topical use or if ingested.

DIAGNOSIS

Clinical Presentation

- Nausea, vomiting, tinnitus, tachypnea, hyperpnea, and malaise are common. Hyperthermia results uncoupled mitochondrial oxidative phosphorylation and suggests a poor prognosis.
- Severe intoxications may include lethargy, convulsions, and coma which may result from cerebral edema and energy-depletion in the CNS.

- Noncardiogenic pulmonary edema may occur and is more common with chronic ingestion, cigarette smoking, neurologic symptoms, and older age.
- Severe overdoses may include tachypnea, dehydration, pulmonary edema, altered mental status, seizures, coma, or a total dose > 300 mg/kg.

Diagnostic Testing

Laboratories
- Obtain electrolytes, BUN, creatinine, glucose, and salicylate concentration.
- Obtain either ABGs or VBGs.
- ABGs may reveal an early respiratory alkalosis, followed by metabolic acidosis.
  - Approximately 20% of patients exhibit either respiratory alkalosis or metabolic acidosis alone (*J Crit Illness 1986;1:77*).
  - Most adults with pure salicylate overdose have a primary metabolic acidosis and a primary respiratory alkalosis.
  - After mixed overdoses, respiratory acidosis may become prominent (*Arch Intern Med 1978;138:1481*).
- Serum salicylate concentrations drawn after acute ingestion of salicylates assist in prediction of severity of intoxication and patient disposition. However, **do not rely upon the Done nomogram.**
  - Salicylate concentrations > 70 mg/dL at any time represent moderate to severe intoxication.
  - Salicylate concentrations > 100 mg/dL are very serious and often fatal. This information is useful only for acute overdoses of nonenteric-coated aspirin.
  - Enteric-coated aspirin may have delayed absorption and delayed peak concentration.
  - Chronic ingestion can cause toxicity with lower salicylate concentrations.
  - Bicarbonate concentrations and pH are more useful than salicylate concentrations as prognostic indicators in chronic intoxication.

Imaging
- Repeated blood salicylate concentrations that fail to decline should prompt contrast radiography of the stomach. Salicylate concretions may require endoscopy, multiple-dose AC, or bicarbonate lavage.
- Consider whole-bowel irrigation with polyethylene glycol.

TREATMENT

Medications
- Administer 50 to 100 g **AC** if presentation is within 1 hour of ingestion.
- **Multidose charcoal** may be useful in severe overdose (*Pediatrics 1990;85:594*), or in cases in which salicylate concentrations fail to decline (due to possible gastric bezoar formation).
- **Alkaline diuresis** is indicated for symptomatic patients with salicylate blood concentrations > 40 mg/dL.
  - Administer 150 mEq (three ampules) sodium bicarbonate in 1,000 mL D_5W at a rate of 10 to 15 mL/kg/hr if the patient is clinically volume depleted until urine flow is achieved.
  - Maintain alkalinization using the same solution at 2 to 3 mL/kg/hr, and monitor urine output, urine pH (target pH, 7 to 8), and serum potassium. Successful alkaline diuresis requires the simultaneous administration of potassium chloride.

- Give **40 mEq potassium chloride IVPB** over 4 to 5 hours. Give additional potassium chloride either orally or intravenously as needed to maintain serum potassium concentration above 4 mEq/L.
- **Use caution with alkaline diuresis in older patients,** who may have cardiac, renal, or pulmonary comorbidity, as pulmonary edema is more likely to occur in this population.
- **Do not use acetazolamide** (carbonic anhydrase inhibitor). Although acetazolamide alkalinizes the urine, it increases salicylate toxicity because it also alkalinizes the CNS (trapping more salicylate in the brain) and worsens acidemia.
- **Hyperventilate any patient requiring endotracheal intubation.** In salicylate-poisoned patients with tachypnea and hyperpnea, the respiratory alkalosis partially compensates for the metabolic acidosis. Mechanical ventilation with neuromuscular paralysis, sedation, and "normal" ventilator rates will remove the respiratory alkalosis, will worsen acidosis, and will cause rapid deterioration or death.
- **Treat altered mental status with IV dextrose,** despite normal blood glucose.
- Treat cerebral edema with hyperventilation and osmotic diuresis.
- Treat **seizures** with a **benzodiazepine** (diazepam, 5 to 10 mg IV q15min up to 50 mg) followed by **phenobarbital,** 15 mg/kg IV. Give **dextrose** 25 g IV immediately following seizure control.

Other Nonoperative Therapies

- **Hemodialysis** is indicated for blood concentrations > 100 mg/dL after acute intoxication. Hemodialysis rapidly removes salicylate and corrects acidosis. Hemodialysis may be useful with chronic toxicity when salicylate concentrations are as low as 40 mg/dL in patients with any of the following: persistent acidosis, severe CNS symptoms, progressive clinical deterioration, pulmonary edema, or renal failure.
- Treatment of pulmonary edema may also require mechanical ventilation with a high fraction of inspired oxygen concentration and PEEP (in addition to high respiratory rate).

SPECIAL CONSIDERATIONS

- Patients with minor symptoms (nausea, vomiting, tinnitus), an acute ingestion of <100 mg/kg, and a first blood concentration of <50 mg/dL may be treated in the emergency department. Blood concentrations should be repeated every 2 hours until they show a decline. These patients often are medically stable for discharge, and their disposition can be determined based on psychiatric evaluation.
- Admit moderately symptomatic patients for at least 24 hours. Repeat serum salicylate concentration, electrolytes, BUN, creatinine, and glucose at least every 6 hours to confirm declining salicylate concentration, improving bicarbonate concentration, and stable potassium concentration. Measure urine pH at least every 6 hours (if patient has urinary bladder catheter) or with each spontaneous void to confirm urinary alkalinization.
- Admit patients with severe overdoses to an ICU. Monitor laboratory studies as with moderately ill patients. Closely monitor ABGs. Arrange for immediate hemodialysis. Use great caution with mechanical ventilation, and hyperventilate any patient who requires mechanical ventilation.

Phenytoin and Fosphenytoin

GENERAL PRINCIPLES

Classification

There are four major mechanisms by which anticonvulsants exert therapeutic activity—sodium channel blockade, GABA agonism, calcium channel antagonism, and inhibition of excitatory amino acids. In overdose, these features are enhanced.

Pathophysiology

- Phenytoin has been a first-line treatment for seizures since its introduction. Fosphenytoin was developed as a response to some of the toxicity associated with intravenous phenytoin administration. Fosphenytoin is a prodrug that is converted to phenytoin after IV or IM injection and therefore will be referred to as phenytoin below.
- **Neither of these drugs is indicated for the treatment of toxin-induced seizures** (*NEJM 1985;313:145–151*), **including ethanol withdrawal seizures** (*Ann Emerg Med 1991;20:520–522*).
- Phenytoin exerts therapeutic activity by binding to sodium channels and inhibiting reactivation (*J Neural Transm 1988;72:173–183*). Phenytoin exhibits saturable kinetics, and at plasma levels above 20 mcg/mL, toxic effects become rapidly apparent.
- Acute toxicity is associated with the development of a **neurologic syndrome** that appears to be cerebellar in origin. **Cardiotoxicity** is **not** associated with phenytoin **ingestion** (*Heart Lung 1997;26:325–328*); however, it has been **reported with IV administration** of phenytoin. Rapid IV administration slows cardiac conduction and decreases systemic vascular resistance and myocardial contractility. The cardiac toxicity associated with intravenous phenytoin administration is due in part to the presence of propylene glycol and ethanol in the diluent, which are known myocardial depressants and vasodilators (*Am J Cardiol 1966;17:332–338*). The introduction of fosphenytoin has decreased the incidence of cardiac complications.

Risk Factors

Other than overdose, risk factors for developing phenytoin toxicity are associated with the coadministration of drugs that affect the **cytochrome P450** system.

DIAGNOSIS

There are several classic clinical findings that point to the diagnosis of phenytoin toxicity.

Clinical Presentation

History

Patients exhibiting toxicity from phenytoin will often be brought in by family members who will describe the patient as **ataxic** and increasingly **confused.** There is usually a history of seizure disorder and the medication list will include phenytoin. In intentional overdoses, the patient may be lethargic with slurred speech and an extrapyramidal movement disorder (*Ann Emerg Med 1989;7:61–67*).

Physical Examination

- At plasma concentrations of >15 mcg/mL, patients will exhibit **nystagmus. Ataxia** develops at levels of 30 mcg/mL. **Confusion** and **frank movement disorders** occur at levels of 50 mcg/mL or greater. Chronic phenytoin ingestion is also associated with **gingival hyperplasia,** which is a very useful clinical finding when uncertain of the diagnosis. **Ingestions** are **not** associated with **cardiotoxicity** or vital sign abnormalities (*Ann Emerg Med 1991;20:508–512*). Rapid **intravenous** administration of phenytoin results in **hypotension** and **bradycardia. Death** has been reported (*JAMA 1968;20:2118–2119*).
- **Extravasation** injury is a serious complication of intravenous phenytoin administration and can result in severe tissue injury described as **the purple glove syndrome.** This injury will occasionally require surgical debridement (*Neurology 1998; 51(4):1034–1039*).

Differential Diagnosis

Phenytoin toxicity is similar in presentation to carbamazepine poisoning; however, carbamazepine tends to exhibit cardiotoxicity. Other considerations include a convulsive status epilepticus, meningitis, encephalitis, or other intracerebral lesion.

Diagnostic Testing

Laboratories

- **Serial phenytoin concentrations** should be obtained on any patient with a potential history of exposure.
- **CBC:** Phenytoin has been reported to occasionally cause agranulocytosis.
- **HFP:** Phenytoin is associated with the occasional development of hepatotoxicity.

Electrocardiography

ECGs and telemetry are generally not needed in oral overdoses (*Ann Emerg Med 1991;20:508–512*). However, in IV infusions, it is necessary to have the patient in a monitored setting.

TREATMENT

- Admission is warranted for patients with ataxia, and serial levels should be obtained while in the hospital.
- Supportive care is the mainstay of treatment for acute or chronic phenytoin toxicity. **Multidose activated charcoal** (MDAC) is useful in decreasing the serum half-life; however, given the pharmacokinetic profile of this drug, it is possible to rapidly lower the serum concentration below therapeutic levels and precipitate a seizure.
- **Benzodiazepines** are the mainstay of treatment for seizures.
- Hypotension and bradycardia in the setting of IV administration is usually self-limiting and will resolve with supportive care. In refractory bradycardia or hypotension, ACLS principles apply.
- Cases of agranulocytosis are responsive to **G-CSF** administration.
- Hepatotoxicity usually resolves with the **discontinuation** of the drug.

Surgical Management

In cases of extravasation, it is important to have a surgical evaluation in order to determine the need for operative debridement.

SPECIAL CONSIDERATIONS

Phenytoin is generally of limited use in the treatment of active seizures. Since the mainstay of treatment is benzodiazepine administration and IV phenytoin is associated with significant toxicity, it is better to orally load patients whenever possible.

OUTCOME/PROGNOSIS

Phenytoin overdoses tend to be benign and self-limiting with supportive care. Deaths are exceedingly unusual even in the setting of massive overdose.

Carbamazepine/Oxcarbazepine

GENERAL PRINCIPLES

Definition

Carbamazepine and oxcarbazepine are structurally related to TCAs. Like fosphenytoin, oxcarbazepine is a prodrug that is metabolized to an active metabolite. An anticonvulsant.

Pathophysiology

- The therapeutic efficacy of carbamazepine and oxcarbazepine are due to **sodium channel blockade,** which prevents the propagation of an abnormal focus. The therapeutic serum concentration of carbamazepine is 4 to 12 mg/L. There is no routine laboratory testing for oxcarbazepine; however, the carbamazepine assay will detect the presence of oxcarbazepine.
- The toxicity associated with carbamazepine is likely due to its chemical structure. TCA-like effects include sodium channel blockade, QT prolongation, and anticholinergic features.
- In overdose, carbamazepine is erratically absorbed and may form concretions in the GI tract causing prolonged toxicity.
- Persistently high levels of carbamazepine have been reported to increase antidiuretic hormone secretion leading to syndrome of inappropriate antidiuretic hormone release (SIADH) (*Prog Neuropsychopharmacol Biol Psychiatry 1994;18:211–233*).

Risk Factors

Carbamazepine toxicity may be enhanced by concomitant use of drugs that are metabolized by the CYP450 system.

DIAGNOSIS

There are several key features of carbamazepine toxicity.

Clinical Presentation

History

Toxicity should be suspected in individuals who present with a history of a seizure disorder and altered mental status. **Delayed toxicity** has been reported after an acute overdose given the variability in GI absorption (*J Toxicol Clin Toxicol 1979;14:263–269*). Patients may exhibit a relapsing syndrome of coma and altered consciousness due to bezoar formation and enterohepatic recirculation.

Physical Examination
- The predominant clinical findings in carbamazepine toxicity are neurologic and cardiovascular effects. In mild to moderate toxicity, patients may present with ataxia, nystagmus, and mydriasis. In serious overdose, patients may develop **coma** and **seizures,** including status epilepticus. Vital sign abnormalities include **tachycardia** due to the anticholinergic effects of the drug as well as **hypotension** and **bradycardia** due to direct myocardial depressant effects.
- The combination of cerebellar findings on exam, in conjunction with an anticholinergic toxidrome, should prompt the clinician to consider carbamazepine as a potential toxicant.

Differential Diagnosis

Mild to moderate carbamazepine toxicity resembles phenytoin toxicity. Other considerations include a convulsive status epilepticus, meningitis, encephalitis, or other intracerebral lesion.

Diagnostic Testing

Serum carbamazepine concentrations should be obtained on any patient who presents with a history of ingestion. The therapeutic range is from 4 to 12 mg/L. Serial levels should be obtained every 4 to 6 hours to evaluate for delayed toxicity or prolonged absorption. Concentrations of >40 mg/L are associated with the development of cardiotoxicity (*J Toxicol Clin Toxicol 1993;31:449–458*).

Electrocardiography
Patients with carbamazepine overdoses will often develop signs of cardiac toxicity. ECG findings include QRS ant QT_c prolongation and AV conduction delays. Cardiotoxicity will occasionally be delayed, so all patients should be admitted with telemetry.

TREATMENT

Medications

Maintain airway protection at all times, treat seizures with **benzodiazepines.** Although there is a paucity of data regarding the efficacy of **sodium bicarbonate** in this setting, its use should be considered if the QRS duration is >100 milliseconds, given the structural similarity to TCAs.

Other Nonoperative Therapies

Like phenytoin, carbamazapine's half-life is reduced by the administration of **MDAC** by decreasing enterohepatic recirculation of the drug (*Eur J Clin Pharmacol 1980;17:51–57*).

Lamotrigine

GENERAL PRINCIPLES

Definition

Lamotrigine is widely prescribed as a mood stabilizer as well as for the treatment of partial complex seizures. An anticonvulsant.

Pathophysiology

Lamotrigine exerts its therapeutic effects by blocking pre- and postsynaptic sodium channels. In overdose, excess sodium channel blockade may result in widening of the QRS on the ECG and conduction blocks. Idiopathic cases of dermatologic pathology including Steven–Johnson syndrome and toxic epidermal necrolysis have been reported with the therapeutic administration of lamotrigine.

DIAGNOSIS

Clinical Presentation

History

Suspect lamotrigine toxicity in patients with a seizure disorder and altered mental status.

Physical Examination

Patients with lamotrigine toxicity present with lethargy, ataxia, and nystagmus. Overdose may present with seizures as well.

Differential Diagnosis

Lamotrigine toxicity is similar to other sodium channel blocking anticonvulsant agents.

Diagnostic Testing

Laboratories

Therapeutic concentrations range from 3 to 14 mg/L; concentrations greater than 15 mg/L are associated with the development of toxicity.

Electrocardiography

Lamotrigine overdose has been associated with the development of conduction delays and QRS widening. Patients should be admitted on telemetry.

TREATMENT

AC should be administered to alert patients with an intact airway. Seizures should be treated with **benzodiazepines**. There are theoretical benefits of administering **sodium bicarbonate,** 150 mEq in 1 L of 5% dextrose, in patients with a QRS > 100 milliseconds; however, there is a paucity of experimental data to support this practice. In the setting of bicarbonate administration, close monitoring of **serum potassium** levels is required in order to avoid life-threatening hypokalemia.

Levetiracetam

GENERAL PRINCIPLES

Levetiracetam is becoming increasingly used in the management of several of the different subtypes of epilepsy. An anticonvulsant.

Pathophysiology

The mechanism by which levetiracetam exerts its therapeutic effect is not well described; however, it does block N-type calcium channels on the presynaptic terminals of neurons.

DIAGNOSIS

Clinical Presentation

Very little data exist on levetiracetam overdoses. Lethargy and respiratory depression have been reported in the setting of overdose.

Differential Diagnosis

In patients with a seizure disorder and lethargy, intoxication, infectious, and metabolic disorders should be considered.

Diagnostic Testing

Although a test is available for measuring serum levels this assay is not routinely available.

TREATMENT

Medications

Generally, **supportive care** is required. In cases where respiratory depression is evident, the patient should be intubated and ventilated. Avoid AC in patients with an altered mental status and an unprotected airway.

Valproic Acid

GENERAL PRINCIPLES

Valproic acid (VPA) is widely used for the management of seizures and mood disorders and exerts its effects by inhibiting the function of voltage-gated sodium and calcium channels as well as enhancing the function of GABA. An anticonvulsant.

Pathophysiology

VPA is metabolized by the hepatocytes through a complicated biochemical process that involves β-oxidation in the mitochondria. This drug may result in fatty infiltrates in the liver and accumulation of ammonia.

Risk Factors

Hepatic dysfunction can occur even at therapeutic levels and therefore should be monitored. The therapeutic range runs from 50 to 100 mg/L. In overdose, the risk of hepatic dysfunction and hyperammonemia increases.

DIAGNOSIS

Clinical Presentation

Patients with valproate overdoses may present with tremor, ataxia, sedation, altered sensorium, or coma. Occasionally, patients will present with abdominal pain.

Diagnostic Testing

Laboratories
- Therapeutic concentrations range from 50 to 100 mg/L. Patients who present with overdoses should have a **BMP** drawn to evaluate for hyponatremia and metabolic acidosis.

- In cases of massive overdose, a **CBC** should be sent as cases of pancytopenia have been reported in the literature (*Scott Med J 1987;32:85–86*). Hemopoietic disturbances may occur up to 5 days after overdose.
- Chronic VPA therapy has been associated with the development of hepatotoxicity and may result in a fatal hepatitis. In cases of chronic toxicity, an **HFP** should be sent to evaluate for transaminitis. Likewise, any patient with VPA toxicity should have an **ammonia** level sent.
- There have been occasional reports of pancreatitis (*J Toxicol Clin Toxicol 1995;33:279–284*); therefore in massive overdose, consider sending **lipase** as well.

TREATMENT

Medications

- Most cases of toxicity resolve with supportive care. In patients who are awake with adequate airway protection, **AC** is warranted.
- In patients with hyperammonemia > 35 mcgmol/L (>80 mcg/dL) **l-carnitine** therapy should be instituted. In awake patients, oral carnitine is the preferred route at 50 to 100 mg/kg/d divided every 6 hours up to 3 g/d. In cases where patients are not able to tolerate PO, intravenous l-carnitine may be administered at 100 mg/kg IV up to 6 g as a loading dose, and then 15 mg/kg every 4 hours. Therapy may be discontinued when the patient's ammonia level declines to <35 mcgmol/L.

Monoamine Oxidase Inhibitors

GENERAL PRINCIPLES

Although several different classes of monoamine oxidase inhibitors (MAOIs) exist, the drugs most frequently implicated in toxicity are the first-generation drugs: **phenelzine, isocarboxazid,** and **tranylcypromine. Clorgyline,** a later-generation drug, is also associated with a similar toxic profile. The third-generation drugs including **moclobemide** have a better safety profile. Antidepressants.

Pathophysiology

Monoamine oxidase is an enzyme responsible for the inactivation of biogenic amines such as **epinephrine, norepinephrine, tyramine, dopamine,** and **serotonin.** Inhibition of this enzyme results in an increase of synaptic concentrations of biogenic amines. An increase in norepinephrine and serotonin, in particular, is thought to be responsible for mood elevation. MAOIs are structurally similar to amphetamine. In overdose, a significant amount of neurotransmitter is released resulting in a **sympathomimetic** toxidrome. Phenelzine and isocarboxazid are also hydrazine derivatives and in overdose have been associated with the development of **seizure** activity. As neurotransmitters become depleted, patients develop cardiovascular collapse, which is often refractory to therapy. Given the fact that MAOIs affect an enzymatic pathway, there is often a **significant delay** in the development of toxicity after overdose, with most cases occurring in a **24-hour** period post ingestion, although there are cases of toxicity occurring **up to 32 hours** after overdose (*Ann Emerg Med 1984;13:1137–1144*). This effect may occur with seemingly small overdoses of five or six pills (*J Clin Psychiatry 1983;44:280–288*).

Risk Factors

The classic risk factors for developing toxicity include increasing a prescribed dose or eating foods rich in **tyramine**, such as aged cheddar cheese or red wine. Drug–drug interactions occur when a new antidepressant (often a selective serotonin reuptake inhibitor [SSRI]) is introduced without an adequate **washout period** of several weeks after discontinuing the MAOI.

Prevention

Patients should be well educated on the risk associated with these drugs. The **duration of action in these drugs significantly outlasts their half-lives;** therefore, physicians should always use a reference guide or consult a pharmacist prior to prescribing a new drug in addition to or as a replacement for the MAOI.

Associated Conditions

- MAOIs have been associated with severe **hypertensive crises** in the setting of coingestions of **tyramine**-containing foods such as **aged cheddar and red wine.** Likewise, coingestion of **indirect-acting sympathomimetics,** which cause presynaptic release of norepinephrine, may precipitate a hypertensive crisis. Agents included in this category are **amphetamine-based drugs, dopamine, and pseudoephedrine.**
- **Serotonin syndrome** is also associated with the coingestion of **SSRIs, St. John's Wort, meperidine,** and **dextromethorphan.**

DIAGNOSIS

Clinical Presentation

MAOI overdose is associated with a considerable risk of mortality and morbidity.

History

- In overdose, there may be a **significant delay** in the development of symptoms. Anyone who presents with normal vital signs and history of MAOI overdose must be **admitted and monitored** for at least 24 hours.
- Overdose should be suspected in patients who are taking MAOIs and present in extremis with a florid **sympathomimetic** toxidrome.

Physical Examination

Patients may initially present with minimal signs of toxicity. Subsequently, they will develop **agitation, diaphoresis, tachycardia, severe hypertension, and dilated pupils, and headache.** As their illness progresses, they may develop **hyperthermia, rigidity, and seizures.** Ultimately, there is depletion of neurotransmitter stores and the patient develops refractory cardiovascular collapse.

Differential Diagnosis

MAOI overdose produces a clinical picture that is similar to severe serotonin syndrome and severe sympathomimetic toxicity. Serotonin syndrome has a relatively faster onset of action and occurs within minutes to hours of ingestion.

Diagnostic Testing

Laboratories

These include routine labs such as a **BMP,** looking for metabolic acidosis, hyper-kalemia, and renal failure. A **CK** is useful in overdose patients as they may develop rhabdomyolysis. In severe cases, **troponins** should be obtained to evaluate for myocardial infarction. **Coagulation studies** are important as these patients may develop disseminated intravascular coagulopathy.

Electrocardiography
ECG analysis may reveal a range of disorders from a simple sinus tachycardia to a wide complex dysrhythmia.

Imaging
A **head CT** should be obtained on altered patients and patients complaining of a headache in order to evaluate for intracranial hemorrhage.

TREATMENT

- The management of first-generation MAOI overdose can be very difficult as the patient may have dramatically variable vital signs. Patients with MAOI overdose should be aggressively managed with **orogastric lavage,** even if they are asymptomatic on arrival to the hospital.
- In hyperthermic patients, **rapid cooling measures** should be instituted.

Medications
First Line
- **AC** (1 g/kg) should be administered to the patient after the airway is secured. Many patients will be awake and alert and may not need immediate intubation; however, these patients should receive AC as well.
- Given the propensity for wildly fluctuating BP, titratable and short-acting agents are the mainstay of treatment in these patients. Hypertension should be managed with **nitroglycerin, nitroprusside, or phentolamine.** If the patient develops hypotension, a direct-acting α-agonist such as **norepinephrine** should be used. **Avoid dopamine** in the setting of MAOI overdose as it often fails to improve BP due to catecholamine depletion.
- **Benzodiazepines** should be used for seizures and agitation. Rigidity that does not respond to benzodiazepine administration may be managed with **nondepolarizing** paralytics. There are case reports describing the resolution of rigidity after the administration of **cyproheptadine** (*J Clin Psychopharmacol 1993;13:312–320*).

Second Line
In patients with refractory seizures, early administration of **pyridoxine** is warranted. Doses of 70 mg/kg not to exceed 5 g should be administered early as an IV infusion of 0.5 g/min.

SPECIAL CONSIDERATIONS

- Patients with MAOI overdoses require admission with monitoring for at least 24 hours, given the propensity for delayed toxicity. Aggressive decontamination measures should be taken, even if the patient seems to be asymptomatic as decompensation is rapid and frequently fatal.
- The **exception** to this is an overdose of **moclobemide,** which has a much better safety profile and tends to have a benign course because of its short duration of MAO inhibition.

PATIENT EDUCATION

- Patients who are placed on MAOIs should be educated about food and drug interactions and warned about the risk of interactions with herbal supplements, including St. John's Wort.
- A washout period of at least 2 weeks after discontinuation of an MAOI should be observed before starting another antidepressant.

Tricyclic Antidepressants

GENERAL PRINCIPLES

Multiple TCAs are on the market, including amitriptyline, clomipramine, doxepin, imipramine, trimipramine, desipramine, nortriptyline, and amoxapine.

Pathophysiology

- TCAs interact with a wide variety of receptors with many consequent effects in the setting of an overdose. The primary antidepressant effect is due to the inhibition of serotonin and norepinephrine reuptake. Additionally, TCAs modulate the function of central sympathetic and serotonergic receptors, which is thought to contribute to their antidepressant effects.
- In toxicity, other effects become apparent as well. TCAs have antimuscarinic effects, resulting in tachycardia, dry mucous membranes and skin, urinary retention, and decreased GI motility. Patients will also have dilated pupils (*Psychopharmacology 1994;114:559–565*). Sedation is likely due to antihistamine effects. Furthermore, these agents are potent α_1-antagonists leading to the development of hypotension and a reflex tachycardia. Cardiac toxicity is due to sodium channel blockade, resulting in a wide complex rhythm on the ECG (*Annu Rev Med 1984;35:503–511*). TCAs also exhibit a complex interaction with the GABA receptor, which in overdose likely contributes to seizure activity (*Life Sci 1988;43:303–307*).

DIAGNOSIS

TCA overdose exhibits its own toxidrome due to the widespread effects on various receptors as outlined above. Patients with an acute overdose may present to the emergency department with a normal mental status and vital signs, but then rapidly decompensate.

Clinical Presentation

History
As with any overdose, a history is often unreliable. The clinical picture in serious toxicity is fairly stereotypical and a careful physical examination can help establish the diagnosis.

Physical Examination
Patients with TCA overdose often present with a rapid onset of **CNS depression.** They will be **tachycardic** and **hypotensive** due to vasodilatation and antimuscarinic effects. They will have **dilated pupils, dry mucous membranes,** and **urinary retention** due to the anticholinergic effects of the drug. Patients with significant overdoses may present with **seizure** activity.

Diagnostic Criteria

The CA toxidrome is a fairly consistent constellation of signs including hypotension, tachycardia, coma, and seizures.

Diagnostic Testing

Laboratories
- **Serum TCA concentrations** have a **limited role** in the management of acute TCA toxicity as they are **not predictive of severity of illness** (*NEJM 1985;313:474–479*). Qualitative measurements of TCA concentrations in the urine are unreliable as there are many common drugs that cross-react on the assay, including diphenhydramine and cyclobenzaprine.
- Serial **VBG**s should be measured in patients undergoing alkalinization. As bicarbonate treatment can cause profound hypokalemia, serial K^+ should be followed and repleted.
- **Dextrose** should be checked in any patient with an altered mental status.

Electrocardiography
The ECG has proved to be a valuable tool in predicting the degree of morbidity in TCA overdose. In one classic study, one-third patients with a **QRS of ≥100 milliseconds** developed **seizures.** Fifty percent of patients with a QRS of ≥160 milliseconds developed **ventricular dysrhythmias** (*NEJM 1985;313:474–479*). A terminal 40-millisecond axis of greater than 120° is found in patients who are taking TCAs and may help narrow the diagnosis in patients with an altered mental status of unknown etiology. Simply put, the ECG will show an **R′ in aVR,** and an S wave in leads I and aVL. An R′ in aVR of >3 mm has been demonstrated to be predictive of neurologic and cardiac complications in TCA-poisoned patients (*Ann Emerg Med 1995;26(2):195–201*).

TREATMENT

Patients with TCA overdose require early aggressive intervention. In patients with altered mental status, early **intubation, resuscitation,** and **GI decontamination** are warranted. Orogastric lavage may be beneficial in patients who are intubated with large ingestions because of decreased GI motility. Avoid this in small children as they only typically take one to two pills. **Hyperventilation** to achieve rapid serum alkalinization may be used as a bridge until bicarbonate therapy is started.

Medications

First Line
- **After the patient's airway is protected,** a dose of **AC** 1 g/kg is warranted even in delayed presentations.
- **Sodium bicarbonate** has been demonstrated to narrow the QRS, decrease the incidence of ventricular arrhythmias, and improve hypotension (*Emerg Med 2001;13:204–210*). A bolus of 1 to 2 mEq/kg every 3 to 5 minutes should be given with continuous ECG monitoring until the QRS narrows or the BP improves. Serial VBGs should be obtained with a goal of maintaining the blood pH at 7.50 to 7.55.
  - A bicarbonate drip should be titrated to the QRS narrowing and resolution of hypotension. The patient should be monitored in an ICU with serial pH and serum potassium measurements as well as monitoring for fluid overload.

- Alkalinization should continue for 12 to 24 hours until the clinical picture and the ECG improves.
- **Norepinephrine** is the pressor of choice in hypotensive patients who do not respond to alkalinization because of its direct effects on the vasculature.
- **Lidocaine** may be considered in the presence of ventricular dysrhythmias precipitated by TCA toxicity. However, class **Ia and Ic antidysrhythmics are contraindicated in the management of TCA-poisoned patients.**
- **Benzodiazepines** are the mainstay of treatment for seizures. **Phenytoin should be avoided.**

Second Line
Propofol and barbiturates may be beneficial in refractory seizures.

Other Nonoperative Therapies
Cardiopulmonary bypass and extracorporeal membrane oxygenation have been used in critically ill patients with refractory hypotension (*Ann Emerg Med 1994;23:480–486; Am J Emerg Med 1994;12:456–458*).

Selective Serotonin Reuptake Inhibitors

GENERAL PRINCIPLES

Classification
This class of drugs includes **fluoxetine, fluvoxamine, paroxetine, sertraline, citalopram, and escitalopram**. These drugs have a much better safety profile than the earlier drugs marketed for the management of depressive disorders and as such, have largely supplanted MAOIs and TCAs in the treatment of depression.

Pathophysiology
These drugs enhance serotonergic activity by preventing its reuptake into the presynaptic terminal of the neuron, which may partially explain their antidepressant effects. Unlike other antidepressants, SSRIs have limited effects on other receptors and therefore tend to be less toxic in overdose.

DIAGNOSIS

Clinical Presentation
The vast majority of these overdoses have a benign clinical course. However, patients may present with signs of serotonin excess. Patients who have ingested **citalopram** or **escitalopram** may develop delayed toxicity.

History
Overdose histories are unreliable. Many patients who claim to have taken an overdose yet who look well actually took SSRIs.

Physical Examination
Signs of toxicity are usually absent unless the patient has taken a massive overdose. In these cases, patients may present with nausea, vomiting, and tachycardia. Patients with **citalopram** or **escitalopram** ingestions may present with **seizures.**

Diagnostic Testing

Laboratories
- SSRIs have been implicated in the development of **SIADH;** therefore, a **BMP** should be obtained.
- **Dextrose** should be checked in patients with an altered mental status or seizures.
- In patients with **serotonin syndrome,** a **CPK** and **lactate** should be checked as well as a **coagulation profile.**

Electrocardiography
Patients will occasionally present with a sinus tachycardia. In patients with citalopram or escitalopram, ingestions may develop QT_c widening as late as 24 hours after an overdose (*J Toxicol Clin Toxicol 1997;35:237–240*).

TREATMENT

The vast majority of overdoses require only 6 hours of observation and supportive care. Patients with intentional **citalopram** and **escitalopram** overdoses should be admitted to the floor with 24 hours of telemetry to monitor for QT_c widening.

Medications
- In patients who are awake and alert, 1 g/kg of **AC** may be administered.
- Treat seizures with **benzodiazepines.**
- Treat torsades with **magnesium,** correction of electrolytes, **lidocaine,** and **overdrive pacing.**

Serotonin Syndrome

GENERAL PRINCIPLES

Definition
Serotonin syndrome is a disorder that can be precipitated by the introduction of a serotonergic agent and has been reported to occur even after ingestion of a single pill (*Ann Emerg Med 1999;33 457–459*).

Pathophysiology
Serotonin syndrome is thought to occur secondary to excess stimulation of $5HT_{2A}$ receptors (*J Psychopharmacol 1999;13:100–109*). This syndrome can result from the coadministration of two or more serotonergic agents including SSRIs, MAOIs, meperidine, amphetamines, cocaine, TCAs, and various other drugs.

DIAGNOSIS

Clinical Presentation
History
Suspect serotonin syndrome in any patient who presents with a rapid onset of tremor and clonus after administration of a serotonergic agent. It is important to avoid the addition of other serotonergic agents in the management of these patients.

Physical Examination

Patients with serotonin syndrome will present with signs of excess serotonergic activity including restlessness, shivering, diaphoresis, and diarrhea. As the syndrome progresses, patients develop myoclonus, ocular clonus, and muscle rigidity. Vital sign abnormalities include tachycardia and hyperpyrexia.

Diagnostic Criteria

- Serotonin syndrome is diagnosed by the presence of four of the following major criteria: alteration of consciousness, coma, or mood elevation; shivering, myoclonus, rigidity, or hyperreflexia; pyrexia or sweating.
- Additional minor criteria include restlessness or insomnia; mydriasis or akathisia; tachycardia, diarrhea, respiratory or BP abnormalities (*Med Hypotheses 2000;55:218–224*).

Differential Diagnosis

Patients who present with altered mental status, rigidity, and hyperpyrexia may be misdiagnosed with NMS. NMS tends to develop over days to weeks, whereas serotonin syndrome has a fast onset, usually manifesting over a 24-hour period.

Diagnostic Testing

Serotonin syndrome is diagnosed by a constellation of symptoms and signs rather than any specific laboratory findings; however, as the disease evolves, laboratory abnormalities develop.

Laboratories

Patients who present early with a mild form of the syndrome may have no lab abnormalities. On the other hand, more severe presentations may develop complications from psychomotor agitation and muscle rigidity including elevated **CK, metabolic acidosis,** and an **elevated lactate. Renal failure** may occur in the presence of rhabdomyolysis as well. Additionally, patients with hyperthermia may develop a **coagulopathy.** Therefore, a **BMP** and **coagulation studies** should be obtained. As with any critical illness, patients may succumb to multiorgan failure, and therefore, laboratory studies should be obtained on the basis of the presentation.

Electrocardiography

The typical ECG will show a sinus tachycardia; however, there are no specific diagnostic electrocardiographic criteria associated with serotonin syndrome.

TREATMENT

The treatment of serotonin syndrome is largely supportive and requires the removal of the offending agent. Aggressive cooling and hydration measures should be taken in the hyperthermic patient.

Medications

- **Benzodiazepines** should be used liberally to treat psychomotor agitation and myoclonus. In severe cases, **nondepolarizing paralytics** should be used to limit the degree of rhabdomyolysis.

- In patients with mild to moderate symptoms, **cyproheptadine,** an antihistamine with $5HT_{1A}$ and $5HT_{2A}$ antagonism should be considered. A **4 to 8 mg** initial dose should be given orally, which often results in a rapid reversal of symptoms. If there is no response, the dose may be repeated in 2 hours. Subsequent dosing is 2 to 4 mg orally every 6 hours until the patient improves or a maximum dose of 32 mg/d is reached.

Lithium

GENERAL PRINCIPLES

Classification

Toxicity may be classified as **acute, chronic, or acute on chronic.** Lithium has a low therapeutic index, and therefore, risk of toxicity is high in patients on chronic therapy. The therapeutic range is approximately 0.6 to 1.2 mmol/L. An antidepressant.

Pathophysiology

The mechanism by which lithium exerts its antimanic properties is not well understood. There is some evidence that lithium enhances serotonin function, which may contribute to its mood-stabilizing properties (*Science 1981;213:1529–1531*). Acute toxicity is associated with the development of a GI illness as lithium is a metal. On the other hand, chronic toxicity is primarily associated with neurologic dysfunction. Although serum levels are helpful in the management of these patients, the clinical picture should be the basis for therapy. Generally speaking, in **chronically** exposed patients, levels of less than 2.5 mEq/L are associated with tremulousness, ataxia, and nystagmus. Levels greater than 2.5 mEq/L are associated with a deteriorating neurologic syndrome and are an indication for aggressive intervention including dialysis. A serum concentration of 4.0 mEq/L in an **acute** overdose is also an indication for dialysis (*Q J Med 1978;47:123–144*).

Risk Factors

Lithium has peripheral effects, which may enhance its toxicity, including the development of nephrogenic diabetes insipidus. This phenomenon is thought to occur through the reduction in the binding of aquaporins in the collecting duct of the kidney (*Annu Rev Physiol 1996;58:619–648*). This development enhances toxicity by creating dehydration, which leads to an increase in proximal tubular reabsorption of lithium (*J Physiol 1991;437:377–391*). Other dehydration states may enhance toxicity as well.

Prevention

Patients on chronic lithium therapy should have serum levels monitored and regular follow-up with their psychiatrist which should include evaluation for the clinical signs of toxicity.

Associated Conditions

Lithium therapy has been associated with the development of chronic tubulointerstitial nephropathy (*J Am Soc Nephrol 2000;11:1439–1448*), thyroid dysfunction (*J Toxicol Clin Toxicol 2000;38:333–337*), serotonin syndrome (*Medicine 2000;79:201–209*), and other endocrine effects.

DIAGNOSIS

Clinical Presentation

History

Although the history is often unreliable in overdose patients, acutely intoxicated patients may present complaining of nausea and abdominal discomfort. In chronic toxicity, patients may present with worsening confusion.

Physical Examination

- **Acute overdose** presents with a predominately GI syndrome of nausea, vomiting, diarrhea, and abdominal pain. As the illness progresses, patients may develop signs of volume depletion with tachycardia and hypotension. Severe toxicity is associated with neurologic dysfunction including altered mental status, nystagmus, ataxia, or coma.
- **Chronic toxicity** is associated with tremor, nystagmus, and ataxia. Confusion, dysarthria, fasciculations, and myoclonus are frequent physical findings. Seizures are reported in the literature (*Biol Psychiatry 1987;22:1184–1190*).

Diagnostic Testing

Laboratories

- Obtain serial lithium levels in patients who present with evidence of toxicity. A high initial level may be due to the timing of the last dose; therefore, the clinical picture should guide therapy. **Obtain the serum sample in a lithium-free tube.**
- Other laboratories should include a **BMP** to evaluate electrolyte levels, renal function, and hydration status.
- Lithium induces an elevation in the **white cell count.**

Electrocardiography

The ECG may show nonspecific T-wave flattening or QT_c prolongation; however, cardiac dysfunction is unusual in this overdose.

TREATMENT

AC does not bind to lithium and therefore has no role in the management of these overdoses.

Medications

First Line

- Whole-bowel irrigation with **polyethylene glycol** at a rate of 2 L/hr is indicated for overdoses of sustained-release preparations (*Ann Emerg Med 1991;20:536–539*).
- The mainstay of therapy is the infusion of **0.9% saline solution** at twice maintenance. Closely monitor fluid status in these patients to avoid overload.

Second Line

There are reports that suggest **sodium polystyrene sulfonate** may be a useful adjunct for lithium elimination (*Ann Emerg Med 1993;22:1911–1915*). However, the doses needed may result in significant hypokalemia (*Acad Emerg Med 1996;3:333–337*), so this treatment should be approached with caution.

Other Nonoperative Therapies

Consider **dialysis** for patients unable to tolerate the required fluid load for enhanced elimination, signs of severe toxicity with altered mental status, or other neurologic dysfunction. In patients with acute overdose and a serum lithium concentration of >4.0 mEq/L or chronic overdose and a serum level of >2.5 mEq/L, dialysis should be considered.

Venlafaxine

GENERAL PRINCIPLES

Venlafaxine inhibits norepinephrine reuptake and overdose, although generally benign in most cases, may reflect excess sympathetic tone including tachycardia and hyperthermia as well as nausea, vomiting, and seizures.

DIAGNOSIS

Diagnostic Testing
Electrocardiography
Occasionally, QRS widening reflecting sodium channel blockade may be apparent on the ECG (*Hum Exp Toxicol 1999;18:309–313*).

TREATMENT

Treatment is supportive; consider bicarbonate if there is evidence of QRS widening on the ECG.

Trazodone

GENERAL PRINCIPLES

Trazodone overdose results in CNS depression and hypotension due to α-receptor antagonism. Priapism and SIADH have been reported in therapeutic dosing.

TREATMENT

Management is supportive, hypotension is usually responsive to fluids, and severe cases may require the administration of direct acting vasopressors such as norepinephrine.

Mirtazapine

GENERAL PRINCIPLES

Mirtazapine overdose may cause altered mental status and tachycardia. Significant overdoses may result in the prolongation of the QT_c and respiratory depression.

TREATMENT

Supportive care with close airway monitoring is often all that is required in this overdose.

Bupropion

GENERAL PRINCIPLES

Bupropion has been associated with more severe symptoms than the other atypical agents. Seizures have been reported at therapeutic doses (*J Clin Psychiatry 1991;52:450–456*). **QRS prolongation** has also been described in overdose. Symptoms may be **delayed for up to 10 hours** after ingestion of sustained-release pills.

TREATMENT

Treatment of bupropion overdose includes airway protection. **Whole-bowel irrigation** and **MDAC** should be considered in patients who present early with a normal mental status and ingestion of a sustained-release preparation. This modality is **contraindicated** in seizing patients. Seizures should be treated with **benzodiazepines.** Barbiturates and propofol should be considered in patients with status epilepticus.

Antipsychotics, General

GENERAL PRINCIPLES

Epidemiology

According to the AAPCC 2007 report, antipsychotic/sedative hypnotic agents were the fourth leading cause of fatal overdoses in the United States (*Clin Toxicol Clin Toxicol 2008;46:927–1057*).

Pathophysiology

Antipsychotic agents exert their therapeutic effect largely by binding to dopamine receptors in the CNS, which tends to mitigate the positive symptoms of schizophrenia. Dopamine receptor blockade is also associated with the development of movement disorders, and the newer neuroleptic agents attempt to address this by modulating serotonergic tone. In general, all of the antipsychotics affect multiple receptors in the nervous, endocrine, and cardiovascular system, which accounts for a wide range of toxic symptoms. Generally speaking, the older "typical" agents in the phenothiazine class tend to have more cardiac toxicity, with varying degrees of sodium channel blockade (wide QRS) and potassium channel blockade (QT_c prolongation). Furthermore, these agents tend to have more significant extrapyramidal effects. The newer or "atypical" antipsychotics were developed to address these issues and although they tend to exhibit less cardiac toxicity, they often have pronounced α_1-antagonism reflected by hypotension. The atypicals are also associated with the idiosyncratic development of other medical problems. For example, olanzapine has been associated with the development of fatal DKA (*Am J Psychiatry 2003;12:2241*), and clozapine was briefly withdrawn from the market as a small percentage of patients developed agranulocytosis (*J Clin Psychiatry 2000;61:14–17*).

Phenothiazines

GENERAL PRINCIPLES

Definition

These are the prototypic antipsychotic drugs and include chlorpromazine, thioridazine, prochlorperazine, perphenazine, trifluoperazine, fluphenazine, mesoridazine, haloperidol (a butyrophenone), and thiothixene.

DIAGNOSIS

Clinical Presentation

History

The history is often difficult to obtain in these patients.

Physical Examination

- Overdoses are characterized by agitation or delirium, which may progress rapidly to coma. Pupils may be mydriatic and deep tendon reflexes are depressed. Seizures may occur.
- Vital sign abnormalities may include hyperthermia, hypotension (due to strong α-adrenergic antagonism), tachycardia, arrhythmias (including torsades de pointes), and depressed cardiac conduction occur.

Diagnostic Testing

Laboratories

- Serum concentrations are generally not available or useful.
- Dextrose and a BMP should be checked on all patients with altered mentation.

Imaging

Abdominal radiographs may reveal pill concretions.

TREATMENT

- Assess airway and breathing, place an IV, and institute cardiac monitoring.
- Hypotensive patients should receive a 20 mL/kg bolus of NS.
- Consider whole-bowel irrigation for ingestion of sustained-release formulations.

Medications

- Treat ventricular arrhythmias with lidocaine. Class Ia agents (e.g., procainamide, quinidine, disopyramide) are contraindicated; avoid sotalol.
- Treat hypotension with IV fluid administration and α-adrenergic vasopressors (norepinephrine). Vasodilation may occur in response to epinephrine administration because of unopposed β-adrenergic response in the setting of strong α-adrenergic antagonism.
- Torsades de pointes may require magnesium, isoproterenol, or overdrive pacing (see Chapter 5, Cardiac Arrhythmias).
- Treat seizures with benzodiazepines.

- Treat dystonic reactions with benztropine, 1 to 4 mg, or diphenhydramine, 25 to 50 mg, IM or IV.
- Treat hyperthermia with cooling.

SPECIAL CONSIDERATIONS

- NMS, which may complicate use of these agents, is characterized by rigidity, hyperthermia, altered mental status, and elevated CPKs. NMS should be treated with aggressive cooling measures, benzodiazepines, and bromocriptine 2.5 to 10 mg IV tid until the patient improves, then taper the dose over several days to avoid recrudescence of symptoms.
- Admit those patients who have ingested a significant overdose for cardiac monitoring for at least 48 hours.

Clozapine

GENERAL PRINCIPLES

Definition
An atypical neuroleptic.

DIAGNOSIS

Clinical Presentation
- Overdose is characterized by altered mental status, ranging from somnolence to coma.
- Anticholinergic effects occur, including blurred vision, dry mouth (although hypersalivation may occur in overdose), lethargy, delirium, and constipation. Seizures occur in a minority of overdoses. Coma may occur.
- Vital sign abnormalities include hypotension, tachycardia, fasciculations, tremor, and myoclonus.

Diagnostic Testing
Laboratories
- Obtain WBC and LFTs; follow the WBC weekly for 4 weeks.
- Clozapine levels are not useful.

TREATMENT

As always, support ABCs. Place an IV, institute cardiac monitoring.

Medications
- Consider AC 1 g/kg if the patient presents within an hour of ingestion.
- Treat hypotension with 20 mL/kg of IVF; if resistant, treat with norepinephrine or dopamine.
- Treat seizures with benzodiazepines.
- Consider filgrastim for agranulocytosis.
- Forced diuresis, hemodialysis, or hemoperfusion are not beneficial.
- Admit and monitor patients with severely symptomatic overdoses for 24 hours or more.

Olanzapine

DIAGNOSIS

Clinical Presentation

- Overdose is characterized by somnolence, slurred speech, ataxia, vertigo, nausea, and vomiting (*Ann Emerg Med 1999;34:279*).
- Anticholinergic effects occur, including blurred vision, dry mouth, and tachycardia.
- Seizures are uncommon. Coma may occur.
- Vital sign abnormalities include hypotension and tachycardia. Serious dysrhythmias rarely occur.
- Pinpoint pupils are unresponsive to naloxone.

TREATMENT

Pay attention to ABCs, place an IV, and institute cardiac monitoring.

- Give AC if presentation is within 1 hour of ingestion.
- Treat hypotension with fluids and, if ineffective, norepinephrine.
- Give benzodiazepines for seizures.

Risperidone, Ziprasidone, and Quetiapine

GENERAL PRINCIPLES

Definition

These are newer neuroleptic agents and reports of overdoses have increased significantly. Quetiapine overdose is associated with more adverse outcomes than other neuroleptic agents (*Ann Emerg Med 2008;52:541–547*) and requires aggressive therapy.

DIAGNOSIS

Clinical Presentation

- Clinical effects include CNS depression, tachycardia, hypotension, and electrolyte abnormalities.
- Clinically significant ventricular dysrhythmias are uncommon.
- Quetiapine overdose is associated with respiratory depression (*Ann Emerg Med 2008;52:541–547*).
- Miosis is a common finding.

Diagnostic Testing

Diagnostic Procedures
Electrophysiology. QRS and QT_c prolongation have been reported (*Ann Emerg Med 2003;42:751–758*).

TREATMENT

- Scrupulous attention should be paid to ventilatory and circulatory support.
- Treat hypotension with 20 mL/kg fluid boluses, and if severe and persistent, consider a direct-acting pressor such as norepinephrine.

- Replete electrolytes as needed.
- Diuresis, hemodialysis, and hemoperfusion do not appear to be useful.

β-Adrenergic Antagonists

GENERAL PRINCIPLES

Definition

Of all of the agents available, propranolol tends to exhibit the most toxicity because it is lipophilic and widely distributed throughout the body and possesses significant membrane-stabilizing activity. Sotalol, which is classically thought of as a class III antiarrhythmic, also has some β-adrenergic antagonist activity and in toxic doses can result in a prolonged QT_c and torsades.

Classification

Cardiovascular agents are a frequent cause of serious poisonings and according to the 2007 annual report of the National Poison Data System were the fifth leading cause of fatal drug exposures (*Clin Toxicol 2008;46:927–1057*). Patients with these overdoses require aggressive intervention and close monitoring.

Pathophysiology

The toxicity associated with an overdose of β-blockers is largely due to the effects of antagonism at catecholamine receptors. In general, selectivity is lost in overdose, so bronchospasm may occur in the setting of $β_1$-selective antagonists.

DIAGNOSIS

Clinical Presentation

- Patients with a significant ingestion of an immediate-release product will exhibit signs of toxicity within 6 hours. The exception to this rule is sotalol, which in overdose, can have delayed toxicity and prolonged effects with one report of QT_c prolongation persisting up to 100 hours post ingestion (*Eur Clin J Pharmacol 1981;20:85–89*).
- With the exception of propranolol and sotalol, β-blocker overdose in healthy people tends to be benign, with significant number of patients remaining asymptomatic after ingestion (*J Toxicol Clin Toxicol 1993;31:531–551*).

History

Suspect β-antagonist overdose in patients with altered mental status, bradycardia, and hypotension.

Physical Examination

Patients with significant ingestions present with bradycardia and CHF. Patients with propranolol ingestions may develop coma, seizures, and hypotension. Propranolol overdoses have a high mortality (*J Toxicol Clin Toxicol 1997;35:353–359*).

Differential Diagnosis

In patients with symptomatic bradycardia also consider overdose of CCB, clonidine, or digoxin.

Diagnostic Testing

Laboratories

Patients with β-antagonist overdoses occasionally become hypoglycemic; therefore, a **fingerstick glucose** should be obtained. Likewise any patient with an altered mental status should have a **BMP** sent. Consider obtaining a **lactate** as patients with profound hypotension may develop mesenteric ischemia.

Electrocardiography

The ECG may reveal sinus bradycardia or atrioventricular block. In propranolol ingestions, a wide QRS manifesting sodium channel blockade may be present. With sotalol, QT_c prolongation may appear as a delayed presentation and torsades de pointes may develop.

TREATMENT

The treatment of β-blocker overdose is largely supportive in mild to moderate cases. The patient should have an IV placed, and continuous cardiac monitoring should be instituted. **Hypoglycemia** should be treated with 50 mL of 50% **dextrose.** Consider **AC** if patients present within 1 hour of ingestion. Intubation and ventilation should be instituted in patients with altered mental status. Likewise, consider **orogastric lavage** in patients with potential for severe toxicity such as propranolol overdoses.

Medications

- Patients with significant toxicity, propranolol, or sotalol ingestions should be treated more aggressively.
- **Atropine** 1 mg IV may be given up to 3 mg for symptomatic bradycardia; however, this is usually ineffective as the bradycardia is not vagally mediated.
- **A fluid bolus** of 20 mL/kg should be given and may be repeated; monitor for the development of fluid overload.
- **Glucagon** 2 to 4 mg IV may be given over 1 to 2 minutes. Then start infusion of 2 to 5 mg/hr—not to exceed 10 mg/hr. One of the significant side effects of glucagon administration is nausea and vomiting; monitor for vagally mediated bradycardia.
- **Calcium gluconate** 3 to 9 g IV may be given through a peripheral line in patients with hypotension. Alternatively, consider **calcium chloride** 1 to 3 g through a central line slow IV push over 10 minutes. Calcium chloride is sclerosing and can cause severe extravasation injury.
- Any patient with hypotension is a candidate for **high-dose insulin euglycemia therapy.** Although the mechanism for improvement is unclear, this is routinely used in the management of severe CCB overdose (*J Toxicol Clin Toxicol 1999;37:463–474*). Animal studies of severe propranolol overdose have shown a survival benefit (*Ann Emerg Med 1997;29:748–757*). This involves a bolus of **1 U/kg of regular insulin, followed by an infusion of 0.5 to 1 U/kg/hr of regular insulin.** This should be accompanied by a dose of **50 mL of 50% dextrose and a dextrose drip at 1 g/kg/hr of dextrose.** That calculates to 10 mL/kg/hr of 10% dextrose or 2 mL/kg/hr of 50% dextrose (*Goldfrank's Toxicologic Emergencies. 8th Ed. 2006:933*). Glucose should be obtained every 30 minutes, and potassium levels should be followed every 2 hours with repletion as **profound hypokalemia** may complicate this treatment modality. The BP response tends to be delayed by 15 to 30 minutes.
- **Catecholamines** should be approached with caution in these patients because α-stimulation in conjunction with β-blockade may precipitate acute heart failure. Therefore, **hemodynamic monitoring** should be instituted with careful titration of

epinephrine at 0.02 mcg/kg/min or norepinephrine at 0.1 mcg/kg/min. Isopro-terenol at 0.1 mcg/kg/min may be useful as well; however, monitor closely for the development of hypotension. It is important to note that high doses of these agents may be required.

Other Nonoperative Therapies

- In cases of refractory hypotension and bradycardia, it is reasonable to consider intra-aortic balloon pump (*Ann Emerg Med 1987;16:1381–1383*) and extracorporeal membrane oxygenation (*Arch Mal Coeur Vaiss 2001;94:1386–1392*).
- Transvenous pacing may be attempted, but it is generally difficult to achieve capture, given the degree of myocardial depression.

Calcium Channel Blockers

GENERAL PRINCIPLES

Definition
Calcium channel blockers (CCB) are widely used for the management of tachyarrhyth-mias and hypertension. Generally speaking, the overdoses of dihydropyridines, such as amlodipine, nimodipine, nicardipine, and nifedipine, tend to be more benign although in massive overdose, selectivity may be lost and result in significant symptoms. Vera-pamil and diltiazem can produce severe toxicity, even in the setting of a small overdose.

Pathophysiology
CCBs exert their effects by blocking L-type calcium channels on the smooth muscle of the vasculature and the myocardium. This decreases inotropy and chronotropy and results in a decrement of BP and heart rate. In overdose, these effects are accentuated. L-type calcium channels are also involved in the release of insulin from the β-islet cells of the myocardium. In CCB overdose, patients will often present with elevated blood sugars.

DIAGNOSIS

Clinical Presentation
Patients with diltiazem or verapamil overdoses should be considered critically ill and require aggressive intervention.

History
Patients will often present with an unintentional ingestion where they missed a dose and attempt to "catch up" by doubling their next dose. Intentional ingestions will often not be accurately reported.

Physical Examination
Patients with verapamil or diltiazem overdoses will present with profound **hypoten-sion, bradycardia, and generally have a NORMAL mental status until they arrest.** It is thought that CCBs have somewhat of a neuroprotective effect that may explain the preservation of mentation. In the setting of dihydropyridine overdoses, patients usually present with hypotension and a reflex tachycardia.

Differential Diagnosis
CCB toxicity may resemble β-antagonist or clonidine overdoses.

Diagnostic Testing

This is a clinical diagnosis; serum concentrations are not useful in the management of CCB overdose.

Laboratories
- **Dextrose** should be checked and is elevated in the setting of CCB toxicity. This is part of the toxidrome associated with this particular overdose.
- A **BMP** should be obtained as well to follow serum calcium levels. In patients on a calcium drip, ionized calcium should be followed.

Electrocardiography
The ECG may show sinus bradycardia, conduction delays, or even complete heart block. With dihydropyridine overdose, a sinus tachycardia may be present.

TREATMENT

The treatment of dihydropyridine CCB overdose is largely supportive in mild to moderate cases. The patient should have an IV placed, and continuous cardiac monitoring should be instituted. Consider **AC** if patients present within 1 hour of ingestion. Intubation and ventilation should be instituted in unstable patients. Likewise, consider **orogastric lavage** in patients with potential for severe toxicity. **Whole-bowel irrigation** with polyethylene glycol should be instituted for sustained-release preparations.

Medications

Patients with significant toxicity, verapamil or diltiazem ingestions, should be treated more aggressively.

- **Atropine** 1 mg IV may be given up to 3 mg for symptomatic bradycardia; however, this is usually ineffective as the bradycardia is not vagally mediated.
- **A fluid bolus** of 20 mL/kg should be given and may be repeated; monitor for the development of fluid overload.
- **Calcium gluconate** 3 to 9 g IV may be given through a peripheral line in patients with hypotension. Alternatively, consider **calcium chloride** 1 to 3 g through a central line slow IV push over 10 minutes. A calcium gluconate drip may be started and run up to 2 g/hr. Close monitoring of calcium is required. Calcium chloride is sclerosing and can cause severe extravasation injury.
- Any patient with hypotension is a candidate for **high-dose insulin euglycemia therapy.** See discussion of this topic under treatment of β-blocker overdose.
- **Catecholamines** should be approached with caution in these patients because α stimulation may precipitate acute heart failure. Therefore, **hemodynamic monitoring** should be instituted with careful titration of **epinephrine starting at 0.02 mcg/kg/min or norepinephrine at 0.1 mcg/kg/min.**

Other Nonoperative Therapies

- In cases of refractory hypotension and bradycardia, it is reasonable to consider intra-aortic balloon pump (*Clin Cardiol 1991;14:933–935*) and cardiopulmonary bypass (*Ann Emerg Med 1989;18:984–987*).
- Transvenous pacing may be attempted but it is generally difficult to achieve capture, given the degree of myocardial depression.

SPECIAL CONSIDERATIONS

Patients with ingestions of a sustained-release preparation should be monitored in an intensive care setting. Immediate-release preparations should be monitored for 6 to 8 hours prior to discharge or psychiatric evaluation.

Clonidine

GENERAL PRINCIPLES

Clonidine is an orally administered agent used in the management of hypertension.

Pathophysiology

Clonidine is an imidazoline drug with centrally acting antihypertensive effects related to α_2-agonism, which decreases sympathetic outflow from the CNS (*NEJM 1975;293:1179–1180*). Other drugs in this family include oxymetazoline and tetrahydrozoline, nasal decongestants that exhibit similar toxicity when orally administered. In overdose, peripheral effects include an initial release of norepinephrine with a **transient increase** in BP, followed by hypotension (*Clin Pharmacol Ther 1976;21:593–601*).

DIAGNOSIS

Clinical Presentation

Although the clinical presentation of these overdoses can be quite concerning, most patients recover with supportive care. Patients tend to develop symptoms within 30 minutes to an hour after their overdose.

History

The history is unreliable in these patients as they are often somnolent or comatose on arrival to the hospital.

Physical Examination

Suspect clonidine overdose in patients with hypotension, bradycardia, and CNS depression. Occasionally, patients may develop hypoventilation, which is usually responsive to vocal or tactile stimulation (*Ann Emerg Med 1981;10:107–112*). Pupillary examination reveals miosis, and this finding in the setting of hypotension and bradycardia is highly suggestive of clonidine overdose.

Differential Diagnosis

β-Antagonists, digoxin, and CCB overdose should be included in the differential.

Diagnostic Testing

Laboratories

Serum clonidine concentrations are not routinely used in the management of these patients. A **dextrose** and **BMP** should be obtained on any patient with altered mental status.

Electrocardiography

The ECG generally shows a sinus bradycardia.

TREATMENT

- Patients generally respond with supportive care. In severely poisoned patients, consider intubation and ventilation; however, this is rarely needed.
- **Avoid GI decontamination and AC in these patients as they tend to develop altered mental status quickly.**
- **Atropine** 1 mg IV may be given up to 3 mg for symptomatic bradycardia; however, this is usually not necessary as the bradycardia tends to resolve on its own.
- **A fluid bolus** of 20 mL/kg should be given and may be repeated; monitor for the development of fluid overload.
- An initial dose of 0.4 mg of **naloxone** may be useful in reversing the hypotension and bradycardia associated with clonidine overdose (*Hypertension 1984;69:461–467*). Occasionally high doses may be required with redosing every 2 to 3 hours as naloxone has a shorter duration of action than clonidine.

SPECIAL CONSIDERATIONS

Withdrawal syndromes have been reported in patients who have stopped taking clonidine. It is usually manifested as rebound severe hypertension, agitation, and palpitations. Treatment is to administer clonidine, and taper the dose gradually. Benzodiazepines are also useful in this situation.

Other Antihypertensives

GENERAL PRINCIPLES

- These agents include **diuretics, α_1-antagonists, ACE inhibitors, and angiotensin II receptor blockers.**
- **Diuretics** tend to be benign in overdose. Occasionally, they cause dehydration and electrolyte imbalances. Laboratory studies should include a BMP. Management usually only requires gentle fluid hydration.
- **α_1-Antagonists** cause peripheral vasodilation, which usually responds to hydration. Occasionally, they cause enough hypotension to require vasopressors. In these cases, norepinephrine should be administered.
- **ACE inhibitors** rarely cause significant toxicity although there are case reports of fatal overdoses. Treatment is supportive. In patients with hypotension, naloxone may be useful (*Clin Pharmacol Ther 1985;38:560–565*).
- **Angiotensin II receptor blockers** may cause hypotension in overdose. Treatment is supportive.

Parasympathetic Agents

GENERAL PRINCIPLES

Definition

Acetylcholine (ACh) is a common neurotransmitter of the peripheral and central nervous system, acting on nicotinic and muscarinic receptors.

Anticholinergics

GENERAL PRINCIPLES

Anticholinergic effects are primarily due to blockade of muscarinic receptors (i.e., antimuscarinic effects), and therefore affect mainly parasympathetic functions.

Epidemiology

Anticholinergic poisoning occurs either from intentional ingestion of certain plants or OTC medications (e.g., Jimson weed, diphenhydramine) (*CJEM 2007;9(6):467–468*), or from accidental overdosing (e.g., medical noncompliance, polypharmaceutical regimens) (*Rev Neurol 2006;43(10):603–609*).

Etiology

Drugs and medications with anticholinergic effects include the following:

- **Anticholinergics:** atropine, scopolamine, benztropine, glycopyrrolate, ipratropium.
- **Antihistamines:** diphenhydramine, promethazine, doxylamine.
- **Antipsychotics:** chlorpromazine, clozapine, olanzapine, quetiapine.
- **Antidepressants:** amitriptyline, nortriptyline, imipramine, desipramine.
- **Antiparkinson drugs:** benztropine, trihexyphenidyl.
- **Mydriatics:** cyclopentolate, homatropine, tropicamide.
- **Muscle relaxants:** cyclobenzaprine.
- **Plants:** Belladonna, Jimson weed, *Amanita* mushrooms.

Pathophysiology

- Blockade of muscarinic receptors (i.e., parasympathetic ANS, except for the sympathetically innervated sweat glands) leads to the so-called **anticholinergic toxidrome.**
- **Tachycardia** is one of the main symptoms in anticholinergic poisoning. Vagal blockade of cardiac muscarinic receptors leads to unopposed sympathetic stimulation of the myocardium.
- Some anticholinergic drugs can also cross the blood–brain barrier and interact with muscarinic receptors in the cortex and subcortical regions of the brain causing anticholinergic **CNS manifestations.**

Associated Conditions

- Antihistamines and cyclic antidepressants also block sodium channels and cause additional cardiac symptoms such as dysrhythmias and QRS prolongations.
- Potassium channel blockade may result in QT_c prolongation and torsades de pointes.

DIAGNOSIS

Clinical Presentation

Anticholinergic toxidrome

- **Central effects:** confusion, agitation, euphoria/dysphoria, hallucinations, incoherent thoughts and speech, lethargy, ataxia, choreoathetoid movements, rarely seizures or coma.

- **Peripheral effects:** tachycardia, mouth dryness, decreased perspiration with flushed skin and hyperthermia, dilated pupils with photophobia and blurred vision, decreased bowel sounds, urinary retention.
- A helpful mnemonic for antimuscarinic effects is "RED as a beet, DRY as a bone, BLIND as a bat, MAD as a hatter, and HOT as a hare."

TREATMENT

- All patients presenting with an anticholinergic toxidrome need **cardiovascular monitoring.** Serial evaluation of vital signs and serial physical exams are essential to address sudden worsening of the patient's condition (dysrhythmia, seizure).
- GI decontamination is only indicated if the patient is fully awake and cooperative due to the high risk of aspiration or loss of airway control in unconscious or combative patients. **Gastric lavage** for GI decontamination may be appropriate, given decreased stomach emptying and slowed GI motility from the anticholinergic effect.
- Patients with hyperthermia may benefit from cooling measures.

Medications

- **Physostigmine** is a reversible **anticholinesterase,** which leads to increased ACh in synapses to overcome receptor blockade. It is useful in the management of severe anticholinergic poisoning with delirium, hallucinations, and seizures (*Int J Clin Pharmacol Ther Toxicol 1980 Dec;18(12):523–535*).
- In the emergency department setting, the use of physostigmine as a diagnostic tool in patients with high suspicion of anticholinergic agitation or delirium has been found to be relatively safe (*Ann Emerg Med 2003;42(1):14–19*).
- Contraindications: underlying cardiovascular disease, wide QRS complex or AV block on ECG, asthma, bowel or bladder obstruction, PVD or gangrene. Its use is also contraindicated in the setting of cyclic antidepressant overdose.
- **Adult dosing:** 0.5 mg IV over 5 minutes every 5 minutes up to 2 mg total or until improved level of consciousness.
- Physostigmine has a short duration of action (20 to 60 minutes) and redosing might be necessary if agitation recurs.
- NOTE: Always have **atropine** at bedside for reversal if needed, that is, in case of severe bradycardia or asystole from unopposed cholinergic stimulation, or other dysrhythmias from sodium channel blockade (e.g., in TCA overdose) (*J Emerg Med 2003;25(2):185–191*).
- **Benzodiazepines** should be used as adjuncts to treat anticholinergic agitation or delirium. There is no benefit in benzodiazepine monotherapy in anticholinergic central symptoms (*Ann Emerg Med 2000;35(4):374–381*).

Cholinesterase Inhibitors

GENERAL PRINCIPLES

Definition

Cholinesterase inhibitors are chemical compounds that inhibit the enzyme cholinesterase. Blockade of **AChE** function leads to excess of ACh in synapses of the ANS and SNS.

Classification

Cholinesterase inhibitors are divided into two classes:

- **Organophosphates** (i.e., esters of phosphoric acid)
- **Carbamates**

Organophosphates

GENERAL PRINCIPLES

Epidemiology

- Organophosphates (OPs) are commonly used as pesticides and insecticides (e.g., parathion). Some of them also have medical indications (e.g., malathion in lice shampoo).
- In the developing world, OP and other pesticide poisonings represent the most common causes of death from intoxications (*QJM 2000;93(11):715–731*).
- OPs are also potent chemical terrorist and warfare agents (so-called "nerve gas" agents) (*Anesthesiology 2002;97(4):989–1004*) and have been used in the past in various settings (e.g., Sarin in the Tokyo subway attack, Tabun in the Iraq–Iran war).
- Although self-inflicted OP poisoning with suicidal intent occurs, exposure is primarily occupational or accidental (*Intern Med 2007;46(13):965–969*). Since absorption occurs through skin and airways, the handling of organophosphates requires appropriate protective gear.

Pathophysiology

- Inhibition of ACh breakdown through blocked AChE leads to accumulation of ACh at nicotinic and muscarinic receptors resulting in **excessive cholinergic stimulation.**
- The severity of symptoms varies depending on the route of exposure (dermal, inhalation, oral, parenteral), dose, lipid solubility of OP, and enzyme affinity (*Lancet 2008;371(9612):597–607*).
- Most OPs bind AChE initially in a reversible way. Some OPs, however, become permanently bound over time, a phenomenon known as **"aging."** If aging occurs, the only way to overcome the inhibitory effect is for the body to synthesize new enzyme.
- OPs are hepatically metabolized. Some OPs become active toxins after liver metabolism (e.g., Parathion) (*Bull World Health Organ 1971;44(1):289–307*).
- In severe poisoning, symptoms occur usually within 6 hours after exposure and are unlikely to occur if an exposed person remains free of symptoms for 12 hours or more (*Bull World Health Organ 1971;44(1):289–307*).

DIAGNOSIS

Clinical Presentation

The cholinergic toxidrome is a result of overstimulation of nicotinic and muscarinic receptors (*Bull World Health Organ 1971;44(1):289–307; Lancet 2008;371(9612):597–607*).

- **Muscarinic effects:**
  - **SLUDGE syndrome:** **S**alivation, **L**acrimation, **U**rination, **D**iarrhea, **GI** cramping, **E**mesis.

- **Bradycardia, bronchorrhea, bronchoconstriction** (NOTE: asphyxia and cardiovascular collapse are lethal features of OP poisoning).
- **Other effects:** miosis, diaphoresis.
- NOTE: intoxicated patients may present with tachycardia instead of bradycardia due to hypoxia (bronchoconstriction, bronchorrhea).
- **Nicotinic effects:**
  - **Ganglionic:** tachycardia, hypertension, diaphoresis, mydriasis.
  - **Neuromuscular:** neuromuscular depolarization, fasciculations, motor weakness, paralysis with respiratory failure (analogous to succinylcholine, which is related to ACh).
  - **Central:** confusion, agitation, lethargy, seizures, coma.

Diagnostic Testing

- **Cholinesterase levels:** There are two different cholinesterases that are routinely measured in red blood cells and plasma (*Bull World Health Organ 1971;44(1):289–307*).
- Both assays are relatively useless in assessing the severity of exposure in acute intoxications because of their wide ranges of normal values.
- They are mostly used as sensitivity markers to compare changes from baseline enzyme activity (e.g., in chronic occupational exposure or after OP elimination) (*Lancet 2008;371(9612):597–607*).

TREATMENT

- **Protection:** OP-intoxicated patients pose a significant risk for further contamination of others through direct contact. Health care personnel should use special **personal protective equipment** (PPE) (gowns, gloves, masks) until the patient is properly externally decontaminated (*Lancet 2008;371(9612):597–607*).
  - PPE should not consist of latex or vinyl, since OPs are lipophilic and might penetrate such materials.
- **Decontamination:** Remove patient from potential source of poisoning (*Crit Care Med 2002;30(10):2346–2354*).
  - All clothing, especially leather, should be removed from the patient and discarded in a ventilated area (*Crit Care Med 2002;30(10):2346–2354*).
  - Skin and hair decontamination requires thorough irrigation with water and might be enhanced through use of alcohol-based soaps (*Crit Care Med 2002;30(10):2346–2354*).
  - Ocular decontamination should be irrigated with water only (*Crit Care Med 2002;30(10):2346–2354*).
  - Gastric lavage might be indicated in stable patients who ingested contaminated fluids (*Clin Toxicol 2009;47(3):179–192*).
  - NOTE: All lavaged/aspirated fluids need to be safely discarded.
- **Stabilization:**
  - ABCs: Have a low threshold for early intubation in order to obtain airway protection.
  - AVOID mouth-to-mouth resuscitation because of contamination risk.
  - Start IV fluids as an initial bolus of 20 mL/kg (*Crit Care 2004;8(6):R391–R397*).
- **Atropine** is an antimuscarinic agent which competes with ACh for receptor binding.

- GOAL: **atropinization,** that is, drying of bronchial secretions with normalized oxygen saturation (which may require 10 to 100 times of usually common atropine doses), a heart rate > 80 bpm, and a systolic BP > 80 mm Hg (*Lancet 2008;371(9612):597–607*).
- The initial **adult dose** is 1 to 3 mg IV as a bolus. Then titrate according to persistence of bronchorrhea by giving the double of the previously used dose every 5 minutes until atropinization achieved (*Lancet 2008;371(9612):597–607*).
- The initial **pediatric dose** is 0.02 mg/kg IV. Titrate as in adults (*BMJ 2007 Mar 24;334(7594):629–634*).
- Once the patient is stabilized an infusion of atropine should be started with 10% to 20% of the initial atropinization dose per hour and should be held once anticholinergic effects occur (absent bowel sounds, urinary retention, agitation) (*Lancet 2008;371(9612):597–607*). Adults and children may develop paradoxical bradycardia through central anticholinergic mechanisms. NOTE: atropine has no effect on NMJs, therefore pralidoxime needs to be added as early as possible in order to reverse muscle weakness.
- **Pralidoxime** (2-PAM): Pralidoxime forms a complex with OPs that are bound to AChE. The pralidoxime–OP complex is then released from the enzyme and thus regenerates AChE function.
  - Once the AChE bound OPs start aging, pralidoxime is rendered ineffective. Therefore it is crucial to start pralidoxime therapy early.
  - Pralidoxime also binds to some degree to free OPs and so prevents further AChE binding.
  - **Adult dosing** used to be administered as boluses given over time. New evidence, however, is favoring an infusion regimen (*Lancet 2006;368(9553):2136–2141*): 1 to 2 g of pralidoxime in 100 mL NS IV over 20 minutes, then infusion of 500 mg/hr (*Lancet 2008;371(9612):597–607*).
  - NOTE: Pralidoxime use longer than 24 hours might be indicated if unaged OPs are redistributed from fat tissue. In such cases infusions should be continued until patient remained symptom-free for at least 12 hours without additional atropine doses, or until the patient is extubated (*Lancet 2008;371(9612):597–607*).
  - Cardiac and respiratory failure have been reported after administration of pralidoxime (*Crit Care Med 2006;34(2):502–510*).
  - Though pralidoxime might not be effective in all cases of OP poisoning due to the aging effect, it is still recommended to be used routinely in order to decrease the total atropine requirements (*Crit Care Med 2002;30(10):2346–2354*).
- **Benzodiazepines** are the first-line agents for OP-induced seizures (*BMJ 2007 Mar 24;334(7594):629–634*).

COMPLICATIONS

- **Intermediate syndrome (IMS):**
  - This syndrome is a post-acute paralysis from persistent ACh excess after the acute cholinergic phase has been controlled.
  - Weakness of proximal extremity muscles and muscles supplied by cranial nerves that occurs hours to days after treatment of acute OP poisoning and often leads to respiratory failure if unnoticed (*PLoS Med 2008;5(7):e147*).
- **OP-induced delayed neurotoxicity (OPIDN):**
  - Besides AChE some OPs also inhibit other neurotoxic esterases, resulting in polyneuropathy or spinal cord damage due to demyelination of the long nerve fibers.

- OPIDN usually occurs several days to weeks after acute OP poisoning leading to temporary, chronic or recurrent motor or sensory dysfunctions (*Annu Rev Pharmacol Toxicol 1990;30:405–440*).

MONITORING/FOLLOW-UP

- All patients with severe or moderate poisoning should be admitted to an ICU after initial stabilization for further monitoring and treatment (*Crit Care 2004;8(6): R391–R397*).
- Asymptomatic patients presenting with a history of unintentional poisoning or patients with only mild symptoms do not always require hospital admission, but should be observed for 6 to 12 hours. In these patients, consider measuring cholinesterase activity 6 hours after ingestion to evaluate for major ingestion (*BMJ 2007 Mar 24;334(7594):629–634*).

Carbamates

GENERAL PRINCIPLES

Epidemiology

Carbamates are reversible AChE inhibitors that also lead to ACh excess in the synaptic junction. They are occasionally found in pesticides. However, their most common use in this country is medicinal.

- **Physostigmine** is a naturally occurring methyl carbamate found in the Calabar bean. Other common carbamates are pyridostigmine and neostigmine.
- **Pyridostigmine** has been administered to US soldiers while under nerve agent attack to prevent anticholinergic symptoms after possible exposure (*JAMA 1991;266(5): 693–695*).

Pathophysiology

- Inhibition of ACh breakdown through AChE block leads to accumulation of ACh at nicotinic and muscarinic receptors with **excess cholinergic stimulation.**
- Carbamates are reversible enzyme inhibitors, they release AChE spontaneously. There is no "aging" phenomenon with carbamates.

DIAGNOSIS

Clinical Presentation

The clinical picture of the carbamate induced cholinergic toxidrome is analogous to the one seen in OP poisoning since nicotinic and muscarinic receptors of the ANS and SNS are affected.

- Look for **SLUDGE** syndrome, **bradycardia, bronchorrhea,** and **bronchoconstriction** as well as neuromuscular depolarization, and be aware of the risk of cardiovascular or respiratory failure.
- Symptoms from carbamate poisoning are generally milder compared to OP poisoning and of shorter duration.

Diagnostic Testing

Cholinesterase levels are used to compare changes from baseline enzyme activity in mild exposures or to assess treatment success after acute exposure (*Clin Chem 1995;41:1814–1818*).

TREATMENT

* The same measures of **protection** and **decontamination** as with OP poisoning apply to carbamates.
* **Stabilization:**
  * ABCs: Have a low threshold for early intubation in order to obtain airway protection.
  * Avoid mouth-to-mouth resuscitation because of contamination risk.

Medications
First Line
* **Atropine** is an antimuscarinic agent which competes with ACh for receptor binding.
  * GOAL: **atropinization.** See treatment of Organophosphate poisoning for dosing guidelines.
* Adults and children may develop paradoxical bradycardia through central anticholinergic mechanisms.

Second Line
Given the reversible action of carbamates, pralidoxime should only be given if more than 2 mg atropine has been required for bronchorrhea control (*Am J Emerg Med 1990;8(1):68–70*).

* Pralidoxime should be given if there is no clear evidence for isolated carbamate poisoning since additional OP exposure should always be suspected.
* **Benzodiazepines** are the first-line agents for carbamate-induced seizures.

Barbiturates

GENERAL PRINCIPLES

The use of barbiturates has largely fallen by the wayside as safer drugs are now available. Barbiturates are still used as induction agents for anesthesia as well as second-line agents for seizure control.

DIAGNOSIS

Suspect barbiturate overdose in patients who present with CNS and respiratory depression.

Clinical Presentation
History
It is often difficult to elicit a history as these patients are generally comatose on arrival.

Physical Examination

Typical examination findings include **respiratory depression** and **coma.** Other vital sign abnormalities may include hypothermia. Patients may develop cutaneous bullae known as **"barb blisters"** (*Cutis 1990;45:43*). **Miosis** may be present.

Differential Diagnosis

The differential diagnosis includes benzodiazepine overdose, hypoglycemia, ethanol intoxication, CNS, and other metabolic causes of coma.

Diagnostic Testing

Laboratories

This should include routine testing for any presentation of coma: **dextrose, BMP, hepatic and thyroid function tests.**

Electrocardiography

In barbiturate overdose, EEG recordings may show no electrical activity.

Imaging

- **A CXR** should be obtained on all of these patients to evaluate for aspiration.
- **Head CT** may help evaluate for the presence of CNS lesions contributing to coma.

Diagnostic Procedures

Consider **lumbar puncture** in patients with undifferentiated coma to evaluate for meningitis or subarachnoid hemorrhage.

TREATMENT

The most important management strategy in barbiturate overdose is airway and breathing protection. Patients with respiratory depression should be intubated.

Medications

First Line

- Consider **MDAC** in patients with a protected airway and bowel sounds.
- Hypotension should be treated with 20 mL/kg bolus of NS. If this fails, consider a direct-acting vasopressor such as norepinephrine.

Second Line

Urine alkalinization with sodium bicarbonate is reserved for phenobarbital overdoses refractory to MDAC. It is inferior to MDAC (*J Toxicol Clin Toxicol 2004;42:1–26*).

Other Nonoperative Therapies

Consider **hemoperfusion** in the setting of life-threatening phenobarbital overdose that is refractory to conventional management (*Chest 2003;123:897–922*). **Hemodialysis** has been reported to be useful as well (*Am J Kid Dis 2000;36:640–643*).

Benzodiazepines

GENERAL PRINCIPLES

Generally speaking, benzodiazepines have a wide safety margin. Deaths are usually related to the presence of a coingestant or ethanol.

DIAGNOSIS

Clinical Presentation

History
This is often difficult to elicit as patients are frequently comatose.

Physical Examination
The typical presentation of a pure oral benzodiazepine overdose is **coma with normal vital signs.** Respiratory depression is exceedingly unusual in oral overdose of benzodiazepines.

Differential Diagnosis
The differential diagnosis includes barbiturate overdose, hypoglycemia, ethanol intoxication, CNS, and other metabolic causes of coma.

Diagnostic Testing

Laboratories
- This should include routine testing for any presentation of coma: **dextrose, BMP, hepatic and thyroid function tests.** Consider **lumbar puncture** in patients with undifferentiated coma to evaluate for meningitis or subarachnoid hemorrhage.
- **Urine drug screens** are unreliable in the setting of benzodiazepine overdose as the target metabolite, oxazepam or desmethyldiazepam, is not produced by the metabolism of many of the benzodiazepines. Classically, clonazepam, flunitrazepam, alprazolam, and lorazepam are not detected. Therefore, routine screening is not recommended (*Clin Chem 2003;49:357–379*).

Imaging
- **A CXR** should be obtained on all of these patients to evaluate for aspiration.
- **Head CT** may help evaluate for the presence of CNS lesions contributing to coma.

TREATMENT

Supportive care with observation is the mainstay of therapy. In patients with coingestions and respiratory depression, intubation and ventilation may be required. Since this is a benign overdose, **gastric lavage and AC are not necessary.** These interventions may cause aspiration in an otherwise stable patient.

Medications
- Traditional recommendations include the use of **flumazenil**; however, given the propensity to precipitate seizures and acute benzodiazepine withdrawal in patients on long-term benzodiazepine therapy, this therapy should be **avoided.** Other **contraindications** include a seizure history, coingestion of a cardiotoxic or epileptogenic drug, or ECG evidence of cyclic antidepressant ingestion.
- In **special cases** such as reversal of iatrogenically induced respiratory depression, reversal of sedation, or pediatric benzodiazepine ingestion, flumazenil may be given as a 0.1 mg/min dose intravenously. Repeat injections may be given as resedation occasionally reoccurs.

Zolpidem and Other Hypnotics

GENERAL PRINCIPLES

- These drugs were developed to mitigate the abuse and withdrawal problems associated with earlier sedative hypnotics.
- In overdose, patients present with drowsiness and ataxia. Vital signs remain normal. Treatment is supportive.

SPECIAL CONSIDERATIONS

- Certain sedative hypnotics are used as "date rape" drugs. This includes flunitrazepam and γ-hydroxybutyrate. Neither of these substances routinely appears in the urine drug screen. GHB may cause respiratory depression and myoclonus. On occasion, respiratory depression in the setting of GHB may require intubation and ventilation. Generally speaking, the patient recovers within 6 to 8 hours and may be extubated.
- Precipitous benzodiazepine withdrawal may be life threatening and occasionally produces a syndrome similar to delirium tremens. The treatment includes benzodiazepine replacement and gradual weaning.

Sympathomimetics, General

GENERAL PRINCIPLES

Definition

Patients who overdose on sympathomimetic agents exhibit a syndrome of excess adrenergic tone due to direct stimulation of adrenergic receptors or the effects of norepinephrine and epinephrine. Many of the agents in this category are drugs of abuse, although several therapeutic agents can produce a similar toxidrome.

Classification

Agents that fall into this category include amphetamines, cocaine, vasopressors, methylxanthines, and β-agonists.

Epidemiology

Stimulants and street drugs were the sixth leading cause of fatal exposures according to the AAPCC in 2007, with 188 fatalities reported (*Clin Toxicol 2007;46(10):927–1057*).

Pathophysiology

- Agents that stimulate the sympathetic nervous system generally do so by either causing the release or preventing the reuptake of **endogenous catecholamines,** or **directly stimulating** α- and/or β-**receptors.**
- **Methylxanthines** (theophylline, caffeine) and β-**agonists** (albuterol, dobutamine, isoproterenol) enhance chronotropy and inotropy by **facilitating calcium entry into the myocardium.** They furthermore enhance the function of β_2-receptors leading to **bronchodilatation.** Stimulation of the β_2-rich vascular beds to skeletal muscle results in **vasodilatation** as well. Therefore in a pure β-agonist overdose, **hypotension and tachycardia** predominate.

- **Epinephrine, norepinephrine, cocaine, and amphetamines** have both α and βeffects resulting in **hypertension and tachycardia.**
- Other α-receptors are found on the **iris** which when stimulated results in **pupillary dilatation.**
- Sympathetic stimulation of **sweat glands** is a **cholinergic** effect.

Amphetamines

GENERAL PRINCIPLES

Drugs of abuse in this class include **amphetamine, methamphetamine, and 3,4-methylenedioxymethamphetamine (MDMA).**

DIAGNOSIS

Clinical Presentation
- Suspect amphetamines in any patient presenting with a sympathomimetic toxidrome of **hypertension, tachycardia, dilated pupils, and diaphoresis.**
- Severely intoxicated patients may develop **hyperthermia, seizures, coma, and cardiovascular collapse.**

History
Drug abusers will often deny illicit use; therefore, the history is often unreliable.

Physical Examination
Patients may have **agitation** and **altered mental status** depending upon the degree of intoxication.

Differential Diagnosis
The differential includes anything that may result in a sympathomimetic toxidrome including cocaine, ephedrine, pseudoephedrine, and various amphetamine-derived designer drugs.

Diagnostic Testing
Laboratories
Patients with a sympathomimetic toxidrome should be evaluated for end-organ dysfunction.

- A **BMP** is useful to assess the degree of hydration and renal function.
  - MDMA is also associated with the development of hyponatremia.
- A **CPK** should be checked to evaluate for rhabdomyolysis in agitated patients.
- Patients complaining of chest pain should have a **troponin** drawn.
- **Urine drug screens** are often associated with false-negative and false-positive results, are expensive, and **do not contribute to the management of this syndrome.**

Electrocardiography
An ECG should be obtained to evaluate for ischemia and electrolyte disturbances.

Imaging

In select cases imaging may be useful.

- Obtain a **head CT** in patients complaining of a headache or altered mental status.
- Obtain a **CXR** in patients complaining of chest pain.
- In patients with severe chest pain that radiates to the back or is associated with marked agitation, consider obtaining a **chest CT** to evaluate for aortic dissection.

TREATMENT

Mild to moderate cases usually respond to supportive care including IV hydration. In hyperthermic cases, aggressive cooling measures should be taken. As always, priority should be given to airway protection, breathing, and circulation.

Medications

First Line

- Treat agitation and seizures with **benzodiazepines.** In refractory seizures, consider **barbiturates and propofol.**
- Hypertension and tachycardia may be managed with **CCBs. AVOID β-antagonists as they may be associated with the development of a hypertensive crisis.**
- **Nitroglycerin, nitroprusside,** and **phentolamine** may be used in the setting of severe hypertension.
- Ventricular arrhythmias should be treated with **lidocaine** or **amiodarone.**

Second Line

- Some data suggest that antipsychotics are useful in the management of agitated delirium in these patients (*NEJM 1968;278:1361–1365*). Consider administration of **haloperidol 5 mg IV or droperidol 2.5 mg IV** in patients with hallucinations (*Eur J Emerg Med 1997;4:130*).
- In hyperthermic agitated patients consider **paralysis** with a nondepolarizing agent to prevent rhabdomyolysis.

Other Nonoperative Therapies

Patients with renal failure and rhabdomyolysis may require **hemodialysis.**

SPECIAL CONSIDERATIONS

MDMA may cause hyponatremia and serotonin syndrome (see above).

REFERRAL

Obtain a chemical dependency consult in patients hospitalized as a result of drug abuse.

Cocaine

GENERAL PRINCIPLES

Pathophysiology

- Cocaine exerts its effects by inhibiting the reuptake of norepinephrine, serotonin, epinephrine, and dopamine. Excess adrenergic tone in the setting of toxicity is

reflected by the development of hypertension and tachycardia. Drug-seeking behavior is likely modulated by dopaminergic effects in the ventral tegmental area of the brain.
- Cocaine has also been implicated in the development of early cardiovascular disease (*Circulation 2001;103:502–506*), likely due to a combination of vasospastic (*NEJM 1989;321:1557–1562*), prothrombotic (*Heart 2000;83:688–695*), and atherogenic effects (*J Am Coll Cardiol 2006;47:2120–2122*).

DIAGNOSIS

Clinical Presentation
- Patients with cocaine intoxication often present with complaints of ischemic chest pain.
- Suspect cocaine in any patient presenting with a sympathomimetic toxidrome of **hypertension, tachycardia, dilated pupils, and diaphoresis.**
- Severely intoxicated patients may develop **hyperthermia, seizures, coma, and cardiovascular collapse.**

History
Drug abusers will often deny illicit use; therefore, the history is often unreliable.

Physical Examination
Patients may have **agitation** and **altered mental status** depending upon the degree of intoxication.

Differential Diagnosis
The differential includes anything that may result in a sympathomimetic toxidrome including amphetamines, ephedrine, pseudoephedrine, and various amphetamine-derived designer drugs.

Diagnostic Testing
Laboratories
Patients with a sympathomimetic toxidrome should be evaluated for end-organ dysfunction.

- A **BMP** is useful to assess the degree of hydration and renal function.
- A **CPK** should be checked to evaluate for rhabdomyolysis in agitated patients.
- Patients complaining of chest pain should have a **troponin** drawn.
- **Urine drug screens,** although reliable in determining recent use, should not modify the acute management of these patients.

Electrocardiography
- An ECG should be obtained to evaluate for ischemia and electrolyte disturbances.
- Cocaine is a known sodium channel blocker which may be reflected as a wide complex rhythm on the ECG (*JPET 1992;261:910–917*).
- Cocaine has been reported to increase the QT_c (*Emerg Med J 2004;21:252–253*).

Imaging
In select cases imaging may be useful:

- Obtain a **head CT** in patients complaining of a headache or altered mental status.
- Obtain a **CXR** in patients complaining of chest pain.

- In patients with severe chest pain that radiates to the back or is associated with marked agitation, consider obtaining a **chest CT** to evaluate for aortic dissection.

TREATMENT

Mild to moderate cases usually respond to supportive care including IV hydration. In hyperthermic cases, aggressive cooling measures should be taken. As always, priority should be given to airway protection, breathing, and circulation.

Medications
First Line
- Treat agitation and seizures with **benzodiazepines.** In refractory seizures, consider **barbiturates and propofol.**
- Hypertension and tachycardia may be managed with **CCBs.**
- **AVOID β-antagonists as they may be associated with the development of a hypertensive crisis.**
- **Nitroglycerin, nitroprusside,** and **phentolamine** may be used in the setting of severe hypertension.
- Sodium channel blockade should be treated with **sodium bicarbonate** (*Circulation 1991;83:1799–1807*). Give **1 to 2 mEq/kg** as an IV bolus, may repeat. Monitor for QRS narrowing.
- Ventricular arrhythmias should be treated with **lidocaine.**

Second Line
In hyperthermic agitated patients, consider **paralysis** with a nondepolarizing agent to prevent rhabdomyolysis.

Other Nonoperative Therapies
Patients with renal failure and rhabdomyolysis may require **hemodialysis.**

SPECIAL CONSIDERATIONS

- Body packers with suspected cocaine toxicity or obstructive symptoms should have emergent surgical intervention.
- Consider whole-bowel irrigation in patients who present without signs of toxicity.

Theophylline

GENERAL PRINCIPLES

Definition
Theophylline is a methylxanthine agent used in the treatment of obstructive pulmonary diseases such as asthma and emphysema. Its use has largely fallen by the wayside as alternative less toxic medications have been developed. However, patients with refractory pulmonary disease may still be prescribed this drug.

Classification
Toxicity is classified **acute** or **chronic.** The management strategy is different depending on whether the drug is an **immediate-** or **sustained-release** preparation.

Pathophysiology

Theophylline exerts its therapeutic effects by promoting catecholamine release, which results in enhanced β-agonism (*Circulation 1983;67:162–171*). Additionally, at high doses, theophylline is a phosphodiesterase inhibitor, which prolongs the effects of β-agonism by preventing the breakdown of cAMP. Theophylline is also an adenosine antagonist, which in therapeutic doses enhances bronchodilatation. However, in toxic doses, adenosine antagonism is associated with the development of tachydysrhythmias and seizures.

DIAGNOSIS

Clinical Presentation

- **Acute toxicity:** Patients with serum concentrations of >**20 mcg/mL** will present complaining of **nausea** and multiple episodes of **vomiting.** On examination, the patient will be **tremulous** and **tachycardic. Hyperventilation** is often present. In more severe cases, **hypotension** and **seizures** occur. **Refractory status epilepticus** is due to adenosine antagonism in the CNS (*Neuroscience 1994;58:245–261*). These effects are most often present at serum concentrations of >**90 mcg/mL** in the acutely intoxicated patient.
- **Chronic toxicity** usually occurs in patients with a large body burden of theophylline who develop a concurrent illness, or are administered a drug that delays the P450 metabolism and theophylline clearance. Subtle symptoms such as nausea and anorexia may occur; tachycardia is usually present. Severe toxicity may occur at serum levels of **40 to 60 mcg/mL.** Patients with these serum concentrations may present with seizures.

Diagnostic Testing

Laboratories

- **Acute toxicity** usually occurs at levels of >90 to 100 mcg/mL and is associated with the development of **hypokalemia** and **hyperglycemia.** In severe cases, expect a **metabolic acidosis.** Obtain a **BMP and dextrose.**
- **Serial theophylline** concentrations should be obtained every 1 to 2 hours until a downward trend is present; remember with sustained-release preparations, a peak may not be evident for 16 hours or later post ingestion.
- **Calcium, magnesium, and CPKs** should be checked as well.
- **Chronic toxicity** may occur at levels of >40 mcg/mL and is usually associated with normal laboratory values unless seizures are present. In these cases, obtain the laboratories mentioned above. **Serial theophylline** concentrations are also warranted in these patients.

Electrocardiography

Adenosine antagonism and increased catecholamines may result in a sinus tachycardia or **SVT** on the ECG. In overdose, **PVCs** may be apparent.

TREATMENT

Patients with theophylline toxicity do not require gastric lavage as they tend to vomit. Sustained-release preparations occasionally form bezoars. Severely intoxicated patients require intubation and ventilation. Sustained-release formulations should be treated with **whole-bowel irrigation.** Replete potassium and electrolytes as needed.

Medications

- Administer **AC 1 g/kg.** Consider **MDAC** as theophylline clearance is increased by this modality (*Clin Pharmacol Ther 1983;33:351–354*). Ensure patients have adequate airway protection as vomiting and aspiration may occur.
- **Vomiting** should be managed with **ondansetron** or **metoclopramide. Phenothiazines are contraindicated as they lower the seizure threshold.**
- **Seizures** are often refractory and should initially be treated with **benzodiazepines.** If this modality fails, consider moving to **Phenobarbital** as a 10 mg/kg loading dose at a rate of 50 mg/min, followed by up to a total of 30 mg/kg at a rate of 50 mg/min, followed by 1 to 5 mg/kg/d to maintain therapeutic plasma levels. **Propofol** is a reasonable alternative if these fail. Monitor for hypotension.
- **Hypotension** should be treated with 20 mL/kg bolus of IVF, which may be repeated. Direct pressors such as **phenylephrine** and **norepinephrine** may be added if fluid boluses are not sufficient. Since much of the hypotension is mediated by β_2-agonism, **avoid epinephrine.** Consider using short-acting β-antagonists such as **esmolol,** which although counterintuitive, may reverse β_2-mediated vasodilatation. Monitor for bronchospasm.
- **Arrhythmias** should be treated with β-antagonists. Use short-acting agents such as **esmolol** and monitor for bronchospasm.

Other Nonoperative Therapies

Hemoperfusion (charcoal or resin) or **hemodialysis** is indicated for the following:

- Intractable seizures or life-threatening cardiovascular complications, regardless of drug level.
- A theophylline level of ≥ 100 mg/mL after an **acute** overdose.
- A theophylline level > 60 mg/mL in acute intoxication, with worsening symptoms, or inability to tolerate oral charcoal administration.
- A theophylline level > 60 mg/mL in **chronic** intoxication without life-threatening symptoms.
- A theophylline level > 40 mg/mL in a patient with chronic intoxication and CHF, respiratory insufficiency, hepatic failure, or age older than 60 years (*J Emerg Med 1993;11:415*).

Toxic Alcohol, General

GENERAL PRINCIPLES

- High alcohol concentrations increase the measured plasma osmolality and subsequently widen the osmolar gap. A normal gap is <10 mmol/dL and varies from -14 to $+10$ mmol/dL (*NEJM 1984;310(2):102–105*).
- In presence of a widened gap, the actual serum alcohol level can be estimated if done early after ingestion (*BMC Emerg Med 2008 Apr 28;8:5*) with the following calculation:

$$\text{Osmol gap} \times \frac{\text{Molecular weight of alcohol}}{10} = [\text{Serum alcohol}](\text{mg/dL})$$

- Soon after ingestion, alcohol metabolization begins, the osmol gap falls, and the anion gap rises (*CJASN 2008;3(1):208–225*). Therefore, the osmol gap should only be used to support the diagnosis of toxic alcohol poisoning, and not to draw conclusions about the actual amount of ingested toxin.

$$\textbf{Calculated osmolarity} = 2\,Na^+ + \frac{BUN}{2.8} + \frac{Glucose}{18} + \frac{Alcohol/Molecular\ weight\ of\ alcohol}{10}$$

- The specific molecular weights for each alcohol can be found in the sections below.

TREATMENT

The general treatment approach to toxic alcohol ingestions (*Clin Toxicol 2002;40(4): 415–446*):

- Prevent the formation of toxic metabolites by inhibiting alcohol dehydrogenase (in methanol and ethylene glycol poisoning only).
- Eliminate the toxic alcohol and toxic metabolites from the blood.
- Correct acid–base imbalance.
- Replenish cofactors

Methanol

GENERAL PRINCIPLES

Definition

Methanol is used in gasoline antifreeze, de-icers, windshield washer fluid, paint and varnish removers, fuel, photocopy fluid, embalming fluids; is found in "moonshine" liquor; and is used as a denaturant for ethanol.

Classification
- First level list item 1
  - Second level list item 1

Etiology
- Ingestions are mostly intentional as suicide attempts.
- Another common cause of poisoning is the use of methanol as ethanol substitute.

Pathophysiology

Methanol is oxidized to toxic formic acid and this product is responsible for the anion gap metabolic acidosis in methanol poisoning (*Intern Med 2004;43(8):750–754*).

DIAGNOSIS

Clinical Presentation
- **Early stage:**
  - Early after ingestion, mild CNS depression or headache evolves, but profound obtundation or inebriation can occur as well.
  - These early symptoms are directly caused by methanol prior to metabolization.
- **Late stage:**
  - After a latent period of about 14 to 18 hours, severe anion gap metabolic acidosis without significant lactate or ketone concentrations develops.

- Formate accumulation within the retina and optic nerve fibers causes "snow field vision," blurred vision, visual field defects, or blindness (*AMA Arch Ophthalmol 1991;109(7):1012–1016*).
- Other CNS symptoms during the late phase are lethargy, convulsion, delirium, and coma. Basal ganglia hemorrhage with dyskinesia or hypokinesia has been observed (*IJCP 2004;58(11):1042–1044*).
- Abdominal complaints include nausea, vomiting, pain, and acute pancreatitis (*Clin Toxicol 2000;38(3):297–303*).

History

Obtain history of what, when, how, and how much of the toxic substance was ingested.

Physical Examination

- Assess mental status and respiratory and cardiovascular stability.
- Kussmaul respirations may indicate underlying metabolic acidosis.
- Visual field testing may reveal central scotoma or other visual field defects. A thorough funduscopic exam may show hyperemia, disk edema, or atrophy (*MJA 1978;2(10):483–485*).

Diagnostic Testing

Laboratories

- Address possible causes of an anion gap acidosis:
  - BMP: acidosis, anion gap, renal function
  - UA: ketones
  - Serum lactate
- Accu-Cheks.
- Serum osmolality: if toxic alcohol ingestion is suspected.
- ABG or VBG: to assess acid/base status and treatment success.
- Ethanol level: if elevated, toxic methanol manifestations may be delayed; if elevated in presence of acidosis, the acidosis is unlikely to be related to a toxic alcohol ingestion, since ethanol blocks the metabolism of the parent compound (unless the toxic alcohol ingestion occurred hours before ethanol ingestion).
- Serum methanol level: usually not readily available; therefore, clinically not useful.

TREATMENT

- ABCs and supportive care, monitor urine output.
- GI decontamination:
  - Nasogastric lavage is only indicated in patients who present <30 minutes after ingestion or who ingested large amounts of methanol while maintaining a normal mental status.
- **Do not use AC** since the GI tract rapidly absorbs methanol. AC bears a high risk of aspiration in acutely intoxicated patients.
- Sodium bicarbonate: Give 50 mg IV every 4 hours for arterial pH < 7.30 (*NEJM 2009;360(21):2216–2223*).
  - Serum alkalinization limits the amount of undissociated formic acid, which prevents CNS toxicity.

- Urine alkalinization enhances clearance of formate. CAVEAT: watch for fluid overload if giving large amounts of bicarbonate.
- Ethanol therapy: EtOH serum levels of 100 mg/dL block ADH sufficiently to inhibit formation of toxic metabolites.
  - Loading dose of **7.6 mL/kg of 10% ethanol** solution IV (correlates with an EtOH serum level of 100 to 200 mg/dL).
  - Maintenance dose of **0.8 mL/kg/hr (nondrinker), or 2.0 mL/kg/hr (drinker), or 2.0 to 3.3 mL/kg/hr (on hemodialysis)** of 10% ethanol solution IV (*CJASN 2008;3(1):208–225*).
- Fomepizole therapy: 4-Methylpyrazole (Antizol) is an FDH-approved competitive inhibitor of ADH for the treatment of methanol poisoning (*Intensive Care Med 2005;31(2):189–195*).
  - Loading dose of **15 mg/kg IV,** maintenance dose of **10 mg/kg IV** every 12 hours for 48 hours, then 15 mg/kg IV every 12 hours until methanol level < 20 mg/dL.
  - Dose adjustment may be needed for patients on hemodialysis (*NEJM 2009; 360(21):2216–2223*).
  - Continue treatment until methanol levels < 20 mg/dL and acidosis resolves (*Curr Opin Nephrol Hypertens 2000;9(6):695–701*).
- Indication: Ethanol or fomepizole therapy should be started early if:
  - Strong evidence of methanol ingestion
  - Methanol serum level > 20 mg/dL
  - Osmol gap > 10 mmol/dL
  - Arterial pH < 7.3
  - Serum CO_2 < 20 mmol/L
  - Or unexplained anion gap metabolic acidosis is present (*NEJM 2009;360(21): 2216–2223*)

Other Nonoperative Therapies

- **Hemodialysis** should be used in addition to above therapies in order to prevent end-organ toxicity.
- **Hemodialysis** corrects metabolic abnormalities and eliminates nonmetabolized methanol.
  - Indications for hemodialysis are a methanol level > 50 mg/dL, severe acidemia (bicarbonate < 15 mmol/L, pH < 7.30), and/or optic injury from toxicity (*Hum Exp Toxicol 2005;24(2):55–59*).
- Folic acid 1 mg/kg (up to 50 mg) IV every 4 to 6 hours and folinic acid (leucovorin) 1 mg/kg (up to 50 mg) IV every 4 to 6 hours enhance formate metabolism and should be given until metabolic acidosis resolves (*Alcoholism 1980;4(4):378–383*).

SPECIAL CONSIDERATIONS

- Coingestion of ethanol might delay the onset of initial symptoms because of ethanol's higher affinity to ADH.
- Ethanol therapy has significant disadvantages, for example, complex dosing regimen, hard to titrate therapeutic levels, intensive care requirements, severe side-effect profile). Although very expensive ($500/dose), fomepizole has become the preferred agent in the treatment of methanol intoxication (*Ann Emerg Med 2009;53(4):451–453*).

- Admit all patients on ethanol infusions to the ICU (risk of hypotension, tachycardia, hypoglycemia, CNS and respiratory depression).
- Stable patients on fomepizole infusion can be safely admitted to the floor. Adverse effects of fomepizole are usually mild and include headache, nausea, dizziness, but not sedation (*Alcoholism 1988;12(4):516–522; Lancet 1999;354(9181):831*).
- Report all cases of methanol intoxication to the local poison control center (1-800-222-1222).
- Get a clinical toxicologist involved early.
- Consult ophthalmology or neurology service if signs of optic injury or other neurologic deficits present.

Ethylene Glycol

GENERAL PRINCIPLES

Etiology

- Ingestions are mostly intentional suicide attempts.
- Another common cause of poisoning is the use of ethylene glycol as ethanol substitute.

Pathophysiology

- Ethylene glycol is oxidized to glycolic acid and oxalic acid.
- Glycolate accumulation is responsible for the anion gap metabolic acidosis in ethylene glycol poisoning.
- Oxalate accumulation is responsible for the development of acute renal failure in ethylene glycol poisoning (*Clin Toxicol 1986;24(5):389–402*).

DIAGNOSIS

Clinical Presentation

- Neurologic stage (30 minutes to 12 hours):
  - CNS depression with altered mental status, hallucinations, ataxia, slurred speech, and cranial nerve palsies are directly caused by ethylene glycol prior to metabolization.
  - Seizures, coma, and respiratory depression can occur in severe intoxications.
- Cardiovascular stage (12 to 24 hours):
  - Glycolate affects the cardiopulmonary system and causes tachycardia, hypotension, heart failure, pulmonary edema, and ARDS.
- Renal stage (24 to 72 hours post ingestion):
  - Glycolic acid is further metabolized to oxalic acid. Oxalate is a calcium chelator and accumulation of oxalate leads to **hypocalcemia.**
  - Calcium oxalate can precipitate in the renal tubules, which subsequently causes acute tubular necrosis with flank pain and acute renal failure (*Acta Clin Belg 1999;54(6):351–356*).
- Within 4 to 6 hours after ingestion, development of an anion gap metabolic acidosis with absence of significant lactate or ketone concentrations occurs.
- Abdominal complaints (nausea, vomiting, pain) are also common.

History

Obtain history of what, when, how, and how much of the toxic substance was ingested.

Physical Examination
- Assess mental status and respiratory and cardiovascular stability.
- Kussmaul respiration may indicate severe metabolic acidosis.

Diagnostic Testing

Laboratories
- Address causes of a high anion gap metabolic acidosis:
  - BMP: acidosis, anion gap, renal function
  - UA: ketones, oxalate crystals (usually a late sign during intoxication)
  - Serum lactate
  - **Glycolic acid may also be misinterpreted as a high lactic acid on a point-of-care blood gas analyzer.** Serum levels should be obtained in these cases.
- Serum osmolality—if toxic alcohol ingestion is suspected.
- ABG or VBG—to assess acid/base status and treatment success.
- Ethanol level—if elevated, toxic ethylene glycol manifestations may be delayed; if elevated in presence of acidosis, unlikely to be toxic alcohol ingestion (unless toxic alcohol ingestion occurred hours before ethanol ingestion).
- Serum ethylene glycol level—usually not readily available, therefore clinically often not useful.
- Serum calcium level—low if increased formation of calcium oxalate.
- Repeated renal function testing—increased risk of ARF.
- Urine microscopy—calcium oxalate might be visible as envelope-shaped crystals (*EMJ 2007;24(4):310*).
- NOTE: Wood's lamp examination of urine to detect fluorescence after assumed antifreeze ingestion is not a reliable screening tool (*Am J Emerg Med 2005;23(6):787–792*).

TREATMENT

- ABCs and supportive care, monitor urine output.
- GI decontamination:
  - Nasogastric lavage is only indicated in patients who present <30 minutes after ingestion or who ingested large amounts of ethylene glycol while maintaining a normal mental status.
- **Do not use AC** since the GI tract rapidly absorbs ethylene glycol. AC bears a high risk of aspiration in acutely intoxicated patients.
- **Thiamine** (Vitamin B_1) 100 mg IV every 4 to 6 hours and **pyridoxine** (Vitamin B_6) 50 mg IV every 6 to 12 hours enhance glycolate metabolism and should be given until metabolic acidosis resolves (*Eur J Emerg Med 2005;12(2):78–85*).
- Sodium bicarbonate: Give 50 mg IV every 4 hours for arterial pH < 7.30 (*NEJM 2009;360(21):2216–2223*).
  - Serum alkalinization limits the amount of undissociated glycolic acid, which prevents CNS toxicity.
  - Urine alkalinization enhances clearance of glycolate. CAVEAT: Watch for fluid overload if giving large amounts of bicarbonate.
- Ethanol therapy: EtOH serum levels of 100 mg/dL block ADH sufficiently to inhibit formation of toxic metabolites. See discussion of methanol overdose treatment for dosing.

- **Fomepizole** therapy: 4-Methylpyrazole (Antizol) is an FDH-approved competitive inhibitor of ADH for the treatment of ethylene glycol poisoning (*Intensive Care Med 2005;31(2):189–195*). See discussion of methanol overdose treatment for dosing.
- **Indications:** Ethanol or fomepizole therapy should be started early if:
  - Strong evidence of ethylene glycol ingestion
  - Ethylene glycol serum level > 20 mg/dL
  - Osmol gap > 10 mmol/dL
  - Arterial pH < 7.3
  - Serum CO_2 < 20 mmol/L
  - Or unexplained anion gap metabolic acidosis is present (*NEJM 2009;360(21): 2216–2223*)

Other Nonoperative Therapies

- **Hemodialysis** should be used in addition to above therapies in order to prevent end-organ toxicity.
- **Hemodialysis** corrects metabolic abnormalities and eliminates nonmetabolized ethylene glycol.
  - Indications for hemodialysis are an ethylene glycol level > 50 mg/dL, severe acidemia (bicarbonate < 15 mmol/L, pH < 7.30), and/or optic injury from toxicity (*Hum Exp Toxicol 2005;24(2):55–59*).

Ethanol

GENERAL PRINCIPLES

- Elimination rate: 20 to 25 mg/dL/hr (zero-order kinetics, faster in chronic alcoholics).
- Ethanol is present in all alcoholic beverages, some food extracts, mouthwash, cold syrups, but is also industrially used as a solvent in its denatured form.

Pathophysiology

Ethanol is oxidized to acetic acid (acetate), which is further metabolized to nontoxic intermediates.

DIAGNOSIS

Clinical Presentation

- CNS depression with ataxia, drowsiness, and confusion are common symptoms at blood levels of >100 mg/dL. Respiratory depression can occur at higher concentrations (*Emerg Med 1984;2(1):47–61*).
- Chronic alcohol abuse induces tolerance and patients appear asymptomatic even with high blood levels (*J Emerg Med 1997;15(5):687–692*).
- Hypoglycemia is due to an altered NADH/NAD ratio with the development of a reduced redo state. Pyruvate is then shunted off the gluconeogenesis pathway and lactate production is favored. Severe hypoglycemia is common in chronic alcoholics and in children.
- Chronic intoxication causes further gluconeogenesis disturbances, an increase in ketogenesis (β-hydroxybutyrate), and eventually the development of alcoholic ketoacidosis (AKA) (*Hum Exp Toxicol 1996;15(6):482–488*).

Diagnostic Testing

Laboratories
- Obtain glucose levels and BMP (especially in chronic alcoholics).
- Serum ethanol levels are only relevant to rule out poisoning with other alcohols, in presence of coma or altered mental status, or to proof incapacity in an intoxicated patient.
- Serum osmolality (if coingestion with other alcohols is suspected).

TREATMENT

Treatment is mainly supportive; however, hemodialysis may be indicated in severe poisoning.

SPECIAL CONSIDERATIONS

- Increased morbidity and mortality result from chronic toxicity (liver and GI injuries) and alcoholic ketoacidosis.
- Traumatic injuries and severe hypothermia are frequent findings due to risky behavior or decreased judgment capability during acute intoxication.
- Ethanol withdrawal can lead to life-threatening conditions and requires special attention.
- Patients should be observed until signs of clinical intoxication resolve.

Appendix A

Immunizations and Postexposure Therapies

Carlos A. Q. Santos and Victoria J. Fraser

MANAGEMENT OF RABIES

- **Pre-exposure vaccination** is indicated for persons in high-risk groups, including laboratory workers, veterinarians, animal handlers, and international travelers.[1]
  - The **dose** is three 1-mL injections of human diploid cell vaccine (HDCV), or purified chick embryo cell vaccine (PCECV) IM (deltoid) on days 0, 7, and 21 or 28.
  - **Research laboratory and vaccine production workers** should have serum rabies antibody testing every 6 months; spelunkers, veterinarians and staff, animal control and wildlife officers in areas where rabies is enzootic, and laboratory workers who perform rabies diagnostic testing should have serum rabies antibody testing every 2 years.
  - **Pre-exposure booster vaccination** should be given to people in the above groups to maintain their serum rabies antibody titer at a level corresponding with complete neutralization of challenge virus at a 1:5 serum dilution by the rapid fluorescent focus inhibition test (RFFIT).
- **Postexposure rabies therapy** (see Table 6).
  - For **bats and wild animals,** capturing and sacrificing the animal and performing immunofluorescence for rabies on brain tissue provides definitive determination of the animal's rabies status. Except in cases of bites or scratches on the head or neck or bat exposure, it is reasonable to wait for diagnostic testing on the source animal before instituting postexposure therapy. If diagnostic testing on animal brain tissue is negative, no postexposure therapy is necessary.
  - For **bites or scratches on the head or neck,** postexposure therapy should be instituted immediately because of proximity to the central nervous system and potentially shorter incubation period.
  - **All direct bat exposure warrants post exposure therapy.** Potential bat exposures also warrant therapy if there is any possibility of an unobserved bite or scratch (i.e., bat found with person sleeping in a room, unattended child, mentally disabled, or intoxicated adult).

[1] If contact with potentially rabid animals and limited access to medical care are likely.

Postexposure Prophylaxis Resources	
National Clinicians' Post-exposure Hotline	Telephone: 1-888-448-4911 http://www.ucsf.edu/hivcntr
CDC (for reporting HIV seroconversions in health care workers with and without postexposure prophylaxis)	Telephone: 1-800-893-0485
Antiretroviral Pregnancy Registry	Telephone: 1-800-258-4263 http://www.apregistry.com
U.S. FDA (for reporting unusual or severe toxicity to antiretroviral agents)	Telephone: 1-800-332-1088 http://www.fda.gov/medwatch
Hepatitis Hotline	Telephone: 1-800-232-4636 http://www.cdc.gov/hepatitis

Table 1 Routine Adult Immunizations

Vaccine *Brand Name* (Type)	Persons for Whom Indicated	Dose	Contraindications
Hepatitis A *Havrix* *Vaqta* *Twinrix* (Inactivated)	Travelers to endemic areas; men who have sex with men; illegal drug users; persons with clotting factor deficiencies, chronic liver disease, occupational risk for infection (e.g., researchers)	1 mL IM, repeated in 6–12 mo (*Havrix*), or 6–18 mo (*Vaqta*) If combined hepatitis A and hepatitis B vaccine (*Twinrix*) is used, administer 3 doses at 0, 1, and 6 mo; alternatively, a 4-dose schedule administered on days 0, 7, and 21 to 30, followed by a booster dose at month 12 may be used	Severe allergic reaction to vaccine or to vaccine component
Hepatitis B *Engerix* *Recombivax* *Twinrix* (Inactivated plasma or recombinant DNA derived)	Everyone	1 mL IM (in the deltoid) at 0, 1, and 6 mo (*Engerix, Recombivax*) If combined hepatitis A and hepatitis B vaccine (*Twinrix*) is used, administer 3 doses at 0, 1, and 6 mo; alternatively, a 4-dose schedule administered on days 0, 7, and 21 to 30 followed by a booster dose at month 12 may be used For adult patients receiving hemodialysis or with other immunocompromising conditions: 1 dose of 40 µg/mL (*Recombivax*) administered on a 3-dose schedule or 2 doses of 20 µg/mL (*Engerix*) administered simultaneously on a 4-dose schedule at 0, 1, 2, and 6 mo	Severe allergic reaction to vaccine or to vaccine component

Vaccine	Indications	Dose/Schedule	Contraindications
Influenza *Fluarix* *FluLaval* *Fluvirin* *Fluzone* (Inactivated) *FluMist* (Live attenuated)	Everyone ≥50 yr, high-risk patients,[a] women who will be in second or third trimester of pregnancy during influenza season, health care workers (consider offering to everyone)	0.5 mL IM prior to influenza season (inactivated vaccine) Healthy, nonpregnant adults <50 yr without high-risk medical conditions, who are not contacts of severely immunocompromised persons in special care units can receive either intranasally administered live, attenuated influenza vaccine (*FluMist*) or inactivated vaccine	Severe allergic reaction to vaccine or to vaccine component, including egg protein (inactivated vaccine)
Pneumococcus *Pneumovax* (23-Valent polysaccharide)	Everyone ≥65 yr, high-risk patients[a] ≥2 yr old, anatomic or functional asplenia, CSF leak	0.5 mL IM once, repeated after ≥5 yr for highest-risk patients	Severe allergic reaction to vaccine or to vaccine component
Tetanus, diphtheria, acellular pertussis booster Td Tdap (Toxoid)	Everyone	0.5 mL IM q10 yr, or a single booster at age 50 (Td) Tdap should replace a single dose for Td for adults aged 19 through 64 yr who have not received a dose of Tdap previously	Severe allergic reaction to vaccine or to vaccine component
Varicella *Varivax* (Live attenuated)	All susceptible persons, especially (i) health care workers, (ii) persons who live/work in environments where VZV transmission is likely,[b] (iii) adolescents and adults living with children, (iv) non-pregnant women of childbearing age, (v) international travelers	0.5 mL SC, repeated in 4–8 wk	Severe allergic reaction to vaccine or to vaccine component; pregnancy; severe immunosuppression[c]

(continued)

Table 1 Routine Adult Immunizations (*Continued*)

Vaccine *Brand Name* (Type)	Persons for Whom Indicated	Dose	Contraindications
Zoster *Zostavax* (Live attenuated)	Persons ≥60 yr	0.65 mL SC	Severe allergic reaction to vaccine or to vaccine component; severe immunosuppression[c]
Measles, mumps, rubella MMR (Live attenuated)	Measles/mumps: Adults born after 1957 unless medically contraindicated or immune. Rubella: Women whose rubella vaccination history is unreliable or who lack laboratory evidence of immunity	0.5 mL SC. Second dose should be given to adults who are exposed or are in outbreak settings, students in post-secondary educational institutions, persons who work in a health-care facility, persons who plan to travel internationally	Pregnancy; history of sensitivity to eggs or neomycin; severe immunosuppression[c]
Meningococcus *Menactra* (4-Valent conjugated polysaccharide)	During outbreaks of serogroup C,[d] consider for college freshmen living in dormitories; indicated for patients with terminal complement component deficiencies, functional	0.5 mL SC	Severe allergic reaction to vaccine or to vaccine component

| | or anatomic asplenia, travelers to countries where *Neisseria meningitides* is hyperendemic (i.e., sub-Saharan Africa), microbiologists routinely exposed to isolates of *N. meningitides*, military recruits | | |
| Human papillomavirus *Gardasil* (Recombinant inactive protein) | Females aged 11–26 yr | 0.5 mL IM, repeated 2 and 6 mo after first dose | Severe allergic reaction to vaccine or to vaccine component |

CSF, cerebrospinal fluid; VZV, varicella zoster virus.

[a]High-risk patients are those with chronic pulmonary, cardiovascular, metabolic, or renal diseases or hemoglobinopathies, or immunosuppressed or institutionalized persons.

[b]Teachers of young children, day care employees, residents/staff in institutional settings, college students, correctional institution inmates/staff members, military personnel.

[c]Individuals with leukemia, lymphomas, or other malignant neoplasms affecting the bone marrow or lymphatic systems; primary and acquired immunodeficiency states including advanced HIV; those receiving immunosuppressive therapy

[d]Outbreak is defined as ≥3 probable or confirmed cases within ≤3 months for a primary attack rate of ≥10 cases/100,000 population.

Table 2	Vaccination Schedule for Adult Stem Cell Transplant Recipients	
Time (Months Post-SCT)	**Vaccine**	**Dose**
6	HIB vaccine (*HibTITER*) #1	0.5 mL IM
	Neisseria meningitidis types A and C (*Menactra*)	0.5 mL IM
	Not routinely recommended but may be given in situations where risk of disease is increased	
	Diphtheria, tetanus, acellular pertussis (*Tdap*) #1	0.5 mL IM
	Influenza	0.5 mL IM, yearly before influenza season
	Vaccination of family members before the first influenza season is recommended	
	Inactivated polio (*IPOL*) # 1	0.5 mL IM
8	HIB vaccine (*HibTITER*) #2	0.5 mL IM
	Diphtheria, tetanus, acellular pertussis (*Tdap*) #2	0.5 mL IM
	Inactivated polio (*IPOL*) #2	0.5 mL IM
10	HIB vaccine (*HibTITER*) #3	0.5 mL IM
	Diphtheria, tetanus, acellular pertussis (*Tdap*) #3	0.5 mL IM
	Inactivated polio (*IPOL*) # 3	0.5 mL IM
12	Pneumococcal vaccine (*Pneumovax*)	0.5 mL IM
24	Measles, mumps, rubella (*MMR*)	0.5 mL SC
	Should not be given in patients with chronic GVHD or ongoing immunosuppression	
	Rubella vaccine is recommended in female patients who have retained the potential for pregnancy	
	Varicella (*Varivax*)	0.5 mL SC
	Should not be given in patients with chronic GVHD or ongoing immunosuppression. Do not confuse with zoster vaccine (Zostavax)	

SCT, stem cell transplant; HIB, *Hemophilus influenzae* type B; GVHD, graft-versus-host disease.

Table 3	Recommended Vaccines for Adult Solid-Organ Transplant Recipients		
	Recommended		**Contraindicated**
Pretransplant	**Posttransplant**	**Special Circumstances**	**After Transplant**
Pneumococcus (*q3–yr*)	Pneumococcus (*q3–5yr*)	Haemophilus influenzae type B	Bacille Calmette-Guerin
Tetanus, diphtheria, pertussis	Tetanus, diphtheria, pertussis	Meningococcus[a]	Smallpox
Oral polio		Inactivated polio[b]	Oral polio[c]
Influenza[d] (*yearly*)	Influenza[d] (*yearly*)	Typhoid Vi[e]	Live oral typhoid
Hepatitis B[f]		Hepatitis B	Yellow fever
Hepatitis A		Hepatitis A[g]	Live Japanese B encephalitis
Human papillomavirus[h]		Inactivated Japanese encephalitis	Zoster
Varicella			Varicella
Measles, mumps, rubella			Measles, mumps, rubella

[a]Recommended for specific high-risk groups: college-age patients, travelers to or residents of endemic areas and areas with active outbreaks, military recruits, patients with asplenia, and those with complement deficiencies.
[b]A booster may be given if more than 10 yr have elapsed since the last polio vaccine dose.
[c]Causes vaccine-induced paralytic disease in immunosuppressed patients. Household contacts and medical staff should likewise only be immunized with the inactivated polio vaccine.
[d]Also vaccinate household contacts and medical staff.
[e]An inactive parenteral vaccine, Typhim Vi (Aventis Pasteur) should be given to transplant recipients several months prior to travel to endemic areas.
[f]Doses (40 μg/dose) given at 0, 1, and 2 months are generally sufficient. Quantitative levels of hepatitis B surface antigen antibody (anti-HBs IgG) should be determined 4 months after the last dose. Patients who do not develop protective titers should have another dose administered and titers rechecked.
[g]Two doses of the vaccine, 6 to 12 months apart should be given to transplant recipients who are at least 1 yr beyond transplant, and being treated with only modest doses of immunosuppressive medications. If there is not enough time to provide active vaccination, intramuscular hepatitis A immunoglobulin may be given prior to travel.
[h]All females between the ages of 9–26 yr.

Table 4	Passive Immunization

Disease	Indications and Dosage
Diphtheria	Suspected respiratory tract diphtheria: diphtheria antitoxin (DAT–equine source), 20,000–120,000 units IM (IV for serious illness) after cultures taken (given in addition to antibiotics). Not routinely recommended for household contacts given significant risk of anaphylaxis (7%) and serum sickness (5%) and equivalent efficacy of antimicrobial prophylaxis (benzathine penicillin, 1.2 million units IM × 1, or erythromycin, 1 g daily in divided doses × 7–10 days). Not currently commercially available in the United States, but may be obtained from the CDC (404-639-2889)
Hepatitis A	**Postexposure:** within 14 days of known exposure in high-risk persons [unvaccinated household and sexual contacts of infected individual; coworkers of infected food handlers; all staff and children at day care centers where ≥1 case has occurred or when cases occur in ≥2 households of center attendees; consider for family members of diapered children who attend such day care centers during outbreaks (cases in ≥3 families)]—IG, 0.02 mL/kg IM.[a] IG not indicated for casual contacts (e.g., office coworkers)
Hepatitis B	**Preexposure:** vaccine prophylaxis preferred (Table 1) **Postexposure:** see Table 7
Measles	For nonimmune contacts within 6 days of exposure: IG, 0.25 mL/kg (maximum 15 mL) for normal host; 0.5 mL/kg (maximum 15 mL) for immunocompromised patients. MMR vaccine may provide some protection if given within 72 hr of initial exposure[b]
Rabies	See Table 6
Tetanus	See Table 5
Varicella	Vaccine, 0.5 mL SC within 3 days of exposure (possibly effective up to 5 days of postexposure) or varicella zoster IG (*VariZIG*), 1 vial (125 units) IM for each 10-kg body weight (minimum, 125 units; maximum, 625 units) within 96 hr of exposure[b,c]

DAT, direct antiglobulin test; MMR, measles, mumps, rubella.
[a]Can be ordered from the following distributors; delivery within 24 hr can be arranged: Alternative Site Distributors (1-800-837-5403), BioCare Division, Blood Systems, Inc. (1-800-304-3064), Health Coalition (1-800-456-7283), Chapin Medical (1-800-221-7180), FFF Enterprises (1-800-843-7477), Nationwide (1-800-997-8846), NHS (1-800-344-6087). Anaphylaxis has been reported after injection of IG in IgA-deficient persons.
[b]Live attenuated vaccines [MMR, varicella zoster virus (VZV)] should be delayed after administration of IG (3 mo for MMR, 5 mo for VZV). Patients who received MMR within 2 wk before IG or VZV within 3 wk before IG should be revaccinated.
[c]Available through expanded access protocol sponsored by Cangene Corporation/FFF Enterprises (1-800-843-7477; delivery within 24 hr can be arranged.

Table 5   Tetanus Prophylaxis

History of Tetanus Immunization (Doses)	Clean, Minor Wounds		Other Wounds	
	Give Td[a]	**Give TIG**[b]	**Give Td**	**Give TIG**
Unknown or <3 doses	Yes	No	Yes	Yes
≥3 doses	Only if last dose given ≥10 yr	No	Only if last dose given ≥5 yr	No

[a]Td, adult tetanus-diphtheria booster.
[b]TIG, tetanus immune globulin, 250 units IM, given concurrently with Td at a separate site.

Table 6   Postexposure Rabies Therapy

Species	Condition of Animal at Time of Attack	Treatment of Exposed[a] Persons
Domestic cats, dogs, ferrets	Healthy and available for 10 days of observation	None unless animal develops rabies
	Rabid or suspected rabid	HRIG and vaccine[b]
	Unknown (e.g., escaped)	Contact public health department
Bats[a]	Any	HRIG and vaccine[b]
Skunks, foxes, coyotes, raccoons, or other wild terrestrial carnivores	Regarded as rabid unless proven negative by laboratory testing	HRIG and vaccine[b]
Wild or domestic rodents (squirrels, chipmunks, rats, mice, hamsters, guinea pigs, gerbils) and lagomorphs (rabbits, hares)	Consider individually; rarely infected with rabies	Contact local health department

HRIG, human rabies immunoglobulin.
[a]Exposure: bites or scratches, or animal saliva contaminating abrasions, open wounds, or mucous membranes *except for bats*. **Any bat exposure or potential bat exposures warrant therapy.**
[b]HRIG: Administer once to previously unvaccinated persons, 20 IU/kg; best if done immediately (can be given through seventh day after first dose of vaccine administered). As much of the product as is anatomically feasible should be infiltrated around wound(s); any remaining product should be administered IM in the deltoid or quadriceps at a location other than that used for vaccine administration. **Do not** administer HRIG in same syringe or at same anatomic site as vaccine. Previously vaccinated persons (those who received one of the recommended regimens of human diploid cell vaccine or purified chick embryo cell vaccine and had a documented rabies antibody titer): two IM 1-mL doses of vaccine, days 0 (immediately) and 3. Vaccine: Four 1-mL doses on days 0, 3, 7, and 14 IM in deltoid (anterolateral aspect of thigh acceptable for children). Gluteal area should not be used, as this results in lower neutralizing antibody titers.

Table 7	Blood-borne Pathogen Postexposure Guidelines[a]
Pathogen	Treatment
HIV[b,c]	For percutaneous injury (e.g., bloody needlestick) or prolonged, excessive exposure of mucous membrane or nonintact skin to blood, blood-contaminated fluids, or potentially infectious material (e.g., cerebrospinal fluid, amniotic fluid), one of the following drug regimens for 4 wk (determine based on resistance in source patient and geographic area): (i) Combivir (zidovudine 300 mg/lamivudine 300 mg) PO bid, (ii) Truvada (tenofovir 300 mg/emtricitabine 200 mg) PO daily, (iii) lamivudine 300 mg PO daily, plus stavudine 40 mg PO bid, (iv) emtricitabine 200 mg PO daily, plus stavudine 40 mg twice daily, (v) lamivudine 300 mg PO daily, or 150 mg PO bid, plus didanosine 400 mg PO daily, or 200 mg PO bid, (vi) emtricitabine 200 mg PO daily, plus didanosine 400 mg PO daily, or 200 mg PO bid. For highest-risk exposure (e.g., large blood volumes, high HIV viral load, hollow-bore needle), one of the following drugs should be added: (i) lopinavir/ritonavir 400/100 mg three capsules twice daily with food, (ii) atazanavir 300 mg PO daily, plus ritonavir 100 mg PO daily, (iii) efavirenz 600 mg PO daily at bedtime [*MMWR Morb Mortal Wkly Rep 2005; 54(RR09): 1–17*] For exposures to other material (e.g., urine), therapy is not recommended
Hepatitis B	For percutaneous injury with blood or blood-contaminated fluids: Unvaccinated health care worker: Administer hepatitis B immunoglobulin (HBIG), 0.06 mL/kg IM, within 96 hr of exposure; start hepatitis B vaccine series Vaccinated health care worker: Check anti-HBs titer. If ≥10 IU/mL, no therapy. If <10 IU/mL, give HBIG, 0.06 mL/kg, and booster dose of vaccine, or 2 doses of HBIG 1 mo apart (this is preferred for health care workers known not to have responded to second vaccine series)
Hepatitis C	Immunoglobulin not effective. Ensure occupational health follow-up for baseline and subsequent follow-up testing

[a]All blood and body fluid exposures should be reported to the occupational health department. Source patients should be tested for HIV (with consent), hepatitis B surface antigen (HbsAg), and hepatitis C antibody (anti-HCV).

[b]For exposure to patients with known HIV or at high risk for HIV, postexposure prophylaxis should be started as soon as possible (preferably within 1–2 hr, because there is less evidence for efficacy in preventing transmission after 24–36 hr).

[c]Other antiretrovirals may be indicated if there is a high likelihood that the source patient has drug resistance to components of the standard regimen. If therapy is started for a patient with suspected HIV, it can be stopped if the patient's HIV antibody test is negative, unless there is a high suspicion of acute HIV illness.

Table 8	Postexposure Prophylaxis for Centers for Disease Control and Prevention (CDC) Class A Bioterrorism Agents[a]
Pathogen	**Treatment**
Anthrax	Adults: ciprofloxacin 500 mg PO bid, or doxycycline 100 mg PO bid, or levofloxacin 500 mg PO daily for 60 d Children: ciprofloxacin 15 mg/kg PO bid (not to exceed 500 mg/dose), or doxycycline 100 mg PO bid (>8 yr and >45 kg), 2.2 mg/kg PO bid (>8 yr and $\leq$45 kg, or $\leq$8 yr), or levofloxacin 500 mg PO daily (>50 kg), 8 mg/kg PO bid, not to exceed 500 mg/d ($\geq$6 mo and <50 kg) for 60 d
Botulinum toxin	Close observation of exposed person, treat with equine antitoxin or human-derived botulism IG at first sign of illness
Pneumonic plague	For close contacts (<2 m), doxycycline, 100 mg PO bid, or ciprofloxacin, 500 mg PO bid for 7 days is preferred (see above for pediatric dosing); chloramphenicol, 25 mg/kg/dose q6h is alternative (not used in children <2 yr old); watch closely for fever or cough, promptly initiate parenteral therapy with streptomycin, 1 g IM q12h, or gentamicin in symptomatic patients
Tularemia	If attacks identified during early incubation period: ciprofloxacin or doxycycline PO for 14 days (see above for dosing); if attack unrecognized until multiple people ill, observe exposed persons closely, initiate parenteral therapy at first sign of illness
Smallpox	Vaccinate[b] ideally within 3 d of exposure; vaccination 4–7 d after exposure may offer some protection

[a] In the event of a bioterrorism attack, the latest recommendations can be accessed via the U.S. Centers for Disease Control and Prevention internet site: http://www.bt.cdc.gov.
[b] An individualized assessment of risks and benefits of vaccination must be made. In general, vaccination for contacts of smallpox cases is recommended even in the presence of usual contraindications (history of or presence of eczema; atopic dermatitis; other acute, chronic, or exfoliative skin conditions; immunosuppression; pregnancy or intent to become pregnant within 4 wk; breast-feeding; age <1 yr). If an exposed person declines vaccination, the alternative strategy is isolation for 19 d.

Infection Control and Isolation Recommendations

Carlos A. Q. Santos and Victoria J. Fraser

- **Standard precautions** (previously called *body substance isolation* or *universal precautions*) should be practiced on **all patients at all times** to minimize the risk of nosocomial infection.
  - **Perform hand hygiene,** preferably with an alcohol-based rub or foam before and after direct patient contact, after contact with the environment, between caring for different patients, and after removing gloves. Soap and water should be used for visibly contaminated hands.
  - **Wear gloves** when direct contact with moist body substances (e.g., blood, sputum, urine, pus, stool) is anticipated.
  - **Wear a gown** when clothing is likely to be soiled by a body fluid.
  - **Wear a mask and goggles or glasses** when splashes of a body fluid are anticipated (e.g., during most invasive procedures).
- **Specific isolation categories.** In addition to precautions that should be followed for all patients, certain diseases, depending on their mode of spread, **require additional isolation precautions.** Categories and indications for their use may vary slightly among different hospitals. Contact an infection control specialist if there is any uncertainty about what type of isolation a patient might need. The following categories are those suggested by the Centers for Disease Control and Prevention.
  - Airborne precautions
    - Use a negative-pressure room.
    - Keep doors closed.
    - Wear a **respirator, grade N95 or better,** certified by the National Institute for Occupational Safety and Health **(not a surgical mask)** if entering the room of a patient who is suspected of having tuberculosis.
    - For patients with measles or varicella (e.g., chickenpox) infections, immune persons may enter the room without a mask. Nonimmune persons ideally should not enter the room of such patients, but, if it is absolutely necessary that they enter, they should wear a mask.
    - If patient transport is absolutely necessary, the patient should wear a **surgical** mask.
    - Instruct the patient to cover his or her mouth when coughing or sneezing, even if alone.
  - **Droplet precautions**
    - Keep doors closed.
    - Wear a surgical mask if entering the room.
    - Discard mask **after** leaving the room.
    - If patient transport is absolutely necessary, the patient should wear a **surgical** mask.
  - **Contact precautions**
    - Wear a gown and gloves to enter the room.
    - Use a dedicated stethoscope and thermometer.
    - Remove gown and gloves before leaving the room.
- Perform hand hygiene with an alcohol-based rub or foam or antimicrobial soap before leaving the room.
- **Isolation for specific infections and duration of isolation.** See Tables 1 and 2.

| Table 1 | Isolation for Specific Infections and Duration of Isolation |

Isolation Type and Diseases	Duration of Isolation
Airborne	
Tuberculosis (TB)	Until TB is ruled out with three negative acid-fast bacilli smears on consecutive days. (If patient has documented or strongly suspected TB, isolation for hospitalized patients should continue for at least 2 wk of therapy with a good clinical response; however, patients can be discharged during this time if proper follow-up has been arranged with the local health department.)
Measles	4 d after start of rash or for duration of illness if patient is immunocompromised
Chickenpox[a]/disseminated zoster[a]	Until all lesions are crusted. (Note: Nonimmune persons are potentially contagious days 8–21 after exposure to varicella zoster virus.)
SARS-associated coronavirus	Duration of illness
Droplet	
Adenovirus (pneumonia)	Duration of illness
Diphtheria (pharyngeal)	Until cultures are negative (at least 24 hr after stopping antibiotics)
Seasonal influenza, pandemic H1N1 influenza,[b] avian influenza[b]	Duration of illness
Meningitis	24 hr after start of therapy for known or suspected *Neisseria meningitidis* or *Haemophilus influenzae*; this is prudent for all meningitis initially
Mumps[a]	9 d after onset of swelling
Mycoplasma	Duration of illness
Parvovirus B19[c]	7 d for aplastic crisis or for duration of illness if patient is immunosuppressed
Pertussis	5 d after start of therapy
Plague (pneumonic)	72 hr after start of therapy
Rubella[c]	7 d after onset of rash; for congenital rubella, place infant on contact precautions during any admission until 1 yr of age unless nasopharyngeal and urine cultures are negative after age 3 mo
Streptococcal pharyngitis, pneumonia, or scarlet fever in infants and young children	24 hr after start of therapy

(*continued*)

| Table 1 | Isolation for Specific Infections and Duration of Isolation (*Continued*) |

Isolation Type and Diseases	Duration of Isolation
Contact	
Acute infectious diarrhea	Duration of illness
Abscess[d]	Duration of illness
Clostridium difficile	Until diarrhea resolves or treatment is completed
Enterovirus	Duration of illness
Herpes simplex (neonatal, primary or disseminated mucocutaneous, severe)	Duration of illness
Hepatitis A	Until 1 wk after onset of symptoms
Parainfluenza	Duration of illness
Respiratory syncytial virus (infants, young children, and immunocompromised adults)	Duration of illness
Scabies	24 hr after start of therapy
Viral conjunctivitis ("pink eye")	Duration of illness
Methicillin-resistant *Staphylococcus aureus*	Duration of hospitalization and future hospitalizations[e]
Vancomycin-resistant or intermediate-sensitive *S. aureus*	Duration of hospitalization and future hospitalizations[e]
Vancomycin-resistant enterococci	Duration of hospitalization and future hospitalizations[e]
Multidrug-resistant gram-negative bacteria	Duration of hospitalization and future hospitalizations[e]

[a]Nonimmune persons should stay out of room if possible.
[b]Subject to change because of evolving nature of the virus. Consult hospital infection control specialists for latest recommendations.
[c]Nonimmune pregnant women should stay out of room (Barnes-Jewish Hospital policy, not an official Centers for Disease Control and Prevention recommendation).
[d]If community-acquired MRSA is suspected.
[e]Unless criteria for discontinuing isolation have been met; consult hospital infection control specialists for specific criteria.

Table 2   Isolation for Centers for Disease Control and Prevention Class A[a] Agents of Bioterrorism

Isolation Type and Agent	Duration of Isolation
Airborne	
Smallpox[b]	Duration of hospitalization or until scabs fall off
Viral hemorrhagic fevers[c]	Duration of hospitalization
Droplet	
Pneumonic plague (*Yersinia pestis*)	Until 72 hr after start of antimicrobial therapy
Contact	
Cutaneous anthrax	Until lesions resolve
Standard precautions	
Inhalational anthrax	Duration of hospitalization
Botulism	Duration of hospitalization
Tularemia	Duration of hospitalization

[a]Six class A agents have been identified by the Centers for Disease Control and Prevention. Criteria for inclusion in class A are easily disseminated or transmitted person to person, high mortality, potential for major public health impact, potential for public panic and social disruption, and requirement for special action for public health preparedness.
[b]Contact precautions should be used in handling items potentially contaminated by infectious lesions.
[c]Lassa, Marburg, Ebola, Congo-Crimean. Droplet isolation can be used if the patient does not have prominent coughing, vomiting, diarrhea, or hemorrhaging. Private rooms with potential for conversion of air flow to negative pressure are recommended at admission to avoid later patient transport to negative-pressure isolation.

Appendix C

Advanced Cardiac Life Support Algorithms

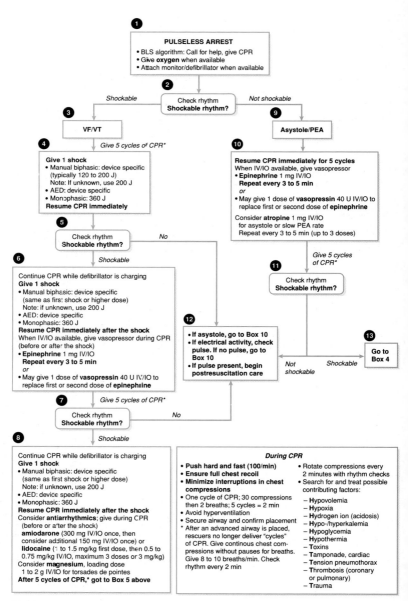

PULSELESS ARREST
- BLS algorithm: Call for help, give CPR
- Give **oxygen** when available
- Attach monitor/defibrillator when available

Check rhythm
Shockable rhythm?

Shockable — **VF/VT**

Not shockable — **Asystole/PEA**

Give 5 cycles of CPR*

Give 1 shock
- Manual biphasic: device specific (typically 120 to 200 J)
  Note: If unknown, use 200 J
- AED: device specific
- Monophasic: 360 J
Resume CPR immediately

Resume CPR immediately for 5 cycles
When IV/IO available, give vasopressor
- **Epinephrine** 1 mg IV/IO
  Repeat every 3 to 5 min
  or
- May give 1 dose of **vasopressin** 40 U IV/IO to replace first or second dose of **epinephrine**

Consider **atropine** 1 mg IV/IO
for asystole or slow PEA rate
Repeat every 3 to 5 min (up to 3 doses)

Check rhythm
Shockable rhythm? *No*

Shockable

Give 5 cycles of CPR*

Check rhythm
Shockable rhythm?

Continue CPR while defibrillator is charging
Give 1 shock
- Manual biphasic: device specific (same as first shock or higher dose)
  Note: if unknown, use 200 J
- AED: device specific
- Monophasic: 360 J
Resume CPR immediately after the shock
When IV/IO available, give vasopressor during CPR
(before or after the shock)
- **Epinephrine** 1 mg IV/IO
  Repeat every 3 to 5 min
  or
- May give 1 dose of **vasopressin** 40 U IV/IO to replace first or second dose of **epinephrine**

- If asystole, go to Box 10
- If electrical activity, check pulse. If no pulse, go to Box 10
- If pulse present, begin postresuscitation care

Go to Box 4

Not shockable — *Shockable*

Give 5 cycles of CPR*

Check rhythm
Shockable rhythm? *No*

Shockable

Continue CPR while defibrillator is charging
Give 1 shock
- Manual biphasic: device specific (same as first shock or higher dose)
  Note: if unknown, use 200 J
- AED: device specific
- Monophasic: 360 J
Resume CPR immediately after the shock
Consider **antiarrhythmics**; give during CPR
(before or after the shock)
  amiodarone (300 mg IV/IO once, then consider additional 150 mg IV/IO once) or
  lidocaine (1 to 1.5 mg/kg first dose, then 0.5 to 0.75 mg/kg IV/IO, maximum 3 doses or 3 mg/kg)
Consider **magnesium**, loading dose
1 to 2 g IV/IO for torsades de pointes
After 5 cycles of CPR,* got to Box 5 above

During CPR

- **Push hard and fast (100/min)**
- **Ensure full chest recoil**
- **Minimize interruptions in chest compressions**
- One cycle of CPR; 30 compressions then 2 breaths; 5 cycles = 2 min
- Avoid hyperventilation
- Secure airway and confirm placement
- After an advanced airway is placed, rescuers no longer deliver "cycles" of CPR. Give continous chest compressions without pauses for breaths. Give 8 to 10 breaths/min. Check rhythm every 2 min

- Rotate compressions every 2 minutes with rhythm checks
- Search for and treat possible contributing factors:

  – Hypovolemia
  – Hypoxia
  – Hydrogen ion (acidosis)
  – Hypo-/hyperkalemia
  – Hypoglycemia
  – Hypothermia
  – Toxins
  – Tamponade, cardiac
  – Tension pneumothorax
  – Thrombosis (coronary or pulmonary)
  – Trauma

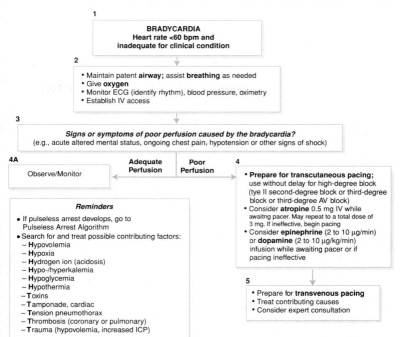

1
BRADYCARDIA
Heart rate <60 bpm and
inadequate for clinical condition

2
- Maintain patent **airway**; assist **breathing** as needed
- Give **oxygen**
- Monitor ECG (identify rhythm), blood pressure, oximetry
- Establish IV access

3
Signs or symptoms of poor perfusion caused by the bradycardia?
(e.g., acute altered mental status, ongoing chest pain, hypotension or other signs of shock)

4A
Observe/Monitor

Adequate Perfusion | Poor Perfusion

4
- **Prepare for transcutaneous pacing;**
  use without delay for high-degree block
  (tye II second-degree block or third-degree
  block or third-degree AV block)
- Consider **atropine** 0.5 mg IV while
  awaitng pacer. May repeat to a total dose of
  3 mg. If ineffective, begin pacing
- Consider **epinephrine** (2 to 10 μg/min)
  or **dopamine** (2 to 10 μg/kg/min)
  infusion while awaiting pacer or if
  pacing ineffective

5
- Prepare for **transvenous pacing**
- Treat contributing causes
- Consider expert consultation

Reminders
- If pulseless arrest develops, go to
  Pulseless Arrest Algorithm
- Search for and treat possible contributing factors:
  – **H**ypovolemia
  – **H**ypoxia
  – **H**ydrogen ion (acidosis)
  – **H**ypo-/hyperkalemia
  – **H**ypoglycemia
  – **H**ypothermia
  – **T**oxins
  – **T**amponade, cardiac
  – **T**ension pneumothorax
  – **T**hrombosis (coronary or pulmonary)
  – **T**rauma (hypovolemia, increased ICP)

Figure 2. Bradycardia algorithm. AV, atrioventricular; bpm, beats per minute; ECG, electrocardiogram; ICP, intracranial pressure; IV, intravenous. (From American Heart Association in collaboration with the International Liaison Committee on Resuscitation. Guidelines 2005 for cardiopulmonary resuscitation and emergency cardiovascular care. Part 7.2: Management of symptomatic bradycardia and tachycardia. *Circulation* 2005;112(24 Suppl):IV67–IV87.)

Figure 1. Advanced cardiac life support pulseless arrest algorithm. AED, automated external defibrillator; BLS, basic life support; CPR, cardiopulmonary resuscitation; IO, intraosseous; IV, intravenous; PEA, pulseless electrical activity; VF, ventricular fibrillation; VT, ventricular tachycardia. (From American Heart Association in collaboration with the International Liaison Committee on Resuscitation. Guidelines 2005 for cardiopulmonary resuscitation and emergency cardiovascular care. Part 7.2: Management of cardiac arrest. *Circulation* 2005;112(24 Suppl):IV58–IV66.)

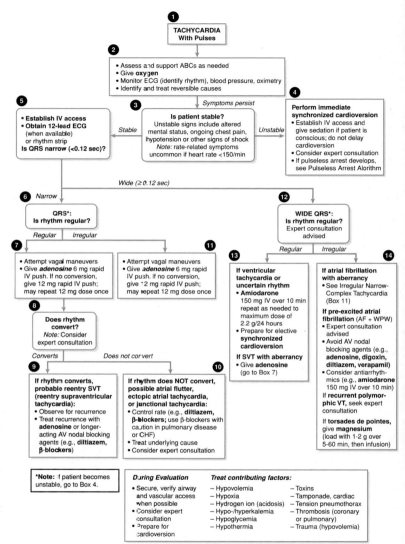

①

TACHYCARDIA
With Pulses

②
- Assess and support ABCs as needed
- Give **oxygen**
- Monitor ECG (identify rhythm), blood pressure, oximetry
- Identify and treat reversible causes

Symptoms persist

⑤
- **Establish IV access**
- **Obtain 12-lead ECG**
  (when available)
  or rhythm strip
- **Is QRS narrow (<0.12 sec)?**

③
Is patient stable?
Unstable signs include altered
mental status, ongoing chest pain,
hypotension or other signs of shock
Note: rate-related symptoms
uncommon if heart rate <150/min

Stable ← → *Unstable*

④
**Perform immediate
synchronized cardioversion**
- Establish IV access and
  give sedation if patient is
  conscious; do not delay
  cardioversion
- Consider expert consultation
- If pulseless arrest develops,
  see Pulseless Arrest Alorithm

Wide (≥0.12 sec)

⑥ *Narrow*

**QRS*:
Is rhythm regular?**

Regular | *Irregular*

⑫

**WIDE QRS*:
Is rhythm regular?**
Expert consultation
advised

Regular | *Irregular*

⑦
- Attempt vagal maneuvers
- Give **adenosine** 6 mg rapid
  IV push. If no conversion,
  give 12 mg rapid IV push;
  may repeat 12 mg dose once

⑪
- Attempt vagal maneuvers
- Give **adenosine** 6 mg rapid
  IV push. If no conversion,
  give 12 mg rapid IV push;
  may repeat 12 mg dose once

⑬
**If ventricular
tachycardia or
uncertain rhythm**
- **Amiodarone**
  150 mg IV over 10 min
  repeat as needed to
  maximum dose of
  2.2 g/24 hours
- Prepare for elective
  **synchronized
  cardioversion**

If SVT with aberrancy
- Give **adenosine**
  (go to Box 7)

⑭
**If atrial fibrillation
with aberrancy**
- See Irregular Narrow-
  Complex Tachycardia
  (Box 11)

**If pre-excited atrial
fibrillation** (AF + WPW)
- Expert consultation
  advised
- Avoid AV nodal
  blocking agents (e.g.,
  **adenosine, digoxin,
  diltiazem, verapamil**)
- Consider antiarrhyth-
  mics (e.g., **amiodarone**
  150 mg IV over 10 min)

If recurrent polymor-
phic VT, seek expert
consultation

If torsades de pointes,
give **magnesium**
(load with 1-2 g over
5-60 min, then infusion)

⑧
**Does rhythm
convert?**
Note: Consider
expert consultation

Converts | *Does not convert*

⑨
**If rhythm converts,
probable reentry SVT
(reentry supraventricular
tachycardia):**
- Observe for recurrence
- Treat recurrence with
  adenosine or longer-
  acting AV nodal blocking
  agents (e.g., **diltiazem,
  β-blockers**)

⑩
**If rhythm does NOT convert,
possible atrial flutter,
ectopic atrial tachycardia,
or junctional tachycardia:**
- Control rate (e.g., **diltiazem,
  β-blockers**; use β-blockers with
  caution in pulmonary disease
  or CHF)
- Treat underlying cause
- Consider expert consultation

*Note: if patient becomes
unstable, go to Box 4.

During Evaluation
- Secure, verify airway
  and vascular access
  when possible
- Consider expert
  consultation
- Prepare for
  cardioversion

Treat contributing factors:
– Hypovolemia
– Hypoxia
– Hydrogen ion (acidosis)
– Hypo-/hyperkalemia
– Hypoglycemia
– Hypothermia

– Toxins
– Tamponade, cardiac
– Tension pneumothorax
– Thrombosis (coronary
  or pulmonary)
– Trauma (hypovolemia)

Figure 3. Advanced cardiac life support tachycardia algorithm. AF, atrial fibrillation; AV, atrioventricular; ECG, electrocardiogram; IV, intravenous; SVT, supraventricular tachycardia; WPW, Wolff-Parkinson-White syndrome. (From American Heart Association in collaboration with the International Liaison Committee on Resuscitation. Guidelines 2005 for cardiopulmonary resuscitation and emergency cardiovascular care. Part 7.2: Management of symptomatic bradycardia and tachycardia. *Circulation* 2005;112(24 Suppl):IV67–IV87.)

Index

Note: Italicized *f* and *t* refer to figures and tables